MAYO CLINIC INTERNAL MEDICINE BOARD REVIEW

TENTH EDITION

MAYO CLINIC SCIENTIFIC PRESS

Mayo Clinic Atlas of Regional Anesthesia and Ultrasound-Guided Nerve Blockade
Edited by James R. Hebl, MD, and Robert L. Lennon, DO

Mayo Clinic Preventive Medicine and Public Health Board Review
Edited by Prathibha Varkey, MBBS, MPH, MHPE

Mayo Clinic Internal Medicine Board Review, Ninth Edition
Edited by Amit K. Ghosh, MD

Mayo Clinic Challenging Images for Pulmonary Board Review
Edited by Edward C. Rosenow III, MD

Mayo Clinic Gastroenterology and Hepatology Board Review, Fourth Edition
Edited by Stephen C. Hauser, MD

Mayo Clinic Infectious Diseases Board Review
Edited by Zelalem Temesgen, MD

Mayo Clinic Antimicrobial Handbook: Quick Guide, Second Edition
Edited by John W. Wilson, MD, and Lynn L. Estes, PharmD

Just Enough Physiology
By James R. Munis, MD, PhD

Mayo Clinic Cardiology: Concise Textbook, Fourth Edition
Edited by Joseph G. Murphy, MD, and Margaret A. Lloyd, MD

MAYO CLINIC INTERNAL MEDICINE BOARD REVIEW

TENTH EDITION

EDITOR-IN-CHIEF

Robert D. Ficalora, MD

CONSULTANT,
DIVISION OF GENERAL INTERNAL MEDICINE
MAYO CLINIC, ROCHESTER, MINNESOTA
ASSOCIATE PROFESSOR OF MEDICINE
COLLEGE OF MEDICINE, MAYO CLINIC

EDITOR

Paul S. Mueller, MD

ASSOCIATE EDITORS

Thomas J. Beckman, MD

Margaret Beliveau, MD

Mark C. Lee, MD

Nicole P. Sandhu, MD, PhD

Amy T. Wang, MD

Christopher M. Wittich, MD

MAYO CLINIC SCIENTIFIC PRESS

OXFORD UNIVERSITY PRESS

MAYO
CLINIC

The triple-shield Mayo logo and the words MAYO, MAYO CLINIC, and MAYO CLINIC SCIENTIFIC PRESS
are marks of Mayo Foundation for Medical Education and Research.

OXFORD
UNIVERSITY PRESS

Oxford University Press is a department of the University of Oxford.
It furthers the University's objective of excellence in research, scholarship,
and education by publishing worldwide.

Oxford   New York
Auckland   Cape Town   Dar es Salaam   Hong Kong   Karachi
Kuala Lumpur   Madrid   Melbourne   Mexico City   Nairobi
New Delhi   Shanghai   Taipei   Toronto

With offices in
Argentina   Austria   Brazil   Chile   Czech Republic   France   Greece
Guatemala   Hungary   Italy   Japan   Poland   Portugal   Singapore
South Korea   Switzerland   Thailand   Turkey   Ukraine   Vietnam

Oxford is a registered trademark of Oxford University Press in the UK and certain other
countries.

Published in the United States of America by
Oxford University Press
198 Madison Avenue, New York, NY 10016

Catalogue record is available from the Library of Congress
ISBN 978-0-19-994894-9

9 8 7 6 5 4 3 2 1
Printed in China on acid-free paper

Dedicated to all the patients who help us, as internists, learn, practice, and master internal medicine.

Robert D. Ficalora, MD

FOREWORD

One of the Department of Medicine's strategic goals is to provide premier education in the science and art of medicine. Established goals include leading the nation in the development of lifelong learning programs and educating physician and nonphysician learners at all levels and along all points of the education continuum. These goals are attained by providing state-of-the-art graduate medical education. The rapid pace at which medical knowledge is being discovered necessitates frequent updates. *Mayo Clinic Internal Medicine Board Review*, Tenth Edition, reflects changes in the science of medicine and contains features that facilitate retention of the knowledge imparted. The chapters have been completely revised to correspond to American Board of Internal Medicine objectives and include evidence-based recommendations. Bulleted points allow easy access to key points. The questions and their answers have been placed in a companion volume to make this text more portable and user-friendly. New questions

and answers simulate the types of questions included on the American Board of Internal Medicine examination. The editors and associate editors added their depth of experience to ensure that this edition is the finest in the long history of this book. The text is not only informational but also of great assistance in preparing for board certification and recertification, and it allows for the practical application of knowledge to serve our patients.

Morie A. Gertz, MD
Chair, Department of Internal Medicine
Mayo Clinic, Rochester, Minnesota
Professor of Medicine
College of Medicine
Mayo Clinic

PREFACE

Mayo Clinic Internal Medicine Board Review, Tenth Edition, is the result of the combined efforts of Mayo Clinic physicians who practice in all the various subspecialties of Internal Medicine. Many have achieved certificates in medical education and thus understand how to communicate information to our readers—physicians who are in training and practicing clinicians who are preparing for the American Board of Internal Medicine (ABIM) certification and maintenance-of-certification examinations in internal medicine.

Our annual Mayo Clinic Board Review Course, now in its 27th year, gives the authors and editors the unique opportunity to interact with our readers and tailor our approach to the way the current generation of learners prepares for a high stakes examination. With the ABIM Certification Examination Blueprint in mind, we prepared each chapter to be not only readable but also scannable by the reader. Key review points are bulleted in context. We thoroughly updated the information and used state-of-the-art guidelines and algorithms whenever possible. Bullets, tables, and figures throughout each chapter highlight and summarize important clinical information. The book is comprehensive and yet easy to study.

The book chapters reflect the ABIM medical subject and cross-content categories and percentages. Authors with wide clinical expertise composed the chapters or subsections of chapters that reflect the key information. Interesting but extraneous information that was not likely to be included on the examination was removed. To facilitate study, questions are now in a separate volume for easy reference and portability. More than 300 ABIM-format multiple-choice questions with a single answer and explanation are keyed to each chapter.

I am grateful to the current and past authors for their careful attention and hard work. This book would not exist without the dedication of the associate editors who labored in isolation over the chapter drafts. We are all indebted to staffs of the Department of Medicine; Section of Scientific Publications, Joseph G. Murphy, MD, Chair; LeAnn M. Stee and Randall J. Fritz, DVM (editors), Kenna Atherton (manager), Jane M. Craig (editorial assistant), and Alissa K. Baumgartner (proofreader); and Section of Illustration and Design, Deb Veerkamp and Ryan Ledebuhr, at Mayo Clinic for their contributions to this edition. I gratefully acknowledge the support and cooperation of the publisher, Oxford University Press. In particular, I am indebted to my administrative partner, Michael O'Brien, whose unfailing support helped me through some very difficult times.

In the spirit of the previous editions, I trust that *Mayo Clinic Internal Medicine Board Review,* Tenth Edition, will serve our readers well in preparation for the primary certification or maintenance-of-certification examination.

About the cover: The images for the cover were selected to convey both the content and the purpose of this text. Three content areas (dermatology, pulmonary medicine, and hematology) and the collaborative learning environment of medicine are represented. Panel descriptions: upper left, erythema multiforme (Figure 47.4); upper right, bronchial carcinoid (Figure 17.20B); lower left, original artwork depicting Mayo Clinic's group practice and educational excellence; lower right, ring sideroblasts (Figure 34.3).

Robert D. Ficalora, MD
Editor-in-Chief

CONTENTS

CONTRIBUTORS

Charles F. Abboud, MB, ChB
Consultant, Division of Endocrinology, Diabetes,
    Metabolism, & Nutrition
Mayo Clinic, Rochester, Minnesota; and
Associate Professor of Medicine
College of Medicine, Mayo Clinic

Haitham S. Abu-Lebdeh, MD
Consultant, Division of General Internal Medicine
Mayo Clinic, Rochester, Minnesota; and
Assistant Professor of Medicine
College of Medicine, Mayo Clinic

Timothy R. Aksamit, MD
Consultant, Division of Pulmonary and Critical Care Medicine
Mayo Clinic, Rochester, Minnesota; and
Associate Professor of Medicine
College of Medicine, Mayo Clinic

Thomas J. Beckman, MD
Consultant, Division of General Internal Medicine
Mayo Clinic, Rochester, Minnesota; and
Professor of Medicine and of Medical Education
College of Medicine, Mayo Clinic

Margaret Beliveau, MD
Consultant, Division of General Internal Medicine
Mayo Clinic, Rochester, Minnesota; and
Assistant Professor of Medicine
College of Medicine, Mayo Clinic

Eduardo E. Benarroch, MD
Consultant, Department of Neurology
Mayo Clinic, Rochester, Minnesota; and
Professor of Neurology
College of Medicine, Mayo Clinic

Elie F. Berbari, MD
Consultant, Division of Infectious Diseases
Mayo Clinic, Rochester, Minnesota; and
Associate Professor of Medicine
College of Medicine, Mayo Clinic

Peter A. Brady, MB, ChB, MD
Consultant, Division of Cardiovascular Diseases
Mayo Clinic, Rochester, Minnesota; and
Associate Professor of Medicine
College of Medicine, Mayo Clinic

Robert D. Brown Jr, MD
Chair, Department of Neurology
Mayo Clinic, Rochester, Minnesota; and
Professor of Neurology
College of Medicine, Mayo Clinic

John B. Bundrick, MD
Consultant, Division of General Internal Medicine
Mayo Clinic, Rochester, Minnesota; and
Assistant Professor of Medicine
College of Medicine, Mayo Clinic

Maria L. Collazo-Clavell, MD
Consultant, Division of Endocrinology, Diabetes,
    Metabolism, & Nutrition
Mayo Clinic, Rochester, Minnesota; and
Associate Professor of Medicine
College of Medicine, Mayo Clinic

C. Scott Collins, MD
Senior Associate Consultant, Division of
    General Internal Medicine
Mayo Clinic, Rochester, Minnesota; and
Instructor in Medicine
College of Medicine, Mayo Clinic

Brian A. Crum, MD
Consultant, Department of Neurology
Mayo Clinic, Rochester, Minnesota; and
Assistant Professor of Neurology
College of Medicine, Mayo Clinic

Lisa A. Drage, MD
Consultant, Department of Dermatology
Mayo Clinic, Rochester, Minnesota; and
Assistant Professor of Dermatology
College of Medicine, Mayo Clinic

J. Christopher Farmer, MD
Consultant, Division of Pulmonary and
    Critical Care Medicine
Mayo Clinic, Rochester, Minnesota; and
Professor of Medicine
College of Medicine, Mayo Clinic

Fernando C. Fervenza, MD, PhD
Consultant, Division of Nephrology & Hypertension
Mayo Clinic, Rochester, Minnesota; and
Professor of Medicine
College of Medicine, Mayo Clinic

Robert D. Ficalora, MD
Consultant, Division of General Internal Medicine
Mayo Clinic, Rochester, Minnesota; and
Associate Professor of Medicine
College of Medicine, Mayo Clinic

William W. Ginsburg, MD
Consultant, Division of Rheumatology
Mayo Clinic, Jacksonville, Florida; and
Associate Professor of Medicine
College of Medicine, Mayo Clinic

C. Christopher Hook, MD
Consultant, Division of Hematology
Mayo Clinic, Rochester, Minnesota; and
Associate Professor of Medicine
College of Medicine, Mayo Clinic

Lyell K. Jones Jr, MD
Consultant, Department of Neurology
Mayo Clinic, Rochester, Minnesota; and
Assistant Professor of Neurology
College of Medicine, Mayo Clinic

Henna Kalsi, MD
Consultant, Division of Cardiovascular Diseases
Mayo Clinic, Rochester, Minnesota; and
Assistant Professor of Medicine
College of Medicine, Mayo Clinic

Kianoush B. Kashani, MD
Consultant, Division of Nephrology & Hypertension
Mayo Clinic, Rochester, Minnesota; and
Assistant Professor of Medicine
College of Medicine, Mayo Clinic

Mary J. Kasten, MD
Consultant, Divisions of General Internal Medicine
and Infectious Diseases
Mayo Clinic, Rochester, Minnesota; and
Assistant Professor of Medicine
College of Medicine, Mayo Clinic

Kyle W. Klarich, MD
Consultant, Division of Cardiovascular Diseases
Mayo Clinic, Rochester, Minnesota; and
Associate Professor of Medicine
College of Medicine, Mayo Clinic

Mark C. Lee, MD
Consultant, Division of General Internal Medicine
Mayo Clinic, Rochester, Minnesota; and
Assistant Professor of Medicine
College of Medicine, Mayo Clinic

Scott C. Litin, MD
Consultant, Division of General Internal Medicine
Mayo Clinic, Rochester, Minnesota; and
Professor of Medicine
College of Medicine, Mayo Clinic

Conor G. Loftus, MD
Consultant, Division of Gastroenterology and Hepatology
Mayo Clinic, Rochester, Minnesota; and
Assistant Professor of Medicine
College of Medicine, Mayo Clinic

Fabien Maldonado, MD
Consultant, Division of Pulmonary and Critical Care Medicine
Mayo Clinic, Rochester, Minnesota; and
Assistant Professor of Medicine
College of Medicine, Mayo Clinic

Karen F. Mauck, MD, MSc
Consultant, Division of General Internal Medicine
Mayo Clinic, Rochester, Minnesota; and
Assistant Professor of Medicine
College of Medicine, Mayo Clinic

Robert D. McBane, MD
Consultant, Division of Cardiovascular Diseases
Mayo Clinic, Rochester, Minnesota; and
Professor of Medicine
College of Medicine, Mayo Clinic

Bryan McIver, MB, ChB, PhD
Consultant, Division of Endocrinology, Diabetes,
    Metabolism, & Nutrition
Mayo Clinic, Rochester, Minnesota

Clement J. Michet, MD
Consultant, Division of Rheumatology
Mayo Clinic, Rochester, Minnesota; and
Associate Professor of Medicine
College of Medicine, Mayo Clinic

Kevin G. Moder, MD
Consultant, Division of Rheumatology
Mayo Clinic, Rochester, Minnesota; and
Associate Professor of Medicine
College of Medicine, Mayo Clinic

Timothy J. Moynihan, MD
Consultant, Division of Medical Oncology
Mayo Clinic, Rochester, Minnesota; and
Associate Professor of Oncology
College of Medicine, Mayo Clinic

Paul S. Mueller, MD
Chair, Division of General Internal Medicine
Mayo Clinic, Rochester, Minnesota; and
Professor of Biomedical Ethics and of Medicine
College of Medicine, Mayo Clinic

Michelle A. Neben Wittich, MD
Senior Associate Consultant, Department of Radiation Oncology
Mayo Clinic, Rochester, Minnesota; and
Instructor in Radiation Oncology
College of Medicine, Mayo Clinic

James S. Newman, MD
Consultant, Division of Hospital Internal Medicine
Mayo Clinic, Rochester, Minnesota; and
Assistant Professor of History of Medicine
College of Medicine, Mayo Clinic

Suzanne M. Norby, MD
Consultant, Division of Nephrology & Hypertension
Mayo Clinic, Rochester, Minnesota; and
Assistant Professor of Medicine
College of Medicine, Mayo Clinic

Amy S. Oxentenko, MD
Consultant, Division of Gastroenterology and Hepatology
Mayo Clinic, Rochester, Minnesota; and
Associate Professor of Medicine
College of Medicine, Mayo Clinic

Brian A. Palmer, MD
Senior Associate Consultant, Division of Psychiatry
    and Psychology
Mayo Clinic, Rochester, Minnesota; and
Assistant Professor of Psychiatry
College of Medicine, Mayo Clinic

John G. Park, MD
Consultant, Division of Pulmonary and Critical Care Medicine
Mayo Clinic, Rochester, Minnesota; and
Assistant Professor of Medicine
College of Medicine, Mayo Clinic

Naveen L. Pereira, MD
Consultant, Division of Cardiovascular Diseases
Mayo Clinic, Rochester, Minnesota; and
Assistant Professor of Medicine
College of Medicine, Mayo Clinic

Axel Pflueger, MD, PhD
Consultant, Division of Nephrology & Hypertension
Mayo Clinic, Rochester, Minnesota; and
Professor of Medicine
College of Medicine, Mayo Clinic

John J. Poterucha, MD
Consultant, Division of Gastroenterology and Hepatology
Mayo Clinic, Rochester, Minnesota; and
Professor of Medicine
College of Medicine, Mayo Clinic

Abhiram Prasad, MD
Consultant, Division of Cardiovascular Diseases
Mayo Clinic, Rochester, Minnesota; and
Professor of Medicine
College of Medicine, Mayo Clinic

Rajiv K. Pruthi, MBBS
Consultant, Division of Hematology
Mayo Clinic, Rochester, Minnesota; and
Associate Professor of Medicine
College of Medicine, Mayo Clinic

Qi Qian, MD
Consultant, Division of Nephrology & Hypertension
Mayo Clinic, Rochester, Minnesota; and
Associate Professor of Medicine and of Physiology
College of Medicine, Mayo Clinic

Nicole P. Sandhu, MD, PhD
Consultant, Division of General Internal Medicine
Mayo Clinic, Rochester, Minnesota; and
Assistant Professor of Medicine
College of Medicine, Mayo Clinic

Majid Shafiq, MD
Associate Consultant, Division of Hospital Internal Medicine
Mayo Clinic, Rochester, Minnesota; and
Assistant Professor of Medicine
College of Medicine, Mayo Clinic

Neel B. Shah, MB, BCh
Senior Associate Consultant, Division of Hospital
    Internal Medicine
Mayo Clinic, Rochester, Minnesota; and
Instructor in Medicine
College of Medicine, Mayo Clinic

Pankaj Shah, MD
Consultant, Division of Endocrinology, Diabetes,
    Metabolism, & Nutrition
Mayo Clinic, Rochester, Minnesota; and
Assistant Professor of Medicine
College of Medicine, Mayo Clinic

Lynne T. Shuster, MD
Consultant, Division of General Internal Medicine
Mayo Clinic, Rochester, Minnesota; and
Assistant Professor of Medicine
College of Medicine, Mayo Clinic

M. Rizwan Sohail, MD
Consultant, Division of Infectious Diseases
Mayo Clinic, Rochester, Minnesota; and
Assistant Professor of Medicine
College of Medicine, Mayo Clinic

Marius N. Stan, MD
Consultant, Division of Endocrinology, Diabetes,
    Metabolism, & Nutrition
Mayo Clinic, Rochester, Minnesota; and
Assistant Professor of Medicine
College of Medicine, Mayo Clinic

Karen L. Swanson, DO
Consultant, Division of Pulmonary and Critical Care Medicine
Mayo Clinic, Rochester, Minnesota; and
Associate Professor of Medicine
College of Medicine, Mayo Clinic

Seth R. Sweetser, MD
Consultant, Division of Gastroenterology and Hepatology
Mayo Clinic, Rochester, Minnesota; and
Assistant Professor of Medicine
College of Medicine, Mayo Clinic

Keith M. Swetz, MD
Consultant, Division of General Internal Medicine
Mayo Clinic, Rochester, Minnesota; and
Assistant Professor of Medicine
College of Medicine, Mayo Clinic

Zelalem Temesgen, MD
Consultant, Division of Infectious Diseases
Mayo Clinic, Rochester, Minnesota; and
Professor of Medicine
College of Medicine, Mayo Clinic

Carrie A. Thompson, MD
Consultant, Division of Hematology
Mayo Clinic, Rochester, Minnesota; and
Assistant Professor of Medicine
College of Medicine, Mayo Clinic

Pritish K. Tosh, MD
Mayo Clinic Scholar in Infectious Diseases
Mayo Clinic, Rochester, Minnesota; and
Assistant Professor of Medicine
College of Medicine, Mayo Clinic

Gerald W. Volcheck, MD
Consultant, Division of Allergic Diseases
Mayo Clinic, Rochester, Minnesota; and
Associate Professor of Medicine
College of Medicine, Mayo Clinic

Amy T. Wang, MD
Senior Associate Consultant, Division of General
    Internal Medicine
Mayo Clinic, Rochester, Minnesota; and
Assistant Professor of Medicine
College of Medicine, Mayo Clinic

Carilyn N. Wieland, MD
Senior Associate Consultant, Department of Dermatology
Mayo Clinic, Rochester, Minnesota; and
Assistant Professor of Dermatology
College of Medicine, Mayo Clinic

Christopher M. Wittich, MD
Consultant, Division of General Internal Medicine
Mayo Clinic, Rochester, Minnesota; and
Assistant Professor of Medicine
College of Medicine, Mayo Clinic

Alexandra P. Wolanskyj, MD
Consultant, Division of Hematology
Mayo Clinic, Rochester, Minnesota; and
Associate Professor of Medicine
College of Medicine, Mayo Clinic

1.

PREPARING FOR THE ABIM EXAMINATION

Robert D. Ficalora, MD

GOALS

- Review the content and format of the American Board of Internal Medicine (ABIM) examination.

- Provide strategies for preparation for the examination.

- Utilize techniques to improve test-taking skills.

OVERVIEW

Since 2006, more than 7,000 individuals per year have taken the ABIM initial certification examination, and between 3,000 and 5,000 individuals per year have taken the Maintenance of Certification (MOC) examination. Pass rates have ranged from 79% to 94%. Pass rates for first-time takers on both examinations exceed those of repeat takers. There is no doubt that careful and serious preparation for the examination is valuable and necessary. Although some individuals can take and pass the examination with minimal preparation, most takers need rigorous preparation. In recent years, board certification has assumed greater importance in the minds of patients. In a 2003 Gallup poll of 1,001 US adults aged 18 years or older, 98% wanted their physicians to be board-certified, 79% thought that the recertification process was very important, and 54% would choose a new internist if their physicians' board certification had expired.

EXAMINATION: BASIC INFORMATION

The ABIM website (www.abim.org) has a wealth of information for test takers. No one should approach the examination without reading the ABIM Information and Statistics (http://www.abim.org/exam/prepare.aspx) and the ABIM Certification and Recertification Exam Guide (http://www.abim.org/exam/default.aspx). The "Exam Day: What to Expect" section, http://www.abim.org/exam/exam-day.aspx, has up-to-date information about changes to and navigation of the ABIM approach to computer-based testing, such as the following:

How do I answer questions?

How do I change answers?

How do I make notes?

How do I mark questions for review?

- Review the ABIM website materials to understand the testing approach.

EXAMINATION FORMAT

Almost all of the questions are clinical and based on correct diagnosis and management. Because there is no penalty for guessing, candidates should answer every question. Most questions are based on clinical cases. Among these, 75% are related to the outpatient and emergency department settings, and the remainder are related to the inpatient setting, including the critical care unit and nursing home. Increasing emphasis is placed on patient safety and evidence-based quality of care. Selecting the correct answer to these questions requires integration of information provided from several sources (eg, history, physical examination, laboratory test results, and consultations), prioritization of alternatives, or use of clinical judgment. Up to one-third of questions are experimental and included to test question quality. They are not scored and cannot be identified during the examination. Patient management with a cost-effective, evidence-based approach is stressed. Very few questions require simple recall of medical facts. There are no intentional trick questions.

- The ABIM examination has a uniform question approach that stresses clinical reasoning over simple recall.

EXAMINATION CONTENT

The questions in the examination cover a broad area of internal medicine. They are divided into primary and cross-content groups (http://www.abim.org/pdf/blueprint/im_cert.pdf). Each session (4 for initial certification and 3 for maintenance of certification) contains 60 multiple-choice questions. The question may include a case history, a brief statement, a radiograph, a graph, or a photograph (such as a blood smear or Gram stain). Each question has 5 possible answers, and the candidates should identify the single-best answer. More than 1 answer may appear correct or partially correct for a question. Sample questions are included in the ABIM tutorial, http://www.abim.org/exam/prepare.aspx.

COMPUTER-BASED TESTING

Candidates currently take a computer-based certification examination that has been designed to provide a flexible, quiet, and professional environment for examination. The computer-based test is administered by about 200 centers in the United States. Candidates schedule their examination date according to the updated instructions on the ABIM website, http://www.abim.org/exam/. Candidates are well advised to access the online tutorial at http://www.abim.org/exam/prepare.aspx. This tutorial allows the candidate to become familiar with answering questions, changing answers, making notes electronically, accessing the table of normal laboratory values, and marking questions for review.

- Candidates are advised to familiarize themselves with the computer-based testing format by accessing the online tutorial.

MAINTENANCE OF CERTIFICATION

The diplomate certificates issued to candidates who have passed the ABIM examination in internal medicine since 1990 are valid for 10 years. The total number of candidates who took the ABIM MOC examination for the first time in 2007 was 3,837. Of these, 83% passed.

ENHANCEMENTS TO MOC PROGRAM

In January 2006, the ABIM enhanced the MOC program to increase flexibility and assess performance in clinical practice. The 3 retained general components (credentialing, self-evaluation, and secure examination) and the added self-evaluation module each have a point value.

Every candidate must complete a total of 100 points in self-evaluation modules. Unlike the previous system, renewal of more than 1 certificate does not necessitate taking additional self-evaluation modules (ie, the same number of points, 100, satisfies the requirement to sit for these examinations). Candidates must complete at least 20 points in medical knowledge and at least 20 points in practice performance. The remaining 60 points may be obtained from completion of modules developed by ABIM or other organizations that meet the ABIM standards. Thus, one could combine an ABIM knowledge module (20 points) and an ABIM practice improvement module (20 points) with the American College of Physicians Medical Knowledge Self-assessment Program (MKSAP) (3 modules, 60 points), or one could combine an ABIM practice improvement module (20 points) with 6 annual-update ABIM knowledge modules (60 points) and the ABIM peer and patient feedback module (20 points). All points are valid for 10 years. Further refinements to this process are likely. Thus, candidates should check for updates on the ABIM website.

- MOC is a multistep process in addition to the examination.
- Always check the ABIM website for information and updates.

The self-evaluation modules evaluate performance in clinical skills, preventive services, practice performance, fund of medical knowledge, and feedback from patients and colleagues. Successfully completed self-evaluation modules are valid for 10 years. Candidates may apply to begin the MOC process any time after initial certification. The ABIM recommends that completion of the self-evaluation modules be spread out over the certification period. A candidate should complete 1 self-assessment module every 1 to 2 years. The ABIM encourages candidates to enroll within 4 years of certification in order to have adequate time to complete the program.

- Candidates who passed the ABIM certification examination in internal medicine in 1990 and thereafter have a certificate that is valid for 10 years.
- The MOC process is called continuous professional development and consists of a 3-step process.

10 TIPS FOR EFFECTIVE EXAMINATION PREPARATION

1. HAVE A STUDY PLAN

We all have busy lives. Successful candidates stress that the most valuable preparation strategies must include scheduling *a time to study*. Preparing in small, discrete pieces improves recall, facilitates review, and makes the overall task less onerous. Spending 3 or 4 hours a week, using various approaches such as directed reading, practice questions, and group review, is enough to stay focused. Simply reading by itself is usually a bad strategy. You may not be able to retain much of the ABIM material by reading without focus. Start with a question, a problem to solve, or a patient scenario in mind. This approach to a study session will help you and your group understand what you are studying, the clinical context, pathophysiology, and management and the reasons for it. Keep asking yourself "why?" and "why not?"

How can I study such a large mass of material?

Plan a pace of no more than 3 major topics per hour.

Survey the material.

Consider the major subsections as potential questions.

Review the material in each subsection carefully to answer the question.

Recite in your own words.

Revise in your notes.

Take notes! Even if you never look at them again, the act of synthesizing the information in writing will help you retain it.

- To study, use active learning approaches to maximize efficiency.

- Simply reading, no matter how much, is generally an ineffective preparation strategy.

2. FORM A STUDY GROUP

If possible, form a study group. You will be more likely to make and stay on a schedule if individuals feel a responsibility to the group's progress. A group will boost everyone's morale and give a common sense of purpose. A group size of only 2 to 5 candidates permits study of different textbooks, board review materials, and review articles in journals. Make sure that you have a committed, available group of study partners. Individuals who push ahead on their own and those who don't keep their commitments can sabotage an otherwise productive group. Schedule regular meetings and assign individuals specific topics. This approach saves time, covers more topics per session, and allows everyone to retain more from the discussion. Take turns acting as group moderator, to keep to the topic and schedule. The moderator should be responsible, congratulating productive members and offering a friendly word to someone who might be slacking off. If everyone has a turn, no one person has to be the "bad guy." Selected review articles on common and important topics, such as represented by the ABIM objectives, should be included in every session. Avoid indiscriminate reading of articles from many journals.

Remember that questions are tested for several examination cycles before they are included in the examination. It is unlikely that new information or current controversies will be represented on your examination. Notes and other materials the candidates have gathered during residency training can be good sources of information. Finding the justification for these "pearls" can cement one's command of a particular topic. These clinical "pearls" gathered from mentors will be of help in remembering certain important points. Always save some time each session to review questions and discuss the answers and their rationales. Don't forget to discuss each of the options in detail. This will develop your thought process and sharpen your test-taking skills.

- Keep your study group small and stay focused.

- Make a schedule and read ahead of the discussion.

- Discuss study material.

- Do multiple-choice questions in groups.

- Indiscriminate reading of articles from many journals should be avoided.

- Information in recent journals is unlikely to be included in the examination.

3. DETERMINE WHAT YOU NEED TO STUDY

For recent graduates attempting primary certification, let your in-training examination subsection score results guide your study choices. In general, if your score in a given area was below the fifth decile, or fiftieth percentile, you should consider that an area for intensive review and preparation. Use the section called "educational objectives," which gives your performance by content area, to guide your choice of preparation topics.

MOC candidates should use practice questions to guide your study choices. Do as many questions as you can, and monitor your performance by the ABIM blueprint section, http://www.abim.org/pdf/blueprint/im_cert.pdf.

Serious preparation for the examination actually starts at the beginning of residency training. In addition to daily reading and achieving subspecialty-based proficiency, most candidates require a minimum of 6 to 8 months of intense preparation for the examination. Cramming before the examination, whether by yourself or at a review course, is unlikely to be successful.

Use a standard textbook of internal medicine. Ideally, you should use one good textbook and not jump from one to another. Although online, just-in-time resources may be useful for fact checking, they rarely give an inclusive, case-based review. The most effective way to use the textbook is with patient-centered reading. Read the descriptions of the symptoms and signs carefully because often they are part of the questions in the examination. Table 1.1 provides several examples of the common descriptions of symptoms and signs that could be part of the examination. Rather than reading chapters at random, read the literature in a structured manner to assist in future recall of facts. This book and similar books are excellent tools for brushing up on important board-relevant information several weeks to months before the examination. They, however, cannot take the place of comprehensive textbooks of internal medicine. This book is designed as a study guide rather than a comprehensive textbook of medicine. Therefore, it should not be used as the sole source of medical information for the examination.

- Study first with a standard textbook of internal medicine.

- This book is designed as a study guide and should not be used as the sole source of information for preparation for the examination.

- Pay attention to the descriptions of signs and symptoms.

Table 1.1 COMMON DESCRIPTIONS OF SIGNS AND SYMPTOMS IN EXAMINATION QUESTIONS

HISTORY (SYMPTOMS)	PHYSICAL FINDINGS (SIGNS)	LIKELY DIAGNOSIS
Cardiology		
Shortness of breath or asymptomatic	Late peaking systolic murmur, intensity decreases with handgrip & increases with squatting	Hypertrophic obstructive cardiomyopathy
Asymptomatic, headache	Hypertension, diminished or absent lower extremity pulses, systolic murmur, bruit over chest wall	Coarctation of aorta
Neurology		
Gait impairment, falls, dysphagia, dysarthria	Inability to look up & side to side	Progressive supranuclear palsy
Diplopia, oscillating images, reading fatigue, loss of depth perception	Impaired adduction on lateral gaze, with nystagmus in the contralateral abducting eye	Internuclear ophthalmoplegia (consider multiple sclerosis, cerebrovascular disease)
Fluctuating memory, confusion, visual hallucinations	Mild parkinsonism, dementia	Lewy body dementia
Inappropriate behavior, dementia, poor social skills	Dementia	Frontotemporal dementia
Paroxysmal pain affecting the side of the face	Usually normal	Trigeminal neuralgia affecting 1 of the branches of cranial nerve V
Muscle stiffness, clumsiness, occasional emotional lability	Brisk reflexes, spasticity (upper motor neuron signs), atrophy, fasciculation (lower motor neuron signs)	Amyotrophic lateral sclerosis
Altered mental status, fever, headache	Flaccid paralysis, neck rigidity ±, altered mental status	West Nile virus encephalitis
Infectious disease		
Recurrent sinusitis, skin, or pulmonary infections due to *Staphylococcus aureus*	Sinus tenderness, abnormal lung sounds	Chronic granulomatous disorder
Recurrent *Neisseria* infections	Neck rigidity ±, altered mental status	Inherited deficiencies of complement (C5, 6, 7, 8, 9), factor D, or properdin
Recurrent episodes of bacterial pneumonia, sinusitis, diarrhea due to *Streptococcus pneumoniae*	Malnourished, abnormal lung sounds	Common variable immunodeficiency
Gastroenterology		
Cirrhosis of liver, ingestion of raw oysters	Fever, hypotension, hemorrhagic bullae, signs of cirrhosis of liver	*Vibrio vulnificus*
Diarrhea	Pruritus, grouped vesicles over the elbow, knee, scalp, or back of neck	Dermatitis herpetiformis due to celiac sprue
Hepatitis C, photosensitivity	Skin fragility, erosions, blisters on dorsum of hand, hyperpigmentation	Porphyria cutanea tarda
Dermatology		
Facial rash, photosensitivity	Papules & pustules on bridge of nose & face, telangiectasia	Rosacea
Rash	Sharply demarcated erythematous papules, silvery white scales over scalp, extensor surfaces of extremities, & nails	Psoriasis
Cough with sore throat	Tender, erythematous pretibial nodules	Erythema nodosum
Ulcerative colitis	Irregular, undermined ulcer with violaceous border or scarring in lower extremities	Pyoderma gangrenosum
Flushing, diarrhea, rapid heart rate	Brown-red macules, urticaria on stroking skin	Systemic mastocytosis

4. CREATE AND DEVOTE TIME

Board preparation should be part of your daily routine, like exercising, showering, or brushing your teeth. If you don't regularly do some preparation, it will fall off your routine, and your preparation just won't happen. You can spend as little or as much time as you want on a particular activity. Often you can review familiar topics in small discrete time periods (eg, before or after lunch). Less familiar topics may require an hour in a quiet room, and this time may be best reserved for early in the morning or on a weekend. Keep in mind that the more time and energy you spend actively learning a topic, the better your command, and the less dependent you will be on rote memorization.

Some people can study effectively while on a treadmill, on a train, or in a car. If you can do this, you can incorporate this into your studying routine. How much time it takes to perform these tasks varies from person to person and will improve as you solidify your study habits. Regardless, every learning task takes time, and you must budget for that time. Only you can decide how much time you want to spend in solitary study, in groups, or in summary objective review. You can make great plans, but life and work aren't predictable, so you should build in some catch-up time for unexpected distractions.

You also have to consider how much time it takes to organize your studying. Review of cardiology may go quickly, whereas glomerulopathies may take a pad and pencil to figure out. You may have to travel to study sessions or spend time looking for information to ensure your command of a given objective. Many candidates try to set aside large blocks of time. With our busy lives, that may be laudable but impractical. Many shorter sessions not only allow for study and catch-up but also can be worked in around standing commitments more effectively than large blocks, and thus a missed session won't be a major setback for that week. The time you spend will come back to you when you pass, and a failure only means you have to devote the time all over again.

Certifying or recertifying board examinations can be stressful. The sheer mass of information can be overwhelming to some. The press of occupational and personal responsibilities makes finding the time to study very difficult, so many opt to take a review course. A review course should be the final integrating activity once you have completed your own primary preparation. To be successful you should go to the review course prepared and ready to "fill in" objectives you may have missed or to learn from experts' objectives that you couldn't understand on your own. Don't expect a course to substitute for primary preparation. Attending a highly focused, no-fluff course that delivers the information in a concentrated, high-yield manner right before the examination may seem like an easy way out, but it is unlikely to be the difference between success and failure.

- Residents: Prepare for the boards during residency.
  You will not find that kind of quality time after your residency.
  Once residency is over and you start fellowship or a job, *you will not find time to study*.

- MOC: Schedule the time.

- Schedule multiple short preparation sessions rather than fewer long ones.

- Do not rely solely on a review course; they are not a substitute for primary preparation.

5. PREPARE A PLAN AND SCHEDULE IT

All ABIM objectives are not equal. Review the relative percentage of the contents of the examination and the number of questions per objective (http://www.abim.org/pdf/blueprint/im_cert.pdf). Note that some areas may have an estimated number of questions of 11 to 15, whereas many will range from 5 to 10 with some estimated to have 0 to 2. Pace your preparation by subject:

Subjects with a large estimated number of questions are very likely to be there. Master them.

Subjects with a medium to low estimated number of questions will be there in some form. Review them.

Subjects with a very low estimated number of questions may be tangential or favorite board *zebras*. Depending on your available study time, it may be worthwhile for you to consider them only for last-minute review.

Plot out your objectives review on a calendar, mixing more and less complex objectives. Leave time for discussion, literature and online searches, and follow-up for problem items from previous study sessions. Always plan to cover new material and to periodically cycle back to previously reviewed difficult or detailed information. Imagine cases that might go with the material at hand.

The most effective way to manage your study time is to periodically assess your progress through practice tests and test questions. It is impossible to overemphasize the importance of this point. "Boardsmanship" is a real skill, and there is no substitute for familiarity with the form and content of the ABIM-type questions. Therefore, you are strongly encouraged to take at least a few mock examinations and simulate the actual testing environment (ie, no breaks, snacks, music, phones, pagers). Taking mock questions is an effective use of a board review or board questions book. Practice material at intervals during your long-term test preparation schedule. Your schedule should be the most intense in the 3 months before the test. After that, focus on review, consolidating key points, and resolving previously difficult problems.

Once you or your group has a schedule, stick to it. Add sessions, but never delete any. Stick to your start and stop times.

- Schedule your progress and build in assessment sessions.

- Make changes, but no deletions.

- Plan to review material that you have chosen several times (minimum twice).

- Stay focused throughout the months before the examination.

- Board review preparation must be at its peak by 3 months before the examination. If you have not yet formed a study group, now is your last chance.

6. ANSWER QUESTIONS SIMILAR TO EXAMINATION CONTENT

The purpose of standardized testing is to measure a candidate's command of the material so that scores from different test dates can be reliably compared with one another. The results must correlate statistically with the results of all the test-takers who have answered the same questions. Persons who construct board review materials and questions go to great pains to build them for the same content and content level as on the actual board examination. The good ones are validated and have been tested to make sure that they perform in a reliable, predictable manner and that they adequately test the content they purport to test. Any questions prepared for other courses, local residency, fellowship rotations, or other venues that cover similar material likely won't test the material in a way that predicts your performance on the board examination. Read a board review book, go to a board review course, and always practice answering questions. When you practice answering questions, do it as you would during the examination; just reading the book and reading the answers likely will not prepare you for the actual test. For every question, identify in your own mind the concept being tested. Make sure you read all the wrong answers and make sure you understand why they weren't the best answer for the question asked.

Sometimes candidates try to prepare by studying materials that are harder than the real test, such as subspecialty board–level review courses and practice tests. The idea is that becoming familiar with something harder will make the real thing easier by comparison. Preparing with something more challenging can be a good idea in some types of athletic or endurance preparation, but it is a bad idea for the ABIM examination. Because the objectives are specific and public, preparing by using objectives for another examination may cause you to misinterpret or overinterpret what is being asked. Reliably finding the easiest approach to a test question requires being aware that the test can't require you to use a certain higher-level data set or decision tree. Because the harder material is testing a different skill set, reviewing this may lead to incorrect answers.

As silly as this piece of advice may seem, **read the questions carefully!** Doing so can make a big difference in your score. If you read questions hastily, there is a high likelihood that you will misinterpret them. Some questions offer incorrect choices that are designed to answer a common misinterpretation of the actual question. Be particularly careful with answers that have more than one part. Only one part may be correct. Other distraction techniques include 2 responses that are similar except for a word or phrase. Watch for responses that contradict others; usually, both of these can be ruled out. What if you read a question and the traditional correct answer isn't an option? What if more than one answer *could be* correct? Then select the best option available. Be very careful of responses that are the longest or the unique answer. They are no more likely or unlikely to be correct despite prevailing wisdom.

- Don't try to read the board review material from cover to cover.

- The best way to prepare is to review and always practice answering questions.

- To improve your understanding, read the explanation, and look up additional information related to each of the choices—both correct and incorrect.

- Familiarize yourself with the teaching principle and the testing objective, which may give you insight into the questions and the possible responses.

7. DON'T FORGET ABOUT IMAGES

Every image-based question will also include text or a clinical case or both. Don't simply focus on the image without reading the text. Familiarize yourself with the image and its details after you have read the case, and then read it again. Photographs of skin disorders, radiographs, electrocardiograms, and other images given in board questions are generally easy ways to score points. Reading the ABIM question stem last helps put the pieces of the puzzle in place. Methodically review a radiograph as you would in a patient encounter. Immediately focusing on an obvious abnormality can distract you from a more subtle finding that may alert you to the correct answer. You may miss the pneumothorax as the cause of the dyspnea if you focus only on the heart size and the small pleural effusion. Likewise for skin findings; use your clinical skills to interpret the finding. Is it flat or raised, erythematous or pigmented?

- Approach an image question as you would a patient.

- Methodically examine the image.

- Use the text and the stem to focus your inquiry.

8. SPEND SOME TIME BECOMING EXPERT IN "BOARDSMANSHIP"

Some candidates fail the examination despite intense preparation and the clinical competence necessary to pass the examination. Failing usually happens because they don't understand or interpret the questions properly. The ability to understand the nuances of the question format is sometimes referred to as "boardsmanship." Intelligent interpretation of the questions is very important for candidates who are not well versed in the format of multiple-choice questions. Answer the questions whose answers you know first, making sure you understand what is being asked to ensure that they are answered correctly. It is easy to become overconfident with such questions, and thus you may fail to read the questions or the answer options carefully. Make sure you never make mistakes on easy questions. Read the final sentence (that appears just before the multiple answers) several times to understand how an answer should be selected. Recheck the question format before selecting the correct answer. Read each answer option completely.

Occasionally, a response may be only partially correct. At times, the traditionally correct answer is not listed. In these situations, select the best alternative listed. Watch for qualifiers such as next, immediately, or initially. Avoid answers that contain absolute or very restrictive words such as always, never, or must. Answer options that contain absolutes are likely incorrect. Try to think of the correct answer to the question before looking at the list of potential answers. Assume you have been given all the necessary information to answer the question. If the answer you had formulated is not among the list of answers provided, you may have interpreted the question incorrectly. When a patient's case is presented, think of the diagnosis before looking at the list of answers. If you do not know the answer to a question, very often you are able to rule out one or several answer options. Determine whether your diagnosis is supported by any of the answers. If you can eliminate any answers as clearly wrong, you will improve your odds at guessing. Occasionally, you can use information presented in one question to help you answer other, difficult questions. Many questions are on the test for trial or validation purposes and are not scored. If a question seems to you to be a bad or confusing question, it may be in this category. It is best not to spend an inordinate amount of time trying to second guess this type of question. Come back to it after you have finished, if you still have time.

- When reading long multiple-choice cases:

  First read the actual "lead line" of the question

- Once you understand what the question is asking:

  Stay focused and look for clues in the long stem of the question.

- As you read through the questions:

  Note the key facts and abnormal findings

  Skip questions about which you have no idea, and come back after a complete first pass

9. USE YOUR REFLEXES

Associations, causes, complications, and other relationships between a phenomenon or disease and clinical features are important to remember and recognize. Each subspecialty has many common connections, and candidates for the ABIM and other examinations may want to prepare lists like this for different areas. For example, a case that presents a patient with health care–associated pneumonia should immediately bring to mind antipseudomonal antibiotics, not antibiotics traditionally used for community-acquired pneumonia. Combined knee and hip pain should have you considering a gait abnormality rather than abnormality in 2 joints simultaneously.

Use the basic fund of knowledge accumulated from clinical experience and reading to solve the questions. Approaching the questions as real-life encounters with patients is far better than trying to second-guess the examiners or trying to analyze whether the question is tricky. As indicated above, the questions are never tricky, and there is no reason for the ABIM to trick the candidates into choosing wrong answers.

Use examination techniques to your advantage. Look for target populations in questions. Start with a basic premise in mind, then modify it as the information warrants. Examples are as follows:

For young patients, aim for aggressive management.

For elderly patients, aim for less aggressive alternatives, especially in those with multisystem disease.

Beware of adverse medication effects and polypharmacy.

For asymptomatic healthy patients, do nothing and observe.

- Use your existing fund of knowledge of internal medicine and your previous clinical experience.

- Approach each question as a real-life patient encounter.

- There are *no* trick questions.

10. PLAN FOR THE DAY OF THE EXAMINATION

You should have adequate time to read and answer all the questions; therefore, there is no need to rush or become anxious. Watch the time to ensure that you are at least halfway through the examination when half of the time has elapsed. Start by answering the first question and continue sequentially. Almost all of the questions follow a case-presentation format. At times, subsequent questions will give you information that may help you answer a previous question. Do not be alarmed by lengthy questions; look for the question's salient points. When faced with a confusing question, do not become distracted by that question. Mark it so you can find it later, then go to the next question and come back to the unanswered ones at the end. Extremely lengthy stem statements or case presentations are intended to test the candidate's ability to separate the essential from the unnecessary or unimportant information. You may want to highlight important information presented in the question in order to review this information after reading the entire question and the answer options. There is no penalty for guessing, so you should never leave an answer blank. Every time you can eliminate just one choice you increase your chance of choosing a correct answer by 20%, so it's best to guess among the remaining choices. If you truly have no idea about any of the choices, the "B" answer has been statistically more likely to be correct. It is better to choose "B" if you truly don't know the answer.

- Look for the salient points in each question.

- If a question is confusing, mark it to find it and come back to the unanswered questions at the end.

- If you must guess, choose "B"; statistically, it is more likely to be correct.

It's really not productive to discuss the questions or answers after the examination with other candidates. Such discussions usually cause more consternation, although some candidates may derive a false sense of having performed well on the examination. In any case, the candidates are bound by their oath to the ABIM not to discuss or disseminate the questions. Do not study between examination sessions. To minimize stress, stick to your daily routine; don't start or stop exercising or using caffeine, and don't skip meals or load up on carbohydrates. Be as rested and refreshed as you can be. Forget about your electronic devices such as pagers and cell phones.

- Don't study the day before the examination or between the examination sessions.

- Discussing the examination questions with others raises anxiety and can adversely affect your performance in the next session.

- Maintain your normal routine.

SUMMARY

Preparation for the ABIM examination requires a serious and organized approach. Devote adequate time. Familiarize yourself with the examination format and objectives. Use commonsense test-taking strategies, including practice tests and question analysis. Treat the examination day as you would for any competitive event by preparing physically.

PART I

CARDIOLOGY

2.

ARRHYTHMIAS AND SYNCOPE

Nicole P. Sandhu, MD, PhD, Peter A. Brady, MB, ChB, MD,

and Robert D. Ficalora, MD

GOALS

- Discuss the evaluation and management of cardiac arrhythmias.

- Explain the different types of syncope.

- Describe the evaluation and management of syncope.

MECHANISM OF ARRHYTHMIAS

Abnormal cardiac arrhythmias may be due to reentry, abnormal automaticity, or triggered activity. Reentry is the most common mechanism for cardiac arrhythmias. Reentrant rhythms may be microreentrant (eg, a small circuit around an area of myocardial fibrosis, as in sinus node reentry or atrioventricular [AV] node reentry) or macroreentrant (eg, around an area of myocardial infarction or scar and reentry within the atrium, as in atrial flutter or an accessory pathway, such as in Wolff-Parkinson-White syndrome). Three conditions are needed for reentry to occur: 1) more than 2 anatomically or functionally distinct pathways (eg, AV nodal reentry), 2) a unidirectional block in 1 pathway, and 3) slowed conduction in the second pathway.

Automatic rhythms are more common in enhanced sympathetic tone, hypoxia, acid-base and electrolyte disturbances, or atrial or ventricular stretch (eg, exacerbations of congestive heart failure). Digoxin toxicity is the most common cause of arrhythmias due to triggered activity.

- Reentry is the most common mechanism of cardiac arrhythmias.

- Automatic rhythms are more common in settings of enhanced sympathetic tone, hypoxia, acid-base and electrolyte disturbances, or atrial or ventricular stretch.

- Arrhythmias due to triggered activity are most often due to digoxin toxicity (Figures 2.1 and 2.2).

EVALUATION OF SUSPECTED RHYTHM DISORDERS

ELECTROCARDIOGRAPHY

Electrocardiography (ECG) is the most simple and cost-effective tool for evaluating rhythm disorders. It can provide important clues to the diagnosis (eg, ventricular pre-excitation in Wolff-Parkinson-White syndrome). Whenever possible, a current ECG should be compared with previous recordings.

AMBULATORY ECG MONITORING

Ambulatory ECG (Holter) monitoring allows evaluation of rhythm disturbances and their relationship to daily activities. It is useful to have a patient who is undergoing ambulatory ECG monitoring keep a diary and correlate symptoms with the recorded heart rhythm during symptoms. Normal results on Holter monitoring do not rule out a heart rhythm abnormality as a cause of symptoms unless symptoms occur during the monitoring period. Ambulatory ECG monitoring is also useful for assessing impact of medical and pacemaker therapy.

- Ambulatory ECG monitoring allows evaluation of rhythm disturbances and their relationship with daily activities.

- Normal results on Holter monitoring do not rule out a heart rhythm abnormality unless symptoms occur during monitoring and the rhythm is normal.

EVENT RECORDING

Transtelephonic event recording is similar to ambulatory ECG monitoring but is more useful for documenting heart rate and rhythm when symptoms are less frequent (<1 episode per 24–48 hours). The device is activated during symptoms

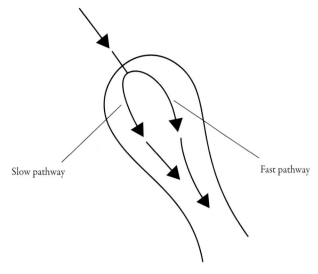

Figure 2.1 Reentry Within the Atrioventricular (AV) Node. The 2 limbs of reentrant circuit are shown. Recent evidence suggests that a portion of the reentrant pathway is separate from the AV node.

by the patient. Continuous loop recorders record the ECG obtained 30 seconds to 4 minutes before the activation button is depressed. This study is useful in patients whose symptoms are brief or sudden in onset.

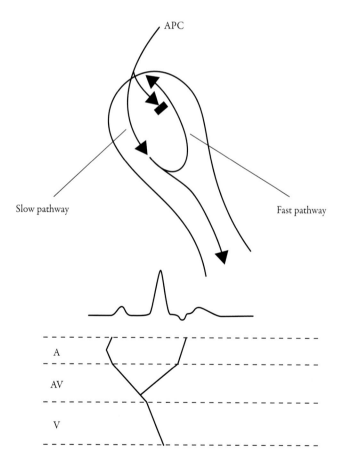

Figure 2.2 Atrioventricular (AV) Nodal Reentrant Tachycardia. An atrial premature complex (APC) blocks in fast pathway but conducts over slow pathway to ventricle. Impulse then returns to atria over recovered fast pathway and can reenter slow pathway and initiate tachycardia. The A indicates atrium; V, ventricle.

Implantable loop event recording is used when symptoms are infrequent or are of sudden onset. These devices can be programmed to provide information regarding rhythm disturbances over several months.

- Transtelephonic event recorders are useful in patients whose symptoms are brief or sudden in onset because continuous loop recorders store the ECG for a certain time before activation by the patient.

ELECTROPHYSIOLOGIC TESTING

Electrophysiologic (EP) testing is an invasive method that is useful for assessing the cardiac conduction system. Indications for EP testing include syncope suggestive of a cardiogenic mechanism and palpitations likely due to a cardiac rhythm disorder (premature supraventricular tachycardia or ventricular tachycardia). It can be used in combination with tilt-table testing for the evaluation of patients with syncope when no obvious cause is immediately identified and conduction or structural heart disease is suspected. EP testing is not required in most patients with symptomatic bradycardia for whom a permanent pacemaker is indicated, nor is it useful in patients with cardiac conditions such as long QT syndrome or hypertrophic cardiomyopathy unless another arrhythmia is suspected. It is most useful for inducing a sustained ventricular tachycardia in a patient with a myocardial scar due to myocardial infarction. EP testing is less commonly used to assess sinus node function or the effects of antiarrhythmic drug therapy. Complications are infrequent (<0.5% to 1.0% of cases) and usually minor.

- Syncope suggestive of a cardiogenic mechanism and palpitations likely due to a rhythm disorder are common indications for EP testing.

- When no obvious cause is identified and the patient is at high risk of cardiogenic syncope, EP testing may be used in combination with tilt-table testing to evaluate syncope.

- EP testing is not necessary in most patients with symptomatic bradycardia for whom a pacemaker is indicated or for patients with long QT syndrome, hypertrophic cardiomyopathy, or others without a defined substrate.

THERAPY FOR HEART RHYTHM DISORDERS

Several therapeutic options are available for heart rhythm disorders. These include drug therapy, radiofrequency ablation, and device therapy (pacing for bradyarrhythmias and implantable cardioverter-defibrillators [ICDs] for tachyarrhythmias).

ANTIARRHYTHMIC DRUGS

With the increasing efficacy of radiofrequency ablation (RFA), antiarrhythmic drugs for supraventricular arrhythmias are less commonly used. However, they still have a role

Table 2.1 PROPERTIES OF ANTIARRHYTHMIC DRUGS

DRUG	THERAPEUTIC RANGE, MCG/ML	HALF-LIFE, H	ROUTE OF METABOLISM Hepatic, %	Renal, %
Class IA				
Quinidine	2–5	6–8	80	20
Procainamide	4–10	3–6	50	50
Disopyramide	2–5	4–8	50	50
Class IB				
Lidocaine	1.5–5	1–4	100	0
Mexiletine	1–2	8–16	100	0
Phenytoin	10–20	24	~100	0
Class IC				
Flecainide	0.2–1	12–27	75	25
Propafenone	Not helpful[a]	2–10	100	0
Class III				
Amiodarone	1–2.5	25–110 days	80	0
Sotalol	~2.5	7–18	0	100
Ibutilide	Not established	2–12	0	80
Dofetilide	1–3.5	10	0	80

[a] Therapeutic effects for propafenone are generally associated with a QRS width increase of 10% above baseline.

Adapted from MKSAP IX: Part C, Book 1, 1992. American College of Physicians. Used with permission.

Table 2.2 RELATIVE EFFECTIVENESS OF ANTIARRHYTHMIC DRUGS

DRUG	EFFECTIVENESS[a] PVCs	VT	PSVT	AF
Quinidine	2+	2+	2+	2+
Procainamide	2+	2+	2+	2+
Disopyramide	2+	2+	2+	2+
Lidocaine	2+	2+	0	0
Mexiletine	2+	2+	0	0
Ibutilide[b]	NI	NI	NI	2+
Flecainide	4+	2+	3+	2+
Propafenone	4+	2+	3+	2+
Dofetilide[c]	2+	2+	NI	2+
Amiodarone	4+	3+	3+	3+
Sotalol	3+	2–3+	3+	2+

Abbreviations: AF, atrial fibrillation (prevention of paroxysmal AF); NI, not indicated; PSVT, paroxysmal supraventricular tachycardia that uses atrioventricular node as part of reentrant circuit; PVCs, premature ventricular complexes; VT, ventricular tachycardia.

[a] Effectiveness: 0, not effective; 1+, least effective; 4+, most effective.

[b] Only intravenous form available; approved for acute cardioversion.

[c] An option to maintain sinus rhythm in patients with atrial fibrillation and underlying heart disease.

in treatment of many ventricular arrhythmias, usually as an adjunct to ICD therapy. Table 2.1 lists the therapeutic range, half-life, and routes of metabolism of antiarrhythmic drugs. Table 2.2 outlines the relative effectiveness of these drugs for treating premature ventricular contractions, ventricular tachycardia, paroxysmal supraventricular tachycardia that uses the AV node as part of the reentrant circuit, and atrial fibrillation. Table 2.3 provides the toxicity and adverse effect profiles of antiarrhythmic drugs. The predominant target of specific antiarrhythmic drugs is shown in Figure 2.3. Antiarrhythmic drugs are less commonly used because RFA has become increasingly effective.

Amiodarone

Amiodarone is highly effective, but its use is limited by multiple noncardiac effects, including those involving the thyroid (hyperthyroidism and hypothyroidism), liver, and lungs. Nevertheless, amiodarone has been shown to be effective and relatively safe in high-risk patients. In patients with congestive heart failure (CHF), amiodarone has an essentially neutral effect on survival. It is not indicated as prophylaxis, however, against sudden death in patients who have CHF. Amiodarone does not increase mortality in patients with symptomatic premature ventricular contractions or ventricular tachycardia and is most often used as an adjunct to an ICD. Routine use of amiodarone after myocardial infarction or in unselected patients with CHF is not recommended.

- The use of amiodarone is limited by its noncardiac effects.
- Amiodarone is not indicated for prevention of sudden death in patients with CHF.

Adenosine

Adenosine can terminate reentrant tachycardia that relies on conduction through the AV node by slowing AV node conduction. It has a half-life of 10 seconds. It is indicated for termination of rapid reentrant supraventricular tachycardia (SVT) that uses the AV node as part of the reentrant circuit. Adenosine will not terminate arrhythmias such as atrial fibrillation or flutter in which the AV node is not a critical part of the reentrant circuit, but it may help in diagnosis of these arrhythmias (eg, by slowing AV conduction to allow visualization of flutter waves). Because of adenosine's short half-life, approximately 10% of patients have recurrent SVT after its administration, whereas recurrent SVT is less common after termination by verapamil. Adenosine may terminate some ventricular arrhythmias (adenosine-sensitive ventricular tachycardia) that originate from the right ventricular outflow tract. Adenosine (and verapamil) are contraindicated in patients presenting with a wide QRS tachycardia and atrial fibrillation associated with Wolff-Parkinson-White syndrome because of the risk of hemodynamic collapse as atrial fibrillation transitions to ventricular fibrillation.

Table 2.3 TOXICITY AND ADVERSE EFFECTS OF ANTIARRHYTHMIC DRUGS

DRUG	FREQUENCY OF ADVERSE EFFECTS, %	ORGAN TOXICITY	% PROARRHYTHMIA DURING TREATMENT FOR VT	RISK OF CONGESTIVE HEART FAILURE[a]		ADVERSE EFFECTS
				EF >30%	*EF ≤30%*	
Quinidine	30	Moderate	3	0	0	Nausea, abdominal pain, diarrhea, thrombocytopenia, hypotension, ↓ warfarin clearance
Procainamide	30	High	2	0	1+	Lupuslike syndrome, rash, fever, headache, nausea, hallucinations, diarrhea
Disopyramide	30	Low	2	1+	4+	Dry mouth, urinary hesitancy, blurred vision, constipation, urinary retention
Lidocaine	40	Moderate	2	0	0	L-H, seizure, tremor, confusion, memory loss, nausea
Mexiletine	40	Low	2	0	0	L-H, tremor, ataxia, confusion, memory loss, altered liver function
Ibutilide[b]	25	Low	4	0	0	Nausea, headache
Flecainide	30	Low	5	1+	3+	L-H, visual disturbance, headache, nausea
Propafenone	30	Low	5	0–1+	2+	L-H, headache, nausea, constipation, metallic taste, ↓ warfarin clearance
Dofetilide	20	Low	4	0	0	Headache, chest pain, dizziness
Amiodarone	65	High	4	0	1+	Corneal deposits, photosensitivity, sleep disturbance, nausea, anorexia, tremor, ataxia, neuropathy, pulmonary fibrosis, thyroid disorders, hepatotoxicity, ↓ warfarin clearance
Sotalol	30	Low	5	1+	3+	L-H, fatigue, dyspnea, nausea

Abbreviations: EF, ejection fraction; L-H, light-headedness; VT, sustained ventricular tachycardia.

[a] Congestive heart failure risk: 0, no risk; 4+, high risk.

[b] Intravenous therapy for acute cardioversion in patients with atrial fibrillation.

Adapted from MKSAP IX: Part C, Book 1, 1992. American College of Physicians. Used with permission.

- Adenosine slows AV conduction and has a half-life of 10 seconds.

- It is indicated for termination of rapid SVT using the AV node.

- Adenosine is contraindicated in patients with atrial fibrillation associated with Wolff-Parkinson-White syndrome because of the risk of hemodynamic collapse as atrial fibrillation transitions to ventricular fibrillation.

Adverse Effects of Antiarrhythmic Drugs

Proarrhythmic effect (Table 2.3), a common and important problem of all antiarrhythmic drugs, occurs when the drug creates an adverse rhythm disturbance, including sinus node suppression and sinus bradycardia, AV block, or increased frequency of or new-onset atrial or ventricular arrhythmias. An example, quinidine syncope due to polymorphic ventricular tachycardia, is shown in Figure 2.4. All antiarrhythmic agents can be proarrhythmic. The frequency of proarrhythmia is higher in patients with decreased ventricular function and a history of sustained ventricular tachycardia or ventricular fibrillation. Proarrhythmia can occur in structurally normal hearts.

- All antiarrhythmic drugs can cause arrhythmias.

TRANSCATHETER RFA

Transcatheter RFA using a radiofrequency energy source to heat tissue has revolutionized the treatment of almost all heart rhythm disorders. Narrow complex tachycardias such as AV nodal reentrant tachycardia or tachycardia due to an accessory pathway (eg, Wolff-Parkinson-White syndrome) are curable with RFA in more than 95% of cases. Atrial tachycardias are curable in more than 90% of cases. Table 2.4 lists arrhythmias amenable to catheter ablation therapy. Atrial fibrillation (especially paroxysmal atrial fibrillation) and ventricular tachycardia due to reentry around a scar after myocardial infarction can also be treated with RFA. RFA prevents further conduction

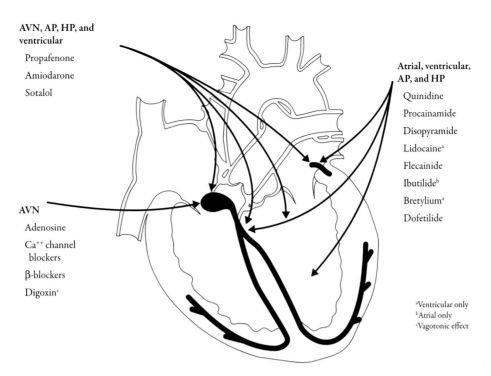

AVN, AP, HP, and ventricular

Propafenone

Amiodarone

Sotalol

Atrial, ventricular, AP, and HP

Quinidine

Procainamide

Disopyramide

Lidocaine[a]

Flecainide

Ibutilide[b]

Bretylium[a]

Dofetilide

AVN

Adenosine

Ca^{++} channel blockers

β-blockers

Digoxin[c]

[a]Ventricular only
[b]Atrial only
[c]Vagotonic effect

Figure 2.3 The Predominant Targets of Frequently Used Antiarrhythmic Agents. AP indicates accessory pathway; AVN, atrioventricular node; HP, His-Purkinje system.

of electrical impulses and prevents the abnormal rhythm from occurring. Complications include vascular injury, cardiac perforation, and infection and occur in 1% to 2% of patients. There is a 5% risk of creating complete heart block requiring permanent pacing if the ablated area is close to the normal conduction system or if AV nodal reentrant tachycardia is ablated.

Catheter ablation also may be used to achieve complete heart block in 95% of patients with difficult-to-control atrial fibrillation or atrial flutter–associated heart rates that are refractory to medications. After ablation, permanent pacing is required. This approach results in substantial improvement in symptoms and exercise capacity with use of rate-responsive pacing. The major disadvantage is that patients are pacemaker-dependent and it is irreversible. This approach is reserved for very elderly patients or when other approaches fail. Catheter ablation techniques aimed at removing the

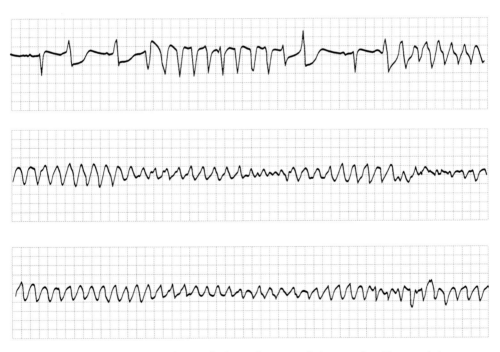

Figure 2.4 Proarrhythmic Response to Quinidine. Quinidine resulted in prolongation of QT interval, and late-coupled premature ventricular complex initiated polymorphic ventricular tachycardia, termed *torsades de pointes*.

Table 2.4 HEART RHYTHMS AMENABLE TO CATHETER ABLATION

RHYTHM	CURABLE	TREATABLE
SVT	AVNRT AVRT (bypass tract) EAT AFL (without fibrillation)	AF
Ventricular	RV outflow tract tachycardia Idiopathic LV tachycardia	VT due to coronary disease & scar after MI

Abbreviations: AF, atrial fibrillation; AFL, atrial flutter; AVNRT, atrioventricular node reentry tachycardia; AVRT, atrioventricular reentry tachycardia; EAT, ectopic atrial tachycardia; LV, left ventricular; MI, myocardial infarction; RV, right ventricular; SVT, supraventricular tachycardia; VT, ventricular tachycardia.

triggers that cause atrial fibrillation and flutter are used with increasing success.

- Narrow complex tachycardia due to AV nodal reentrant tachycardia, accessory pathway in Wolff-Parkinson-White syndrome, focal atrial tachycardia, atrial flutter, and, often, atrial fibrillation and ventricular tachycardia can be cured with RFA.

- In patients with atrial fibrillation or flutter whose heart rates are refractory to medications, catheter ablation may be used to achieve complete heart block. After ablation, permanent pacing is required.

Current therapeutic interventions available to patients with symptoms due to tachycardia are summarized in Table 2.5.

DEVICE THERAPY

Device therapy is appropriate for symptomatic bradycardia, ventricular tachycardia, or prevention of sudden cardiac death in patients with high-risk cardiac disease. Indications for a

Table 2.5 SUMMARY OF TACHYARRHYTHMIA THERAPY

SUPRAVENTICULAR TACHYCARDIA	DRUG	ABLATION	ICD
AVNRT	+	++	–
AVRT	+	++	–
EAT	+	+	–
IAST	++	o	–
Typical A flutter	+	++	–
Afib	++	+	o

Symbols: +, effective; ++, preferred; o, investigational; –, no indication.
Abbreviations: A, atrial; Afib, atrial fibrillation; AVNRT, atrioventricular nodal reentry tachycardia; AVRT, atrioventricular reentry tachycardia; EAT, ectopic atrial tachycardia; IAST, inappropriate sinus tachycardia; ICD, implantable cardioverter-defibrillator.

Box 2.1 INDICATIONS FOR PACEMAKER IMPLANTATION

Sinus node dysfunction
  Class I
    Documented symptomatic bradycardia
  Class II
    HR <40 bpm, symptoms present but not clearly correlated with bradycardia
  Class III
    Asymptomatic bradycardia (<40 bpm)
AV block
  Class I
    Symptomatic 2° or 3° AV block, permanent or intermittent
    Congenital 3° AV block with wide QRS
    Advanced AV block 14 days after cardiac surgery
  Class II
    Asymptomatic type II 2° or 3° AV block with ventricular rate >40 bpm
  Class III
    Asymptomatic 1° & type I 2° AV block
Myocardial infarction
  Class I
    Recurrent type II 2° AV block & 3° AV block with wide QRS
    Transient advanced AV block in presence of BBB
  Class II
    Persistent advanced AV block with narrow QRS
    Acquired BBB in absence of AV block
  Class III
    Transient AV block in absence of BBB

Abbreviations: AV, atrioventricular, BBB, bundle branch block; bpm, beats per minute; HR, heart rate.

permanent pacemaker implantation in specific conduction system diseases are listed in Box 2.1.

Permanent Cardiac Pacemaker Implantation

An internationally used 4-letter system is used to classify different types of implantable pacemakers and ICDs (Table 2.6). The choice of device used depends on the clinical circumstances.

Physiologic pacing attempts to maintain heart rate with normal AV synchrony and to increase heart rate in response to physical activity. Patients fitted with this type of pacemaker have increased exercise endurance during treadmill testing. A sensor that responds to body motion, respiratory rate, blood temperature, or some other variable can be used to drive the pacemaker so that the rate at which pacing occurs is appropriate to metabolic demands. Patients with both sinus node dysfunction and AV conduction system disease benefit most from DDDR pacing.

- Rate-modulated pacing increases exercise endurance during treadmill testing.

Table 2.6 CODE OF PERMANENT PACING

CHAMBER(S) PACED	CHAMBER(S) SENSED	MODE(S) OF RESPONSE	PROGRAMMABLE CAPABILITIES
V = Ventricle	V = Ventricle	T = Triggered	R = Rate modulated
A = Atrium	A = Atrium	I = Inhibited	
D = Dual (atrium & ventricle)	D = Dual (atrium & ventricle)	D = Dual (triggered & inhibited)	
	O = None	O = None	

Early complications (within 30 days of implantation) are usually related to vascular injury, hematoma, pneumothorax, dislodgment of the lead, and extracardiac stimulation. *Late complications* include lead fracture or insulation defect, infection, pacemaker syndrome, and pacemaker-mediated tachycardia.

Pacemaker-mediated tachycardia is a well-recognized complication of dual-chamber pacemakers (DDD pacing). Pacemaker-mediated tachycardia occurs during DDD pacing when there is intact retrograde conduction between the ventricle and atrium. A spontaneous premature ventricular contraction occurs that conducts retrogradely to the atrium. The tachycardia rate is typically close to the upper rate limit of the device. Most pacemakers can recognize and attempt to abort pacemaker-mediated tachycardia. Pacemaker-mediated tachycardia is corrected by programming changes of the pacemaker generator.

- Early complications occur within 30 days of implantation and are related to vascular injury, lead displacement, pneumothorax, and extracardiac stimulation.

- Late complications are related to lead fracture or insulation defects, infection, pacemaker syndrome, or pacemaker-mediated tachycardia.

Implantable Cardioverter-Defibrillators

An ICD continuously monitors heart rhythm and can detect and treat abnormal ventricular arrhythmia with overdrive pacing (antitachycardia pacing), low-energy cardioversion, or up to 30- to 40-J shocks. ICDs have been shown to improve mortality outcomes among patients who survive sudden cardiac death. An ICD is superior for reducing overall mortality in comparison with empiric amiodarone therapy in patients with a history of out-of-hospital cardiac arrest or symptomatic sustained ventricular tachycardia.

Indications for ICD implantation include the following:

1. Documented episode of cardiac arrest caused by ventricular fibrillation not due to a transient or reversible cause, documented sustained ventricular tachyarrhythmia (spontaneous or induced by an electrophysiology study) not associated with an acute myocardial infarction and not due to a transient or reversible cause

2. Documented familial or inherited conditions with a high risk of life-threatening ventricular tachycardia (eg, long QT syndrome or hypertrophic cardiomyopathy)

3. Ischemic and nonischemic cardiomyopathy (left ventricular ejection fraction [LVEF] <35%) plus congestive heart failure (New York Heart Association [NYHA] class II or III)

4. Ischemic cardiomyopathy due to prior myocardial infarction and LVEF <30%

5. ICDs provide greater overall mortality reduction in patients with a history of out-of-hospital arrest or symptomatic sustained ventricular tachycardia than amiodarone.

SUMMARY OF THERAPY FOR HEART RHYTHM DISORDERS

Table 2.5 summarizes the roles of drug therapy, ablation therapy, and ICD therapy for different supraventricular tachyarrhythmias.

SPECIFIC ARRHYTHMIAS

THE BRADYCARDIAS

Bradycardia is defined as a heart rate less than 60 beats per minute at rest or a decreased heart rate response to exercise. Causes of bradycardia include high vagal tone (most cases occur in asymptomatic and often fit and healthy persons), sinus node dysfunction, drug therapy, heart block, and myocardial infarction.

Sinus Node Dysfunction

Sinus node dysfunction includes sinus bradycardia, sinus pauses, tachycardia-bradycardia syndrome (Figure 2.5), sinus arrest, and chronotropic incompetence. In most cases, sinus node dysfunction is diagnosed on the basis of the history and results of ECG and Holter monitoring. EP testing is usually not necessary. Prolonged monitoring with an event recorder may be required to correlate symptoms with bradycardia. Treadmill testing can distinguish true sinus node dysfunction, in which a blunted heart rate occurs in response to exercise, from high vagal tone, in which the heart rate increases appropriately during exercise to meet metabolic need. EP testing is reserved for a minority of patients in whom the arrhythmia mechanism cannot be determined by ECG or Holter monitoring.

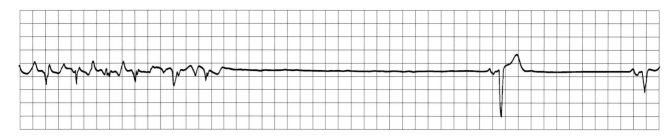

Figure 2.5 Tachycardia-Bradycardia Syndrome. In this case, episode of atrial fibrillation terminated spontaneously, followed by a 4.5-second pause until the sinus node recovered. (Adapted from MKSAP IX: Part C, Book 1, c1992. American College of Physicians. Used with permission.)

Asymptomatic patients with sinus node dysfunction do not require specific therapy, whereas symptomatic patients usually receive a pacemaker. Patients with tachycardia-bradycardia often have atrial fibrillation that can present with rapid ventricular rates or with symptomatic bradycardia. Pacemakers are used to prevent the bradycardia. Drugs can be used to slow conduction through the AV node and to prevent episodes of rapid ventricular rate.

- Sinus node dysfunction includes sinus bradycardia, sinus pause, tachycardia-bradycardia syndrome, sinus arrest, and chronotropic incompetence.

- History and results of ECG and ambulatory ECG monitoring are sufficient to allow diagnosis in the majority of patients.

- EP testing is rarely needed for the diagnosis of sinus node dysfunction.

- Patients with tachycardia-bradycardia often have atrial fibrillation that can present with rapid ventricular rates or with symptomatic bradycardia.

Conduction System Disorders

A conduction system disorder occurs when there is a delay in impulses from the sinus node reaching the ventricles or when some impulses do not reach the ventricles because of an AV node or distal conduction system (His-Purkinje system) block. Conduction system disorders can be divided into first-degree, second-degree, and third-degree (complete) heart block.

First-Degree AV Block

In first-degree AV block, the PR interval on the ECG is prolonged (>200 milliseconds). If the QRS is narrow, the conduction delay is most likely within the AV node. In the setting of an associated bundle branch block, the conduction delay may be in the His-Purkinje system or bundle branches.

- First-degree AV block is diagnosed from a prolonged PR interval on the ECG.

- If the QRS is narrow, the conduction delay is likely in the AV node.

Second-Degree AV Block

There are 2 subtypes of second-degree AV block: Mobitz I and Mobitz II. Mobitz I block (Wenckebach) manifests as gradual prolongation of the PR interval before a nonconducted P wave. The PR interval after the nonconducted P wave is shorter than the PR interval before the nonconducted P wave (Figures 2.6 and 2.7). The RR interval that encompasses the nonconducted P wave is shorter than 2 RR intervals between conducted beats. Wenckebach conduction often occurs after an inferior myocardial infarction as a result of AV node ischemia. Wenckebach conduction does not require pacing unless hemodynamic problems are associated with the slow heart rate.

Mobitz II second-degree AV block usually is caused by conduction block within the His-Purkinje system and frequently is associated with bundle branch block. The ECG shows a sudden failure of conduction of a P wave, with no change in the PR

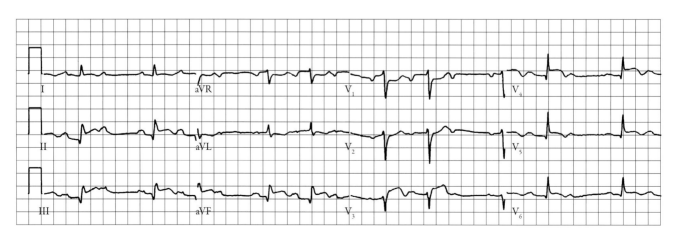

Figure 2.6 3:2 Mobitz I (or Wenckebach) Second-Degree Atrioventricular Block. Patient had acute inferior myocardial infarction.

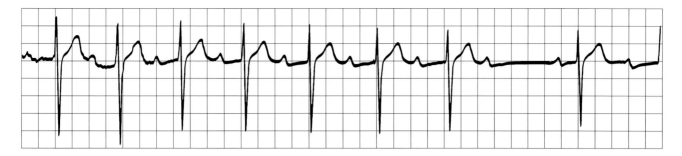

Figure 2.7 Mobitz I Second-Degree Atrioventricular Block. Note gradual PR prolongation. The PR interval after a nonconducted P wave is shorter than the PR interval preceding the nonconducted P wave.

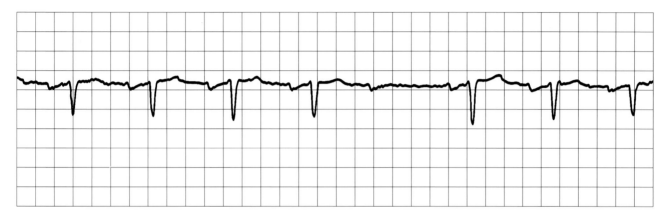

Figure 2.8 Mobitz II Second-Degree Atrioventricular Block. There was no change in the PR interval before or after a nonconducted P wave.

interval either before or after the nonconducted P wave (Figure 2.8). The ventricular escape rhythm is either a junctional escape focus, with a conduction pattern similar to that seen during normal rhythm, or a ventricular escape focus, with a wide QRS conduction pattern. Mobitz II block is usually due to conduction disease in the His-Purkinje system. It often heralds complete heart block, and permanent pacing should be considered.

- Mobitz I block is identified by gradual prolongation of the PR interval before a nonconducted P wave, and the PR interval after the nonconducted P wave is shorter than the PR interval before the nonconducted P wave.

- Mobitz II block is diagnosed from the sudden nonconduction of a P wave without alteration in any PR interval.

- Mobitz II block often heralds complete heart block, and permanent pacing should be considered.

Third-Degree (Complete) Heart Block

Complete heart block is diagnosed when there is no relation between atrial rhythm and ventricular rhythm, and atrial rhythm is faster than ventricular escape rhythm (Figure 2.9). Treatment is with permanent pacing.

- Complete heart block is treated with permanent pacing.

Bifascicular block refers to left bundle branch block (both fascicles blocked), right bundle branch block with left anterior fascicular block (marked left axis deviation), or right bundle branch block with left posterior fascicular block (right axis deviation). Patients presenting with syncope and bifascicular block may have intermittent complete heart block due to conduction system disease or ventricular tachycardia caused by underlying myocardial disease. Permanent pacing can be used to treat syncope due to complete heart block.

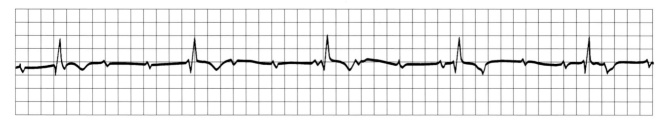

Figure 2.9 Complete Heart Block. Atrial rate was 70 beats per minute and ventricular escape rhythm was 30 beats per minute.

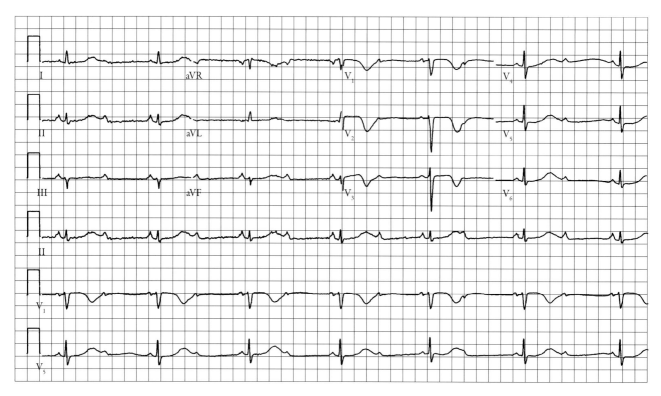

Figure 2.10 High-Grade 2:1 Atrioventricular Conduction Block.

- Bifascicular block usually is associated with structural heart disease and progresses to complete heart block in about 1% of asymptomatic persons.

  High-degree (high-grade) AV block is diagnosed when there is a 2:1 or higher AV conduction block (Figure 2.10). It can be due to a Wenckebach or Mobitz II mechanism. A Wenckebach mechanism is more likely if QRS conduction (duration) is normal, whereas a Mobitz II mechanism is more likely if the QRS complex demonstrates additional conduction disease, such as bundle branch block.

- High-grade AV block is diagnosed when the ECG shows a 2:1 or higher AV conduction block.

Carotid Sinus Hypersensitivity Syndrome

Approximately 40% of patients older than 65 years have a hyperactive carotid sinus reflex (a 3-second pause or a decrease in systolic blood pressure of 50 mm Hg) (Figure 2.11). Rarely, neck abnormalities, such as lymph node enlargement, prior neck surgery, or a regional tumor, can cause carotid sinus hypersensitivity syndrome. Most patients do not have spontaneous syncope. Carotid sinus massage may be performed over the carotid bifurcation at the angle of the jaw for 5 seconds while monitoring heart rate and blood pressure to test for this cause, but only in patients without a carotid bruit or a history of cerebrovascular disease. One-third of patients with a hyperactive carotid sinus reflex have a pure cardioinhibitory component manifested only by a pause in ventricular activity exceeding 3 seconds. Fifteen percent of patients have a pure vasodepressor component, with a normal heart rate maintained but a decrease in systolic blood pressure of more than 50 mm Hg. Sixty percent of patients have a combined response of both cardioinhibitory and vasodepressor components. Permanent pacing may prevent the cardioinhibitory response, but the vasodepressor response continues to produce symptoms.

AV sequential pacing is the primary form of therapy for the cardioinhibitory component, and elastic stockings are used to

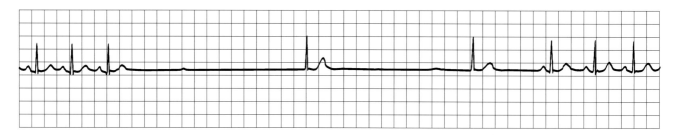

Figure 2.11 Sinus Pause With Junctional Escape Beats Before Sinus Rhythm Returns. Test was done during carotid sinus massage.

treat the vasodepressor component. Occasionally, the condition responds to anticholinergic medications. Surgical techniques to treat this condition are often unsuccessful.

- Patients with a hyperactive carotid sinus reflex experience a 3-second pause or a decrease of 50 mm Hg in systolic blood pressure.

- The cardioinhibitory component is treated with AV sequential pacing, and elastic stockings are used to treat the vasodepressor component.

- Anticholinergics are occasionally helpful, and surgical procedures are usually unsuccessful.

THE TACHYCARDIAS

Atrial Flutter

Atrial flutter is identified on the ECG by the characteristic sawtooth pattern of atrial activity at a rate of 240 to 320 beats per minute. Patients with normal conduction systems maintain 2:1 AV conduction; the ventricular rate is often close to 150 beats per minute. Higher degrees of AV block (3:1 or higher) in the absence of drugs that slow AV nodal conduction (digoxin, β-adrenergic blockers, calcium channel antagonists) suggest the presence of intrinsic AV conduction disease (Figure 2.12). In patients with 2:1 AV conduction and a heart rate of 150 beats per minute, 1 of the flutter waves is often buried in the QRS complex. Carotid sinus massage (or transient AV node blockade with adenosine) may help reveal the flutter waves to establish the diagnosis.

Pharmacologic therapy for atrial flutter is used to slow AV node conduction and control the ventricular rate or to control the flutter itself. The same medications used to treat atrial fibrillation are used to treat atrial flutter. Success rates for the control of atrial flutter are 30% to 50%. Catheter ablation has a success rate of more than 90%. A permanent pacemaker is needed after AV node ablation. The atria continue to flutter or fibrillate but symptoms are improved.

- Catheter ablation of atrial flutter has a success rate of >90%.

- Atrial flutter is associated with the same risk of thromboembolism as atrial fibrillation and should be treated similarly to atrial fibrillation with regard to anticoagulation.

- In atrial flutter, the ECG shows a characteristic sawtooth pattern with an atrial rate of 240–320 beats per minute.

- AV node conduction rate and ventricular rate control are achieved with the pharmacologic therapy used in atrial fibrillation; success rates for control of atrial flutter are 30%–50%.

Atrial Fibrillation

Atrial fibrillation is characterized by continuous and irregular activity of the ECG baseline caused by swarming electric currents in the atria and is the most common arrhythmia encountered in clinical practice. Its prevalence increases with age; 5% of patients 65 or older are affected. Common associated conditions include hypertension, cardiomyopathy, valvular heart disease (particularly mitral stenosis), sleep-disordered breathing, sick sinus syndrome, Wolff-Parkinson-White syndrome (especially in young patients), alcohol use ("holiday heart"), and thyrotoxicosis. Atrial fibrillation should be distinguished from atrial flutter (uniform flutter waves) and multifocal atrial tachycardia (isoelectric interval between premature atrial contractions that have 3 or more different morphologic forms).

- Atrial fibrillation is the most common arrhythmia in clinical practice; its prevalence increases with age.

- Hypertension, cardiomyopathy, valvular heart disease, sleep apnea, sick sinus syndrome, Wolff-Parkinson-White syndrome, excess alcohol intake, and thyrotoxicosis are commonly associated with atrial fibrillation.

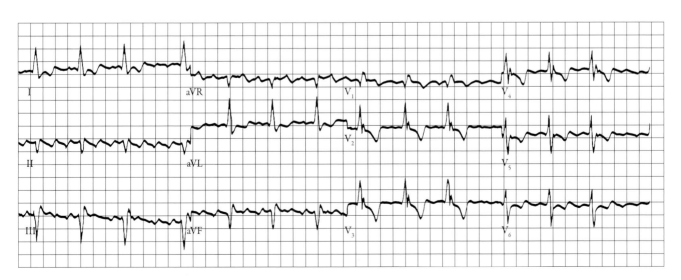

Figure 2.12 Atrial Flutter With 3:1 Conduction. Patient had atrioventricular conduction disease.

- Atrial fibrillation should be distinguished from atrial flutter and multifocal atrial tachycardia.

Therapy for Atrial Fibrillation

The therapeutic approach to patients with atrial fibrillation is determined by the severity of symptoms and comorbid conditions. Therapeutic options include rate control (pharmacologic agents or ablation to slow AV node conduction), stroke prophylaxis in patients at risk of stroke, and rhythm control (treatment aims to restore and maintain sinus rhythm). Rhythm control is essential in patients with symptoms despite adequate rate control. Symptoms associated with atrial fibrillation include palpitations, shortness of breath, fatigue, chest pain, and, rarely, presyncope or syncope. Separate from rhythm evaluation, assessment of stroke risk is necessary. Several risk scores are available, but the most clinically useful is the CHADS2 scoring system (congestive heart failure, hypertension, age >75 years, diabetes, and previous stroke). Rhythm control is most appropriate in patients with symptoms due to atrial fibrillation. In asymptomatic patients, rate control has mortality outcomes similar to those with rhythm control. In all patients, initial management should be rate control using AV nodal blocking agents and an assessment of stroke risk and need for anticoagulation before deciding on a long-term strategy. Pharmacologic agents useful for rate control and rhythm control are shown in Table 2.7. In patients at risk of stroke based on the CHADS2 score, the use of drug therapy or ablative therapy to maintain and restore sinus rhythm may not reduce stroke risk.

- Therapy for atrial fibrillation is based on the presence or absence of symptoms and comorbid conditions.

- Adequate rate control (with anticoagulation therapy if risk of stroke is increased) has outcomes similar to those of rhythm control.

- Restoration of sinus rhythm may not reduce stroke risk.

The 3 main categories of drugs used to blunt the AV node response in atrial fibrillation are digitalis glycosides, β-blocking agents, and calcium channel blockers. These are summarized in Table 2.7. None of these agents prevent recurrent atrial fibrillation.

Digoxin acts indirectly by increasing vagal tone and at therapeutic concentration has no direct effect in slowing AV node conduction. Because of its mechanism of action, digoxin is less effective than β-blockers or calcium channel blockers, particularly with exercise, when an increase in sympathetic tone results in more rapid AV node conduction. The optimal role for digoxin in atrial fibrillation is therapy for patients with left ventricular dysfunction (because of the drug's positive inotropy) or as adjunctive therapy for patients receiving β-blockers or calcium channel blockers. Digoxin alone is no better than placebo for terminating atrial fibrillation.

- Digoxin is less effective than β-blockers or calcium channel blockers for controlling ventricular rate and is best used as an adjunctive agent because of its inotropic effect in patients with impaired ventricular function.

β-Blockers (eg, propranolol, metoprolol, atenolol) slow AV node conduction and may be particularly useful when atrial fibrillation complicates hyperthyroidism or myocardial infarction. β-Blockers also decrease the risk of postoperative myocardial infarction and are useful for postoperative atrial fibrillation. Carvedilol decreases mortality of patients with chronic heart failure. Esmolol, because of its intravenous formulation and short half-life, is particularly useful for acute management of atrial fibrillation.

- β-Blockers slow the ventricular rate in atrial fibrillation, but they do not terminate atrial fibrillation (although they may prevent it postoperatively).

Calcium channel blockers are divided into 2 groups: dihydropyridines (eg, nifedipine, amlodipine, and felodipine)

Table 2.7 **PHARMACOLOGIC THERAPY FOR ATRIAL FIBRILLATION**

AGENTS	COMMENTS
Control of ventricular rate	
β-Blockers (eg, atenolol, metoprolol, propranolol, carvedilol)	Ideal postoperatively & in hyperthyroidism, acute MI, & chronic CHF (especially carvedilol)
Calcium channel blockers (eg, verapamil, diltiazem)	Nifedipine, amlodipine, & felodipine are not useful for slowing AV conduction
Digoxin	Less effective than β-blockers & calcium channel blockers, especially with exercise
	Useful in heart failure
Maintenance of sinus rhythm	
Class IA: quinidine, disopyramide, procainamide	Enhance AV conduction—rate must be controlled before use
	Monitor QTc
Class IC: propafenone, flecainide	Slow AV conduction
	Often first choice for patients with normal heart
	Monitor QRS duration
Class III: sotalol, amiodarone	Amiodarone is agent of choice for ventricular dysfunction & after MI

Abbreviations: AV, atrioventricular; CHF, congestive heart failure; MI, myocardial infarction.

and nondihydropyridines (eg, diltiazem and verapamil). Dihydropyridine agents have little or no effect on AV node conduction and no role in the management of atrial fibrillation. Verapamil and diltiazem are both available as intravenous and oral preparations and are well suited for acute and chronic rate control. Both agents have negative inotropic effects and must be used cautiously in CHF.

- Diltiazem and verapamil are the only effective calcium channel blockers for rate control in atrial fibrillation.

Adenosine has no role in the treatment of atrial fibrillation but can be useful diagnostically by transiently slowing the ventricular rate and thus permitting visualization of atrial activity.

When pharmacologic rate control fails (due to persistent symptoms or intolerance of medications), catheter ablation of the AV junction may be considered. This approach is more than 95% effective for controlling symptoms and carries minimal risk. The major disadvantage is creation of pacemaker dependence. In patients with paroxysmal atrial fibrillation a dual-chamber pacemaker is implanted, whereas in patients with persistent atrial fibrillation a single-chamber ventricular pacemaker (programmed to VVIR mode) is implanted. Dual-chamber pacemakers have a mode-switching function that permits tracking of P waves during sinus rhythm and reverts to VVIR (or DDIR) mode pacing when atrial fibrillation recurs.

- Catheter ablation of the AV node should be considered when pharmacologic rate control fails.

Rhythm control (maintenance of sinus rhythm) controls symptoms effectively. Common types of pharmacologic rhythm control include class IC antiarrhythmic agents (eg, propafenone and flecainide), which are good first choices and often can be given safely in the outpatient setting (with ECG and treadmill testing at 3 days to exclude proarrhythmic effect). These drugs should be avoided in patients with structural heart disease. Amiodarone and dofetilide (class III agents) are generally safe in patients with prior myocardial infarction and those with systolic dysfunction. Other class I drugs (IA and IB) are rarely used.

- Avoid class IC drugs in patients with structural heart disease.
- Amiodarone is generally safe in patients with a history of myocardial infarction or systolic dysfunction.

For acute stroke risk, electrical cardioversion from atrial fibrillation is commonly used to control atrial fibrillation. Patients with atrial fibrillation lasting more than 2 days should receive anticoagulation before cardioversion. Three weeks of warfarin therapy before cardioversion substantially decreases the incidence of cardioversion-associated thromboembolism to 0% to 1.6% (compared with up to 7% in the absence of anticoagulation). Anticoagulation

should be continued for a minimum of 4 weeks after cardioversion because of the increased risk of thromboembolism in the weeks after cardioversion or indefinitely in select patients with other risk factors for stroke. Current guidelines do not mandate anticoagulation in the setting of cardioversion for atrial fibrillation of recent onset (<48 hours). Anticoagulation guidelines for atrial flutter are identical to those for atrial fibrillation. An alternative approach for patients with atrial fibrillation for more than 2 days is heparin therapy with transesophageal echocardiography and cardioversion if no thrombus is found followed by anticoagulation for 3 to 4 weeks.

- To reduce stroke risk, patients with atrial fibrillation of >2 days should receive anticoagulation with warfarin for 3 weeks before cardioversion and for 4 weeks after.

- An alternative approach is heparin therapy and transesophageal echocardiography to exclude left atrial appendage thrombus followed by anticoagulation for 3–4 weeks after cardioversion.

For chronic stroke prevention, warfarin therapy should be used in patients with atrial fibrillation due to rheumatic valvular disease because they have a markedly increased risk of stroke. Most patients have nonrheumatic atrial fibrillation. Warfarin decreases the incidence of thromboembolism by close to 80% in this population. Risk of thromboembolism can be determined using the CHADS2 score (Table 2.8). For patients in whom warfarin therapy is indicated, an international normalized ratio should be maintained in the range of 2.0 to 3.0.

- Clinical risk factors for stroke in nonrheumatic atrial fibrillation include CHF, hypertension, age >75 years, diabetes mellitus, and previous transient ischemic attack or stroke.

Table 2.8 RISK FACTORS FOR THROMBOEMBOLISM IN NONRHEUMATIC ATRIAL FIBRILLATION

CHADS2 CRITERIA	POINTS	STROKE RISK SCORE	RECOMMENDED THERAPY
Congestive heart failure	1	Low=0	Aspirin 100–300 mg daily
Hypertension	1	Moderate	Warfarin or aspirin
Age ≥75 years	1		
Diabetes mellitus	1		
Previous stroke or TIA	2	High=2–6	Warfarin (INR 2–3)

Abbreviations: INR, international normalized ratio; TIA, transient ischemic attack.

Data from Gage BF, Waterman AD, Shannon W, Boechler M, Rich MW, Radford MJ. Validation of clinical classification schemes for predicting stroke: results from the National Registry of Atrial Fibrillation. JAMA. 2001 Jun 13;285(22):2864–70.

- Echocardiographic risk factors for stroke are depressed ventricular function and left atrial enlargement.

- Patients <60 years of age with structurally normal hearts and no history of hypertension are at low risk for thromboembolism and require no specific therapy other than aspirin.

- There is no difference in stroke risk between paroxysmal and chronic atrial fibrillation.

- Warfarin substantially decreases the risk of thromboembolism in patients with atrial fibrillation.

Other Supraventricular Tachycardias

Tachycardia (rate >100 beats per minute) should be characterized as a narrow complex or a wide complex tachycardia.

Paroxysmal Supraventricular Tachycardia

Paroxysmal supraventricular tachycardia (PSVT) is due to a reentrant mechanism with an abrupt onset and termination, a regular rate, and a narrow QRS complex (Figure 2.13), unless there is a rate-related or preexisting bundle branch block. Acutely, PSVT responds to vagal maneuvers; adenosine (or verapamil if PSVT is recurrent) terminates the arrhythmia in 90% of patients. PSVT generally is not a life-threatening arrhythmia; it often occurs in an otherwise normal heart. It is more serious and can lead to cardiac decompensation when it is associated with underlying heart disease. The preferred method for management of symptomatic PSVT is catheter ablation, which has success rates of more than 90%. For patients with PSVT and other comorbidities (eg, hypertension), in whom catheter ablation is not feasible or preferred, β-blockers or calcium channel blockers may be useful for treating both conditions.

- Catheter ablation is preferred for management of symptomatic PSVT; it has a high success rate.

- β-Blockers or calcium channel blockers may be useful in patients with PSVT and comorbid conditions such as hypertension.

Multifocal atrial tachycardia is an automatic atrial rhythm diagnosed when 3 or more distinct atrial foci (P waves of different morphology) are present and the rate exceeds 100 beats per minute (Figure 2.14). This rhythm occurs primarily in patients with decompensated lung disease and associated hypoxia, increased catecholamines (exogenous and endogenous), atrial stretch, and local tissue acid-base and electrolyte disturbances. Digoxin worsens multifocal atrial tachycardia (shortens atrial refractoriness). Multifocal atrial tachycardia is best treated with calcium channel blockers and correction of the underlying medical illnesses, including increasing oxygenation.

- Multifocal atrial tachycardia is diagnosed when 3 or more distinct atrial foci are present and the heart rate exceeds 100 beats per minute. The P waves all have a different morphology.

- Multifocal atrial tachycardia is best treated with nondihydropyridine calcium channel blockers and treatment of underlying medical conditions.

Differentiating Supraventricular Tachycardia With Aberrancy From Ventricular Tachycardia

Wide QRS tachycardia may be due to supraventricular tachycardia with aberrancy or to ventricular tachycardia (Figure 2.15). Findings useful for identifying ventricular tachycardia are listed in Box 2.2.

Wide QRS tachycardias are ventricular in origin in more than 85% of cases and are often well tolerated. The absence of hemodynamic compromise during tachycardia does not prove the tachycardia is supraventricular in origin.

A simple approach to a wide complex tachycardia is to review the morphologic features of the complex in lead V_1 and decide whether the pattern is that of right or left bundle

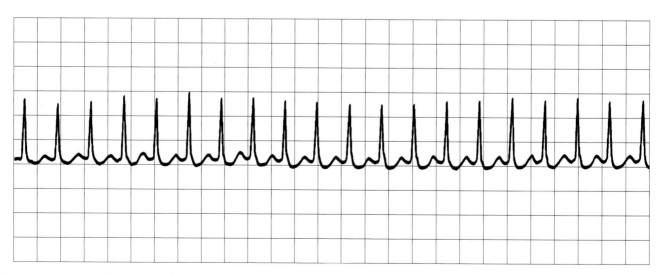

Figure 2.13 Paroxysmal Supraventricular Tachycardia.

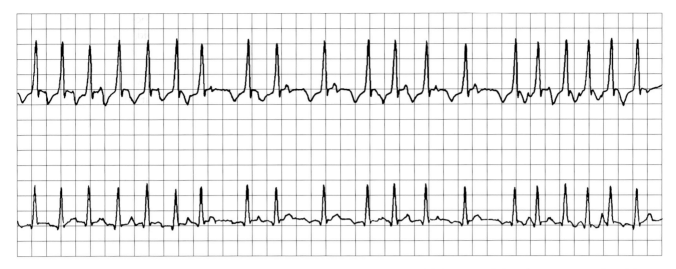

Figure 2.14 Multifocal Atrial Tachycardia. Simultaneous recordings show 3 or more P waves of different morphology. (Lower tracing, adapted from MKSAP IX: Part C, Book 1, c1992. American College of Physicians. Used with permission.)

branch block. If the morphologic pattern exactly matches a normal right or left bundle branch block, then it might be supraventricular with rate-related aberrant conduction. The safest approach to any wide complex tachycardia is to assume that it is due to ventricular tachycardia and treat it accordingly.

- It is safest to treat all wide complex tachycardias as ventricular in origin.

Wolff-Parkinson-White Syndrome

Wolff-Parkinson-White syndrome is defined as symptomatic tachycardia with a short PR interval (<0.12 second), a delta wave, and a prolonged QRS interval (>0.12 second). A portion of the ventricular activation is due to conduction over the accessory pathway, with the remaining activation due to conduction via the normal His-Purkinje conduction system. Not all patients with preexcitation have a short PR interval.

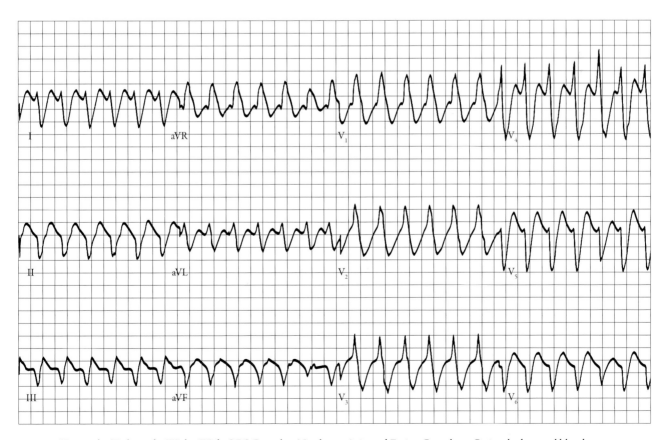

Figure 2.15 Ventricular Tachycardia With a Wide QRS Complex, Northwest Axis, and Fusion Complexes. Patient had normal blood pressure.

Normal PR conduction may occur if the accessory pathway is distant from the AV node.

Ventricular activation is abnormal in patients with Wolff-Parkinson-White syndrome. Infarction, ventricular hypertrophy, and ST-T wave changes should not be interpreted after the diagnosis is established, because these changes are usually due to the abnormal pattern of ventricular activation. Preexcitation occurs in about 2 of 1,000 patients; tachycardia subsequently develops in 70%. The most serious rhythm disturbance is atrial fibrillation with rapid ventricular conduction over the accessory pathway leading to ventricular fibrillation (Figure 2.16). Patients who are asymptomatic have a negligible chance of sudden death. For patients who are symptomatic, the incidence of sudden death is 0.0025 per patient-year.

In most cases during tachycardia, conduction from the atria to the ventricles occurs over the normal conduction system and therefore results in a normal (narrow) QRS complex (unless there is rate-related bundle branch block) (Figure 2.17). Up to 5% of patients may have reentrant tachycardia that goes in the reverse direction, in which ventricular activation over the accessory pathway activates the ventricle from an ectopic location (Figure 2.18).

EP testing and RFA of the accessory pathway are indicated in patients with symptomatic Wolff-Parkinson-White syndrome. Patients who have Wolff-Parkinson-White syndrome can safely take drugs that block the AV node, but digoxin should be avoided. AV nodal blocking drugs can be safely

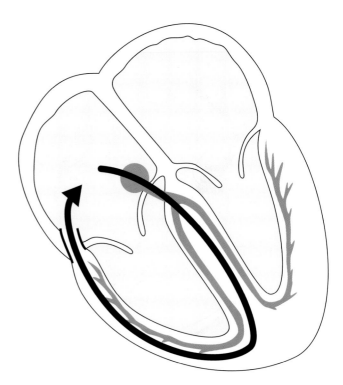

Figure 2.17 Typical Mechanism of Supraventricular Tachycardia in Wolff-Parkinson-White Syndrome (Orthodromic Atrioventricular Reentry). Result is a narrow QRS complex because ventricular activation is over the normal conduction system.

prescribed for attempted termination of PSVT (when the QRS complex is narrow, ie, <100 milliseconds).

- Reentrant tachycardia may occur in up to 5% of patients who have Wolff-Parkinson-White syndrome with ventricular activation occurring over the accessory pathway and activating the ventricle from an ectopic location.

- In patients with symptomatic Wolff-Parkinson-White syndrome, the accessory pathway is treated with RFA.

- Digoxin should be avoided, but AV node blocking agents are safe.

- PSVT termination can be attempted safely using AV nodal blocking drugs if the QRS complex is narrow.

Wolff-Parkinson-White syndrome is associated with an increased frequency of atrial fibrillation related to the presence of the accessory pathway (Figure 2.16). After successful catheter ablation of the accessory pathway, atrial fibrillation resolves in most cases. During "preexcited" atrial fibrillation, wide, irregular, and rapid ventricular complexes are seen because activation down the accessory pathway does not use the normal His-Purkinje system (Figure 2.19). In preexcited atrial fibrillation, the drug of first choice is procainamide, which slows the accessory pathway and intra-atrial conduction. Acute administration of digoxin, adenosine, β-blockers, or calcium channel blockers in patients who present with atrial fibrillation

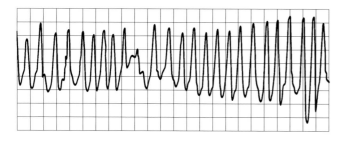

Figure 2.16 Atrial Fibrillation in Wolff-Parkinson-White Syndrome. Recording shows a wide QRS complex and irregular RR intervals.

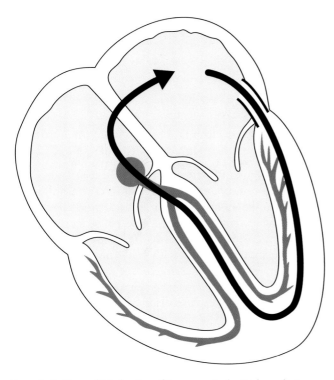

Figure 2.18 Unusual Mechanism of Supraventricular Tachycardia in Wolff-Parkinson-White Syndrome. Result is a wide QRS complex because ventricular activation is over an accessory pathway. This arrhythmia is difficult to distinguish from ventricular tachycardia.

and Wolff-Parkinson-White syndrome is contraindicated because of the risk of ventricular fibrillation. If the heart rate is rapid and there is hemodynamic compromise, cardioversion should be performed.

- Avoid acute administration of digoxin, adenosine, β-blockers, or calcium channel blockers for atrial fibrillation and Wolff-Parkinson-White syndrome because of the risk of ventricular fibrillation.

- Cardioversion should be performed if the heart rate is rapid and hemodynamic compromise is present.

Narrow complex tachycardia (whether due to an accessory pathway or other mechanism) often is terminated with vagal maneuvers or intravenously administered adenosine or verapamil. Recurrence can be prevented with a β-blocker, a calcium antagonist, and class IA (eg, quinidine, procainamide, and disopyramide), class IC (eg, propafenone and flecainide), and class III (eg, amiodarone and sotalol) antiarrhythmic drugs. RFA is used to cure tachycardia and should be strongly considered for symptomatic patients.

- Vagal maneuvers or intravenously administered adenosine or verapamil usually terminates narrow complex tachycardia.

- Recurrence can be prevented with β-blockers, calcium channel blockers, and class IA drugs (eg, procainamide and disopyramide).

Ventricular Ectopy and Nonsustained Ventricular Tachycardia

Management of frequent ventricular ectopy and nonsustained ventricular tachycardia is based on the underlying cardiac lesion. In symptomatic patients, management includes reassurance, β-blockers or calcium channel blockers for disturbing symptoms, and, in rare cases of frequent monomorphic symptomatic ventricular ectopy, catheter ablation. Patients with a structurally normal heart and complex ectopy or nonsustained ventricular tachycardia have an excellent prognosis. Management includes reassurance or, if bothersome symptoms persist, calcium channel blockers or β-blockers.

- Frequent ventricular ectopy and nonsustained ventricular tachycardia should be treated on the basis of the underlying lesion.

- Reassurance, β-blockers, or calcium channel blockers may be used.

Ventricular Tachycardia and Fibrillation

Survivors of sudden cardiac death have a risk of death approaching 30% in the first year after hospital dismissal. Antiarrhythmic drug therapy has not been shown to have benefit. ICD therapy, however, improves survival outcomes.

- Sudden cardiac death survivors have a high 1-year risk of death after hospital dismissal.

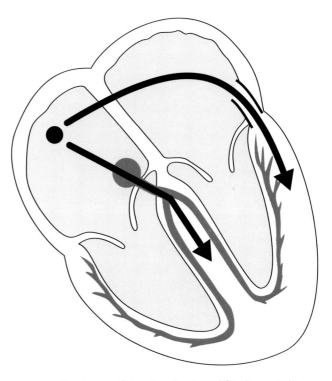

Figure 2.19 Conduction of Sinus Impulses in Wolff-Parkinson-White syndrome. The ventricles are activated over the normal atrioventricular node–His-Purkinje system and accessory pathway; the result is a fusion complex (QRS and delta wave).

- Drug therapy has no demonstrated benefit.
- Survival outcomes are improved with ICD therapy.

Torsades de Pointes

Torsades de pointes is a form of ventricular tachycardia with a characteristic polymorphic morphologic pattern described as a "twisting of the points" (torsades de pointes) (Figure 2.20).

It is related to ventricular fibrillation and occurs in the setting of QT interval prolongation and acute myocardial ischemia or infarction. Common causes include medications that prolong the QT interval (eg, quinidine, procainamide, disopyramide, sotalol, and tricyclic antidepressants), electrolyte disturbance (hypokalemia), or bradycardia (especially after myocardial infarction). Acute treatment options include temporary overdrive pacing (if due to bradycardia) and correction of electrolyte abnormality. QT interval prolongation may be due to an inherited disorder of cardiac ion channels. Patients with this abnormality require evaluation and, in some cases, implantation of a cardioverter-defibrillator.

- Torsades de pointes occurs in the setting of QT prolongation and acute myocardial infarction or ischemia.
- Patients with cardiac ion channel abnormalities require evaluation and consideration of ICD implantation.

Tachycardia-Mediated Cardiomyopathy

Persistent atrial fibrillation with a rapid ventricular rate may lead to progressive ventricular dysfunction (termed *tachycardia-mediated cardiomyopathy*). It is reversible in most cases because control of the ventricular rate improves ventricular function. In patients presenting with tachycardia and congestive heart failure, or found to have left ventricular dysfunction during evaluation, it can be difficult to determine whether heart failure is causing tachycardia or tachycardia has caused the heart failure. In a patient with heart failure and a rhythm with an abnormal P-wave axis, tachycardia-mediated cardiomyopathy should be suspected.

- Progressive ventricular dysfunction may result from persistent atrial fibrillation with a rapid ventricular rate.
- This condition is often reversible because control of the ventricular rate leads to improved ventricular function.

Ventricular Arrhythmias During Acute Myocardial Infarction

Prevention of myocardial ischemia and the use of β-blockers are essential during and after acute myocardial infarction to decrease the frequency of life-threatening ventricular arrhythmias. Asymptomatic complex ventricular ectopy, including nonsustained ventricular tachycardia, should not be treated empirically with lidocaine or amiodarone in the acute phase because the risk of proarrhythmia outweighs the potential benefit of therapy for reducing the incidence of sudden cardiac death after hospital dismissal. Ventricular tachycardia and fibrillation occurring within 24 hours after myocardial infarction are independent risk factors for in-hospital mortality but not for subsequent total mortality or mortality due to an arrhythmic event after hospital dismissal and do not require antiarrhythmic therapy. Ventricular tachycardia and fibrillation occurring more than 24 hours after an acute myocardial infarction (without ongoing ischemia or reinfarction) are independent risk factors for increased total mortality and death due to an arrhythmic event after hospital dismissal. Patients may be assessed with EP testing; treatment is usually with an ICD. Use of a prophylactic ICD after myocardial infarction is not supported by available data. Refractory ventricular tachycardia and fibrillation during acute myocardial infarction should be treated with intravenously administered lidocaine or amiodarone.

- Life-threatening arrhythmias are reduced with use of β-blockers during and after an acute myocardial infarction.
- Ventricular tachycardia and fibrillation occurring >24 hours after an acute myocardial infarction are independent risk factors for increased total mortality and death due to arrhythmia after dismissal.

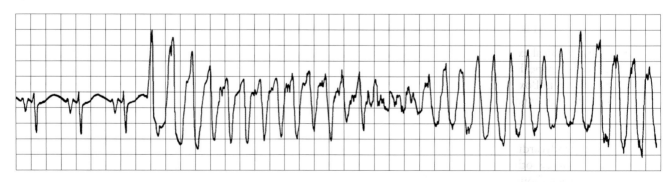

Figure 2.20 Torsades de Pointes in a Patient With Long QT Syndrome. (Adapted from Hammill SC. Electrocardiographic diagnoses: criteria and definitions of abnormalities. In: Murphy JG, Lloyd MA, editors. Mayo Clinic cardiology: concise textbook. 4th ed. Rochester [MN]: Mayo Clinic Scientific Press and New York [NY]: Oxford University Press; c2013. p. 205–38. Used with permission of Mayo Foundation for Medical Education and Research.)

- There is no evidence for the prophylactic use of an ICD after myocardial infarction.

- Treat refractory ventricular tachycardia and fibrillation during acute myocardial infarction with intravenously administered lidocaine or amiodarone.

Role of Pacing in Acute Myocardial Infarction

Among patients with an acute inferior myocardial infarction, 5% to 10% have Mobitz I second-degree or third-degree block in the absence of bundle branch block. This finding usually is transient, tends not to recur, and requires pacing only if there are symptoms due to bradycardia. Bundle branch block occurs in 10% to 20% of patients with an acute myocardial infarction. The appearance of a new bundle branch block is an indication for prophylactic temporary pacing. Patients in whom transient complete heart block develops in association with a bundle branch block are at risk for recurrent complete heart block and should undergo permanent pacing. A new bundle branch block that never progresses to complete heart block is not an indication for permanent pacing. Death of patients with myocardial infarction and bundle branch block usually is due to advanced heart failure, not complete heart block. Second-degree (Mobitz II) block with bilateral bundle branch block and third-degree (complete) AV block warrant pacing.

- Bundle branch blocks develop in up to 20% of patients after acute myocardial infarction.

- Pacing is only required in the setting of symptomatic bradycardia.

SYNCOPE

Syncope is defined as a transient loss of consciousness with spontaneous recovery. It can be categorized as cardiogenic (about 30% of cases are due to bradycardia or tachycardia), noncardiogenic (about 35% vasovagal and 10%–25% orthostatic, situational, seizures, drug-related, for example), or unknown (10%–25%) (Box 2.3).

EVALUATION OF SYNCOPE

The history and physical examination are highly valuable for the evaluation of syncope. Risk factors for a cardiogenic cause of syncope are listed in Box 2.4. Recommendations for evaluation of patients with syncope are outlined in Figure 2.21. Consider EP testing in patients at increased risk for cardiogenic syncope. EP testing is usually not indicated if an arrhythmogenic cause (bradycardia or tachycardia) of syncope has been established unless other arrhythmias are suspected. A noninvasive approach should be considered in patients at low risk for cardiogenic syncope. Tilt-table testing is effective in suspected vasovagal syncope. Tilt-table testing is also indicated for patients with recurrent syncope without structural heart disease or patients with structural heart disease after other causes of syncope have been excluded. Tilt-table testing is not indicated after a single episode of syncope without injury or in a high-risk setting with obvious vasovagal clinical features.

Box 2.3 MAJOR CAUSES OF SYNCOPE

CARDIOGENIC	NONCARDIOGENIC
Cardiogenic syncope	Neurologic
Structural heart disease	Metabolic
Coronary artery disease	Psychiatric
Rhythm disturbances	
Reflex syncope	
Vasovagal	
Carotid sinus hypersensitivity	
Situational	
Micturition	
Deglutition	
Defecation	
Glossopharyngeal neuralgia	
Postprandial	
Tussive	
Valsalva maneuver	
Oculovagal	
Sneeze	
Instrumentation	
Diving	
After exercise	
Orthostatic hypotension	

Adapted from Shen W-K, Gersh BJ. Fainting: approach to management. In: Low PA, editor. Clinical autonomic disorders: evaluation and management. 2nd ed. Philadelphia (PA): Lippincott-Raven; c1997. p. 649–79. Used with permission of Mayo Foundation for Medical Education and Research.

Box 2.4 RISK STRATIFICATION IN PATIENTS WITH UNEXPLAINED SYNCOPE[a]

HIGH-RISK FACTORS	LOW-RISK FACTORS
Coronary artery disease, previous myocardial infarction	Isolated syncope without underlying cardiovascular disease
Structural heart disease	Younger age
Left ventricular dysfunction	Symptoms consistent with a vasovagal cause
Congestive heart failure	Normal ECG
Older age	
Abrupt onset	
Serious injuries	
Abnormal ECG (presence of Q wave, bundle branch block, or atrial fibrillation)	

Abbreviation: ECG, electrocardiogram.

[a] In patients who present with a prodrome (eg, nausea, diaphoresis), a neurocardiogenic mechanism is likely. Patients who experience rapid recovery (less than 5–10 minutes) rarely have a neurologic cause for syncope and are most likely to have syncope due to seizure or "brain hypoperfusion" because recovery in such circumstances takes hours. Thus, for cases in which recovery from syncope is rapid and no residual neurologic signs or symptoms are present, detailed (and expensive) neurologic evaluation should be avoided.

Adapted from Shen W-K, Gersh BJ. Fainting: approach to management. In: Low PA, editor. Clinical autonomic disorders: evaluation and management. 2nd ed. Philadelphia (PA): Lippincott-Raven; c1997. p. 649–79. Used with permission of Mayo Foundation for Medical Education and Research.

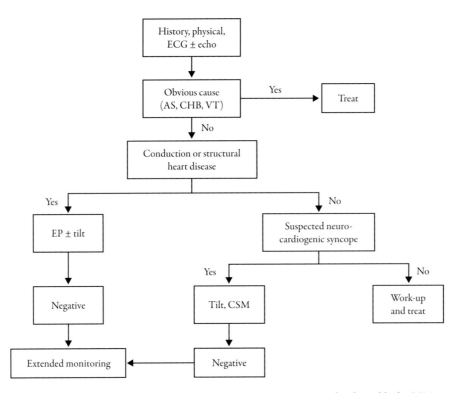

Figure 2.21 Diagnostic Pathway for Evaluation of Syncope. AS indicates aortic stenosis; CHB, complete heart block; CSM, carotid sinus massage; ECG, electrocardiography; echo, echocardiography; EP, electrophysiologic study; tilt, tilt-table testing; VT, ventricular tachycardia.

- History and physical examination provide key information needed to diagnose the cause of syncope.

- Tilt-table testing is effective in patients with suspected vasovagal syncope, recurrent syncope without structural heart disease, or structural heart disease in whom other causes of syncope have been excluded.

MANAGEMENT OF SYNCOPE

Pacemaker therapy is appropriate for sinus node dysfunction and AV conduction disease. Management of recurrent neurocardiogenic syncope (vasovagal syncope) includes education about the mechanism and triggering factors, instruction regarding appropriate action (eg, sitting or lying down to avert episodes), instruction regarding maintenance of increased intravascular volume, and instruction on maneuvers to prevent venous pooling. Midodrine, which promotes increased venous return, may be considered. Serotonin reuptake blockers may be effective in a subgroup of patients. β-Blockers have limited or no benefit. Pacemaker therapy has a limited role in preventing vasovagal syncope.

- β-Blockers and pacemakers have limited or no benefit in patients with vasovagal syncope.

SUMMARY

- Reentry is the most common mechanism of cardiac arrhythmias.

- Ambulatory ECG monitoring allows evaluation of rhythm disturbances and their relationship with daily activities.

- Syncope suggestive of a cardiogenic mechanism and palpitations likely due to a rhythm disorder are common indications for EP testing.

- Sinus node dysfunction includes sinus bradycardia, sinus pause, tachycardia-bradycardia syndrome, sinus arrest, and chronotropic incompetence.

- Syncope is categorized as cardiogenic, noncardiogenic, or unknown.

3.

CARDIAC EXAMINATION, VALVULAR HEART DISEASE, AND CONGENITAL HEART DISEASE

Kyle W. Klarich, MD

GOALS

- Review the clinical cardiac examination.
- Discuss diagnosis and management of valvular heart disease.
- Summarize congenital heart disease.

Accurate bedside assessment is essential and allows appropriate, cost-effective, and efficient ordering of tests. This chapter presents the salient features of the clinical cardiac examination, cardiac imaging techniques, and the diagnosis and management of valvular and congenital heart diseases.

CARDIAC PHYSICAL EXAMINATION

JUGULAR VENOUS PRESSURE

Jugular venous pressure reflects right atrial pressure and the relationship between right atrial filling and emptying into the right ventricle (Figure 3.1). Changes in wave amplitude may indicate structural disease and rhythm changes. Normal jugular venous pressure is 6 to 8 cm H_2O. It is best evaluated with the patient supine at an angle of at least 45°. The right atrium lies 5 cm below the sternal angle, and thus the estimated jugular venous pressure equals the height of the jugular venous pressure above the sternal angle + 5 cm (Figure 3.1). The normal venous profile contains 3 positive waves and 2 negative waves. *Positive* waves are *a*, atrial contraction; *c*, closure of tricuspid valve; and *v*, atrial filling. *Negative* waves are the *x* descent (the downward motion of the right ventricle) and the *y* descent (the early right ventricular filling phase). The *a* wave comes just before the first heart sound, and the *v* wave comes during the ejection phase of the left ventricle.

The examiner must distinguish jugular venous pressure from carotid pulsations: jugular venous pressure varies with respiration, is nonpalpable, and can be eliminated by applying gentle pressure at descent (diastole). When the pressure is increased, consider biventricular failure, constrictive pericarditis, pericardial tamponade, cor pulmonale (especially pulmonary embolus), and superior vena cava syndrome.

- Jugular venous pressure reflects atrial pressure and the relationship between right atrial filling and emptying.
- Jugular venous pressure varies with respiration, is nonpalpable, and can be obstructed with gentle pressure.
- Biventricular failure, constrictive pericarditis, pericardial tamponade, cor pulmonale, and superior vena cava syndrome increase jugular venous pressure.

Abnormalities of the venous waves suggest various cardiac conditions. Increased jugular venous pressure indicates possible fluid overload (common in congestive heart failure). The likelihood of congestive heart failure is increased 4 times if jugular venous pressure is increased. Large *a* waves may indicate tricuspid stenosis, right ventricular hypertrophy, pulmonary hypertension (ie, increased right ventricular end-diastolic pressure). Cannon *a* waves are due to atria contracting intermittently against a closed atrioventricular valve (atrioventricular dissociation). Rapid *x* + *y* descent indicates constrictive pericarditis. Kussmaul sign (paradoxical increase in jugular venous pressure with inspiration) occurs in pericardial tamponade, constriction, and right ventricular failure. Large, fused *cv* waves are due to tricuspid regurgitation. Increased jugular venous pressure can be associated with pulmonary embolus, superior vena cava syndrome, tamponade, and constrictive pericarditis.

- Venous wave abnormalities can help identify the underlying cardiac condition.
- Increased jugular venous pressure can be associated with pulmonary embolus, superior vena cava syndrome, tamponade, and constrictive pericarditis.

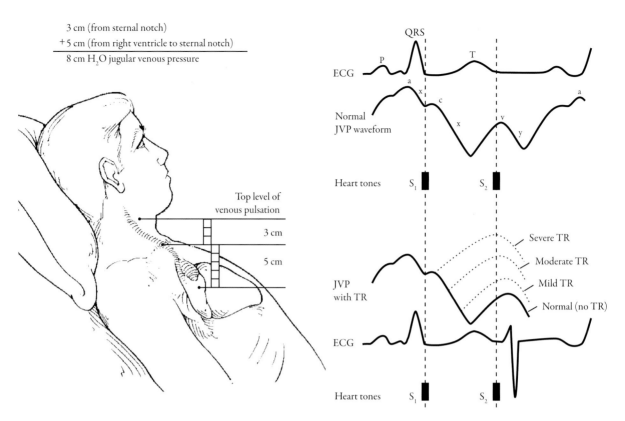

3 cm (from sternal notch)

+5 cm (from right ventricle to sternal notch)

8 cm H$_2$O jugular venous pressure

Top level of venous pulsation

3 cm

5 cm

QRS

P

T

ECG

a

x

c

Normal JVP waveform

x

v

y

a

Heart tones

S$_1$

S$_2$

Severe TR

Moderate TR

Mild TR

Normal (no TR)

JVP with TR

ECG

Heart tones

S$_1$

S$_2$

Figure 3.1 Evaluation of Jugular Venous Pressure (JVP). ECG indicates electrocardiogram; S$_1$, first heart sound; S$_2$, second heart sound; TR, tricuspid regurgitation.

ARTERIAL PULSES

Palpation of the radial pulse is useful for heart rate. The brachial or carotid pulse is checked for contour and timing. It is important to assess the upstroke and volume. Tardus is the timing and rate of rise of upstroke, and parvus is the pulse volume. Assess for radial- or brachial-femoral delay in patients with hypertension by checking radial, or brachial, and femoral pulses simultaneously. A delay is consistent with aortic coarctation.

• Assess pulse contour and timing using the radial pulse; assess contour and timing with the brachial or carotid pulse.

• Tardus refers to timing and rate of rise, and parvus refers to pulse volume.

Abnormalities of the arterial pulse and their associated conditions are as follows:

1. Parvus (low volume) and tardus (delayed and slowed upstroke): aortic stenosis

2. Parvus only: low output, cardiomyopathy

3. Bounding upstroke: aortic regurgitation or atrioventricular fistulas and shunts

4. Bifid (2 systolic peaks): hypertrophic obstructive cardiomyopathy (from midsystolic obstruction)

5. Bisferiens (2 systolic peaks and a distinct systolic dip, occurs when a large volume is ejected rapidly): aortic regurgitation

6. Dicrotic (a systolic peak followed by diastolic pulse wave): left ventricular failure with hypotension, low output, and increased peripheral resistance

7. Pulsus paradoxus (exaggerated inspiratory decrease [>10 mm Hg] in pulse pressure): tamponade

8. Pulsus alternans (alternating strong and weak pulse): severely reduced left ventricular function

APICAL IMPULSE

This is normally a discrete area of localized contraction, usually maximal at the fifth intercostal space in the midclavicular line and the size of a quarter (25-cent piece). Abnormalities of the apical impulse and their associated conditions are as follows:

1. Displaced (laterally, downward, or both) with a weak, diffuse impulse: cardiomyopathy

2. Sustained (may not be displaced): left ventricular hypertrophy, aortic stenosis (often with large *a* wave)

3. Trifid (or multifid): hypertrophic cardiomyopathy

4. Hyperdynamic, descended, and enlarged with rapid filling wave: mitral regurgitation, aortic regurgitation

5. Tapping quality, localized, nondisplaced: normal but may indicate mitral stenosis

ADDITIONAL CARDIAC PALPATION

A palpable aortic valve component (A_2) at the right upper sternum suggests a dilated aorta (eg, aneurysm, dissection, severe aortic regurgitation, poststenotic dilatation in aortic stenosis, hypertension). Severe tricuspid regurgitation may cause a pulsatile liver palpable in the right epigastrium. Hepatojugular reflux (distention of the external jugular vein 3 or 4 beats after compression of the liver) may also occur. The apical impulse rotates medially and may be appreciated in the epigastrium (which can be confused with a pulsatile liver) in patients with severe emphysema. Right ventricular hypertrophy results in sustained lift, best appreciated in the fourth intercostal space along the left parasternal border. Diastolic overload (eg, atrial septal defect, anomalous pulmonary venous return) results in a vigorous outward and upward motion but may not be sustained. The pulmonary valve component (P_2) may be palpable in the second right intercostal space in marked pulmonary hypertension. This may be physiologic in slender people with a small anteroposterior diameter.

- Pressure overload of the right ventricle usually results in sustained lift of the sternum and a palpable pulmonary closure.

- Volume overload (eg, regurgitant lesions, atrial septal defect) usually is appreciated as dynamic and forceful but not sustained impulses.

THRILLS

Thrills indicate marked turbulent flow (eg, aortic stenosis, severe mitral regurgitation, and ventricular septal defect) and distinction of a grade 4 murmur.

HEART SOUNDS

Knowledge of how the heart sounds are related to the cardiac cycle allows an understanding of cardiac auscultation (Figure 3.2). The cardiac cycle starts with atrial contraction; this increases ventricular pressure just before closure of the atrioventricular valves, which generates the first heart sound (S_1). There is a period of time while the left ventricle generates pressure, known as the isovolumic contraction time, when the atrioventricular and semilunar valves are closed. Normally silent semilunar valve openings then occur, followed by blood ejection from the left ventricle to the aorta (creating the pulse). As the ventricle relaxes, aortic pressure decreases; this decrease closes the

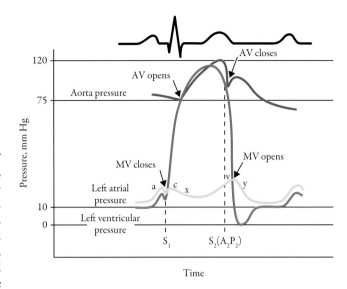

Figure 3.2 The Normal Cardiac Cycle. A_2 indicates the aortic valve component of S_2; AV, aortic valve; MV, mitral valve; P_2, pulmonary valve component of S_2; S_1, first heart sound; S_2, second heart sound.

semilunar valves, creating the second heart sound (S_2). Another period follows when both sets of valves are closed. Pressure decreases below the left atrial pressure, leading to the usually silent opening of the atrioventricular valves. Early rapid filling followed by slow filling of the ventricles is followed by atrial contraction. The mnemonic for valve sequence—S_1-S_2 (right ventricular-left ventricular sequence—is "Many Things Are Possible" [MTAP]: S_1 = *m*itral opens before *t*ricuspid; S_2 = *a*ortic closes before *p*ulmonary) under normal conditions.

- S_1: closure of the atrioventricular valves due to increased left ventricular pressure after atrial contraction.

First Heart Sound

S_1 consists of audible mitral valve closure followed by tricuspid valve closure. A loud S_1 occurs with mitral stenosis and short PR intervals (the mitral valve is open when the left ventricle begins to contract and then slaps shut). S_1 also is augmented in hypercontractile states (eg, fever, exercise, thyrotoxicosis, pheochromocytomas, anxiety, and anemia). Conversely, S_1 is decreased if the mitral valve is heavily calcified and immobile (severe mitral stenosis) and with a long PR interval, poor left ventricular function, and rapid diastolic filling (due to premature mitral valve closure) as in aortic regurgitation.

- S_1 is loud with a short PR interval, mitral stenosis, and hypercontractile states.

- S_1 is quiet with a heavily calcified mitral valve, long PR interval, left ventricular dysfunction, and aortic regurgitation.

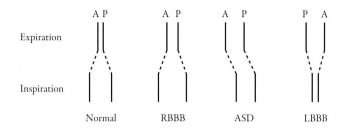

Figure 3.3 Effects of Respiration and Conduction on the Second Heart Sound. The A indicates aortic closure; ASD, atrial septal defect; LBBB, left bundle branch block; P, pulmonary closure; RBBB, right bundle branch block.

Second Heart Sound

S_2 consists of aortic valve closure (A_2) followed by pulmonary valve closure (P_2). Intensity is increased by hypertension (ie, loud or tympanic A_2 with systemic hypertension; loud P_2 with pulmonary hypertension, with P_2 audible at apex). Intensity is decreased with heavily calcified valves (severe aortic stenosis). Normally, the split between A_2 and P_2 widens on inspiration and narrows on expiration due to relatively increased blood return to the right heart during inspiration and greater capacitance of the lungs, such that A_2 moves slightly closer to S_1 and P_2 moves farther away (Figure 3.3). This is reversed during expiration. This is normal physiologic splitting of S_2. This is best heard in the left second intercostal space with the patient seated.

- The intensity of S_2 is increased by hypertension.

- The intensity of S_2 is decreased with heavily calcified valves.

- Physiologic splitting of S_2 occurs in inspiration due to increased blood return to the right heart.

The interplay of multiple factors can affect the timing of the closure of semilunar valves: electrical activation, duration of ventricular ejection, gradient across semilunar valves, and elastic recoil properties of the great vessels. Common types of splitting of the S_2 and their indicated conditions are as follows:

1. Physiologic splitting: normal splitting due to respiratory variation of blood flow; on inspiration, A moves to the "left" closer to S_1, and P moves to the "right" away from S_1

2. Fixed split: atrial septal defect. The widest split occurs with a combination of atrial septal defect and pulmonary stenosis

3. Paradoxic split (delayed aortic closure, the pulmonary valve closes first): left bundle branch block

4. Persistent splitting: right bundle branch block. A_2 and P_2 are separated because of delayed electromechanical activation of the right ventricle. Inspiration accentuates the effect

Third Heart Sound

The third heart sound (S_3) occurs in early diastole, coinciding with maximal early diastolic left ventricular filling. It is low-pitched and best heard with the stethoscope bell. S_3 is associated with left ventricular volume overload (eg, aortic regurgitation, mitral regurgitation, and cardiomyopathy). It is a normal variant in very fit young adults.

- An S_3 indicates left ventricular volume overload.

Fourth Heart Sound

The fourth heart sound (S_4) is low-pitched, best heard with the stethoscope bell and loudest at the apex. This sound occurs with the atrial "kick" as blood is forced into the left ventricle by atrial contraction against a stiff and noncompliant left ventricle. An S_4 may be heard in aortic stenosis, systemic hypertension, hypertrophic cardiomyopathy, and ischemia. It cannot occur in atrial fibrillation because of the loss of atrial contraction.

- An S_4 indicates cardiac disease such as aortic stenosis or ischemia.

- Atrial fibrillation precludes an S_4.

Opening Snap

Opening snap is an early diastolic sound caused by opening of the pathologic rheumatic mitral valve. It is virtually always caused by mitral stenosis. With severe mitral stenosis, the left atrial pressure is very high and thus the valve opens earlier, and the interval is less than 60 m/s.

- Opening snap is virtually always caused by mitral stenosis.

MURMURS

The specific murmurs are discussed with the individual valvular lesions described later in this chapter, but some broad guidelines are presented here.

A systolic ejection murmur begins after S_1 and ends before S_2. It may have a diamond-shaped quality with crescendo and decrescendo components. In general, a more severe obstruction (a narrower valve orifice) causes a louder, later-peaking murmur. An *ejection click* may precede a bicuspid (aortic or pulmonary) valve murmur if the valve pliability is preserved. A holosystolic murmur engulfs S_1 and S_2 and occurs when blood moves from a very high-pressure to a low-pressure system, such as in mitral regurgitation and ventricular septal defect. Diastolic murmurs are always abnormal. Echocardiography should be considered in this setting if a systolic murmur of grade 3 or higher is heard or if there are other signs or symptoms of cardiac disease (Figure 3.4).

- Systolic ejection murmurs occur when semilunar valves are stenotic, and, in general, the more severe the obstruction, the louder the murmur and the later the peak.

- Diastolic murmurs are always abnormal.

Certain maneuvers alter cardiac murmurs. *Inspiration* increases venous return, increasing right-sided sounds (S_3 and S_4) and murmurs (tricuspid and pulmonary stenosis,

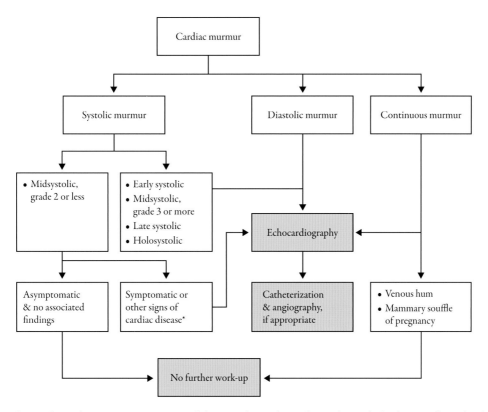

Figure 3.4 Recommendations for Evaluating Heart Murmurs. *If electrocardiography or chest radiography has been performed and the results are abnormal, echocardiography is recommended. (Adapted from Bonow RO, Carabello BA, Chatterjee K, de Leon AC Jr, Faxon DP, Freed MD, et al; American College of Cardiology/American Heart Association Task Force on Practice Guidelines. 2008 Focused update incorporated into the ACC/AHA 2006 guidelines for the management of patients with valvular heart disease: a report of the American College of Cardiology/American Heart Association Task Force on Practice Guidelines [Writing Committee to revise the 1998 guidelines for the management of patients with valvular heart disease]. Endorsed by the Society of Cardiovascular Anesthesiologists, Society for Cardiovascular Angiography and Interventions, and Society of Thoracic Surgeons. J Am Coll Cardiol. 2008 Sep 23;52[13]:e1–142 and Bonow RO, Carabello BA, Chatterjee K, de Leon AC Jr, Faxon DP, Freed MD, et al; 2006 Writing Committee Members; American College of Cardiology/American Heart Association Task Force. 2008 Focused update incorporated into the ACC/AHA 2006 guidelines for the management of patients with valvular heart disease: a report of the American College of Cardiology/American Heart Association Task Force on Practice Guidelines [Writing Committee to Revise the 1998 Guidelines for the Management of Patients With Valvular Heart Disease]: endorsed by the Society of Cardiovascular Anesthesiologists, Society for Cardiovascular Angiography and Interventions, and Society of Thoracic Surgeons. Circulation. 2008 Oct 7;118[15]:e523–661. Epub 2008 Sep 26. Used with permission.)

and tricuspid and pulmonary regurgitation). The *Valsalva maneuver* increases intrathoracic pressure, inhibiting venous return and thus decreasing preload. Most cardiac murmurs and sounds diminish in intensity during the Valsalva maneuver because of decreased ventricular filling and cardiac output. The exception is hypertrophic obstructive cardiomyopathy, in which the murmur increases because of dynamic left ventricular outflow obstruction accentuated by decreased preload. The Valsalva maneuver is the classic way to distinguish between the murmurs of aortic stenosis and hypertrophic cardiomyopathy. *Handgrip* increases cardiac output and systemic arterial pressure, decreasing the gradient across a stenotic aortic valve. A *change in posture* from supine to upright causes decreased venous return, reducing stroke volume and thus a reflex increase in heart rate and peripheral resistance. *Squatting* and the Valsalva maneuver have opposite hemodynamic effects. Squatting increases peripheral resistance and venous return. *Amyl nitrite* pharmacologically decreases afterload. The amyl nitrite is inhaled and transiently lowers blood pressure, increasing the murmurs of hypertrophic cardiomyopathy and aortic stenosis. Its main use is to determine the gradient in patients with dynamic left ventricular outflow obstruction due

to hypertrophic cardiomyopathy. The effects of maneuvers are shown in Table 3.1.

- Bedside maneuvers that alter cardiac murmurs are as follows:

    Inspiration

    Valsalva maneuver

    Handgrip

    Change in posture

    Squatting

    Inhalation of amyl nitrite

- The Valsalva maneuver distinguishes between aortic stenosis and hypertrophic cardiomyopathy.

IMAGING IN CARDIOLOGY

Appropriate choice of an imaging method aids in the diagnosis, quantification, and prognosis of various diseases.

Table 3.1 EFFECTS OF PHYSICAL MANEUVERS AND OTHER FACTORS ON VALVULAR DISEASES

MANEUVER OR FACTOR	RESULT	MITRAL REGURGITATION	MVP	AORTIC STENOSIS	HOCM
Amyl nitrite	↓ afterload	↓	↑/0	↑	↑
Valsalva	↓ preload	↓	↑	↓	↑
Handgrip	↑ afterload	↑	↓/0	↓	↓
Post-PVC	↑ contractility ↓ afterload	=	↓	↑	↑[a]

Abbreviations: HOCM, hypertrophic obstructive cardiomyopathy; MVP, mitral valve prolapse; PVC, premature ventricular complex.

[a] Although the murmur increases, the peripheral pulse decreases because of the increase in outflow obstruction.

Left ventricular function is the most commonly ordered assessment. Various techniques are available, as outlined in Table 3.2. Focused clinical questioning allows selection of the most appropriate technique.

Coronary Angiography

This was the first imaging method to permit visualization of the cardiac chambers and direct assessment of left ventricular size and function. It is an invasive technique. Risks include the use of ionizing radiation, iodine allergy, and impaired renal function. Coronary angiography is considered the standard technique to assess the location and extent or quantity of coronary artery stenosis. Left ventricular function assessment by contrast ventriculography can be performed during coronary angiography.

Echocardiography

Echocardiography generates images and gives temporal-spatial resolution for timing the motion of heart structures during the cardiac cycle. Left ventricular volumes in end-diastole and end-systole and thus stroke volume, ejection fraction, cardiac output, and muscle mass can be determined. Echocardiography is noninvasive, lending itself to serial image acquisition. It is easily available and the most widely used imaging technology in cardiology.

Regional wall motion abnormalities are identified by assessing endocardial motion and wall thickening. Valve morphology (eg, pliability, degree of calcification, morphologic abnormalities, and flail segments) and intracardiac and pericardial structures can be analyzed. With exercise or pharmacologic (usually dobutamine) stress, regional wall motion can be assessed at rest and with stress.

The use of Doppler with echocardiography allows direct measurements of blood velocities across valves and conduits (eg, left ventricular outflow tract and vessels), permitting calculation of stroke volume, cardiac output, valve gradients, and severity of regurgitant lesions and semiquantitation of intracardiac and extracardiac shunts. Obesity, severe cachexia, and extensive lung disease (eg, smoking-related disorders, chronic obstructive pulmonary disease, and restrictive lung disease) reduce the ability to obtain adequate images in transthoracic echocardiography in a small percentage of cases.

Table 3.2 CARDIAC IMAGING METHODS

METHOD	VARIABLE ASSESSED				COST-EFFECTIVENESS[a]
	LVEF	RV Function	LV Mass	RWMA	
Contrast angiography	Yes	No	No	Yes	++++[b]
Two-dimensional echocardiography	Yes	Yes	Yes	Yes	++
First-pass RNA	Yes	Yes, quantitative[c]	No	No	+
Blood pool RNA	Yes	No	No	Yes	+
Magnetic resonance imaging	Yes	Yes, quantitative[c]	Yes	Yes	+++/+
Electron beam computed tomography	Yes	Yes, quantitative[c]	Yes	Yes	+++

Abbreviations: LV, left ventricular; LVEF, left ventricular ejection fraction; RNA, radionuclide angiography; RV, right ventricular; RWMA, regional wall motion abnormalities.

[a] +, Least expensive; ++++, most expensive.

[b] If performed without coronary angiography.

[c] Quantitative, absolute measurements of global ventricular volumes possible to facilitate measure of RV ejection fraction.

Transesophageal echocardiography minimizes the interference of bones, muscle, and obesity, but it requires sedation and the most operator experience and is more operator-dependent. Echocardiography cannot visualize the coronary arteries like angiography.

Contrast echocardiography enhances the echocardiographic signal using an enhancing agent. Some of these agents are smaller than red blood cells and cross the pulmonary vascular bed. Clinical applications include better endocardium visualization.

Radionuclide Imaging

Radionuclide imaging uses 2 techniques: labeling erythrocytes with an isotope to assess endocardial motion or using perfusion tracers (thallium, sestamibi) to assess differences between resting and stress blood flow.

Radionuclide Angiography

Erythrocytes are labeled with technetium, and images are acquired over multiple cardiac cycles. This imaging technique is not suitable for patients with atrial fibrillation and markedly variable RR intervals. Left ventricular function can be quantified very accurately. Excellent discrimination between low ejection fractions, particularly during serial assessment, is possible. In contrast, echocardiography is less accurate for quantification of left ventricular function in severely dysfunctional ventricles.

Myocardial Perfusion Imaging

Thallium and sestamibi are the most commonly used isotopes. They distribute to the myocardium according to blood flow and are avidly taken up by myocytes. Imaging can be performed at rest and after exercise (Figure 3.5). During stress (exercise or pharmacologic), uptake is usually reduced (hypoperfusion) in damaged myocardium. At rest, thallium redistributes and there is preferential washout of the normal myocardium and preferential uptake of the hypoperfused myocardium. Sestamibi is irreversibly taken up by the myocardium and a repeat resting injection is needed to show resting flow conditions. The extent and severity of the perfusion defect provide information about the disease prognosis. It is also used to assess residual ischemia after a myocardial infarction and to assess therapeutic efficacy in patients treated medically or by intervention. Imaging study results should be viewed along with the data available from the exercise or stress electrocardiogram.

Gated Sestamibi Imaging

With this technique, myocardium motion is imaged throughout the cardiac cycle, allowing regional wall motion analysis similar to that of echocardiography. Post-stress images are acquired with a considerable time delay and mainly reflect resting contractility.

Magnetic Resonance Imaging

Magnetic resonance imaging is a noninvasive, 3-dimensional imaging technique that allows assessment of left ventricular

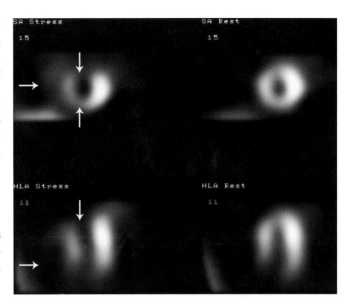

Figure 3.5 Myocardial Perfusion Image for a Patient With Exertional Angina (Class III) of Recent Onset. Low-level exercise with 1-mm ST-segment depression at 2 minutes into exercise. The left column depicts the stress images with a representative short-axis tomogram (upper left panel) and the horizontal long axis (lower left panel). In the right column are the rest images, with corresponding short-axis tomogram in the right upper panel and the corresponding horizontal long-axis tomogram in the right lower panel. Note the severely reduced uptake in the apical, septal, anterior, and inferior segments (arrows). At rest, there is nearly complete normalization in all segments. Subsequent angiography indicated complete occlusion of the right coronary artery and 80% stenosis in the proximal left anterior descending coronary artery. The circumflex coronary artery did not show a critical lesion.

size, function, and muscle mass and of cardiac chamber size. It can assess anatomical structure, distinguish viable myocardium from scarred myocardium, and characterize tissue. It can differentiate plaque composition and may be able to identify vulnerable plaques.

Electron Beam Computed Tomography

Electron beam computed tomography allows high-fidelity, high-resolution, 3-dimensional images of the entire heart. It requires only 1 heartbeat to complete a scan cycle. It is ideally suited for serial studies in left ventricular remodeling because of its high precision and accuracy. Drawbacks are the requirements for a contrast agent and use of ionizing radiation. It is currently the most widely used technique in the field of early detection of coronary atherosclerosis because of its ease of application (rapid acquisition time, no contrast agent) and standardization. It detects coronary calcium, a component of coronary plaque.

Positron Emission Tomography

Positron emission tomography allows high-spatial and temporal resolution imaging and currently is the reference standard for the assessment of myocardial viability. However, the complexity of the technology and the cost currently limit its use to tertiary academic centers.

AORTIC STENOSIS

The pathophysiologic effect of aortic stenosis on the heart is pressure overload, leading to left ventricular hypertrophy. The vast majority of cases of aortic stenosis are due to valvular stenosis.

Types

The *congenital bicuspid* type of aortic stenosis occurs in 2% of the population; the male to female ratio is 3:1. It is inherited in an autosomal dominant pattern. First-degree relatives should be screened. Bicuspid aortic valve is the most common cause of aortic stenosis in adults younger than 55 years. Frequently, when a patient is young and the valve is still pliable, the auscultation is different from that of degenerative aortic valve disease. An ejection click classically precedes the systolic murmur and may be heard even in the absence of murmur or before the murmur is present. This is a high-pitched sound that comes early in systole, right after S_1. The ejection click represents opening of the less pliable bicuspid valve and is heard best in the aortic listening post, the second intercostal space. It is a high-pitched sound that is best heard with the diaphragm of the stethoscope. As aortic stenosis worsens, aortic valve closure is delayed; when aortic stenosis is severe, there may even be paradoxic splitting of S_2.

Bicuspid aortic valve may be associated with coarctation of the aorta in about 10% of patients. Conversely, if coarctation is noted, there is a 30% to 50% chance of bicuspid aortic valve. Even with a normally functioning aortic valve, the ascending aorta may not be normal. The aortopathy associated with bicuspid aortic valve can cause dilatation of the sinus of Valsalva and the ascending aorta. Both of these phenomena should be specifically screened for with imaging of the aorta. If bicuspid aortic valve is suspected, the diagnosis usually can be made with 2-dimensional and Doppler echocardiography without the need for cardiac catheterization in young people. If the diagnosis is confirmed, the aorta should be imaged with ultrasonography, magnetic resonance imaging, or computed tomography to rule out coarctation and aortic dilatation or aneurysm. *Degenerative aortic valve disease* due to calcification is the most common cause of aortic stenosis in adults older than 55 years. The valve is tricuspid. When calcification is extensive, A_2 becomes inaudible.

- Congenital bicuspid valvular aortic stenosis occurs in 2% of the population, affects males more than females, and is the most common cause of aortic stenosis in adults younger than 55 years.

- Bicuspid aortic valve is associated with ascending aortic aortopathy that can lead to aneurysm formation. Screening of relatives is important.

- Degenerative aortic valve disease is the most common cause of aortic stenosis in adults older than 55 years.

- When calcification is extensive, A_2 becomes inaudible.

The *rheumatic* type of aortic valve disease is less common. It is associated with thickening and fusion of the aortic cusps at the commissures. It always occurs with a rheumatic mitral valve, although considerable mitral stenosis or regurgitation may not always be evident. It usually occurs in adulthood (age 40–60 years), usually 15±5 years after acute rheumatic fever.

- The rheumatic type of aortic valve disease is a less common cause of valvular aortic stenosis.

Symptoms

The classic symptoms of the valvular type of aortic stenosis (regardless of type) include exertional dyspnea, syncope, angina, and sudden cardiac death. The onset of symptoms is an ominous sign and portends a very poor prognosis. Patients with symptomatic aortic stenosis need rapid surgical intervention (Figure 3.6). The presence of angina does not necessarily indicate coexisting coronary disease; rather, it is related to increased left ventricular filling pressure causing subendocardial ischemia. The chest pain syndrome, in absence of coronary artery disease, is due to supply-demand mismatch.

- Symptoms of aortic stenosis are exertional dyspnea, syncope, angina, and sudden cardiac death.

- Angina does not necessarily indicate coexisting coronary disease.

Physical Examination

The arterial pulse is parvus (minimal) and tardus (delayed) in hemodynamically significant aortic stenosis. The left ventricular impulse is localized, lateralized, and sustained. Arterial thrills may be palpable at the carotid artery, suprasternal notch, second intercostal space, or left and right sternal borders. An audible and palpable S_4 may be present. A_2 is diminished and delayed and may even become absent with decreasing pliability

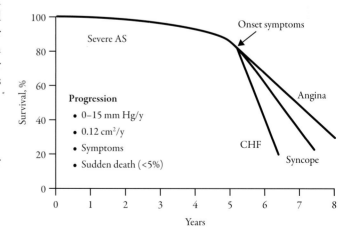

Figure 3.6 Natural History of Aortic Stenosis (AS). CHF indicates congestive heart failure. (Adapted from Ross J Jr, Braunwald E. Aortic stenosis. Circulation. 1968 Jul 1;38 Suppl 1:61–7. Used with permission.)

of the aortic cusps. The ejection systolic murmur becomes louder and peaks later with increasing severity, radiating to the carotid arteries and the apex.

- The pulse is parvus (minimal) and tardus (delayed) in hemodynamically significant aortic stenosis.
- The ejection systolic murmur becomes louder with increasing severity.
- A_2 is diminished, delayed, or absent with progressive aortic stenosis.

Diagnosis

Electrocardiography in aortic stenosis may show left ventricular hypertrophy; echocardiography is more sensitive and specific. Left bundle branch block is common; in later stages of the condition, conduction abnormalities may develop (eg, complete heart block) if calcium impinges on the conducting system. On chest radiography, the heart size is usually normal even when the stenosis is severe and the left ventricle fails; enlargement of the heart may not be evident until left ventricular remodeling occurs in the late stages. The aortic root may show "poststenotic" dilatation, now recognized as an aortopathy. In degenerative aortic valve disease, calcium may be seen in the valve leaflets and in the intervalvular fibrosa, especially on a lateral view.

- Echocardiography is the best way to diagnose aortic stenosis and assess its severity.

The differential diagnosis of aortic stenosis includes 1) hypertrophic cardiomyopathy (note different carotid upstroke and change in murmur with Valsalva maneuver) and 2) mitral regurgitation (murmur may radiate anteriorly and upward along the aorta, particularly if there is rupture of chordae of the posterior mitral valve leaflet; no radiation to the carotid arteries).

Aortic stenosis can be diagnosed with bedside physical examination. The most important physical finding is the parvus and tardus pulse contour. The degree of aortic stenosis can be difficult to determine, particularly in older patients. Noninvasive Doppler echocardiography is useful for assessing aortic valve area and gradients and correlates well with invasive catheter-based assessment of the same. Severe aortic stenosis is present when the mean Doppler gradient is more than 40 mm Hg, the valve area is less than 1.0 cm^2, and the valve index is 0.6 cm^2/m^2 or less. Progression of aortic stenosis is highly variable; on average, it is about 0.12 cm^2 per year. Progression to symptoms can be insidious; the onset of clinical symptoms is an ominous prognostic sign. Survival after symptom onset is 1 to 3 years (Figure 3.6).

Treatment

All patients should be educated about worrisome symptoms that may develop. Dyspnea, chest pain, angina, syncope, or newly diagnosed congestive heart failure are important clinical evidence for surgical intervention and should be promptly evaluated (Table 3.3). Aortic valve replacement is the only

effective treatment for patients with severe obstruction (Figure 3.7).

- Aortic stenosis can be diagnosed with bedside physical examination.
- The most important physical finding is observation of parvus and tardus pulse contour.
- Dyspnea, chest pain, angina, syncope, or newly diagnosed congestive heart failure may herald progression to severe aortic stenosis.
- Aortic valve replacement is the only effective treatment of symptomatic aortic stenosis.

AORTIC REGURGITATION

The pathophysiology of aortic regurgitation is that of volume and pressure overload on the left ventricle, leading to hypertrophy and dilatation. It can be related to either the aortic valve or the aortic root, and the condition can be acute or chronic (Table 3.4). Acute aortic regurgitation may be associated with an aortic dissection.

Valvular

Causes of valvular aortic regurgitation include 1) congenital bicuspid valve, 2) rheumatic fever, 3) endocarditis, 4) degenerative aortic valve disease, 5) seronegative arthritis, 6) ankylosing spondylitis, and 7) rheumatoid arthritis.

Aortic Root Dilatation

Various conditions have been associated with aortic root dilatation. Advancing age is one factor; hypertension accelerates this process. Aortic regurgitation associated with age or hypertension is common and usually mild. Marfan syndrome may cause progressive dilatation of the aortic root and sinuses (cystic medial necrosis). Prophylactic β-adrenergic blocker therapy slows the rate of aortic dilatation and reduces the development of aortic complications in some patients with Marfan syndrome. When the aortic root reaches 5 to 5.5 cm or more in diameter, it should be replaced. Syphilis is an uncommon cause of aortic regurgitation and usually causes aortic root dilatation above the sinuses, sparing the sinuses. Syphilis is associated with aortic root calcium on chest radiography.

- Marfan syndrome can be associated with aortic root dilatation.
- Hypertension and advancing age are common causes of aortic regurgitation (usually mild).

Symptoms

The symptoms of *acute* aortic regurgitation are extreme: pulmonary edema, shock, and, often, chest pain (in the setting of aortic dissection). The symptoms of *chronic* aortic regurgitation can develop insidiously because of compensatory mechanisms of the heart. The most common symptoms of *severe*

Table 3.3 **QUANTITATION OF THE SEVERITY OF AORTIC STENOSIS AND TREATMENT GUIDELINES**

SEVERITY	AVA, CM²	AVA INDEX, CM²/M²	GRADIENT, MM HG	FOLLOW-UP OR TREATMENT
Normal	3.0–4.0		<10	
Mild	>1.5	>0.8	<30	Echo every 5 y or if symptoms
Moderate	1.0–1.5	0.5–0.8	30–40	Monitor for symptoms Echo every 1–2 y
Severe	<1.0	<0.6	>40	Symptoms: operate No symptoms: echo every 6–12 mo

Abbreviations: AVA, aortic valve area; echo, echocardiography.

Data from Bonow RO, Carabello BA, Chatterjee K, de Leon AC Jr, Faxon DP, Freed MD, et al; American College of Cardiology/American Heart Association Task Force on Practice Guidelines. 2008 focused update incorporated into the ACC/AHA 2006 guidelines for the management of patients with valvular heart disease: a report of the American College of Cardiology/American Heart Association Task Force on Practice Guidelines (Writing Committee to revise the 1998 guidelines for the management of patients with valvular heart disease). Endorsed by the Society of Cardiovascular Anesthesiologists, Society for Cardiovascular Angiography and Interventions, and Society of Thoracic Surgeons. J Am Coll Cardiol. 2008 Sep 23;52(13):e1–142 and Bonow RO, Carabello BA, Chatterjee K, de Leon AC Jr, Faxon DP, Freed MD, et al; 2006 Writing Committee Members; American College of Cardiology/American Heart Association Task Force. 2008 Focused update incorporated into the ACC/AHA 2006 guidelines for the management of patients with valvular heart disease: a report of the American College of Cardiology/American Heart Association Task Force on Practice Guidelines (Writing Committee to Revise the 1998 Guidelines for the Management of Patients With Valvular Heart Disease): endorsed by the Society of Cardiovascular Anesthesiologists, Society for Cardiovascular Angiography and Interventions, and Society of Thoracic Surgeons. Circulation. 2008 Oct 7;118(15):e523–661. Epub 2008 Sep 26.

aortic regurgitation include fatigue, dyspnea, palpitations, and exertional angina.

Physical Examination

Severe aortic regurgitation is associated with physical findings that include a bounding, rapidly collapsing Corrigan pulse resulting from wide pulse pressure; bisferiens pulse (may be present); de Musset head nodding; Duroziez sign (systolic and diastolic ["to-and-fro"] murmur on gentle compression with stethoscope) over the femoral artery; and Quincke sign (pulsatile capillary nail bed). Müller sign (systolic pulsations of the uvula) is often noted. The left ventricular impulse is diffuse and hyperdynamic. The apical impulse is often displaced downward. A diastolic decrescendo murmur is heard at either the left or the right sternal border, and the S$_2$ may be paradoxically split because of increased left ventricular volume.

Murmur duration is related to the rate of pressure equilibration between the aorta and the left ventricle. Aortic regurgitation with physiologic diastolic pressures results in a holodiastolic murmur. The shorter the aortic regurgitation murmur, the faster the pressure equilibration, thus the more severe the aortic regurgitation (higher left ventricular end-diastolic pressure). The loudness of the murmur does not correlate with the severity of aortic regurgitation, particularly in acute aortic regurgitation (such as with dissection). A systolic flow murmur is common, because of the increased ejection volume. It does not necessarily indicate aortic stenosis.

Diagnosis

Acute aortic regurgitation may not be identified on bedside examination if a patient presents with little or no murmur. Electrocardiography often shows left ventricular hypertrophy.

Echocardiography is best suited to gather the important functional and hemodynamic data needed to make management decisions in patients with aortic regurgitation.

Because chronic aortic regurgitation has a long, silent, well-compensated natural history, left ventricular size, aortic root size and morphology, valve morphology, and left ventricular function (ejection fraction) should be followed with echocardiography.

Chest radiography shows an enlarged cardiac shadow and prominence of the left ventricle in a leftward and inferior pattern. The aorta also may be enlarged, especially in Marfan syndrome. Table 3.5 outlines the natural history of severe aortic regurgitation.

- Findings indicative of aortic regurgitation are a bounding, rapidly collapsing Corrigan pulse, diastolic decrescendo murmur, and an S$_2$ that may be paradoxically split.

- In aortic regurgitation, electrocardiography may show left ventricular hypertrophy.

- Echocardiography is useful to confirm the diagnosis and guide therapy.

Treatment

Acute severe aortic regurgitation is a surgical emergency. If untreated, severe pulmonary congestion, arrhythmias, and circulatory collapse will develop. As a bridge to operation, nitroprusside to reduce peripheral resistance and encourage forward flow or inotropic agents to augment cardiac output may be considered. An intra-aortic balloon pump is contraindicated because it will worsen regurgitation.

- Acute aortic regurgitation is a surgical emergency.

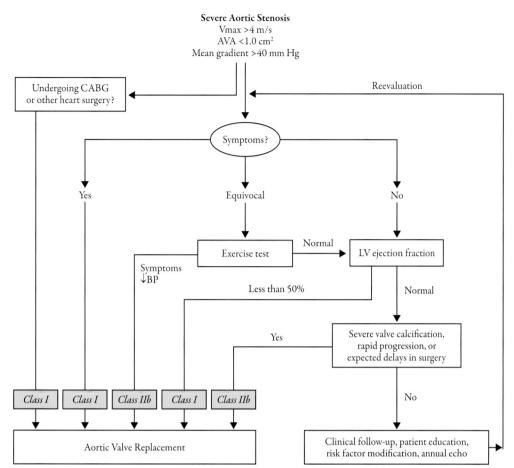

Figure 3.7 Management Strategy for Patients With Severe Aortic Stenosis. Preoperative coronary angiography should be performed routinely as determined by age, symptoms, and coronary risk factors. Cardiac catheterization and angiography may also be helpful when there is discordance between clinical findings and those on electrocardiography. AVA indicates aortic valve area; BP, blood pressure; CABG, coronary artery bypass graft surgery; echo, echocardiography; LV, left ventricular; Vmax, maximal velocity across aortic valve by Doppler echocardiography. (Adapted from Bonow RO, Carabello BA, Chatterjee K, de Leon AC Jr, Faxon DP, Freed MD, et al; American College of Cardiology/American Heart Association Task Force on Practice Guidelines. 2008 focused update incorporated into the ACC/AHA 2006 guidelines for the management of patients with valvular heart disease: a report of the American College of Cardiology/American Heart Association Task Force on Practice Guidelines [Writing Committee to revise the 1998 guidelines for the management of patients with valvular heart disease]. Endorsed by the Society of Cardiovascular Anesthesiologists, Society for Cardiovascular Angiography and Interventions, and Society of Thoracic Surgeons. J Am Coll Cardiol. 2008 Sep 23;52[13]:e1–142 and Bonow RO, Carabello BA, Chatterjee K, de Leon AC Jr, Faxon DP, Freed MD, et al; 2006 Writing Committee Members; American College of Cardiology/American Heart Association Task Force. 2008 Focused update incorporated into the ACC/AHA 2006 guidelines for the management of patients with valvular heart disease: a report of the American College of Cardiology/American Heart Association Task Force on Practice Guidelines [Writing Committee to Revise the 1998 Guidelines for the Management of Patients With Valvular Heart Disease]: endorsed by the Society of Cardiovascular Anesthesiologists, Society for Cardiovascular Angiography and Interventions, and Society of Thoracic Surgeons. Circulation. 2008 Oct 7;118[15]:e523–661. Epub 2008 Sep 26. Used with permission.)

Chronic aortic regurgitation is a combined volume and pressure overload on the left ventricle. The left ventricle compensates by dilating and increasing compliance. Patients with aortic regurgitation may remain asymptomatic for decades. The development of symptoms usually reflects left ventricular dysfunction, and survival is limited (10% annual mortality) unless surgical intervention is prompt. Medical management (eg, angiotensin-converting enzyme inhibitor or nifedipine) slows ventricular dilatation in patients with severe aortic regurgitation and may help delay operation. Compensation is not maintained indefinitely, and eventually left ventricular filling pressure increases, coronary flow reserve diminishes, and left ventricular dysfunction develops insidiously. Angina, even in the absence of epicardial coronary stenosis, may be present as a result of supply-and-demand mismatch.

Asymptomatic left ventricular dysfunction may develop in a subset of patients. Several factors have been suggested to prompt surgical intervention before left ventricular dysfunction develops: an end-systolic dimension more than 55 mm, an end-diastolic dimension more than 75 mm, or an ejection fraction of 50% or less (Figure 3.8). Asymptomatic patients with a dilated left ventricle must be followed carefully. Evidence of left ventricular systolic dysfunction at rest, progressive diastolic dysfunction, or rapidly progressive left ventricular dilatation should prompt surgical treatment. The ability to repair (rather than replace) the valve may favor earlier operation (before left ventricular dilatation has occurred).

- Asymptomatic patients with a dilated left ventricle should be carefully followed for progression.

Table 3.4 AORTIC REGURGITATION: SYMPTOMS AND FINDINGS ON EXAMINATION

	ACUTE	CHRONIC
Symptoms	Pulmonary edema Shock Arrhythmia Chest pain Dissection, RCA infarct	Dyspnea Fatigue Exercise intolerance Night sweats Palpitations
Examination	Faint, short murmur	Peripheral pulses Quincke and Duroziez signs, pistol-shot pulse Enlarged, diffuse, hyperdynamic LV Murmur LSB—valve etiology RSB—root etiology
Chest radiography	Wide mediastinum Pulmonary edema	Enlarged heart Enlarged aorta
Electrocardiography	Low voltage (if pericardial effusion) ST elevation II, III, F (if aortic dissection into RCA)	LVH

Abbreviations: LSB, left sternal border; LV, left ventricle; LVH, left ventricular hypertrophy; RCA, right coronary artery; RSB, right sternal border.

Table 3.5 NATURAL HISTORY OF SEVERE AORTIC REGURGITATION

STATUS OF PATIENT	% OF PATIENTS/Y
Asymptomatic with normal LV systolic function	
Progression to symptoms or LV dysfunction	<6
Progression to asymptomatic LV dysfunction	<3.5
Sudden death	<0.2
Asymptomatic with LV dysfunction	
Progression to cardiac symptoms	>25
Symptomatic	
Mortality rate	>10

Abbreviation: LV, left ventricular.

Adapted from Bonow RO, Carabello BA, Chatterjee K, de Leon AC Jr, Faxon DP, Freed MD, et al; American College of Cardiology/American Heart Association Task Force on Practice Guidelines. 2008 focused update incorporated into the ACC/AHA 2006 guidelines for the management of patients with valvular heart disease: a report of the American College of Cardiology/American Heart Association Task Force on Practice Guidelines (Writing Committee to revise the 1998 guidelines for the management of patients with valvular heart disease). Endorsed by the Society of Cardiovascular Anesthesiologists, Society for Cardiovascular Angiography and Interventions, and Society of Thoracic Surgeons. J Am Coll Cardiol. 2008 Sep 23;52(13):e1–142 and Bonow RO, Carabello BA, Chatterjee K, de Leon AC Jr, Faxon DP, Freed MD, et al; 2006 Writing Committee Members; American College of Cardiology/American Heart Association Task Force. 2008 Focused update incorporated into the ACC/AHA 2006 guidelines for the management of patients with valvular heart disease: a report of the American College of Cardiology/American Heart Association Task Force on Practice Guidelines (Writing Committee to Revise the 1998 Guidelines for the Management of Patients With Valvular Heart Disease): endorsed by the Society of Cardiovascular Anesthesiologists, Society for Cardiovascular Angiography and Interventions, and Society of Thoracic Surgeons. Circulation. 2008 Oct 7;118(15):e523–661. Epub 2008 Sep 26. Used with permission.

- If ejection fraction decreases below normal, operation is indicated.

MITRAL STENOSIS

Etiology and Pathophysiology

Rheumatic fever is the cause of rheumatic heart disease, which leads to leaflet thickening with fusion of the commissures and later calcification. These effects result in mitral stenosis, and prophylaxis against rheumatic fever is therefore strongly recommended. Mitral stenosis results in obstruction of blood flow from the left atrium to the left ventricle, preventing proper diastolic filling and leading to pulmonary congestion.

Symptoms

Symptoms of mitral stenosis usually develop decades after rheumatic fever. The murmur of mitral stenosis is apparent on physical examination about 10 years after rheumatic fever. After another decade, symptoms develop, usually dyspnea and later orthopnea with paroxysmal nocturnal dyspnea, which can be insidious. Atrial fibrillation leads to deterioration of clinical status. Hemoptysis and pulmonary hypertension with signs of right-sided failure (ie, ascites and peripheral edema) are late manifestations. Systemic emboli also may result from atrial fibrillation (about 20% without anticoagulation) due to left atrial clot.

- Mitral stenosis is almost always due to rheumatic heart disease.

- Symptoms are dyspnea and orthopnea with paroxysmal nocturnal dyspnea.

Physical Examination

The S_1 in mitral stenosis is loud as long as the leaflets remain pliable. The shorter the interval from A_2 to the opening snap, the more severe the mitral stenosis. An opening snap occurs only with a pliable valve, and it disappears if the valve calcifies. The stenosis is mild if this interval is more than 90 milliseconds, moderate if it is 80 milliseconds, and severe if it is less than 60 milliseconds. The diastolic murmur is a low-pitched, holodiastolic rumble, heard best at the apex with the bell of the stethoscope and with the patient in the left lateral decubitus position. The murmur may have presystolic accentuation if sinus rhythm is present. Right ventricular lift and increased P_2 are associated with pulmonary hypertension.

- Findings on physical examination in mitral stenosis include a loud S_1 if the mitral valve leaflets are pliable and a diastolic murmur that is a low-pitched, holodiastolic rumble.

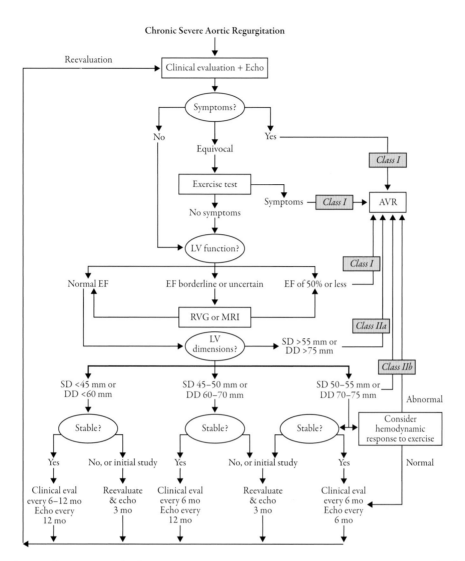

Figure 3.8 Management Strategy for Patients With Chronic Severe Aortic Regurgitation. Preoperative coronary angiography should be performed routinely as determined by age, symptoms, and coronary risk factors. Cardiac catheterization and angiography may also be helpful when there is discordance between clinical findings and those on echocardiography. "Stable" refers to stable echocardiographic measurements. In some centers, serial follow-up may be performed with radionuclide ventriculography (RVG) or magnetic resonance imaging (MRI) rather than echocardiography (Echo) to assess left ventricular (LV) volume and systolic function. AVR indicates aortic valve replacement; DD, end-diastolic dimension; EF, ejection fraction; eval, evaluation; SD, end-systolic dimension. (Adapted from Bonow RO, Carabello BA, Chatterjee K, de Leon AC Jr, Faxon DP, Freed MD, et al; American College of Cardiology/American Heart Association Task Force on Practice Guidelines. 2008 focused update incorporated into the ACC/AHA 2006 guidelines for the management of patients with valvular heart disease: a report of the American College of Cardiology/American Heart Association Task Force on Practice Guidelines [Writing Committee to revise the 1998 guidelines for the management of patients with valvular heart disease]. Endorsed by the Society of Cardiovascular Anesthesiologists, Society for Cardiovascular Angiography and Interventions, and Society of Thoracic Surgeons. J Am Coll Cardiol. 2008 Sep 23;52[13]:e1–142 and Bonow RO, Carabello BA, Chatterjee K, de Leon AC Jr, Faxon DP, Freed MD, et al; 2006 Writing Committee Members; American College of Cardiology/American Heart Association Task Force. 2008 Focused update incorporated into the ACC/AHA 2006 guidelines for the management of patients with valvular heart disease: a report of the American College of Cardiology/American Heart Association Task Force on Practice Guidelines [Writing Committee to Revise the 1998 Guidelines for the Management of Patients With Valvular Heart Disease]: endorsed by the Society of Cardiovascular Anesthesiologists, Society for Cardiovascular Angiography and Interventions, and Society of Thoracic Surgeons. Circulation. 2008 Oct 7;118[15]:e523–661. Epub 2008 Sep 26. Used with permission.)

Diagnosis

Electrocardiography can show left atrial enlargement, P mitrale (notched P wave in leads I and II with a duration of ≥0.12 millisecond due to characteristic left atrial enlargement), and right ventricular hypertrophy. Chest radiography (Figure 3.9) shows straightening of the left heart border with a large left atrial shadow and dilated upper lobe pulmonary veins. With pulmonary hypertension, the central pulmonary arteries become prominent. In severe stenosis, pulmonary congestion characterized by Kerley B lines may be present, indicating a pulmonary wedge pressure of more than 20 mm Hg.

Two-dimensional and Doppler echocardiography is the test of choice to diagnose mitral stenosis and determine its severity. Information is gained about valve gradient and valve area (Table 3.6), and pulmonary artery pressures can be non-invasively assessed. Cardiac catheterization is usually unnecessary unless the coronary arteries need to be studied or the echocardiographic findings do not concur with the clinical

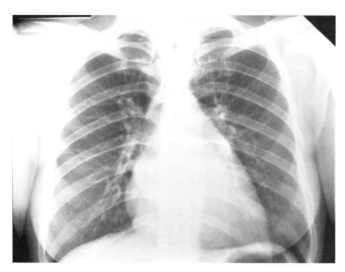

Figure 3.9 Chest Radiograph From a Patient With Severe Mitral Stenosis. The straight left heart border, prominent pulmonary artery, large left atrium, right ventricular contour, and pulmonary venous hypertension are typical findings.

Table 3.6 SEVERITY OF MITRAL STENOSIS, BY VALVE AREA, GRADIENT, AND PULMONARY PRESSURE

SEVERITY	VALVE AREA, CM²	MEAN GRADIENT, MM HG	SYSTOLIC PAP, MM HG
Mild	1.5–2	<6	Normal
Moderate	1–1.5	6–11	≤50
Severe	<1	≥12	>50

Abbreviation: PAP, pulmonary artery pressure.

situation. Severe stenosis usually correlates with a mean gradient of 12 mm Hg or more.

- In mitral stenosis, electrocardiography shows P mitrale and right ventricular hypertrophy.

- Chest radiography shows straightening of the left heart border, a large left atrial shadow, and dilated upper lobe pulmonary veins.

- For diagnosis of mitral stenosis, cardiac catheterization is usually unnecessary.

- Severe stenosis correlates with a mean gradient >12 mm Hg.

Treatment

Because mitral stenosis represents obstruction to diastolic filling, anything that shortens diastolic filling time will worsen the severity and symptoms of the disease (eg, tachycardia, atrial fibrillation, and exercise). Therefore, β-adrenergic blockers and calcium channel blockers can be used to slow heart rate and improve left ventricular filling. Salt restriction and diuretic therapy are useful for early symptoms.

The left ventricle is unaffected in mitral stenosis. It is small, vigorous, and possibly underfilled (reduced preload) in late mitral stenosis. Intervention on the mitral valve is not recommended until there are symptoms of exertional dyspnea, pulmonary edema, or moderate pulmonary hypertension. Marked volume overload of the left atrium leads to increased stroke risk as a result of stagnation of blood flow and thrombus formation. Atrial fibrillation is frequent and intermittent in the early stages. Intermittent screening may be warranted, and anticoagulation should be considered early.

Once symptoms are present, treatment is with either surgical valve replacement or percutaneous balloon valvuloplasty. Percutaneous mitral valve balloon valvuloplasty is first-line therapy when mitral valve leaflets are pliable and noncalcified and when regurgitation is minimal; valve replacement may be delayed for at least 10 years with this approach. Intervention for mitral stenosis is indicated with exertional dyspnea, pulmonary edema, or moderate pulmonary hypertension (>50 mm Hg).

MITRAL REGURGITATION

Etiology and Pathophysiology

The mitral valve is a complex structure, and regurgitation can result from abnormalities of 3 anatomical locations: leaflet, tensor apparatus (chordal and papillary muscles), and myocardium. Common causes of mitral regurgitation include mitral valve prolapse syndrome and myxomatous degeneration, infective endocarditis, left ventricular dilatation in congestive heart failure, collagen vascular disease, ischemia, rheumatic heart disease, and left ventricular dilatation due to cardiomyopathy

Table 3.7 TYPES OF MITRAL REGURGITATION

ANATOMICAL TYPE	CLINICAL PRESENTATION	
	Chronic	*Acute or Subacute*
Leaflets	Rheumatic Prolapse Annular calcification Connective tissue disease Congenital cleft Drug-related	Infective endocarditis
Tensor apparatus (chordal & papillary muscles)	Prolapse	Rupture of chordae Myocardial infarction Papillary muscle rupture
Myocardium	Regional ischemia or infarctions Dilated cardiomyopathy Hypertrophic cardiomyopathy	

Adapted from McGoon MD, Schaff HV, Enriquez-Sarano M, Fuster V, Callahan MJ. Mitral regurgitation. In: Guiliani ER, Gersh BJ, McGoon MD, Hayes DL, Schaff HV, editors. Mayo Clinic practice of cardiology. 3rd ed. St. Louis (MO): Mosby; c1996. p. 1450–69. Used with permission of Mayo Foundation for Medical Education and Research.

(Table 3.7). In the case of ischemic mitral regurgitation, the posterior medial papillary muscle with its single blood supply (compared with anterolateral, which has a dual blood supply) is more susceptible.

Symptoms

Chronic mitral regurgitation causes left ventricular volume overload with reduced afterload. Given time, the left ventricle compensates by increasing stroke volume. A long asymptomatic phase is thus possible. The most common symptoms include fatigue, dyspnea (due to increased left atrial pressure), and pulmonary edema. Symptoms often worsen with atrial fibrillation.

- Common causes of mitral regurgitation are mitral valve prolapse and myxomatous degeneration, ischemia, and infective endocarditis.
- Fatigue, dyspnea, and pulmonary edema are the most common symptoms and are worsened by atrial fibrillation.

Physical Examination

Findings of mitral regurgitation include a diffuse and hyperdynamic left ventricular impulse, which may be visible, and a palpable rapid filling wave. The S_2 may be obliterated, and there is a holosystolic murmur. There may be an S_3 (or S_3 and a flow rumble) and an S_4. An S_3 with a low-pitched early diastolic rumble indicates severe regurgitation; it represents a volume murmur, but coexisting mitral stenosis needs to be ruled out.

In acute mitral regurgitation, the murmur may be short because of increased left atrial pressure. In severe mitral regurgitation, the carotid upstroke may appear parvus, because of the low forward stroke volume, but not tardus. The left atrium may be palpable with systole, and the left ventricle, with diastole. The cause of mitral regurgitation may be suspected by the radiation of the auscultated murmur. A murmur that is due to a rupture of the anterior leaflet chordae leads to a posteriorly directed jet of mitral regurgitation and a murmur that radiates to the axilla and back. When posterior leaflet chordae rupture, the murmur radiates to the sternum and possibly the carotid arteries.

- A diffuse, hyperdynamic left ventricular impulse, holosystolic murmur, lack of S_2, and an S_3 are findings on examination.
- A murmur radiating to the axilla and back is due to anterior chord rupture, whereas posterior chord rupture leads to a murmur heard at the sternal border and the carotid arteries.

Diagnosis

Chest radiography may first show a dilated left atrium and then, as mitral regurgitation increases, dilatation of the left ventricle. A low or low-normal ejection fraction suggests substantial ventricular dysfunction. It is important to follow patients closely to determine the optimal timing of surgical intervention.

Treatment

There is no universally accepted medical treatment for mitral regurgitation. The onset of clinical symptoms warrants intervention (mitral valve repair or replacement). Asymptomatic patients with a normal or hyperdynamic ejection fraction can continue to have regular observation. Operation should be considered for symptomatic patients (preoperative left ventricular function considerably influences the postoperative outcome), and, because afterload is increased when the mitral valve is replaced, left ventricular function may actually deteriorate after mitral valve repair or replacement. In most patients, ejection fraction decreases approximately 10% after mitral valve repair or replacement.

In mildly symptomatic patients, operation may be considered, particularly if serial examinations show progressive cardiac enlargement. Earlier operation may be indicated in patients who are suitable for mitral valve repair rather than replacement, especially when the ejection fraction is less than 60% or the left ventricular end-systolic dimension is more than 40 mm (Figure 3.10).

- In symptomatic patients with severe mitral regurgitation, operation should be considered.
- In asymptomatic patients with an ejection fraction <60% or left ventricular end-systolic dimension >40 mm, operation may be considered, especially if mitral valve repair is possible and surgical risk is relatively low.

MITRAL VALVE PROLAPSE

Pathophysiology and Natural History

Mitral valve prolapse is the most common cause of both valvular heart disease and mitral regurgitation in the United States. Mitral valve prolapse refers to a systolic billowing of one or both mitral leaflets into the left atrium with or without mitral regurgitation. In patients with mitral valve prolapse, as with other causes of mitral regurgitation, the degree of left atrial and left ventricular dilatation depends on the severity of mitral regurgitation. Mitral valve prolapse is associated with secundum atrial septal defect and supraventricular arrhythmias.

- Valvular heart disease and mitral regurgitation are most often due to mitral valve prolapse.

In Marfan syndrome, the supporting apparatus is often involved with dilatation of the mitral annulus in addition to elongated chordae and redundant leaflets, abnormalities leading to mitral valve prolapse. Other valves also may be involved with the same myxomatous degeneration, which leads to tricuspid valve prolapse (occurring in approximately 40% of patients with mitral valve prolapse), pulmonic valve

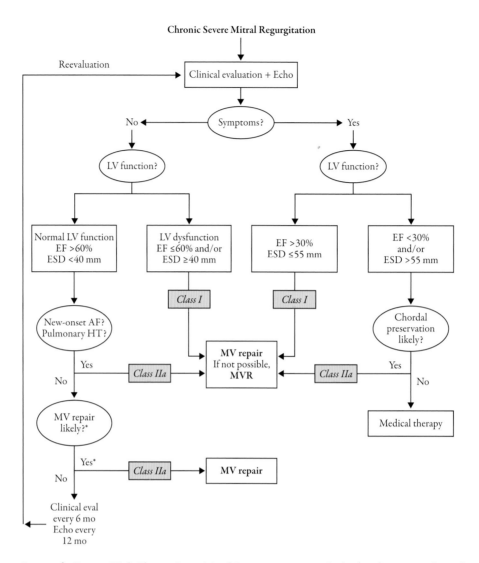

Figure 3.10 Management Strategy for Patients With Chronic Severe Mitral Regurgitation. *Mitral valve (MV) repair may be performed in asymptomatic patients with normal left ventricular (LV) function if performed by an experienced surgical team and if the likelihood of successful MV repair is greater than 90%. AF indicates atrial fibrillation; Echo, echocardiography; EF, ejection fraction; ESD, end-systolic dimension; eval, evaluation; HT, hypertension; MVR, mitral valve replacement. (Adapted from Bonow RO, Carabello BA, Chatterjee K, de Leon AC Jr, Faxon DP, Freed MD, et al; American College of Cardiology/American Heart Association Task Force on Practice Guidelines. 2008 focused update incorporated into the ACC/AHA 2006 guidelines for the management of patients with valvular heart disease: a report of the American College of Cardiology/American Heart Association Task Force on Practice Guidelines [Writing Committee to revise the 1998 guidelines for the management of patients with valvular heart disease]. Endorsed by the Society of Cardiovascular Anesthesiologists, Society for Cardiovascular Angiography and Interventions, and Society of Thoracic Surgeons. J Am Coll Cardiol. 2008 Sep 23;52[13]:e1–142 and Bonow RO, Carabello BA, Chatterjee K, de Leon AC Jr, Faxon DP, Freed MD, et al; 2006 Writing Committee Members; American College of Cardiology/American Heart Association Task Force. 2008 Focused update incorporated into the ACC/AHA 2006 guidelines for the management of patients with valvular heart disease: a report of the American College of Cardiology/American Heart Association Task Force on Practice Guidelines [Writing Committee to Revise the 1998 Guidelines for the Management of Patients With Valvular Heart Disease]: endorsed by the Society of Cardiovascular Anesthesiologists, Society for Cardiovascular Angiography and Interventions, and Society of Thoracic Surgeons. Circulation. 2008 Oct 7;118[15]:e523–661. Epub 2008 Sep 26. Used with permission.)

prolapse (about 10%), and aortic valve prolapse (2%). Other connective tissue disorders may be associated with mitral valve prolapse.

Mitral valve prolapse syndrome has a benign course in most patients. Patients with diagnostic findings of click-murmur on auscultation, thickened mitral leaflets on echocardiography, and left ventricular and atrial enlargement are at high risk for future complications, including atrial fibrillation, systemic embolism, and pulmonary hypertension. There is also a life-long risk for ruptured mitral valve chordae, which may lead to acute decompensation. Infective endocarditis is a serious complication of mitral valve prolapse, although the overall incidence is low. There is a low risk for sudden cardiac death (Figure 3.11).

- Mitral valve prolapse and other valvular prolapse can occur in Marfan syndrome and other connective tissue disorders.

- Risks for mitral valve prolapse include infective endocarditis (low risk), ruptured chordae leading to acute decompensation, and sudden cardiac death (low risk).

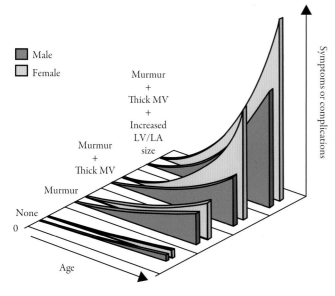

Figure 3.11 Risk Factors for Complications in Mitral Valve Prolapse. LA indicates left atrial; LV, left ventricular; MV, mitral valve. (Adapted from Boudoulas H, Kolibash AJ Jr, Wooley CF. Mitral valve prolapse: a heterogeneous disorder. Primary Cardiol. 1991;17[2]:29–43. Used with permission.)

Physical Examination

Mitral valve prolapse is usually diagnosed with cardiac auscultation in asymptomatic patients or incidentally on echocardiography. The classic auscultatory finding is the midsystolic click, a high-pitched sound of short duration. There may be multiple clicks. According to Bonow et al clicks result from sudden tensing of the mitral valve apparatus as the leaflets prolapse into the left atrium during systole. The midsystolic click(s) is frequently followed by a mid-late systolic murmur that is high-pitched, musical, or honking and often loudest at the cardiac apex. The character and intensity of the clicks and the murmur vary with left ventricle loading conditions. Dynamic auscultation helps establish the diagnosis. Changes in left ventricular end-diastolic volume result in changes in the timing of the click(s) and murmur. When end-diastolic volume is decreased (eg, with standing), the critical volume is achieved earlier in systole and the click-murmur complex occurs earlier after S_1. By contrast, any maneuver that augments the volume of blood in the ventricle (eg, squatting), reduces myocardial contractility, or increases left ventricular afterload lengthens the time from onset of systole to initiation of mitral valve prolapse, and the systolic click or murmur moves toward S_2 (Figure 3.12).

- Classically, in mitral valve prolapse, a midsystolic click(s) caused by sudden tensing of the mitral valve apparatus during prolapse, often followed by a mid-late systolic high-pitched murmur, is heard.

Diagnosis

Results of electrocardiography most often are normal, although 24-hour ambulatory electrocardiographic recordings or event monitors may be useful for documenting arrhythmias. Echocardiography is the most useful noninvasive test for defining mitral valve prolapse. The definition includes more than 2 mm of posterior displacement of 1 or both leaflets into the left atrium. All patients with mitral valve prolapse should have an initial echocardiogram to establish the diagnosis, stratify risk, and define possible associated lesions (eg, atrial septal defect). Serial echocardiograms are not necessary in asymptomatic patients with mitral valve prolapse. Echocardiographic follow-up should be done if there are clinical indications of progression.

Treatment

Reassurance is a major part of the management of patients with mitral valve prolapse because most are asymptomatic and lack a high-risk profile. A normal lifestyle and regular exercise are encouraged. Patients should be educated about when to seek medical advice (worsening symptoms). Subacute bacterial endocarditis prophylaxis is no longer indicated for mitral valve prolapse without a history of endocarditis.

According to Bonow et al, common symptoms include palpitations, chest pain that rarely resembles classic angina pectoris, dyspnea, and fatigue. Patients should be advised to discontinue caffeine, alcohol, and tobacco use. Patients with recurrent palpitations often respond to β-adrenergic blockers or calcium channel blockers. Orthostatic symptoms due to postural hypotension and tachycardia are treated with volume expansion, preferably by liberalizing fluid and salt intake. Transient cerebral ischemic episodes occur with increased incidence in patients with mitral valve prolapse, and some patients need long-term anticoagulation (Table 3.8).

- Serial echocardiograms are not necessary in asymptomatic patients with mitral valve prolapse.

- Most patients with mitral valve prolapse can be reassured and encouraged to lead a normal lifestyle.

- Palpitations, chest pain, dyspnea, and fatigue are common symptoms.

- Transient ischemic attacks may occur, and long-term anticoagulation may be indicated.

According to Bonow et al, asymptomatic patients with mitral valve prolapse and no serious mitral regurgitation can be evaluated clinically every 3 to 5 years. Serial echocardiography is necessary only in patients who have high-risk features on the initial echocardiogram.

Surgery may be required in a small subset of patients. The thickened, redundant mitral valve often can be repaired rather than replaced; repair has a low operative mortality rate and excellent short- and long-term results. Repair is often sufficient in patients who have a flail mitral leaflet due to rupture or marked elongation of the chordae tendineae. Recommendations for surgery in patients with mitral valve prolapse and mitral regurgitation are the same as those for patients with other forms of severe mitral regurgitation.

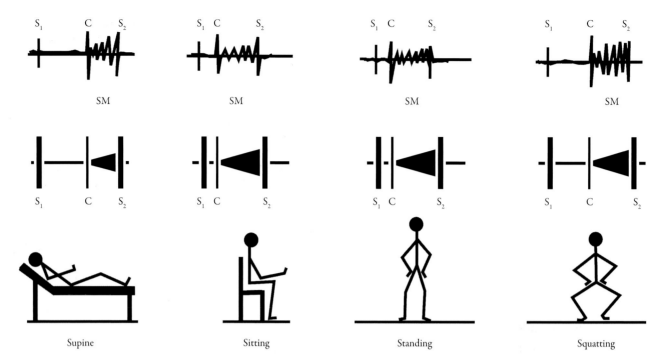

Figure 3.12 Auscultation Findings in Mitral Valve Prolapse. C indicates click; S$_1$, S$_2$, heart sound (first, second); SM, systolic murmur; ◀, murmur.

- Asymptomatic, low risk patients with mitral valve prolapse can be evaluated every 3–5 years.
- Repair, rather than replacement, of the valve has low operative mortality rate and excellent results.

TRICUSPID STENOSIS

The cause of tricuspid stenosis is almost always rheumatic, and it is never an isolated lesion. Carcinoid syndrome may cause tricuspid valve retraction and a relative stenosis (usually causes worse tricuspid regurgitation), and in rare cases atrial tumors may be the cause.

- The cause of tricuspid stenosis is almost always rheumatic.
- Tricuspid stenosis is never an isolated lesion.

TRICUSPID REGURGITATION

Mild tricuspid regurgitation is relatively common, occurring in up to 85% to 90% of patients. Significant tricuspid regurgitation is usually caused by right ventricle dilatation. Tricuspid regurgitation often accompanies mitral valve disease, but it may be related to 1) right ventricular infarction, 2) primary pulmonary hypertension (common), 3) congenital heart disease (eg, Ebstein anomaly), or 4) carcinoid syndrome—more commonly associated with tricuspid regurgitation than tricuspid stenosis.

- Tricuspid regurgitation often accompanies mitral valve disease, but it is associated with other conditions, including carcinoid syndrome, pulmonary hypertension, and congenital heart disease.

TRICUSPID VALVE PROLAPSE

This may occur in isolation or be associated with other connective tissue abnormalities. The tricuspid valve may prolapse or become flail as a result of trauma or endocarditis (commonly fungal or staphylococcal in drug addicts).

Physical Examination

Findings on physical examination include jugular venous distention with a prominent *v* wave, a prominent right ventricular impulse, a pansystolic murmur at the left sternal edge, possibly a right-sided S$_3$, and peripheral edema, ascites, and hepatomegaly.

Surgical Therapy

Tricuspid annuloplasty may be helpful if regurgitation is caused by right ventricular dilatation. However, if there is considerable pulmonary hypertension, tricuspid valve replacement is usually required with either a biologic or a mechanical valve. Biologic prostheses in the tricuspid position do not degenerate as quickly as left-heart prostheses. In patients with endocarditis, the tricuspid valve can be removed completely, and patients may tolerate this well for several years.

PROSTHETIC VALVES

Bioprosthetic Valves

These are made of animal or human tissue, which may be mounted in a frame. Different types include homograft (human tissue, either aortic or pulmonary), heterograft (porcine valve, eg, Hancock or Carpentier-Edwards), and

Table 3.8 **RECOMMENDATIONS FOR USE OF ASPIRIN AND ORAL ANTICOAGULANTS IN MITRAL VALVE PROLAPSE**

INDICATIONS	CLASS
1. Aspirin therapy for cerebral transient ischemic attacks	I
2. Warfarin therapy for patients aged ≥65 years, in atrial fibrillation with hypertension, mitral regurgitation murmur, or history of heart failure	I
3. Aspirin therapy for patients aged <65 years, in atrial fibrillation with no history of mitral regurgitation, hypertension, or heart failure	I
4. Warfarin therapy after stroke	I
5. Warfarin therapy for transient ischemic attacks despite aspirin therapy	IIa
6. Aspirin therapy after stroke in patients with contraindications to anticoagulants	IIa
7. Aspirin therapy for patients in sinus rhythm with echocardiographic evidence of high-risk mitral valve prolapse	IIb

Data from Bonow RO, Carabello BA, Chatterjee K, de Leon AC Jr, Faxon DP, Freed MD, et al; American College of Cardiology/American Heart Association Task Force on Practice Guidelines. 2008 focused update incorporated into the ACC/AHA 2006 guidelines for the management of patients with valvular heart disease: a report of the American College of Cardiology/American Heart Association Task Force on Practice Guidelines (Writing Committee to revise the 1998 guidelines for the management of patients with valvular heart disease). Endorsed by the Society of Cardiovascular Anesthesiologists, Society for Cardiovascular Angiography and Interventions, and Society of Thoracic Surgeons. J Am Coll Cardiol. 2008 Sep 23;52(13):e1–142 and Bonow RO, Carabello BA, Chatterjee K, de Leon AC Jr, Faxon DP, Freed MD, et al; 2006 Writing Committee Members; American College of Cardiology/American Heart Association Task Force. 2008 Focused update incorporated into the ACC/AHA 2006 guidelines for the management of patients with valvular heart disease: a report of the American College of Cardiology/American Heart Association Task Force on Practice Guidelines (Writing Committee to Revise the 1998 Guidelines for the Management of Patients With Valvular Heart Disease): endorsed by the Society of Cardiovascular Anesthesiologists, Society for Cardiovascular Angiography and Interventions, and Society of Thoracic Surgeons. Circulation. 2008 Oct 7;118(15):e523–661. Epub 2008 Sep 26.

pericardial (bovine valve, eg, Ionescu-Shiley). Because tissue valves are not as thrombogenic as mechanical valves, most patients in sinus rhythm do not require anticoagulation after the first 3 to 6 months. Patients with atrial fibrillation have increased risk for systemic embolism, particularly with a mitral prosthesis. Tissue valves degenerate and calcify, and approximately 50% of patients need valve replacement at 10 to 15 years. Tissue valves may calcify very rapidly in patients aged 20 years or younger. Tissue valves last longer in the tricuspid position than in left heart positions. Aortic valves are more durable than mitral valves. Prosthesis failure can be detected by clinical evaluation and 2-dimensional and Doppler echocardiography.

- Tissue valves are not as thrombogenic as mechanical valves.
- Most patients with tissue valves in sinus rhythm do not require anticoagulation.

- About 50% of patients need valve replacement 10–15 years after original valve placement due to degeneration and calcification.

Mechanical Valves

Newer-generation mechanical valves (eg, the bileaflet St. Jude valve) are less thrombogenic than prior models, but all mechanical valves have risk for thromboembolism and necessitate long-term anticoagulation (Table 3.9). Hemolysis may occur with mechanical prostheses, especially if there is a perivalvular leak. Anticoagulation complications include hemorrhage and thrombosis (when anticoagulation is subtherapeutic). The rate of minor hemorrhages is 2% to 4% per year, and that of major hemorrhages is 1% to 2% per year. Risk for complications, including endocarditis, is approximately 1% per year. All patients with a valvular prosthesis require antibiotic prophylaxis for endocarditis.

- Mechanical valves have risk for thromboembolism, and systemic anticoagulation is required.
- Anticoagulation can be associated with hemorrhage and thrombosis; therapeutic range must be strictly managed.
- All patients with a valvular prosthesis require antibiotic prophylaxis for endocarditis.

CONGENITAL HEART DISEASE

ATRIAL SEPTAL DEFECT

There are multiple types of atrial septal defects (Table 3.10).

Secundum Atrial Septal Defect

Patients with secundum atrial septal defect often survive to adulthood and may be asymptomatic. If the defect has gone undetected, atrial fibrillation frequently develops in the sixth decade of life along with onset of symptoms, usually dyspnea with subsequent tricuspid regurgitation and right-sided heart failure. Stroke may occur as a result of paradoxic embolism.

- Secundum atrial septal defect is found on routine examination with "fixed" split S_2.
- Stroke may occur as a result of paradoxic embolism.

Electrocardiography characteristically shows right bundle branch block and right axis deviation. Chest radiography shows pulmonary plethora, a prominent pulmonary artery, and right ventricular enlargement (Figure 3.13). Echocardiography is warranted for definitive diagnosis.

Sinus Venosus Atrial Septal Defect

An uncommon condition, this occurs in the superior portion of the atrial septum. It is often associated with anomalous pulmonary veins, usually the right upper. If echocardiography shows

Table 3.9 RECOMMENDATIONS FOR ANTITHROMBOTIC THERAPY IN PATIENTS WITH PROSTHETIC HEART VALVES[a]

VALVE TYPE	THERAPY			
	Aspirin, 75–100 mg/day	*Warfarin, INR 2.0–3.0*	*Warfarin, INR 2.5–3.5*	*No Warfarin*
Mechanical valve				
AVR, low risk				
<3 mo	Yes, class I	Yes, class I	Yes, class IIa	
>3 mo	Yes, class I	Yes, class I		
AVR, high risk	Yes, class I		Yes, class I	
MVR	Yes, class I		Yes, class I	
Biologic prosthetic valve				
AVR, low risk				
<3 mo	Yes, class I	Yes, class I		Class IIb
>3 mo	Yes, class I			Class IIa
AVR, high risk	Yes, class I	Yes, class I		
MVR, low risk				
<3 mo	Yes, class I	Yes, class IIa		
>3 mo	Yes, class I			Class IIa
MVR, high risk	Yes, class I	Yes, class I		

Abbreviations: AVR, aortic valve replacement; INR, international normalized ratio; MVR, mitral valve replacement.

[a] Depending on a patient's clinical status, antithrombotic therapy must be individualized. Aspirin is recommended in virtually all patients receiving warfarin. Risk factors are atrial fibrillation, left ventricular dysfunction, previous thromboembolism, and hypercoagulable condition. The international normalized ratio should be maintained between 2.5 and 3.5 for aortic disk valves and Starr-Edwards valves.

Adapted from Bonow RO, Carabello BA, Chatterjee K, de Leon AC Jr, Faxon DP, Freed MD, et al; American College of Cardiology/American Heart Association Task Force on Practice Guidelines. 2008 focused update incorporated into the ACC/AHA 2006 guidelines for the management of patients with valvular heart disease: a report of the American College of Cardiology/American Heart Association Task Force on Practice Guidelines (Writing Committee to revise the 1998 guidelines for the management of patients with valvular heart disease). Endorsed by the Society of Cardiovascular Anesthesiologists, Society for Cardiovascular Angiography and Interventions, and Society of Thoracic Surgeons. J Am Coll Cardiol. 2008 Sep 23;52(13):e1–142 and Bonow RO, Carabello BA, Chatterjee K, de Leon AC Jr, Faxon DP, Freed MD, et al; 2006 Writing Committee Members; American College of Cardiology/American Heart Association Task Force. 2008 Focused update incorporated into the ACC/AHA 2006 guidelines for the management of patients with valvular heart disease: a report of the American College of Cardiology/American Heart Association Task Force on Practice Guidelines (Writing Committee to Revise the 1998 Guidelines for the Management of Patients With Valvular Heart Disease): endorsed by the Society of Cardiovascular Anesthesiologists, Society for Cardiovascular Angiography and Interventions, and Society of Thoracic Surgeons. Circulation. 2008 Oct 7;118(15):e523–661. Epub 2008 Sep 26. Used with permission.

Table 3.10 TYPES OF ATRIAL SEPTAL DEFECTS

TYPE	%	LOCATION	ASSOCIATED FINDINGS	ECG FINDINGS
Ostium secundum	75	Fossa ovalis	None	Incomp RBBB, R axis
Sinus venosus	10	Vena cava	Anomalous PV	Incomp RBBB, ectopic P wave, R axis
Ostium primum	10–15	Lower septum	Cleft MV, Down syndrome	Incomp RBBB, L axis (LAHB)

Abbreviations: ECG, electrocardiography; Incomp, incomplete; L axis, left axis deviation; LAHB, left anterior hemiblock; MV, mitral valve; P wave, atrial depolarization wave on ECG; PV, pulmonary veins; R axis, right axis deviation; RBBB, right bundle branch block.

right ventricular volume overload and no secundum defect (surface echocardiography can miss the sinus venosus area), consider sinus venosus atrial septal defect or anomalous pulmonary veins.

Primum Atrial Septal Defect (Partial Atrioventricular Canal)

This is a defect in the lower portion of the septum due to partial atrioventricular canal defect. The mitral valve is often congenitally cleft and produces various degrees of mitral regurgitation.

Diagnosis

On electrocardiography, findings are different from those of secundum type; left axis deviation and right bundle branch block are evident. More than 75% of patients have first-degree atrioventricular block. The chest radiographic findings are the same as those for secundum atrial septal defect, but there

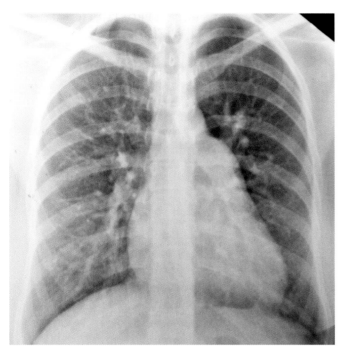

Figure 3.13 Chest Radiograph From a Patient With a Large Left-to-Right Shunt Due to a Secundum Atrial Septal Defect. Note cardiac enlargement with right ventricular contour, prominent pulmonary artery, and pulmonary plethora.

may be left atrial enlargement due to mitral regurgitation. Atrioventricular canal defects are the most common cardiac anomaly associated with Down syndrome.

- Electrocardiography shows left axis deviation with right bundle branch block and often first-degree atrioventricular block.

- Atrioventricular canal defects are the most common cardiac anomaly associated with Down syndrome.

Treatment

Antibiotic prophylaxis is not recommended unless there is associated complex congenital heart disease. Patients with atrial septal defect have variable symptoms depending on the size of the shunt. Intervention should be considered in the setting of hemodynamic compromise (left-to-right shunting of more than 30% or evidence of right-sided chamber enlargement). Surgical treatment has a very low complication rate. Percutaneous closure with an occluder device was recently approved for use. Although the duration of follow-up is short, results indicate that this is a viable approach in certain cases.

- In primum atrial septal defect, antibiotic prophylaxis is not recommended unless there is associated complex congenital heart disease.

VENTRICULAR SEPTAL DEFECT

Ventricular septal defect occurs in different parts of the ventricular septum, most commonly classified as either in the membranous septum or in the muscular septum. A small ventricular septal defect generally presents with a loud holosystolic murmur in an asymptomatic patient, and often a thrill at the left sternal edge, usually around the fourth interspace, is heard. Large defects may produce a mitral diastolic flow rumble (due to increased volume) at the apex, especially when the shunt is more than 2.5:1, and may cause considerable symptoms early in life. Ventricular septal defects are usually detected in early childhood, and in developed countries they are usually closed when discovered. If undiscovered until late childhood or adulthood, a large ventricular septal defect often has progressed to Eisenmenger syndrome (severe pulmonary hypertension) and cannot be closed (see "Eisenmenger Syndrome" below). Patients may present with symptoms of subacute bacterial endocarditis; thus, endocarditis prophylaxis is essential if Eisenmenger syndrome develops. Affected women of childbearing age should be advised against pregnancy.

- Ventricular septal defects are most common in the membranous septum or the muscular septum.

- If undiscovered until adulthood, a large ventricular septal defect may have progressed to Eisenmenger syndrome.

PATENT DUCTUS ARTERIOSUS

This condition is associated with maternal rubella. It produces the equivalent of an arteriovenous fistula. A small ductus is compatible with a normal lifespan. The ductus may calcify in adult life. A continuous "machinery" murmur envelops the S_2 heard at the second interspace beneath the left clavicle and anteriorly along the left second intercostal space. A large patent ductus arteriosus may produce ventricular failure. Surgical ligation is curative; subsequently, patients do not need prophylaxis for endocarditis.

- Patent ductus arteriosus is associated with maternal rubella.

- In the absence of surgical ligation, endocarditis prophylaxis is essential.

EISENMENGER SYNDROME

Eisenmenger syndrome develops in the first few years of life when a large shunt (usually a ventricular septal defect or patent ductus arteriosus, less often atrial septal defect) produces pulmonary hypertension and irreversible pulmonary vascular disease. This condition causes the shunt to reverse so that blood flows from the right to the left, and subsequent cyanosis occurs. The condition is then inoperable. Death commonly occurs in the third or fourth decade of life. Exercise-induced syncope, arrhythmias, hemoptysis, or stroke can all lead to death. Cyanosis produces marked erythrocytosis, often with markedly increased hemoglobin values. Phlebotomy is not needed when the hemoglobin value is less than 20 g/dL or the hematocrit value is less than 65%. Repeated phlebotomy leads to iron deficiency, and, because iron-deficient erythrocytes are more rigid, the risk for stroke is increased. The decision about phlebotomy ideally should be guided by a specialist in adult congenital heart disease. Fluid should be replaced concomitantly in patients with Eisenmenger syndrome because hypotension and syncope may be fatal as a result of exacerbation of right-to-left shunting and hypoxia. Volume depletion, considerable exercise, and vasodilation should be avoided.

- Eisenmenger syndrome typically develops in the first few years of life when there is a large shunt or later if a small shunt enlarges.

- Conditions associated with Eisenmenger syndrome include exercise-induced syncope, arrhythmia, hemoptysis, and stroke, any of which can be fatal.

PULMONARY STENOSIS

Pulmonary stenosis may occur as an isolated lesion or in association with a ventricular septal defect. Valvular pulmonary stenosis often causes few or no symptoms. The valve is frequently pliable, and it may be bicuspid. Thickened dysplastic valves, often stenotic, occur in association with the Noonan syndrome.

- Thickened dysplastic valves, often stenotic, occur with the Noonan syndrome.

Physical Examination

A late P_2 may be heard; with severe stenosis, the P_2 becomes inaudible. The pulmonary opening click is the only right-sided sound that gets softer with inspiration as the pulmonary valve partially opens with the inspiratory increase in venous return. Later in life, the valve may become so thick, calcified, and immobile that the ejection click disappears. Findings of pulmonary stenosis include a prominent *a* wave in the jugular venous pulse and an ejection systolic click.

Diagnosis

Electrocardiography shows right ventricular hypertrophy. Poststenotic pulmonary dilatation, especially of the left pulmonary artery (Figure 3.14), is the chest radiographic hallmark.

The diagnosis is reliably made with 2-dimensional echocardiography, and Doppler echocardiography reliably predicts the gradient and estimates right ventricular pressure. In asymptomatic patients, treatment is indicated when the right ventricular systolic pressure approaches more than two-thirds the systemic blood pressure. The treatment of choice for a pliable noncalcified valve is percutaneous balloon valvuloplasty.

- Two-dimensional and Doppler echocardiography establish the diagnosis of pulmonary stenosis.

COARCTATION OF THE AORTA

This condition is usually either a discrete or a long segment of narrowing adjacent to the left subclavian artery. It is more

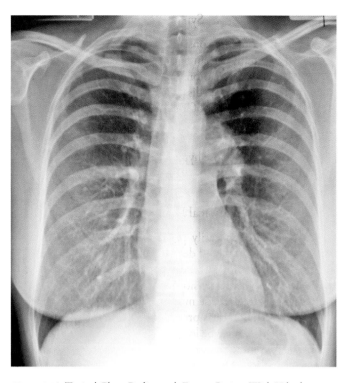

Figure 3.14 Typical Chest Radiograph From a Patient With Valvular Pulmonary Stenosis. Normal cardiac size and marked prominence of main and left pulmonary arteries represent poststenotic dilatation. This does not occur with infundibular pulmonary stenosis. Lung fields appear mildly oligemic.

common in males and frequently is associated with a bicuspid aortic valve. Only about 20% of cases are diagnosed in adulthood. This is the most common cardiac anomaly associated with Turner syndrome. Other associations include aneurysms of the circle of Willis and aortic dissection or rupture. There is an increased incidence of aortic dissection or rupture in Turner syndrome, even in the absence of coarctation. As a result of the coarctation, systemic collateral vessels develop from the subclavian and axillary arteries through the internal mammary, scapular, and intercostal arteries and may be identified by rib notching on the chest radiograph.

- Coarctation of the aorta is more common in males.

- The condition is frequently associated with a bicuspid aortic valve.

- Only 20% of cases are diagnosed in adulthood.

- It is the most common cardiac anomaly associated with Turner syndrome.

There are 5 major complications of coarctation of the aorta: 1) cardiac failure, 2) aortic valve disease, 3) aortic rupture or dissection, 4) endarteritis, and 5) rupture of an aneurysm of the circle of Willis. The risk for aneurysmal rupture is increased by hypertension. Systemic hypertension may be the presenting clinical finding in adults younger than 50 years. Some patients complain of pain and fatigue in the legs on exercise, reminiscent of claudication.

Symptoms

Coarctation should be considered in patients with hypertension who are younger than 50 years. There may be coexistent lower extremity claudication. Patients may present with symptoms of aortic rupture, dissection, congestive heart failure, or associated conditions of Turner syndrome, circle of Willis aneurysm, or bicuspid valve.

- Coarctation may cause hypertension in adults younger than 50 years.

Physical Examination

Findings include an easily palpable brachial pulse, but the femoral pulse is weak and delayed. There are systolic pressure differences between the upper and the lower extremities, and upper extremity hypertension and lower extremity hypotension are possible. Exercise may exaggerate systemic hypertension. An ejection click is present when there is an associated bicuspid valve. A_2 may be loud as a result of hypertension. An S_4 may be present with associated left ventricular hypertrophy and hypertension. Murmurs may originate from 1) the coarctation, which can produce a systolic murmur over the left sternal edge and over the spine in the midthoracic region, and it sometimes extends into diastole in the form of a continuous murmur; 2) arterial collateral vessels, which are spread widely over the thorax; and 3) the bicuspid aortic valve, which may generate a systolic murmur.

- Physical findings of coarctation of the aorta include brachial-femoral delay and systolic blood pressure differences between the upper and lower extremities.

Diagnosis

The electrocardiogram may be normal. Left ventricular hypertrophy with or without repolarization changes is more likely when coarctation stenosis and hypertension are more severe. Chest radiography may show rib notching from the dilated and pulsatile intercostal arteries and a "3" configuration of the aortic knob, due to the coarctation site with proximal and distal dilatation.

- The electrocardiogram may be normal in coarctation of the aorta.
- Chest radiographic findings in coarctation of the aorta are rib notching and a "3" configuration of the aortic knob.

Treatment

Surgical treatment is an accepted approach. Balloon angioplasty has been performed in some patients, but it has been associated with aneurysm formation and re-coarctation. Even after surgical repair, there is a considerable rate of hypertension. Up to 75% of patients are hypertensive at 30-year follow-up. Surgically treated patients still often die prematurely of coronary artery disease, heart failure, stroke, or ruptured or dissected aorta. Age at operation is important. The 20-year survival rate is 91% in patients who have operation when they are younger than 14 years and 79% in patients who have operation when they are older than 14 years.

- Surgical repair is the accepted treatment of coarctation of the aorta.

EBSTEIN ANOMALY

This is a congenital lesion of the right side of the heart with a variable clinical spectrum. Inferior displacement of the tricuspid valve ring into the right ventricular cavity causes a sail-like elongated anterior cusp or tricuspid valve on echocardiography. The degree of displacement is variable, as is the degree of abnormality of the tricuspid valve. The inferior displacement of the tricuspid valve results in "atrialization" of the right ventricle. This anomaly has been associated with maternal lithium ingestion during pregnancy.

- Ebstein anomaly involves inferior displacement of the tricuspid valve ring into the right ventricular cavity with a sail-like tricuspid valve on echocardiography.
- Ebstein anomaly has been associated with maternal lithium ingestion during pregnancy.

Symptoms

Ebstein anomaly has a protracted natural history. Most patients present with cyanosis and dyspnea with or without atrial arrhythmias.

Physical Examination

The extremities are usually cool, often with peripheral cyanosis (due to low cardiac output). A prominent a wave and v wave (if tricuspid regurgitation is present) are present; this finding is variable because the large right atrium may accommodate a large tricuspid regurgitant volume. A right ventricular lift is noted. The S_1 has a loud tricuspid (T_1) component. A holosystolic murmur increases on inspiration at the left sternal edge from tricuspid regurgitation. One or more systolic clicks are noted. Common associated conditions are secundum atrial septal defect, preexcitation syndrome, and bundle of Kent (atrioventricular accessory pathway). Patients with secundum atrial septal defects are often very cyanotic as a result of increased right-to-left shunting, and they may present with neurologic events due to paradoxic embolism. Tachycardia often occurs as a result of the high frequency of accessory atrioventricular pathways.

Diagnosis

Chest radiography shows a narrow pedicle with an enlarged globular silhouette and right atrial enlargement. The lung fields are normal or oligemic. Electrocardiographic findings include tall P waves (so-called Himalayan P waves) and right bundle branch block. Two-dimensional and Doppler echocardiography precisely delineate the anatomy. Cardiac catheterization is unnecessary. Electrophysiologic study may be necessary to delineate a bypass tract.

Treatment

The long asymptomatic phase supports postponing surgical intervention until the patient has significant symptoms. Patients may require anticoagulation if an atrial septal defect is present and paradoxical emboli have occurred.

- Conditions associated with Ebstein anomaly are secundum atrial septal defect, preexcitation syndrome, and bundle of Kent.

- Tachycardia may be an indication for an electrophysiologic study to identify an accessory atrioventricular pathway.

- Anticoagulation should be considered in the setting of an atrial septal defect if paradoxical emboli have occurred.

SUGGESTED READING

Bonow RO, Carabello BA, Chatterjee K, de Leon AC Jr, Faxon DP, Freed MD, et al; American College of Cardiology/American Heart Association Task Force on Practice Guidelines. 2008 focused update incorporated into the ACC/AHA 2006 guidelines for the management of patients with valvular heart disease: a report of the American College of Cardiology/American Heart Association Task Force on Practice Guidelines (Writing Committee to revise the 1998 guidelines for the management of patients with valvular heart disease). Endorsed by the Society of Cardiovascular Anesthesiologists, Society for Cardiovascular Angiography and Interventions, and Society of Thoracic Surgeons. J Am Coll Cardiol. 2008 Sep 23;52(13):e1–142.

Bonow RO, Carabello BA, Chatterjee K, de Leon AC Jr, Faxon DP, Freed MD, et al; 2006 Writing Committee Members; American College of Cardiology/American Heart Association Task Force. 2008 Focused update incorporated into the ACC/AHA 2006 guidelines for the management of patients with valvular heart disease: a report of the American College of Cardiology/American Heart Association Task Force on Practice Guidelines (Writing Committee to Revise the 1998 Guidelines for the Management of Patients With Valvular Heart Disease): endorsed by the Society of Cardiovascular Anesthesiologists, Society for Cardiovascular Angiography and Interventions, and Society of Thoracic Surgeons. Circulation. 2008 Oct 7;118(15):e523–661. Epub 2008 Sep 26.

Lucas RV Jr, Edwards JE. The floppy mitral valve. Curr Probl Cardiol. 1982 Jul;7(4):1–48.

O'rourke RA, Crawford MH. The systolic click-murmur syndrome: clinical recognition and management. Curr Probl Cardiol. 1976 Mar-Apr;1(1):1–60.

Task Force on Practice Guidelines (Committee on Management of Patients with Valvular Heart Disease). ACC/AHA guidelines for the management of patients with valvular heart disease: a report of the American College of Cardiology/American Heart Association. J Am Coll Cardiol. 1998 Nov;32(5):1486–588.

4.

THE HEART AND SYSTEMIC DISEASE, PREGNANCY AND HEART DISEASE, AND MISCELLANEOUS CARDIAC DISORDERS

Kyle W. Klarich, MD

GOALS

- Describe the cardiac manifestations of systemic diseases.
- Review normal cardiac changes of pregnancy and the interaction of cardiac conditions with pregnancy.
- Summarize miscellaneous cardiac disorders.

Many systemic diseases may have manifestations in the heart. This section describes those that are most likely to be included on the board examination.

THE HEART AND SYSTEMIC DISEASE

HYPERTHYROIDISM

Effects

Cardiovascular manifestations of hyperthyroidism include increased heart rate, stroke volume, and cardiac output. Peripheral vascular resistance is decreased, and thus pulse pressure is widened. As a result, myocardial oxygen consumption increases, which may precipitate angina. Other symptoms include palpitations, presyncope or syncope, and exertional dyspnea. Arrhythmias may occur.

Symptoms

Common symptoms include weight loss, weakness (especially in the elderly), and tachycardia or palpitations.

Physical Examination

Common physical findings are tachycardia and a bounding pulse with a wide pulse pressure, a forceful apical impulse, and a systolic ejection murmur due to increased flow. Supraventricular tachycardia and atrial fibrillation are the most common arrhythmias. Angina may be present. Atrial fibrillation occurs in 10% to 20% of patients. Indeed, thyrotoxicosis should be excluded in patients with atrial

fibrillation. Examination may also show tremor; a goiter may be present.

Treatment

Treatment of hyperthyroidism usually leads to reversal of cardiac symptoms. If atrial fibrillation is present, the risk of embolization is high and anticoagulation should be instituted. Cardioversion should not be attempted until a euthyroid state is achieved.

- Hyperthyroidism may lead to increased myocardial work and oxygen consumption and precipitate angina and arrhythmias, especially atrial fibrillation.
- Thyrotoxicosis should be excluded in patients with atrial fibrillation.
- Cardiac symptoms are reversed with treatment of hyperthyroidism.
- Anticoagulation is necessary in patients with thyrotoxicosis-associated atrial fibrillation.

HYPOTHYROIDISM

Effects

Mucoprotein infiltration of the myocardium due to hypothyroidism leads to cardiac enlargement and decreased function. Hypothyroidism decreases metabolic rate and circulatory demand and causes bradycardia, decreased contractility and stroke volume, and increased peripheral resistance. One-third of patients have pericardial effusion. The cardiomyopathy is reversible if detected early. Hypothyroidism is associated with increased cholesterol levels and atherosclerosis.

Symptoms

Patients may present with depression, lethargy, and slowed mentation. Hair loss on the scalp and lateral aspect of the eyebrows and a thick tongue may occur. Many patients report constipation and weight gain.

Physical Examination

Cardiac enlargement can be caused by myocardial disease or a pericardial effusion. The pulse volume is decreased as a result of reduced contractility. Sinus bradycardia usually is present. Other findings may include macroglossia, thinning or loss of the lateral third of the eyebrows, coarse hair and dry skin, and myxedema. Chest radiography shows increased cardiac size. Electrocardiography shows low voltage of QRS with prolonged intervals of QRS, PR, and QT.

Hypothyroidism-related cardiomyopathy can be reversed with early treatment.

- Physical findings in hypothyroidism include cardiac enlargement, reduced myocardial contractility, and pericardial effusion (in one-third of patients).

- Atherosclerosis is accelerated.

- Hypothyroidism may lead to a reversible dilated cardiomyopathy.

Treatment

Reversal of cardiac involvement occurs with early treatment of hypothyroidism.

DIABETES MELLITUS

Effects

Diabetes mellitus is associated with premature atherosclerosis, which is twice as prevalent in diabetic men and 3 times more prevalent in diabetic women than in a nondiabetic population. Patients with diabetes have a higher prevalence of hypertension and hyperlipidemia. Angina and myocardial infarction manifest with nonclassic symptoms, or patients may have silent ischemia. Congestive heart failure may be the first manifestation of coronary artery disease among diabetics. Cardiomyopathy not associated with coronary atherosclerosis may also exist; this may be caused by small-vessel disease. Fatal myocardial infarction is more common in patients with diabetes than in those who do not have diabetes.

Treatment

Aggressive management of traditional risk factors for coronary artery disease lowers mortality. Diabetic-specific risk factors for coronary artery disease include glycemic control and urinary protein excretion. The use of antihypertensive agents for aggressive blood pressure lowering (systolic pressure ≤120 mm Hg, diastolic pressure ≤80 mm Hg) reduces mortality. Statins and fibrates are effective for primary and secondary prevention of coronary artery disease in patients with both diabetes and hyperlipidemia. Aspirin also is effective for primary and secondary prevention. Angiotensin-converting enzyme inhibitors reduce cardiovascular events and mortality in patients with diabetes who are older than 55 years and have additional risk factors. To date, glycemic control has not been shown to lower the incidence of cardiovascular events.

- Patients with diabetes may present with nonclassic symptoms or silent ischemia; congestive heart failure may be the first clinical manifestation of diabetic coronary disease.

- Aggressive risk factor modification reduces cardiovascular events and mortality in patients with diabetes.

- Blood pressure and lipid management and monitoring for urinary protein excretion are cornerstones of care.

Coronary artery bypass grafting was previously shown to reduce the death rate more than percutaneous transluminal coronary angioplasty in patients with diabetes or those with multivessel coronary artery disease. However, stents and glycoprotein IIb/IIIa inhibitors were not routinely used in prior studies. Therefore, diabetes is not an absolute indication for the use of coronary artery bypass grafting.

AMYLOIDOSIS

Effects

Amyloidosis leads to extracellular deposition of insoluble proteins in organs and is classified by the precursor plasma proteins forming the extracellular fibril deposits. The primary systemic type, AL, is due to monoclonal immunoglobulin free light chains. The hereditary (familial) type is due to mutant transthyretin deposition, and its inheritance is autosomal dominant. The wild-type transthyretin type (wild-type TTR, senile type) is due to normal wild-type transthyretin deposition. The secondary type (AA type) is related to amyloid A protein, usually the result of multiple myeloma. The heart is frequently involved, especially by the AL type. Nearly 90% of patients with primary amyloidosis have clinical manifestations of cardiac dysfunction.

Cardiomyopathy may result from protein infiltration, which causes thickened ventricular myocardium. Amyloid deposition in the atrioventricular cardiac valves may occur. Amyloid can also deposit in small vessels and lead to ischemia.

Cardiac involvement may occur in secondary amyloidosis, but it is usually not a prominent feature. Secondary amyloidosis occurs in association with chronic diseases such as rheumatoid arthritis, tuberculosis, chronic infection, neoplasm (especially multiple myeloma), and chronic renal failure. In senile amyloidosis, the heart is the most commonly involved organ, and prevalence increases after age 60 years.

Clinical Features

Cardiac amyloidosis may cause congestive heart failure, arrhythmias, sudden death, angina, chest pain, pericardial effusion (usually not hemodynamically significant), and regurgitant murmurs. The natural history is usually intractable because of ventricular failure. Diastolic abnormalities are common early in the disease process and are classic for restrictive cardiomyopathy, which indicates a poor prognosis.

- Cardiac involvement in primary amyloidosis is common, particularly in the AL (primary systemic) type.
- Cardiac involvement in secondary amyloidosis is not a prominent feature but may occur.
- Senile amyloidosis frequently involves the heart.
- Amyloid heart disease can cause multiple cardiac abnormalities, ranging from regurgitant murmurs and arrhythmias to sudden death.

Symptoms and Findings

Amyloidosis should be considered when a patient (usually age 40–70 years) presents with dyspnea and progressive edema of the lower extremities. Associated conditions such as vocal hoarseness, carpal tunnel syndrome, or peripheral neuropathy may be present and point to the systemic nature of the disease. The patient often has received treatment with digoxin (contraindicated in cardiac amyloid) and a diuretic but has had little improvement. The key finding is a low-voltage QRS complex with or without other conduction abnormalities (such as increased PR interval or bundle branch block) coupled with echocardiographic findings of thick walls and usually preserved ventricular function.

Diagnosis

Cardiac involvement is suggested by the classic electrocardiographic findings of a low-voltage QRS complex. However, this is a nonspecific finding, and 20% to 25% of patients with cardiac amyloid may have normal electrocardiographic findings. Echocardiography is particularly useful, showing increased left ventricular wall thickness, in contradistinction to the small (or normal) voltage on electrocardiography (Figure 4.1). Echocardiographic tissue characteristics are often described as having a granular or speckled appearance. The atria generally are dilated. The cardiac valves may show some thickening and regurgitation. A small pericardial effusion may be present. Diastolic function generally is abnormal; in the early stages of the disease, findings consistent with prolonged relaxation are found, whereas restrictive filling (consistent with high left ventricular filling pressures) is found in later stages.

Treatment

If an underlying cause can be identified, treatment may lead to a better prognosis. However, once cardiac amyloidosis is diagnosed, the prognosis generally is poor. Referral to a tertiary center with expertise in amyloidosis is warranted because prior experimental protocols have evolved into treatment options, such as stem cell transplant in primary amyloidosis or chemotherapy.

- Hallmark findings of cardiac amyloidosis are normal to low QRS voltage on electrocardiography and thick ventricular walls on echocardiography.
- Echocardiographic features are helpful for evaluating and monitoring progression of cardiac amyloidosis.
- Liver or heart transplant or other therapies such as stem cell transplant or chemotherapy may be warranted.

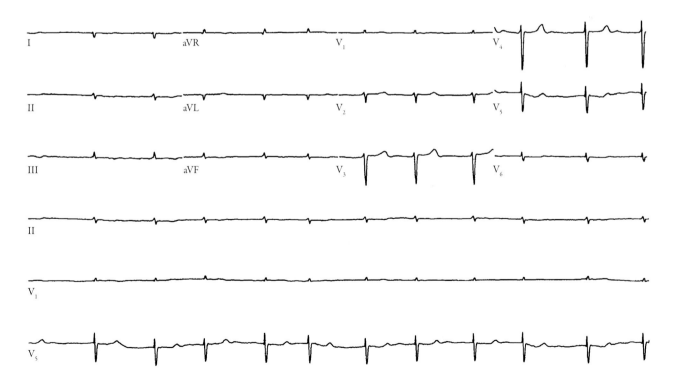

Figure 4.1 Electrocardiography in Cardiac Amyloidosis. Classic finding is low-voltage complexes.

HEMOCHROMATOSIS

Effects

Hemochromatosis, an iron-storage disease, may be primary or secondary (related to exogenous iron, usually from repeated transfusions). Iron deposits within the cardiac cells may occur. Cardiac hemochromatosis is usually accompanied by other organ involvement, primarily pancreas, liver, and skin, leading to the classic tetrad of diabetes, liver disease, brown skin pigmentation, and congestive heart failure. Affected patients may present with cardiomegaly, congestive heart failure (with features of systolic and diastolic dysfunction), and arrhythmias. Once clinical cardiac symptoms appear, the prognosis is very poor unless treatment is initiated with a combination of phlebotomy and iron chelation.

Symptoms and Findings

Patients may present with bronze-colored skin, diabetes or glucose intolerance, arthralgias, and loss of libido. Symptoms and signs of heart failure may be present. Increased transferrin saturation and increased serum ferritin values establish the diagnosis of hemochromatosis.

- Iron deposition may result in substantial cardiac disease and, once symptomatic, patients have a poor prognosis.
- The key to the diagnosis of hemochromatosis is the tetrad of diabetes, liver disease, skin hyperpigmentation, and congestive heart failure.

CARCINOID HEART DISEASE

Effects

Liver or lung metastases from carcinoid tumors can produce a classic syndrome (in only about 4% of patients) due to production of serotonin-like substances. These substances cause cutaneous flushing, wheezing, and diarrhea (the carcinoid syndrome) and are toxic to cardiac valves. Cardiac involvement occurs in approximately 50% of patients with hepatic or pulmonary metastasis; toxic effects generally affect right-sided cardiac valves. Left-sided valves can be affected if a cardiac shunt is present; such a shunt allows right-to-left movement of serotonin-like substances via the bloodstream. Carcinoid lesions are fibrous plaques that form on valvular endocardium. The valve leaflets become thickened, relatively immobile, and retracted. Regurgitation results, with some stenosis of the tricuspid and the pulmonary valves.

- Serotonin-like substances produced by metastatic carcinoid tumors are toxic to heart valves and may lead to regurgitation and stenosis.
- Right-sided valves are most commonly affected.

Symptoms

Patients may complain of weight loss, fatigue, watery diarrhea (>10 stools daily), dyspnea on exertion, and intermittent hot flashes.

Physical Examination

Typical findings on examination are an increased jugular venous pressure profile, a prominent *v* wave, a cardiac murmur, a pulsatile liver that may be enlarged, ascites, and usually peripheral edema. Audible wheezes may be present, and patients may have a ruddy complexion.

Diagnosis

Electrocardiography typically shows right ventricular hypertrophy and right bundle branch block. Diagnosis is made by identification of a thickened tricuspid valve and pulmonary valve (left-sided valves only if a shunt is present). Lung and liver metastasis may be found if computed tomography is performed. The diagnosis is confirmed by a 24-hour urine measurement of 5-hydroxyindoleacetic acid. Acquired tricuspid and pulmonary stenosis with or without regurgitation is rare and should always raise the possibility of carcinoid heart disease.

- Right ventricular hypertrophy due to pulmonary valve regurgitation and stenosis may be identified in carcinoid heart disease.
- Acquired tricuspid and pulmonary stenosis with or without regurgitation is rare and should always raise the possibility of carcinoid heart disease.

Treatment

Treatment of the underlying tumor is important for symptom relief. In the setting of right heart failure (eg, intractable edema, ascites, and dyspnea), surgery may be warranted. Surgical therapies include tricuspid valve replacement and pulmonary valve resection.

HYPEREOSINOPHILIC SYNDROME

Effects

This syndrome, with persistent eosinophil concentrations of more than 1.5×10^9/L, typically affects young, usually male, patients. Causes include idiopathic hypereosinophilia, Löffler endocarditis, reactive or allergic eosinophilia, leukemic or neoplastic eosinophilia, and Churg-Strauss syndrome. All of these may have cardiac manifestations.

Clinical Features

Patients typically present with weight loss, fatigue, dyspnea, syncope, and systemic embolization. Pulmonary involvement should prompt consideration of Churg-Strauss syndrome. Cardiac manifestations include arrhythmias, myocarditis, conduction abnormalities, and thrombosis. Cardiac eosinophilic deposition may occur, with clot formation in the ventricular apices and the inflow surfaces of the mitral and tricuspid valves. Matting down of the atrioventricular valves occurs, causing considerable regurgitation. Scarring occurs where the clot formed, leading to endomyocardial fibrosis and restrictive cardiomyopathy.

- Arrhythmias, myocarditis, conduction abnormalities, and thrombosis may occur in hypereosinophilic syndrome.

- Valve involvement may lead to regurgitation, fibrosis, and restrictive cardiomyopathy.

- Churg-Strauss syndrome should be considered if pulmonary involvement is present.

SYSTEMIC LUPUS ERYTHEMATOSUS

Systemic lupus erythematosus may involve any of the cardiac structures. Special features of involvement include the antiphospholipid syndrome and Libman-Sacks endocarditis. Cardiac involvement may include pericarditis, characterized by a positive antinuclear antibody in the pericardial fluid, myocarditis (more common in patients with anti-Ro antibody), valvulopathy, and coronary arteritis. Libman-Sacks endocarditis, which results in noninfective vegetations, occurs in up to 50% of patients with systemic lupus erythematosus. The vegetations do not generally embolize or interfere with valvular function. Congenital heart block may occur in newborns of mothers with lupus with anti-La and anti-Ro antibodies due to myocarditis and to inflammation and fibrosis of the conduction system (neonatal lupus).

- The vegetations of Libman-Sacks endocarditis generally do not cause clinical problems.

- Offspring of mothers with SS-a and SS-b antibodies are at risk for congenital heart block.

SCLERODERMA

Cardiac involvement is manifested by intramural coronary involvement and immune-mediated endothelial injury, which is often associated with the Raynaud phenomenon clinically (due to peripheral small vessel involvement). Other systemic features include sclerotic skin changes and esophageal abnormalities. Cardiac involvement is the third most common cause of mortality in patients with scleroderma. Conduction defects occur in up to 20% of patients, and a usually asymptomatic pericardial effusion is found in a third of patients. Indirect cardiac involvement due to pulmonary hypertension and cor pulmonale is frequent.

- Cardiac involvement is the third most common cause of mortality in patients with scleroderma.

- Conduction defects may occur in up to 20% of patients, and pericardial effusions are also common.

RHEUMATOID ARTHRITIS

Nearly all cardiac components, including pericardium, myocardium, valves, coronary arteries, and aorta, may be affected in patients with rheumatoid arthritis. Granulomatous inflammation and nongranulomatous inflammation of valve leaflets occur but rarely lead to severe valvular incompetence. Associated pericarditis is typically associated with a low glucose level and complement depletion in the pericardial fluid. Rheumatoid nodules in the conduction system can lead to heart block. Aortitis and pulmonary hypertension due to pulmonary vasculitis are very rare complications.

- Pericardial fluid is low in glucose and complement.

- Rheumatoid nodule involvement in the conduction system may lead to heart block.

- Nongranulomatous and granulomatous involvement of valvular tissue may lead to valve incompetence.

ANKYLOSING SPONDYLITIS

Approximately 10% of patients with ankylosing spondylitis have aortic dilatation and aortic regurgitation. Aortic valve cusp distortion and retraction also may cause considerable aortic regurgitation. Fibrosis and inflammation of the conduction system may occur.

- Cardiac abnormalities of ankylosing spondylitis include aortic dilatation, aortic valve regurgitation, and conduction system abnormalities.

MARFAN SYNDROME

Degeneration of elastic tissues occurs in this autosomal dominant condition. Features include arachnodactyly, tall stature, pectus excavatum, kyphoscoliosis, and lenticular dislocation. Cardiac involvement is common, including mitral valve prolapse, aortic regurgitation due to aortic dilatation, and increased risk of aortic dissection. Long-term β-adrenergic blockade decreases the rate of aortic dilatation and the risk of aortic dissection. Dissection occurs rarely in an aorta less than 55 mm in diameter. When dissection occurs, it tends to start in the ascending aorta and extend along the entire aorta.

- Degeneration of elastic tissues results in considerable risk of aortic regurgitation and aortic dissection. Mitral valve prolapse may occur.

FRIEDREICH ATAXIA

This autosomal recessive neurologic disorder involves the heart in up to 90% of cases. It usually manifests as a symmetric hypertrophy of the myocardium and less commonly as a dilated cardiomyopathy.

- Cardiac involvement is very common in Friedreich ataxia.

OSTEOGENESIS IMPERFECTA

The hallmarks of this condition are brittle bones, blue sclera, and deafness. The underlying problem is a lack of collagen-supporting matrix. Ultimately, degeneration of elastic tissue occurs, including aortic root dilatation, aortic regurgitation, annular dilatation, and chordal stretch leading to marked atrioventricular regurgitation.

- Absence of a collagen-supporting matrix leads to degeneration of elastic tissues and the resulting cardiac complications.

LYME DISEASE

Lyme disease is caused by *Borrelia burgdorferi* infection. Clinical cardiac involvement occurs in up to 10% of affected patients. Atrioventricular block is the most common manifestation of Lyme carditis, but myopericarditis can also occur. The diagnosis is generally made in the setting of consistent clinical features and positive Lyme serologic testing. Right ventricular myocardial biopsy or gallium scanning establishes the diagnosis, but these procedures are rarely necessary. Treatment is with antimicrobial agents and supportive measures. If a conduction block is present or patients have concerning cardiac symptoms, monitoring should be started. Temporary pacing may be needed.

- Atrioventricular conduction blocks and Lyme carditis occur in up to 10% of patients with Lyme disease.

ACQUIRED IMMUNODEFICIENCY SYNDROME

Clinically apparent cardiac involvement may occur in up to 10% of patients with AIDS. Myocarditis may be associated with ventricular arrhythmias, dilated cardiomyopathy, pericarditis, or infectious or malignant invasion of the cardiac structures. Up to 50% of patients have myocarditis at autopsy.

- Clinically evident cardiac involvement occurs in up to 10% of patients with AIDS, but up to 50% of autopsies identify myocarditis.

CARDIAC TRAUMA

Cardiac contusion may lead to arrhythmia, increased cardiac enzyme values, transient regional wall motion abnormalities, and pericardial effusion or tamponade. It may also cause disruption of the aorta or valves (tricuspid valve most often) or right ventricular rupture. Commotio cordis is sudden cardiac death due to trauma, characteristically mild trauma to the chest wall. This is generally due to a nonpenetrating blow (eg, by a baseball or softball) leading to instantaneous cardiac arrest. Cardiac disease is often absent. The trauma must be delivered during the vulnerable phase of the cardiac cycle, described as the 15 to 30 milliseconds before and after the T wave.

- Cardiac contusion, such as a sudden deceleration injury, may cause various types of cardiac injury that may be life-threatening.

PREGNANCY AND HEART DISEASE

PHYSIOLOGIC CHANGES OF PREGNANCY

A relative anemia occurs due to nonparallel increases in plasma volume and red cell mass. Cardiac output increases by 30% to 50%, peripheral resistance decreases, and heart rate increases. Increased venous pressure in the lower extremities leads to pedal edema in 80% of healthy pregnant women. To the unaware examiner, these normal changes may suggest cardiac abnormalities. A healthy pregnant woman is expected to have increased jugular venous pressure, bounding carotid pulses, and an ejection systolic murmur in the pulmonary area (not more than grade 3/6). The second heart sound (S_2) is loud, and there is often a third heart sound (S_3) or diastolic filling sound. A fourth heart sound (S_4) occasionally may be heard.

- Clinical findings can be easily misinterpreted by examiners who are unfamiliar with normal changes of pregnancy.

PREGNANCY AND CARDIAC DISEASE

Although an S_3 or diastolic filling sound is common, a long diastolic rumble should raise concern for mitral stenosis. Decreased peripheral resistance and increased output changes result in poor tolerance of valvular stenosis compared with regurgitation. An example is that a patient with aortic stenosis has exaggeration of the aortic valve gradient, whereas a patient with mitral regurgitation experiences "afterload reduction" due to peripheral vasodilatation and tolerates pregnancy better. The functional class of the patient is an important consideration for determining whether pregnancy is contraindicated. New York Heart Association functional class III or IV is associated with a maternal mortality rate approaching 7%.

- An S_3 or diastolic filling sound is common in pregnancy, but a long rumble should raise the possibility of mitral stenosis.
- For patients in New York Heart Association functional class III or IV, the maternal mortality rate approaches 7%.

Pregnancy is *absolutely* contraindicated in patients with the following conditions: 1) Marfan syndrome with a dilated aortic root (hormonal changes soften the connective tissue, resulting in an unpredictable risk of dissection and rupture, even with a normal aortic root size), 2) Eisenmenger syndrome (maternal mortality rate is 50% and fetal mortality rate approaches 100%), 3) primary pulmonary hypertension, 4) symptomatic severe aortic stenosis, 5) symptomatic severe mitral stenosis, and 6) symptomatic dilated cardiomyopathy.

Although not absolute contraindications, the following conditions are of concern in pregnancy: 1) atrial septal defect (deep venous thrombosis may lead to paradoxic embolus) and 2) coarctation (increased risk of dissection and rupture). Patients at risk during pregnancy should minimize physical activity to prevent increased cardiac output, reduce dietary sodium, and minimize anemia with iron and vitamin supplements.

- Absolute contraindications to pregnancy include Marfan syndrome, Eisenmenger syndrome, primary pulmonary hypertension, symptomatic severe aortic or mitral valve stenosis, and symptomatic dilated cardiomyopathy.

Bed rest is indicated if congestive heart failure develops. Arrhythmias such as atrial fibrillation must be treated promptly. Cardioversion can be performed with apparently low risk to the fetus. Fetal cardiac monitoring should also be performed. Occasionally patients require surgery. Operation during the first trimester is associated with a markedly increased rate of fetal loss. Percutaneous aortic, mitral, and pulmonary balloon valvuloplasty have been performed during pregnancy and may obviate cardiopulmonary bypass. Careful lead shielding of the fetus is necessary because of the use of ionizing radiation.

- Arrhythmias must be promptly treated and cardioversion can be safely performed in pregnant patients.

MEDICAL THERAPY DURING PREGNANCY

Many cardiac drugs cross the placenta but can be used safely when necessary. These include digoxin, quinidine, procainamide, β-adrenergic blockers, and verapamil. β-Adrenergic blockers are associated with fetal growth retardation, neonatal bradycardia, and hypoglycemia and should be used cautiously. Patients with hypertrophic cardiomyopathy may require high doses, and fetal growth must be monitored.

Angiotensin-converting enzyme inhibitors (which cause fetal renal dysgenesis), phenytoin (which causes hydantoin syndrome and teratogenicity), and warfarin (which causes teratogenicity and abortion) should be avoided in pregnancy.

- Drugs to avoid in pregnancy include angiotensin-converting enzyme inhibitors, phenytoin, and warfarin.

DELIVERY IN THE SETTING OF CARDIAC DISEASE

Rapid hemodynamic swings occur during delivery. About 500 mL of blood is released into the circulation with each uterine contraction. Cardiac output increases with advancing labor, and oxygen consumption increases 3-fold. High-risk patients need careful monitoring (possibly with Swan-Ganz catheterization to maintain preload at an optimal level), maternal and fetal electrocardiographic monitoring, careful analgesia and anesthesia to avoid hypotension,

delivery in the left lateral position, and a short second stage of labor. Facilitated delivery may be needed if labor progresses slowly.

- Pregnant women with cardiac disease require careful monitoring during delivery.

Vaginal delivery is safer for most women with cardiac disease; with vaginal delivery, average blood loss is 500 mL, as opposed to cesarean section, with an average blood loss of 800 mL. Cesarean section is typically performed only for obstetric indications. American Heart Association guidelines state that there is no need for antibiotic prophylaxis in an uncomplicated vaginal delivery.

- Vaginal delivery is safer for the majority of patients with cardiac disease; cesarian section is typically used for obstetric indications only.

MANAGEMENT OF PROSTHETIC VALVES DURING PREGNANCY

Most women of childbearing age who want to bear children and who also need a valve replacement elect to have a biologic valve. Anticoagulants are usually not required in the setting of sinus rhythm. A biologic valve obligates patients to additional heart surgery. Women with mechanical valves require warfarin, posing a problem with teratogenicity (first trimester) and increased risk of spontaneous abortion. Pregnancy should be diagnosed as soon as possible, therapy should be switched to unfractionated subcutaneous heparin, and the activated partial thromboplastin time should be monitored. High-risk pregnancy teams adept at management are essential to early management.

- In pregnant patients with mechanical valves, therapy should be switched from warfarin to unfractionated subcutaneous heparin.

HYPERTENSION AND PREGNANCY

High blood pressure during pregnancy is defined as a systolic blood pressure increase of >30 mm Hg, a diastolic blood pressure increase of 15 mm Hg or more, or an absolute diastolic blood pressure of 90 mm Hg or more. It may be due to 1) chronic hypertension (blood pressure ≥140/80 mm Hg before pregnant state), 2) transient hypertension (develops during pregnancy), 3) preeclampsia (starts at ≥20 weeks of pregnancy), or 4) a combination. Methyldopa is the most extensively studied drug for hypertension during pregnancy and is safe. β-Adrenergic blockers are safe and efficacious but may cause growth retardation and fetal bradycardia. Angiotensin-converting enzyme inhibitors are contraindicated. Hydralazine is used if dual therapy is indicated, but it may cause fetal thrombocytopenia. Calcium channel blockers have been used more commonly in recent years.

Diuretics are effective because the hypertension of pregnancy is "salt-sensitive." The Working Group on Hypertension in Pregnancy allows continuation of the use of diuretics if they had been prescribed before gestation.

- Methyldopa is the first-line drug to manage hypertension during pregnancy.

- β-Blockers, hydralazine, and diuretics are overall safe to use. Fetal growth must be monitored when using β-adrenergic blockers.

PERICARDIAL DISEASE

The space between the visceral and parietal pericardium normally contains 15 to 25 mL of clear fluid. The pericardium functions to prevent cardiac distention, limit cardiac displacement (by its attachment to neighboring structures), and protect the heart from inflammation.

ACUTE OR SUBACUTE INFLAMMATORY PERICARDITIS

Symptoms

The chest pain of pericarditis is aggravated by movement of the trunk, inspiration, and coughing. The pain can be relieved by sitting up. Low-grade fever and malaise may occur.

Diagnosis

Pericardial friction rub may be variable. Chest radiography is usually normal, but globular enlargement may be found if the effusion is marked (>250 mL). A pulmonary infiltrate or small pleural effusion may be present. Left pleural effusion predominates for unknown reasons. Electrocardiography shows acute, concave ST elevation in all ventricular leads. The PR segment is depressed in the early stages. Echocardiography is diagnostic and helps determination of hemodynamic significance.

- Chest pain is the presenting symptom of pericarditis, and a friction rub may be heard on examination.

Causes

Causes include viral or idiopathic pericarditis, autoimmune and collagen vascular diseases, and postmyocardial infarction. Postcardiotomy syndrome may occur weeks to months after open heart procedures. It presents with pyrexia, increased sedimentation rate, and pleural or pericardial chest pain. Incidence decreases with age. Management is with anti-inflammatory agents. Pericarditis is also associated with radiation and neoplasm (especially Hodgkin disease, leukemia, and lymphoma). Melanoma and breast, thyroid, and lung tumors can metastasize to the pericardium and cause pericarditis or pericardial effusion. Uremia and tuberculosis also can cause pericarditis. Idiopathic viral pericarditis is the most likely diagnosis in the absence of a definable cause, and treatment with high-dose aspirin or other nonsteroidal anti-inflammatory agents usually resolves the condition.

- Causes of pericarditis include autoimmune and collagen vascular diseases, postmyocardial infarction, radiation, neoplasm, uremia, and tuberculosis.
- Management includes treatment of the underlying cause and anti-inflammatory drugs.

PERICARDIAL EFFUSION

The pericardium exudes fluid, fibrin, and blood cells in response to inflammation, causing a pericardial effusion. It cannot be seen on chest radiography until the effusion is 250 mL. With slow fluid accumulation, the pericardial sac distends slowly with no cardiac compression. With rapid accumulation (eg, bleeding), tamponade can occur with relatively small amounts of fluid. Tamponade restricts ventricular filling, decreasing ventricular volume. Increased intrapericardial pressure increases ventricular end-diastolic pressure, and increased mean atrial pressure increases the venous pressure. Decreased ventricular volume and filling diminish cardiac output. Any cause of pericarditis can cause tamponade, but acute causes of hemopericardium should be considered (eg, ruptured myocardium after infarction, aortic dissection, ruptured aortic aneurysm, and sequelae of cardiac operation).

- Tamponade can occur with small amounts of fluid.

Clinical Features

Tamponade produces a continuum of features, depending on severity. Typical findings are low blood pressure, a small and quiet heart, tachycardia, increased jugular venous pressure, and pulsus paradoxus (enhanced systemic blood pressure drop during inspiration due to decreased left ventricular filling). Kussmaul sign (increased distention of the neck veins during inspiration) may occur, as with constrictive pericarditis.

- Tamponade leads to multiple clinical findings, including pulsus paradoxus and Kussmaul sign.

Treatment

Emergency pericardiocentesis guided by echocardiography is necessary in hemodynamically compromised patients.

CONSTRICTIVE PERICARDITIS

Constrictive pericarditis is characterized by dissociation of respiratory-induced changes in intrathoracic and intracardiac pressures. Ventricular filling is limited by the constraining pericardium, an effect leading to lower ventricular volume, higher end-diastolic pressures, and decreased cardiac output. The most common causes are recurrent viral pericarditis, irradiation, previous open heart operation, tuberculosis, and neoplastic disease.

- Constriction causes decreased ventricular filling.

Symptoms

Symptoms of constrictive pericarditis are predominantly right-sided failure, peripheral edema, ascites, and often dyspnea and fatigue.

Physical Examination

In constrictive pericarditis, the jugular venous pressure is increased (best observed when the patient is sitting or standing), and inspiratory distention of neck veins (Kussmaul sign) is present. The jugular venous pressure may show rapid descents; a pericardial knock is present in fewer than 50% of cases. Ascites and peripheral edema are usually present. Chest radiography may show pericardial calcification and cardiac enlargement. No specific changes are found on electrocardiography.

- Typical examination findings in constrictive pericarditis are Kussmaul sign and signs consistent with right-sided heart failure.

Diagnosis

A high degree of clinical suspicion is necessary because the diagnosis of constrictive pericarditis can be challenging. Echocardiography, particularly with Doppler, shows the hemodynamic effects of respiratory changes in mitral and tricuspid inflow velocities and other classic changes. Pericardial thickness may be delineated by computed tomography and magnetic resonance imaging, but up to 20% of constraining pericardium may not be thickened according to computed tomographic criteria. Magnetic resonance scanning can show pericardial inflammation. Restrictive cardiomyopathy is the main differential diagnosis and differentiation can be difficult. Myocardial disease is likely if pulmonary artery systolic pressure is more than 50 mm Hg or if end-diastolic pulmonary artery pressure is more than 30% of systolic pressure, but both are nonspecific findings. In very difficult cases, cardiac catheterization for hemodynamic measurements may be necessary to show the intraventricular dependence and dissociation of intracardiac and intrathoracic pressures.

- Constrictive pericarditis is diagnosed from respiratory changes noted on Doppler echocardiography.
- The major confounding diagnosis is restrictive cardiomyopathy.
- Diastolic pressure is increased and equal in all 4 chambers.

Treatment

The treatment of choice for constrictive pericarditis is pericardiectomy.

CARDIAC TUMORS

Metastatic tumors are far more common than primary cardiac tumors (>20-fold). The most frequent metastases to the heart are melanoma, lymphoma, and breast, lung, and esophageal tumors. More than half of patients with malignant melanoma have metastases to the heart.

The most common primary benign tumors of the adult heart are cardiac myxoma, fibroma, and papillary fibroelastoma. Primary tumors are extremely rare. Cardiac tumors may cause circulatory problems, valve dysfunction, myocardial infiltration–related complications, invasion into local structures, or embolization.

- Primary cardiac tumors are much rarer than metastatic tumors.

The the most common primary cardiac tumor is myxoma, a benign tumor. Most cardiac myxomas are sporadic, but a subset of these tumors is familial. The majority (75%–85%) are located in the left atrium, 18% are in the right atrium, and the rest are ventricular. Most atrial tumors arise from the atrial septum, usually adjacent to the fossa ovalis. About 95% are solitary. Most have a short stalk, are gelatinous and friable, and tend to embolize. They occasionally calcify and may be visible on chest radiography.

A familial syndrome, Carney complex, involves multiple, often recurrent, cardiac and extracardiac myxomas, lentiginosis (spotty pigmentation) and other pigmentation abnormalities, endocrine tumors, and schwannomas. Myxomas present at a young age compared with sporadic myxomas.

- Myxomas are the most common primary cardiac tumor.

Blood flow obstruction, embolization, and systemic effects are the most common complications. Systemic emboli may occur in 30% to 60% of patients with left-sided myxoma, frequently to the brain and lower extremities. Coronary embolization is rare, but it should be considered in a young patient with no known previous cardiac disease. Systemic effects are fatigue, fever, weight loss, and arthralgia. Systemic effects may be associated with an increased sedimentation rate, leukocytosis, hypergammaglobulinemia, and anemia. Increased immunoglobulins are usually of immunoglobulin G class.

Left atrial tumors prolapse into the mitral valve orifice, producing symptoms of mitral stenosis (dyspnea, orthopnea, cough, pulmonary edema, and hemoptysis). Classically, symptoms occur with a change in body position. Physical findings suggest mitral stenosis. Pulmonary hypertension may occur. An early diastolic sound, the tumor "plop," may be heard, with the timing of an S_3. The later timing and lower frequency differentiate it from an opening snap.

Echocardiography allows accurate diagnosis. Once diagnosed, myxomas should be surgically excised.

- Clinical features of cardiac myxoma include blood flow obstruction and embolization.
- An early diastolic sound, the tumor "plop," may be heard.
- Systemic embolism is common in left-sided myxoma.
- Carney complex involves recurrent myxomas and systemic and skin abnormalities and is familial.

SUMMARY

- Hyperthyroidism may lead to increased myocardial work and oxygen consumption and precipitate angina and arrhythmias, especially atrial fibrillation.
- Physical findings in hypothyroidism include cardiac enlargement, reduced myocardial contractility, and pericardial effusion (in one-third of patients).
- Patients with diabetes may present with nonclassic symptoms or silent ischemia; congestive heart failure may be the first clinical manifestation of diabetic coronary disease.
- Amyloid heart disease can cause multiple cardiac abnormalities, ranging from regurgitant murmurs and arrhythmias to sudden death.
- Iron deposition may result in substantial cardiac disease and, once symptomatic, patients have a poor prognosis.
- Cardiac involvement is the third most common cause of mortality in patients with scleroderma.
- Absolute contraindications to pregnancy include Marfan syndrome, Eisenmenger syndrome, primary pulmonary hypertension, symptomatic severe aortic or mitral valve stenosis, and symptomatic dilated cardiomyopathy.
- Chest pain is the presenting symptom of pericarditis, and a friction rub may be heard on examination.
- Primary cardiac tumors are much rarer than metastatic tumors.
- Clinical features of cardiac myxoma include blood flow obstruction and embolization.

5.

HEART FAILURE AND CARDIOMYOPATHIES

Nicole P. Sandhu, MD, PhD, Naveen L. Pereira, MD,

and Robert D. Ficalora, MD

GOALS

- Review the presentation, evaluation, and management of heart failure.

- Describe the various types of cardiomyopathy.

- Distinguish the presentations and management of the different types of cardiomyopathy.

- Explain the roles of medical and device therapy and identify the indications for cardiac transplant.

HEART FAILURE

Heart failure is a clinical syndrome characterized by inability of the heart to maintain adequate cardiac output to meet the metabolic demands of the body while still maintaining normal or near-normal ventricular filling pressures. Heart failure may be present at rest, but often it is present only during exertion because of the dynamic nature of cardiac demands. For correct treatment of heart failure, the mechanism, underlying cause, and any reversible precipitating factors must be identified. Typical manifestations of heart failure are dyspnea and fatigue limiting activity tolerance and fluid retention leading to pulmonary or peripheral edema. These abnormalities do not always occur simultaneously. Dyspnea may be due to impaired cardiac output, increased filling pressures, or both.

- Heart failure is the inability of the heart to maintain adequate cardiac output to meet the metabolic demands of the body while still maintaining normal filling pressures.

- Heart failure may manifest at rest or only with exertion.

- Cardinal symptoms of heart failure are fatigue (related to impaired output) and fluid retention (resulting in pulmonary or peripheral edema).

- Dyspnea may be due to impaired output or increased filling pressures or both.

Heart failure, the symptomatic expression of cardiac disease, usually arises some time after cardiac disease is established. The American College of Cardiology and the American Heart Association stages of heart failure (Figure 5.1) emphasize that symptoms follow an asymptomatic phase of cardiac dysfunction. It is often challenging to determine whether symptoms are cardiac due to structural disease or whether they are coincidental noncardiac symptoms coexisting with asymptomatic structural disease.

- Asymptomatic cardiac dysfunction precedes heart failure, the symptomatic expression of cardiac disease.

- It may be difficult to determine whether symptoms are cardiac or noncardiac coincident with asymptomatic cardiac structural disease.

Heart failure may result from abnormalities of the pericardium, myocardium, endocardium, cardiac valves, or vascular or renal systems. Most commonly it is due to impaired left ventricular myocardial function. In approximately 50% of cases, the left ventricle is enlarged and there is abnormal contractile function with reduced ejection fraction. This type is referred to as dilated cardiomyopathy. The ejection fraction is normal in the remaining 50%. This type is referred to as heart failure with preserved ejection fraction. Isolated right ventricular failure can occur; however, the majority of cases of heart failure involve either the left ventricle alone or the left ventricle with associated right ventricular dysfunction. High ventricular filling pressures can cause dyspnea and edema.

- The most common cause of heart failure is left ventricular myocardial dysfunction, but other cardiac abnormalities may also lead to heart failure.

- High ventricular filling pressures cause dyspnea and edema.

- Myocardial dysfunction with preserved ejection fraction is as important as dilated cardiomyopathy in causing heart failure.

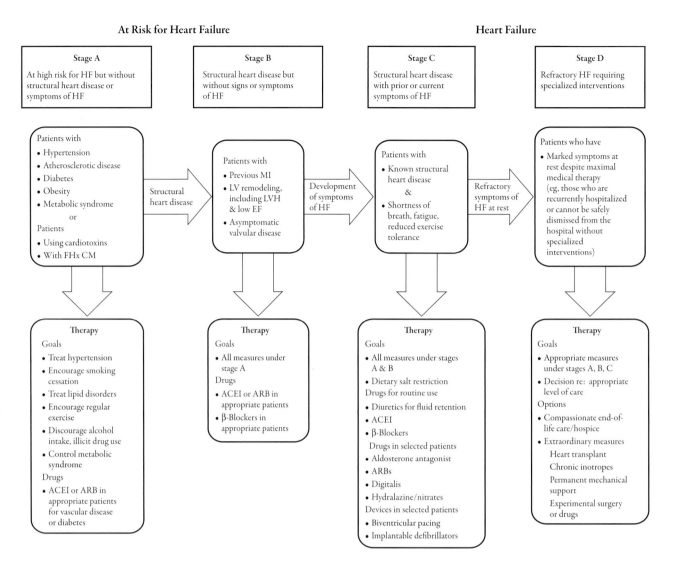

At Risk for Heart Failure

Heart Failure

Stage A
At high risk for HF but without structural heart disease or symptoms of HF

Stage B
Structural heart disease but without signs or symptoms of HF

Stage C
Structural heart disease with prior or current symptoms of HF

Stage D
Refractory HF requiring specialized interventions

Patients with
- Hypertension
- Atherosclerotic disease
- Diabetes
- Obesity
- Metabolic syndrome
  or
Patients
- Using cardiotoxins
- With FHx CM

Structural heart disease →

Patients with
- Previous MI
- LV remodeling, including LVH & low EF
- Asymptomatic valvular disease

Development of symptoms of HF →

Patients with
- Known structural heart disease
  &
- Shortness of breath, fatigue, reduced exercise tolerance

Refractory symptoms of HF at rest →

Patients who have
- Marked symptoms at rest despite maximal medical therapy (eg, those who are recurrently hospitalized or cannot be safely dismissed from the hospital without specialized interventions)

Therapy
Goals
- Treat hypertension
- Encourage smoking cessation
- Treat lipid disorders
- Encourage regular exercise
- Discourage alcohol intake, illicit drug use
- Control metabolic syndrome
Drugs
- ACEI or ARB in appropriate patients for vascular disease or diabetes

Therapy
Goals
- All measures under stage A
Drugs
- ACEI or ARB in appropriate patients
- β-Blockers in appropriate patients

Therapy
Goals
- All measures under stages A & B
- Dietary salt restriction
Drugs for routine use
- Diuretics for fluid retention
- ACEI
- β-Blockers
  Drugs in selected patients
- Aldosterone antagonist
- ARBs
- Digitalis
- Hydralazine/nitrates
Devices in selected patients
- Biventricular pacing
- Implantable defibrillators

Therapy
Goals
- Appropriate measures under stages A, B, C
- Decision re: appropriate level of care
Options
- Compassionate end-of-life care/hospice
- Extraordinary measures
  Heart transplant
  Chronic inotropes
  Permanent mechanical support
  Experimental surgery or drugs

Figure 5.1 Stages in the Development of Heart Failure and Recommended Therapy by Stage. ACEI indicates angiotensin-converting enzyme inhibitor; ARB, angiotensin receptor blocker; EF, ejection fraction; FHx CM, family history of cardiomyopathy; HF, heart failure; LV, left ventricular; LVH, left ventricular hypertrophy; MI, myocardial infarction. (Adapted from Hunt SA, Abraham WT, Chin MH, Feldman AM, Francis GS, Ganiats TG, et al; American College of Cardiology Foundation; American Heart Association. 2009 Focused update incorporated into the ACC/AHA 2005 guidelines for the diagnosis and management of heart failure in adults: a report of the American College of Cardiology Foundation/American Heart Association Task Force on Practice Guidelines Developed in Collaboration With the International Society for Heart and Lung Transplantation. J Am Coll Cardiol 2009 Apr 14;53[15]:e1–90. Erratum in: J Am Coll Cardiol. 2009 Dec 15;54[25]:2464 and Hunt SA, Abraham WT, Chin MH, Feldman AM, Francis GS, Ganiats TG, et al. 2009 Focused update incorporated into the ACC/AHA 2005 Guidelines for the Diagnosis and Management of Heart Failure in Adults: a report of the American College of Cardiology Foundation/American Heart Association Task Force on Practice Guidelines: developed in collaboration with the International Society for Heart and Lung Transplantation. Circulation. 2009 Apr 14;119[14]:e391–479. Epub 2009 Mar 26. Erratum in: Circulation. 2010 Mar 30;121[12]:e258. Used with permission.)

PRESENTATION

Patients may present with asymptomatic ventricular dysfunction (usually dilated ventricles with reduced ejection fraction). These patients do not have heart failure, and they can usually be managed as outpatients; their treatment is discussed later in this chapter. Patients with heart failure (ie, symptoms and signs) may present either as outpatients or to acute care facilities, often depending on the severity of their symptoms. This heterogeneous group is said to have acute decompensated heart failure and includes both patients presenting for the first time with heart failure and patients presenting with a decompensation of known heart failure.

- Patients may present with asymptomatic ventricular dysfunction or may be in heart failure at presentation (symptoms and signs of cardiac dysfunction).

- Patients may present with acute decompensated heart failure, either for the first time or with known cardiac disease.

Hospitalization is advisable when hypotension, worsening renal function, altered mentation, dyspnea at rest, significant arrhythmias (eg, new atrial fibrillation), or other complications such as disturbed electrolytes or lack of outpatient care options are present (Box 5.1). Patients without these factors

Box 5.1 CONDITIONS THAT PROMPT HOSPITALIZATION IN HEART FAILURE

Hypotension
Worsening renal function
Altered mentation
Dyspnea at rest
Significant arrhythmias
Disturbed electrolytes
Lack of outpatient care

who have exclusively exertional symptoms, are not severely congested on examination, and have adequate vascular perfusion (warm extremities, adequate blood pressure) may receive treatment as outpatients. The stages of heart failure development and management are outlined in Figure 5.1.

- Patients with significant symptoms and signs of acute decompensated heart failure should be hospitalized.

- Outpatient management may be reasonable in the setting of exertional symptoms only, minimal congestion, and good vascular perfusion.

DIAGNOSIS

Heart failure is a clinical diagnosis based on symptoms, physical findings, and chest radiography. The symptoms typically include some combination of dyspnea, fatigue, and fluid retention. The dyspnea may be with exertion or with recumbency. Physical findings include evidence of low output, volume overload, or both. These include narrow pulse pressure, poor peripheral perfusion, jugular venous distention, hepatojugular reflux, peripheral edema, ascites, and dull lung bases suggestive of pleural effusions. Lung crackles usually represent atelectatic compression rather than fluid in the alveoli, the latter being more common in *acute* heart failure. Edema usually affects the lower extremities but can also affect the abdomen. Cardiac findings include abnormalities of the cardiac apex (enlarged, displaced, sustained point of maximal impulse) and gallop rhythms. The liver may be enlarged, pulsatile, and tender if there is right heart failure. Clinical signs indicating high- and low-output heart failure could aid in patient management (Table 5.1). Both the symptoms and the signs of heart failure described above are nonspecific and can occur in other conditions. Use of the modified Framingham criteria (Box 5.2) for the clinical diagnosis of congestive heart failure retains an important place in the practice of clinical cardiology.

- Heart failure is a clinical diagnosis based primarily on symptoms and physical findings.

- Symptoms include dyspnea, fatigue, and fluid retention; dyspnea may be exertional or with recumbency.

- Physical examination findings are consistent with low cardiac output, volume overload, or both.

Table 5.1 MANAGEMENT OF HIGH-OUTPUT AND LOW-OUTPUT HEART FAILURE

PERFUSION AT REST	CONGESTION AT REST	
	NO	YES
Normal	Warm & dry PCWP normal CI normal (compensated)	Warm & wet PCWP increased CI normal ↓ Hospitalize ± Nesiritide or vasodilators[a] Diuretics
Low	Cold & dry PCWP low or normal CI decreased ↓ Hospitalize Cautious hydration Inotropic drugs[b]	Cold & wet PCWP increased CI decreased ↓ Hospitalize Nesiritide or vasodilators[a] Diuretics

Abbreviations: CI, cardiac index; PCWP, pulmonary capillary wedge pressure; ±, patient may or may not require hospitalization, depending on clinical assessment.

[a] Vasodilators: nitroglycerin or nitroprusside.

[b] Inotropic drugs: milrinone or dobutamine.

Box 5.2 FRAMINGHAM CRITERIA FOR CLINICAL DIAGNOSIS OF CONGESTIVE HEART FAILURE[a]

MAJOR CRITERIA	MINOR CRITERIA
PND	Peripheral edema
Orthopnea	Night cough
Increased JVP	DOE
Rales	Hepatomegaly
Third heart sound	Pleural effusion
Chest radiography	Heart rate >120 beats per minute
Cardiomegaly	Weight loss ≥4.5 kg in 5 days with diuretic
Pulmonary edema	

Abbreviations: DOE, dyspnea on exertion; JVP, jugular venous pressure; PND, paroxysmal nocturnal dyspnea.

[a] Validated congestive heart failure if 2 major or 1 major and 2 minor criteria are present concurrently.

Adapted from Ho KK, Anderson KM, Kannel WB, Grossman W, Levy D. Survival after the onset of congestive heart failure in the Framingham Heart Study subjects. Circulation. 1993 Jul;88(1):107–15. Used with permission.

According to the modified Framingham criteria, the simultaneous presence of 2 major or of 1 major and 2 minor criteria satisfies the clinical diagnosis of congestive heart failure. Exertional dyspnea does not have the same weight as paroxysmal nocturnal dyspnea or orthopnea, and edema does not have the same weight as increased venous pressure. Patients with low-output heart failure may not have findings of volume overload (congestion) and thus may not satisfy Framingham criteria.

- Two major criteria or 1 major plus 2 minor modified Framingham criteria present simultaneously allow a clinical diagnosis of congestive heart failure.

- Paroxysmal nocturnal dyspnea and orthopnea have greater diagnostic weight than exertional dyspnea, and increased venous pressure has greater diagnostic weight than edema.

- Use of the modified Framingham criteria can assist in diagnosing heart failure but will not be as helpful in patients with low-output heart failure without associated congestion.

Increased intracardiac pressure or chamber dilatation leads to increased production of natriuretic peptides, substances produced by the heart. Accordingly, measurement of B-type natriuretic peptide or N-terminal pro-brain natriuretic peptide complements the clinical diagnosis of heart failure. In general, the degree of increase reflects the degree of myocardial dysfunction. Increased levels of these peptides do not distinguish systolic from diastolic, left from right, or acute from chronic cardiac dysfunction. Interpreting these levels has caveats (Box 5.3). In addition, there is substantial variability of levels in stable patients, up to 50%.

The utility of the natriuretic peptide values for diagnosing heart failure has been best shown in patients without prior known cardiac disease. Interpretation of intermediately increased levels can be difficult in patients with a prior history of ventricular dysfunction or heart failure who are receiving medical treatment. The negative predictive value of normal natriuretic peptide levels (in the absence of constriction, morbid obesity, or mitral stenosis) is more powerful than their positive predictive value. Natriuretic peptide values are most useful in patients without a prior diagnosis of heart failure and in patients not receiving treatment for heart failure.

- Natriuretic peptide levels are increased in the setting of increased intracardiac pressure or chamber dilatation.

- The type of cardiac dysfunction cannot be distinguished using natriuretic peptide values.

- The negative predictive value of normal natriuretic peptide levels is generally greater than their positive predictive value.

MANAGEMENT OF ACUTE HEART FAILURE

At the time of initial diagnosis, the common alternative diagnoses of pulmonary embolism or chronic obstructive pulmonary disease exacerbation must be excluded. Clinical stratification guides initial treatment (usually parenteral) (Figure 5.2).

Once clinical improvement begins, treatment is adjusted to optimize hemodynamics, minimize symptoms, and allow transition to oral medications. The mechanism of heart failure and precipitating factors are defined, patient and family education are provided, and dismissal (including follow-up) is planned.

- Consideration of common alternate diagnoses (pulmonary embolism and chronic obstructive pulmonary disease) is important when heart failure is diagnosed.

MECHANISMS OF HEART FAILURE

Selection of proper therapy depends on correctly identifying the mechanism of heart failure. A simple categorical framework is given in Table 5.2. Left ventricular myocardial dysfunction is the most common cause of heart failure. Accurate diagnosis is essential because treatment and prognosis are based on the cause of heart failure. Diagnosis is initially based on physical examination and noninvasive testing, such as echocardiography or radionuclide angiography.

- The most common cause of heart failure is left ventricular myocardial dysfunction.

- Therapy depends on the mechanism of heart failure.

PRECIPITATING FACTORS

New-onset or worsening heart failure symptoms may represent only natural disease progression. However, 1 or more precipitating factors may be responsible for symptomatic deterioration (Box 5.4). If these factors are not identified and corrected, heart failure symptoms often return after initial therapy. The most common precipitants are dietary indiscretion (eg, sodium, excess fluid, and alcohol), medication nonadherence due to cost, regimen complexity, lack of patient understanding, and suboptimally controlled hypertension.

Evaluation should follow these steps: 1) a medical history, which includes sodium and fluid intake, medication use and compliance, and sleep history from bedroom partners; 2) chest radiography to look for pneumonitis; 3) electrocardiography and measurement of cardiac biomarkers to document heart rhythm and identify myocardial ischemia or injury; and 4) cultures of blood, urine, and sputum on the basis of the history. Other tests should include determination of complete blood count and thyroid-stimulating hormone and creatinine levels.

- Precipitating factors must be sought and treated.

- Dietary indiscretion, medication noncompliance, regimen complexity, and uncontrolled hypertension are common precipitants of heart failure decompensation.

CARDIOMYOPATHIES

Cardiomyopathies are divided into primary and secondary cardiomyopathies, and the primary disorders are further

---

Box 5.3 PITFALLS IN THE INTERPRETATION OF NATRIURETIC PEPTIDE VALUE

NP HIGHER THAN EXPECTED	NP LOWER THAN EXPECTED
Women	Obesity
Elderly	Acute heart failure
Renal failure	Heart failure due to mitral stenosis
	Constriction

Abbreviation: NP, natriuretic peptide.

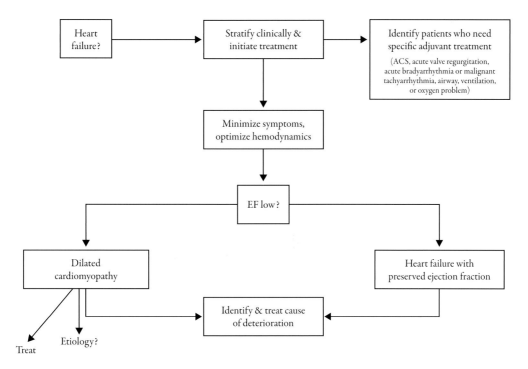

Figure 5.2 Approach to Acute Heart Failure. ACS indicates acute coronary syndrome; EF, ejection fraction.

subdivided as genetic, acquired, or mixed. This classification scheme accounts for progressive understanding of this heterogeneous group of disorders. However, the previous phenotypic classification scheme of dilated, hypertrophic, and restrictive diseases is more useful in clinical understanding and management. The different anatomical and pathophysiologic processes for each cardiomyopathy are listed in Table 5.3.

DILATED CARDIOMYOPATHY

Pathology and Etiology

The major abnormality in dilated cardiomyopathy is a remodeled left ventricle characterized by dilatation and reduced ejection fraction. Left ventricular end-diastolic pressure is typically increased. The increased filling pressures and low cardiac output cause dyspnea and fatigue. *Idiopathic* dilated

Table 5.2 **CAUSES OF HEART FAILURE AND TREATMENT**

CAUSE	TREATMENT
Myocardial	
Dilated cardiomyopathy (including ischemic)	Angiotensin-converting enzyme inhibitors, angiotensin receptor blockers, β-adrenergic blockers (eg, carvedilol, metoprolol succinate, bisoprolol), diuretics, aldosterone antagonists, nitrates, digoxin, nitrates & hydralazine in combination, transplant, coronary revascularization, left ventricular aneurysmectomy (surgical ventricular remodeling), cardiac resynchronization therapy, cardiac defibrillator
Hypertrophic cardiomyopathy	β-Adrenergic blockers, verapamil, disopyramide, surgical myectomy, septal alcohol ablation, dual-chamber pacing
Restrictive cardiomyopathy	Diuretics, heart transplant, treatment of underlying systemic disease
Pericardial	
Tamponade	Pericardiocentesis
Constrictive pericarditis	Pericardiectomy
Valvular	Valve repair or replacement
Hypertension	Antihypertensive treatment
Pulmonary hypertension	Prostacyclin infusion, calcium channel blockers, heart-lung transplant, endothelin antagonists, phosphodiesterase type 5 inhibitor
High output	
Hyperthyroidism, Paget disease, arteriovenous fistula	Correction of underlying cause

Box 5.4 **PRECIPITATING FACTORS IN HEART FAILURE**

Diet (excessive sodium or fluid intake, alcohol)
Noncompliance with medication or inadequate dosing
Sodium-retaining medications (NSAIDs)
Infection (bacterial or viral)
Myocardial ischemia or infarction
Arrhythmia (atrial fibrillation, bradycardia)
Breathing disorders of sleep
Worsening renal function
Anemia
Metabolic (hyperthyroidism, hypothyroidism)
Pulmonary embolus

Abbreviation: NSAIDs, nonsteroidal anti-inflammatory drugs.

cardiomyopathy indicates left ventricular dysfunction without any known cause. The right ventricle may be normal, hypertrophied, or dilated.

- A dilated left ventricle is the major abnormality in dilated cardiomyopathy.

- The right ventricle may be normal, hypertrophied, or dilated.

Many cases of dilated cardiomyopathy are genetic with at least 1 identifiable affected family member in up to 30% of cases. Other causes of left ventricular dysfunction include severe coronary artery disease—the most common cause in the United States—(hibernating myocardium), previous infarction, uncontrolled hypertension, ethanol abuse, myocarditis, hyperthyroidism or hypothyroidism, postpartum cardiomyopathy, toxins and drugs (including doxorubicin and trastuzumab), tachycardia-induced cardiomyopathy, infiltrative cardiomyopathy (ie, hemochromatosis, sarcoidosis), AIDS, and pheochromocytoma.

- The most common cause of dilated cardiomyopathy in the United States is coronary artery disease.

- Other causes of left ventricular dysfunction include uncontrolled hypertension, ethanol abuse, thyroid

disease, myocarditis, postpartum cardiomyopathy, toxins and drugs, and tachycardia-induced cardiomyopathy.

Clinical Presentation

The presentation is highly variable. The patient may be asymptomatic and the diagnosis prompted by examination, chest radiography, electrocardiography (ECG), or imaging findings. Patients may have symptoms of mild to severe heart failure (New York Heart Association [NYHA] functional class II-IV). Atrial and ventricular arrhythmias are common in dilated cardiomyopathy. Physical examination may indicate increased jugular venous pressure, a right ventricular lift (if there is right heart involvement), low-volume upstroke of the carotid artery, displaced and sustained left ventricular impulse (possibly with a rapid filling wave), audible third or fourth heart sounds, and an apical systolic murmur of mitral regurgitation. Pulsus alternans may occur in patients with advanced heart failure. Pulmonary examination may have normal results or indicate crackles or evidence of pleural effusion.

- The clinical presentation of dilated cardiomyopathy is highly variable.

- Atrial and ventricular arrhythmias are common.

The ECG is almost always abnormal and frequently indicates left ventricular hypertrophy, intraventricular conduction delay, or bundle branch block. Rhythm abnormalities may include premature atrial contractions, atrial fibrillation, premature ventricular contractions, or short bursts of ventricular tachycardia. The chest radiograph often shows left ventricular enlargement and pulmonary venous congestion. The diagnosis is based on the findings of left ventricular enlargement and reduced ejection fraction, which can be measured with echocardiography, radionuclide angiography, left ventriculography, cine computed tomography, or magnetic resonance imaging.

- The diagnosis of dilated cardiomyopathy requires evidence of left ventricular enlargement and reduced ejection fraction by cardiac imaging.

Table 5.3 **ANATOMICAL AND PATHOPHYSIOLOGIC PROCESSES FOR EACH CARDIOMYOPATHY**

TYPE	LEFT VENTRICULAR CAVITY SIZE	LEFT VENTRICULAR WALL THICKNESS	EJECTION FRACTION	DIASTOLIC FUNCTION	OTHER
Dilated cardiomyopathy	↑	N/↑	↓	↓	
Hypertrophic cardiomyopathy	↓/N	↑	↑	↓	Left ventricular outflow obstruction
Restrictive cardiomyopathy	N/↑	N	N	↓	

Abbreviation and symbols: ↓, decreased; N, normal; ↑, increased.

Evaluation

After diagnosis, treatable secondary causes of left ventricular dysfunction should be sought. Tests of thyroid function should be done to exclude hyperthyroidism or hypothyroidism. Transferrin levels should be measured to screen for hemochromatosis. Measurement of the serum angiotensin-converting enzyme level should be considered if sarcoidosis is a possibility. Metanephrine levels should be measured if there is a history of severe labile hypertension or unusual spells. Ethanol or drug abuse history should be obtained.

In severe coronary artery disease, reversible left ventricular dysfunction can be caused by hibernating myocardium. With revascularization, left ventricular function may improve gradually. Identifying affected patients is difficult. Currently, the reference standard is positron emission tomography to evaluate metabolic activity. Viability protocols used in stress echocardiography and radionuclide perfusion imaging are more widely available than positron emission tomography and are useful for identifying hibernating myocardium.

- Treatable secondary causes of left ventricular dysfunction, such as thyroid disease and hemochromatosis, should be sought.

- Hibernating myocardium in the setting of severe coronary artery disease can lead to reversible left ventricular dysfunction.

Tachycardia-induced cardiomyopathy can occur in patients with prolonged periods of tachycardia (usually atrial fibrillation or flutter or prolonged atrial tachycardia). Because systolic dysfunction can be completely reversed with treatment of tachycardia, identifying these causes is important.

Acute myocarditis may cause left ventricular dysfunction; the natural history is unknown. Many patients have development of persistent left ventricular dysfunction, whereas others have improvement with time. Thus, it is necessary to remeasure left ventricular function 3 to 6 months after diagnosis and treatment. Endomyocardial biopsy may help diagnose myocarditis. Immunosuppressive therapy does not improve outcome and should be reserved for patients with giant cell myocarditis, concomitant skeletal myositis, or clinical deterioration despite standard pharmacologic therapy.

- Myocarditis often leads to persistent left ventricular dysfunction, but some patients may have improvement over time. Left ventricular function should be reassessed 3 to 6 months after diagnosis and treatment.

Pathophysiology

The hemodynamic, pathophysiologic, and biologic aspects of heart failure must be appreciated to understand treatment of dilated cardiomyopathy. Preload is the ventricular volume at the end of diastole (end-diastolic volume). Typically, when it is increased, stroke volume increases. The relationship of stroke volume to preload is illustrated by the

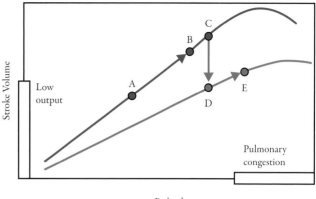

Figure 5.3 Starling Curve. Blue line is patient with normal contractility, and red line is one with depressed systolic function. Normally, stroke volume depends on preload of the heart. Increasing preload increases stroke volume (A to B). Myocardial dysfunction causes a shift of the curve downward and to the right (C to D), causing a severe decrease in stroke volume, which leads to symptoms of fatigue and lethargy. The compensatory response to decrease in stroke volume is an increase in preload (D to E). Because the diastolic pressure-volume relationship is curvilinear, increased left ventricular volume produces increased left ventricular end-diastolic pressure, causing symptoms of pulmonary congestion. Note flat portion of the curve at its upper end; here, there is little increase in stroke volume for increase in preload.

Starling curve (Figure 5.3). Afterload is the tension, force, or stress on the ventricular wall muscle fibers after fiber shortening begins. Left ventricular afterload is increased by aortic stenosis and systemic hypertension but is decreased by mitral regurgitation. Ventricular enlargement increases afterload.

Figure 5.4 illustrates the neurohormonal response to decreased myocardial contractility. Decreased cardiac output activates baroreceptors and the sympathetic nervous system. Sympathetic nervous system stimulation causes increased heart rate and contractility. α-Stimulation of the arterioles causes increases in afterload. The renin-angiotensin system is activated by sympathetic stimulation, decreased renal blood flow, and decreased renal sodium, in turn activating aldosterone, causing increased renal retention of sodium, which leads to pulmonary congestion. Low renal blood flow causes renal sodium retention. Increased angiotensin II causes vasoconstriction and increased afterload. In congestive heart failure, the compensatory mechanisms that increase preload eventually cause a malcompensatory increase in afterload, in turn causing further decrease in stroke volume.

In the subacute and chronic stages of heart failure, neurohormonal (adrenergic, angiotensin II) and other signaling pathways lead to myocyte dysfunction and cell death. Increased collagen production results in progressive cardiac fibrosis. Progressive myocardial dysfunction and remodeling are the natural history of untreated myocardial disease.

- Initial compensatory neurohormonal mechanisms lead to long-term mal-compensatory increases in afterload and subsequent decreased stroke volume.

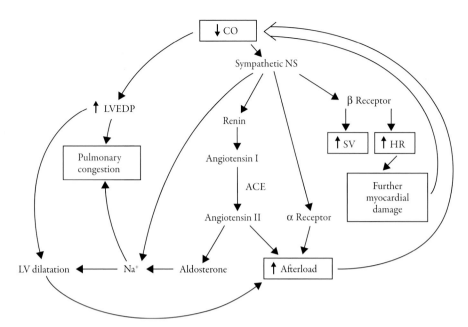

Figure 5.4 Neurohormonal Response to Decreased Myocardial Contractility. ACE indicates angiotensin-converting enzyme; CO, cardiac output; HR, heart rate; LV, left ventricular; LVEDP, left ventricular end-diastolic pressure; NS, nervous system; SV, stroke volume.

Treatment

Nonpharmacologic Treatment

For adequate treatment of dilated cardiomyopathy, precipitating factors must be identified and addressed. Nonpharmacologic treatment is crucial and includes sodium and fluid restriction, alcohol avoidance, daily weight monitoring, and regular aerobic exercise. Ongoing patient and family education and regular outpatient follow-up reduce heart failure exacerbations, emergency department visits, and hospitalizations.

Pharmacologic Treatment

Angiotensin-converting enzyme (ACE) inhibitors, β-adrenergic blockers, and diuretics are the mainstays of pharmacologic therapy. ACE inhibitors decrease afterload, decrease sodium retention by inhibiting aldosterone formation, and

directly affect myocyte growth and myocardial remodeling (Figure 5.5).

ACE inhibitors provide symptomatic improvement in patients with NYHA functional class II-IV failure and improve mortality in patients with moderate and severe heart failure. In asymptomatic patients, ACE inhibitors prevent onset of heart failure and reduce the need for hospitalization. The dose of the ACE inhibitor used should be titrated up as tolerated based on symptoms and blood pressure. Upward dose adjustment as tolerated is beneficial even in clinically compensated patients receiving low to intermediate doses. Common adverse effects include hypotension, hyperkalemia, azotemia, cough, angioedema (mild or severe), and dysgeusia. The benefits and potential side effects of ACE inhibitors are thought to be a class effect.

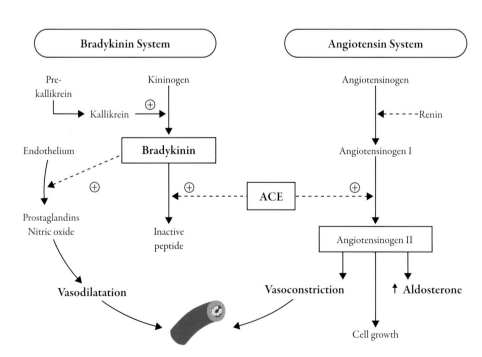

Figure 5.5 Action of Angiotensin-Converting Enzyme (ACE) on the Bradykinin and Angiotensin Systems.

- Nonpharmacologic management is essential and includes sodium and fluid restriction, alcohol avoidance, daily weight monitoring, and regular aerobic exercise.

- Medications augment nonpharmacologic therapy.

- ACE inhibitor use decreases mortality in patients with moderate and severe heart failure, provides symptomatic improvement in patients with NYHA class II-IV heart failure symptoms, and reduces the need for hospitalization.

Angiotensin II receptor blockers provide hemodynamic benefits similar to those of ACE inhibitors in patients with dilated cardiomyopathy. They can be used in patients who have cough and angioedema with use of ACE inhibitors because they do not inhibit the breakdown of bradykinin (the cause of cough and angioedema). They are less beneficial than ACE inhibitors in the reverse remodeling of the myocardium, and thus they remain second-line treatment.

- Angiotensin II receptor blockers provide hemodynamic benefits similar to those of ACE inhibitors.

- They remain second-line agents for patients who cannot tolerate ACE inhibitors.

β-Adrenergic blockers (β-blockers) improve symptoms and ejection fraction and decrease hospitalizations and mortality in patients with systolic heart failure. They may have unwanted hemodynamic effects in the acute setting (negative inotropic effects, attenuation of heart rate response that may be maintaining cardiac output in the setting of reduced stroke volume), but they provide long-term benefit by modifying the unfavorable biologic effects of enhanced adrenergic tone. This benefit may take up to 6 months to observe. These drugs are most useful for patients with asymptomatic left ventricular dysfunction after myocardial infarction and NYHA class II or III symptoms. They can be given cautiously to patients with class IV symptoms but should *not* be given to patients with substantial volume overload and cardiogenic shock. Initial dosing should be low, with close clinical follow-up. Upward titration of the β-blocker dose should be slow and cautious. The likelihood of patients continuing treatment with β-blockers is much higher when treatment is initiated during a hospitalization for heart failure. Well-studied β-blockers with established benefit for patients with heart failure include metoprolol succinate, carvedilol, and bisoprolol.

- β-Blockers are effective and essential therapy in patients with dilated cardiomyopathy.

- Initiation of β-blocker therapy should be avoided in heart failure when there is substantial volume overload.

Diuretics are part of the routine management of symptoms and signs of systemic and pulmonary congestion. Diuretic doses should be minimized when possible because of associated neurohormonal activation and electrolyte imbalance. Fluid overload can be treated initially with thiazide or loop diuretics. Occasionally, a combination of thiazides and loop diuretics is needed for severe fluid retention. The addition of spironolactone can help in patients with hypokalemia and may provide additional benefit by blocking aldosterone-mediated effects.

- Diuretics should be used for patients with heart failure and volume overload.

- Diuretic doses should be minimized to avoid unwanted metabolic adverse effects.

Drugs directly affecting myocardial contractility include digoxin, phosphodiesterase inhibitors (milrinone), and β-agonists (dopamine and dobutamine). Digoxin provides symptomatic relief when the ejection fraction is less than 40%, but it does not improve survival. It is useful for ventricular rate control and atrial fibrillation and in patients who are symptomatic despite treatment with ACE inhibitors and β-blockers. Because digoxin is excreted by the kidneys, dosage must be decreased in older patients and patients with renal dysfunction. Because of drug-drug interactions, digoxin dosage should be decreased with concomitant administration of amiodarone, verapamil, and quinidine. Short-term parenteral inotropic agents (milrinone and dobutamine) may improve symptoms, but long-term use *increases* mortality, and therefore these drugs should be used transiently in the hospital for low-output states and occasionally for palliative purposes in refractory end-stage heart failure.

- Digoxin, phosphodiesterase inhibitors (milrinone), and β-agonists (dopamine and dobutamine) directly affect myocardial contractility.

- Digoxin dosage needs to be decreased in azotemic and older patients.

Aldosterone antagonists may provide additional benefit by inhibiting fibrosis and combating mechanical and electrical remodeling. Significant survival benefit has been shown in patients with NYHA class III-IV heart failure. Eplerenone, a selective aldosterone inhibitor, provides survival benefit at 30 days and 1 year in patients after infarction and who have left ventricular dysfunction and either heart failure or diabetes. However, eplerenone has a considerable risk of hyperkalemia and thus must be given carefully with cautious follow-up, avoidance of nonsteroidal anti-inflammatory drugs, and prompt attention to illnesses predisposing patients to dehydration.

- Aldosterone antagonists can be used in highly symptomatic patients already receiving baseline therapy or in patients with either heart failure or diabetes early after infarction.

- Patients with hyperkalemia or renal dysfunction should not receive these drugs.

High-dose nitrates and hydralazine in combination provide symptomatic improvement and improved mortality in patients with heart failure, but this approach is inferior to ACE inhibitors when used alone. It is used in patients who are unable to tolerate ACE inhibitors or angiotensin receptor blockers because of renal insufficiency or hyperkalemia. The combination has been shown to increase survival in African-American patients when given as adjunctive therapy to ACE inhibitors and β-blockers.

- The combination of nitrates and hydralazine improves symptoms and mortality, especially in the African-American population with dilated cardiomyopathy.

Amlodipine and felodipine are safe in patients with dilated cardiomyopathy. They can be used to treat hypertension that persists despite optimal dosages of ACE inhibitors and β-blockers, but they do not provide a survival benefit. First-generation calcium channel blockers (verapamil, diltiazem, nifedipine) are *contraindicated* because of their negative inotropic effects.

- First-generation calcium channel blockers (verapamil, diltiazem, nifedipine) are contraindicated because of their negative inotropic effects.

Anticoagulation with warfarin is recommended for patients in atrial fibrillation and those with intracardiac thrombus or a history of systemic or pulmonary thromboembolism. Retrospective studies have suggested that aspirin may diminish the benefits of ACE inhibitors by blocking prostaglandin-induced vasodilatation. An increased incidence of hospitalizations for heart failure in patients with dilated cardiomyopathy receiving aspirin was also observed. The most common recommendation is to use low-dose aspirin in patients with heart failure and coronary artery disease.

- Anticoagulation with warfarin is recommended in patients with atrial fibrillation, intracardiac thrombus, or a history of thromboembolism.
- Aspirin therapy (low dose) should be reserved for patients with heart failure and coronary artery disease.

Device Therapy

Implanted defibrillators improve survival when used at least 40 days after a myocardial infarction in patients with ischemic and nonischemic dilated cardiomyopathies who have ejection fractions less than 35% despite optimal medical therapy. They should be offered to patients who have a reasonable functional status with at least 1 year of survival. Patients in sinus rhythm with ventricular dyssynchrony may benefit from biventricular pacing (cardiac resynchronization therapy). Current implantation criteria are sinus rhythm, QRS duration more than 120 milliseconds, NYHA class III-IV, ejection fraction less than 35%, and optimal medical management. Cardiac resynchronization therapy results in improvement in symptoms, exercise capacity, and left ventricular ejection fraction and survival in well-selected patients.

- Implanted defibrillators improve survival in patients with both ischemic and nonischemic dilated cardiomyopathy who have ejection fractions less than 35% despite optimal medical therapy.

Cardiac Replacement Therapy

Heart transplant is the procedure of choice for patients with dilated cardiomyopathy and severe, refractory symptoms. With a successful transplant, the 1-year survival rate can exceed 90%. Early referral to a heart transplant center is recommended for patients with refractory heart failure. Long-term complications include rejection, infection, hypertension, hyperlipidemia, malignancy, and accelerated coronary vasculopathy. Donor availability is the major limiting factor. In selected patients, left ventricular assist devices have now been approved by the US Food and Drug Administration and are used either as a bridge to transplant or as final (destination) therapy.

- The procedure of choice for patients with severely symptomatic dilated cardiomyopathy despite optimal medical management is heart transplant.
- With a successful transplant, the 1-year survival rate can exceed 90%.

HEART FAILURE WITH PRESERVED EJECTION FRACTION

Approximately half of hospitalized patients with newly diagnosed heart failure have a normal ejection fraction. Many of these patients have contractile abnormalities that could be identified by more sophisticated evaluation techniques, but ejection fraction is the most widely available measure of systolic function and remains the standard. This is a heterogeneous group of disorders and includes hypertrophic and restrictive cardiomyopathies, infiltrative cardiac disorders, and constrictive pericarditis.

- Approximately half of patients with newly diagnosed heart failure have a normal ejection fraction.

Many patients have a history of hypertension. Some have fairly normal diastolic filling properties at rest, but exertional hypertension, ischemia, or both cause deterioration of diastolic filling properties, resulting in increased filling pressure. Others have abnormal baseline diastolic compliance with superimposed volume overload, which increases diastolic filling pressures. Other patients have exuberant heart rate responses to exercise with inadequate diastolic filling periods, and others rely on the atrial contribution to ventricular filling and suffer when atrial fibrillation develops. Some have low output due to severe regurgitant valve disease (including severe tricuspid regurgitation) or bradycardia. Severe occult renal insufficiency is also a common finding in this condition. It is important to try to understand the mechanism of diastolic dysfunction in any given patient to tailor the most effective treatment, which might include some combination of antihypertensive or coronary revascularization strategies, diuretic treatment, ventricular rate slowing or support (pacemaker), restoration of sinus rhythm, valvular intervention, or renal replacement therapy. Morbidity and mortality in this group of patients are high, approaching the rates in patients with reduced ejection fraction.

HYPERTROPHIC CARDIOMYOPATHY

Hypertrophic cardiomyopathy is a rare (approximately 0.2% prevalence in the general population) heterogeneous group of disorders characterized by increased thickness of the ventricle and preserved ejection fraction. The hypertrophy may be regional (involving the septum, mid left ventricle, or apex) or concentric. Obstruction in the left ventricular outflow tract or mid-ventricular cavity may occur. Diagnosis is based on increased myocardial wall thickness on echocardiogram in the absence of an underlying cause such as hypertension, aortic stenosis, chronic renal failure, or infiltrative disease. Because of its hereditary nature, first-degree relatives of patients should be screened, and genetic counseling is advised for patients considering childbearing.

- Hypertrophic cardiomyopathy is a heterogeneous family of genetic disorders characterized by increased ventricular thickness.
- Diagnosis is based on increased myocardial wall thickness in the absence of a cause on the echocardiogram.

SYMPTOMS

Hypertrophic cardiomyopathy appears to have a bimodal distribution of age at presentation. Affected young males (typically teens or early 20s) often present with syncope and sudden death. Recently, an X-linked variant known as *LAMP2* cardiomyopathy (Danon disease) was described in younger patients. Affected older patients (sixth and seventh decades of life) typically present with shortness of breath and angina and may have a better prognosis than young patients. The classic presentation in the younger group is a young athlete undergoing a physical examination found to have a heart murmur or left ventricular hypertrophy on electrocardiography. The classic presentation in the older group is an older woman who has development of pulmonary edema after noncardiac surgery and worsening with diuresis, afterload reduction, and inotropic support (due to worsening dynamic left ventricular outflow tract obstruction). The classic symptom triad is syncope, angina, and dyspnea. The symptoms are similar to those of valvular aortic stenosis. The per-year frequency of evolution from hypertrophic to dilated cardiomyopathy is 1.5%. This may reflect either the natural history or a superimposed secondary process such as ischemia. The treatment of a "burnt-out hypertroph" is then the same as that of other dilated cardiomyopathies.

- The classic presentation of hypertrophic cardiomyopathy is the triad of angina, syncope, and dyspnea.
- The prognosis for older patients may be better than that for younger patients.
- Affected patients have a 1.5% per-year risk of progression to dilated cardiomyopathy.

PATHOPHYSIOLOGY

Signs and symptoms of hypertrophic cardiomyopathy are caused by 4 major abnormalities: diastolic dysfunction, left ventricular outflow tract obstruction, mitral regurgitation, and ventricular arrhythmias.

Diastolic dysfunction is caused by many mechanisms, including marked abnormalities in calcium metabolism (abnormal ventricular relaxation), high afterload due to left ventricular tract obstruction (also delays ventricular relaxation) and severe hypertrophy and increased muscle mass (decreased compliance). Diastolic dysfunction leads to increased left ventricular diastolic pressure, angina, and dyspnea. Coronary microvascular dysfunction also contributes to angina and dyspnea. In many patients, dynamic left ventricular tract obstruction is caused by the hypertrophied septum encroaching into the left ventricular outflow tract. Subsequently, the anterior leaflet of the mitral valve is "sucked in" (systolic anterior motion), and left ventricular outflow tract obstruction is created. Because of this pathophysiologic process, dynamic outflow tract obstruction increases dramatically with decreased preload, decreased afterload, or increased contractility. Systolic anterior motion of the mitral valve distorts the mitral valve apparatus during systole and may cause considerable mitral regurgitation. Thus, the degree of mitral regurgitation is also dynamically influenced by the degree of left ventricular outflow tract obstruction. Patients with severe mitral regurgitation usually have severe symptoms of dyspnea. Cellular disorganization leads to abnormalities in the conduction system; thus, patients are prone to ventricular arrhythmias. Frequent ventricular arrhythmias may cause sudden death or syncope.

- Diastolic dysfunction is caused by abnormal ventricular relaxation or decreased compliance.
- Abnormal ventricular relaxation may be due to abnormal calcium metabolism or high afterload (due to outflow tract obstruction).

Left ventricular outflow tract obstruction and mitral regurgitation are caused by distortion of the mitral valve apparatus (systolic anterior motion), and they are dynamically influenced by preload, afterload, and contractility.

EXAMINATION

The carotid artery upstroke and left ventricular impulse are abnormal in patients with hypertrophic cardiomyopathy. The carotid artery upstroke is more rapid than that in aortic stenosis.

If left ventricular outflow tract obstruction is extensive, the carotid artery upstroke has a bifid quality. In the setting of considerable left ventricular hypertrophy, the left ventricular impulse is sustained and there is often a palpable *a* wave. The first heart sound is normal, but the second heart sound is paradoxically split. Patients with excessive left ventricular outflow tract obstruction may have a triple apical impulse and a loud systolic ejection murmur. The murmur changes in intensity with changes in loading conditions (Box 5.5). A holosystolic murmur of mitral regurgitation may be present; it increases in intensity with increases in the dynamic left ventricular outflow tract obstruction. Maneuvers affect the mitral regurgitant murmur of hypertrophic obstructive cardiomyopathy differently than other mitral regurgitant murmurs. When mitral regurgitation is *not* due to hypertrophic obstructive cardiomyopathy, the murmur increases with increasing afterload and varies little with changes in contractility and preload. When mitral regurgitation *is* due to hypertrophic cardiomyopathy, increased afterload decreases the dynamic left ventricular outflow obstruction and thus the degree of mitral regurgitation. In patients with hypertrophic cardiomyopathy with obstruction, the intensity of the ejection murmur increases, whereas the arterial pulse volume *decreases* on the beat following a premature ventricular contraction (the Brockenbrough sign) as a result of postectopic increased contractility and decreased afterload, resulting in more dynamic obstruction. These changes differ from those in patients with fixed left ventricular outflow tract obstruction (eg, aortic stenosis) in whom *both* the murmur intensity and the pulse volume increase with the beat following a premature ventricular contraction.

- The diagnosis of hypertrophic cardiomyopathy is suspected by palpating a sustained left ventricular impulse and rapid upstroke of the carotid artery.

- The outflow murmur intensity and carotid upstroke change with changes in loading conditions of the heart.

DIAGNOSTIC TESTING

A marked left ventricular hypertrophy pattern on electrocardiography (Figure 5.6) is usually seen in patients with hypertrophic cardiomyopathy, whereas patients with apical hypertrophy have deep, symmetric T-wave inversions across the precordium (Figure 5.7). Electrocardiographic abnormalities may precede echocardiographic abnormalities; thus, surveillance echocardiography is appropriate in patients with suspicious electrocardiographic results.

- In hypertrophic cardiomyopathy, electrocardiography shows marked left ventricular hypertrophy.

Echocardiography shows severe hypertrophy of the myocardium (left ventricular wall thickness >16 mm in diastole) without any other identified cause. Hypertrophy may be in any part of the myocardium. Doppler echocardiography can be used to diagnose left ventricular outflow tract obstruction, measure its severity, and detect mitral regurgitation. Cardiac catheterization is no longer necessary to diagnose dynamic left ventricular outflow tract obstruction.

- Presence of outflow tract obstruction, its severity, and presence of mitral regurgitation may be assessed with echocardiography, and cardiac catheterization is no longer needed.

Patients with hypertrophic cardiomyopathy may have sudden death. Because of the strong association between ventricular arrhythmias and sudden death, 48- to 72-hour Holter monitoring is recommended for all patients with hypertrophic cardiomyopathy. Predictors of sudden death include a personal or family history of sudden death, severe left ventricular hypertrophy, ventricular tachycardia on Holter monitoring or electrophysiologic study, and history of syncope. Genetic markers may identify patients with a strong propensity for sudden death. In some patients, carefully supervised stress testing may be indicated to search for induced ventricular tachycardia, to determine exercise tolerance, and to evaluate the variables contributing to symptoms.

- Predictors of sudden death in hypertrophic cardiomyopathy are personal or family history of sudden death, history of syncope, ventricular tachycardia on Holter monitoring or electrophysiologic study, and severe left ventricular hypertrophy.

Box 5.5 **DYNAMIC LEFT VENTRICULAR OUTFLOW TRACT OBSTRUCTION**

Increased obstruction
Decreased afterload
    Amyl nitrite
    Vasodilators
Increased contractility
    Postpremature ventricular contraction beat
    Digoxin
    Dopamine
Decreased preload
    Squat-to-stand
    Nitrates
    Diuretics
    Valsalva maneuver (strain phase)
Decreased obstruction
Increased afterload
    Handgrip
    Stand-to-squat
Decreased contractility
    β-Adrenergic blockers
    Verapamil
    Disopyramide
Increased preload
    Fluids

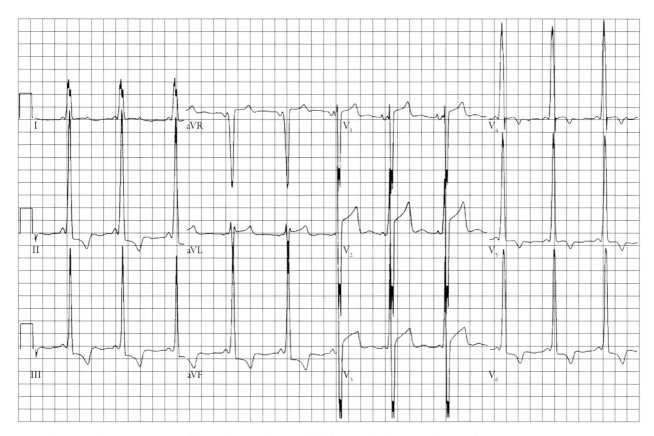

Figure 5.6 Electrocardiogram in Hypertrophic Cardiomyopathy. Marked left ventricular hypertrophy is noted.

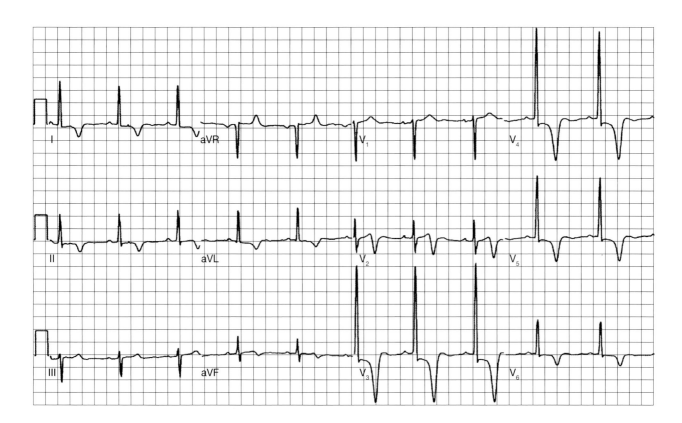

Figure 5.7 Electrocardiogram in Apical Hypertrophic Cardiomyopathy. Deep, symmetric T-wave inversions are shown in precordial leads.

- 48- to 72-Hour Holter monitoring is recommended for all patients with hypertrophic cardiomyopathy.

TREATMENT

Symptomatic Patients

For symptomatic patients, initial treatment is with drugs that decrease contractility in an attempt to decrease left ventricular outflow tract obstruction (Figure 5.8). The most effective medication is a high dose of β-blockers (equivalent of >240 mg propranolol/day). Although verapamil may be used if β-adrenergic blockade fails, it may cause sudden hemodynamic deterioration in patients with high resting left ventricular outflow tract gradients because of its vasodilating properties. Disopyramide may improve symptoms by decreasing left ventricular outflow tract obstruction, but anticholinergic adverse effects limit its use. All drugs that reduce afterload or preload and those that increase contractility *must* be avoided in patients with hypertrophic cardiomyopathy. Diuretics may be cautiously used for volume-overloaded states.

- Treat symptomatic patients initially with β-blockers.

- Verapamil may be used if β-blockade fails, but it may cause sudden hemodynamic collapse in patients with high resting outflow tract gradients and must be used cautiously.

- Avoid any drug that reduces preload or afterload or increases contractility.

Asymptomatic Patients

Asymptomatic patients should be assessed for risk of sudden cardiac death. Treatment of asymptomatic patients with

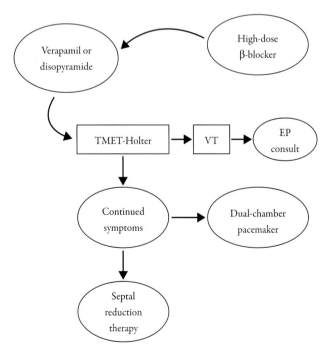

Figure 5.8 Treatment of Symptomatic Hypertrophic Cardiomyopathy. EP indicates electrophysiologic; TMET, treadmill exercise test; VT, ventricular tachycardia.

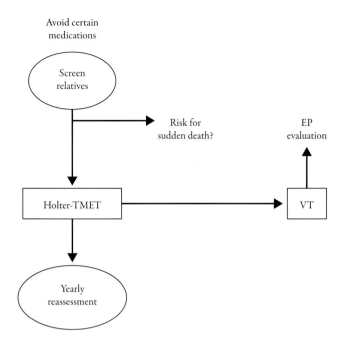

Figure 5.9 Treatment of Asymptomatic Hypertrophic Cardiomyopathy. EP indicates electrophysiologic; TMET, treadmill exercise test; VT, ventricular tachycardia.

nonsustained ventricular tachycardia is controversial (Figure 5.9). No antiarrhythmic agent is uniformly effective, and any agent may make the arrhythmia worse. In select patients with multiple risk factors for sudden death, empiric amiodarone or an implantable cardiac defibrillator might be chosen. In patients who have had an out-of-hospital arrest, the treatment of choice is an implantable cardiac defibrillator.

- An implantable cardiac defibrillator is the treatment of choice for patients with out-of-hospital arrest and for certain patients at high risk for sudden cardiac death.

RESTRICTIVE CARDIOMYOPATHY

Diastolic dysfunction is the primary abnormality in restrictive cardiomyopathy and is usually due to abnormal relaxation, abnormal ventricular filling, and ineffectual atrial contribution to filling, which in turn affect the pulmonary and systemic circulations, causing shortness of breath and edema. In addition, because the ventricle cannot fill adequately to meet its preload requirements, low cardiac output (Starling mechanism), fatigue, and lethargy result. Normal or near-normal left ventricular ejection fraction and volumes are present in most patients with restrictive cardiomyopathy.

- In restrictive cardiomyopathy, the primary abnormality is diastolic dysfunction.

The cause of primary restrictive cardiomyopathy is unknown. The 2 major categories are idiopathic restrictive cardiomyopathy and endomyocardial fibrosis. Progressive fibrosis of the myocardium is seen in idiopathic restrictive cardiomyopathy. Familial cases, often with associated peripheral myopathy, have been reported. Endomyocardial fibrosis is probably an end stage of eosinophilic syndromes in which there is intracavitary thrombus filling of the left ventricle. This restricts filling and causes increased diastolic pressures. Fibrosis also may involve the mitral valve, causing severe mitral regurgitation. There may be 2 different forms of endomyocardial fibrosis: active inflammatory eosinophilic myocarditis (temperate zones) and chronic endomyocardial fibrosis (tropical zones).

- The 2 major categories of primary restrictive cardiomyopathy are idiopathic and endomyocardial fibrosis.

- Fibrosis may involve the mitral valve, leading to mitral regurgitation.

Infiltration diseases involving the myocardium (eg, amyloidosis) have a presentation and pathophysiology similar to those of primary restrictive cardiomyopathy. Signs and symptoms similar to those of restrictive cardiomyopathy also may develop after radiation therapy and anthracycline chemotherapy. Although other infiltrative diseases (eg, sarcoidosis, hemochromatosis) initially may mimic restrictive cardiomyopathy, they usually progress to a dilated cardiomyopathy by the time they cause cardiac symptoms.

- Infiltrative diseases (eg, amyloidosis) may cause restrictive cardiomyopathy.

- Radiation therapy and anthracycline therapy may cause cardiac syndromes with signs and symptoms similar to those of restrictive cardiomyopathy.

SIGNS AND SYMPTOMS

Patients with restrictive cardiomyopathy usually present with symptoms of right heart failure such as edema, dyspnea, and ascites. Atrial arrhythmias due to passive atrial enlargement are frequently present, and the patient may present with atrial fibrillation. Jugular venous pressure is almost always increased, with rapid x and y descents. The precordium is quiet, and heart sounds are soft. There may be an apical systolic murmur of mitral regurgitation and a left sternal border murmur of tricuspid regurgitation. A third heart sound may be present. Dullness at the bases of the lungs is consistent with bilateral pleural effusions. Electrocardiography is usually low or normal voltage with atrial arrhythmias. Chest radiography may show pleural effusions with a normal cardiac silhouette or atrial enlargement.

- Restrictive cardiomyopathy frequently presents as right heart failure with dyspnea, edema, and ascites.

- Atrial arrhythmias are common.

- Jugular venous pressure is increased, with rapid x and y descents.

DIAGNOSIS

Restrictive cardiomyopathy is diagnosed with echocardiography. Typical findings are normal left ventricular cavity size, preserved ejection fraction, and marked biatrial enlargement. In the setting of right heart failure, the inferior vena cava is enlarged. In amyloid heart disease, echocardiography demonstrates thickened myocardium with a scintillating appearance, a pericardial effusion, and thickened regurgitant valves. In endomyocardial fibrosis, there is an apical thrombus (without underlying apical akinesis) or thickening of the endocardium under the mitral valve, which often tethers the valve, causing mitral regurgitation. Other causes of restrictive cardiomyopathy have nonspecific echocardiographic features. Cardiac catheterization shows increase and end-equalization of all end-diastolic pressures. A typical "square-root sign" or "dip-and-plateau" pattern consistent with early rapid filling is present. Endomyocardial biopsy usually is not helpful, except to confirm the diagnosis of amyloidosis.

- Restrictive cardiomyopathy is diagnosed with echocardiography.

TREATMENT

Treatment of idiopathic restrictive cardiomyopathy is usually symptom-based. Diuretics decrease filling pressures and give symptomatic relief, but these effects may be at the expense of further decreasing cardiac output. Heart transplant is the only proven therapy for patients with severe restrictive cardiomyopathy. Corticosteroids are appropriate during the early stages of eosinophilic endocarditis. Endomyocardial fibrosis can be surgically resected and the mitral valve can be replaced, although mortality is significant.

- Treatment of idiopathic restrictive cardiomyopathy is symptom-based.

- Diuretics decrease filling pressures.

- Heart transplant is the only proven therapy for severe restrictive cardiomyopathy.

It is important to differentiate restrictive cardiomyopathy from constrictive pericarditis. Both have similar presentations and findings on clinical examination and diagnostic studies. However, in constrictive pericarditis, pericardiectomy produces symptomatic improvement and, frequently, survival. Therefore, exploratory thoracotomy may be indicated in patients with normal left ventricular systolic function, large atria, and severe increase of diastolic filling pressures if doubt remains after anatomical (computed tomography or magnetic resonance imaging) and other tests (echocardiography, cardiac catheterization).

- Differentiate restrictive cardiomyopathy from constrictive pericarditis.

6.

ISCHEMIC HEART DISEASE

Abhiram Prasad, MD

GOALS

- Identify risk factors for and clinical presentations of ischemic heart disease.

- Review primary and secondary prevention of ischemic heart disease.

- Define the various tests for ischemic heart disease and recognize their roles.

- Review the roles of medical management, percutaneous intervention, and surgical management in ischemic heart disease.

- Describe acute coronary syndromes, their evaluation, and management.

- Identify the mechanical complications of myocardial infarction.

Ischemic heart disease may be asymptomatic or present with stable angina, non–ST-elevation acute coronary syndrome, ST-elevation myocardial infarction (MI), or sudden death. Ischemic heart disease causes nearly 800,000 deaths annually. Notably, about a third of deaths annually in the United States are due to MI. Primary prevention and new treatments have led to a substantial decrease in death from acute MI since 1970 (Figure 6.1).

PREVENTION

The Framingham risk score is the most commonly used model to calculate the 10-year risk for development of ischemic heart disease (http://hp2010.nhlbihin.net/atpiii/calculator.asp). The score is derived from a the patient's risk factors: age, sex, low-density lipoprotein (LDL) cholesterol level, high-density lipoprotein (HDL) cholesterol level, systemic blood pressure, diabetes mellitus, and smoking history (Circulation. 1998 May 12;97[18]:1837–47).

Ischemic heart disease risk factors for which interventions have been proved to reduce cardiac events include tobacco use, serum LDL cholesterol level, serum HDL level, and hypertension (Box 6.1). Factors that clearly increase the risk of ischemic heart disease and for which therapeutic interventions are likely to be effective include diabetes mellitus, physical inactivity, obesity, metabolic syndrome, and serum triglyceride levels. Factors for which intervention may improve subsequent risk include psychosocial factors (eg, anxiety and depression).

- The Framingham risk score is derived from a patient's risk factors for ischemic heart disease.

- Therapeutic interventions for tobacco abuse, serum LDL cholesterol level, serum HDL level, and hypertension are known to reduce cardiac events.

- Therapeutic interventions for diabetes mellitus, physical inactivity, obesity, metabolic syndrome, and serum triglyceride levels are likely to be effective.

Smoking more than doubles the risk of ischemic heart disease and increases mortality by 50%. The relative risk of smokers who quit smoking decreases rapidly, approaching the levels of nonsmokers within 2 to 3 years. Plasma levels of total and LDL cholesterol are important risk factors for ischemic heart disease. A 1% decrease in total serum cholesterol reduces risk by 2% to 3%. Lowering the LDL level slows progression and may result in regression of coronary atherosclerosis. Lowering the LDL level also prevents coronary events, possibly due to atherosclerotic plaque stabilization.

For every 1-mm-Hg decrease in diastolic blood pressure, the risk for MI is reduced by 2% to 3%. The risk for MI is decreased 35% to 55% with maintenance of an active vs sedentary lifestyle. Adjusted mortality rates for ischemic heart disease are 2 to 3 times higher in men and 3 to 7 times higher in women with diabetes mellitus compared with the rates in men and women without diabetes. Heavy alcohol use increases the risk of ischemic heart disease, but moderate consumption decreases risk. Metabolic syndrome is present in 20% of the US population, and it is associated with a twofold to threefold increase in mortality from cardiovascular disease. Aspirin is recommended for persons at intermediate risk for ischemic heart disease and at low risk for bleeding. This

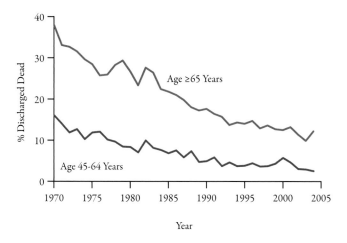

Figure 6.1 Case-Fatality Rate for Acute Myocardial Infarction in the United States, 1970–2004. (Adapted from National Heart, Lung, and Blood Institute. Morbidity and mortality: 2007 chart book on cardiovascular, lung, and blood diseases. Bethesda [MD]: National Institutes of Health; 2007.)

includes patients with an absolute risk of more than 15% over 10 years by Framingham score or patients with diabetes with a risk of more than 10% over 10 years. The role of aspirin in the primary prevention of stroke or overall cardiovascular *mortality* is uncertain. Estrogen replacement therapy is *not* indicated in women with cardiovascular disease, and it may be harmful.

- Smoking is a major risk factor for ischemic heart disease, and smoking cessation leads to a rapid reversal in imposed risk.

- Management of hyperlipidemia and hypertension are essential for reducing the risk of ischemic heart disease.

- Aspirin is recommended for patients at high or intermediate risk of ischemic heart disease. Estrogen therapy should not be used in women with cardiovascular disease because it may be harmful.

Secondary prevention aims to prevent recurrent ischemic events in patients with known ischemic heart disease. Smoking cessation and optimum treatment of hyperlipidemia, hypertension, and diabetes mellitus are essential. Statin drugs reduce

ischemic events after MI more than would be expected from their effect on atherosclerosis progression alone, possibly due to stabilization of lipid-rich, rupture-prone plaques. Statins decrease overall mortality by 30% and coronary event-related mortality by 42% in patients with a prior MI and high cholesterol (>220 mg/dL). Statins reduce the risk for fatal heart disease or recurrent MI by 24% in patients with a prior MI and average levels of cholesterol (total cholesterol <240 mg/dL; LDL, >125 mg/dL).

The following are indications for cholesterol-lowering therapy:

1. Known coronary artery disease (or diabetes mellitus, peripheral vascular disease, multiple risk factors that confer a 10-year risk for coronary artery disease of more than 20% calculated using a modified Framingham risk score) and LDL level more than 100 mg/dL. Goal LDL level is less than 100 mg/dL (optimal <70 mg/dL)

2. Two or more risk factors for coronary artery disease and level more than 130 mg/dL

3. 0 or 1 risk factor for coronary artery disease and LDL level more than 160 mg/dL

Therapeutic targets include treatment of metabolic syndrome, increased triglyceride levels, and low HDL level. Therapeutic lifestyle changes, including a low-fat, low-cholesterol diet, weight management, and physical activity are essential for cholesterol lowering. Soluble fiber (10–25 g/day) and plant stanols or sterols (2 g/day) should be considered as therapeutic options.

Novel risk factors proposed for ischemic heart disease, especially in patients who do not have the conventional risk factors, include increased blood levels of lipoprotein(a), homocysteine, small dense LDL particle (phenotype B), and fibrinogen. Additionally, acute and chronic inflammation and possibly lifetime exposure to pathogens (eg, *Chlamydia*, cytomegalovirus, and *Helicobacter*) have been proposed as potential factors in the pathophysiology of atherosclerosis.

- Secondary prevention refers to therapeutic interventions to prevent recurrent ischemic events.

Box 6.1 RISK FACTORS FOR ISCHEMIC HEART DISEASE

MODIFIABLE FACTOR	NONMODIFIABLE FACTOR	NOVEL FACTOR
Increased LDL cholesterol level	Age	Inflammatory markers (eg, C-reactive protein)
Low HDL cholesterol level	Male sex	Small, dense LDL
Cigarette smoking	Family history of premature CAD[a]	Lipoprotein (a)
Hypertension		Homocysteine
Diabetes mellitus		Fibrinogen
Sedentary lifestyle		
Obesity		
Metabolic syndrome		
Stress & depression		
Socioeconomic factors		

Abbreviations: CAD, coronary artery disease; HDL, high-density lipoprotein; LDL, low-density lipoprotein.

[a] Age at onset less than 55 years in men and less than 65 years for primary relatives.

- Considerable attempts at risk factor modification (diabetes mellitus, tobacco use, hyperlipidemia, hypertension, dietary changes, weight management, physical activity) are warranted.

- Statins reduce ischemic heart disease–related events.

MECHANISM OF ATHEROSCLEROSIS

The response-to-injury hypothesis is the most prevalent explanation of atherosclerosis. The stages of the process are as follows:

Stage I: Chronic injury to the arterial endothelium due to risk factors such as hypercholesterolemia, hypertension, diabetes mellitus, tobacco abuse, inflammation, and possibly infections

Stage II: Release of toxic products by macrophages, leading to platelet adhesion and smooth muscle cell migration and proliferation resulting in formation of fibrointimal lesions or lipid plaques

Stage III: Disruption of the lipid-rich plaque leads to thrombus formation. Acute coronary syndrome (unstable angina or myocardial infarction) results from thrombus organization and atherosclerosis or vessel occlusion (Figure 6.2).

The most frequent site of atherosclerotic plaque disruption is lipid-laden coronary artery lesions with mild to moderate angiographic stenosis—not severely stenotic lesions. The culprit lesion is at a site with less than 50% stenosis in up to two-thirds of cases of unstable angina or MI.

- Modifiable (and possibly some nonmodifiable) risk factors lead to chronic endothelial injury that may progress through endogenous changes to more advanced changes in the coronary vessel wall.

- These changes may lead to unstable angina or MI.

- The most frequent site of plaque disruption is an artery with less than 50% stenosis.

CHRONIC STABLE ANGINA

PATHOPHYSIOLOGY

A mismatch between myocardial oxygen demand and supply causes myocardial ischemia. Demand is determined by heart rate, afterload, contractility, and wall tension. With a dilated, poorly contractile left ventricle, the contribution of wall tension to myocardial oxygen consumption outweighs the other factors.

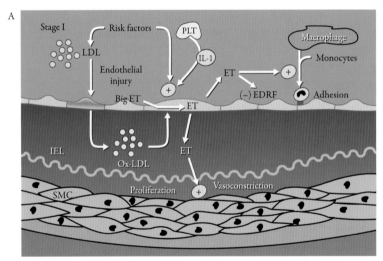

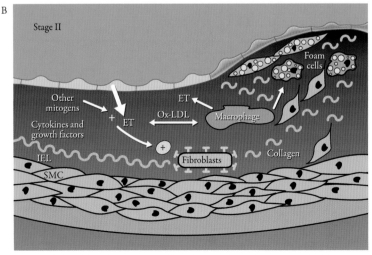

Figure 6.2 Stages of Vascular Injury. A, Stage I. B, Stage II. Interaction of endothelin (ET) and the atherosclerotic plaque. EDRF indicates endothelium-derived relaxing factor; IEL, internal elastic lamina; IL-1, interleukin 1; LDL, low-density lipoprotein particles; Ox-LDL, oxidized LDL particles; PLT, platelet; SMC, smooth muscle cell. "+" indicates stimulation. (Adapted from Lerman A. The endothelium. In: Murphy JG, editor. Mayo Clinic cardiology review. 2nd ed. Philadelphia [PA]: Lippincott Williams & Wilkins; c2000. p. 99–112. Used with permission of Mayo Foundation for Medical Education and Research.)

Normally, coronary blood flow can increase up to 5 times to meet effort-related increases in myocardial oxygen demands. The double product [(heart rate) × (systolic blood pressure)] is a useful index for quantifying myocardial oxygen demand. Ischemia occurs when flow reserve is inadequate, usually the result of fixed coronary artery disease.

Restriction of resting blood flow sufficient to cause resting ischemia does not occur unless vessel stenosis is more than 95%. However, decreased overall flow reserve begins to occur at about 60% vessel stenosis, and symptoms of exercise-induced ischemia may begin. The temporal sequence of events during ischemia are diastolic dysfunction→abnormal perfusion→regional wall motion abnormalities→electrocardiographic (ECG) changes→pain.

- Mismatched oxygen demand and supply lead to myocardial ischemia.

- Heart rate, afterload, contractility, and wall tension are the factors that determine myocardial oxygen consumption and demand.

- When the left ventricle is dilated and contracts poorly, wall tension plays a larger role in myocardial oxygen consumption than other factors.

- Vessel stenosis >95% leads to resting ischemia, but decreased flow reserve begins with about 60% stenosis, leading to exertional ischemia.

CLINICAL PRESENTATION

Symptomatic Chronic Stable Coronary Artery Disease

Typical angina is characterized by retrosternal pain occurring with cardiovascular stress and relieved by rest or nitroglycerin. Atypical angina is defined by the presence of 2 of these 3 features. Noncardiac chest pain is defined by the presence of 1 or none of these features.

Angina may be precipitated by any activity that increases myocardial oxygen consumption. The pain has various descriptions such as pressure, burning, stabbing, ache, hurt, or heaviness, or it may be described as shortness of breath. It can be substernal or epigastric, and it may radiate to the neck, jaw, shoulder, back, elbow, or wrist. In stable angina, the pain lasts 2 to 30 minutes and is usually relieved by rest. Uncommon findings that may occur with ischemia include a fourth heart sound and mitral regurgitant murmur due to papillary muscle dysfunction. ST-segment depression may be found on the ECG, indicating subendocardial ischemia.

- Angina can have typical or atypical symptoms and may be described in various ways by patients.

- Stable angina pain is usually relieved by rest or nitroglycerin.

- A fourth heart sound and mitral regurgitant murmur due to papillary muscle dysfunction are uncommon.

- Subendocardial ischemia may be manifested by ST-segment depression on ECG.

Silent Ischemia

Silent ischemia is common in patients with chronic stable coronary artery disease, with unstable angina, or after myocardial infarction. Patients with diabetes may have silent ischemia, possibly due to neuropathy. Silent ischemia is also more common in the elderly. It is defined as the presence of dynamic ST-segment depression in the absence of symptoms. Medical therapy is similar to that for symptomatic ischemia. Whether percutaneous coronary intervention or coronary artery bypass grafting should be performed for silent ischemia in the absence of other markers of high risk is unknown. The prognosis for this condition is the same as that for symptomatic ischemia.

NONINVASIVE TESTING FOR ISCHEMIA

Ancillary tests for ischemic heart disease include measurement of left ventricular function, stress testing, and coronary angiography.

Left Ventricular Function

Left ventricular function is the most important predictor of prognosis and should be measured in all patients with 2-dimensional echocardiography, radionuclide angiography, or left ventricular angiography.

Stress Testing

Exercise stress testing to identify ischemia is performed using ECG monitoring, thallium or technetium-sestamibi scanning (to assess myocardial perfusion), or echocardiography (to assess left ventricular function). Heart rate, blood pressure, and the onset of subjective symptoms are monitored.

The stress ECG is positive for ischemia if there is a flat or downsloping ST-segment depression of 1 mm or more with exertion, whereas it is uninterpretable when there is more than 1 mm of *resting* ST-segment depression, left bundle branch block, left ventricular hypertrophy, paced rhythm, or preexcitation (Wolff-Parkinson-White syndrome). Digoxin therapy results in an uninterpretable stress ECG. A stress imaging test (eg, sestamibi or echocardiography) is indicated in patients with an uninterpretable ECG.

- Exercise stress testing identifies ischemia and is used with ECG monitoring, perfusion scanning, or echocardiography.

- Careful attention to patient and ECG characteristics is important for determining whether the stress ECG is interpretable.

- Stress imaging should be used in patients who have or are anticipated to have an uninterpretable stress ECG.

Treadmill exercise testing can identify high-risk patients. A patient is at high risk if the following results are obtained:

1. A positive ECG in stage I of the Bruce protocol or at a heart rate less than 120 beats per minute

2. ST-segment depression more than 2 mm

3. ST-segment depression more than 6 minutes in duration after stopping exercise

4. Decrease in blood pressure

5. Multiple perfusion or wall motion defects (>25% of segments with exercise) and an increase in left ventricular end-systolic volume with exercise

Patients who achieve a good workload with appropriate blood pressure and heart rate responses without marked ST-segment depression have an excellent prognosis; therefore, medical management may be preferred in these patients.

Imaging-based stress testing slightly increases the sensitivity and specificity of ECG exercise testing. In nuclear perfusion imaging, the tracer is injected at peak exercise and labels areas of hypoperfusion as a defect or "cold spot." Scanning is repeated a few hours later at rest, and persistent cold spots indicate infarction, whereas reperfused areas indicate areas of inducible ischemia. In patients with left bundle branch block or severe left ventricular hypertrophy, thallium and sestamibi scanning give false-positive results during exercise stress.

- Stress imaging modestly improves sensitivity and specificity of ECG exercise stress testing.

- Left bundle branch block and severe left ventricular hypertrophy lead to false-positive exercise thallium and sestamibi stress tests.

In exercise echocardiography, 2-dimensional echocardiography is performed at rest and at peak exercise. The test is positive for ischemia if new regional wall motion abnormalities develop, global systolic function decreases, or left ventricular end-systolic volume increases.

- In exercise echocardiography, new regional wall motion abnormalities, decline in global systolic dysfunction, or increased left ventricular end-systolic volume indicate ischemia.

Exercise stress testing should *not* be performed for patients with high-risk unstable angina, patients who have had acute MI in the prior 2 days, or patients with symptomatic severe aortic stenosis, uncontrolled heart failure, or uncontrolled arrhythmia. Consider invasive angiography to define coronary artery anatomy and evaluate the need for revascularization in patients with poor prognostic factors.

- Patients at high risk for an adverse event during exertion should not undergo exercise stress testing.

Imaging stress tests are considerably more expensive than the ECG exercise test and should not be routinely used instead of ECG exercise testing for diagnostic purposes, except when the result of resting ECG is uninterpretable, the ECG result is possibly false-positive, or specific regions of ischemia need to be localized (for planning revascularization procedures).

- Only when the resting ECG is uninterpretable, the ECG result is thought to be false-positive, or mapping of ischemic regions is necessary should imaging stress testing be used instead of ECG exercise stress testing.

Pharmacologic stress tests are used for patients who cannot exercise. These tests include the use of vasodilators such as adenosine and dipyridamole (redistribute flow away from ischemic myocardium). The tests are generally performed with perfusion agents such as thallium or sestamibi. Alternatively, dobutamine is used as a chronotropic and inotropic agent to increase myocardial oxygen demand, and imaging is performed with echocardiography.

- Pharmacologic stress testing is used when patients are unable to exercise.

Stress tests should not be used for the diagnosis of ischemic heart disease in patients at high or low risk. Stress testing is appropriate for patients at intermediate risk to rule in or rule out ischemia. The pretest probability of ischemic heart disease is estimated using the following criteria: age (men >40 years and women >60 years), male sex, and symptom status (in decreasing order of risk: typical angina, atypical angina, noncardiac chest pain, asymptomatic) (Table 6.1 and Figure 6.3).

- Stress testing of low-risk and high-risk patients is not recommended.

Noninvasive Coronary Angiography

Computed tomography and magnetic resonance imaging can be used for noninvasive coronary angiography. However, the diagnostic accuracy and applicability to clinical practice of these novel imaging methods have not been established, and they should not be considered an alternative to invasive coronary angiography. Computed tomography requires the use of contrast media and produces suboptimal images in patients with greater than mild coronary calcification or an irregular rhythm. Noninvasive imaging may have a role in symptomatic patients with a low to moderate pretest probability of ischemic heart disease given its high negative predictive value. A useful role for noninvasive angiography is for imaging coronary anomalies. It is *not* recommended for screening asymptomatic patients or patients with established ischemic heart disease. In addition, the clinical utility of coronary calcium scores derived by computed tomography is not established.

- Noninvasive coronary imaging is useful for imaging coronary artery anomalies.

- The clinical role of noninvasive angiography is otherwise unclear.

- The clinical use of coronary calcium scores has not been established.

AGE, Y	SEX	TYPICAL/DEFINITE ANGINA PECTORIS	ATYPICAL/PROBABLE ANGINA PECTORIS	NON-ANGINAL CHEST PAIN	ASYMPTOMATIC
30–39	Males	Intermediate	Intermediate	Low (<10%)	Very low (<5%)
	Females	Intermediate	Very low (<5%)	Very low	Very low
40–49	Males	High (>90%)	Intermediate	Intermediate	Low
	Females	Intermediate	Low	Very low	Very low
50–59	Males	High (>90%)	Intermediate	Intermediate	Low
	Females	Intermediate	Intermediate	Low	Very low
60–69	Males	High	Intermediate	Intermediate	Low
	Females	High	Intermediate	Intermediate	Low

[a] High indicates more than 90%; intermediate, 10% to 90%; low, less than 10%; very low, less than 5%.

Data from Gibbons RJ, Balady GJ, Bricker JT, Chaitman BR, Fletcher GF, Froelicher VF, et al; American College of Cardiology/American Heart Association Task Force on Practice Guidelines (Committee to Update the 1997 Exercise Testing Guidelines). ACC/AHA 2002 guideline update for exercise testing: summary article: a report of the American College of Cardiology/American Heart Association Task Force on Practice Guidelines (Committee to Update the 1997 Exercise Testing Guidelines). Circulation. 2002 Oct 1;106(14):1883–92 and Gibbons RJ, Balady GJ, Bricker JT, Chaitman BR, Fletcher GF, Froelicher VF, et al; American College of Cardiology/American Heart Association Task Force on Practice Guidelines. Committee to Update the 1997 Exercise Testing Guidelines. ACC/AHA 2002 guideline update for exercise testing: summary article. A report of the American College of Cardiology/American Heart Association Task Force on Practice Guidelines (Committee to Update the 1997 Exercise Testing Guidelines). J Am Coll Cardiol. 2002 Oct 16;40(8):1531–40. Erratum in: J Am Coll Cardiol. 2006 Oct 17;48(8):1731.

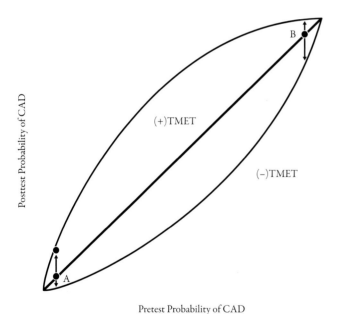

Figure 6.3 The Effect of Bayes Theorem on the Ability of Treadmill Exertion Testing (TMET) to Diagnose Coronary Artery Disease (CAD). Patient A, a young patient with atypical chest pain and no risk factors. Pretest probability (5%) of coronary artery disease is low. If the test results are negative, the probability decreases to 3%. However, if the results are positive, the probability is less than 15%. Patient B, an older man with typical chest pain and multiple risk factors. Pretest probability of coronary artery disease is high (90%), and even with negative test results the probability is higher than 70%. Thus, stress tests should not be used for the diagnosis of coronary artery disease in patients at high or low risk.

Invasive Coronary Angiography

Although coronary angiography has limitations, it is the standard for defining the severity and extent of coronary artery disease. Subjective visual estimation of the percentage of stenosis may underestimate the severity of disease, especially if it is diffuse, because angiography outlines the vessel lumen. The risk of serious complications of coronary angiography is approximately 0.1%, including myocardial infarction, stroke, and death. Patients with advanced age, severe left ventricular dysfunction, left main coronary artery disease, or other comorbidities have a somewhat higher risk of complications. Other complications include vascular complications (0.5%) and contrast nephropathy.

- Invasive coronary angiography is the standard for defining extent and severity of coronary artery disease but may underestimate severity.

- The risk of serious complications is very low.

MEDICAL THERAPY OF ANGINA

Medical therapy for chronic stable angina includes risk factor modification, antiplatelet therapy, and medication-based therapy of myocardial ischemia. Antiplatelet agents are essential. Aspirin reduces the likelihood of acute MI and mortality, but it does not prevent progression of atherosclerosis. Aspirin therapy provides greater benefit for secondary than for primary prevention. Treatable underlying factors that contribute to ischemia (eg, anemia, thyroid abnormalities, and hypoxia) should always be sought.

A stepwise approach should be used when introducing a pharmacologic strategy to treat myocardial ischemia. Medications should be titrated according to symptoms. The dose of a first-line drug should be optimized before adding additional agents.

- Medical therapy includes risk factor modification, antiplatelet therapy, and medications to relieve ischemia.
- A stepwise approach should be used for pharmacological treatment of myocardial ischemia.

β-Adrenergic blockers (β-blockers) are the most effective and are first-line drugs for ischemic heart disease. They relieve angina by decreasing heart rate, reducing contractility, and decreasing afterload (blood pressure). They are the most effective drugs for reducing the double product (heart rate × blood pressure) with exercise. β-Blockers may improve survival for some patients with ischemic heart disease, particularly those with prior MI or depressed left ventricular systolic function. β-Blockers should not be used in the setting of *marked* bronchospastic disease, decompensated heart failure, or bradycardia. However, they should be given to patients with left ventricular systolic dysfunction in the absence of overt heart failure. The target resting heart rate is 70 beats per minute or less and dose should be titrated to effect.

- β-Blockers should be considered first-line therapy for ischemic heart disease.
- Contraindications include severe bronchospastic disease, decompensated heart failure, or bradycardia in which additional heart rate reduction cannot be tolerated.
- Target heart rate <70 beats per minute; titrate dose to effect.

Nitrates should be added if symptoms continue despite optimal β-blocker therapy. Nitrates cause venodilatation and decreasing wall tension, thus relieving angina. Nitrate tolerance can develop with continuous exposure. Thus, a nitrate-free interval is important, particularly when using short-acting preparations. Sublingual nitroglycerin should be given to all symptomatic patients for use as needed.

- Nitrates should be added if symptoms continue despite optimal β-blocker therapy.
- Include a nitrate-free interval to avoid nitrate tolerance.
- All patients with ischemic heart disease should carry sublingual nitroglycerin for as-needed use.

Calcium channel blockers decrease afterload, heart rate, and contractility. Short-acting calcium channel blockers, specifically the dihydropyridines (eg, amlodipine, nifedipine), may cause reflex tachycardia and increased mortality; therefore, they are relatively contraindicated in patients with ischemic heart disease. This detrimental effect probably does not occur with the longer-acting calcium channel blockers or in patients with normal systolic function, but they should be avoided in patients with left ventricular systolic dysfunction. If a calcium channel blocker is required for patients with left ventricular systolic dysfunction, amlodipine is preferred.

- Because short-acting calcium channel blockers may cause reflex tachycardia, they are relatively contraindicated.
- However, if a short-acting calcium channel blocker is required in a patient with left ventricular systolic dysfunction, amlodipine is preferred.

Ranolazine (Ranexa) is a second-line drug used as an adjunct to one of the aforementioned drugs. Experience with its use is limited. The mode of action is unknown.

For patients with left ventricular dysfunction or nocturnal angina, diuretics and angiotensin-converting enzyme inhibitors decrease wall tension. They may be beneficial for secondary prevention in ischemic heart disease regardless of the degree of systolic function.

Diuretics and angiotensin-converting enzyme inhibitors decrease wall tension in patients with left ventricular dysfunction or nocturnal angina.

- Angiotensin-converting enzyme inhibitors may be beneficial for secondary prevention for all patients with ischemic heart disease.

PERCUTANEOUS CORONARY INTERVENTION

Percutaneous coronary intervention (PCI) for chronic stable angina relieves symptoms but does not reduce the risk of MI or death. It is indicated for treatment in symptomatic patients, particularly those who remain symptomatic despite optimized medical therapy. An initial medical strategy is reasonable for most patients at low to moderate risk of an event (based on symptoms and the findings on stress testing or angiography). There is no clear role for PCI in management of asymptomatic disease.

- PCI relieves symptoms, but it does not alter the risk of MI or death.
- PCI is indicated for patients who remain symptomatic despite optimal medical therapy.
- PCI should not be used to treat asymptomatic disease.

PCI is performed at the time of coronary angiography. During percutaneous transluminal coronary angioplasty (PTCA), the device is placed across a coronary stenosis and a balloon is inflated to increase the area of the lumen. This procedure "splits" the atheroma and stretches the vessel. The major problem is restenosis, occurring in 30% to 40% of patients within 6 months. Antiplatelet agents may decrease the rate of acute closure, but they do not prevent restenosis.

Other catheter-based therapies such as atherectomy and laser have high restenosis rates and are infrequently used.

- PCI uses an intracoronary balloon to open a coronary stenosis.

- Restenosis is a common problem.

- Antiplatelet agents may decrease vessel closure rate, but they do not prevent restenosis.

Intracoronary stent placement at the time of PCI decreases restenosis. Stents are used in approximately 90% of PCIs. The restenosis rate after successful bare-metal stent implantation is 20% to 30%. Stents also are used to treat acute complications of PTCA such as acute dissection and have decreased the need for emergency coronary artery bypass grafting (CABG). However, for patients who have restenosis within a stent, the rate of recurrent restenosis is high (>60%) if another procedure is performed.

- Intracoronary stent placement decreases restenosis.

- Acute complications of PTCA (eg, coronary artery dissection) can be treated with stents.

- The rate of recurrent stenosis is high when another procedure is performed to treat restenosis.

Drug-eluting stents are coated with and release drugs that considerably decrease restenosis (5%–10%). They are the most commonly used stents. They are associated with a higher risk for very late (>1 year) stent thrombosis than bare-metal stents.

Dual antiplatelet therapy is initiated at the time of stent deployment to prevent early restenosis. Duration varies according to the type of stent (Table 6.2). Recommendations regarding discontinuation of dual antiplatelet therapy for noncardiac surgery are outlined in Box 6.2.

Table 6.2 **ANTIPLATELET THERAPY USED WITH CORONARY STENTS**

THERAPY	DURATION
Aspirin	Indefinitely
Clopidogrel (Plavix) or prasugrel (Effient)	
Bare-metal stent	At least 1 month for patient with stable disease. At least 12 months for an acute coronary syndrome (unstable angina & myocardial infarction). If the risk of substantial bleeding outweighs the anticipated benefit, earlier discontinuation should be considered
Drug-eluting stent	12 months (a subset of patients may require long-term therapy). If the risk of morbidity because of bleeding outweighs the anticipated benefits afforded by thienopyridine therapy, earlier discontinuation should be considered

The success rate for PCI is greater than 95%. Potential complications include myocardial infarction (<5%), vascular complications (1%), emergency CABG (0.2%), and mortality (<0.5%). The risks of the procedure are higher during emergency procedures, in the elderly, and in patients with severely reduced ejection fraction, acute coronary syndromes, or severe diffuse coronary artery disease.

- Drug-eluting stents considerably decrease the likelihood of restenosis after angioplasty.

- Very late stent thrombosis is higher with drug-eluting stents than with bare-metal stents.

- Long-duration dual antiplatelet therapy is used in the setting of drug-eluting stents.

- Caution must be exercised when considering discontinuation of dual anti-platelet therapy for a surgical procedure.

PCI is the preferred revascularization strategy for single-vessel disease, young patients (age <50 years), elderly patients with significant comorbid conditions, and patients who are not surgical candidates.

SURGICAL TREATMENT

CABG uses the saphenous vein (occlusion rate of 20% at 1 year and 50% at 5 years) and internal mammary artery (occlusion rate <10% at 10 years). CABG provides excellent symptom relief (partial relief in >90%, complete relief in >70%).

The indications for CABG (over medical therapy or PCI) are symptom relief in patients whose limiting symptoms are unresponsive to other management strategies and prolonging the life of patients with severe disease.

- Internal mammary artery grafting results in better long-term patency than saphenous vein grafting.

- Indications for CABG include symptom relief in patients not responding to other management approaches and decreasing mortality due to severe disease.

CABG reduces mortality in patients with severe disease, including left main coronary artery disease, 3-vessel disease with moderately depressed left ventricular function, 3-vessel disease with severe ischemic symptoms at a low workload, and multivessel disease with proximal left anterior descending artery involvement. CABG does not prevent myocardial infarction, improve left ventricular function, or decrease ventricular arrhythmias. Recommendations for surgery are derived from randomized trials of CABG vs medical therapy. In meta-analyses, a survival benefit in favor of CABG compared with medical therapy has been observed for all patients with 3-vessel disease.

- CABG reduces mortality in patients with defined severe coronary artery disease and offers a survival benefit compared to medical management in patients with 3-vessel disease.

In-hospital mortality after CABG varies widely (about 1% in most elective cases to 30% in high-risk cases). Mortality increases with age, female sex, reduced left ventricular function, diffuse multivessel disease, recent acute coronary syndrome, diabetes mellitus, repeat CABG, and emergency surgery. Complications of CABG include sternal wound infection (especially in patients with diabetes mellitus), severe left ventricular dysfunction (from perioperative myocardial infarction or inadequate cardioprotection), and late constrictive pericarditis.

- CABG is associated with a widely varying in-hospital mortality rate depending on underlying patient risk factors.

- Mortality is higher in patient with diabetes, women, and patients who are older, have diffuse multivessel disease, have reduced left ventricular function, have had a recent acute coronary syndrome, had prior CABG, or are undergoing emergency surgery.

- Complications include wound infection, severe left ventricular dysfunction, and constrictive pericarditis.

POSTCARDIOTOMY SYNDROME

Postcardiotomy syndrome occurs 2 weeks to 2 months postoperatively and consists of fever, pericarditis, and increased erythrocyte sedimentation rate. Rarely, it presents as pericardial tamponade. It is likely an autoimmune process. Treatment is with aspirin and other nonsteroidal anti-inflammatory drugs. Rarely, constrictive pericarditis may be a late complication. The diagnosis should be suspected in patients presenting months to years after cardiac surgery with congestive heart failure with predominantly right-sided signs of fluid overload, including increased jugular venous pressure but normal left ventricular ejection fraction.

- Postcardiotomy syndrome may occur 2 weeks to 2 months after surgery.

- It is defined by fever, pericarditis, and increased erythrocyte sedimentation rate.

- Treatment is with aspirin and other nonsteroidal anti-inflammatory drugs.

- Constrictive pericarditis is a rare late complication.

MEDICAL VS CATHETER-BASED VS SURGICAL THERAPY

The decision about which therapy to use for a patient with chronic stable angina must be individualized. Factors to consider include disease severity, ischemia, and symptoms, and the patient's age, lifestyle, and personal preference. The incidence of MI and emergency CABG with PCI is similar to that with medical management. PCI neither decreases risk for MI nor improves resting left ventricular function or survival. Procedure-related mortality is lower with PCI than with CABG.

- PCI and medical management have a comparable incidence of MI and emergency CABG.

- PCI neither decreases risk for MI nor improves resting left ventricular function or survival.

There are more procedure-related infarctions and strokes with CABG than with PCI, and the duration of hospitalization is longer after CABG. The overall rates of death or myocardial infarction at 5-year follow-up are similar for PCI and CABG (85%–90% free of death and 80% free of myocardial infarction), except for patients with severe disease. This subgroup includes patients with left main coronary artery disease, 3-vessel disease with moderately depressed left ventricular function, 3-vessel disease with severe ischemic symptoms at a low workload, and multivessel disease with proximal left anterior descending artery involvement. CABG offers a survival benefit in these patients. Patients with multivessel or anatomically complex disease who have CABG have less angina, require less antianginal medication, and are less likely to need a repeat revascularization procedure. For patients with diabetes mellitus and diffuse multivessel disease, survival is higher with CABG than with PCI. Increased survival is related to having a patent internal mammary artery graft to the left anterior descending artery.

- CABG is related to more procedure-related infarctions and strokes.

- CABG offers a survival benefit in patients with defined severe coronary artery disease.

- CABG offers a survival benefit in patients with diabetes and in patients with diffuse multivessel disease.

CORONARY ARTERY SPASM

The vasomotor tone of coronary arteries is important in the pathogenesis of coronary artery disease. Arterial injury leads to coronary artery vasoconstriction. The vascular endothelium regulates vasomotor tone by releasing relaxing factors (eg, prostacyclin and nitric oxide), preventing vasoconstriction and platelet deposition. Endothelial dysfunction leads to depletion of these factors and the coronary arteries become prone to spasm. Most clinical episodes of coronary artery spasm are superimposed on atherosclerotic plaques. However, coronary artery spasm may also develop in patients with angiographically normal coronary arteries.

Coronary artery spasm classically consists of recurrent episodes of rest pain with associated ST-segment elevation, which reverses with administration of nitrates (Prinzmetal angina). However, many patients present with atypical chest pain without ECG changes. Coronary angiography with acetylcholine provocation is used to diagnose coronary artery spasm, but the sensitivity and specificity are not known. Coronary artery spasm is treated with long-acting nitrates or calcium channel blockers.

- Coronary artery spasm may occur in the setting of arterial injury and endothelial dysfunction.

- Although coronary artery spasm usually occurs in the setting of atherosclerosis, it also occurs in angiographically normal coronary arteries.

- Spasm usually presents as recurrent chest pain with ECG changes, but it may have an atypical clinical presentation.

- Coronary catheterization-based testing is needed to diagnose spasm.

- Long-acting nitrates or calcium channel blockers are used for treatment.

ACUTE CORONARY SYNDROMES

Acute coronary syndromes include unstable angina and acute MI (both ST-segment elevation and non–ST-segment elevation MI). At the time of initial presentation, the differentiation of these patients from those with noncardiac chest pain is based on clinical assessment.

The resting ECG is essential for the evaluation and triage of a patient presenting with an acute coronary syndrome. Those without ST-segment elevation have unstable angina or non–ST-segment elevation MI, usually the result of subtotal coronary artery occlusion. Patients with ST-segment elevation generally have complete coronary artery occlusion leading to transmural injury.

- Acute coronary syndromes include unstable angina and acute MI.

- Clinical assessment is used to differentiate acute coronary syndrome from noncardiac chest pain.

- The resting ECG is essential for evaluation and management of patients with acute coronary syndrome.

Patients presenting with a suspected acute coronary syndrome require prompt evaluation. Patients with ST-segment elevation must be treated on an emergency basis. Patients without ST-segment elevation can be evaluated in an emergency department chest pain unit allowing discharge of low-risk patients, observation of intermediate-risk patients, and admission of high-risk patients (Box 6.3 and Figures 6.4 and 6.5).

- Early risk stratification and care of patients presenting with chest pain or other symptoms potentially due to an acute coronary syndrome are essential.

UNSTABLE ANGINA AND NON–ST-SEGMENT ELEVATION MI

Pathophysiology

These conditions are due to mismatched myocardial oxygen demand and supply, most often precipitated by conditions of decreased myocardial oxygen supply—usually due to coronary stenosis from nonocclusive thrombus at the site of a disrupted atherosclerotic plaque. Episodes may also be caused by increased myocardial oxygen demand in the presence of a fixed myocardial oxygen supply. Coronary spasm may also precipitate episodes.

Box 6.3 **BASELINE CHARACTERISTICS ANALYZED FOR TIMI RISK SCORE FOR UNSTABLE ANGINA AND NON–ST-SEGMENT ELEVATION MYOCARDIAL INFARCTION**

- Age ≥65 y

- ≥3 CAD risk factors

- Known CAD (stenosis ≥50%)

- Aspirin use in past 7 days

- Recent (≤24 h) severe angina

- ↑ Cardiac markers

- ST deviation ≥0.5 mm

Abbreviations: CAD, coronary artery disease; TIMI, Thrombolysis in Myocardial Infarction trial.

Adapted from Antman EM, Cohen M, Bernink PJLM, McCabe CH, Horacek T, Papuchis G, et al. The TIMI risk score for unstable angina/non–ST elevation MI: a method for prognostication and therapeutic decision making. JAMA. 2000 Aug 16;284(7):835–42. Used with permission.

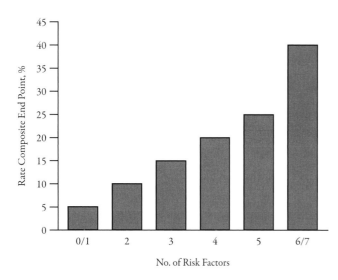

Figure 6.4 The 14-Day Risk of Death, Myocardial Infarction, and Severe Ischemia Requiring Urgent Revascularization. Rates are based on number of risk factors present (Thrombolysis in Myocardial Infarction [TIMI] trial cohort). (Adapted from Antman EM, Cohen M, Bernink PJLM, McCabe CH, Horacek T, Papuchis G, et al. The TIMI risk score for unstable angina/non–ST elevation MI: a method for prognostication and therapeutic decision making. JAMA. 2000 Aug 16;284[7]:835–42. Used with permission.)

Nocturnal ischemic symptoms are generally due to unstable angina and may be due to altered coronary tone or increased wall tension in patients with left ventricular dysfunction.

- Unstable angina and non–ST-segment elevation MI are due to mismatched myocardial oxygen demand and supply, most often precipitated by conditions of decreased myocardial oxygen supply.

- Increased myocardial oxygen demand in the presence of a fixed myocardial oxygen supply can cause unstable angina and non–ST-segment elevation MI.

Biomarkers

Cardiac biomarkers are used to differentiate unstable angina from non–ST-segment elevation MI. Cardiac-specific troponin T and I are the preferred biomarkers. MI is defined by increased troponin T and I levels in the presence of symptoms of ischemia, and biomarker increases identify patients at high risk for future events.

- Increased levels of cardiac biomarkers can be used to differentiate unstable angina from non–ST-segment elevation MI.

- Biomarker increases can help identify patients at risk for future events.

Management

All patients with a possible acute coronary syndrome should have continuous ECG monitoring and treatment to improve the myocardial oxygen demand-supply mismatch. Sedation may decrease anxiety and catecholaminergic stimulation of the heart. β-Adrenergic blockade is the treatment of choice to decrease myocardial oxygen demand.

Antiplatelet agents, such as aspirin, are given immediately and decrease the incidence of progression to ST-segment elevation MI. Clopidogrel is an alternative in patients with aspirin allergy or intolerance. Clopidogrel is usually given in addition to aspirin. However, in many hospitals where patients with an acute coronary syndrome undergo diagnostic catheterization within 24 hours of admission, clopidogrel use is not started until it is clear that CABG will not be needed within 4 to 5 days. However, in clopidogrel-treated patients, urgent CABG may have an acceptable bleeding risk when performed by experienced surgeons.

- Continuous ECG monitoring and treatment to improve myocardial oxygen supply (oxygen therapy, pain management, β-adrenergic blockade, and appropriate sedation) should be used in all patients with possible acute coronary syndrome.

- Antiplatelet therapy decreases progression to ST-segment elevation MI and is essential unless contraindicated.

- Clopidogrel is recommended (in addition to aspirin) unless CABG is anticipated.

Anticoagulation decreases the incidence of progression to MI and should be given to all patients without contraindications. Continuous intravenous administration of unfractionated heparin or subcutaneous injections of low-molecular-weight heparin may be used. Bivalirudin (direct thrombin inhibitor) and fondaparinux (activated factor X inhibitor) are alternative anticoagulants.

- Anticoagulation should be initiated in patients without contraindications to decrease progression to MI.

Conservative vs Invasive Strategy

There are 2 accepted therapeutic pathways for patients presenting with unstable angina or non–ST-segment elevation MI, depending on risk stratification. Patients at high risk should undergo an early invasive strategy (within 4–48 hours of admission) with revascularization (PCI or CABG) performed when appropriate. High-risk patients include those with a Thrombolysis in Myocardial Infarction trial (TIMI) risk score of more than 3, ongoing chest pain, ST-segment depression on the resting ECG, and an increase in troponin levels. Use of clopidogrel or a glycoprotein IIb/IIIa inhibitor should be initiated before coronary angiography (Box 6.3 and Figure 6.6A and 6.6B).

A conservative (or selective invasive) strategy is indicated for non–high-risk patients. Initially, medical management is used for treatment. Coronary angiography is indicated if 1) recurrent ischemia occurs despite optimal medical therapy, 2) results of the pre-discharge stress test are positive, 3) there is left ventricular dysfunction (ejection fraction ≤40%) or heart failure, or 4) serious arrhythmias occur.

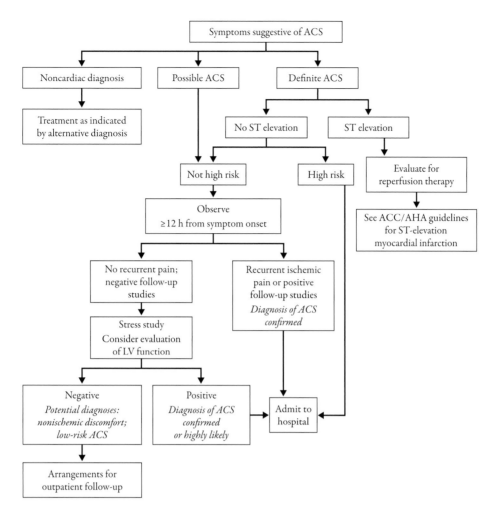

Figure 6.5 Algorithm for Evaluation and Management of Patients Suspected of Having Acute Coronary Syndrome (ACS). ACC indicates American College of Cardiology; AHA, American Heart Association; LV, left ventricular. (Adapted from Anderson JL, Adams CD, Antman EM, Bridges CR, Califf RM, Casey DE Jr, et al. ACC/AHA 2007 guidelines for the management of patients with unstable angina/non–ST-elevation myocardial infarction: a report of the American College of Cardiology/American Heart Association Task Force on Practice Guidelines [Writing Committee to Revise the 2002 Guidelines for the Management of Patients With Unstable Angina/Non–ST-Elevation Myocardial Infarction]. J Am Coll Cardiol. 2007 Aug 14;50[7]:e1–157 and Anderson JL, Adams CD, Antman EM, Bridges CR, Califf RM, Casey DE Jr, et al; American College of Cardiology; American Heart Association Task Force on Practice Guidelines [Writing Committee to Revise the 2002 Guidelines for the Management of Patients With Unstable Angina/Non ST-Elevation Myocardial Infarction]; American College of Emergency Physicians; Society for Cardiovascular Angiography and Interventions; Society of Thoracic Surgeons; American Association of Cardiovascular and Pulmonary Rehabilitation; Society for Academic Emergency Medicine. ACC/AHA 2007 guidelines for the management of patients with unstable angina/non ST-elevation myocardial infarction: a report of the American College of Cardiology/American Heart Association Task Force on Practice Guidelines [Writing Committee to Revise the 2002 Guidelines for the Management of Patients With Unstable Angina/Non ST-Elevation Myocardial Infarction]: developed in collaboration with the American College of Emergency Physicians, the Society for Cardiovascular Angiography and Interventions, and the Society of Thoracic Surgeons: endorsed by the American Association of Cardiovascular and Pulmonary Rehabilitation and the Society for Academic Emergency Medicine. Circulation. 2007 Aug 14;116[7]:e148–304. Epub 2007 Aug 6. Erratum in: Circulation. 2008 Mar 4;117[9]:e180. Used with permission.)

- High-risk patients should undergo invasive strategy, whereas non–high-risk patients can receive more conservative treatment, which can be switched to an invasive strategy if high-risk factors emerge.

ST-SEGMENT ELEVATION MYOCARDIAL INFARCTION

Pathophysiology

An ST-segment elevation MI is the result of events occurring after rupture of an intracoronary plaque. Plaque rupture causes platelet adhesion and aggregation, thrombus formation, and sudden, complete occlusion of the artery. Without collateral circulation, 90% of the myocardium supplied by the occluded coronary artery is infarcted within 3 hours. Transmural MI develops if the condition is untreated. Patients with ST-segment elevation MI require urgent diagnosis and therapy to preserve the myocardium because prompt reperfusion therapy improves survival.

- Plaque rupture may ultimately lead to sudden, complete occlusion of a coronary artery, resulting in an ST-segment elevation MI.

- Rapid reperfusion leads to improved myocardial preservation and survival.

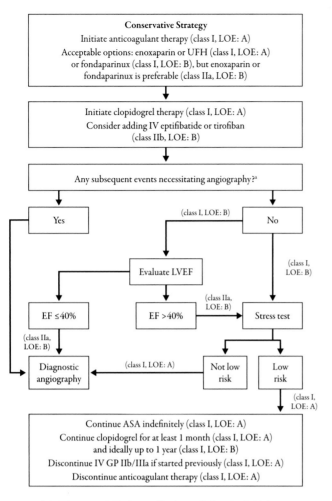

Conservative Strategy

Initiate anticoagulant therapy (class I, LOE: A)

Acceptable options: enoxaparin or UFH (class I, LOE: A) or fondaparinux (class I, LOE: B), but enoxaparin or fondaparinux is preferable (class IIa, LOE: B)

↓

Initiate clopidogrel therapy (class I, LOE: A)
Consider adding IV eptifibatide or tirofiban (class IIb, LOE: B)

↓

Any subsequent events necessitating angiography?[a]

Yes   No (class I, LOE: B)

Evaluate LVEF (class I, LOE: B)

EF ≤40%   EF >40% (class IIa, LOE: B) Stress test

Diagnostic angiography (class I, LOE: A)   Not low risk   Low risk

(class IIa, LOE: B)   (class I, LOE: A)

Continue ASA indefinitely (class I, LOE: A)
Continue clopidogrel for at least 1 month (class I, LOE: A) and ideally up to 1 year (class I, LOE: B)
Discontinue IV GP IIb/IIIa if started previously (class I, LOE: A)
Discontinue anticoagulant therapy (class I, LOE: A)

Figure 6.6A Therapeutic Pathways for Acute Ischemia. Initial conservative strategy. [a] Recurrent symptoms/ischemia, heart failure, or serious arrhythmia. Abbreviations are defined in the legend for Figure 6.6B.

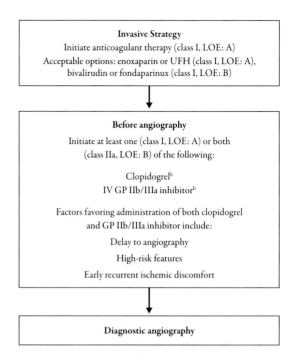

Invasive Strategy

Initiate anticoagulant therapy (class I, LOE: A)

Acceptable options: enoxaparin or UFH (class I, LOE: A), bivalirudin or fondaparinux (class I, LOE: B)

↓

Before angiography

Initiate at least one (class I, LOE: A) or both (class IIa, LOE: B) of the following:

Clopidogrel[b]
IV GP IIb/IIIa inhibitor[b]

Factors favoring administration of both clopidogrel and GP IIb/IIIa inhibitor include:

Delay to angiography
High-risk features
Early recurrent ischemic discomfort

↓

Diagnostic angiography

Figure 6.6B Therapeutic Pathways for Acute Ischemia. Initial invasive strategy. [b] Evidence exists that GP IIb/IIIa inhibitors may not be necessary if a patient received a preloading dose of at least 300 mg of clopidogrel at least 6 hours earlier (class I, LOE B for clopidogrel administration) and bivalirudin is selected as the anticoagulant (class IIa, LOE B). ASA indicates acetylsalicylic acid; EF, ejection fraction; GP, glycoprotein; IV, intravenous; LOE, level of evidence; LVEF, left ventricular ejection fraction; UFH, unfractioned heparin. (Both A and B adapted from Anderson JL, Adams CD, Antman EM, Bridges CR, Califf RM, Casey DE Jr, et al. ACC/AHA 2007 guidelines for the management of patients with unstable angina/non–ST-elevation myocardial infarction: a report of the American College of Cardiology/ American Heart Association Task Force on Practice Guidelines [Writing Committee to Revise the 2002 Guidelines for the Management of Patients With Unstable Angina/Non–ST-Elevation Myocardial Infarction]. J Am Coll Cardiol. 2007 Aug 14;50[7]:e1–157 and Anderson JL, Adams CD, Antman EM, Bridges CR, Califf RM, Casey DE Jr, et al. ACC/AHA 2007 guidelines for the management of patients with unstable angina/non–ST-elevation myocardial infarction: a report of the American College of Cardiology/American Heart Association Task Force on Practice Guidelines [Writing Committee to Revise the 2002 Guidelines for the Management of Patients With Unstable Angina/ Non–ST-Elevation Myocardial Infarction]. Circulation. 2007 Aug 14;116[7]:e148-e304. Epub 2007 Aug 6. Erratum in: Circulation. 2008 Mar 4;117[9]:e180. Used with permission.)

MI is a major public health problem in the United States—about 1 million patients annually are admitted for an acute coronary syndrome, including MI. ST-segment elevation accounts for 20% of these cases. More than 30% of patients with MI die before reaching a hospital. With improved cardiac care, mortality from MI has declined, primarily due to treatment of ventricular arrhythmias. β-Adrenergic blockade has also decreased in-hospital and post-hospital mortality by 30% to 40%. Reperfusion therapy has contributed to improved survival. Currently, the overall in-hospital mortality for patients with an ST-segment elevation MI is 5% to 10%.

- Plaque rupture leads to sudden occlusion of the coronary artery; when untreated, it results in myocardial death.

- Prompt arterial reperfusion improves survival.

- The advent of improved cardiac care has improved survival.

Stunned myocardium occurs when reversible systolic dysfunction of the myocardium follows transient, nonlethal ischemia. With early reperfusion, contraction of the affected myocardium may be decreased and the myocardium remains viable. Systolic contraction returns hours to days later.

- Myocardial stunning may occur due to ischemia, but with early reperfusion the myocardium remains viable and systolic contraction returns.

Infarct remodeling occurs mainly after a large anteroapical MI. An area of infarction may undergo thinning, dilatation, and dyskinesis. Myocardial remodeling may lead to congestive heart failure and increased mortality. Adverse infarct remodeling may be reduced with early initiation of therapy with angiotensin-converting enzyme inhibitors or angiotensin receptor blockers (if angiotensin-converting enzyme inhibitors are contraindicated).

- Myocardial remodeling after an MI increases the risk of heart failure and death.

- Early initiation of therapy with angiotensin-converting enzyme inhibitors or angiotensin receptor blockers can reduce myocardial remodeling.

Presentation and Diagnosis

Patients with ST-segment elevation MI commonly present with angina-like pain lasting longer than 20 minutes associated with typical ECG changes and increased levels of cardiac biomarkers (Figure 6.7). However, more than 25% to 30% of MIs are silent, and silent MIs often occur in patients with diabetes mellitus and in the elderly. In addition, women having an MI often present without "typical" angina-like pain. Symptoms such as nausea, jaw pain, upper back pain, and shortness of breath should be considered possible indicators of ischemia, in addition to chest pain or pressure.

- An ST-segment elevation MI may present with typical angina-like chest pain but often does not.

- Women, persons with diabetes, and the elderly are less likely to experience typical angina-like pain during an MI; thus, a high degree of clinical suspicion is essential.

- Persons with diabetes and the elderly are more likely to suffer a silent MI.

An acute MI is usually diagnosed on the basis of ECG changes (ST elevation or depression or pathologic Q-wave development that meets criteria for diagnosis) in the setting of ischemic symptoms, biochemical markers of myocardial damage, or other evidence of myocardial damage not due to another potential cause.

Management

Bed rest, pain management, and sedation are essential and beneficial in the acute stage of myocardial infarction to decrease myocardial oxygen demand. Oxygen has little benefit after 2 or 3 hours unless hypoxia (oxygen saturation <90%) is present. Modest hypoxemia is common as a result of ventilation-perfusion lung mismatch, even with uncomplicated MI. Continuous ECG monitoring is required to detect tachyarrhythmias and bradyarrhythmias.

- Measures to reduce myocardial oxygen demand are essential.

- Oxygen has some benefit but little beyond 2–3 hours of presentation unless hypoxemia is present.

Aspirin (325 mg) reduces recurrent MI and mortality when given in addition to thrombolytic therapy and

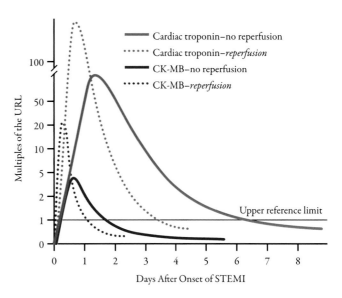

Figure 6.7 Cardiac Biomarkers in ST-Segment Elevation Myocardial Infarction (STEMI). Typical cardiac biomarkers that are used to evaluate patients with STEMI include the MB isoenzyme of creatine kinase (CK-MB) and cardiac-specific troponins. The horizontal line depicts the upper reference limit (URL) for the cardiac biomarker in the clinical chemistry laboratory. The URL is that value representing the 99th percentile of a reference control group without STEMI. The kinetics of release of CK-MB and cardiac troponin in patients who do not undergo reperfusion are shown in the solid blue and red curves as multiples of the URL. Note that when patients with STEMI undergo reperfusion, as depicted in the dotted blue and dotted red curves, the cardiac biomarkers are detected sooner, increase to a higher peak value, but decline more rapidly, resulting in a smaller area under the curve and limitation of infarct size. (Adapted from Antman EM, Anbe DT, Armstrong PW, Bates ER, Green LA, Hand M, et al. ACC/AHA guidelines for the management of patients with ST-elevation myocardial infarction: a report of the American College of Cardiology/American Heart Association Task Force on Practice Guidelines [Committee to Revise the 1999 Guidelines for the management of patients with acute myocardial infarction]. J Am Coll Cardiol. 2004 Aug 4;44[3]:E1-E211 and Antman EM, Anbe DT, Armstrong PW, Bates ER, Green LA, Hand M, et al; American College of Cardiology; American Heart Association Task Force on Practice Guidelines; Canadian Cardiovascular Society. ACC/AHA guidelines for the management of patients with ST-elevation myocardial infarction: a report of the American College of Cardiology/American Heart Association Task Force on Practice Guidelines [Committee to Revise the 1999 Guidelines for the Management of Patients with Acute Myocardial Infarction]. Circulation. 2004 Aug 31;110[9]:e82–292. Errata in: Circulation. 2005 Apr 19;111[15]:2013–4. Circulation. 2007 Apr 17;115[15]:e411. Circulation. 2010 Jun 15;121[23]:e441. Used with permission.)

should be administered upon admission. Clopidogrel (75 mg daily) is an alternative in patients with aspirin allergy or intolerance. Clopidogrel therapy is also indicated in patients given thrombolytics and should be started on day 1 and continued during the hospitalization and possibly up to 4 weeks.

- Aspirin in combination with thrombolytic therapy leads to decreased recurrent MI and improved survival.

- Dual antiplatelet therapy (aspirin and clopidogrel) is indicated.

Anticoagulation prevents recurrent infarction (especially after thrombolytic therapy, when it should be administered for at least 24 hours), deep vein thrombosis, and intracardiac thrombus formation. Long-duration anticoagulation is indicated for higher-risk patients (large anterior myocardial infarction for which reperfusion therapy was not given or was unsuccessful, atrial fibrillation, previous embolus). Thromboembolism is uncommon in patients in whom reperfusion therapy is successful. Unfractionated heparin or low-molecular-weight heparin can be used.

- Anticoagulation reduces recurrent infarction and other complications of an ST-segment elevation MI.

- If thrombolytic therapy was not used or was unsuccessful, atrial fibrillation is present, or the patient had a prior embolic event, anticoagulation should be used for a longer duration.

Nitroglycerin is useful for certain patients with MI: those with pulmonary edema, severely increased blood pressure, or persistent myocardial ischemia. Intravenous nitroglycerin should be given instead of long-acting oral nitrates. Nitrate intolerance develops with infusions of more than 24 hours in duration. Intravenous nitroglycerin should not be given in the setting of low blood pressure (systolic <90 mm Hg) or right ventricular infarction or in patients who have used a phosphodiesterase inhibitor (eg, sildenafil) within the previous 24 hours (48 hours for tadalafil).

- Nitroglycerin should be used in the setting of pulmonary edema, severe hypertension, or persistent ischemia.

- Nitroglycerin tolerance develops when infusions are used for longer than 24 hours.

- Intravenous nitroglycerin should be avoided in the setting of hypotension, right ventricular infarct, or recent use of phosphodiesterase inhibitors.

β-Adrenergic blockade during and after MI lowers mortality in the hospital and after discharge. Oral β-adrenergic blockers should be administered at presentation to patients who do not have contraindications. Intravenous administration may be considered in hypertensive patients. Contraindications to β-adrenergic blockers are bradycardia (heart rate <60 beats per minute), second- or third-degree atrioventricular block, hypotension (systolic blood pressure <100 mm Hg), acute heart failure, cardiogenic shock, and cocaine-induced myocardial infarction. The need for continued treatment should be reassessed periodically. Beneficial effects include decreased pain, decreased myocardial oxygen demand, reduced ventricular fibrillation, decreased platelet aggregability, and decreased sympathetic effects on the myocardium. β-Adrenergic blockers are most beneficial for patients with a large infarction who are at higher risk for complications.

- β-Adrenergic blockers improve survival.

- Exercise caution with the use of β-adrenergic blockers in the setting of contraindications.

- β-Adrenergic blockade leads to decreased pain, myocardial oxygen demand, ventricular fibrillation, platelet aggregation, and sympathetic effects on heart muscle.

Calcium channel blockers are generally not used in patients with an acute MI. However, diltiazem may be used to control ventricular rate in atrial fibrillation, especially if β-adrenergic blockers are contraindicated. Amlodipine may be used to treat hypertension after the acute phase.

Angiotensin-converting enzyme inhibitors prevent ventricular remodeling, especially after a large anterior myocardial infarction. Oral therapy may be initiated within the first 24 hours if blood pressure and renal function are stable. Angiotensin-converting enzyme inhibitors are absolutely indicated in patients with anterior infarction, congestive heart failure, or left ventricular ejection fraction less than 40%. It is reasonable to treat all patients after ST-segment elevation myocardial infarction in the absence of hypotension or contraindications. Angiotensin-receptor blockers are recommended as an alternative in patients who are intolerant of or allergic to angiotensin-converting enzyme inhibitors.

- Avoid calcium channel blockers during an acute MI.

- Consider diltiazem for rate control in atrial fibrillation if β-adrenergic blockers cannot be used.

- Angiotensin-converting enzyme inhibitors prevent ventricular remodeling after an MI and should be considered for all patients after ST-segment elevation MI unless contraindicated.

Long-term aldosterone blockade (spironolactone or eplerenone) is indicated for patients without renal dysfunction (creatinine, <2.0 mg/dL for women and <2.5 mg/dL for men) or hyperkalemia (potassium, <5.0 mEq/L) who are receiving therapeutic doses of angiotensin-converting enzyme inhibitors and have a left ventricular ejection fraction of less than 40% with either symptomatic heart failure or diabetes mellitus.

- Consider aldosterone blockade when the left ventricular ejection fraction is less than 40% in patients with diabetes mellitus or symptomatic heart failure when therapeutic doses of angiotensin-converting enzyme inhibitors are being used.

- Renal dysfunction and hyperkalemia are contraindications to use of aldosterone blockade agents.

Glycoprotein IIb/IIIa inhibitors are given only if primary PCI is performed, and their use is generally initiated in the cardiac catheterization laboratory. They are not indicated in patients treated with thrombolytics.

- Glycoprotein IIb/IIIa inhibitors should be used when PCI is performed.

- Glycoprotein IIb/IIIa inhibitors are not indicated with thrombolysis.

Magnesium does not seem to have a therapeutic role after MI and should be given only for the treatment of torsades de pointes or if a patient has documented hypomagnesemia of potential clinical significance.

- Avoid magnesium unless treating torsades de pointes or hypomagnesemia.

Reperfusion Therapy

Early reperfusion therapy decreases mortality by approximately 25%. The extent of myocardial salvage and degree of beneficial effect on mortality are measurably improved the earlier reperfusion occurs. Mortality is as low as 1% when fibrinolysis is given less than 90 minutes after the onset of pain. The majority of delays to reperfusion lie in time to patient presentation, transport, and in-hospital institution of therapy. Reperfusion at 2 to 6 hours results in a lesser effect on myocardial salvage but still has an important effect on survival.

- Early reperfusion decreases mortality considerably.
- When reperfusion occurs 2–6 hours after onset of symptoms, less myocardium is salvaged but survival is still improved.

Reperfusion therapy with fibrinolytics (thrombolytics) or primary PCI is indicated for patients presenting within 12 hours of onset of symptoms with the following findings: 1+ mm of ST-segment elevation in 2 adjacent leads, a new (or presumably new) left bundle branch block, or a true posterior myocardial infarction.

PCI is more effective than fibrinolysis for restoring normal coronary blood flow (TIMI grade 3) (90% vs 65%–70%). However, intravenous fibrinolysis allows faster administration and is more widely available. The preferred strategy depends on time since the onset of symptoms, transportation time to a skilled PCI laboratory, risk profile of the patient, and contraindications to fibrinolytics. Primary PCI is indicated for patients with immediate access to a high-volume catheterization laboratory, a contraindication to intravenous fibrinolysis, high-risk ST-segment elevation MI (eg, cardiogenic shock or pulmonary edema), or continued ischemia after thrombolytic therapy (rescue PCI).

- PCI is more effective than fibrinolysis for restoring normal coronary blood flow but is less widely available and in most settings cannot be initiated as quickly.
- Several factors determine the preferred strategy.
- PCI is indicated in the setting of high-risk ST-segment elevation MI, ongoing or recurrent ischemia after fibrinolytic therapy, or contraindications to fibrinolytic therapy.
- Consider PCI rather than fibrinolysis when a skilled, high-volume PCI laboratory is immediately available.

Routine immediate PCI after successful fibrinolytic therapy is not indicated in the absence of ongoing symptoms or

ischemia. Reperfusion therapy is not indicated for patients with ST-segment depression or those who present late (>12 hours after symptom onset) and are asymptomatic without hemodynamic compromise or serious arrhythmia. Fibrinolytic therapy is less beneficial for patients 75 years or older.

- PCI is not indicated after successful fibrinolytic therapy (no evidence of ongoing ischemia or symptoms).
- ST-segment depression, late presentation (>12 hours after symptoms started), and lack of symptoms with normal hemodynamics and normal cardiac rhythm are contraindications to reperfusion therapy.
- Fibrinolysis is less beneficial in elderly patients.

Major complications of intravenous fibrinolysis include major bleeding (5%–6%), intracranial bleeding (0.5%), major allergic reaction (0.1%–1.7%), and hypotension (2%–10%). The incidence of myocardial rupture may be higher in patients who are given thrombolytic therapy late (>12 hours after pain onset). Several agents are available for intravenous fibrinolysis, including streptokinase (a nonselective thrombolytic agent) and tissue plasminogen activator (selectively binds to and lyses preformed fibrin). Tissue plasminogen activator has the fastest onset of action. The dosage is 100 mg over 90 minutes. Newer thrombolytic agents such as reteplase and tenecteplase offer better selectivity for active thrombus, but their efficacy is equivalent to that of tissue plasminogen activator in clinical trials. Their greatest advantage is the ability to administer them as a bolus, which reduces drug errors and speeds delivery. Streptokinase is rarely used in the United States, and tenecteplase and reteplase are now the most commonly used fibrinolytics.

- Major complications of fibrinolysis are bleeding (including intracranial), allergic reaction, and hypotension.
- Late fibrinolysis may increase the incidence of myocardial rupture.

After intravenous fibrinolytic administration, a high-grade residual lesion is usually present. Reocclusion or ischemia occurs in 15% to 20% of patients and reinfarction occurs in 2% to 3%. Heparin should be given in conjunction with intravenous fibrinolysis with tissue-specific plasminogen activators used to prevent reinfarction. The indications for coronary angiography or PCI after intravenous fibrinolysis are spontaneous or inducible ischemia, cardiogenic shock, pulmonary edema, ejection fraction less than 40%, and serious arrhythmias.

- Reocclusion or ischemia occur in 15% to 20% of patients after fibrinolysis.
- Heparin should be used with a tissue plasminogen activator to prevent reinfarction.
- Spontaneous or inducible ischemia, cardiogenic shock, pulmonary edema, ejection fraction <40%, and serious

arrhythmias are indications for angiography (and possible PCI) after fibrinolysis.

Acute Mechanical Complications of ST-Segment Elevation MI

Mechanical complications are relatively uncommon in patients who receive reperfusion therapy and include cardiogenic shock, myocardial free wall rupture, papillary muscle rupture, and ventricular septal defects. Right ventricular infarct may also occur after an inferior MI.

- Mechanical complications are relatively uncommon after reperfusion therapy.

Most cases of cardiogenic shock are due to extensive left ventricular dysfunction. Echocardiography is helpful to determine the mechanism of cardiogenic shock. The mortality from cardiogenic shock is 50% (Table 6.3).

- Severe left ventricular dysfunction is the most common cause of cardiogenic shock after ST-segment elevation MI.

Right ventricular infarction occurs in up to 40% of patients with inferior myocardial infarction, can present hours to days after the infarction, and is diagnosed from increased jugular venous pressure in the presence of clear lung fields. ST-segment elevation in lead V_4R is diagnostic of a large right ventricular infarction and portends increased mortality. In extreme circumstances, right ventricular infarction can cause cardiogenic shock due to compromised left ventricle filling. Treatment includes intravenous fluid resuscitation and dobutamine infusion. When right ventricular infarction is recognized early, reperfusion therapy is indicated.

- Right ventricular infarction is relatively common after an inferior ST-segment elevation MI and causes increased jugular venous pressure with clear lung fields. ST elevation in lead V_4R is diagnostic.

- Cardiogenic shock may occur in extreme circumstances; treat with fluid resuscitation and dobutamine.

- Reperfusion therapy is indicated.

Myocardial free wall rupture causes abrupt decompensation. Free wall rupture occurs in 85% of all ruptures. It usually occurs 2 to 14 days after transmural MI, most commonly in elderly hypertensive women, and usually presents as electromechanical dissociation or death. Tamponade may occur if the rupture is contained in the pericardium. If the diagnosis can be made with emergency echocardiography, surgery should be performed. If the rupture is sealed off, a pseudoaneurysm may occur. Surgical treatment is required because of the high incidence of further rupture.

Papillary muscle rupture usually occurs 2 to 10 days after MI. It is associated with inferior myocardial infarction because of the single blood supply to the posteromedial papillary muscle. Rupture of papillary muscle is heralded by the sudden onset of dyspnea and hypotension. Although a murmur may be present, it may not be audible because of equalization of left atrial and left ventricular pressures. The diagnosis is made with echocardiography. The treatment is intra-aortic balloon pump and emergency surgery.

Ventricular septal defects usually occur 1 to 20 days after MI and are equally frequent in inferior and anterior MIs. Ventricular septal defects associated with inferior MIs have a poorer prognosis because of the serpiginous nature of the rupture and associated ventricular infarction. They are indicated by the abrupt onset of dyspnea and hypotension. A loud murmur and systolic thrill are almost always present. The diagnosis is made with echocardiography. Treatment is intra-aortic balloon pump and an emergency operation.

Pre–Hospital-Discharge Evaluation

Risk stratification for long-term outcomes is required before hospital discharge and should include left ventricular function determination, assessment of risk for arrhythmias, and identification of inducible ischemia. A submaximal treadmill test can be performed before discharge, 4 to 6 days after MI.

Table 6.3 **DIAGNOSIS OF CAUSE OF CARDIOGENIC SHOCK**

| CAUSE | PULMONARY ARTERY CATHETERIZATION | | | CATHETERIZATION FINDINGS | TWO-DIMENSIONAL ECHOCARDIOGRAPHY |
	RA	PAWP	CO		
Left ventricular dysfunction	↑	↑↑	↓↓	NA	Poor left ventricle
Right ventricular infarction	↑↑	↓	↓↓	NA	Dilated right ventricle
Tamponade	↑↑	↑↑	↓↓	End-equalization	Pericardial tamponade
Papillary muscle rupture	↑	↑↑	↓↓	Large V	Severe mitral regurgitation
Ventricular septal defect	↑	↑↑	↑	Step-up	Defect seen
Pulmonary emboli	↑↑	=	↓	PADP >PAWP	Dilated right ventricle

Abbreviations: CO, cardiac output; NA, not applicable; PADP, pulmonary artery diastolic pressure; PAWP, pulmonary artery wedge pressure; RA, right atrial pressure.

Alternatively, a symptom-limited treadmill test can be performed safely 10 to 21 days after MI. If a submaximal treadmill test is performed before discharge, a late symptom-limited treadmill test should be performed at follow-up evaluation 3 to 6 weeks after MI. High-risk patients identified by treadmill exertion testing have an ST-segment depression greater than 1 mm, a decrease in blood pressure, or an inability to achieve 4 metabolic equivalents on the exercise test. Imaging exercise tests may identify additional high-risk patients by demonstrating multiple areas of ischemia. Pharmacologic stress tests (dobutamine echocardiography, dipyridamole thallium scanning, or adenosine thallium scanning) may be useful for patients unable to exercise.

- Risk stratification is required before hospital discharge.
- Risk stratification includes determination of left ventricular function, arrhythmia risk assessment, and identification of inducible ischemia.

Increasingly, rather than a stress test, a delayed invasive (pharmacoinvasive) strategy is being practiced in which coronary angiography is performed at least 4 hours after fibrinolysis and before hospital discharge. PCI is performed in the majority of patients, and few undergo CABG or medical therapy alone. The choice between PCI and CABG is based on factors similar to those used to make the decision in patients with stable coronary artery disease. This strategy is associated with lower recurrent ischemia and infarction compared with the ischemia-guided approach described above.

Optimal risk factor modification is essential, including an exercise program, weight loss, and dietary modifications. The goal of treatment is to decrease the low-density lipoprotein cholesterol level to 100 mg/dL or less (optimal <70). If the level is more than 100 mg/dL, statin treatment should be initiated before discharge. All tobacco users should be counseled and nicotine cessation must be stressed.

Aspirin and statins decrease recurrent MI and mortality and should be given to all patients unless contraindicated. β-Adrenergic blockers improve survival after MI and are most effective in high-risk patients (ie, decreased left ventricular function and ventricular arrhythmias). Chronic therapy may not be required for low-risk patients. Antiarrhythmic agents are associated with increased mortality and should not be used to suppress ventricular ectopy. Angiotensin-converting enzyme inhibitors decrease mortality after anterior MI and depressed left ventricular function, presumably by inhibiting infarct remodeling. A rehabilitation program is essential for the patient's well-being and cardiovascular fitness. An automatic implantable cardioverter-defibrillator should be considered if the ejection fraction is less than 35% 1 month after MI in patients with an expected survival of at least 1 year.

- Optimize risk factors, including exercise program, weight loss, and dietary modifications.
- Tobacco users must be counseled to quit and assistance offered.
- Provide aspirin and statins to decrease recurrent MI and mortality.
- β-Adrenergic blockers improve survival after MI, particularly in high-risk patients.
- Angiotensin-converting enzyme inhibitors decrease remodeling and are recommended.
- Antiarrhythmic agents are *not* recommended.
- Consider an automatic implantable cardioverter-defibrillator in patients with an ejection fraction <35% 1 month after MI if the life expectancy is at least 1 year.

SUMMARY

- The Framingham risk score is derived from a patient's risk factors for ischemic heart disease.
- Modifiable (and possibly some nonmodifiable) risk factors lead to chronic endothelial injury that may progress through endogenous changes to more advanced changes in the coronary vessel wall.
- Mismatched oxygen demand and supply lead to myocardial ischemia.
- Coronary artery spasm may occur in the setting of arterial injury and endothelial dysfunction.
- Acute coronary syndromes include unstable angina and acute MI.

7.

VASCULAR DISEASES

Henna Kalsi, MD, and Robert D. McBane, MD

GOALS

- Review the pathogenesis and clinical presentation of common arterial diseases.

- Describe the evaluation and treatment of these common arterial diseases.

- Identify atypical vascular diseases on the basis of clinical presentation.

DISEASE OF THE AORTA

ANEURYSMAL DISEASE

Thoracic Aortic Aneurysm

The histopathologic features of thoracic aortic aneurysms (TAA) depend on aneurysm location. Ascending aorta aneurysm is typically due to medial degeneration, whereas descending thoracic aorta aneurysm is primarily due to atherosclerosis. Men and women are equally affected, and the prevalence of TAA increases with advancing age. Overall incidence is approximately 1 per 10,000 individuals, and 20% of patients with TAA have at least 1 affected first-degree relative. Typical risk factors include history of tobacco exposure, chronic systemic hypertension, infection, and trauma.

- Ascending TAA is typically due to medial degeneration, whereas descending TAA is usually due to atherosclerosis.

- Men and women are equally affected.

- The prevalence of TAA increases with age. Other common risk factors include smoking history and hypertension.

- Trauma is an important risk factor to consider.

- A familial tendency to develop TAA exists.

Uncommon causes to consider include arteritis and connective tissue disorders, including temporal arteritis (age >50 years) or Takayasu arteritis (age <50 years), Behçet

disease, ankylosing spondylitis, syphilitic aortitis, Marfan syndrome, Loeys-Dietz syndrome, and Ehlers-Danlos syndrome. Clinical clues include young age at onset or diagnosis (<40 years), ascending aortic involvement (especially the root), and family history of aortic dissection or sudden death. Specific clinical clues may include ectopia lentis (Marfan syndrome); bifid uvula (Loeys-Dietz syndrome); visceral perforation such as gastrointestinal, uterine, or pneumothorax (Ehlers-Danlos syndrome); and coarctation, bicuspid aortic valve, webbed neck, and short stature (Turner syndrome).

- TAA may occur in patients with arteritis and connective tissue diseases. Consider these causes with ascending aortic involvement or other clinical features.

Most TAAs are asymptomatic and incidentally discovered on chest radiography (Figure 7.1). If symptomatic, patients may report chest or back pain, vocal hoarseness, cough, dyspnea, stridor, or dysphagia. Hemoptysis or hematemesis may occur in the setting of erosion into adjacent structures. Findings on physical examination may include hypertension or fixed distention of a neck vein(s). Findings on cardiac examination may include mid systolic clicks (bicuspid aortic valve), and systolic or diastolic murmurs (aortic regurgitation). Other examination findings may include a fixed vocal cord, signs of cerebral or systemic embolism, or other aneurysmal disease (ie, abdominal aortic aneurysm [AAA]), and synchronous aneurysms should be sought (AAA, femoral and popliteal aneurysms).

- TAA may be asymptomatic and incidentally discovered on imaging or may be symptomatic.

- Symptoms and physical examination findings may assist with identification of TAA.

- Synchronous other aneurysmal disease should be sought.

Complications of TAA include rupture, dissection, or, rarely, thromboembolism. There is a direct correlation

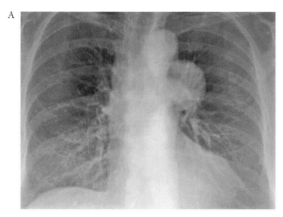

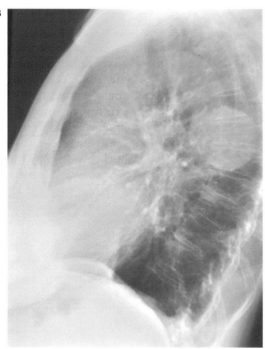

Figure 7.1 Chest Radiographs Show a Large Mass in Left Posterior Aspect of Chest. A, Anteroposterior. B, Lateral.

between aneurysm size and risk of rupture (diameter <4.0 cm, 0%; 4.0–5.9 cm, 16%; ≥6.0 cm, 31%).

The diagnosis is confirmed with magnetic resonance imaging (MRI) (Figure 7.2A), computed tomography (CT) (Figure 7.2B), or transesophageal echocardiography (TEE).

Diastolic hypertension, large aneurysm size (critical hinge point for rupture: >6 cm at the ascending aorta and >7 cm at the descending thoracic aorta), traumatic aneurysm, and associated coronary and carotid artery disease worsen prognosis. The cumulative risk of rupture after 5 years is 20%, but rupture risk is a function of aneurysm size at recognition.

- Confirm the diagnosis of TAA with CT, MRI, or TEE.

- Complications of TAA include rupture, dissection, and rarely thrombosis.

- Aneurysmal size is an important factor in determining risk of rupture.

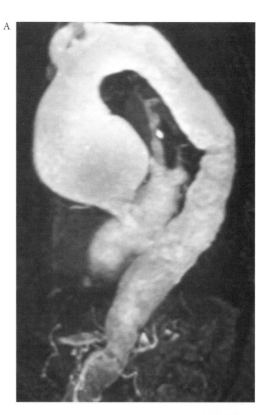

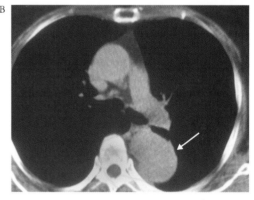

Figure 7.2 Imaging of Thoracic Aortic Aneurysm. A, Magnetic resonance angiogram (longitudinal view) shows a large ascending aortic aneurysm and moderate aortic regurgitation. B, Computed tomogram shows a saccular aneurysm in the mid descending thoracic aorta (arrow).

- Diastolic hypertension, traumatic aneurysm, and associated vascular disease worsen prognosis.

Medical management places strong emphasis on control of systemic hypertension with a goal blood pressure of less than 140/90 mm Hg (130/80 mm Hg if there is coexisting diabetes mellitus). Preferred antihypertensive agents include β-adrenergic blockers or angiotensin receptor blockers; blood pressure should be reduced to the lowest point tolerable. β-Adrenergic blocking drugs should be administered to all patient with Marfan syndrome who have aortic aneurysm to reduce the growth rate of aortic dilatation unless contraindicated. Statin therapy to achieve a target low-density lipoprotein cholesterol value of 70 mg/dL or less is warranted (class IIa).

Smoking cessation is warranted. Unless surgical repair is already indicated, serial follow-up of patients combines clinical assessment with noninvasive imaging tests. Elective surgical repair is indicated for ascending TAA of 5.5 cm or more and for descending TAA of 6.0 cm or more or if the growth rate exceeds 0.5 cm per year in either. Elective repair is indicated in patients with Marfan syndrome, Loeys-Dietz syndrome, or Ehlers-Danlos syndrome when size is more than 4.5 cm. Elective repair is indicated in patients with bicuspid aortic valves if the diameter of the aortic root or ascending aorta is 5.0 cm or more or if growth rate exceeds 0.5 cm per year.

- Medical management of TAA with aggressive risk factor modification is strongly advised.

- Unless surgical repair is already indicated, follow patients with clinical assessment in combination with noninvasive imaging to assess for changes in aneurysm diameter.

- Elective repair is indicated when the aneurysm size reaches 5.5 cm for ascending TAA, 6 cm for descending TAA, or ≥5.0 cm in patients with bicuspid aortic valve; when growth rate of any TAA exceeds 0.5 cm per year; or in patients with Marfan, Loeys-Dietz, or Ehlers-Danlos syndrome and an aneurysm size >4.5 cm (Circulation. 2010 Apr 6;121[13]:e266–369. Epub 2010 Mar 6).

Abdominal Aortic Aneurysm

The abdominal aorta is the commonest site of aneurysm. Men are 5 times more commonly affected than women, and the incidence increases with age. The prevalence of AAA is 3% among persons 50 years or older. Most aneurysms are due to atherosclerosis. Tobacco use is a considerable risk factor. However, other diseases must be considered, including connective tissue diseases (Marfan syndrome, Ehlers-Danlos syndrome, pseudoxanthoma elasticum), infection, trauma, or vasculitis (Takayasu arteritis and temporal arteritis). Twenty-five percent of patients with AAA have an affected relative; thus, a familial predisposition is suspected. Most AAAs are infrarenal. Suprarenal AAAs (2%–5%) are usually due to distal extension of a thoracic aneurysm (thoracoabdominal aneurysm).

- AAA is 5 times more likely to develop in men than women.

- Atherosclerosis (and its risk factors) is a major risk factor for AAA.

- Patients with certain connective tissue diseases or vasculitides are at higher-than-average risk to develop AAA.

- Twenty-five percent of patients with AAA have an affected relative.

Most patients with AAA are asymptomatic. Livedo reticularis, blue toes with palpable pulses, hypertension, renal insufficiency, increased erythrocyte sedimentation rate, and transient eosinophilia imply AAA-associated atheroembolism (Figure 7.3). Abdominal or low back pain suggests aneurysm instability. The triad of severe abdominal pain, hypotension, and a tender abdominal mass characterize AAA rupture. The annual risk of rupture is directly related to aneurysm size: 4.0 cm, <2%; 5.0 cm, 5%; 6.0 cm, 10%; and 7.0 cm or more, 20%.

- Most patients with AAA are asymptomatic.

- History and physical examination features are important for identifying AAA instability, rupture, and associated atheroembolism.

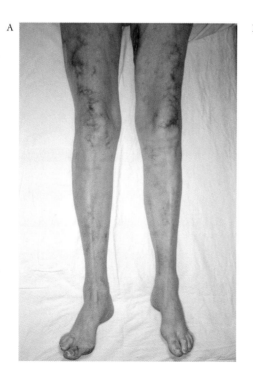
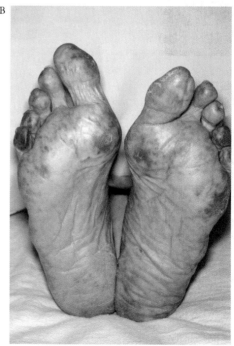

Figure 7.3 Findings in a Patient With Atheroembolism. A and B, Livedo reticularis (upper aspect of thighs, plantar surface of feet) and multiple blue toes.

- Severe abdominal pain, hypotension, and a tender abdominal mass should increase suspicion of AAA rupture.
- Annual risk of rupture is related to aneurysm size.

The most common physical examination finding is a pulsatile abdominal mass. The sensitivity of abdominal palpation for the detection of AAA is relatively low: 43% overall (57% for aneurysms >4.0 cm in diameter and 29% for aneurysms <4.0 cm in diameter). A 1-time screening ultrasonography for men 65 to 75 years old who have ever smoked is recommended, and AAA screening is indicated for men 60 years or older who have a first-degree family history of AAA. Ultrasonography, CT and CT angiography, or MRI and MR angiography are reliable for diagnosis (Figure 7.4).

- A pulsatile abdominal mass is the most common physical finding of AAA, but the sensitivity of abdominal palpation for AAA detection is low.

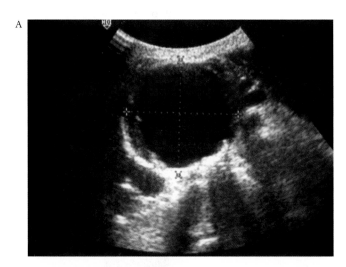

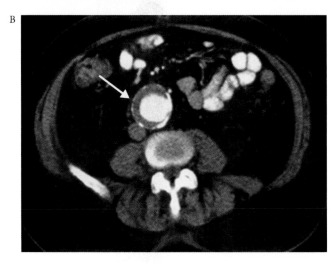

Figure 7.4 Imaging of Abdominal Aortic Aneurysm. A, Ultrasonogram (transverse view) shows a 4.7-cm aneurysm. B, Computed tomogram (contrast-enhanced) shows aneurysm (arrow).

- One-time screening is advised for men 65 to 75 years old who have any smoking history and men older than 60 years who have an affected first-degree relative (http://www.uspreventiveservicestaskforce.org/uspstf/uspsaneu.htm).

Medical management includes modification of atherosclerotic risk factors, including blood pressure control (preferably with a β-adrenergic blocker), tobacco cessation, and statin therapy. Patients should be followed with serial imaging of the aneurysm every 6 to 12 months if the aneurysm is more than 4.0 cm and every 2 to 3 years if it is less than 4.0 cm.

Endovascular repair of AAA with stent grafts is an alternative to open surgical repair. Endovascular and surgical repair are associated with similar risks of overall and aneurysm-related mortality. Graft-related complications are higher for endovascular AAA repair. An endoleak (ie, persistent flow into the aneurysm sac, most often due to patent branch vessels feeding the aneurysm sac) is the most common graft-related complication. It is usually repaired by catheter-based techniques. Because of the risk of endovascular leak, serial CT angiography surveillance is required indefinitely. For this reason, endovascular repair is often reserved for older patients with increased surgical risk, whereas open repair is recommended for younger patients at low to average surgical risk.

- Aggressive risk factor modification is recommended for AAA, including blood pressure control, tobacco cessation, and lipid management. β-Adrenergic blockers and statins are advised.
- The frequency of serial imaging depends on aneurysm size (every 6–12 months if >4.0 cm and every 2–3 years if <4.0 cm).
- Endovascular and open surgical repair have similar overall and aneurysm-related mortality. Open repair is indicated for patients at low to average operative risk (including young patients), whereas endovascular repair is generally reserved for older patients because of the risk of endoleak and the need for serial CT imaging indefinitely.

THORACIC AORTIC DISSECTION

Aortic dissection begins with a tear through the arterial intima that allows pulsating blood to penetrate along the media longitudinally, separating the arterial wall. The dissection extends before either reentering the lumen through a second intimal tear or exiting the artery through an adventitial tear. Dissection can be catastrophic, leading to occlusion of the affected artery or its branch vessels or to arterial rupture with varying degrees of blood loss. Causes include atherosclerosis (and its risk factors), hypertension, cystic medial necrosis (ascending aorta, including connective tissue disease processes such as Marfan syndrome), bicuspid or unicuspid aortic valve, or trauma (blunt or penetrating). Dissection may also be iatrogenic, such as cardiac surgery or invasive angiography. Aortic dissection may complicate pregnancy in at-risk women; when this occurs, it is usually in the third trimester. An intramural hematoma (10% of dissection cases) may also occur if bleeding develops within the media without intimal tear or flowing blood within a false lumen. A penetrating aortic ulcer (10% of dissection cases) results from an area of aortic ulceration that penetrates through the internal elastic lamina with bleeding into the media, often in a segment of atheromatous plaque. Incomplete rupture of the thoracic aorta (in the region of the aortic isthmus) results from a sudden deceleration injury, frequently a motor vehicle crash (Figure 7.5).

- Aortic dissection may be due to atherosclerosis, aortic valve anomalies, connective tissue diseases, or trauma or may be iatrogenic.

- Catastrophic outcomes may result from aortic dissection.

- Penetrating aortic ulcers and intramural hematomas may occur in 10% of dissections.

- Sudden deceleration injuries, usually due to motor vehicle accidents, may cause incomplete aortic rupture.

Symptoms of aortic dissection include sudden-onset, severe, often migratory pain in the anterior aspect of the chest, back, or abdomen; these occur in 70% to 80% of patients (sensitivity 90%, specificity 84%). The pain is often described as "ripping," "tearing," or "stabbing." Hypertension is present in 70% of patients. Additional findings include a diastolic murmur due to aortic regurgitation (from disruption of the aortic annulus; 20%), pulse deficits (30%), neurologic changes (20%), and syncope (13%). A pulse deficit portends a worse outcome; when it is present, in-hospital mortality increases to 45% (compared with 15% if absent). Focal neurologic deficits imply carotid transection. Hypotension, tachycardia, jugular venous distension, systemic vascular congestion, and pulsus paradoxus suggest pericardial tamponade due to rupture into the pericardium. Congestive heart failure is usually due to acute, severe aortic regurgitation. Acute myocardial infarction, pericarditis, and complete heart block may also occur.

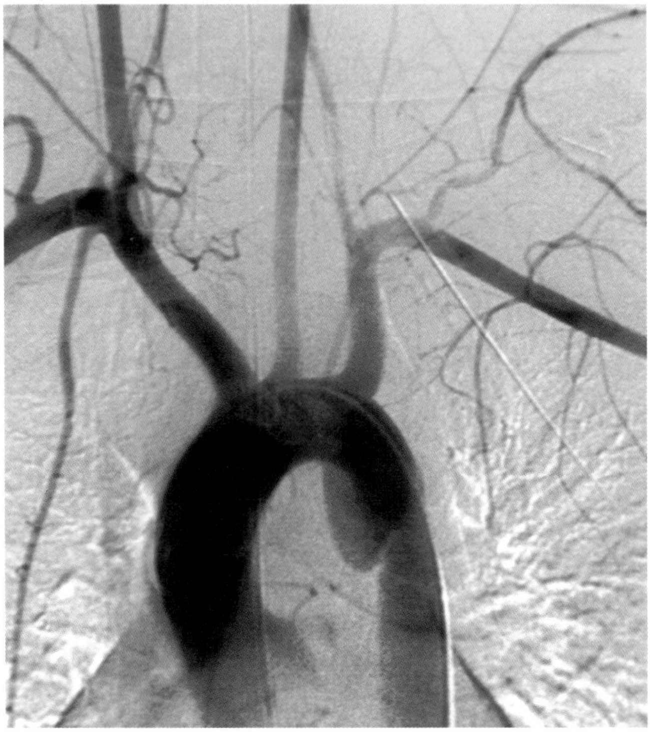

- The majority of patients with aortic dissection report sudden severe chest, back, or abdominal pain. The pain is often described as "ripping," "tearing," or "stabbing."

- In-hospital mortality is increased in the setting of a pulse deficit.

- Pericardial tamponade due to rupture into the pericardium is a potentially devastating result of dissection.

- Severe aortic regurgitation due to aortic annulus disruption may lead to congestive heart failure.

- Other cardiac consequences include acute myocardial infarction, pericarditis, and complete heart block.

- Focal neurologic deficits imply transection of the carotid artery.

Chest radiography may show widening of the superior mediastinum (Figure 7.6) and supracardiac aortic shadow, deviation of the trachea from the midline, a discrepancy in diameter between the ascending aorta and the descending aorta, and pleural effusion. Electrocardiography most commonly shows left ventricular hypertrophy, but ST-segment depression, ST-segment elevation, T-wave changes, and the changes of acute pericarditis and complete heart block occur in up to 55% of patients. Diagnosis is readily and accurately

Figure 7.5 Aortogram of Contained Rupture of Proximal Descending Thoracic Aorta Just Distal to Origin of Left Subclavian Artery. Patient was involved in a severe motor vehicle crash.

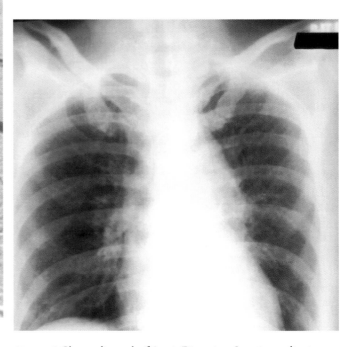

Figure 7.6 Chest radiograph of Aortic Dissection. Superior mediastinum is widened.

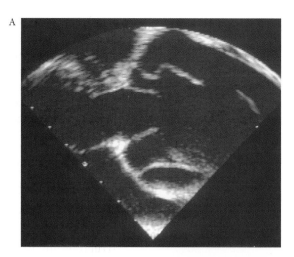

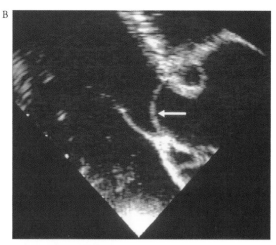

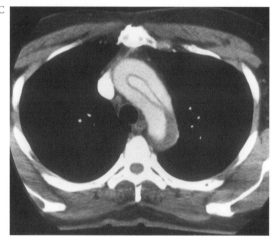

Figure 7.7 Imaging of Aortic Dissection. A and B, Multiplane transesophageal echocardiograms. Longitudinal view (A) shows an intimal flap in the ascending aorta. In diastole (B), the intimal flap prolapses through the aortic valve (arrow). C, Computed tomogram (contrast-enhanced) shows a spiraling intimal flap in the transverse aortic arch.

confirmed with TEE, CT angiography, and MR angiography, all of which are both sensitive and specific (Figure 7.7). Test choice is determined by availability and local expertise.

- Chest radiographic findings may include superior mediastinal widening, a supracardiac aortic shadow, tracheal deviation, pleural effusion, or discrepant ascending and descending aortic diameter.

- Left ventricular hypertrophy is a common electrocardiographic finding, but ST- and T-wave changes, electrical changes due to pericarditis, and complete heart block may also occur.

- TEE or angiography (by CT or MRI) provides an accurate diagnosis, but test choice is determined by availability, the patient's hemodynamic stability, and radiology expertise.

Aortic dissections are classified by location relative to the ascending aorta (Figure 7.8). Aortic dissection involving the ascending aorta is designated as type I or II (proximal, type A), and dissection confined to the descending thoracic aorta is designated as type III (distal, type B). Clinical clues to type I and type II (ascending) aortic dissection include substernal pain, aortic valve incompetence, decreased pulse or blood pressure in the right arm, decreased right carotid pulse, pericardial friction rub, syncope, and ischemic electrocardiographic changes. Patients with Marfan syndrome typically have type A dissections. Clinical clues to type III aortic dissection include interscapular pain, hypertension, and left pleural effusion.

- Type I and II dissections involve the ascending thoracic aorta. They are also known as proximal or type A dissections.

- Type III dissections are confined to the descending aorta. They are also called distal or type B dissections.

- Various clinical findings can provide clues to the dissection location and classification.

Acute dissections of the ascending thoracic aorta require urgent surgical repair because of the high mortality, whereas acute dissections of the descending thoracic aorta should be managed medically with aggressive blood pressure and heart rate control. Intravenous β-adrenergic blockers (goal heart

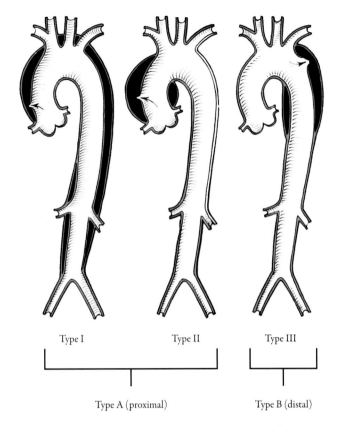

Type I   Type II   Type III

Type A (proximal)   Type B (distal)

Figure 7.8 Classification System for Aortic Dissection.

rate <70 beats per minute) are indicated in the acute setting. Pharmacologic therapy should be instituted as soon as the diagnosis of any aortic dissection is suspected (Box 7.1). If systolic blood pressure remains more than 120 mm Hg, angiotensin-converting enzyme inhibitors or other vasodilators should be administered.

Indications for surgical repair for a descending thoracic aortic dissection include organ malperfusion, progression of the dissection despite aggressive heart rate and blood pressure control, aneurysm enlargement, and inability to control blood pressure or symptoms of the dissection.

Factors predicting a poor prognosis for descending thoracic aortic dissections and the need for surgical repair include aortic diameter more than 4.0 cm or a persistently patent false lumen. Preoperative coronary angiography in acute ascending aortic dissection is *not* indicated because of an association with an increased mortality rate. Treatment of an intramural hematoma or penetrating aortic ulcer is similar to treatment of dissection of the corresponding thoracic aortic segment (surgical if ascending, medical if descending). Once the patient is stabilized, serial imaging is necessary to monitor progression and development of aneurysmal disease.

The management of acute aortic dissection is summarized in Figure 7.9.

- Acute dissections of the ascending aorta require urgent surgical repair.

- Coronary angiography before surgery for acute ascending aortic dissection is *not* recommended because of associated increased mortality.

- Acute dissections of the descending thoracic aorta should initially be managed medically unless indications for surgical repair become evident.

- Any suspected thoracic aortic rupture should lead to immediate aggressive blood pressure control with β-adrenergic blockers; once the patient is hemodynamically

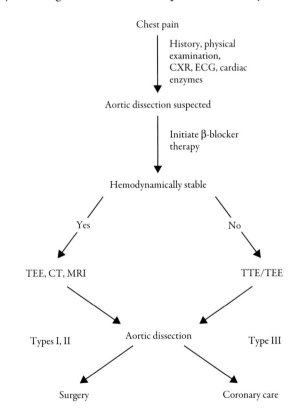

Figure 7.9 Algorithm for Initial Management of Suspected Acute Aortic Dissection. CT indicates computed tomography; CXR, chest radiography; ECG, electrocardiography; MRI, magnetic resonance imaging; TEE, transesophageal echocardiography; TTE, transthoracic echocardiography.

stable, investigations and patient status should direct further management.

- Surgical repair of dissections of the descending thoracic aorta is needed when organ malperfusion is present, aneurysm enlargement occurs, blood pressure or symptoms cannot be controlled, or the dissection progresses despite best medical management.

- Surgical repair of dissections of the descending thoracic aorta should be considered when aortic diameter is greater than 4.0 cm or there is a persistently patent false lumen.

THORACIC AORTIC ATHEROSCLEROSIS

The presence of thoracic aortic atheroma or thrombus (including at the arch) is a considerable risk factor for ischemic stroke and systemic embolization. Treatment with a statin and antiplatelet therapy is recommended for patients with aortic arch atheroma to reduce the risk of stroke, unless contraindicated. Anticoagulation with warfarin (goal international normalized ratio, 2.0–3.0) may be a reasonable option and can be considered in patients with prior stroke. TEE accurately assesses aortic atheromatous disease. Aortic arch atheroma larger than 4.0 mm and mobile thrombus of any are substantial risk factors for embolization.

Other complications of thoracic aortic atherosclerosis include subclavian stenosis leading to intermittent arm claudication or subclavian steal syndrome. When these occur, reversal of blood flow (eg, during arm exercise) may lead to transient cerebral ischemia. Physical findings may include reduced upper extremity pulses or blood pressure differential between arms. Delayed pulsation in an arm may be noted (Circulation. 2010 Apr 6;121[13]:e266–369. Epub 2010 Mar 6).

- Atheromatous disease of the thoracic aorta is a considerable risk factor for stroke and systemic embolization.

- Statins and antiplatelet therapy are recommended.

- Anticoagulation should be considered in patients with a prior history of stroke.

- Intermittent arm claudication due to subclavian stenosis or subclavian steal syndrome may occur with thoracic aortic atherosclerosis.

- Subclavian steal syndrome may lead to transient cerebral ischemia due to blood flow reversal.

- Reduced arm pulses, blood pressure discrepancy between arms, or delayed pulsation in an arm should raise suspicion of subclavian steal syndrome.

PERIPHERAL ARTERIAL CONDITIONS

PERIPHERAL ARTERY ANEURYSMS

Peripheral artery aneurysms are most common in men older than 60 years because they are most often due to atherosclerosis.

Coronary and carotid artery disease are common comorbid conditions. Hypertension, tobacco use, trauma, infection, familial tendency, and some connective tissue diseases and vasculitides are additional risk factors. Although most peripheral artery aneurysms are asymptomatic, rupture, infection, embolization, and pressure on surrounding structures can also occur. Rupture is less common in peripheral artery aneurysms than embolization.

- Men >60 years old are more likely than younger men or women to have peripheral artery aneurysms due to atherosclerosis.

- Additional risk factors include trauma, infection, familial tendency, and some connective tissue diseases and vasculitides.

- Most peripheral artery aneurysms are asymptomatic.

- Rupture is less common than embolization.

Iliac artery aneurysms are usually associated with AAA, but they may occur as an isolated finding. Obstructive urologic symptoms, iliac vein obstruction, and unexplained groin or perineal pain can be caused by iliac artery aneurysm and should be investigated. Repair is indicated when the aneurysm size is 3.5 cm or more. Femoral artery aneurysm repair is indicated at a size of 3.0 cm or more. Popliteal artery aneurysm may lead to thromboembolization, neuropathy, or thrombophlebitis in the popliteal distribution, venous obstruction, infection, or rupture. Repair is indicated when the aneurysm is more than 2 cm or when thrombus is present. The greatest concern for popliteal aneurysm is thromboembolism to distal arteries. Popliteal artery aneurysm is bilateral in 50% of patients, and 40% of patients have 1 or more aneurysms at other sites, most commonly the abdominal aorta.

- Iliac and popliteal artery aneurysms can occur in the setting of AAA but may occur in isolation.

- Carotid and coronary artery disease are common comorbid conditions in the setting of iliac artery aneurysms.

- Embolism is the most common complication of femoral and popliteal artery aneurysms.

- Repair is indicated at an aneurysm size of >3.5 cm for the iliac artery, >3.0 cm for the femoral artery, and >2 cm for the popliteal artery, or when an aneurysm is symptomatic.

PERIPHERAL ARTERY DISEASE

Peripheral artery disease of the legs may be symptomatic at presentation (50%) or may be found incidentally (50%). Of symptomatic patients, 40% have intermittent claudication and 10% have critical limb ischemia at diagnosis. Intermittent claudication is the most common symptom and is defined as "exertional pain involving the calf that impedes walking, resolves within 10 minutes of rest, and neither begins at rest nor resolves on walking" (Monogr Ser World Health Organ. 1968;56:

Table 7.1 DIFFERENTIAL DIAGNOSIS OF INTERMITTENT CLAUDICATION AND PSEUDOCLAUDICATION

	CLAUDICATION	PSEUDOCLAUDICATION
Onset	Walking	Standing & walking
Character	Cramp, ache	"Paresthetic"
Bilateral	±	+
Walking distance	Fairly constant	More variable
Cause	Atherosclerosis	Spinal stenosis
Relief	Standing still	Sitting down, leaning forward

Table 7.2 GRADING SYSTEM FOR LOWER-EXTREMITY ARTERIAL OCCLUSIVE DISEASE

| GRADE | ABI | |
	Supine Resting	*Postexercise*[a]
Normal	1.0–1.4	No change or increase
Mild disease	0.8–0.9	>0.5
Moderate disease	0.5–0.8	>0.2
Severe disease	<0.5	<0.2

Abbreviation: ABI, ankle-to-brachial systolic pressure index.

[a] After treadmill exercise (1–2 mph, 10% grade for 5 minutes or until limited by symptoms) or active pedal plantar flexion (50 repetitions or until limited by symptoms).

1–188). Pseudoclaudication (due to lumbar spinal stenosis) is the condition most commonly confused with intermittent claudication. Clinical clues suggesting pseudoclaudication include day-to-day variability of distance to symptom onset, symptom onset with prolonged standing (spinal extension), and need to sit for symptom relief (spinal flexion) (Table 7.1). Other clues may include a history of back pain or spinal operations. Lumbar spinal stenosis can be confirmed with a normal or minimally abnormal ankle-to-brachial systolic pressure index (ABI) before and after exercise in combination with characteristic findings on electromyography and CT or MRI of the lumbar spine. Symptoms of walking impairment remain stable in 75% of affected patients, and less than 2% per year require amputation. However, mortality is high (5 years 30%, 10 years 50%, 15 years 70%), reflecting coexisting atherosclerosis: severe coronary artery disease (40%–60%), carotid artery disease (25%–50%), and renal artery disease (25%–40%).

- Peripheral artery disease of the legs may be symptomatic (usually intermittent claudication) or incidentally identified.

- The most common symptom is intermittent claudication (calf pain due to exertion that resolves with rest, does not begin at rest, and does not resolve with walking).

- Pseudoclaudication may mimic peripheral artery disease, but clinical clues can reliably distinguish the 2 conditions.

- Although fewer than 2% of patients require amputation annually and walking symptoms remain stable in the majority, mortality is high due to comorbid atherosclerotic disease.

ABI screening should be performed in patients with exertional leg symptoms, patients 50 to 60 years old with atherosclerosis risk factors (especially diabetes mellitus or smoking), patients older than 70 years, or patients with a Framingham risk score of more than 10%. Patients with diabetes mellitus should be screened every 5 years (TASC II guidelines. Available from: http://www.tasc-2-pad.org/upload/ssrubriqueproduit/fichier2/597.pdf). Supine ABIs before and after exercise testing (treadmill walking or active pedal plantar

flexion) confirm the diagnosis (Table 7.2). If ABIs are normal at rest but symptoms are suggestive of intermittent claudication, ABIs should be determined before and after treadmill exercise. Heavily calcified peripheral arteries may result in a falsely increased Doppler-derived systolic pressure and invalidate the ABI (>1.3). In these cases, an accurate pressure may be obtained by measuring the toe pressure and calculating the toe-brachial index (a pressure gradient of 20–30 mm Hg is normally present between the ankle and the toe). An abnormally high ABI (>1.4) implies arterial calcification, is associated with diabetes, and is associated with an increased cardiovascular risk. Smoking cessation and lipid-lowering, diabetes mellitus, and hypertension treatment according to national treatment guidelines are recommended for all patients with peripheral artery disease. In patients who continue to use tobacco, the risk for major amputation is increased 10-fold and the mortality rate is increased more than 2-fold. Diabetes mellitus accounts for most amputations (12-fold increased risk of below-knee amputation).

- ABIs should be determined in patients with risk factors for peripheral artery disease: exertional leg symptoms, 50–60 years old with atherosclerosis risk factors (diabetes mellitus: diabetes mellitus, smoking), >70 years old, or Framingham risk score >10%.

- Screen patients with diabetes mellitus every 5 years.

- In the setting of suggestive symptoms and normal rest ABIs, test exertional ABIs.

- Calcified peripheral arteries can falsely increase ABIs. Measure toe pressure to calculate toe-brachial index.

- All patients with peripheral artery disease should have aggressive management of lipids, diabetes mellitus, hypertension, and tobacco use.

- Smoking considerably increases the risk of major amputation and the mortality rate.

- Diabetes accounts for the greatest number of amputations among patients with peripheral artery disease.

All patients with peripheral artery disease should receive aspirin (81–325 mg daily) or clopidogrel if they are aspirin-allergic to reduce the risk of limb loss, need for vascular surgery, and incidence of major coronary and cerebrovascular events. Clopidogrel (75 mg daily) has been shown to be more effective than aspirin for preventing major atherosclerotic vascular events in patients with peripheral artery disease (Lancet. 1996 Nov 16;348[9038]:1329–39). Cilostazol can be used for relief of claudication symptoms and improves walking distance to claudication compared with pentoxifylline or placebo, but it is *contraindicated* in patients with heart failure. Although there is no evidence that treatment of hypertension alters the progression of claudication, blood pressure should be controlled to reduce morbidity and death due to cardiovascular and cerebrovascular disease. The angiotensin-converting enzyme inhibitor ramipril reduces the risk of ischemic cardiovascular events in patients with peripheral artery disease and may increase walking distance in select patients, in addition to its renal protective effects in diabetes. Statins reduce cardiovascular events in patients with peripheral artery disease, reduce new or worsening claudication, and improve walking distance and pain-free walking time. All patients with peripheral artery disease should receive treatment to reduce the low-density lipoprotein cholesterol value to less than 100 mg/dL (<70 mg/dL in patients with atherosclerosis in other circulatory beds). Systemic antibiotic therapy should be initiated promptly in patients with critical limb ischemia, skin ulcerations, or evidence of limb infection. Patients at risk of critical limb ischemia (ABI <0.4 in a nondiabetic patient or any diabetic with known lower extremity peripheral artery disease) should undergo regular foot inspection to detect objective signs of critical limb ischemia (J Vasc Surg. 2007 Jan;45[Suppl S]:S5–67). Foot care and protection are of paramount importance in patients with diabetes mellitus who have peripheral artery disease. The combination of peripheral neuropathy, small-vessel disease, and peripheral artery disease in patients with diabetes mellitus makes foot trauma more likely to be associated with a nonhealing wound or ulcer.

- Medical management of peripheral artery disease includes treatment with aspirin or clopidogrel and statin therapy. Lipid levels (low-density lipoprotein) should be lowered, and angiotensin-converting enzyme inhibitor therapy with ramipril should be considered. Blood pressure management is strongly encouraged.

- Cilostazol relieves claudication symptoms and increases walking distance.

- Regular foot inspection for signs of critical limb ischemia is necessary in diabetics and patients with peripheral artery disease who are at risk (ABI <0.4).

- Foot care and foot protection are particularly important in patients with diabetes mellitus because of the increased risk of nonhealing wounds or ulcers in the setting of peripheral neuropathy and small-vessel disease.

Supervised walking should be part of the initial treatment for all patients with peripheral artery disease. Maximal walking distance has been shown to improve 200% to 300% when treadmill or track walking is used to the point of symptom reproduction with rest intervals in 30- to 60-minute sessions, 3 times weekly for 3 months.

- All patients with peripheral artery disease should participate in supervised walking to improve walking distance.

Absolute indications for revascularization (surgical bypass or angioplasty and stenting) include ischemic rest pain and nonhealing ulceration. Ischemic ulcers are typically found at pressure points on the foot (eg, between toes "kissing ulcers") and point of contact with a shoe (eg, medial aspect of great toe, lateral aspect of fifth toe, and heels). A relative indication for revascularization includes lifestyle-limiting intermittent claudication. Duplex ultrasonography, MR angiography, and CT angiography define anatomic localization of disease and provide a roadmap necessary for endovascular or surgical therapeutic planning.

Indications for amputation are severe rest pain with no revascularization option, limb gangrene, or life-threatening infection. Below-knee amputation is associated with a mortality rate of 10% perioperatively and 25% at 1 year. The primary healing rate with below-knee amputation is 60%, and 15% of patients will eventually need above-knee amputation.

- Ischemic rest pain and nonhealing ulcers are *absolute* indications for revascularization (surgical or percutaneous), whereas lifestyle-limiting intermittent claudication is a *relative* indication for revascularization.

- Pressure points and contact points with footwear are common locations for ischemic ulcers.

- Ultrasonography, MR angiography, and CT angiography are used to define location of disease and allow mapping for revascularization.

- Below-knee amputation has a 60% primary healing rate, but it is associated with a 10% perioperative mortality rate and a 25% 1-year mortality rate. Fifteen percent of patients will need above-knee amputation in the future.

ACUTE ARTERIAL OCCLUSION

Acute arterial occlusion is suggested by the sudden onset of extreme pain and paresthesia of the involved limb. It is important to distinguish thrombus due to local plaque rupture from an embolic source because the natural histories of these 2 mechanisms differ. Features suggestive of local thrombus include known arterial occlusive disease of the involved limb, which can be identified by examining the pulse integrity of the limbs. An embolic cause is suggested by the presence of cardiac disease (valvular or ischemic), atrial fibrillation, proximal aneurysm, or proximal atherosclerotic disease.

The 6 *P*s suggestive of acute arterial occlusion include pain, pallor, paresthesia, paralysis, poikilothermy (coldness), and pulselessness.

- The 6 *P*s—pain, pallor, paresthesia, paralysis, poikilothermy, and pulselessness—help distinguish acute arterial occlusion due to plaque rupture from local thrombus.
- An embolic source is suggested by the presence of valvular or ischemic cardiac disease, atrial fibrillation, proximal aneurysms, or proximal atherosclerosis; plaque rupture due to local thrombus is suggested by a history of prior occlusive disease and pulse asymmetry.

Therapeutic results from thrombectomy are much better in embolism than in local thrombus. Amputation rates are considerably higher for patients with local thrombus. Infrequent causes of arterial occlusion include dissection, traumatic transection, vasculitis, sepsis or disseminated intravascular coagulation, compartment syndrome, vasospasm, foreign body embolization, or tumor. Tissue tolerance to ischemia varies by tissue type. Nerve injury occurs within 4 hours, whereas muscle (6 hours) and skin (10 hours) are relatively more resistant to ischemia. Angiography is performed after initiation of intravenous heparin therapy and foot protection. After confirmation of the diagnosis, initial therapeutic options include intra-arterial thrombolysis and surgery (thromboembolectomy). If thrombolysis is the initial treatment, percutaneous treatment or surgical therapy is usually indicated for the underlying stenosis (if present) for improvement of long-term patency rates.

- Thrombectomy is more effective for treating acute arterial occlusion that is due to embolism.
- Patients with acute arterial occlusion due to local thrombus are more likely to require amputation.
- Rarely, arterial occlusion is due to dissection, trauma, vasculitis, sepsis or disseminated intravascular occlusion, compartment syndrome, vasospasm, foreign body embolism, or tumor.

Fluid resuscitation is needed to prevent reperfusion syndrome, including myoglobinuric renal failure, metabolic (lactic) acidosis, and hyperkalemia. Four-compartment fasciotomy is often required to prevent muscle and nerve injury associated with the compartment syndrome. Tissue tolerance to ischemia varies; nerves are affected earlier than muscle and skin.

CAROTID ARTERY DISEASE

Carotid artery disease is present in 5% to 9% of the US population older than 65 years and contributes substantially to transient ischemic attacks and strokes. Large vessel disease, most commonly of the carotid artery, accounts for 30% of ischemic strokes. Carotid disease may initially be detected as a bruit. The prevalence of an asymptomatic bruit may be as high as 13% depending on the population examined. Prevalence increases with age. When carotid artery stenosis is more than 70%, the annual stroke risk is only 3% for medically managed *asymptomatic* disease and more than 15% for medically managed symptomatic disease. Medically managed

carotid artery stenosis of less than 60% is associated with an annual stroke risk of less than 1%.

- Carotid artery disease contributes substantially to ischemic strokes.
- An asymptomatic bruit may lead to the diagnosis of carotid artery disease.
- When carotid artery disease is medically managed, the annual stroke risk is 3% in asymptomatic significant stenosis (>70%) and >15% in symptomatic significant stenosis.
- The annual stroke risk of medically managed carotid artery stenosis of <60% is <1%.

Treatment of hypertension, hyperlipidemia, and diabetes and cessation of tobacco use are strongly recommended. Antiplatelet therapy should be initiated or continued. Carotid endarterectomy reduces the annual risk of stroke to 1.8% for asymptomatic carotid stenosis of 60% or more and to about 4% for symptomatic carotid stenosis of more than 70%. The risk of adverse outcomes (stroke, myocardial infarction, or death) of carotid artery stenting is similar to that of carotid artery surgery in asymptomatic patients with significant carotid artery stenosis. Carotid artery endarterectomy has been shown to be superior to carotid artery stenting in patients with symptomatic severe carotid artery disease.

- Management of hypertension, hyperlipidemia, and diabetes are necessary. Antiplatelet therapy should be started or continued.
- Tobacco cessation should be stressed.
- Patients with symptomatic severe carotid artery disease have better outcomes with carotid endarterectomy than with stenting.

UNCOMMON TYPES OF ARTERIAL OCCLUSIVE DISEASE

The clinical features that suggest an uncommon type of peripheral artery occlusive disease include young age, acute ischemia without a history of arterial occlusive disease, and involvement of the upper extremity or digits.

THROMBOANGIITIS OBLITERANS (BUERGER DISEASE)

Thromboangiitis obliterans (Buerger disease) (Table 7.3) should be considered in young smokers with foot claudication or ulceration of the feet or hands (Figure 7.10). These patients have early symptom onset, typically in the second or fourth decade of life. Foot claudication is nearly universal, and hand or finger involvement occurs in 33% to 63% of patients. All 4 limbs are involved in 40% of patients. Rest pain and ischemic ulceration are typically present in the lower extremity.

Table 7.3 CLINICAL CRITERIA FOR THROMBOANGIITIS OBLITERANS

Age	<40 y (often <30 y)
Sex	Males most often
Habits	Tobacco, cannabis use
History	Superficial phlebitis Claudication of arch or calf Raynaud phenomenon Absence of atherosclerotic risk factors other than smoking
Examination	Small arteries involved Upper extremity involved (positive Allen test) Infrapopliteal artery disease
Laboratory findings	Normal values of glucose, blood cell counts, sedimentation rate, lipids, & screening tests for connective tissue disease & hypercoagulable disorders
Radiography	No arterial calcification

Thromboangiitis obliterans affects distal arteries initially and primarily. Venous involvement (superficial phlebitis) is common. The disease was previously considered a male-dominated disease, but the incidence in women has increased in recent decades. A hallmark of the disease is addiction to tobacco. Smoking cessation ameliorates the course of the disease and reduces the risk of ulcer formation and amputation.

Evaluation must be thorough and distinguish between thromboangiitis obliterans and premature atherosclerosis. Distinguishing features of thromboangiitis obliterans include upper extremity involvement, foot claudication, and a history of superficial thrombophlebitis. Patients may present in their early 20s and 30s; profound premature atherosclerosis usually presents in the fifth decade of life.

- Thromboangiitis obliterans (Buerger disease) should be considered in young smokers with foot claudication. Foot or hand ulceration may be present.

- The incidence in women is increasing.

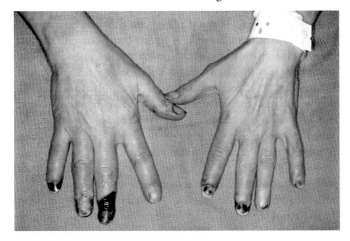

Figure 7.10 Gangrene of the Tips of Multiple Upper Extremity Digits in a Patient With Thromboangiitis Obliterans.

- Patients have a considerable history of tobacco use.

- Smoking cessation ameliorates the disease course, reducing the risk of ulcers and amputation.

- Distinguishing features include upper extremity involvement, foot claudication, and prior or current superficial thrombophlebitis.

Angiographic features include normal proximal vessels, distal artery occlusions, and skip lesions. "Tree root," "spider," and "corkscrew" are adjectives frequently applied to the angiographic appearance of collateral vessels and vasa vasorum; however, these findings are nonspecific and may be present in occlusive disease of other causes. Involved vessels may be thrombosed. Thrombi are infiltrated with inflammatory cells, but inflammatory marker values (ie, erythrocyte sedimentation rate) are nearly always normal.

Treatment is limited to tobacco cessation, wound care, limb protection, and amputation when needed. Arterial bypass grafting and angioplasty with stenting are rarely possible or effective.

- Tobacco cessation, wound care, limb protection, and amputation when necessary are the cornerstones of treatment of thromboangiitis obliterans.

- Bypass grafting and angioplasty with stenting are rarely possible or effective.

- Angiographic features are normal proximal vessels, distal artery occlusions, and skip lesions. Collateral vessels are described as having a "tree root," "spider," or "corkscrew" appearance.

- Inflammatory marker values are typically normal.

THORACIC OUTLET COMPRESSION SYNDROME

The thoracic outlet syndromes are a group of often disabling disorders caused by mechanical compression or irritation of the neurovascular bundle as it leaves the chest cavity through the thoracic outlet. There are 3 unique clinical presentations of the syndromes: 1) neurogenic, 2) venous, and 3) arterial. The thoracic outlet consists of the superior surface of the first rib and the anterior and middle scalene muscles. The neurogenic type is the most common (80% of patients) and presents with numbness, pain, and tingling primarily involving the ulnar nerve. Patients complain of arm symptoms with arm elevation (abduction) such as when working with their arms above their heads. The differential diagnosis of neurogenic thoracic outlet syndrome is broad and includes multiple neurologic, orthopedic, and vascular diagnoses. Electromyographic results will be normal. Cervical spine radiographs may be helpful to show the presence of cervical rib arising from the C7 pedicle (as opposed to T1). Arm lowering (adduction) relieves symptoms. Approximately 15% of patients present with venous symptoms, including subclavian vein thrombosis (Paget-Schroetter syndrome). Approximately 5% of patients have an aneurysm of the subclavian artery as a result of trauma at the point where the artery crosses the outlet. Subclavian artery aneurysms tend to thrombose and embolize, processes that present with embolic digital artery occlusion.

- Mechanical compression or irritation of the neurovascular bundle as it exits the chest cavity through the thoracic outlet results in thoracic outlet syndromes, a group of often disabling disorders.

- The most common thoracic outlet syndrome is neurogenic and presents with ulnar nerve distribution numbness, pain, and tingling. Symptoms are provoked with arm elevation or when patients work with their arms above their heads.

- A cervical rib arising from the C7 pedicle (rather than the T1 pedicle) may be present.

- Symptoms are relieved by arm lowering.

- Paget-Schroetter syndrome (subclavian vein thrombosis) may be present in patients presenting with venous thoracic outlet syndrome.

- Subclavian artery vein aneurysm results from repetitive trauma at the point where the artery crosses the outlet; this occurs in about 5% of patients with thoracic outlet syndrome.

- Subclavian vein aneurysms may thrombose and embolize, processes that lead to digital artery occlusion.

The diagnosis of neurogenic thoracic outlet syndrome (most common presentation) is very complex and is primarily based on clinical presentation and physical findings. Thoracic outlet maneuvers (costoclavicular active, costoclavicular passive, hyperabduction, Adson, and elevated arm stress tests) are performed to aid in the diagnosis. These maneuvers induce dynamic compression of the axillary-subclavian artery, which is identified as dynamic obliteration of the radial pulse. Results of these maneuvers may be positive in up to 30% of the general population; thus, their specificity and positive predictive value are limited. Vascular imaging (ultrasonography, CT angiography, and MR angiography) for neurogenic thoracic outlet syndrome shows dynamic vascular compression with maneuvers in up to 30% of the general population; thus, the usefulness of imaging in diagnostic evaluation is limited.

- Neurogenic thoracic outlet syndrome is difficult to diagnose and is primarily a clinical diagnosis.

- Thoracic outlet maneuvers may assist with diagnosis. Dynamic obliteration of the radial pulse during thoracic outlet maneuvers must be identified to consider results of the maneuver positive.

- Thoracic outlet maneuvers have a high false-positive rate because results are positive in up to 30% of the general population.

- Vascular imaging to demonstrate dynamic vascular compression during thoracic outlet maneuvers has limited usefulness because of the high false-positive rate of maneuvers in the general population.

Treatment for neurogenic thoracic outlet syndrome is primarily and initially conservative with physical therapy. Severe cases in which conservative therapy fails may benefit from thoracic outlet decompression and first rib resection. Patients with upper extremity venous thrombosis related to thoracic outlet syndrome ("effort thrombosis" or Paget-Schroetter syndrome) receive aggressive thrombolytic therapy, anticoagulation, and first rib resection. Patients with upper extremity arterial thrombosis related to thoracic outlet syndrome often present with digital ischemia related to thromboembolism from an axillary-subclavian artery aneurysm. These patients are aggressively treated with surgical repair of the aneurysm, anticoagulation, and thoracic outlet decompression.

- Neurogenic thoracic outlet syndrome is treated with physical therapy. In severe cases, thoracic outlet decompression and first rib resection may be needed.

- Upper extremity venous thrombosis (Paget-Schroetter syndrome) should be aggressively treated with thrombolytics, anticoagulation, and first rib resection.

- Thoracic outlet syndrome–associated upper extremity arterial thrombosis often presents with digital ischemia due to embolism from an axillary-subclavian artery aneurysm. Affected patients should be aggressively treated with surgical repair of the aneurysm, anticoagulation, and thoracic outlet decompression.

VASOSPASTIC DISORDERS

Vasospastic disorders are characterized by episodic color changes of the skin resulting from intermittent spasm of the small arteries and arterioles of the skin and digits. These vascular disorders are important because they may be a clue to another underlying disorder, such as arterial occlusive disease, connective tissue disorders, arterial injury, neurologic disorders, or endocrine disease. Vasospastic disorders may also be caused by toxins and certain medications, particularly β-adrenergic blockers. Ergot preparations, estrogen therapy, chemotherapeutic agents, interferon, cyclosporine, clonidine, narcotics, nicotine, and cocaine use are other possible causes.

RAYNAUD SYNDROME

This syndrome refers to inadequate blood flow to upper and lower extremity digits due to arterial impairment of the digital arteries or the distal arcade. This may be caused by either inappropriate intense vasoconstriction or fixed obstruction. The important thing about this syndrome is to differentiate vasospasm due to primary Raynaud disease from secondary Raynaud phenomenon (due to a fixed obstruction) (Table 7.4). The natural histories of these 2 disorders vary considerably.

Primary Raynaud Disease

Raynaud disease typically involves the digits of the upper and to a lesser extent the lower extremity. Females are more often

Table 7.4 CHARACTERISTIC CLINICAL FEATURES OF PRIMARY AND SECONDARY RAYNAUD SYNDROME

CLINICAL FEATURE	PRIMARY	SECONDARY
Symmetry	Bilateral	Unilateral or bilateral
Pulses	Normal	Abnormal
Skin ulcers	Absent	May be present
Gangrene, tissue loss	Absent	May be present
Vascular laboratory finding	Vasospasm	Fixed obstruction
Other underlying connective tissue disease	Absent	Present
Response to vasodilator or warming	Present	Minimal

affected than males, and the typical patient is young at onset of the disease (<40 years). Vasospasm is induced by cold weather or emotional stress. Involvement is typically bilateral with multiple, if not all, digits involved. The symptoms are usually stable over time. Triphasic color changes (blanching, cyanosis, and hyperemic in response to warming) may be present but are not universal. Other features of connective tissue disease such as systemic lupus erythematosus, rheumatoid arthritis, or scleroderma are absent. Arterial occlusion and digital ulcerations are rare. The cause is unknown. It is considered a benign condition, and treatment emphasizes protection from cold exposure and avoidance of vasoconstrictive triggers. Vasodilator therapy includes calcium channel blockers (dihydropyridine class) and α-adrenergic blockers (doxazosin).

Secondary Raynaud Phenomenon

In contrast to Raynaud disease, patients with secondary Raynaud phenomenon are more commonly male and older than 40 years. It is usually unilateral or asymmetric at onset. There is evidence of fixed digital artery obstruction, which may be due to various causes, including atherosclerosis, vasculitis, connective tissue diseases, hypothenar hammer syndrome, embolism, or drugs (especially β-adrenergic blockers and ergotamine). Distribution of symptoms is asymmetric with involvement of few digits. Associated pulse deficits, ischemic changes (including digital ulcerations), and systemic signs and symptoms are often present. Identification of the underlying cause is essential to allow appropriate treatment.

- Raynaud disease (primary) most commonly affects women, and age at onset is younger than 40 years.
- Secondary Raynaud phenomenon is more common in men older than 40 years.
- Raynaud disease is typically bilateral involving multiple digits. Arterial occlusion and digital ulcerations are rare. Cause is unknown, and typically symptoms and signs of systemic disease are not present. Treatment

focuses on protection from cold and avoidance of vasoconstrictive triggers. Calcium channel blockers and α-adrenergic blockers may be used when not contraindicated.

- Raynaud phenomenon is due to a fixed digital artery obstruction, which may be due to various causes, including connective tissue disease, vasculitis, embolism, atherosclerosis, and drugs. Distribution is typically asymmetric. Associated findings include pulse deficits and ischemic changes.

Evaluation should focus on differentiating primary Raynaud disease from secondary Raynaud phenomenon, including exclusion of connective tissue diseases and vasculitis. Vascular laboratory testing is important to differentiate vasospasm from vaso-occlusion. Baseline laboratory tests include complete blood count, erythrocyte sedimentation rate, serum protein electrophoresis, antinuclear antibody, antiphospholipid antibody, cryoglobulin, cryofibrinogen, and cold agglutinins. Conventional angiography (arch angiogram with upper extremity runoff) is rarely needed for the evaluation of primary Raynaud disease but can often be helpful for the evaluation of secondary Raynaud phenomenon, particularly if the underlying disease is not apparent.

- Evaluation for secondary Raynaud phenomenon should focus on exclusion of an underlying disease process.
- Conventional angiography is rarely needed; however, it may be helpful in certain circumstances.

LIVEDO RETICULARIS

Livedo reticularis is due to spasm or occlusion of dermal arterioles leading to a bluish mottling of the skin in a lacy, reticular pattern (Figure 7.3). Primary livedo reticularis is idiopathic and not associated with an identifiable underlying disorder. Secondary livedo reticularis is suggested by an abrupt, severe onset of symptoms, ischemic changes, and systemic symptoms. Most commonly, it is the result of atheroembolism from a proximal aneurysm or from proximal atheromatous plaques. The appearance of livedo reticularis in a patient older than 50 years should suggest atheroembolism. Other causes of secondary livedo reticularis include connective tissue disease, antiphospholipid antibody syndrome, vasculitis, myeloproliferative disorders, dysproteinemias, reflex sympathetic dystrophy, cold injury, and an adverse effect of amantadine hydrochloride therapy.

- Livedo reticularis is due to spasm or occlusion of dermal arterioles leading to the pathognomonic skin appearance.
- Primary livedo reticularis is idiopathic with no identifiable cause, whereas secondary livedo reticularis is due to an underlying condition and should be further evaluated.

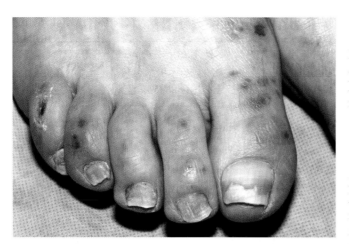

Figure 7.11 Characteristic Lesions of Chronic Pernio.

- Livedo reticularis developing in a patient older than 50 years should prompt consideration of an atheroembolic cause.

CHRONIC PERNIO

Chronic pernio is a vasospastic disorder characterized by sensitivity to cold and predominantly occurs in female patients with a past history of often intense cold exposure and injury. It may result in a blistering process with ulceration, particularly of the toes (Figure 7.11). It typically presents with symmetric blueness of the toes in cooler weather and resolution of the discoloration with warmer weather. Treatment with an α-adrenergic receptor antagonist is quite effective.

ERYTHROMELALGIA

Erythromelalgia is the occurrence of red, hot, painful, burning digits with exposure to warm temperatures or after exercise. It is not a true vasospastic disorder, but it is associated with color change of the skin. It may be primary (idiopathic) or due to an underlying disorder, most commonly myeloproliferative disorders (eg, polycythemia rubra vera), diabetes mellitus, or small-fiber neuropathy.

Treatment of the primary form includes warm temperature avoidance and aspirin therapy. Therapy with a nonselective β-adrenergic blocker is helpful in some patients. Symptoms of secondary erythromelalgia are typically relieved with treatment of the underlying disorder.

- Erythromelalgia is not a true vasospastic disorder, but it presents with skin color changes.

- The primary form is idiopathic and is managed by avoiding warm temperatures and using aspirin therapy. Nonselective β-adrenergic blockers may also be helpful.

- The secondary form is due to an underlying disorder (myeloproliferative disorders, diabetes mellitus, small fiber neuropathies) and typically responds to treatment of these disorders.

EDEMA

Lower extremity edema is commonly encountered in clinical practice and has several potential underlying causes. Noncardiac causes of regional edema usually can be identified from characteristic clinical features.

LYMPHEDEMA

Lymphedema can be primary (idiopathic) or due to an underlying disorder. Primary lymphedema (lymphedema praecox) is more common in women (9-fold greater frequency than in men) and typically begins before age 40 years and often before age 20 years. In women, symptoms often first appear at menarche or with the first pregnancy. Edema is bilateral in about half the cases (Table 7.5).

Secondary lymphedema is broadly classified into obstructive (postsurgical, postradiation, or neoplastic) and inflammatory (infectious) types.

- Primary lymphedema is idiopathic, and secondary lymphedema is due to an underlying obstructive or inflammatory (typically infectious) cause.

- A healthy young woman with painless progressive swelling of one or both legs consistent with lymphedema likely has primary lymphedema.

- Secondary lymphedema may be obstructive or inflammatory.

- Obstructive lymphedema may be due to surgery, radiation therapy, or malignancy.

Obstructive lymphedema due to neoplasm typically begins after age 40 years and often is due to a pelvic neoplasm or non-Hodgkin lymphoma. Initial evaluation should include a complete history and physical examination. CT of the abdomen and pelvis should be done to evaluate for a neoplastic cause of lymphatic obstruction. Women should undergo a pelvic examination and Papanicolaou smear. Men should be evaluated for prostate cancer. Inflammatory lymphedema occurs as a result of chronic or recurring lymphangitis or cellulitis. Dermatophytosis (tinea pedis) is the most common portal of entry for infection, which is often overlooked. The

Table 7.5 **DIFFERENTIAL DIAGNOSIS OF REGIONAL TYPES OF EDEMA**

FEATURE	VENOUS	LYMPHEDEMA	LIPEDEMA
Bilateral	Occasional	±	Always
Foot involved	+	+	−
Toes involved	−	+	−
Thickened skin	−	+	−
Stasis changes	+	−	−

Table 7.6 CLINICAL FEATURES OF THE 4 MOST COMMON TYPES OF LEG ULCER

FEATURE	TYPE OF ULCER			
	Venous	*Arterial*	*Arteriolar*	*Neurotrophic*
Onset	Trauma ±	Trauma	Spontaneous	Trauma
Course	Chronic	Progressive	Progressive	Progressive
Pain	No (unless infected)	Yes	Yes	No
Location	Medial aspect of leg	Toe, heel, foot	Lateral, posterior aspect of leg	Plantar
Surrounding skin	Stasis changes	Atrophic	Normal	Callous
Ulcer edges	Shaggy	Discrete	Serpiginous	Discrete
Ulcer base	Healthy	Eschar, pale	Eschar, pale	Healthy or pale

diagnosis of lymphedema can be evaluated noninvasively with lymphoscintigraphy.

- Patients with obstructive lymphedema should be evaluated for a malignancy.

Medical management of lymphedema includes edema reduction therapy using bandage wrapping, followed by daily use of custom-fitted, graduated compression (usually 40–50 mm Hg) elastic support. Manual lymphatic drainage is a type of massage used in combination with skin care, support and compression therapy, and exercise to manage lymphedema. A combined multimodality approach may substantially reduce excess limb volume and improve quality of life. Dermatophytosis, if present, should be treated with antifungal agents. Weight reduction in obese patients is beneficial. Surgical treatment of lymphedema (eg, lymphaticovenous anastomosis, lymphedema reduction) may be helpful in carefully selected patients.

- Therapy includes edema reduction therapy using wrapping, followed by daily compression elastic support in combination with manual lymphatic drainage, skin care, and exercise.

- Appropriate management of lymphedema leads to reduction in excess limb volume and improved quality of life.

- Treatment of dermatophytosis with antifungal agents is necessary.

- Weight reduction in obese patients is helpful.

LEG ULCER

The cause of lower extremity ulceration usually can be determined by a careful clinical examination. Clinical features of the 4 most common types of leg ulcer are summarized in Table 7.6.

8.

HYPERTENSION

Christopher M. Wittich, MD, and Robert D. Ficalora, MD

GOALS

- Cite the classification of hypertension and list the steps in initial evaluation of a patient with hypertension.

- Define an approach to selecting treatment for a patient with hypertension.

- Identify secondary causes of hypertension, including pheochromocytoma, primary aldosteronism, and renovascular hypertension.

- Recognize special cases of hypertension, including pregnancy and hypertensive crisis.

HYPERTENSION CLASSIFICATION AND INITIAL EVALUATION

MEASUREMENT AND CLASSIFICATION

Hypertension affects 50 million people in the United States. Systolic blood pressure more than 115 mm Hg increases the risk for stroke and coronary artery disease. For every 20 mm Hg increase in systolic blood pressure, the risk doubles.

Blood pressure should be taken with the patient seated with feet on the floor. The arm should be supported at the level of the heart with a properly sized cuff. Two separate measurements should be taken before making a diagnosis or treatment decision. Ambulatory blood pressure monitoring can be useful to determine values outside of the physician's office and response to therapy.

The Seventh Report of the Joint National Commission on the Prevention, Detection, Evaluation, and Treatment of High Blood Pressure (JNC7) defines a normal blood pressure as less than 120/80 mm Hg (Table 8.1). Prehypertension is defined as a blood pressure of 120–139/80–89 mm Hg, stage 1 hypertension as 140–159/90–99 mm Hg, and stage 2 hypertension as 160 or more/100 or more mm Hg.

Isolated systolic hypertension is defined as systolic pressure 140 mm Hg or higher and diastolic pressure less than 90 mm Hg. It is associated with age, disorders of increased cardiac output (anemia, thyrotoxicosis, arteriovenous fistula), and increased cardiac stroke volume (aortic insufficiency, complete heart block). Pseudohypertension is falsely increased systolic and diastolic pressures due to stiff vasculature caused by atherosclerosis. This condition occurs more frequently in elderly patients, and these patients may have marked increases of blood pressure but lack expected target organ injury.

The timing of follow-up of an abnormal blood pressure depends on the stage of the screening blood pressure. JNC7 follow-up recommendations are listed in Table 8.2.

- Systolic blood pressure more than 115 mm Hg increases the risk for stroke and coronary artery disease.

- A normal blood pressure is less than 120/80 mm Hg.

- Prehypertension is defined as a blood pressure of 120–139/80–89 mm Hg, stage 1 hypertension as 140–159/90–99 mm Hg, and stage 2 hypertension as 160 or more/100 or more mm Hg.

INITIAL EVALUATION OF HYPERTENSION

According to JNC7, initial evaluation of hypertension should focus on 1) determining lifestyle and cardiovascular risk factors, 2) identifying and treating secondary causes of hypertension, and 3) identifying target organ damage.

Lifestyle and Cardiovascular Risk Factors

Lifestyle and cardiovascular risk factors include cigarette smoking, obesity, physical activity, dyslipidemia, diabetes mellitus, microalbuminuria, age older than 55 years for men and 65 years for women, family history of premature cardiovascular disease defined for men as less than 55 years and for women as less than 65 years. The *metabolic syndrome* is defined by the presence of 3 or more of the following specific cardiovascular risk factors:

1. Hypertension

2. Obesity (body mass index greater than 30 kg/m²)

Table 8.1 CLASSIFICATION OF BLOOD PRESSURE FOR ADULTS 18 YEARS OR OLDER[a]

CATEGORY	BLOOD PRESSURE, MM HG		
	Systolic		*Diastolic*
Normal	<120	&	<80
Prehypertension	120–139	or	80–89
Hypertension			
Stage 1	140–159	or	90–99
Stage 2	≥ 160	or	≥100

[a] Not taking antihypertensive drugs and not acutely ill. When a patient's systolic and diastolic blood pressures are in different categories, the higher category should be selected to classify the blood pressure status.

Adapted from Chobanian AV, Bakris GL, Black HR, Cushman WC, Green LA, Izzo JL Jr, et al; Joint National Committee on Prevention, Detection, Evaluation, and Treatment of High Blood Pressure. National Heart, Lung, and Blood Institute; National High Blood Pressure Education Program Coordinating Committee. Seventh report of the Joint National Committee on Prevention, Detection, Evaluation, and Treatment of High Blood Pressure. Hypertension. 2003 Dec;42(6):1206–52. Epub 2003 Dec 1. Used with permission.

3. Diabetes mellitus

4. Dyslipidemia

Laboratory testing in the initial evaluation of hypertension should include determinants of cardiovascular risk, including cholesterol, triglycerides, glucose, and urinary microalbumin.

Secondary Causes of Hypertension

Causes of secondary hypertension and key features of each condition are listed in Table 8.3. Physical examination and

Table 8.2 FOLLOW-UP RECOMMENDATIONS BASED ON SCREENING BLOOD PRESSURE IN ADULTS

SCREENING BLOOD PRESSURE	FOLLOW-UP[a]
Normal	Recheck in 2 y
Prehypertension	Recheck in 1 y
Hypertension	
Stage 1	Confirm within 2 mo
Stage 2	Confirm within 1 mo; if blood pressure >180/110 mm Hg, confirm within 1 wk or treat immediately, depending on clinical situation

[a] Modify the follow-up schedule on the basis of knowledge of previous blood pressure measurement, other cardiovascular risk factors, or target organ disease.

Adapted from Chobanian AV, Bakris GL, Black HR, Cushman WC, Green LA, Izzo JL Jr, et al; Joint National Committee on Prevention, Detection, Evaluation, and Treatment of High Blood Pressure. National Heart, Lung, and Blood Institute; National High Blood Pressure Education Program Coordinating Committee. Seventh report of the Joint National Committee on Prevention, Detection, Evaluation, and Treatment of High Blood Pressure. Hypertension. 2003 Dec;42(6):1206–52. Epub 2003 Dec 1. Used with permission.

initial laboratory studies should focus on detection of secondary causes. Medications that can aggravate or cause hypertension are listed in Table 8.4.

Target Organ Damage

Target organ damage that can occur as a result of hypertension is summarized in Table 8.5. Organs typically involved include the heart, brain, kidney, arteries, and eye. Physical examination should focus on these organs, looking for signs of left ventricular hypertrophy, heart failure, atherosclerosis, stroke, peripheral arterial disease, and retinopathy. Initial laboratory evaluation should include identification of target organ damage, including chest radiography, electrocardiography, urinalysis with microalbumin, and determination of serum creatinine, sodium, potassium, and calcium values.

Table 8.3 SECONDARY CAUSES OF HYPERTENSION

CAUSE	KEY FEATURES
Endocrine	
Pheochromocytoma	Presents with headaches, diaphoresis, & palpitations
	If appropriate, screen with plasma metanephrine value
Primary aldosteronism	Presents with hypokalemia & HTN
	If appropriate, screen with aldosterone-renin ratio
Cushing disease	Presents with hyperglycemia, hypokalemia, & HTN
	If appropriate, screen with 24-hour urinary cortisol value
Hyperparathyroidism	Screen with serum calcium value
Hypothyroidism	Presents with diastolic HTN
Cardiac	
Coarctation of the aorta	Examine for weak, delayed, or absent femoral pulse
	Rib notching on chest radiography
Obstructive sleep apnea	Presents in overweight persons with loud snoring, large neck circumference, morning headaches, & daytime sleepiness
	Confirm diagnosis with polysomnography
Renal	
Renal artery stenosis	Presents in smokers, persons with CAD, or new-onset HTN after age 50 years
	Examine for high-pitched systolic-diastolic abdominal bruit
Fibromuscular dysplasia	Presents in females, usually younger than age 30 years without family history of HTN
Renal parenchymal disease	Check creatinine value & results of urinalysis

Abbreviations: CAD, coronary artery disease; HTN, hypertension.

Adapted from Chobanian AV, Bakris GL, Black HR, Cushman WC, Green LA, Izzo JL Jr, et al; Joint National Committee on Prevention, Detection, Evaluation, and Treatment of High Blood Pressure. National Heart, Lung, and Blood Institute; National High Blood Pressure Education Program Coordinating Committee. Seventh report of the Joint National Committee on Prevention, Detection, Evaluation, and Treatment of High Blood Pressure. Hypertension. 2003 Dec;42(6):1206–52. Epub 2003 Dec 1. Used with permission.

Table 8.4 DRUGS THAT CAN INCREASE BLOOD PRESSURE

DRUG	MECHANISM
Oral contraceptives (with high estrogenic activity)	Induce sodium retention & increase renin substrate
	Facilitate action of catecholamines
Alcohol (>30 mL daily)	Activates sympathetic nervous system
	Increases cortisol secretion
	Increases intracellular calcium levels
Sympathomimetics & amphetamine-like substances (eg, cold formulas, allergy medications, diet pills)	Increase peripheral vascular resistance
Nonsteroidal anti-inflammatory drugs	Induce sodium retention
Corticosteroids	Iatrogenic Cushing disease
Tricyclic antidepressants	Block uptake of guanethidine
	Inhibit action of centrally acting drugs such as methyldopa & clonidine
Monoamine oxidase inhibitors (in combination with tyramine—found in aged cheeses & some red wines)	Prevent degradation & metabolism of norepinephrine released by tyramine-containing foods
Cocaine	Vasoconstriction
	Interferes with action of adrenergic inhibitors
Marijuana	Increases systolic blood pressure
Cyclosporine, tacrolimus	Renal & systemic vasoconstriction
Erythropoietin	Systemic vasoconstriction
Serotonin	Systemic vasoconstriction
Glycyrrhizinic acid (eg, chewing tobacco, imported licorice, health food products)	Inhibits renal cortisol catabolism

Table 8.5 HYPERTENSIVE TARGET ORGAN INJURY

TARGET ORGAN	INJURY	CLINICAL MARKER/DIAGNOSIS
Heart	Left ventricular hypertrophy	S_4 gallop, forceful & prolonged apical thrust
		Displacement of point of maximal intensity
		Chest radiography, ECG, echocardiography
	Angina	History, ECG
	Prior myocardial infarction	
	Prior revascularization	
	Heart failure (systolic or diastolic)	History
		Lung rales
		S_3 gallop
		Edema
		Chest radiography, echocardiography
Brain	Stroke	History
	Leukoaraiosis	CT or MRI
	Transient ischemic attack	History
	Dementia	History
		Cognitive testing
Kidney	Chronic kidney disease	Creatinine, serum urea nitrogen, urinalysis, eGFR
Arteries	Peripheral artery disease	History of claudication
		Bruits
		Diminished pulses
Eye	Retinopathy	Funduscopic examination:
		Generalized & focal arteriolar narrowing
		"Copper wiring" of arterioles
		Arteriovenous nicking
		Cotton-wool spots
		Microaneurysms & macroaneurysms
		Flame & blot-shaped retinal hemorrhages
		Retinal vein occlusion
		Optic disc swelling

Abbreviations: CT, computed tomography; ECG, electrocardiography; eGFR, estimated glomerular filtration rate; MRI, magnetic resonance imaging; S_3, third heart sound; S_4, fourth heart sound.

- Initial evaluation of hypertension should focus on 1) determination of lifestyle and cardiovascular risk factors, 2) identifying and treating secondary causes of hypertension, and 3) identifying target organ damage.

TREATMENT OF HYPERTENSION

GOALS OF TREATMENT

The goal of therapy is to eliminate the morbidity and mortality of cardiovascular disease attributable to hypertension. Generally, the goal blood pressure is less than 140/90 mm Hg. However, patients with diabetes mellitus, chronic kidney disease, and high-risk coronary artery disease (carotid artery disease, peripheral arterial disease, abdominal aortic aneurysm, or 10-year Framingham risk

for cardiovascular events greater than 10%) should be treated to achieve a blood pressure less than 130/80 mm Hg. A goal of less than 125/75 mm Hg is appropriate for persons with proteinuria of more than 1 gram per 24 hours. An even lower goal of less than 120/80 mm Hg is advised for persons with reduced left ventricular function due to coronary artery disease.

- For most patients, goal blood pressure is less than 140/90 mm Hg.

- Patients with certain comorbid conditions may have a lower blood pressure goal.

Table 8.6 EFFECT OF LIFESTYLE MODIFICATIONS ON SYSTOLIC BLOOD PRESSURE

MODIFICATION	RECOMMENDATION	EXPECTED DECREASE IN SYSTOLIC BLOOD PRESSURE, mm Hg[a]
Adopt DASH eating plan	Consume a diet rich in fruits, veg-etables, & low-fat dairy products with a reduced content of satu-rated & total fat	8–14
Reduce weight	Normal body weight (BMI, 18.5–24.9)	5–20 (per 10 kg)
Restrict dietary sodium	Restrict daily sodium intake to ≤2.4 g (6 g sodium chloride)	2–8
Increase physical activity	Regular aerobic exercise (eg, brisk walking for 30 min) most days of the week	4–9
Limit alcohol intake	For most men: ≤2 drinks daily (30 mL alcohol) For women: ≤1 drink daily	2–4

Abbreviations: BMI, body mass index; DASH, Dietary Approaches to Stop Hypertension.

[a] Effects on blood pressure may be greater in some individuals.

Adapted from Chobanian AV, Bakris GL, Black HR, Cushman WC, Green LA, Izzo JL Jr, et al; Joint National Committee on Prevention, Detection, Evaluation, and Treatment of High Blood Pressure. National Heart, Lung, and Blood Institute; National High Blood Pressure Education Program Coordinating Committee. Seventh report of the Joint National Committee on Prevention, Detection, Evaluation, and Treatment of High Blood Pressure. Hypertension. 2003 Dec;42(6):1206–52. Epub 2003 Dec 1. Used with permission.

LIFESTYLE MODIFICATION

Lifestyle modifications (Table 8.6) are the initial step for any patient found to have prehypertension, stage 1 hypertension, or stage 2 hypertension. The modifications may be sufficient as initial therapy for some persons. They are adjunctive therapy for those with more severe hypertension.

The Dietary Approaches to Stop Hypertension (DASH) eating plan is effective for lowering blood pressure. The DASH eating plan includes consuming a diet rich in fruits, vegetables (high potassium), and low-fat dairy products (high calcium) with a reduced content of total and saturated fat.

The prevalence of hypertension is higher among obese persons than non-obese persons. An increase in blood pressure often parallels weight gain, and numerous clinical trials have documented the effectiveness of weight loss to decrease blood pressure. Weight reduction to within the normal range (body mass index, 18.5–24.9) is the goal, although losses as small as 4.5 kg may decrease blood pressure.

Restriction of daily sodium intake decreases blood pressure in some but not all hypertensive persons. Although salt sensitivity is more common among persons who are African American, obese, or elderly, the antihypertensive effect of many medications is enhanced by sodium restriction.

Restriction of daily alcohol intake to less than 30 mL of ethanol (15 mL for women) is associated with a decrease in blood pressure. Because complications of coronary artery disease are the most common causes of death in hypertensive persons, all risk factors for cardiovascular disease must be addressed. This includes smoking cessation and treatment of the metabolic syndrome.

- Lifestyle modifications are the initial step for any patient found to have prehypertension, stage 1 hypertension, or stage 2 hypertension.

PHARMACOLOGIC TREATMENT

The JNC7 recommends initiation of medication therapy in patients if lifestyle modifications are inadequate to reach the desired blood pressure goal (Figure 8.1). Thiazide diuretics are the recommended first agents because large studies have shown that they prevent cardiovascular complications of hypertension. However, some data suggest better outcomes with angiotensin-converting enzyme inhibitors as the first agents in white men.

In general, stage 1 hypertension should be treated initially with lifestyle modification and single-drug therapy. Stage 2 hypertension should be treated initially with lifestyle modification and a 2-drug combination. Compelling indications, if present, should be used to guide initial drug choice (Figure 8.1). Compelling indications include heart failure (eg, β-blocker) and diabetes (eg, angiotensin-converting enzyme inhibitor). The goal is to maximize the benefits of pharmacologic therapy (ie, to treat hypertension and the compelling indication).

Additional important factors influencing initial drug selection include age, race, and comorbidities. For example, diuretics and calcium channel blockers are more effective in African Americans and the elderly. Comorbidities such as Raynaud phenomenon (calcium channel blockers) and prostatism (α-blocker) may benefit from specially selected medications.

- Medication therapy should be initiated when lifestyle modifications are not adequate to reach the desired blood pressure goal.

- In most patients, the initial medication for hypertension should be a thiazide diuretic.

- Stage 1 hypertension should be initially treated with a single medication.

- Stage 2 hypertension should be initially treated with a 2-drug combination.

- Comorbidities and compelling indications should be considered when selecting a medication for hypertension.

SECONDARY HYPERTENSION

Secondary causes of hypertension should be considered when there is an unusual age at onset, when there is a sudden change

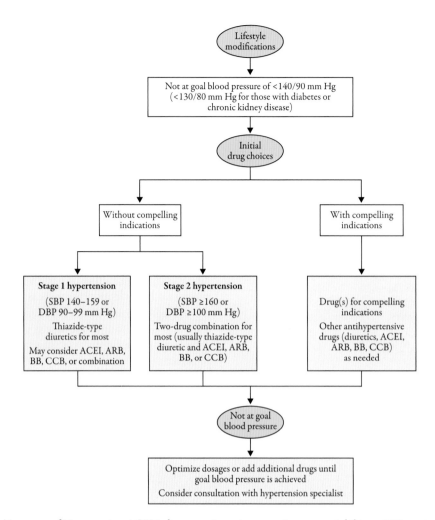

Figure 8.1 Algorithm for Treatment of Hypertension. ACEI indicates angiotensin-converting enzyme inhibitor; ARB, angiotensin receptor blocker; BB, β-blocker; CCB, calcium channel blocker; DBP, diastolic blood pressure; SBP, systolic blood pressure. (Adapted from Chobanian AV, Bakris GL, Black HR, Cushman WC, Green LA, Izzo JL Jr, et al; Joint National Committee on Prevention, Detection, Evaluation, and Treatment of High Blood Pressure. National Heart, Lung, and Blood Institute; National High Blood Pressure Education Program Coordinating Committee. Seventh report of the Joint National Committee on Prevention, Detection, Evaluation, and Treatment of High Blood Pressure. Hypertension. 2003 Dec;42[6]:1206–52. Epub 2003 Dec 1. Used with permission.)

in blood pressure, and when hypertension is refractory to treatment.

RENOVASCULAR HYPERTENSION

Renovascular hypertension is a potentially curable form of secondary hypertension. Generally, renovascular hypertension can be grouped into 1) renal artery stenosis and 2) fibromuscular dysplasia.

Clues that suggest renovascular hypertension include lack of a family history of hypertension, onset of hypertension before age 30 years (consider fibromuscular dysplasia, especially in white women), onset of hypertension after age 50 years (consider atherosclerotic renovascular disease, especially in a smoker or a person with coronary or peripheral arterial disease), or presentation with accelerated hypertension.

The most important physical finding is an abdominal bruit, especially a high-pitched systolic-diastolic bruit in the upper abdomen or flank. However, 50% of persons with renovascular hypertension do not have this finding.

Options for the management of renovascular hypertension include interventional therapies when feasible and medical therapy for persons who are not candidates for interventional therapy. Percutaneous transluminal angioplasty is the treatment of choice for amenable lesions caused by fibromuscular dysplasia and is an option in some cases of atherosclerotic renovascular disease. Stent-supported angioplasty is the best option for most persons with atherosclerotic renal artery stenosis, especially for orificial disease. Recurrent stenosis is common. Surgical intervention is the treatment of choice in patients with aneurysmal or severe atherosclerotic disease of the aorta requiring concomitant aortic reconstruction and in patients in whom percutaneous intervention has failed. The role of interventional therapy for preservation of renal function in ischemic nephropathy is uncertain.

The medical treatment of renovascular hypertension is similar to that of essential hypertension. The presence of severe bilateral renal artery stenosis (ischemic nephropathy) is suggested by an acute decline in renal function either after the initiation of therapy with an angiotensin-converting enzyme inhibitor or an angiotensin receptor blocker.

- Renovascular hypertension can be grouped into 1) renal artery stenosis and 2) fibromuscular dysplasia.

- Think of bilateral renal artery stenosis in a patient with acute decline in renal function after starting therapy with an angiotensin-converting enzyme inhibitor or an angiotensin receptor blocker.

RENAL PARENCHYMAL DISEASE

Renal parenchymal disease is a common secondary cause of hypertension. Moreover, hypertension in patients with renal parenchymal disease is associated with a more rapid loss of renal function. The major mechanisms of hypertension in renal disease include volume expansion from impaired renal elimination of salt and water, oversecretion of renin, and decreased production of renal vasodilators. Angiotensin-converting enzyme inhibitors reduce proteinuria and high glomerular transcapillary pressures, slowing further loss of renal function. However, they can cause hyperkalemia and an acute decline in renal function. Modest acute decreases in renal function (<30%) should be tolerated because they are often followed by stabilization and preservation of renal function. Calcium channel blockers are effective blood pressure–lowering agents in persons with chronic kidney disease. Nondihydropyridine calcium channel blockers reduce proteinuria, but dihydropyridine calcium channel blockers do not.

PRIMARY ALDOSTERONISM

The syndrome of primary aldosteronism is characterized by clinical and laboratory consequences of autonomous overproduction of aldosterone by the adrenal glands. These consequences are hypertension, hypokalemia, alkalosis, hyperglycemia, and increased aldosterone levels. Prevalence estimates range from 2% to 15% of the hypertensive population.

Primary aldosteronism should be suspected in hypertensive patients who have spontaneous hypokalemia or marked hypokalemia precipitated by usual doses of diuretics. However, in many patients with primary aldosteronism, the potassium level is normal. Additionally, it should be suspected in those with an adrenal mass, a history of early-onset hypertension, or a first-degree relative with primary aldosteronism.

Screening for primary aldosteronism is done using the aldosterone-renin ratio. This should be measured when the patient is not taking any aldosterone-blocking medications. In essential hypertension, the average value of the ratio is 5.5. A ratio more than 15 to 20 suggests the diagnosis of primary aldosteronism.

Treatment of primary aldosteronism can involve spironolactone, eplerenone, other antihypertensive medications, or surgery.

- Primary aldosteronism should be suspected in any hypertensive person who presents with spontaneous hypokalemia or marked hypokalemia precipitated by usual doses of diuretics.

- Screening for primary aldosteronism is done using the aldosterone-renin ratio.

PHEOCHROMOCYTOMA

Pheochromocytoma is a tumor that causes hypertension due to excess catecholamines. Tumors can be present in the adrenal medulla (pheochromocytomas) or sympathetic ganglia (extra-adrenal pheochromocytomas or paragangliomas). Pheochromocytoma is rare; its incidence is 2 to 8 cases per million persons per year. The prevalence is 0.5% among persons with hypertension.

A "rule of 10" describes the typical locations of pheochromocytomas: 10% are extra-adrenal; 10% of extra-adrenal gland tumors are extra-abdominal; 10% occur in children; 10% are multiple or bilateral; 10% recur after the initial resection; 10% are malignant; 10% are found in persons without hypertension; and 10% are familial.

Patients can present with paroxysms of hypertension, but most have sustained hypertension. Paroxysms can be associated with headache, diaphoresis, and palpitations. The presentation of pheochromocytoma corresponds to 5 Ps: *pressure, *pain, *palpitations, *perspiration, and *pallor. Patients can also present with symptoms mimicking an anxiety attack. Additionally, pheochromocytomas can be discovered as an incidental adrenal mass on an imaging study.

Pheochromocytoma is associated with multiple endocrine neoplasia (MEN) type 2a (medullary thyroid carcinoma, pheochromocytoma, and parathyroid tumors), MEN type 2b (medullary thyroid cancer, pheochromocytoma, and neuroma), neurofibromatosis, von Hippel-Lindau disease (pheochromocytoma, retinal hemangiomatosis, cerebellar hemangioblastomas, epididymal cystadenoma, renal and pancreatic cysts, and renal cell carcinoma), and familial paraganglioma syndrome.

Investigations for pheochromocytoma should be selective and based on results of history and examination. Initial studies involve measurement of catecholamine metabolites. Plasma or urine measures of catecholamines alone lack diagnostic accuracy. Measurement of plasma free metanephrines is considered the test of choice by some because of its high sensitivity. Measurement of plasma free metanephrines should be strongly considered if a familial syndrome is suspected, if the person has a previous history of pheochromocytoma, or if clinical suspicion is high. A negative result for either the plasma test or the urine test excludes the diagnosis in most cases.

Because of the low prevalence of pheochromocytoma, false-positive results outnumber true-positive results during screening for this disorder. Diet, medications, and physiologic stresses can interfere with the tests.

Computed tomography or magnetic resonance imaging of the abdomen and pelvis is the initial test used to locate a tumor after biochemical testing has confirmed the presence of the disorder. Treatment is surgical. Preoperatively, administration of a phenoxybenzamine is needed to control blood pressure and cardiac rhythm. Because pheochromocytomas can recur in 10% of cases, long-term biochemical follow-up is required.

- Pheochromocytomas are tumors that cause hypertension due to excess catecholamines.

- Investigation should be stepwise, with biochemical testing preceding imaging.

COARCTATION OF THE AORTA

Coarctation of the aorta is a constriction of the vessel usually just beyond the takeoff of the left subclavian artery. It is usually detected in childhood when blood pressure in the upper extremities is increased and blood pressure in the lower extremities is low. Weak or delayed lower extremity pulses can also be present. Patients can experience signs of lower extremity claudication. Dilated collateral vessels can cause bruits and characteristic rib notching on chest radiography. Treatment is surgical repair.

OBSTRUCTIVE SLEEP APNEA

Obstructive sleep apnea is associated with hypertension that may be severe and resistant to control. Upper body obesity is a risk factor for obstructive sleep apnea and is common in hypertensive persons. Consider the diagnosis of obstructive sleep apnea in persons who are overweight, snore loudly, have a large neck circumference, and complain of morning headaches and daytime sleepiness.

OTHER CAUSES OF HYPERTENSION

Cushing syndrome should be considered in the hypertensive person who has impaired fasting glucose and unexplained hypokalemia.

Hypothyroidism is associated with diastolic hypertension due to decreased cardiac output and contractility. Tissue perfusion is maintained by an increase in peripheral vascular resistance mediated by increased activity of the sympathetic nervous system.

Hyperparathyroidism may increase blood pressure directly via hypercalcemia, which increases peripheral vascular resistance, and indirectly by increasing vascular sensitivity to catecholamines.

SPECIAL CASES OF HYPERTENSION

PREGNANCY

Blood pressure typically decreases early in pregnancy (first 16–18 weeks) and then gradually increases. Hypertension during pregnancy is defined as a systolic blood pressure of 140 mm Hg or greater or diastolic blood pressure of 90 mm Hg or greater. Hypertension during pregnancy is associated with increased neonatal morbidity and mortality.

Gestational hypertension is increased blood pressure that develops for the first time during pregnancy without findings of preeclampsia. If gestational hypertension does not evolve into preeclampsia by delivery, and if blood pressure normalizes within 12 weeks post partum, the hypertension is called *transient hypertension of pregnancy*. This is a predictor of the future development of essential hypertension. If blood pressure remains increased, it is recognized retrospectively as *chronic hypertension* that was previously undiagnosed and masked by the decrease in blood pressure that occurs during early pregnancy.

Preeclampsia is defined as a blood pressure greater than 140/90 mm Hg and proteinuria (24-hour urine protein excretion greater than 0.3 g) that develops after the 20th week of gestation. Eclampsia is defined by seizures that occur in the presence of preeclampsia and cannot be attributed to other causes. Patients with preeclampsia can also have headache, blurry vision, epigastric pain, nephrotic-range proteinuria (>3.5 g in 24 hours), oliguria, creatinine level greater than 1.2 mg/dL, low platelet count, evidence of microangiopathic hemolytic anemia (abnormal blood smear or increased lactate dehydrogenase value), increased liver transaminase values, and pulmonary edema.

Preeclampsia occurs more commonly in African American women, the relatively young (<18 years), the relatively old (>35 years), first pregnancies, twin pregnancies, obese women, diabetic patients, and women with a personal or family history of preeclampsia. Preeclampsia that develops before the 20th week of gestation suggests molar pregnancy, fetal hydrops, thalassemia, or renal disease.

The HELLP syndrome (*h*emolysis, *e*levated *l*iver enzymes, and *l*ow *p*latelet count) occurs when intravascular coagulation and liver ischemia develop in preeclampsia. The HELLP syndrome can rapidly develop into a life-threatening disorder of liver failure and worsening thrombocytopenia in the presence of only mild or moderate hypertension. The most serious complication of the HELLP syndrome is liver rupture, which is associated with high maternal and fetal mortality.

The oral agent of choice is methyldopa. If methyldopa is ineffective or not tolerated, other drugs can be considered. Except for angiotensin-converting enzyme inhibitors, angiotensin receptor blockers, and direct renin inhibitors, none of the currently available drugs are known to increase perinatal morbidity or mortality. Magnesium sulfate is the treatment of choice for impending eclampsia or for preventing recurrent seizures. The only definitive treatment of eclampsia and the HELLP syndrome is delivery.

- Blood pressure typically decreases early in pregnancy (first 16–18 weeks) and then gradually increases.

- Preeclampsia is defined as a blood pressure greater than 140/90 mm Hg and proteinuria (24-hour urine protein excretion >0.3 g) that develops after the 20th week of gestation.

- Eclampsia is defined by seizures that occur in the presence of preeclampsia and cannot be attributed to other causes.

- The oral agent of choice for hypertension in pregnancy is methyldopa.

HYPERTENSION AND BREASTFEEDING

Increased blood pressure may persist for 6 to 12 weeks after delivery in women who have preeclampsia or gestational hypertension. Most antihypertensive drugs are compatible with breastfeeding, and all studied drugs are excreted into breast milk. Methyldopa and hydralazine have been shown to be safe. Propranolol and labetalol are the preferred β-blockers. Angiotensin-converting enzyme inhibitors and angiotensin receptor blockers should be avoided because their use may be associated with adverse neonatal renal effects. Diuretics may suppress milk volume. Regardless of the drug chosen, the infant should be carefully monitored for adverse effects.

HYPERTENSIVE CRISIS

Hypertensive crisis can be subdivided into hypertensive urgency and emergency. *Hypertensive urgency* is severe hypertension without evidence of acute target organ injury. It should be treated to decrease blood pressure to safer levels over 24 to 48 hours. This decrease can usually be achieved in the outpatient setting with oral agents. *Hypertensive emergency* is severe hypertension with evidence of acute injury to target organs. It implies the need for hospitalization to immediately lower blood pressure with parenteral therapy.

Sodium nitroprusside is the drug of choice for hypertensive emergency. It is a balanced arterial and venous dilator that decreases both preload and afterload. Toxicity is related to the metabolism of nitroprusside to cyanide in erythrocytes. Thiocyanate levels should be monitored.

Other medications can be used to reduce blood pressure in patients with hypertensive emergency on the basis of the clinical scenario, such as angiotensin-converting enzyme inhibitor in scleroderma renal crisis.

- *Hypertensive urgency* is severe hypertension without evidence of acute target organ injury.
- *Hypertensive emergency* is severe hypertension with evidence of acute injury to target organs.
- Sodium nitroprusside is the drug of choice for hypertensive emergency.

SUMMARY

- Initial evaluation of hypertension should focus on 1) determination of lifestyle and cardiovascular risk factors, 2) identifying and treating secondary causes of hypertension, and 3) identifying target organ damage.

- Treat stage 1 hypertension with a single medication. Treat stage 2 hypertension with a 2-drug combination. Use compelling indications, if present, to help select a medication for hypertension.

- Look for secondary causes of hypertension when there is an unusual age at onset or a sudden change in blood pressure or when hypertension is refractory to treatment.

PART II

GASTROENTEROLOGY AND HEPATOLOGY

9.

COLON

Conor G. Loftus, MD

GOALS

- Review the diagnosis and treatment of inflammatory bowel disease.

- Understand the colonic manifestations of human immunodeficiency virus (HIV) infection.

- Discuss the diagnosis and treatment of ischemic colitis and diverticular disease.

- Review the diagnosis and management of colon cancer.

INFLAMMATORY BOWEL DISEASE

Inflammatory bowel disease refers to 2 disorders of unknown cause: ulcerative colitis and Crohn disease. Other possible causes of inflammation, especially infection, should be excluded before making the diagnosis of inflammatory bowel disease. The presence of chronic inflammation on biopsy is the key factor for making a diagnosis of inflammatory bowel disease.

Ulcerative colitis is mucosal inflammation involving only the colon. *Crohn disease* is transmural inflammation that can involve the gastrointestinal tract anywhere from the esophagus through the anus. The rectum is involved in about 95% of patients with ulcerative colitis and in only 50% of patients with Crohn disease. Ulcerative colitis is a continuous inflammatory process that extends from the anal verge to the more proximal colon (depending on the extent of the inflammation). Crohn disease is segmental inflammation in which inflamed areas alternate with virtually normal areas. Patients with ulcerative colitis usually present with frequent, bloody bowel movements with minimal abdominal pain, whereas patients with Crohn disease present with fewer bowel movements, less bleeding, and, more commonly, abdominal pain. Crohn disease is associated with intestinal fistulas, fistulas from the intestine to other organs, and perianal disease. Ulcerative colitis does not form fistulas, and perianal disease is uncommon. Strictures of the intestine are common with

Crohn disease but rare in ulcerative colitis (when they are present, they suggest cancer).

- Chronic inflammation on biopsy is the key factor for diagnosing inflammatory bowel disease.

- Ulcerative colitis involves only the colon.

- Crohn disease can involve the gastrointestinal tract anywhere from the esophagus through the anus.

- Ulcerative colitis is a continuous process.

- Crohn disease is segmental inflammation.

- Ulcerative colitis is characterized by frequent, bloody bowel movements.

- Crohn disease is characterized by fewer bowel movements, less bleeding, and more abdominal pain.

- Crohn disease is associated with intestinal fistulas, strictures, and perianal disease.

EXTRAINTESTINAL MANIFESTATIONS OF INFLAMMATORY BOWEL DISEASE

Arthritis occurs in 10% to 20% of patients with inflammatory bowel disease, usually as monarticular or pauciarticular involvement of large joints. Peripheral joint symptoms mirror bowel activity: joint symptoms flare when colitis flares and joint symptoms improve as colitis improves. When axial joint symptoms develop, such as those of ankylosing spondylitis (which has a relationship with HLA-B27) and sacroiliitis, they are usually progressive and do not improve when colitis improves.

Skin lesions occur in 10% of patients. The 3 lesions seen most commonly are erythema nodosum, pyoderma gangrenosum, and aphthous ulcers of the mouth. Erythema nodosum and aphthous ulcers usually improve with treatment of colitis, whereas pyoderma gangrenosum has an independent course. Severe, refractory skin disease is an indication for surgical treatment.

Eye lesions occur in 5% of patients. The lesion is usually episcleritis or uveitis (or both). Episcleritis usually mirrors inflammatory bowel disease activity, but uveitis does not. Patients with episcleritis typically present with a painless red eye, whereas those with uveitis often present with a painful red eye. Uveitis is an indication for emergent ophthalmologic evaluation.

Renal lithiasis occurs in 5% to 15% of patients. In Crohn disease with malabsorption, calcium oxalate stones occur. In ulcerative colitis, uric acid stones due to dehydration and loss of bicarbonate in the stool lead to acidic urine.

Liver disease occurs in 5% of patients. Primary sclerosing cholangitis is more common in ulcerative colitis than in Crohn disease. If the alkaline phosphatase level is increased in a patient with inflammatory bowel disease, the evaluation for primary sclerosing cholangitis may include ultrasonography, endoscopic retrograde cholangiopancreatography, and possibly liver biopsy.

- Peripheral joint symptoms mirror bowel activity.

- Axial joint symptoms, such as those of ankylosing spondylitis and sacroiliitis, can develop and have a progressive course independent of bowel activity.

- The skin lesions seen most commonly are erythema nodosum, pyoderma gangrenosum, and aphthous ulcers of the mouth.

- Patients who have inflammatory bowel disease and a painful red eye (uveitis) should be referred to an ophthalmologist without delay.

- If a patient's alkaline phosphatase level increases with inflammatory bowel disease, evaluate for primary sclerosing cholangitis.

- Central (axial) arthritis, pyoderma gangrenosum, primary sclerosing cholangitis, and uveitis usually follow a course that is independent of bowel disease activity.

INDICATIONS FOR COLONOSCOPY

Colonoscopy is indicated for evaluating the extent of the disease, performing biopsies, and evaluating strictures and filling defects. It is also indicated for differentiating Crohn disease from ulcerative colitis when they are otherwise indistinguishable. Another indication is monitoring with surveillance biopsies (typically, a total of 32 biopsies) for the development of dysplasia or cancer in patients who have had ulcerative colitis (involving colon proximal to the rectum) or Crohn colitis for more than 8 years. Patients who have ulcerative colitis limited to the rectum (ulcerative proctitis) are not at increased risk of dysplasia and colon cancer; they do not require surveillance colonoscopy.

TOXIC MEGACOLON

In patients with active inflammation, avoid potential precipitants of toxic megacolon, such as opiates, anticholinergic agents, hypokalemia, and barium enema.

- In patients with active inflammation, avoid potential precipitants of toxic megacolon.

TREATMENT OF ULCERATIVE COLITIS

Sulfasalazine and other aminosalicylates can induce remission in 80% of patients with mild or moderate ulcerative colitis and are effective maintenance therapy for 50% to 75% of patients with ulcerative colitis. The active agent of sulfasalazine, 5-aminosalicylic acid (5-ASA), is bound to sulfapyridine (the vehicle). Colonic bacteria break the bond and release 5-ASA, which is not absorbed but stays in contact with the mucosa and exerts its anti-inflammatory action. The efficacy of 5-ASA may be related to its ability to inhibit the lipoxygenase pathway of arachidonic acid metabolism or to function as an oxygen free radical scavenger. It is effective in acute disease and in maintaining remission. The side effects include reversible sterility in men, malaise, nausea, pancreatitis, rashes, headaches, hemolysis, impaired folate absorption, hepatitis, aplastic anemia, and exacerbation of colitis. They are related to the sulfapyridine moiety and occur in 30% of patients who take sulfasalazine.

The 5-ASAs are a group of drugs that deliver 5-ASA to the intestine in various ways. They eliminate sulfa toxicity but are more expensive than sulfasalazine. Two of these drugs are mesalamine and olsalazine. Mesalamine can be given topically (Rowasa suppositories and Rowasa enema) or orally (Asacol, which is 5-ASA coated with an acrylic polymer that releases 5-ASA in the terminal ileum, and Pentasa, which has an ethylcellulose coating that releases 50% of the 5-ASA in the small bowel). Olsalazine consists of 2 molecules of 5-ASA conjugated with each other. Bacteria break the bond, releasing 5-ASA into the colon.

Aminosalicylates are used for mild to moderately active ulcerative colitis and for Crohn disease. Topical forms are useful for proctitis or left-sided colitis; systemic forms are used for pancolitis. Of the patients who do not tolerate sulfasalazine, 80% to 90% tolerate oral 5-ASA preparations. Side effects include hair loss, pancreatitis (often in patients in whom pancreatitis developed while they were taking sulfasalazine), reversible worsening of underlying renal disease, and exacerbation of colitis.

- Sulfasalazine and other aminosalicylates can induce remission in 80% of patients with mild or moderate ulcerative colitis and are effective maintenance therapy for 50%–75% of patients with ulcerative colitis.

- Sulfasalazine may cause reversible sterility in male patients.

- Other aminosalicylates are equally effective but more expensive; they are useful in 80%–90% of patients intolerant of sulfasalazine.

Topical corticosteroid preparations may be used for patients with active disease that is limited to the distal colon and is unresponsive to topical aminosalicylates. Oral corticosteroids should be added to the regimen of patients with more proximal disease if oral aminosalicylates do not control the attacks. Up to 50% of the dose can be absorbed. Oral preparations (prednisone, 40 mg daily) are indicated in active pancolonic disease that is of moderate severity and is unresponsive to aminosalicylates. Prednisolone, the active metabolite, is the preferred form of drug for patients with cirrhosis (these patients may not be able to convert inactive prednisone to prednisolone). For patients who have a prompt response to oral corticosteroids, the dose may be tapered gradually at a rate not to exceed a 5-mg decrease in the total dose every 7 days. In severely ill patients, intravenous preparations should be given (methylprednisolone, 40–60 mg daily) for up to 7 to 10 days. If improvement occurs at that time, therapy should be converted to oral corticosteroids (40 mg daily). If improvement does not occur, infliximab (discussed in the "Treatment of Crohn Disease" subsection) may be considered for induction of remission. If there is no improvement, surgical intervention (colectomy) is required. Because corticosteroids are not thought to prevent relapse, they should not be prescribed after the patient has complete remission and is free of symptoms.

- Prescribe topical preparations for patients with active mild or moderate disease that is limited to the distal colon.

- Oral corticosteroids should be added to the regimen of patients with more proximal disease if aminosalicylates have not controlled the attacks.

- Oral preparations (corticosteroids) are useful in active pancolonic disease of moderate severity.

- Intravenous corticosteroids are given to severely ill patients.

- Corticosteroids are useful in remission induction for ulcerative colitis but are not effective in maintenance of remission.

Total parenteral nutrition does not alter the clinical course of an ongoing attack. Indications for its use include severe dehydration and cachexia with marked fluid and nutrient deficits, excessive diarrhea that has not responded to standard therapy for ulcerative colitis, and debilitation in patients undergoing colectomy. Use of opiates (or their synthetic derivatives) and anticholinergic agents should be limited in ulcerative colitis because they can contribute to the development of toxic megacolon.

- Total parenteral nutrition does not alter the clinical course of an ongoing attack.

- Use of opiates and anticholinergic agents should be limited in ulcerative colitis.

Surgical treatment is curative in ulcerative colitis. Indications for colectomy include severe intractable disease, acute life-threatening complications (perforation, hemorrhage, or toxic megacolon unresponsive to treatment), symptomatic colonic stricture, and suspected or documented colon cancer. Other indications are intractable moderate or severe colitis, refractory uveitis or pyoderma gangrenosum, growth

retardation in pediatric patients, cancer prophylaxis, or inability to taper a regimen to low doses of corticosteroid (ie, <15 mg daily) over 2 to 3 months.

- Surgical treatment is curative in ulcerative colitis.

TREATMENT OF CROHN DISEASE

The use of sulfasalazine is discussed above (see "Treatment of Ulcerative Colitis" subsection). This drug is more effective for colonic disease than for small-bowel disease, although 5-ASA products designed to be released and activated in the small bowel may prove to be effective in the colon. Sulfasalazine does not have an additive effect or a steroid-sparing effect when given with corticosteroids, nor does it maintain remission in Crohn disease as it does in ulcerative colitis. None of the 5-ASA products are effective for the prophylaxis of Crohn disease.

- Sulfasalazine is more effective for colonic disease than for small-bowel disease.

- It does not have an additive effect or a sparing effect when given with corticosteroids.

- It does not maintain remission in Crohn disease.

The use of corticosteroids is discussed above (see "Treatment of Ulcerative Colitis" subsection). Corticosteroids are the agents that are most effective at controlling an acute exacerbation of Crohn disease. They are the most useful drugs for treating acute small-bowel Crohn disease and for achieving rapid remission. Budesonide is favored for the treatment of mild to moderate small-bowel and proximal colonic Crohn disease since it has limited systemic toxicity owing to first-pass hepatic metabolism. Budesonide is ineffective for more distal colonic Crohn disease.

Azathioprine and 6-mercaptopurine (the active metabolite of azathioprine) have steroid-sparing effects. These immunomodulating medications are effective for maintaining remission but not for treating acute disease flares because they have a gradual onset of action (6–8 weeks). Their use should be reserved for patients who are taking corticosteroids for active disease and whose corticosteroid dose needs to be decreased (or a given dose needs to be maintained in the face of worsening disease activity).

- 6-Mercaptopurine is the active metabolite of azathioprine.

- Azathioprine and 6-mercaptopurine are effective as maintenance therapy for Crohn disease. Both agents have a steroid-sparing effect.

Metronidazole (at a dose of 20 mg/kg) is effective for treating perianal Crohn disease. Six weeks may be needed for the therapeutic effect to become manifest. Recurrences are frequent when the drug dose is tapered or discontinued, leading to long-term therapy. It is less effective for colonic and small-bowel disease. Side effects include glossitis, metallic taste, vaginal and urethral burning sensation, neutropenia, dark urine, urticaria, disulfiram (Antabuse) effect, and paresthesias.

- Metronidazole is effective for treating perianal Crohn disease.

- Recurrences are frequent when the drug dose is tapered or discontinued.

Infliximab (Remicade) is a chimeric monoclonal antibody directed against tumor necrosis factor α. This intravenously administered anti-inflammatory agent is effective in treating moderately or severely active Crohn disease and ulcerative colitis that are refractory to conventional therapy and in treating fistulizing Crohn disease. Infliximab is a steroid-sparing agent that is effective in maintaining remission of Crohn disease. Infusion reactions (pruritus, dyspnea, or chest pain) may occur. The drug is associated with an increased risk of infection, including perianal abscesses, tuberculosis, and other respiratory infections. Rarely, subsequent infusions of infliximab may be associated with delayed hypersensitivity reactions. Additional monoclonal antibody–based therapeutic agents directed against tumor necrosis factor α include adalimumab (Humira) and certolizumab pegol (Cimzia). Adalimumab and certolizumab are generally reserved for patients who no longer have a response to infliximab; these agents are administered by subcutaneous injection rather than intravenous infusion.

- Infliximab is effective in treating moderately or severely active Crohn disease that is refractory to conventional therapy and in treating fistulizing Crohn disease.

- Infliximab is associated with acute infusion reactions, delayed hypersensitivity reactions, and an increased risk of infections.

Bowel rest per se does not have any role in achieving remission in Crohn disease. However, providing adequate nutritional support does help facilitate remission; any form of nutritional support is acceptable as long as the amount is adequate. Adequate nutrition can be essential in maintaining growth in children who have severe Crohn disease.

If Crohn disease is present during exploration for presumed appendicitis, the acute ileitis should be left alone (in many of these patients, chronic Crohn disease does not develop). Appendectomy can be performed if the cecum and appendix are free of disease. Of the patients with Crohn disease who have surgical treatment, 70% to 90% require reoperation within 15 years (many within the first 5 years after the initial operation). The anastomotic site is the most likely location for recurrence of disease. Indications for surgical treatment include intractable symptoms, acute life-threatening complications, obstruction, refractory fistulizing disease, abscess formation, and malignancy.

- Of the patients with Crohn disease who are operated on, 70%–90% require reoperation within 15 years.

- The anastomotic site is the most likely location for disease recurrence.

GASTROINTESTINAL MANIFESTATIONS OF AIDS

Gastrointestinal tract symptoms occur in 30% to 50% of North American and European patients who have AIDS and in nearly 90% of patients in developing countries. The gastrointestinal tract in patients with AIDS is predisposed to a spectrum of viral, bacterial, fungal, and protozoan pathogens. The most frequent gastrointestinal tract symptom is diarrhea, which is often chronic, associated with weight loss, and usually caused by 1 or more identifiable pathogens. Dysphagia, odynophagia, abdominal pain, and jaundice are less frequent, and gastrointestinal tract bleeding is rare. The goal of evaluation is to identify treatable causes of infection or symptoms. When no cause is identified, the condition may be idiopathic AIDS enteropathy or it may be caused by as yet unidentified pathogens.

- The majority of AIDS patients with diarrhea have 1 or more identifiable pathogens.

- Some have no identifiable cause despite extensive evaluation. This may result from idiopathic AIDS enteropathy or as yet unidentified pathogens.

VIRAL PATHOGENS

Cytomegalovirus

Cytomegalovirus is one of the most common and potentially serious opportunistic pathogens. It most commonly affects the colon and esophagus, although the entire gut, liver, biliary tract, and pancreas are susceptible. A patchy or diffuse colitis may progress to ischemic necrosis and perforation. Symptoms include watery diarrhea and fever and, less commonly, hematochezia and abdominal pain. Odynophagia may be present if the esophagus is involved. Diagnosis is based on biopsy specimens that show cytomegalic inclusion cells ("owl's eye" appearance) with surrounding inflammation. Treatment is ganciclovir, 5 mg kg twice daily for 14 to 21 days. If the virus is resistant to ganciclovir, use foscarnet.

Herpes Simplex Virus

The 3 gastrointestinal tract manifestations of herpes simplex virus infection in patients with AIDS are perianal lesions (chronic cutaneous ulcers), proctitis, and esophagitis. As in cytomegaloviral infection, the organs most commonly affected are the colon and esophagus. Symptoms include perianal lesions that are painful; proctitis that causes tenesmus, constipation, and inguinal lymphadenopathy; and esophagitis that causes odynophagia, with or without dysphagia. Diagnosis is based on the cytologic identification of intranuclear (Cowdry type A) inclusions in multinucleated cells and is confirmed with isolation of the virus from biopsies. Treatment is acyclovir given orally or intravenously.

Adenovirus

Adenovirus reportedly causes diarrhea. The organ affected is the colon. The main symptom is watery, nonbloody diarrhea. Diagnosis is based on culture and biopsy. There is no treatment.

BACTERIAL PATHOGENS

Mycobacterium avium-intracellulare

Mycobacterium avium-intracellulare causes infection of the gut in patients with disseminated disease. The small intestine is affected more commonly than the colon. Symptoms include fever, weight loss, diarrhea, abdominal pain, and malabsorption. Diagnosis is based on finding acid-fast organisms in the stool and tissue, with confirmation from culture of stool and biopsy specimens. Treatment is multiple drug therapy with ethambutol, rifampin, and isoniazid.

Other Bacteria

Other important bacteria include the following:

1. *Salmonella* ser Typhimurium and *Salmonella* ser Enteritidis—Treatment is with amoxicillin, trimethoprim-sulfamethoxazole, or ciprofloxacin.

2. *Shigella flexneri*—Treatment is with trimethoprim-sulfamethoxazole, ampicillin, or ciprofloxacin.

3. *Campylobacter jejuni*—Treatment is with erythromycin or ciprofloxacin.

AIDS patients with *Salmonella, S flexneri*, or *C jejuni* have a substantially higher incidence of intestinal infection, bacteremia, and prolonged or recurrent infections because of antibiotic resistance or compromised immune function, or both.

FUNGAL PATHOGENS

Candida albicans

In patients with AIDS, *Candida albicans* causes locally invasive mucosal disease in the mouth and esophagus. Disseminated candidiasis is rare because neutrophil function remains relatively intact. The presence of oral candidiasis in persons at risk of AIDS should alert the physician to possible HIV infection. If oral candidiasis is present, endoscopy is required to confirm esophageal involvement. The symptoms of odynophagia suggest esophageal involvement. Diagnosis is based on histologic examination showing hyphae, pseudohyphae, or yeast forms. However, endoscopy is not necessary for the initial evaluation of odynophagia in a patient who has AIDS and evidence of oral thrush. A trial of empirical antifungal therapy is reasonable. Treatment is with nystatin, ketoconazole, fluconazole, or amphotericin.

Histoplasma capsulatum

Histoplasma capsulatum causes an important opportunistic infection in AIDS patients who reside in areas where the organism is endemic. Colonic involvement is more common than small-bowel involvement. Symptoms include diarrhea, weight loss, fever, and abdominal pain. Diagnosis is established by culture. Colonoscopy may show inflammation and ulcerations, and histologic examination with Giemsa stain shows intracellular yeast-like *H capsulatum* within lamina propria macrophages. Treatment is with amphotericin or itraconazole.

PROTOZOAN PATHOGENS

Cryptosporidium

Cryptosporidium is among the most common enteric pathogens, occurring in 10% to 20% of patients who have AIDS and diarrhea in the United States and in 50% of those in developing countries. The organs affected are the small and large intestines and the biliary tree. Symptoms include voluminous watery diarrhea, severe abdominal cramps, weight loss, anorexia, malaise, and low-grade fever. Biliary tract obstruction has been reported. Diagnosis is based on microscopic identification of organisms in stool specimens with modified acid-fast staining or stains specific for *Cryptosporidium*. Organisms may also be identified in biopsy specimens or in duodenal fluid aspirates. Treatment is with paromomycin, which improves the diarrhea.

Cystoisospora belli

Cystoisospora belli is the most common cause of diarrhea in developing countries. The small intestine is primarily affected, but the organisms can be identified throughout the gut and in other organs. Symptoms include watery diarrhea, cramping abdominal pain, weight loss, anorexia, malaise, and fever. Diagnosis is based on identifying oval oocysts in stool with a modified Kinyoun carbolfuchsin stain. Biopsy specimens from the small intestine may show organisms in the lumen or within cytoplasmic vacuoles in enterocytes. Although *C belli* oocysts resemble *Cryptosporidium* oocysts, *C belli* oocysts contain 2 sporoblasts. *Cryptosporidium* oocysts are small and round and contain 4 sporozoites. Treatment is with trimethoprim-sulfamethoxazole.

Microsporida (*Enterocytozoon bieneusi*)

Organisms in the order Microsporida are emerging as important pathogens; they have been identified in up to 33% of AIDS patients who have diarrhea. The organ affected is the small intestine, and symptoms include watery diarrhea with gradual weight loss but no fever or anorexia. Diagnosis is based on electron microscopic identification of round or oval meront (proliferative) and sporont (spore-forming) stages of Microsporida in the villous but not crypt epithelial cells of the duodenum and jejunum. There are reports of positive stool specimens with Giemsa staining. There is no known treatment.

Other Protozoa

1. *Entamoeba histolytica*—Treatment is with metronidazole.

2. *Giardia lamblia*—Treatment is with metronidazole.

3. *Blastocystis hominis*—Because there is no evidence that *B hominis* is pathogenic, it does not need to be treated.

The rates of symptomatic infection with *E histolytica*, *G lamblia*, or *B hominis* are not markedly higher than in patients who do not have AIDS. In most patients with AIDS, *E histolytica* is a nonpathogenic commensal. Giardiasis may require prolonged treatment, as in other immunocompetent persons.

DIAGNOSTIC EVALUATION OF PATIENTS WITH AIDS WHO HAVE DIARRHEA

When patients with AIDS have diarrhea, initial studies include the following:

a. Examination for stool leukocytes

b. Stool cultures for *Salmonella* species, *S flexneri*, and *C jejuni* (≥3 specimens)

c. Stool examination for ova and parasites (use of saline, iodine, trichrome, and acid-fast preparations)

d. Stool assay for *Clostridium difficile* toxin

Additional studies include the following:

a. Gastroscopy to inspect tissue, to aspirate luminal material, and to obtain biopsy specimens

b. Examination of duodenal aspirate for parasites and culture

c. Culture of duodenal biopsy specimens for cytomegalovirus and mycobacteria

d. Colonoscopy to inspect tissue and to obtain biopsy specimens

e. Culture of biopsy specimens for cytomegalovirus, adenovirus, mycobacteria, and herpes simplex virus

f. Staining biopsy specimens with hematoxylin-eosin for protozoa and viral inclusion cells, with methenamine silver or Giemsa stain for fungi, and with the Fite method for mycobacteria

Whether further evaluation is needed if the studies listed above do not yield a diagnosis is a matter of controversy. Most experts advocate empirical treatment with loperamide (Imodium). Others recommend that biopsy specimens from the duodenum be examined with electron microscopy for Microsporida or from the colon for adenovirus. Empirical treatment with loperamide is favored because there is no treatment for either Microsporida or adenovirus.

PSEUDOMEMBRANOUS ENTEROCOLITIS

Pseudomembranous enterocolitis is a necrotizing inflammatory disease of the intestines characterized by the formation of a membrane-like collection of exudate overlying a degenerating mucosa. Precipitating factors include colon obstruction, uremia, ischemia, intestinal surgery, and all antibiotics (except vancomycin).

ANTIBIOTIC COLITIS

The symptoms of antibiotic colitis are fever, abdominal pain, and diarrhea (mucus and blood), which usually occur 1 to 6 weeks after antibiotic therapy. Sigmoidoscopy shows pseudomembranes and friability. Biopsy specimens show inflammation and microulceration with exudation. The condition usually remits, but it recurs in 15% of patients. Complications include perforation and megacolon. The pathogenesis begins with the antibiotic altering the colonic flora, resulting in an overgrowth of *C difficile*. The toxin produced by *C difficile* is cytotoxic, causing necrosis of the epithelium and exudation (pseudomembranes). Diagnosis is based on a stool toxin assay. Enzyme-linked immunosorbent assay (ELISA)-based stool testing has a sensitivity of 70% when a single stool sample is examined. The sensitivity increases to 90% when 2 stool samples are examined. Polymerase chain reaction (PCR)-based stool testing has a sensitivity of 95% when a single stool sample is examined. Proctoscopic findings may be normal or show classic pseudomembranes. The treatment is to discontinue the use of antibiotics and provide general supportive care (eg, fluids). Avoid use of antimotility agents. Metronidazole (500 mg 3 times daily) is 80% effective and inexpensive and is recommended in patients with mild disease (white blood cell [WBC] count $<15.0\times10^9$/L and normal serum creatinine). Vancomycin (125 mg 4 times daily) is recommended for patients with more severe disease (WBC count $\geq15.0\times10^9$/L and elevated serum creatinine). For a first recurrence, the same antibiotic can be used or the drug can be switched. For multiple recurrences, add cholestyramine and prolong the course of treatment with antibiotics.

- Antibiotic colitis: symptoms include fever, abdominal pain, and diarrhea 1–6 weeks after antibiotic therapy.

- ELISA-based stool testing has a sensitivity of 70%.

- PCR-based stool testing has a sensitivity of 95%.

- Metronidazole is the initial treatment of mild disease.

- Antibiotic colitis recurs in 15% of patients.

- Vancomycin may be used for patients with more severe disease and recurrent disease.

RADIATION COLITIS

Irradiation injury usually affects both the colon and the small bowel. Endothelial cells of the small submucosal arterioles are very radiosensitive and respond to large doses of irradiation by swelling, proliferating, and undergoing fibrinoid degeneration. The result is obliterative endarteritis.

Acute disease occurs during or immediately after irradiation; the mucosa fails to regenerate, and there is friability, hyperemia, and edema. *Subacute disease* occurs 2 to 12 months after irradiation. Obliterative endarteritis produces progressive inflammation and ulceration. *Chronic disease* consists of fistulas, abscesses, strictures, and bleeding from intestinal mucosal vessels. Predisposing factors include other diseases that produce microvascular insufficiency (eg, hypertension, diabetes mellitus, atherosclerosis, heart failure) because they accelerate the development of vascular occlusion, total irradiation dose of 40 to 50 Gy, previous chemotherapy, adhesions, previous surgical procedure and pelvic inflammatory disease, and older age. The elderly are more susceptible. Radiography during acute disease shows fine serrations of the bowel, and radiography during chronic disease shows stricture of the rectum, which is involved most commonly. Endoscopy shows atrophic mucosa with telangiectatic vessels. Endoscopic coagulation is effective treatment for bleeding, but surgery may be required for fistulas, strictures, or abscesses.

- Radiation colitis involves both the colon and the small bowel.

- The endothelial cells of the small submucosal arterioles are very radiosensitive.

- The result is obliterative endarteritis.

- Predisposing factors: hypertension, diabetes mellitus, atherosclerosis, chemotherapy, and >40 Gy of irradiation.

- The rectum is involved most commonly.

ISCHEMIA

REVIEW OF VASCULAR ANATOMY

The *celiac trunk* supplies the stomach and duodenum. The *superior mesenteric artery* supplies the jejunum, ileum, and right colon. The *inferior mesenteric artery* supplies the left colon and rectum.

ACUTE ISCHEMIA

The symptoms of acute ischemia are sudden severe abdominal pain, vomiting, and diarrhea (with or without blood). Early in the course of ischemia, physical examination findings are normal despite complaints of severe abdominal pain. Risk factors include severe atherosclerosis, congestive heart failure, atrial fibrillation (source of emboli), hypotension, and oral contraceptives.

There are several syndromes. *Acute mesenteric ischemia* is due to embolic obstruction of the superior mesenteric artery in 80% of patients. Most emboli (95%) lodge in this artery because of laminar flow, vessel caliber, and the angle it takes off from the aorta. This syndrome may result in a loss of small bowel and produce short-bowel syndrome. Radiography shows ileus, small-bowel obstruction, and, later, gas in the portal vein. The treatment is embolectomy.

Ischemic colitis is due to a transient decrease in perfusion pressure with chronic, diffuse mesenteric vascular disease. This decrease occurs in severe dehydration or shock and results in ischemia of the gastrointestinal tract. It commonly involves areas of the colon between adjacent arteries (ie, "watershed areas") such as the splenic flexure and the rectosigmoid. Patients with this syndrome present with abdominal pain and rectal bleeding. The characteristic radiographic feature is thumbprinting of watershed areas. The treatment is supportive, with administration of intravenous fluids to maintain adequate tissue perfusion and consideration of antibiotics if clinically significant leukocytosis or fever is present. If the condition deteriorates, surgical resection may be necessary.

Nonocclusive ischemia is due to poor tissue perfusion caused by inadequate cardiac output. It can involve both small and large bowels. Its distribution does not conform to an area supplied by a major vessel. It occurs in patients with cardiac failure or anoxia and in patients who are in shock.

- The diagnosis of ischemic colitis is based on the radiographic finding of thumbprinting of watershed areas.

CHRONIC MESENTERIC ISCHEMIA (INTESTINAL ANGINA)

Chronic mesenteric ischemia is uncommon. Symptoms include postprandial pain and fear of eating, with secondary weight loss. At least 2 of 3 major splanchnic vessels must be occluded. Chronic mesenteric ischemia is associated with hypertension, diabetes mellitus, and atherosclerosis. An abdominal bruit is a clue to the diagnosis. Noninvasive imaging may be performed, including duplex ultrasonography or computed tomography (CT) or magnetic resonance angiography. The primary treatment options are angiography with possible stent placement or surgical revascularization.

Occlusion of the superior mesenteric vein accounts for approximately 10% of the cases of bowel ischemia. Risk factors include hypercoagulable states such as polycythemia vera, liver disease, pancreatic cancer, intra-abdominal abscess, and portal hypertension. Patients present with abdominal pain that gradually becomes severe. Diagnosis is based on noninvasive imaging studies such as duplex ultrasonography or CT scan.

- Chronic mesenteric ischemia is associated with hypertension, diabetes mellitus, and atherosclerosis.

- Mesenteric venous thrombosis occurs with hypercoagulable states.

AMEBIC COLITIS

The colon is the usual initial site of amebic colitis. Symptoms vary from none to explosive bloody diarrhea with fever, tenesmus, and abdominal cramps. Proctoscopy shows discrete ulcers with undermined edges and normal adjacent mucosa. If an exudate is present, swab and make wet mount preparations for trophozoites. Indirect hemagglutination is useful for invasive disease. Radiography shows concentric narrowing of the cecum in 90% of the cases. Treat with metronidazole. The only pathogenic ameba in humans is *E histolytica*.

- Proctoscopy shows discrete ulcers with undermined edges.

- Radiography shows concentric narrowing of the cecum in 90% of the cases.

- The only pathogenic ameba in humans is *E histolytica*.

TUBERCULOSIS

Patients with tuberculosis may present with diarrhea, a change in bowel habits, and rectal bleeding. The ileocecal area is the most commonly involved site. Radiography shows a contracted cecum and ascending colon and ulceration. Proctoscopy may demonstrate deep and superficial ulcers. The rectum may be spared. A hypertrophic ulcerating mass may be seen. Biopsy samples stained with Ziehl-Neelsen stain are positive for acid-fast bacilli. All cases are associated with pulmonary or miliary tuberculosis.

- Tuberculosis is associated with diarrhea, change in bowel habits, and rectal bleeding.

- The ileocecal area is commonly involved.

- Deep and superficial ulcers are characteristic findings.

- All cases are associated with pulmonary or miliary tuberculosis.

STREPTOCOCCUS BOVIS ENDOCARDITIS

Streptococcus bovis endocarditis is associated with colon disease (diverticulosis or cancer). The colon should be evaluated.

IRRITABLE BOWEL SYNDROME

The term *irritable bowel syndrome* is used for symptoms that are presumed to arise from the small and large intestines. It refers to a well-recognized complex of symptoms arising from interactions of the intestine, the psyche, and, possibly, luminal factors. Most patients have abdominal pain that is relieved with defecation or associated with a change in the frequency or consistency of the stool. Other associated symptoms include abdominal bloating and passage of excessive mucus with the stool.

Patients with irritable bowel syndrome usually have a long duration of symptoms, symptoms associated with situations of stress, and no weight loss, no intestinal bleeding, and no associated organic symptoms (eg, arthritis or fever). Irritable bowel syndrome is a diagnosis of exclusion: the diagnosis is confirmed by an appropriate medical evaluation that does not reveal any organic illness. Always ask whether the patient's symptoms are related to ingestion of dairy foods because lactase deficiency must be ruled out. Patients who have upper abdominal discomfort and bloating may require an ultrasonographic examination of the abdomen and esophagogastroduodenoscopy. Patients who have lower abdominal discomfort or a change in bowel habits may require stool studies, proctoscopic examination, or colonoscopy.

The treatment of irritable bowel syndrome is reassurance, stress reduction, and a high-fiber diet or the use of fiber supplements. The use of antispasmodics to control abdominal pain or antimotility agents to control diarrhea should be reserved for patients who do not have a response to a high-fiber diet.

NONTOXIC MEGACOLON (INTESTINAL PSEUDO-OBSTRUCTION)

Acute pseudo-obstruction of the colon occurs postoperatively (after nonabdominal operations) and with spinal cord injury, sepsis, uremia, electrolyte imbalance, and drugs (narcotics, anticholinergics, and psychotropic agents). When the cecum diameter is more than 12 cm, the risk of perforation increases. Obstruction should be ruled out with a Hypaque enema. Treatment includes placement of a nasogastric tube, discontinuation of drug therapy, correction of metabolic abnormalities, and, if needed, neostigmine administration, colonoscopic decompression, or cecostomy.

Chronic pseudo-obstruction of the colon occurs with disorders that cause generalized intestinal pseudo-obstruction.

CONGENITAL MEGACOLON

Congenital megacolon (Hirschsprung disease) occurs in 1 in 5,000 births. The incidence is increased with Down syndrome. Congenital megacolon usually becomes manifest in infancy; however, it can occur in adulthood. There is a variable length of aganglionic segment from the rectum to the proximal colon (usually confined to the rectum or rectosigmoid). The diagnosis is usually made at birth because of meconium ileus or obstipation. If the diagnosis is made when the patient is an adult, the patient usually has a history of chronic constipation. Radiography of the colon shows a characteristically narrowed distal segment and a dilated proximal colon. Rectal biopsy shows aganglionosis. Anorectal manometry shows loss of the anorectal inhibitory reflex. Treatment is with sphincter-saving operations.

- Congenital megacolon: increased incidence with Down syndrome.

- If the diagnosis is made when the patient is an adult, the patient usually has a history of chronic constipation.

- Radiography of the colon shows a characteristically narrowed distal segment and a dilated proximal colon.

- Rectal biopsy shows aganglionosis.

- Evaluation of anorectal motility shows an absence of the anorectal inhibitory reflex.

LOWER GASTROINTESTINAL TRACT BLEEDING

The evaluation of acute rectal bleeding should begin with a digital rectal examination, anoscopy, and proctosigmoidoscopy. If a definitive diagnosis cannot be made, colonoscopy is necessary. The inability to cleanse the colon appropriately during active bleeding makes colonoscopy sometimes difficult to perform and interpret. Some advocate the use of nuclear scanning if the extent of bleeding is uncertain. If clinically significant active bleeding cannot be treated endoscopically, angiography may be necessary. Colonoscopy is not useful if bleeding in the lower gastrointestinal tract is torrential, but it may be of some benefit with a slower rate of bleeding. Colonoscopy is valuable for evaluating patients who have unexplained rectal bleeding and persistently positive findings on tests for occult blood in the stool.

Important causes of lower gastrointestinal tract bleeding are the following:

a. Angiodysplasia—usually involves the right colon and small bowel and may respond to endoscopic treatment

b. Diverticular disease—usually bleeding without other symptoms

c. Inflammatory bowel disease (colitis)—5% of patients present with it

d. Ischemic colitis—painful and bloody diarrhea

e. Cancer—rarely causes marked bleeding

f. Meckel diverticulum—the commonest cause of lower gastrointestinal tract bleeding in young patients; it is usually painless

g. Internal hemorrhoids—painless with small volume of "outlet-type" bleeding

h. External hemorrhoids—pain with small volume of "outlet-type" bleeding

i. Anal fissure—very painful defecation associated with small volume of "outlet-type" bleeding and often coexisting with constipation

In the evaluation of lower gastrointestinal tract bleeding, stabilize the patient's condition, perform proctoscopy to rule out rectal outlet bleeding (due to hemorrhoids or anal fissure), and obtain a nasogastric tube aspirate or use esophagogastroduodenoscopy to rule out upper gastrointestinal tract bleeding. A radionuclide-tagged red blood cell scan may help determine whether bleeding is occurring, but it may not precisely localize the bleeding site. If bleeding stops or occurs at a slow rate, perform colonoscopy. If the patient is young, perform a Meckel scan. For persistent bleeding that is not amenable to endoscopic therapy, angiography may be used to localize the bleeding site; infusion of vasopressin or embolization may be useful. If colonoscopy demonstrates bleeding, injection of epinephrine, electrocoagulation, or laser coagulation may be useful. If bleeding is massive or if marked bleeding continues, management is surgical.

ANGIODYSPLASIA

Angiodysplasia is a common cause of lower gastrointestinal tract bleeding, usually involving the cecum and ascending colon, in elderly patients. It is associated with cardiac disease (especially aortic stenosis), advanced age, and chronic renal insufficiency. There are no associated skin or visceral lesions. Colon radiography is of no diagnostic value, but angiography localizes the extent of involvement. Colonoscopy may show lesions, and cautery application may be effective.

- Acquired vascular ectasias are associated with aging, aortic stenosis, and chronic renal insufficiency.

- Angiodysplasia usually involves the cecum and ascending colon.

- Colonoscopy may show lesions. Apply cautery.

DIVERTICULAR DISEASE OF THE COLON

DEFINITIONS

Diverticula are acquired herniations of the mucosa and submucosa through the muscular layers of the colonic wall. *Diverticulosis* is the mere presence of uninflamed diverticula of the colon. *Diverticulitis* is the inflammation of 1 or more diverticula. The diagnosis and management of the complications of diverticular disease are outlined in Table 9.1.

DIVERTICULITIS

Microperforation or macroperforation of the diverticulum with subsequent peridiverticular inflammation is necessary to produce diverticulitis. The severity of the clinical symptoms depends on the extent of the inflammation. Free perforation is infrequent (diverticula are invested with longitudinal muscle and mesentery). Local perforations may dissect along the colonic wall and form intramural fistulas. The clinical presentation is left lower quadrant pain, fever, abdominal distention, change in bowel habits, and, occasionally, a palpable tender

COMPLICATION	SIGNS & SYMPTOMS	FINDINGS	TREATMENT
Diverticulitis	Pain, fever, & constipation or diarrhea (or both)	Palpable tender colon, leukocytosis	Liquid diet (with or without antibiotics) or elective surgery
Pericolic abscess	Pain, fever (with or without tenderness), or pus in stools	Tender mass, guarding, leukocytosis, soft tissue mass on abdominal films or ultrasonograms	Nothing by mouth, intravenous fluids, antibiotics, early surgical treatment with colostomy
Fistula	Depends on site: dysuria, pneumaturia, fecal discharge on skin or vagina	Depends on site: fistulogram, methylene blue	Antibiotics, clear liquids, colostomy; later, resection
Perforation	Sudden severe pain, fever	Sepsis, leukocytosis, free air	Antibiotics, nothing by mouth, intravenous fluids, immediate surgical treatment
Liver abscess	Right upper quadrant pain, fever, weight loss	Tender liver, tender bowel or mass, leukocytosis, increased serum alkaline phosphatase, lumbosacral scan (filling defect)	Antibiotics, surgical drainage, operation for bowel disease
Bleeding	Bright red or maroon blood or clots	Blood on rectal examination, sigmoidoscopy, colonoscopy, angiography	Conservative; blood transfusion if needed, with or without operation

mass. Treatment includes resting the bowel or using a low-fiber diet and antibiotics and obtaining an early surgical consultation. Indications for surgical treatment include generalized peritonitis, an enlarging inflammatory mass, fistula formation, colonic obstruction, inability to rule out carcinoma in an area of stricture, or recurrent episodes of diverticulitis.

- The clinical symptoms of diverticulitis depend on the extent of inflammation.

- Free perforation is infrequent.

- Clinical presentation is left lower quadrant pain, fever, abdominal distention, change in bowel habits, and, occasionally, a palpable tender mass.

- Treatment includes resting the bowel, administering antibiotics, and obtaining a surgical consultation.

COLONIC POLYPS

Three types of epithelial polyps are benign: hyperplastic, hamartomatous, and inflammatory polyps. *Hyperplastic polyps* are metaplastic, completely differentiated glandular elements. *Hamartomatous polyps* are a mixture of normal tissues. *Inflammatory polyps* are an epithelial inflammatory reaction.

The fourth type of epithelial polyp, *adenomatous polyps*, results from failed differentiation of glandular elements. Adenomatous polyps are the only neoplastic (premalignant) polyps. The 3 types of adenomatous polyps are tubular adenoma, mixed (tubulovillous) adenoma, and villous adenoma. The risk of cancer with any adenomatous polyp depends on 2 features: size larger than 1 cm and the presence of villous elements. If a polyp is found on flexible sigmoidoscopy and biopsy shows a hyperplastic polyp, no further work-up is needed. If biopsy shows an adenomatous polyp, perform colonoscopy to look for additional polyps and to perform polypectomy if necessary.

- Adenomatous polyps are the only neoplastic (premalignant) polyp.

- The risk of cancer with any adenomatous polyp depends on 2 features: size >1 cm and the presence of villous elements.

HEREDITARY POLYPOSIS SYNDROMES ASSOCIATED WITH RISK OF CANCER

Only the polyposis syndromes associated with adenomatous polyps carry a risk of cancer.

Familial Adenomatous Polyposis

Familial adenomatous polyposis (FAP) is characterized by adenomatous polyps of the colon. Colorectal carcinoma develops in more than 95% of patients, typically by age 40, if prophylactic colectomy is not performed. There are no extra-abdominal manifestations except for bilateral congenital hypertrophy of the retinal pigment epithelium. Diagnosis is based on family history and documentation of adenomatous polyps. Screening is indicated for all family members, and colectomy is indicated before malignancy develops. The inheritance is autosomal dominant; however, the phenotypic expression may vary considerably. The second most common malignancy in patients with FAP is cancer of the duodenum.

- Colorectal carcinoma develops in more than 95% of patients with FAP.

- There are no extra-abdominal manifestations except for bilateral congenital hypertrophy of the retinal pigment epithelium.

- The second most common malignancy in patients with FAP is cancer of the duodenum.

- Colectomy is indicated before malignancy develops.

Gardner Syndrome

In Gardner syndrome, adenomatous polyps involve the colon, although rarely the terminal ileum and proximal small bowel are involved. Colorectal cancer develops in more than 95% of patients. Extraintestinal manifestations include congenital hypertrophy of the retinal pigment epithelium; osteomas of the mandible, skull, and long bones; supernumerary teeth; soft tissue tumors; thyroid and adrenal tumors; and epidermoid and sebaceous cysts. Screening is indicated for family members, and colectomy should be performed before malignancy develops. The inheritance is autosomal dominant.

- Colorectal cancer develops in more than 95% of patients with Gardner syndrome.

- Gardner syndrome includes extraintestinal manifestations.

- Screening is indicated for family members.

Turcot Syndrome

In Turcot syndrome, adenomatous polyps of the colon are associated with malignant gliomas and other brain tumors. The inheritance is likely autosomal dominant but with variable penetrance.

- Only the polyposis syndromes associated with adenomatous polyps carry a risk of cancer.

- Perform colectomy for diffuse polyposis only if the polyps are adenomatous.

- Screening is indicated for patients with heritable polyposis syndromes only if the polyps are adenomatous.

Peutz-Jeghers Syndrome

In Peutz-Jeghers syndrome, hamartomas occur in the small intestine and, less commonly, in the stomach and colon. Pigmented lesions of the mouth, hands, and feet are associated with ovarian sex cord tumors and tumors of the proximal small bowel. The inheritance is autosomal dominant.

- Peutz-Jeghers syndrome is characterized by hamartomas of the small intestine.

- Pigmented lesions of the mouth, hands, and feet are associated with ovarian sex cord and proximal small-bowel tumors.

COLORECTAL CANCER

EPIDEMIOLOGY

Colorectal cancer is the second most common cancer in the United States, with 100,000 new cases and 60,000 deaths annually. Colon cancer eventually develops in 6% of Americans, and the mortality rate has not decreased since the 1930s. The incidence, which varies widely among different populations, is highest in westernized countries. Compared with past rates, as percentages of the total cases of colorectal cancer, the rates for cancer of the right colon and sigmoid colon have increased, but the rates for cancer of the rectum have decreased: cecum or ascending colon, 25%; sigmoid, 25%; rectum, 20%; transverse colon, 12%; rectosigmoid, 10%; and descending colon, 6%.

- Colorectal cancer is the second most common cancer in the United States.

- Rates for cancer of the right colon and sigmoid colon have increased.

ETIOLOGY

The role of the environment as a cause of colorectal cancer is supported by regional differences and migration studies of incidence. A high-fat diet increases the risk and may enhance the cholesterol and bile acid content of bile, which is converted by colonic bacteria to compounds that may promote tumors. A high-fiber diet is protective. Increased stool bulk may dilute carcinogens and promoters and decrease exposure by decreasing transit time. Fiber components may bind carcinogens or decrease bacterial enzymes that form toxic compounds. Charbroiled meat or fish and fried foods contain possible mutagens. Antioxidants (vitamins A and C), selenium, vitamin E, yellow-green vegetables, and calcium may protect against cancer.

- A high-fat diet increases the risk of colorectal cancer.

- A high-fiber diet has a protective effect.

- Charbroiled meat or fish and fried foods contain possible mutagens.

GENETIC FACTORS

Certain oncogenes amplify or alter gene products in colon cancer cells, and aneuploidy is characteristic of more aggressive tumors. The carbohydrate structure of colonic mucus is altered in colon cancer. Cell-cell interaction possibly has a role in cancer development.

Genetic predisposition has a role in many patients with colon cancer. Inheritance of FAP syndromes is autosomal dominant, and most colon cancer arises in adenomatous polyps. Hereditary nonpolyposis colon cancer (Lynch syndrome) is an autosomal dominant disease that may account for up to 5% of cases of colon cancer. Genetic susceptibility in the general population also has a role; for example, there is a 3-fold increased risk of colorectal cancer in first-degree relatives of patients with sporadic colorectal cancer.

- Aneuploidy is characteristic of more aggressive tumors.
- Genetic predisposition to cancer exists in many patients with colon cancer.
- Inheritance of FAP is autosomal dominant.
- There is a 3-fold increased risk of colorectal cancer in first-degree relatives of patients with sporadic colorectal cancer.

RISK FACTORS FOR COLORECTAL CANCER

The risk factors for colorectal cancer include the following:

a. Age older than 40—The risk increases sharply at age 40, doubles each decade until age 60, and peaks at age 80.

b. Personal history of adenoma or colon cancer—The risk increases with the number of adenomas; 2%–6% of patients with colon cancer have synchronous colon cancer, and 1.1%–4.7% have metachronous colon cancer.

c. Inflammatory bowel disease—Dysplasia precedes cancer; the cancer rate begins to increase after 8 years of ulcerative colitis and increases 10% per decade of disease. After 25 years, the risk is 15%–20%. The risk is greatest for pancolitis. The risk of colon cancer is not increased in patients with ulcerative proctitis (involvement of the rectum only). Cancer risk is not related to the severity of the first attack, disease activity, or age at onset. The rate of colon cancer is also increased 4–20 times in Crohn disease or ileocolitis. A family history of colon cancer is a risk factor, and a personal history of female genital or breast cancer carries a 2-fold increased risk of colon cancer.

- Colorectal cancer risk increases among persons older than 40.
- Risk increases with the number of adenomas.
- Among patients with colon cancer, 2%–6% have synchronous colon cancer, and 1.1%–4.7% have metachronous colon cancer.
- Cancer rate begins to increase after 8 years of chronic ulcerative colitis.
- After 25 years, the risk is 15%–20%.
- The risk is greatest for pancolitis.
- In Crohn disease, the rate of colon cancer is increased 4–20 times.

PATHOLOGY AND PROGNOSTIC INDICATORS

Cancer arises in the epithelium and invades transmurally to penetrate the bowel wall; it then enters the regional lymphatics to reach distant nodes. Hematogenous spread is through the portal vein to the liver. The surgical-pathologic stage of the primary tumor describes the depth of invasion and the extent of regional lymph node involvement, which are important in determining prognosis.

Modified Dukes Classification

Survival is determined by the extent of the invasion, which is categorized according to the modified Dukes classification:

A: mucosa, submucosa (5-year survival, 95%)

B1: into, not through, the muscularis propria without nodal involvement (85%)

B2: through the bowel wall without regional nodal involvement (70%–85%)

C1: as in B1 but with regional nodes involved (45%–55%)

C2: as in B2 but with regional nodes involved (20%–30%)

D: distant metastases (<1%)

Regional Node Involvement and Prognosis

The extent of regional node involvement and prognosis are as follows: 1 to 4 nodes, 35% recur; more than 4 nodes, 61% recur.

Other Pathologic Features and Prognosis

An ulcerating or infiltrating tumor is worse than an exophytic or polypoid tumor. Poorly differentiated histologic features are worse than highly differentiated ones. Venous or lymphatic invasion has a poor prognosis, as does aneuploidy.

Clinical Features and Prognosis

A high preoperative level of carcinoembryonic antigen is associated with a high recurrence rate and a shorter time before recurrence. The prognosis is poor if obstruction or perforation is present. The prognosis is worse for younger patients than for older patients. The depth of invasion and the extent of regional lymph node involvement are important in determining prognosis.

- A high preoperative level of carcinoembryonic antigen is associated with a high recurrence rate and a shorter time before recurrence.
- The prognosis is poor if obstruction or perforation is present.
- The prognosis is worse for younger patients than for older patients.

DIAGNOSIS

The clinical presentation is a slow growth pattern. Disease may be present for 5 years before symptoms appear. The symptoms depend on the location of the disease. Patients with a tumor in the proximal colon may present with symptoms of anemia, abdominal discomfort, or a mass. Patients with a tumor in the left colon, which is narrower, may present with obstructive symptoms, a change in bowel habits, and rectal bleeding. If cancer is suspected, perform a colonoscopy.

A metastatic survey includes physical examination, evaluation of liver-associated enzymes, chest radiography, and CT scan of the abdomen. The preoperative level of carcinoembryonic antigen is helpful for assessing prognosis and for follow-up.

- Symptoms of patients with a tumor in the proximal colon may be related to anemia, abdominal discomfort, or a mass.

- Tumor in the left colon is characterized by obstructive symptoms, change in bowel habits, and rectal bleeding.

- Preoperative level of carcinoembryonic antigen is helpful for assessing prognosis and for follow-up.

TREATMENT

For most cases, surgical resection is the treatment of choice. This includes wide resection of the involved segment (5-cm margins), with removal of lymphatic drainage. In rectal carcinoma, a low anterior resection is performed if an adequate distal margin of at least 2 cm can be achieved; this rectal sphincter–saving operation does not make the prognosis worse in comparison with abdominal perineal resection. The tumor may require resection to prevent obstruction or bleeding even if distant metastases are present.

- For most cases, surgical resection is the treatment of choice.

POSTOPERATIVE MANAGEMENT WHEN THERE ARE NO APPARENT METASTASES

A single colonoscopy either preoperatively or within 6 to 12 months postoperatively is needed to exclude synchronous lesions. If the findings are negative, colonoscopy is repeated at 1 year, 3 years, and every 5 years thereafter if there has been no evidence of recurrence.

Adjuvant chemotherapy with 5-fluorouracil and levamisole decreases recurrence by 41% and mortality by 33% in colonic stage C; it may be beneficial for stage B2. Radiotherapy plus 5-fluorouracil decreases the recurrence rate in rectal cancer stages B2 and C, but it is not clear whether there is any survival advantage.

- A single colonoscopy is preferred to exclude synchronous lesions; if the findings are negative, colonoscopy is performed at 1 year, 3 years, and every 5 years thereafter.

- The use of 5-fluorouracil and levamisole decreases recurrence by 41% and mortality by 33% in colonic stage C.

PREVENTION OF COLORECTAL CARCINOMA

Primary Prevention

The steps to be taken in primary prevention are not known, although epidemiologic data suggest that a high-fiber, low-fat diet is a reasonable recommendation.

Secondary Prevention

Secondary prevention involves identifying and eradicating premalignant lesions and detecting cancer while it is still curable. Screening includes occult blood screening and colonoscopy. With occult blood screening, lesions are detected at an earlier stage, but this has not decreased mortality. The Hemoccult test has a positive predictive value of 20% to 30% for adenomas and 5% to 10% for carcinomas. With colonoscopy, earlier-stage lesions are detected and removed.

Recommendations for Screening

Colon cancer screening recommendations are outlined in Tables 9.2 and 9.3. For average-risk patients (ie, anyone not

Table 9.2 COLON CANCER SCREENING RECOMMENDATIONS: ROUTINE SCREENING

PATIENT RISK	AGE AT INITIAL SCREENING	FREQUENCY OF SUBSEQUENT SCREENING IF FINDINGS ARE NORMAL
Average risk	50 y	Every 10 y
Increased risk		
Family history of colon cancer when younger than 60 y	40 y or 10 y younger than age of relative at cancer diagnosis	Every 5 y
Risk of hereditary nonpolyposis colorectal cancer	25 y or 5 y younger than age of relative at diagnosis	Every 2 y until age 40 y; then annually
Risk of familial adenomatous polyposis	Flexible sigmoidoscopy at 10–12 y	Flexible sigmoidoscopy annually until age 40 y; then colonoscopy every 3–5 y
Ulcerative colitis or Crohn colitis	8–10 y after diagnosis of pancolitis or 15 y after left-sided colitis only; if patient has primary sclerosing cholangitis, start immediately	Colonoscopy every 1–3 y

Data from ASGE guideline: colorectal cancer screening and surveillance. Gastrointest Endosc. 2006 Apr;63(4):546–57 and Winawer SJ, Zauber AG, Fletcher RH, Stillman JS, O'Brien MJ, Levin B, et al. Guidelines for colonoscopy surveillance after polypectomy: a consensus update by the U.S. Multi-Society Task Force on Colorectal Cancer and the American Cancer Society. Gastroenterology. 2006 May;130(6):1872–85.

Table 9.3 COLON CANCER SCREENING RECOMMENDATIONS: FOLLOW-UP INTERVALS FOR AVERAGE-RISK PATIENTS IF POLYPS ARE FOUND

FINDING	NEXT COLONOSCOPY
Hyperplastic polyps only	10 y
1 or 2 diminutive (<1 cm) tubular adenomas	5–10 y
≥3 diminutive polyps; any polyp ≥1 cm; any villous features; high-grade dysplasia	3 y (if normal findings at follow-up, increase interval to every 5 y)
>2 cm; piecemeal resection	2–6 mo

Data from Winawer SJ, Zauber AG, Fletcher RH, Stillman JS, O'Brien MJ, Levin B, et al. Guidelines for colonoscopy surveillance after polypectomy: a consensus update by the U.S. Multi-Society Task Force on Colorectal Cancer and the American Cancer Society. Gastroenterology. 2006 May;130(6):1872–85.

in the high-risk group), colonoscopy every 10 years after age 50 has generally become the diagnostic standard; however, an annual occult blood test plus sigmoidoscopy every 3 to 5 years after age 50 is still an alternative. For patients with 1 or 2 small adenomas (<10 mm), surveillance colonoscopy is recommended in 5 years. For patients with multiple polyps, a polyp larger than 10 mm, or polyps with villous histologic features, surveillance colonoscopy is recommended in 3 years. If a patient has more than 10 polyps, a surveillance colonoscopy is generally recommended in 1 year. For patients with previous colon carcinoma, a single colonoscopy either preoperatively or within 6 to 12 months postoperatively is needed to exclude synchronous lesions. If the findings are negative, colonoscopy is repeated at 1 year, 3 years, and every 5 years thereafter if there has been no evidence of recurrence. For patients with a first-degree relative who has colorectal cancer, colonoscopy should be performed every 5 years beginning at age 40 or at the age that is 10 years younger than the youngest age at which a relative received a diagnosis. For patients

with hereditary nonpolyposis colorectal cancer (HNPCC) syndromes, colonoscopy should be performed at age 25 and then every 2 years until age 40 and then annually thereafter. For patients with FAP, annual sigmoidoscopy should be performed beginning at puberty until polyposis is diagnosed, and then colectomy should be performed. For patients with ulcerative colitis or Crohn colitis, of more than 8 years' duration, colonoscopy and multiple biopsies are recommended every 1 to 2 years; dysplasia indicates the need for more frequent endoscopic follow-up and may lead to colectomy.

SUMMARY

- Chronic inflammation on biopsy is the key factor for diagnosing inflammatory bowel disease.

- Sulfasalazine is more effective for colonic disease than for small-bowel disease, it does not have an additive effect or a sparing effect when given with corticosteroids, and it does not maintain remission in Crohn disease.

- The majority of AIDS patients with diarrhea have 1 or more identifiable pathogens.

- The diagnosis of ischemic colitis is based on the radiographic finding of thumbprinting of watershed areas.

- The clinical symptoms of diverticulitis depend on the extent of inflammation. Clinical presentation is left lower quadrant pain, fever, abdominal distention, change in bowel habits, and, occasionally, a palpable tender mass. Treatment includes resting the bowel, administering antibiotics, and obtaining a surgical consultation.

- Symptoms of patients with a tumor in the proximal colon may be related to anemia, abdominal discomfort, or a mass. Tumor in the left colon is characterized by obstructive symptoms, change in bowel habits, and rectal bleeding. For most cases of colorectal cancer, surgical resection is the treatment of choice.

10.

PANCREAS

Conor G. Loftus, MD

GOALS

- Understand the management of acute and chronic pancreatitis.

- Review other pancreatic diseases.

EMBRYOLOGY

The pancreas develops in the fourth week of gestation as a ventral and dorsal outpouching or bud from the duodenum. Each bud has its own duct. As the duodenum rotates, the buds appose and join, and the ducts anastomose. If the ducts of the dorsal and ventral pancreas do not fuse, the resulting anomaly is called *pancreas divisum*. It is debated whether this condition may predispose to acute or recurrent pancreatitis. If part of the ventral pancreas encircles the duodenum (usually the second part, proximal to the ampulla) and causes obstruction, the anomaly is called *annular pancreas*.

- Pancreas divisum: failure of the dorsal and ventral pancreas to fuse; may predispose to acute or recurrent pancreatitis.

- Annular pancreas: part of the ventral pancreas encircles the duodenum (usually the second part, proximal to the ampulla) and causes obstruction.

CLASSIFICATION OF PANCREATITIS

Acute pancreatitis is a reversible inflammation. The 2 varieties are interstitial pancreatitis and necrotizing pancreatitis. *Interstitial pancreatitis*, in which perfusion of the pancreas is intact, accounts for 80% of cases, with less than 1% mortality. *Necrotizing pancreatitis* is more severe and results when perfusion is compromised. It accounts for 20% of cases, with 10% mortality if sterile and 30% if infected.

Chronic pancreatitis is irreversible (ie, there is structural disease with endocrine or exocrine insufficiency). It is documented by pancreatic calcifications on abdominal radiography,

parenchymal and ductal abnormalities on endoscopic ultrasonography (EUS), ductal abnormalities on endoscopic retrograde cholangiopancreatography (ERCP), scarring on pancreatic biopsy, endocrine insufficiency (diabetes mellitus), or exocrine insufficiency (malabsorption).

- Acute interstitial pancreatitis: perfusion is intact; mortality is <1%.

- Acute necrotizing pancreatitis: perfusion is compromised; mortality is 10% if sterile and 30% if infected.

- Chronic pancreatitis: pancreatic calcifications, ductal abnormalities, endocrine insufficiency (diabetes mellitus), or exocrine insufficiency (malabsorption).

ACUTE PANCREATITIS

In acute pancreatitis, activation of pancreatic enzymes causes autodigestion of the gland. The clinical features are abdominal pain, nausea and vomiting ("too sick to eat"), ileus, peritoneal signs, hypotension, and abdominal mass.

ETIOLOGIC FACTORS

Approximately 80% of acute pancreatitis episodes are due to either gallstones or alcohol ingestion. Significant elevation (>3 times normal) of aspartate aminotransferase (AST) or alanine aminotransferase (ALT) in a patient with acute pancreatitis generally indicates that gallstones are the cause. The third most common cause is idiopathic (approximately 10% of cases). The following drugs have been reported to cause pancreatitis: azathioprine, 6-mercaptopurine, L-asparaginase, hydrochlorothiazide diuretics, sulfonamides, sulfasalazine, tetracycline, furosemide, estrogens, valproic acid, pentamidine (both parenteral and aerosolized), and the antiretroviral drug didanosine.

Evidence that the following drugs cause pancreatitis is less convincing: corticosteroids, nonsteroidal anti-inflammatory drugs, methyldopa, procainamide, chlorthalidone, ethacrynic acid, phenformin, nitrofurantoin, enalapril, erythromycin, metronidazole, and nonsulfa-linked aminosalicylate derivatives such as 5-aminosalicylic acid and interleukin 2.

Other causes include hypertriglyceridemia, which may cause pancreatitis if the triglyceride level is greater than 1,000 mg/dL. Look for types I, IV, and V hyperlipoproteinemia and for associated oral contraceptive use. Hypertriglyceridemia may mask hyperamylasemia. Hypercalcemia may also cause pancreatitis; look for underlying multiple myeloma, hyperparathyroidism, or metastatic carcinoma. In immunocompetent patients, mumps and coxsackievirus cause acute pancreatitis. In AIDS patients, acute pancreatitis has been reported with cytomegalovirus infection. Pancreas divisum, or incomplete fusion of the dorsal and ventral pancreatic ducts, may predispose some people to acute pancreatitis, although this is a controversial matter.

- In nonalcoholic patients with acute pancreatitis, review all medications, check lipid and calcium levels, and rule out gallstones.

- Significant elevation (>3 times normal) of AST or ALT in a patient with acute pancreatitis generally indicates that gallstones are the cause.

- Several medications can cause acute pancreatitis.

CLINICAL PRESENTATION

Pain

Pain may be mild to severe; it is usually sudden in onset and persistent. Typically, the pain is located in the upper abdomen and radiates to the back. Relief may be obtained by bending forward or sitting up. The ingestion of food or alcohol commonly exacerbates the pain. Patients without pain have a poor prognosis because they usually present with shock.

Fever

Fever, if present, is low grade, rarely exceeding 38.3°C in the absence of complications. (Fever >38.3°C suggests infection.)

Volume Depletion

Most patients are hypovolemic because fluid accumulates in the abdomen.

Jaundice

Patients with pancreatitis may have a mild increase in the total bilirubin level, but they usually are not clinically jaundiced. When jaundice is present, it generally results from obstruction of the common bile duct by stones, compression by pseudocyst, or inflamed pancreatic tissue.

Dyspnea

A wide range of pulmonary manifestations may occur. More than half of all patients with acute pancreatitis have some degree of hypoxemia, usually from pulmonary shunting. Patients often have atelectasis and may have pleural effusions.

- Fever >38.3°C suggests infection.

DIAGNOSIS OF ACUTE PANCREATITIS

Serum Amylase

Determining the serum level of amylase is the most useful test for diagnosing acute pancreatitis. The level of amylase increases 2 or 3 hours after an attack and remains increased for 3 or 4 days. The magnitude of the increase does not correlate with the clinical severity of the attack. Serum amylase levels may be normal in some patients (<10%) because of alcohol consumption or hypertriglyceridemia. A persistent increase suggests a complication such as pseudocyst, abscess, or ascites. Serum amylase is cleared by the kidney. The urinary amylase level remains elevated after the serum amylase level returns to normal. Isoenzyme identification may aid in distinguishing between salivary (ie, nonpancreatic) and pancreatic sources. Serum lipase levels may help distinguish between pancreatic hyperamylasemia and an ectopic source (lung, ovarian, or esophageal carcinoma). Lipase levels are also increased for a longer time than amylase levels after acute pancreatitis. Computed tomographic (CT) imaging of the abdomen may be useful. If the amylase level is mildly elevated and there is a history of vomiting but no signs of obstruction, one should consider performing an esophagogastroduodenoscopy to rule out a penetrating ulcer.

- If the presentation for pancreatitis is classic but the amylase value is normal, repeat the amylase test, check urinary amylase and serum lipase levels, and scan the abdomen.

- Persistent hyperamylasemia suggests a complication.

- If the amylase level is mildly elevated and there is a history of vomiting but no signs of obstruction, perform an esophagogastroduodenoscopy to rule out a penetrating ulcer.

Nonpancreatic Hyperamylasemia

Nonpancreatic hyperamylasemia may result from parotitis; renal failure; macroamylasemia; intestinal obstruction, infarction, or perforation; ruptured ectopic pregnancy; diabetic ketoacidosis; drugs (eg, morphine); burns; pregnancy; and neoplasms (lung, ovary, or esophagus).

Physical Findings

Physical findings include tachycardia, orthostasis, fat necrosis, and xanthelasmas of the skin. The Grey Turner sign (flank discoloration) and the Cullen sign (periumbilical discoloration) suggest retroperitoneal hemorrhage. The abdominal findings often are less impressive than the amount of pain the patient is experiencing.

- Look for metastatic fat necrosis.

- The Grey Turner sign and the Cullen sign suggest retroperitoneal hemorrhage.

Imaging Studies

Chest Radiography

An isolated left pleural effusion strongly suggests pancreatitis; infiltrates may indicate aspiration pneumonia or acute respiratory distress syndrome.

Abdominal Plain Film

Look for the sentinel loop sign (a dilated loop of bowel over the pancreatic area) and the colon cutoff sign (abrupt cutoff of gas in the transverse colon); pancreatic calcifications indicate chronic pancreatitis.

Ultrasonography

Ultrasonographic examination is the procedure of choice for helping to determine the cause of acute pancreatitis. Although ultrasonography gives information about the pancreas and is the best method for delineating gallstones, it is not a good method if the patient is obese.

Computed Tomography

CT is indicated for critically ill patients to rule out necrotizing pancreatitis. CT scans are not required for patients with documented mild interstitial acute pancreatitis.

Endoscopic Retrograde Cholangiopancreatography

ERCP has no role in the diagnosis of acute pancreatitis and should be avoided because it may cause infection.

Endoscopic Papillotomy

Endoscopic papillotomy is indicated when acute pancreatitis is associated with jaundice and cholangitis.

- An isolated left pleural effusion on chest radiography is strongly suggestive of acute pancreatitis.

- On an abdominal plain film, look for the sentinel loop sign, the colon cutoff sign, and pancreatic calcifications.

- CT is indicated for critically ill patients to rule out necrotizing pancreatitis.

- ERCP has no role in the diagnosis of acute pancreatitis.

TREATMENT

Supportive care is the backbone of treatment, with monitoring for complications and treating them when they occur.

Fluids

Restore and maintain intravascular fluid volume; usually this can be accomplished with crystalloids and peripheral intravenous catheters. Monitor blood pressure, pulse, urine output, daily intake and output, and weight. Eliminate medications that may cause pancreatitis. The use of a nasogastric tube does not shorten the course or severity of pancreatitis, but it should be used for ileus or severe nausea and vomiting.

Analgesics

Common practice has been to use meperidine (Demerol) (75–125 mg given intramuscularly every 3–4 hours) instead of morphine because meperidine purportedly causes less spasm of the sphincter of Oddi. Meperidine has potentially toxic metabolites, though, so it has been removed from many hospital formularies, and the in vivo link between meperidine and sphincter spasm is unclear. Standard methods of analgesia can generally be used with impunity. The efficacy of antisecretory drugs (eg, H_2 receptor antagonists, anticholinergic agents, somatostatin, glucagon) has not been documented.

Nutrition

Patients with severe pancreatitis may require supplemental nutrition. This should be provided by means of a nasoenteric tube. Total parenteral nutrition is unnecessary in most cases of pancreatitis and should be considered only when enteral feeding has failed or is not feasible.

Antibiotics

Antibiotics are indicated for prophylaxis of gram-negative sepsis in patients with necrotizing pancreatitis but not for patients with nonnecrotizing pancreatitis.

- Supportive care is the backbone of treatment of acute pancreatitis.

- Eliminate medications that may cause pancreatitis.

- The use of a nasogastric tube does not shorten the course or severity of pancreatitis.

- Antibiotics are indicated for patients with necrotizing pancreatitis.

COMPLICATIONS

A local complication is *pancreatic phlegmon*, a mass of inflamed pancreatic tissue. It may resolve. *Pseudocyst*, a fluid collection within a nonepithelial-lined cavity, should be suspected if there is persistent pain and persistent hyperamylasemia. In 50% to 80% of patients, this resolves within 6 weeks without intervention. A pancreatic abscess develops usually 2 to 4 weeks after the acute episode and causes fever (>38.3°C), persistent abdominal pain, and persistent hyperamylasemia. If a pancreatic abscess is not drained surgically, the mortality rate is virtually 100%. Give antibiotics that are effective for gram-negative and anaerobic organisms. Jaundice results from obstruction of the common bile duct. Pancreatic ascites results from disruption of the pancreatic duct or a leaking pseudocyst.

A well-recognized systemic complication of acute pancreatitis is acute respiratory distress syndrome. Circulating lecithinase probably splits fatty acids off lecithin, producing a faulty surfactant. Pleural effusion occurs in approximately 20% of patients with acute pancreatitis. Aspirate analysis shows a high amylase content. Fat necrosis may be due to increased levels of serum lipase.

- A local complication of pancreatitis should be suspected if fever, persistent pain, or persistent hyperamylasemia occurs.
- Acute respiratory distress syndrome is a complication of acute pancreatitis.
- Pleural effusion occurs in approximately 20% of patients with acute pancreatitis; the fluid has a high amylase content.

ASSESSMENT OF SEVERITY

Most patients with acute pancreatitis recover without any sequelae. The overall mortality rate of acute pancreatitis is 5% to 10%, and death is due most often to hypovolemia and shock, respiratory failure, pancreatic abscess, or systemic sepsis. The Ranson criteria (Box 10.1) and the Acute Physiology and Chronic Health Evaluation (APACHE) criteria are reliable for predicting mortality in acute pancreatitis. Predicted mortality is calculated as follows: less than 3 Ranson criteria, 1%; 3 or 4 criteria, 15%; 5 or 6 criteria, 40%; and 7 or more criteria, more than 80%.

- Most patients with acute pancreatitis recover without any sequelae.

CHRONIC PANCREATITIS

Long-term alcohol use (≥10 years of heavy consumption) is the most common cause of chronic pancreatitis. Gallstones and hyperlipidemia usually do not cause chronic pancreatitis.

Box 10.1 RANSON CRITERIA

On admission
    Age > 55 y
    White blood cell count $>15\times10^9$/L
    Serum glucose >200 mg/dL
    Serum aspartate aminotransferase >250 U/L
    Serum lactate dehydrogenase >350 U/L
At 48 h after admission
    Pao$_2$ <60 mm Hg
    Hematocrit decrease >10%
    Serum albumin <3.2 g/dL
    Serum urea nitrogen increase >5 mg/dL
    Serum calcium <8 mg/dL
    Estimated fluid sequestration >4 L

Abbreviation: U, units.

Adapted from Ranson JHC. Acute pancreatitis: surgical management. In: Go VLW, Gardner JD, Brooks FP, Lebenthal E, DiMagno EP, Scheele GA, editors. The exocrine pancreas: biology, pathobiology, and diseases. New York (NY): Raven Press; c1986. p. 503–11. Used with permission.

Hereditary pancreatitis is caused by a mutation in the cationic trypsinogen gene, which is inherited as an autosomal dominant trait with variable penetrance. Onset is before age 20, although 20% of patients may present later than this. Hereditary pancreatitis is marked by recurring abdominal pain, positive family history, and pancreatic calcifications. It may increase the risk of pancreatic cancer.

Trauma with pancreatic ductal disruption causes chronic pancreatitis. Protein calorie malnutrition is the most common cause of chronic pancreatitis in Third World countries.

- Chronic pancreatitis is commonly caused by alcohol but seldom by gallstones or hyperlipidemia.
- Hereditary pancreatitis occurs in young people with a positive family history and pancreatic calcifications.
- Protein calorie malnutrition is the most common cause of chronic pancreatitis in Third World countries.

TRIAD OF CHRONIC PANCREATITIS

Patients with chronic pancreatitis present with abdominal pain. In addition, the triad of chronic pancreatitis consists of pancreatic calcifications, steatorrhea, and diabetes mellitus. Diffuse calcification of the pancreas is due to hereditary pancreatitis, alcoholic pancreatitis, or malnutrition. Local calcification is due to trauma, islet cell tumor, or hypercalcemia. By the time steatorrhea occurs, 90% of the pancreas has been destroyed and lipase output has decreased by 90%.

- Patients with chronic pancreatitis present with abdominal pain, pancreatic calcifications, steatorrhea, and diabetes mellitus.
- For steatorrhea to occur, 90% of the gland must be damaged.

LABORATORY DIAGNOSIS

Serum amylase and lipase levels may be normal, and stool fat may be normal. If malabsorption is present, stool fat is more than 10 g in 24 hours during a 48- to 72-hour stool collection while the patient is consuming a diet with 100 g of fat.

For the secretin-cholecystokinin (CCK) test of pancreatic function, secretin and CCK are injected intravenously and then the contents of the small bowel are aspirated and the concentration of pancreatic enzymes is determined.

In the bentiromide test, p-aminobenzoic acid (PABA) conjugated with N-benzoyl tyrosine (bentiromide) is given orally. If chymotrypsin activity is adequate, the molecule is cleaved and PABA is absorbed and excreted in the urine. This test requires a normal small intestine (normal D-xylose test) and is useful only in severe steatorrhea.

CT shows calcifications, an irregular pancreatic contour, a dilated duct system, or pseudocysts. ERCP shows protein plugs, segmental duct dilatation, and alternating stenosis and dilatation, with obliteration of branches of the main duct.

- Serum amylase and lipase levels may be normal, but evidence for structural disease or endocrine or exocrine insufficiency is present.

PAIN

The mechanism for pain is not clearly defined; it may be due to ductular obstruction. One-third to one-half of patients have a decrease in pain after 5 years. The possibility of coexistent disease, such as peptic ulcer, should be considered. Complications of chronic pancreatitis (eg, biliary stricture, pancreatic ductal stricture, malignancy, vascular thrombosis) should be excluded. Abstinence from alcohol may relieve the pain. Analgesics, aspirin, or acetaminophen is used occasionally with the addition of codeine (narcotic addiction is a frequent complicating factor). Celiac plexus blocks relieve pain for 3 to 6 months, but long-term efficacy is less effective. A trial of pancreatic enzyme replacement for 1 or 2 months should be tried. Women with idiopathic chronic pancreatitis are most likely to have a response. Surgical treatment should be considered only after conservative measures have failed. Patients with a dilated pancreatic duct may have a favorable response to a longitudinal pancreaticojejunostomy (Puestow procedure).

- Abstinence from alcohol may relieve the pain.
- Narcotic addiction is a frequent complicating factor.
- A 1- or 2-month trial of pancreatic enzyme replacement is worthwhile; women are more likely to have a response.
- Surgical treatment should be considered only after conservative measures have failed.

MALABSORPTION

Patients have malabsorption not only of fat but also of essential fatty acids and fat-soluble vitamins. The goal of enzyme replacement is to maintain body weight. Diarrhea will not resolve. Enteric-coated or microsphere enzymes are designed to be released at an alkaline pH, thus avoiding degradation by stomach acid. The advantage is that they contain larger amounts of lipase. The disadvantages are that they are expensive and bioavailability is not always predictable.

PANCREATIC CARCINOMA

Pancreatic carcinoma is more common in men than in women. Patients usually present between the ages of 60 and 80 years. The 5-year survival rate is less than 2%. Risk factors include diabetes mellitus, chronic pancreatitis, hereditary pancreatitis, carcinogens, benzidine, cigarette smoking, and high-fat diet. Patients with pancreatic carcinoma usually present late in the course of the disease. They may have a vague prodrome of malaise, anorexia, and weight loss. Symptoms may be overlooked until pain or jaundice develop. Two signs associated with pancreatic cancer are the Courvoisier sign (painless jaundice with a palpable gallbladder) and the Trousseau sign (recurrent migratory thrombophlebitis). Recent-onset diabetes and nonbacterial (thrombotic) marantic endocarditis may be associated with pancreatic cancer.

- Courvoisier sign: painless jaundice with a palpable gallbladder suggests pancreatic cancer.
- Trousseau sign: recurrent migratory thrombophlebitis is associated with pancreatic cancer.
- Recent-onset diabetes and nonbacterial (thrombotic) marantic endocarditis may be associated with pancreatic carcinoma.

Routine laboratory blood analysis has limited usefulness. Patients may have increased levels of liver enzymes, amylase, and lipase or anemia, although this is variable. Tumor markers are also nonspecific. Abdominal ultrasonography and CT are each approximately 80% sensitive in localizing pancreatic masses. The "double duct" sign on CT scan is a classic presentation, with obstruction of the pancreatic ducts and the bile ducts. Either imaging method may be used in conjunction with fine-needle aspiration or biopsy to make a tissue diagnosis. If a mass in the pancreas is found and deemed resectable on CT scan, surgical consultation should be pursued as the next step (additional testing may not be necessary). ERCP and EUS are used if the abdominal ultrasonographic or CT results are inconclusive. ERCP and EUS each have a sensitivity greater than 90%. At ERCP, brushings and biopsies can be performed in an attempt to confirm the diagnosis.

- Abdominal ultrasonography and CT are each 80% sensitive in localizing pancreatic masses.
- ERCP and EUS each have a sensitivity >90%.

Surgical treatment is the only hope for cure; however, most lesions are not resectable. The criteria for resectability are a tumor smaller than 2 cm, the absence of lymph node invasion, and the absence of metastasis. Survival is the same with total pancreatectomy and with the Whipple procedure: 3-year survival, 33%; 5-year survival, 1%; and operative mortality, 5%.

Radiotherapy may have a role as a radiosensitizer in unresectable cancer. However, survival is unchanged. The results of chemotherapy have been disappointing, and studies have not consistently shown improved survival.

CYSTIC FIBROSIS

Because patients with cystic fibrosis are living longer, internists should know the common intestinal complications of this disease. Exocrine pancreatic insufficiency (malabsorption) is the most important complication, and it is quite common (85%–90% of patients). Endocrine pancreatic insufficiency (diabetes mellitus) occurs in 20% to 30% of patients. Rectal prolapse occurs in 20% of patients, and a distal small-bowel obstruction from thick secretions occurs in 15% to 20%. Focal biliary cirrhosis develops in 20% of patients.

- Exocrine pancreatic insufficiency occurs in 85%–90% of patients with cystic fibrosis.

PANCREATIC ENDOCRINE TUMORS

Zollinger-Ellison syndrome is a non–beta islet cell tumor of the pancreas that produces gastrin and causes gastric acid hypersecretion. This results in peptic ulcer disease (see "Peptic Ulcer Disease" subsection in Chapter 11).

Insulinoma is the most common islet cell tumor. It is a beta islet cell tumor that produces insulin and causes hypoglycemia. The diagnosis is based on finding increased fasting plasma levels of insulin and hypoglycemia. CT, EUS, or arteriography may be useful in localizing the tumor.

Glucagonoma is an alpha islet cell tumor that produces glucagon. Patients present with diabetes mellitus, weight loss, and a classic skin rash (migratory necrolytic erythema). The diagnosis is based on finding increased glucagon levels and on finding that the blood glucose level does not increase after an injection of glucagon.

Pancreatic cholera is a pancreatic tumor that produces vasoactive intestinal polypeptide (VIP), which causes watery diarrhea (see "Secretory Diarrhea" subsection in Chapter 12).

Somatostatinoma is a delta islet cell tumor that produces somatostatin, which inhibits insulin, gastrin, and pancreatic enzyme secretion. The result is diabetes mellitus and diarrhea. The diagnosis is based on finding increased plasma levels of somatostatin.

Octreotide is useful in treating pancreatic endocrine tumors except for somatostatinomas. Octreotide prevents the release of hormone and antagonizes hormonal effects on target organs.

- Zollinger-Ellison syndrome: non–beta islet cell tumor of the pancreas.

- Insulinoma: most common islet cell tumor.

- Pancreatic cholera: pancreatic tumor that produces VIP, which causes secretory diarrhea.

- Octreotide prevents hormone release and antagonizes hormonal effects.

SUMMARY

- If the presentation for pancreatitis is classic but the amylase value is normal, repeat the amylase test, check urinary amylase and serum lipase levels, and scan the abdomen. Persistent hyperamylasemia suggests a complication. If the amylase level is mildly elevated and there is a history of vomiting but no signs of obstruction, perform an esophagogastroduodenoscopy to rule out a penetrating ulcer.

- An isolated left pleural effusion on chest radiography is strongly suggestive of acute pancreatitis. On an abdominal plain film, look for the sentinel loop sign, the colon cutoff sign, and pancreatic calcifications.

- Supportive care is the backbone of treatment of acute pancreatitis. Antibiotics are indicated for patients with necrotizing pancreatitis.

- Patients with chronic pancreatitis present with abdominal pain, pancreatic calcifications, steatorrhea, and diabetes mellitus.

- For patients with chronic pancreatitis, abstinence from alcohol may relieve the pain. A 1- or 2-month trial of pancreatic enzyme replacement is worthwhile; women are more likely to have a response. Surgical treatment should be considered only after conservative measures have failed.

11.

ESOPHAGUS AND STOMACH

Amy S. Oxentenko, MD

GOALS

- Distinguish between the 3 main forms of dysphagia on the basis of clinical history, and recognize the differences in the evaluation of each.

- Describe the stepwise diagnostic evaluation of a patient with gastroesophageal reflux disease (GERD).

- List the common causes of peptic ulcer disease (PUD), and describe the differences between the invasive and noninvasive tests for *Helicobacter pylori* infection.

- Recognize the appropriate order of staging tests for the evaluation of both esophageal cancer and gastric cancer.

ESOPHAGUS

ESOPHAGEAL FUNCTION

The main functions of the esophagus are to transport food and prevent reflux. To transport food from the mouth to the stomach, the esophagus must work against a pressure gradient, with negative pressure in the chest and positive pressure in the abdomen. The lower esophageal sphincter (LES) helps to prevent reflux of gastric contents back into the esophagus.

The upper esophageal sphincter (UES) (or cricopharyngeal muscle) and the muscle of the proximal one-third of the esophagus are striated muscle under voluntary control. A transition from skeletal to smooth muscle occurs in the midesophagus, with the distal one-third of the esophagus composed of smooth muscle under involuntary control. The LES is a zone of circular muscle located in the distal 2 to 3 cm of the esophagus.

- The main functions of the esophagus are to transport food and prevent reflux of gastric contents.

- The esophagus transports food from the mouth to the stomach against a pressure gradient.

NORMAL MOTILITY

Immediately after a person swallows, the UES relaxes, allowing a food bolus to pass from the oropharynx into the esophagus. A peristaltic wave then passes through the body of the esophagus, and within 2 seconds after the swallow, the LES relaxes and stays relaxed until the wave of peristalsis passes through it. The LES then contracts and maintains resting tone. If the esophagus cannot perform its 2 main functions, 2 major symptom complexes result: dysphagia (transport dysfunction) and reflux (LES dysfunction).

- Dysphagia results from oropharyngeal or esophageal transport dysfunction.

- Reflux results from LES dysfunction.

DYSPHAGIA

Dysphagia results from defective transport of food and is usually described as "difficulty swallowing" or "food sticking." The 3 causes of dysphagia must be distinguished: 1) oropharyngeal (faulty transfer of a food bolus from the oropharynx into the esophagus), 2) mechanical (structural abnormality of the esophageal lumen), and 3) motor (motility disorder). Answers to 3 questions frequently suggest the diagnosis (Figure 11.1): 1) What types of food produce the dysphagia (solids or liquids)? 2) What is the time course of the dysphagia (intermittent or progressive)? 3) Is there associated heartburn? Esophagogastroduodenoscopy (EGD) is the first test that should be done in the evaluation of dysphagia unless there are features of oropharyngeal dysphagia (see below).

- The 3 types of dysphagia are oropharyngeal, mechanical, and motor.

- The cause of dysphagia is strongly suggested by the triggering foods, time course, and associated symptoms.

- EGD is the initial test of choice for the evaluation of dysphagia unless oropharyngeal dysphagia is suspected.

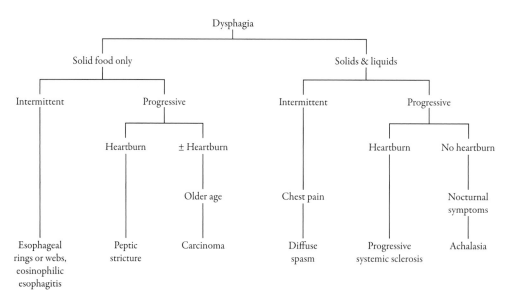

Figure 11.1 Diagnostic Scheme for Dysphagia. The answers to 3 questions (see text) often suggest the most likely diagnosis. (Adapted from MKSAP VI: part 1:44, 1982. American College of Physicians. Used with permission.)

Oropharyngeal Dysphagia

Oropharyngeal dysphagia is the result of faulty transfer of a food bolus from the oropharynx into the esophagus and is most commonly caused by neuromuscular disorders and less commonly by proximal structural abnormalities (Box 11.1). In addition to having difficulty swallowing, patients with oropharyngeal dysphagia present with coughing, choking, aspiration pneumonia, or nasal regurgitation with eating or drinking. The first test in the evaluation of oropharyngeal dysphagia is a video fluoroscopic swallowing test (also called a modified barium swallow). After oropharyngeal dysphagia is diagnosed, an evaluation to determine the underlying diagnosis is needed; there may be associated features that can lead to the diagnosis, such as optic neuritis (with multiple sclerosis) or fatigability (with myasthenia gravis).

- Patients with oropharyngeal dysphagia present with coughing, choking, aspiration pneumonia, or nasal regurgitation.

- The first test in the evaluation of oropharyngeal dysphagia is a video fluoroscopic swallowing test (also called a modified barium swallow).

Motor Dysphagia

Motor (or *motility*) *disorders* are characterized by dysphagia with both solids and liquids. These disorders may follow an intermittent or progressive course. The 3 important motor abnormalities of the esophagus are achalasia, scleroderma, and diffuse esophageal spasm.

- Patients with motor (or motility) disorders present with dysphagia with both solids and liquids; the course may be intermittent or progressive.

Box 11.1 CAUSES OF OROPHARYNGEAL DYSPHAGIA

Muscular disorders
  Amyloidosis
  Dermatomyositis
  Hyperthyroidism
  Hypothyroidism
  Myasthenia gravis
  Myotonia dystrophica
  Oculopharyngeal myopathy
  Stiff man syndrome
Neurologic disorders
  Amyotrophic lateral sclerosis
  Multiple sclerosis
  Parkinson disease
  Polio
  Stroke
  Tabes dorsalis
  Tetanus
Structural causes
  Cervical osteophytes
  Cricopharyngeal dysfunction
  Esophageal webs
  Goiter
  Lymphadenopathy
  Zenker diverticulum

Achalasia, meaning "failure to relax," results from degeneration of Auerbach ganglion cells in the LES. Patients present with years of progressive dysphagia to both solids and liquids. Although they may have regurgitation of undigested food that never passed out of the esophagus, heartburn is typically absent given the tonically contracted LES. Chest radiography may show an air-fluid level within the esophagus in advanced cases. Barium esophagography typically shows a dilated esophagus with a beak-like ("bird beak") tapering at the LES. The motility pattern is characterized by the following: 1) incomplete relaxation of the LES, 2) hypertensive LES, and 3) aperistalsis of the esophageal body. All patients with features of achalasia require an EGD because cancer infiltrating near the esophagogastric junction may have the same radiographic and manometric pattern of achalasia (termed *pseudoachalasia*). Patients with pseudoachalasia tend to be older, have more rapid onset of symptoms (months rather than years), and have more profound weight loss. Treatment of achalasia includes surgical methods (myotomy), injection of botulinum toxin into the LES, or pneumatic dilation. Healthy patients who can undergo surgery should be considered for a myotomy. Botulinum toxin injection into the LES decreases lower esophageal pressure for 3 to 12 months; given the short-term relief of symptoms, it should be considered for elderly patients and for those with high surgical risk. In Brazil, the parasite *Trypanosoma cruzi* (which causes Chagas disease) produces a neurotoxin that destroys the myenteric plexus and leads to esophageal dilatation identical to that of achalasia.

- Clinical features of achalasia include chronic, progressive dysphagia to both solids and liquids with regurgitation of undigested food.

- Radiographic features of achalasia can include an air-fluid level in the esophagus on chest radiography and a dilated esophagus with "bird beak" tapering with barium imaging.

- The manometric pattern in achalasia includes 1) failed LES relaxation, 2) increased or hypertensive LES resting tone, and 3) aperistalsis of the esophageal body.

- All patients with features of achalasia require an EGD to rule out pseudoachalasia.

- Treatment of achalasia includes surgery, pneumatic dilation, or botulinum toxin injection.

Esophageal involvement with scleroderma is associated with the presence of Raynaud phenomenon and is part of the CREST syndrome. Patients have chronic, progressive dysphagia with both solids and liquids, along with severe heartburn and reflux. Barium swallow fluoroscopy may show a rigid esophagus and a widely patent LES. Although motility testing shows aperistalsis in the body of the esophagus similar to achalasia, there is decreased tone of the LES in scleroderma, which differentiates the 2 conditions.

- Although patients with achalasia and scleroderma share some clinical and manometric findings, the presence of decreased LES tone in patients with scleroderma helps to distinguish the condition from achalasia.

Patients with *diffuse esophageal spasm* usually present with chest pain, but they may have intermittent dysphagia with solids or liquids, or both; symptoms may be aggravated by stress, hot or cold liquids, and carbonated beverages. Barium imaging may show a "corkscrew esophagus." Motility

studies may demonstrate simultaneous contractions in the body of the esophagus during symptoms. A trial of acid suppression should be considered because acid reflux may precipitate esophageal spasm in some persons. Medical treatment (nitrates, anticholinergic agents, and nifedipine) has unpredictable results.

- Diffuse esophageal spasm usually causes chest pain.

- Esophageal spasm may be aggravated by stress, hot or cold liquids, and carbonated beverages.

- Barium imaging may show a "corkscrew esophagus" during symptoms.

Mechanical Dysphagia

Dysphagia can result when there is compromise of the esophageal lumen to a diameter of less than 12 mm. This type of dysphagia usually begins with solid foods, but it may progress to involve liquids with further luminal narrowing. Depending on the cause, such as malignancy, weight loss may occur.

- Patients with mechanical abnormalities of the esophagus present with solid food dysphagia, which may progress to involve liquids.

A *peptic stricture* results from esophageal reflux of acid. It is usually a short (<2 cm in length) narrowing in the distal esophagus immediately at or above the esophagogastric junction. Management includes esophageal dilation and acid suppression; proton pump inhibitor (PPI) therapy after dilation of a peptic stricture decreases recurrence.

- A peptic stricture results from acid reflux and is located in the distal esophagus; dilation and acid suppression are recommended.

Alkali is more injurious to the esophagus than acid. *Alkali-induced strictures* can occur in patients after a total gastrectomy (stricture due to alkaline reflux) or after lye ingestion. Inducing emesis after lye ingestion is contraindicated since the caustic substance can further injure the esophagus with subsequent exposure. Lye-induced strictures tend to be long (compared with peptic strictures). Repeated dilation or temporary stenting of the esophagus is often required after an alkali-induced stricture has occurred. Patients with lye-induced strictures have an increased incidence of squamous cell cancer of the esophagus.

- Both postgastrectomy alkaline reflux and lye ingestion can produce alkali-induced strictures.

- Inducing emesis after lye ingestion is contraindicated.

- Lye-induced strictures are associated with an increased incidence of squamous cell cancer of the esophagus.

A *lower esophageal ring* (Schatzki ring) is a constriction at the esophagogastric junction. The rings tend to cause intermittent solid food dysphagia, most notably with foods such as meat and bread. Patients may also present with sudden food impaction, known as "steak house syndrome." Esophageal dilation is the treatment of choice. An *esophageal web* consists of a squamous membrane, which can be found throughout the esophagus, leading to dysphagia. If patients have an esophageal web with a proximal location, they can present with features of oropharyngeal dysphagia. The *Plummer-Vinson syndrome* occurs in females who have iron-deficiency anemia, glossitis, and proximal esophageal webs, with increased risk of esophageal malignancy (squamous cell carcinoma). A *Zenker diverticulum*, an outpouching adjacent to the UES, results from increased tone within the UES. Patients present with dysphagia, regurgitation of small amounts of old food, and halitosis. Fullness in the neck may be apparent. Management includes resection of the diverticulum in combination with UES myotomy.

- Patients with a Schatzki ring present with intermittent solid food dysphagia.

- The Plummer-Vinson syndrome occurs in females who have iron-deficiency anemia, glossitis, and proximal esophageal webs; patients are at increased risk of squamous cell cancer of the esophagus.

Patients with *eosinophilic esophagitis* present with intermittent solid food dysphagia and food impactions. This occurs most commonly in young men, but it may be seen in all ages and in either sex. The patient may have a personal or family history of atopic conditions. Endoscopic findings may include concentric esophageal rings, furrows, or a featureless narrowed esophagus; some patients have normal findings. The diagnosis is established by performing biopsies of the midesophagus and finding more than 15 eosinophils per high-power field. Since esophageal reflux can cause esophageal eosinophilia, initial management is with a PPI trial; for patients who have persistent symptoms despite acid suppression, swallowed, aerosolized fluticasone propionate is recommended. For children, elimination diets may be used. Severe tears can occur in untreated patients, so dilation of any associated strictures should occur after medical therapy has begun.

- Patients with eosinophilic esophagitis present with intermittent solid food dysphagia and food impactions; they may have a personal or family history of atopy.

- Eosinophilic esophagitis is diagnosed by finding >15 eosinophils per high-power field on midesophageal biopsies; treatment is with PPI therapy followed by swallowed, aerosolized corticosteroids in patients who have persistent symptoms.

Squamous cell carcinomas of the esophagus are usually located in the proximal two-thirds of the esophagus, whereas tumors of the distal one-third are more commonly adenocarcinoma. The conditions that predispose to esophageal squamous cell carcinoma include achalasia, lye-induced stricture, Plummer-Vinson syndrome, human papillomavirus, tylosis, smoking, and alcohol consumption. Barrett esophagus is the most recognized risk factor for adenocarcinoma of the esophagus. In the United States, the majority of esophageal cancers are adenocarcinoma. Progressive dysphagia accompanied by weight loss is typical. The diagnosis is established by endoscopy with biopsy. After the diagnosis is confirmed, computed tomography (CT) of the chest and abdomen should be done to evaluate for metastatic disease. Endoscopic ultrasonography may be used to assess locoregional staging after distant metastases have been ruled out. The 5-year survival rate is only 7% to 15% since most patients have advanced disease at presentation.

Surgical resection is the treatment of choice for esophageal cancer that is detected early. For patients with locally advanced disease or lymph node involvement, preoperative chemoradiotherapy may be considered, with restaging thereafter. For patients with extensive nodal or metastatic disease, palliative therapy can be offered, including chemotherapy, radiotherapy, and esophageal stenting.

- Conditions that predispose to esophageal squamous cell cancer include achalasia, lye-induced stricture, Plummer-Vinson syndrome, human papillomavirus, tylosis, smoking, and alcohol consumption.

- Barrett esophagus is the most recognized risk factor for esophageal adenocarcinoma.

- Esophageal malignancies are usually advanced stage at presentation, and patients have poor 5-year survival.

ODYNOPHAGIA

Odynophagia refers to painful swallowing and results most commonly from inflammation (infection or medication induced) or spasm.

Infections of the Esophagus

Patients with immunodeficiency disorders (eg, AIDS), diabetes mellitus, malignancies (especially lymphoma and leukemia), or esophageal motility disorders are susceptible to opportunistic infections of the esophagus and may present with odynophagia. The most important infections to recognize are those caused by *Candida albicans* (the most common cause), herpesvirus, or cytomegalovirus. With candidal infection, endoscopy shows cottage cheese–like plaques adherent to the esophageal mucosa. The diagnosis is made by demonstrating pseudohyphae microscopically from brushings of the mucosa. Treatment is with oral fluconazole for *Candida* esophagitis. For patients presenting with odynophagia who have evidence of thrush, therapy with oral fluconazole may be empirically started for presumed *Candida* esophagitis, reserving endoscopy for those in whom empirical therapy fails. If thrush is not present, patients should undergo endoscopy to establish a diagnosis. With herpesvirus infection, endoscopy may show small discrete ulcers. Diagnosis is based on finding intranuclear inclusions with surrounding halos and multinucleated giant cells in biopsy specimens from an edge of the ulcer. Treatment is with acyclovir. In cytomegaloviral infection, endoscopy may show large, irregular ulcers. Histologic examination of biopsy specimens from the ulcer base shows "owl's eye" intranuclear inclusions and enlarged areas of cytoplasm. Treatment is with ganciclovir or foscarnet (if resistant to ganciclovir).

- Odynophagia in an immunosuppressed patient is typically due to an opportunistic infection with *Candida*, herpesvirus, or cytomegalovirus.

- If a patient presents with odynophagia and has evidence of thrush, empirical therapy with oral fluconazole should be started.

Medication-Induced Esophagitis

Patients with *medication-induced esophagitis* present with odynophagia (or, less frequently, dysphagia). Medication-induced esophagitis may occur if esophageal motility or anatomy is abnormal, but it can happen if medications are not taken with adequate fluids or if patients assume a supine position immediately after taking them. Medications commonly associated with esophagitis include tetracycline, doxycycline, quinidine, potassium supplements, bisphosphonates, ferrous sulfate, and ascorbic acid. The use of these medications should be avoided if possible in patients with known esophageal strictures or symptoms of dysphagia.

- Medicines responsible for medication-induced esophagitis include tetracycline, doxycycline, quinidine, potassium supplements, bisphosphonates, ferrous sulfate, and ascorbic acid.

GASTROESOPHAGEAL REFLUX DISEASE

Reflux

The LES is the major barrier to prevent esophageal reflux of gastric contents. Swallowing causes the sphincter pressure to decrease promptly within 1 to 2 seconds and remain relaxed until the peristaltic wave passes over it. The sphincter then contracts and maintains the increased resting pressure that prevents reflux.

GERD is typically caused by inappropriate relaxation of the LES or by intragastric pressure that exceeds LES pressure. GERD can lead to tissue damage and ulceration, known as *esophagitis*. Factors that determine whether reflux esophagitis occurs include the frequency of transient relaxations of the LES, the rate of gastric emptying (if delayed, reflux may develop), the potency of the refluxate (acid, pepsin, and bile), the efficiency of esophageal clearance (motility and salivary bicarbonate), and the resistance of esophageal tissue to injury. Complications of reflux include esophagitis, bleeding, stricture formation, aspiration, Barrett esophagus, and adenocarcinoma of the esophagus.

Most patients with GERD describe classic heartburn or regurgitation. Atypical symptoms of GERD include noncardiac chest pain, asthma, chronic cough, hoarseness, and enamel defects. Reflux is the most common cause of noncardiac chest pain; however, cardiac status must be evaluated before chest pain is attributed to reflux. Asthmatic patients with coexisting reflux should receive therapy for reflux because it may improve control of respiratory symptoms. Reflux should be considered in asthmatic patients who have postprandial or nocturnal wheezing.

For patients who are younger than 50 years with classic symptoms of reflux and no alarm features (weight loss, anemia, dysphagia, odynophagia, or family history of cancer in the upper gastrointestinal tract), an empirical trial of PPI therapy is warranted. However, testing should be performed if patients have new-onset symptoms after age 50, atypical features, refractory or long-standing symptoms, or alarm features. The initial test in the evaluation of these symptoms would be an EGD; if an EGD does not show esophagitis or other features to support the diagnosis of reflux, a 24-hour ambulatory pH probe can be used to document esophageal acid exposure and symptom correlation.

- For most patients, the medical history is sufficiently typical to warrant a trial of PPI therapy without tests.

- An EGD is recommended for patients with reflux-type symptoms if they have new-onset symptoms after age 50, atypical features, refractory or long-standing symptoms, or alarm features.

- Atypical symptoms of GERD include noncardiac chest pain, asthma, chronic cough, hoarseness, and enamel defects.

- Complications of gastroesophageal reflux include esophagitis, bleeding, stricture formation, aspiration, Barrett esophagus, and adenocarcinoma of the esophagus.

Barrett Esophagus

Barrett esophagus is a complication of chronic gastroesophageal reflux in which the normal esophageal squamous mucosa is replaced by columnar epithelium or intestinal metaplasia. Patients with Barrett esophagus are at increased risk of adenocarcinoma. Although considerable controversy exists about the benefits of performing screening endoscopy to evaluate for Barrett esophagus, most experts recommend screening endoscopy for high-risk patients (obese white men older than 50 years) who have had chronic reflux for more than 5 years. If mucosal changes are seen endoscopically, biopsies are needed to confirm the diagnosis and to look for dysplasia. The surveillance frequency is based on the presence and degree of dysplasia found during the previous study. If there is no dysplasia, surveillance should occur every 3 years. If low-grade dysplasia is identified, surveillance should be yearly. If high-grade dysplasia is identified (and confirmed by 2 pathologists), the patient may elect to undergo an esophagectomy or be considered for an ablative therapy, such as photodynamic therapy.

- Barrett esophagus predisposes to adenocarcinoma.
- EGD to screen for Barrett esophagus should be considered for high-risk patients (obese white men older than 50 years) who have had chronic reflux for more than 5 years.

Tests for Reflux

Barium esophagography is not very helpful in the evaluation of reflux, since reflux of barium occurs in 25% of control subjects. This test can be helpful in clarifying abnormal anatomy (paraesophageal hernia, intrathoracic stomach, complicated strictures) but should not replace upper endoscopy.

- Barium esophagography is not very helpful in the evaluation of reflux, since reflux of barium occurs in 25% of control subjects.

EGD is the test of choice to evaluate for the presence and complications of reflux disease; this test should be done if a PPI trial has failed or if a patient has features that warrant initial evaluation. If esophagitis is present, reflux can be diagnosed with certainty. However, 40% of patients may have symptomatic reflux with no gross inflammation.

- In patients requiring testing to evaluate for esophageal reflux, EGD is the first test indicated.

Monitoring the pH in the distal esophagus during a 24-hour period allows a physiologic evaluation of reflux during daily activities. This test is valuable for patients who have atypical symptoms, reflux symptoms refractory to therapy, or upper endoscopic results that are nondiagnostic (ie, no esophagitis is noted). The test provides objective measurements of acid exposure within the esophagus, with symptom correlation noted.

- Ambulatory 24-hour pH monitoring allows a physiologic evaluation of reflux during daily activities and is valuable for patients who have a nondiagnostic EGD or atypical or refractory symptoms.

Esophageal impedance testing can be used to detect the presence of nonacidic reflux in patients who are receiving PPI therapy or who have achlorhydria or bile reflux, since this test detects the presence of a fluid column, regardless of pH. Esophageal manometry is reserved for patients with suspected esophageal motility disorders; it is not useful for the evaluation of reflux.

- Esophageal impedance testing can be used to evaluate nonacid reflux.
- Esophageal manometry is reserved for suspected esophageal motility disorders.

Treatment of Reflux

The management of GERD is usually stepwise. Patients should be counseled on lifestyle modifications: The head of the patient's bed should be elevated 15 cm to keep the stomach lower than the esophagus, and patients should be advised to not eat for 3 hours before reclining, lose weight if overweight, avoid eating foods that trigger symptoms (eg, fatty foods, chocolate, peppermint, alcohol, citrus juices, tomato products, coffee), and avoid tobacco and alcohol. In addition, drugs that decrease LES pressure should be avoided: anticholinergic agents, sedatives, theophylline, progesterone or progesterone-containing birth control pills, nitrates α-adrenergic agonists, and calcium channel blockers.

Medical therapy for reflux is graduated according to the degree of severity of the patient's symptoms. Over-the-counter antacids or H_2 receptor antagonists may be helpful for the patient who has occasional heartburn and reflux related to a triggering meal. PPIs (eg, omeprazole) are the most effective agents to relieve symptoms and promote mucosal healing. Long-term use of these agents is safe. Patients may take them once or twice daily, optimally 30 to 60 minutes before a meal.

Antireflux surgery can be considered for younger patients who respond to PPI therapy but want to avoid lifelong medical treatment. Those who do not respond to medical therapy are less likely to have relief of symptoms after surgery, and those with dysphagia and bloating should avoid surgery, since both of these symptoms can occur or worsen after antireflux surgery. Nissen fundoplication is the preferred operation.

- Management of reflux disease may include a combination of 1) lifestyle or dietary modifications, 2) avoidance of exacerbating medications, and 3) acid suppression.
- Antireflux surgery is most helpful in patients who have responded well to medical therapy but want to avoid lifelong medical treatment.

NONCARDIAC CHEST PAIN

All patients with chest pain should be thoroughly evaluated to rule out a potential cardiac cause before other diagnoses are considered. GERD is the most common cause of noncardiac chest pain, but esophageal pain may be due to a motor disorder (eg, spasm) or esophageal inflammation (eg, infection or injury). Esophageal spasm can closely mimic angina. EGD is used to rule out mucosal disease (eg, inflammation, neoplasm, or chemical injury). A 24-hour ambulatory pH probe can be used to document the presence of reflux and its correlation with chest pain. Therapy for noncardiac chest pain includes avoidance of precipitants. Antacids, H_2 receptor antagonists, and PPIs may be beneficial for patients with reflux. Sublingual nitroglycerin or calcium channel blockers are sometimes helpful in motor disorders, but their efficacy is unproven. If appropriate, reassurance that cardiac disease is not present may be all that is necessary.

- For all chest pain, first rule out cardiac disease.
- GERD is the most common cause of noncardiac chest pain.

- EGD is useful to detect mucosal disease that may account for chest pain.
- A 24-hour ambulatory pH probe documents reflux and its correlation with symptoms.
- Acid suppression can be helpful in alleviating chest pain by controlling reflux disease.

OTHER ESOPHAGEAL PROBLEMS

Mallory-Weiss Tear

A *Mallory-Weiss tear* is a mucosal laceration at the esophago-gastric junction. It accounts for about 10% of the cases of upper gastrointestinal tract bleeding; most patients have a history of retching or vomiting before the bleeding begins. In 90% of the patients, the bleeding stops spontaneously, but endoscopic hemostatic techniques can be used if needed.

- A Mallory-Weiss tear is a mucosal laceration at the esophagogastric junction; the laceration usually occurs after a bout of retching or vomiting.
- A Mallory-Weiss tear accounts for about 10% of the cases of upper gastrointestinal tract bleeding; bleeding stops spontaneously in 90%.

Esophageal Perforation

Esophageal perforation most commonly occurs after dilation of a strictured area or with stenting of an esophageal cancer. Spontaneous perforation of the esophagus (Boerhaave syndrome) occurs after violent retching, often after an alcohol binge. It has been reported after heavy lifting, seizures, and strenuous childbirth. The most common site of perforation is the left posterior aspect of the distal esophagus. If pleural fluid is present, it may have an increased concentration of amylase. The cervical esophagus may be perforated if a Zenker diverticulum is inadvertently intubated for an EGD.

- Esophageal perforation most commonly occurs after dilation or stenting.
- Boerhaave syndrome occurs after violent retching, often after an alcohol binge.

STOMACH AND DUODENUM

PEPTIC ULCER DISEASE

Peptic ulcers are defects in the gastric or duodenal mucosa that result from an imbalance between acid and pepsin in the gastric juice and the host's protective mechanisms. Stimulators of acid production include acetylcholine, histamine, and gastrin. Inhibitors of gastric acid production include somatostatin and prostaglandin.

Peptic ulcers are categorized as being associated with 3 possible etiologic factors: 1) *Helicobacter pylori*; 2) nonsteroidal anti-inflammatory drugs (NSAIDs), including aspirin; or 3) miscellaneous causes. At least 90% of peptic ulcers are due to either *H pylori* or NSAIDs. Miscellaneous causes include gastrinomas (Zollinger-Ellison syndrome), Crohn disease, malignancy, drugs (cocaine), and viral infections (such as those caused by cytomegalovirus). There is no evidence that smoking or corticosteroids cause PUD, but either can result in decreased ulcer healing and increased complications.

Infection with *H pylori* causes more duodenal ulcers than gastric ulcers. Although NSAIDs tend to cause more gastric ulcers than duodenal ulcers, *H pylori* infection is still more likely to account for gastric ulcer disease in general.

Certain medical conditions may predispose to stress-induced peptic injury; these include ventilator use, underlying coagulopathy, significant burns, and central nervous system injury. Patients with these conditions should be considered candidates for prophylactic therapy.

- More than 90% of peptic ulcers are caused by either *H pylori* infection or NSAID use.
- Risk factors for stress ulcerations include ventilator use, coagulopathy, burns, and central nervous system injury.

HELICOBACTER PYLORI

The Organism

A gram-negative, spiral-shaped bacillus, *H pylori* is commonly acquired through oral ingestion and transmitted among those in close living quarters. This fastidious organism resides and multiplies beneath and within the mucous layer of the gastric mucosa and produces several enzymes, such as urease, important for its survival and pathogenic effects.

Helicobacter pylori infection can lead to a spectrum from acute to chronic gastritis, and it can lead to PUD, atrophic gastritis, mucosa-associated lymphoid tissue (MALT) lymphoma, or gastric malignancy.

Epidemiology

In the United States, *H pylori* has an age-related prevalence, occurring in 10% of the general population younger than 30 years and in 60% of persons older than 60 years. Overall, *H pylori* is more prevalent among blacks and Hispanics, poorer socioeconomic groups, and institutionalized persons. In developing countries such as India and Saudi Arabia, 50% of the population is infected by age 10 years and 70% by age 20; 85% to 95% of the population overall is infected. Evidence of person-to-person transmission exists.

Associated Diseases

Active Chronic Gastritis

The most common cause of chronic active gastritis is *H pylori* infection. The infection is predominantly an antral-based gastritis, although gastritis throughout the gastric body may be seen.

Duodenal Ulcer

In approximately 80% of patients with duodenal ulcers, *H pylori* is present. Among *H pylori*–positive patients with a duodenal ulcer who do not receive treatment targeted at the organism, most have ulcer relapse within 1 year. However, if the infection is successfully eradicated, the rate of relapse approaches zero.

Gastric Ulcer

In more than 50% of patients with gastric ulcers, *H pylori* is present. Eradication of the bacteria decreases the relapse rate of gastric ulcers.

Gastric Tumors

A known carcinogen as identified by the World Health Organization, *H pylori* is the leading cause of gastric malignancy in the world. The gastric cancer that results from *H pylori* infection is due to a progression from chronic gastritis to atrophic gastritis to metaplasia to dysplasia and eventually to gastric adenocarcinoma.

MALT Lymphoma

MALT lymphoma of the stomach is a low-grade B-cell lymphoma. The majority of cases (90%) are related to *H pylori* infection. For early-stage disease, simple eradication of *H pylori* infection can induce complete (50%) or partial (33%) remission. For patients with more advanced disease, traditional lymphoma therapy is recommended.

Nonulcer Dyspepsia

Nonulcer dyspepsia is common, affecting about 20% of the US population. Among persons with functional dyspepsia, up to 50% may be infected with *H pylori*; however, dyspepsia clinically improves with eradication therapy in only a small percentage of patients.

- The most common type of chronic gastritis is *H pylori*–induced gastritis.
- Infection with *H pylori* can lead to a sequence of chronic gastritis, atrophic gastritis, metaplasia, dysplasia, and adenocarcinoma.

- MALT lymphoma is a low-grade B-cell lymphoma associated with *H pylori* infection; eradication of the organism can result in remission of early-stage disease.

Diagnostic Tests for *H pylori* Infection

Various diagnostic tests are available for detecting the presence of *H pylori* infection. The choice of test is determined by the need for endoscopy, the use of certain medications, and cost (Table 11.1).

Serology

Serologic testing is one of the most cost-effective, noninvasive ways to diagnose primary *H pylori* infection, and the results are not affected by medications the patient may be taking.

Urea Breath Test

A radiolabeled dose of urea is given orally to the patient. If *H pylori* is present, the urease activity splits the urea, and radiolabeled carbon dioxide is exhaled.

Stool Antigen Test

The *H pylori* stool antigen test is simple and noninvasive. Unlike serologic testing, stool antigen testing does not depend on disease prevalence.

Rapid Urease Test

For the rapid urease test, a biopsy specimen taken at the time of an EGD is impregnated into agar that contains urea and a pH indicator. As the urea is split by *H pylori*–produced urease, the pH of the medium changes the color of the agar. This test depends on bacterial urease: the more organisms present, the more rapidly the test produces positive results.

Histologic Examination

The *H pylori* organisms can be demonstrated with several specialized stains, including hematoxylin-eosin, Warthin-Starry, and immunostaining.

For patients who need to be assessed for *H pylori* infection but do not require endoscopy, noninvasive evaluation with

Table 11.1 **TESTS FOR DETECTING *HELICOBACTER PYLORI***

TEST	ADVANTAGES	DISADVANTAGES
Noninvasive tests		
Serology	Easy to perform	Prevalence dependent
	Good negative predictive value	Indicates only past infection (not used for eradication testing)
Stool antigen	Indicates active infection	Stool collection
	Useful for primary or eradication testing	
Urea breath test	Indicates active infection	False-negative results with antibiotics, acid suppression, or bismuth
	Useful for primary or eradication testing	
Invasive tests		
Rapid urease test	Quick results	Expense of endoscopy to perform the test
		False-negative results with antibiotics, acid suppression, or bismuth
Histology	Allows evaluation for histologic changes (dysplasia, etc)	Expense of endoscopy to perform the test
		Dependent on expertise of pathologist

serologic antibody, stool antigen, or urea breath testing can be performed. Because many symptomatic patients undergo endoscopy, histologic examination or rapid urease testing can be done. The best tests for determining eradication are the stool antigen test and the urea breath test.

- Serologic tests for *H pylori* infection are prevalence dependent and remain positive over time, which limits their usefulness for previously treated patients.

- Recent therapy with PPIs, antibiotics, or bismuth can lead to false-negative results for most *H pylori* tests except serology.

- The best tests for determining eradication are the stool antigen test and the urea breath test since a positive result indicates active infection.

Treatment

With an *H pylori*–positive duodenal or gastric ulcer, the treatment goal is to heal the ulcer and eradicate the bacteria. All patients who are infected with *H pylori* should receive combination therapy. PPI-based triple therapy (usually in combination with amoxicillin and clarithromycin) for 10 to 14 days is the most commonly used initial therapy; metronidazole can be used in place of amoxicillin in patients who have a penicillin allergy. Because of emerging patterns of resistance to clarithromycin and metronidazole, these agents should be avoided if subsequent treatment is necessary and they were used as initial therapy. If the first course of therapy fails to eradicate the organism, quadruple therapy can be considered (PPI, metronidazole, bismuth, and tetracycline).

- PPI-based triple therapy (usually in combination with amoxicillin and clarithromycin) for 10–14 days is the most commonly used initial therapy for *H pylori* infection.

NSAID-INDUCED ULCERS

NSAIDs inhibit gastroduodenal prostaglandin synthesis, which results in decreased secretion of mucus and bicarbonate, reduced mucosal blood flow, and stimulated acid production. NSAID-induced ulcers occur more commonly in the stomach (typically in the antrum) than in the duodenum.

The risk of PUD with NSAIDs is dose-dependent. Higher doses of NSAIDs or the combination of 2 or more NSAIDs (including low-dose aspirin) increases the risk of gastrointestinal tract injury. Selective cyclooxygenase (COX)-2 inhibition has been shown to decrease the rate of PUD and ulcer complications such as bleeding, perforation, and pain. However, data suggest that even low-dose aspirin can reduce or eliminate any protective benefit of selective COX-2 drugs (celecoxib). In most cases, acetaminophen can be substituted for the NSAID. For patients who require NSAID therapy, the lowest possible dose should be used and combination NSAID therapy avoided. The risk of PUD with NSAID use is maximal in the first month of treatment (ulcers may occur shortly after treatment is begun), and

elderly patients and patients with a previous history of PUD are at highest risk.

The first step in the treatment of an NSAID-induced ulcer is to discontinue use of the drug if feasible. PPIs are most effective in healing and preventing ulcers and have few side effects. H_2 receptor antagonists and sucralfate are less effective in preventing gastric ulcers and in decreasing the frequency of NSAID-induced mucosal erosions. The synthetic prostaglandin agonist misoprostol decreases the incidence of NSAID-induced gastric ulcers; however, its usefulness is limited by the side effect of diarrhea and its role as an abortifacient (avoid using it in women of childbearing age).

- The risk of gastrointestinal tract injury related to NSAID use increases with higher doses of NSAIDs, combinations of 2 or more agents (including low-dose aspirin), elderly patients, and patients with a prior history of PUD.

- For both prevention and treatment of NSAID-induced ulcers, PPI therapy is most often used.

ZOLLINGER-ELLISON SYNDROME

Zollinger-Ellison syndrome is characterized by acid hypersecretion and the triad of peptic ulceration, esophagitis, and diarrhea (since excess acid inactivates pancreatic lipase) caused by a gastrin-producing tumor. The tumor usually is located in the "gastrinoma triangle," which includes the head of the pancreas and the duodenal wall. Two-thirds of gastrinomas are malignant and can metastasize. One-fourth of gastrinomas are related to multiple endocrine neoplasia type 1 (MEN-1) syndrome and are associated with pituitary adenomas and hyperparathyroidism.

Zollinger-Ellison syndrome should be considered in the person with *H pylori*–negative, NSAID-negative PUD, especially when there are multiple ulcers, ulcers in unusual locations (postbulbar duodenum), and refractory ulcers. Increased serum gastrin levels (>1,000 pg/mL) in patients who produce gastric acid are essentially diagnostic of gastrinoma. Increased serum gastrin levels may also be present in patients who are receiving PPI therapy (the most common reason), or who have atrophic gastritis (the next most common reason), pernicious anemia, postvagotomy states, or gastric outlet obstruction. Basal and stimulated gastric acid studies should be performed for all patients who have increased levels of gastrin to see whether there is acid hypersecretion. When the laboratory results are equivocal, a secretin test should be performed; this test produces a paradoxical increase in the serum level of gastrin in patients with gastrinoma.

An octreotide scan (Octreoscan) can be used to localize a gastrinoma owing to the presence of somatostatin receptors. Endoscopic ultrasonography has been very successful in localizing gastrinomas because the pancreas and duodenal wall can be easily viewed with this test.

Since 50% of patients with gastrinomas have metastatic disease, curative surgery is not always feasible. Patients who are not candidates for surgery can be managed with high-dose acid suppression. Those with MEN-1 syndrome are usually not considered for surgical resection because of the multifocality of the disease.

- Zollinger-Ellison syndrome is characterized by acid hypersecretion and the triad of peptic ulceration, esophagitis, and diarrhea due to a gastrin-secreting tumor.

- Rule out Zollinger-Ellison syndrome in patients with *H pylori*–negative, NSAID-negative PUD, especially in those with refractory or multiple postbulbar ulcers.

ULCER DIAGNOSIS AND MANAGEMENT

EGD is the best initial test to establish the diagnosis of PUD. At the time of the endoscopy, any active bleeding can be managed. Histologic evaluation can be performed if an ulcer has malignant features or if testing for *H pylori* infection is desired. If there is concern about perforation, abdominal imaging should be the first test (endoscopy would be contraindicated).

A patient who has active bleeding from suspected ulcer disease needs to be hemodynamically stabilized before endoscopy is performed; endotracheal intubation may be required. PPI therapy should be initiated to stabilize clotting. Endoscopic therapy is selectively used according to stigmata of bleeding. All patients should be assessed for *H pylori* infection and NSAID use.

Angiography may be required for PUD if endoscopic therapy has failed to control active bleeding. Surgical intervention is infrequently needed for bleeding but would be considered if bleeding cannot be controlled angiographically. For perforation, urgent surgical consultation is necessary.

NONEROSIVE NONSPECIFIC CHRONIC GASTRITIS

Chronic gastritis consists of 2 types: type A and type B. *Type A gastritis*, or *autoimmune gastritis*, involves the body and fundus of the stomach (not the antrum). In a subset of patients, atrophic gastritis develops. Pernicious anemia with achlorhydria and megaloblastic anemia may result. Antiparietal cell or anti-intrinsic factor antibodies are found in more than 90% of these patients. Other autoimmune diseases are often present. The serum gastrin level may be markedly increased (given the lack of gastric acid to provide negative feedback) and may give rise to gastric carcinoid tumors, which usually follow an indolent course in these patients. Peptic ulcers do not typically develop in patients with autoimmune gastritis owing to achlorhydria, but the patients are at increased risk of intestinal metaplasia and gastric adenocarcinoma.

- Type A gastritis (autoimmune gastritis): atrophic gastritis may develop with achlorhydria and anemia (pernicious); typically, it does not involve the antrum.

- The serum gastrin level may be markedly increased in patients with atrophic gastritis.

- Type A gastritis is associated with gastric carcinoids and increased risk of gastric adenocarcinoma.

Type B gastritis, the more common type of chronic gastritis, typically involves the antrum and is associated with *H pylori* infection. Serum gastrin levels are normal or mildly increased. Gastric ulcers and duodenal ulcers occur commonly, and the incidence of gastric adenocarcinoma is increased. *Helicobacter pylori*–related gastritis also predisposes to MALT lymphoma.

- Type B gastritis, the more common form of chronic gastritis, is associated with *H pylori* infection.

- Type B gastritis is associated with gastric and duodenal ulcers, gastric adenocarcinoma, and MALT lymphoma.

GASTRIC CANCER

In the 1940s, gastric cancer was the most common malignancy in the United States. Since then, the incidence in the United States has decreased dramatically. Currently, Japan has the highest mortality rate from gastric cancer. Known risk factors for gastric cancer are *H pylori* infection, autoimmune gastritis, and certain hereditary cancer syndromes. Known dietary risk factors include increased consumption of pickled foods, salted fish, processed meat, smoked foods, and products high in nitrates. The male to female ratio is as high as 2:1. Gastric cancer is more common in lower socioeconomic groups.

- The incidence of gastric cancer has decreased dramatically in the United States since the 1940s.

- Risk factors for gastric cancer include *H pylori* infection, autoimmune gastritis, certain hereditary cancer syndromes, and dietary exposures.

Clinical Aspects

Gastric cancer is often asymptomatic in the early stages, becoming symptomatic with advanced disease. The intestinal type of gastric cancer tends to have distinct borders with well-differentiated histology; patients often present with abdominal pain and iron-deficiency anemia. Gastric cancer that is in a diffuse or infiltrating form, also referred to as *linitis plastica*, often causes early satiety and weight loss because the stomach cannot stretch and accommodate food. The diffuse form tends to be poorly differentiated and is associated with signet ring cells and a very poor outcome. EGD is the initial test of choice to obtain a histologic diagnosis. After the diagnosis is established, CT imaging should be performed to evaluate for metastatic disease.

- Patients who have gastric cancer commonly present with abdominal pain, iron-deficiency anemia, weight loss, and early satiety.

- EGD is the initial test of choice to establish the diagnosis.

- After the diagnosis of gastric cancer is made, CT imaging should be performed to evaluate for metastatic disease.

Treatment and Prognosis

For localized disease, resection for tumor-free margins often requires total gastrectomy. For disseminated disease, surgical treatment is necessary only for palliation. Response to chemotherapy is generally poor. Five-year survival is 90% if the tumor is confined to the mucosa and submucosa, 50% if the tumor is through the serosa, and 10% if the tumor involves regional lymph nodes.

GASTRIC POLYPS

Gastric polyps are common and are typically found incidentally. There are 3 types of polyps: cystic fundic gland, hyperplastic, and adenomatous. *Cystic fundic gland polyps* are the most common gastric polyps and are not premalignant except in association with familial adenomatous polyposis (FAP). No additional therapy is needed unless FAP is known or suspected to be present. *Hyperplastic polyps* may occur with chronic gastritis, so patients should be tested for *H pylori*. Hyperplastic polyps rarely have malignant potential. *Adenomatous polyps* are deemed premalignant and need to be fully removed (like colon polyps).

There are 3 types of carcinoid tumors, which may manifest as an incidentally noted gastric polyp. *Type 1 gastric carcinoids* are associated with autoimmune gastritis, whereas *type 2 gastric carcinoids* are associated with MEN-1 syndrome; both forms tend to follow an indolent course. *Type 3 gastric carcinoids* tend to be sporadic and behave aggressively.

- Cystic fundic gland polyps are the most common types of gastric polyps and tend to be benign except in association with FAP.

- Adenomatous polyps are premalignant and need to be removed.

GASTRODUODENAL DYSMOTILITY SYNDROMES

Gastroparesis

Symptoms of delayed gastric emptying, or gastroparesis, may include nausea, vomiting, bloating, early satiety, anorexia, and weight loss. Diabetes mellitus is probably the most common cause of gastroparesis, which can occur with long-standing disease or with dramatic fluctuations in serum glucose levels. Other causes of gastroparesis exist (Box 11.2). After mechanical obstruction has been ruled out (usually with upper endoscopy), the test of choice to assess for gastroparesis is a 4-hour gastric scintigraphic study with a solid meal.

- Nausea, vomiting, bloating, early satiety, anorexia, and weight loss may suggest abnormal gastric motility.

- The test of choice for assessment of gastroparesis (after excluding obstruction) is a 4-hour gastric scintigraphic study with a solid meal.

Box 11.2 **CONDITIONS CAUSING GASTROPARESIS**

Acute conditions
   Anticholinergic drug use
   Hyperglycemia
   Hypokalemia
   Morphine use
   Pancreatitis
   Surgical procedures
   Trauma
Chronic conditions
   Amyloidosis
   Diabetes mellitus
   Gastric dysrhythmias
   Pseudo-obstruction
   Scleroderma
   Vagotomy

Management of gastroparesis includes 1) dietary alterations, 2) antiemetic agents, and 3) prokinetic drugs, if needed. Metoclopramide is a dopamine antagonist and a cholinergic agonist that increases the rate and amplitude of antral contractions. It crosses the blood-brain barrier and can cause drowsiness and galactorrhea (from increased release of prolactin). The most feared complication of this medication is tardive dyskinesia, which can be irreversible. Erythromycin stimulates both cholinergic and motilin receptors, but because tachyphylaxis occurs with long-term use, it is most often used transiently in hospitalized patients.

- Metoclopramide can be used for gastroparesis, but it carries a risk of tardive dyskinesia, which may be irreversible.

- Because long-term use of erythromycin can lead to tachyphylaxis, it is usually used for only short periods.

DUMPING SYNDROME

Patients who have had prior resection of the gastric antrum and pylorus may be predisposed to *dumping syndrome*, which results from hyperosmolar substances rapidly exiting the stomach into the small bowel. Patients may complain of postprandial diarrhea, bloating, sweating, palpitations, and light-headedness. Symptoms can occur within 30 minutes after a meal (*early dumping*) or 1 to 3 hours after a meal (*late dumping*), which is associated with hypoglycemia and neuroglycopenic symptoms. Management includes having patients avoid hyperosmolar nutrient drinks, which aggravate symptoms; patients can modify their diets to include foods that delay gastric emptying (fats and proteins).

- Dumping syndrome results from hyperosmolar substances rapidly exiting the stomach into the small bowel, leading to diarrhea, bloating, sweating, and palpitations.

SUMMARY

- In the evaluation of dysphagia, it is important to determine 1) whether it is oropharyngeal, 2) the types of food that produce the dysphagia (solids or liquids), and 3) whether the symptoms are intermittent or progressive.

- Odynophagia is most commonly from infections or medications.

- Evaluation of GERD is required when patients have new-onset symptoms at an older age, alarm features, or atypical or refractory characteristics.

- *Helicobacter pylori* and NSAIDs account for the majority of peptic ulcers. The type of testing for *H pylori* depends on whether endoscopy is needed, whether the patient has used certain interfering medications, and whether testing is for primary evaluation or for eradication testing.

- For both esophageal cancer and gastric cancer, the initial step is to establish a histologic diagnosis with EGD; the next step is to use CT imaging to evaluate for metastatic disease.

12.

DIARRHEA, MALABSORPTION, AND SMALL-BOWEL DISORDERS

Seth R. Sweetser, MD

GOALS

- Review the causes and mechanisms of diarrhea.
- Understand how malabsorption is caused by diseases of the small intestine.
- Identify the primary disorders of the small intestine.

DIARRHEA

Diarrhea is a symptom or sign, not a disease. As a symptom, it can manifest as a decrease in consistency, an increase in fluidity, an increase in number or volume of stools, or any combination thereof. A stool frequency of 3 or more times daily is considered abnormal; however, most people consider increased fluidity of stool as the essential characteristic of diarrhea. As a sign, diarrhea is an increase in stool weight or volume of more than 200 g or 200 mL per 24 hours for a person eating a Western diet. Although stool weight is often used as the objective definition of diarrhea, diarrhea should not be strictly defined by stool weight because the amount of dietary fiber influences the water content of the stool. Therefore, stool weight can vary considerably depending on fiber intake. In the United States, normal daily stool weight or volume is less than 200 g or 200 mL daily because of lower fiber intake (compared with up to 400 g or 400 mL daily in rural Africa).

Because diarrhea has multiple causes, its evaluation is often complex and time consuming. An understanding of the basic pathogenic mechanisms leading to diarrhea can help facilitate its evaluation and management. The basic mechanism of all diarrheal diseases is incomplete absorption of fluid from luminal contents. Each day, approximately 10 L of fluid passes into the proximal small intestine (2 L from diet; 8 L from endogenous secretions). The small bowel absorbs most of the fluid (9 L), and the colon absorbs about 90% of the remaining 1 L, so that only about 1% of the original fluid entering the small intestine is excreted in the stool. A normal stool is approximately 75% water and 25% solids, with a normal fecal water output of 60 mL daily. An increase in fecal water output of only 100 mL is enough to cause increased stool fluidity

or decreased stool consistency. This volume is approximately 1% of the fluid entering the proximal small intestine each day. Hence, malabsorption of only 1% of the fluid entering the intestine may be sufficient to cause diarrhea. Fortunately, the gut has considerable reserve absorptive capacity, with the small intestine having a maximal absorptive capacity of 12 L daily and the colon, 6 L daily.

MECHANISMS OF DIARRHEA

Osmotic diarrhea occurs when a poorly absorbed substance remains in the intestinal lumen and causes water retention that maintains an intraluminal osmolality equal to that of body fluids (approximately 290 mOsm/kg). This occurs because, unlike the kidney, neither the small intestine nor the colon maintains an osmotic gradient. Osmotic diarrhea follows ingestion of an osmotically active substance and stops with fasting. Stool volume is less than 1 L daily, and the stool osmotic gap (SOG), calculated as follows, is greater than the sum of the measured concentrations of sodium (NA) and potassium (K) (the sum is doubled to account for their associated anions):

$$SOG = 290 \text{ mOsm/kg} - 2 \times (\text{Stool [Na]} + \text{Stool [K]}).$$

A normal stool osmotic gap is less than 50 mOsm/kg. However, with an osmotically active substance in the bowel, sodium and potassium levels will decrease (keeping stool osmotically neutral with the body). The calculated stool osmolality decreases, resulting in a gap (typically >100 mOsm/kg). Clinical causes of osmotic diarrhea include carbohydrate malabsorption, lactase deficiency, sorbitol-sweetened foods, saline cathartics, and magnesium-based antacids. In carbohydrate malabsorption (most commonly lactase deficiency), stool pH is often less than 6.0 because of colonic fermentation of the undigested sugars.

- In osmotic diarrhea, stool volume is <1 L daily.
- Osmotic diarrhea stops with fasting.
- The stool osmotic gap is typically >100 mOsm/kg.

- Causes of osmotic diarrhea: lactase deficiency, sorbitol, and antacids.

The term *secretory diarrhea* is used to indicate disordered intestinal epithelial electrolyte transport (ie, the intestine secretes electrolytes and fluid rather than absorbing them) even though it is more commonly caused by reduced absorption than by net secretion. Stool volume is more than 1 L daily. The stool composition is predominantly extracellular fluid, so there is no stool osmotic gap. Secretory diarrhea persists despite fasting. Causes of secretory diarrhea include bacterial toxins, neuroendocrine tumors, surreptitious ingestion of laxative, bile acid diarrhea, and fatty acid diarrhea.

- In secretory diarrhea, stool volume is >1 L daily.

- There is no stool osmotic gap.

- Secretory diarrhea persists despite fasting.

- Causes of secretory diarrhea: bacterial toxins, neuroendocrine tumors, surreptitious ingestion of laxative, bile acid diarrhea, and fatty acid diarrhea.

A useful method to evaluate chronic watery diarrhea is to distinguish secretory diarrhea from osmotic diarrhea (Table 12.1) by measuring the concentrations of sodium and potassium in stool water (calculate the stool osmotic gap) and observing the patient's response to fasting.

Many disease processes cause diarrhea by more than 1 mechanism. For example, generalized malabsorption, such as in celiac disease, has osmotic components (from carbohydrate malabsorption) and secretory components (unabsorbed fatty acids cause secretion in the colon).

In *exudative diarrhea*, membrane permeability is abnormal and serum proteins, blood, or mucus is exuded into the bowel from sites of inflammation, ulceration, or infiltration.

The volume of feces is small and the stools may be bloody. Examples include invasive bacterial pathogens (eg, *Shigella* and *Salmonella*) and inflammatory bowel disease. In motility disorders, both *rapid transit* (inadequate time for chyme to contact the absorbing surface) and *delayed transit* (bacterial overgrowth) can cause diarrhea. Rapid transit occurs after gastrectomy or intestinal resection and with hyperthyroidism or carcinoid syndrome. Delayed transit occurs with structural defects (strictures, blind loops, and small-bowel diverticula) or with underlying illnesses that cause visceral neuropathy (diabetes mellitus) or myopathy (scleroderma), resulting in pseudo-obstruction.

- Evaluation of chronic watery diarrhea requires distinguishing between secretory diarrhea and osmotic diarrhea.

- Exudative diarrhea: abnormal membrane permeability and a stool volume that is typically small.

- Causes of exudative diarrhea: invasive bacterial pathogens and inflammatory bowel disease.

- Rapid transit: diarrhea results from malabsorption.

- Delayed transit: diarrhea results from bacterial overgrowth.

CLINICAL APPROACH TO DIARRHEA

Knowing the stool volume is potentially useful to distinguish between diarrhea arising from the small bowel or ascending colon ("right-sided diarrhea") and diarrhea arising from the distal colon ("left-sided diarrhea") (Table 12.2). The distal left colon acts as a distensible reservoir that collects stool until defecation. With inflammation of the left colon, the reservoir becomes spastic and its ability to accommodate normal volumes of stool is impaired. As a result, left-sided diarrhea is characterized by frequent, small-volume stools and tenesmus with evidence of inflammation (blood or pus) in the stools.

Table 12.1 FEATURES DIFFERENTIATING OSMOTIC DIARRHEA FROM SECRETORY DIARRHEA

FEATURE	OSMOTIC DIARRHEA	SECRETORY DIARRHEA
Daily stool volume, L	<1	>1
Effect of 48-h fasting	Diarrhea stops	Diarrhea continues
Fecal fluid analysis		
Osmolality, mOsm	290	290
$([Na] + [K]) \times 2$[a], mEq/L	120	280
Solute gap[b]	>100	<50

Abbreviations: K, potassium; Na, sodium.

[a] Multiplied by 2 to account for anions.

[b] Calculated by subtracting $([Na] + [K]) \times 2$ from osmolality.

Adapted from Krejs GJ, Hendler RS, Fordtran JS. Diagnostic and pathophysiologic studies in patients with chronic diarrhea. In: Field M, Fordtran JS, Schultz SG, editors. Secretory diarrhea. Bethesda (MD): American Physiological Society; c1980. p. 141–51. Used with permission.

Table 12.2 FEATURES THAT DISTINGUISH RIGHT-SIDED DIARRHEA FROM LEFT-SIDED DIARRHEA

FEATURE	RIGHT-SIDED (SMALL-BOWEL) DIARRHEA	LEFT-SIDED (COLONIC) DIARRHEA
Reservoir capacity	Intact	Decreased
Stool volume	Large	Small
Increase in number of stools	Modest	Large
Urgency	Absent	Present
Tenesmus	Absent	Present
Mucus	Absent	Present
Blood	Absent	Present

Proctosigmoidoscopic examination usually confirms mucosal inflammation.

Right-sided diarrhea is characterized by large-volume stools (due to normal distensibility of the rectum) and a modest increase in the number of stools. Symptoms attributed to inflammation of the rectosigmoid are absent, and proctoscopic examination findings are normal. Left-sided diarrhea usually suggests an exudative mechanism, whereas the mechanism for right-sided diarrhea is nonspecific.

ACUTE DIARRHEA

Acute diarrhea is abrupt in onset and usually resolves in 3 to 10 days. It is self-limited, and the cause (often viral) usually is not found. No evaluation is necessary unless an invasive infection is suspected (eg, bloody stools, fever, travel history, or a common source outbreak). If these conditions exist, do not treat with antimotility agents. Begin the evaluation with stool studies for bacterial pathogens, ova, and parasites and proctosigmoidoscopy. Recognize the common situations that predispose to specific infections (see "Noninvasive (Toxicogenic) Bacterial Diarrhea" subsection).

- For acute diarrhea, no evaluation is necessary unless an invasive infection is suspected.
- Do not administer antimotility agents if infection is suspected.

CHRONIC DIARRHEA

Chronic diarrhea is defined as diarrhea lasting longer than 4 weeks. The most common cause of chronic diarrhea is irritable bowel syndrome, but lactase deficiency should always be considered. Several features help differentiate organic diarrhea from functional diarrhea (Table 12.3).

- The most common cause of chronic diarrhea is irritable bowel syndrome.

- Always consider lactase deficiency in suspected irritable bowel syndrome.
- Differentiate organic diarrhea from functional diarrhea.

PHYSIOLOGY OF NUTRIENT ABSORPTION

The sites of nutrient, vitamin, and mineral absorption are the following: The duodenum absorbs iron, calcium, folate, water-soluble vitamins, and monosaccharides. The jejunum absorbs fatty acids, amino acids, monosaccharides, and water-soluble vitamins. The ileum absorbs monosaccharides, fatty acids, amino acids, fat-soluble vitamins (A, D, E, and K), vitamin B_{12}, and conjugated bile salts. The distal small bowel can adapt to absorb nutrients. The proximal small bowel cannot adapt to absorb vitamin B_{12} or bile salts.

- The distal small bowel can adapt to absorb nutrients.
- The proximal small bowel cannot adapt to absorb vitamin B_{12} or bile salts.

Fat absorption is the most complex process. Dietary fat consists mostly of long-chain triglycerides that must be digested by pancreatic lipase, which cleaves 2 of the 3 long-chain fatty acids from the glycerol backbone. The resultant free fatty acids and monoglycerides are solubilized by micelles for absorption. The fatty acids and monoglycerides are re-esterified by intestinal epithelial cells into chylomicrons that are absorbed into the circulation via lymphatic vessels. Conversely, medium-chain triglycerides are absorbed directly into the portal venous system and do not require micellar solubilization.

Mechanisms of fat malabsorption are summarized in Table 12.4. Malabsorption should be suspected if the medical history suggests steatorrhea or if diarrhea occurs with weight loss (especially if intake is adequate), chronic diarrhea of indeterminate nature, or nutritional deficiency.

Table 12.3 FEATURES THAT DISTINGUISH ORGANIC DIARRHEA FROM FUNCTIONAL DIARRHEA

FEATURE	ORGANIC DIARRHEA	FUNCTIONAL DIARRHEA
Weight loss	Often present	Absent
Duration of illness	Variable (weeks to years)	Usually long (>6 mo)
Quantity of stool	Variable but usually large (>200 g in 24 h)	Usually small (<200 g in 24 h)
Blood in stool	May be present	Absent (unless from hemorrhoids)
Timing of diarrhea	No special pattern	Usually in the morning or after meals
Nocturnal symptoms	May be present	Absent
Fever, arthritis, skin lesions	May be present	Absent
Emotional stress	No relation to symptoms	Usually precedes or coincides with symptoms
Cramping abdominal pain	Often present	May be present

Adapted from Matseshe JW, Phillips SF. Chronic diarrhea: a practical approach. Med Clin North Am. 1978 Jan;62(1):141–54. Used with permission.

Table 12.4 MECHANISMS OF FAT MALABSORPTION

ALTERATION	MECHANISM	DISEASE STATE
Defective digestion	Inadequate lipase	Pancreatic insufficiency
Impaired micelle formation	Duodenal bile salt concentration	Common duct obstruction or cholestasis
Impaired absorption	Small-bowel disease	Sprue & Whipple disease
Impaired chylomicron formation	Impaired β-globulin synthesis	Abetalipoproteinemia
Impaired lymphatic circulation	Lymphatic obstruction	Intestinal lymphangiectasia & lymphoma

Table 12.5 CAUSES OF SYMPTOMS IN MALABSORPTION

EXTRAGASTROINTESTINAL SYMPTOM	CAUSE
Muscle wasting, edema	Decreased protein absorption
Paresthesias, tetany	Decreased vitamin D & calcium absorption
Bone pain	Decreased calcium absorption
Muscle cramps	Weakness, excess potassium loss
Easy bruisability, petechiae	Decreased vitamin K absorption
Hyperkeratosis, night blindness	Decreased vitamin A absorption
Pallor	Decreased vitamin B_{12}, folate, or iron absorption
Glossitis, stomatitis, cheilosis	Decreased vitamin B_{12} or iron absorption
Acrodermatitis	Zinc deficiency

The causes of symptoms in malabsorption are summarized in Table 12.5, and various features that suggest specific malabsorption conditions are listed in Table 12.6.

The medical history, physical examination, or laboratory results may suggest a possible cause of diarrhea or malabsorption (Tables 12.7 and 12.8). For example, the medical history may include previous surgery (resulting in short-bowel syndrome, dumping syndrome, blind loop syndrome, postvagotomy diarrhea, or ileal resection), irradiation, or systemic disease.

DISEASES CAUSING DIARRHEA

Osmotic Diarrhea

Lactose is normally split by the brush border enzyme lactase into glucose and galactose, which are absorbed in the small bowel. In lactase deficiency, lactose is not split in the small intestine but enters the colon, where it is fermented in the lumen by bacteria, forming lactic acid and liberating hydrogen. The result is diarrhea of low pH and increased intestinal motility. Several other disaccharidase deficiencies can also result in malabsorption of specific carbohydrates; however, the most common disaccharidase deficiency involves lactase.

"Acquired" lactase deficiency (possibly genetic) is common in African Americans, Native Americans, and peoples of Asia and the Middle East. Diarrhea, abdominal cramps, and flatulence occur after ingestion of dairy products. There is improvement with dietary changes. The pH of the stool is less than 6.0. In the lactose tolerance test, blood glucose levels increase less than 20 mg/dL after ingestion of lactose. Results of the hydrogen breath test may be abnormal. Jejunal biopsy results are normal (disaccharidase levels are decreased).

Transient lactose intolerance can occur in any clinical setting in which the intestinal mucosa is damaged, including simple viral gastroenteritis. In patients who eat a weight-reduction diet and drink diet soda or chew sugarless gum, osmotic diarrhea may develop from excessive ingestion of fructose or other artificial sweeteners.

- Lactase deficiency is the most common disaccharidase deficiency; lactose is not split in the small intestine.

- Diarrhea is characterized by stool with low pH and increased intestinal motility.

- Diarrhea, abdominal cramps, and flatulence occur after ingestion of dairy products.

- Results of the hydrogen breath test may be abnormal.

- Artificial sweeteners in diet soda and sugarless gum may cause osmotic diarrhea.

Secretory Diarrhea

VIPoma

The *WDHA* syndrome of *w*atery *d*iarrhea, *h*ypokalemia, and *a*chlorhydria, also called *Verner-Morrison syndrome* or *pancreatic cholera*, is a massive diarrhea (5 L daily) with dehydration and hypokalemia. The patient may have numerous endocrine tumors (with hypercalcemia or hyperglycemia). This diarrhea is associated with a non–beta islet cell tumor of the pancreas. Vasoactive intestinal polypeptide is the most common mediator; other mediators are prostaglandin, secretin, and calcitonin. VIPoma is diagnosed with pancreatic scan or angiography and measurement of hormone levels. Treatment is with somatostatin or surgery.

Carcinoid Syndrome

Carcinoid tumors arise from enterochromaffin cells of neural crest origin. About 90% of the tumors are in the

Table 12.6 FEATURES THAT SUGGEST MALABSORPTION CONDITIONS

FEATURE	CONDITION
Diarrhea with iron deficiency anemia (evaluation for blood loss is negative)	Proximal small-bowel malabsorption (eg, celiac disease)
Diarrhea with metabolic bone disease	Proximal small-bowel malabsorption (from decreased calcium & protein levels)
Hypoproteinemia with normal fat absorption	Protein-losing enteropathy (with eosinophilia, eosinophilic gastroenteritis; with lymphopenia, intestinal lymphangiectasia)
Oil droplets (neutral fat) or muscle fibers (undigested protein) present in stool	Pancreatic insufficiency (maldigestion)
Normal (usually) serum levels of calcium, magnesium, & iron	Pancreatic insufficiency (serum levels of albumin may also be normal)
Howell-Jolly bodies (if there is no history of splenectomy) or dermatitis herpetiformis	Celiac disease
Fever, arthralgia, & neurologic symptoms	Whipple disease

Table 12.7 PATIENT HISTORY FEATURES THAT MAY SUGGEST A POSSIBLE CAUSE OF DIARRHEA OR MALABSORPTION

FEATURE	SUGGESTED CAUSE
Age	Youth: lactase deficiency, inflammatory bowel disease, or sprue
Travel	Parasites or toxicogenic agents (exposure to contaminated food or water)
Drugs	Laxatives, antacids, antibiotics, colchicine, or lactulose
Family history	Celiac sprue, inflammatory bowel disease, polyposis coli, or lactase deficiency

terminal ileum. There is episodic facial flushing (lasting up to 10 minutes), watery diarrhea, wheezing, right-sided valvular disease (endocardial fibrosis), and hepatomegaly. If the gut is normal, look for bronchial tumors or gonadal tumors. Dietary tryptophan is converted into serotonin (which causes diarrhea, abdominal cramps [intestinal hypermotility], nausea, and vomiting), histamine (responsible for flushing), and other chemicals (bradykinin and corticotropin). Persons with intestinal tumors are usually asymptomatic because the mediators have high first-pass clearance in the liver. Carcinoid syndrome arises when these mediators are released into the systemic bloodstream; this suggests that liver metastases or bronchial tumors are present. The diagnosis of carcinoid syndrome is made by finding increased urinary levels of 5-hydroxyindoleacetic acid and by performing liver biopsy. Treatment is with octreotide.

- Pancreatic cholera: massive diarrhea, dehydration, and hypokalemia.

- Patients may have multiple endocrine tumors.

- Diarrhea is associated with a non–beta islet cell tumor of the pancreas.

Table 12.8 ASSOCIATED SIGNS AND SYMPTOMS OF SYSTEMIC ILLNESSES CAUSING DIARRHEA

SIGN OR SYMPTOM	DIAGNOSIS TO BE CONSIDERED
Arthritis	Ulcerative colitis, Crohn disease, Whipple disease, *Yersinia* infection
Marked weight loss	Malabsorption, inflammatory bowel disease, cancer, thyrotoxicosis
Eosinophilia	Eosinophilic gastroenteritis, parasitic disease
Lymphadenopathy	Lymphoma, Whipple disease
Neuropathy	Diabetic diarrhea, amyloidosis
Postural hypotension	Diabetic diarrhea, Addison disease, idiopathic orthostatic hypotension, autonomic dysfunction
Flushing	Malignant carcinoid syndrome
Proteinuria	Amyloidosis
Peptic ulcers	Zollinger-Ellison syndrome
Hyperpigmentation	Whipple disease, celiac disease, Addison disease, pancreatic cholera, eosinophilic gastroenteritis

Adapted from Fine KD. Diarrhea. In: Feldman M, Scharschmidt BF, Sleisenger MH, editors. Sleisenger & Fordtran's gastrointestinal and liver disease: pathophysiology, diagnosis, management. 6th ed. Vol. 1. Philadelphia (PA): WB Saunders Company; c1998. p. 128–52. Used with permission.

Laxative Abuse and Surreptitious Laxative Ingestion

Of the population older than 60 years, 15% to 30% admit that they take laxatives regularly. With the concealed ingestion of laxatives (surreptitious laxative ingestion), patients complain of diarrhea but do not admit that they take laxatives. In referral centers, this is a common cause of chronic watery diarrhea. Colonoscopy may show melanosis coli, which is a brown discoloration of the mucosa due to lipofuscin pigment accumulating in lamina propria macrophages. Melanosis coli is caused by anthraquinone laxatives (senna, cascara, and aloe). This benign condition is reversible with discontinuation of laxative use. A high degree of awareness is required to detect this condition. When surreptitious laxative ingestion is suspected, stool water can be analyzed for laxatives by chemical or chromatographic methods. Patients who ingest laxatives surreptitously often have underlying emotional problems that should be addressed.

- In patients using laxatives, colonoscopy may demonstrate melanosis coli.

- Anthraquinone laxatives cause melanosis coli.

- Address underlying emotional problems.

Bile Acid Malabsorption

Bile acid malabsorption is caused by ileal resection or disease. Diarrhea due to bile acid malabsorption may produce 2 clinical syndromes, each requiring a different treatment.

With a *limited resection* (≤100 cm of small intestine), malabsorbed bile acids enter the colon and stimulate secretion. Liver synthesis can compensate, so bile acid concentration in the upper small bowel is sufficient to achieve the critical micelle concentration and allow for normal fat absorption. The excess bile acids irritate the colon mucosa, causing a secretory diarrhea with minimal fat malabsorption. Treatment of the diarrhea is with cholestyramine, which binds excess bile acids.

With an *extensive resection* (>100 cm of small intestine), bile acid malabsorption is severe and enterohepatic circulation is interrupted. This limits synthesis, and the liver cannot compensate. Bile acid concentration is decreased in the upper small bowel, micelles cannot be formed, and fat malabsorption results. The malabsorbed fatty acids themselves stimulate secretion in the colon. Fat-soluble vitamins (A, D, E, and K) may be malabsorbed. Additionally, excess fatty acids bind intestinal calcium; this allows an increase in oxylate absorption, which increases the risk of oxylate renal stones. The treatment of this bile acid malabsorption is a low-fat diet (<50 g daily) rich in medium-chain triglycerides. Cholestyramine would further decrease bile acid concentration and worsen the steatorrhea.

- Limited resection (≤100 cm of small intestine): treat with cholestyramine.

- Extensive resection (>100 cm of small intestine): treat with a low-fat diet and medium-chain triglycerides.

Bacterial Overgrowth

The proximal small intestine normally has low bacterial counts because it has several major defenses against excess small intestinal bacterial proliferation: intestinal peristalsis (the most important defense), gastric acid, and intestinal IgA. When these defenses are altered, bacterial overgrowth results. The mechanism of steatorrhea in

bacterial overgrowth is the deconjugation of bile acids by bacteria that normally do not occur in the proximal intestine. Deconjugation of bile acids changes the ionization coefficient, and the deconjugated bile acids can then be passively absorbed in the proximal small bowel. Normally, conjugated bile acids are actively absorbed distally in the ileum. As a result, the critical micellar concentration is not reached, and mild steatorrhea results from the intraluminal deficiency of bile acids.

Clinical features of bacterial overgrowth are steatorrhea (typically >20 g daily), vitamin B$_{12}$ malabsorption (macrocytic anemia), increased serum folate levels from bacterial production, and positive duodenal or jejunal cultures. Conditions associated with small intestinal bacterial overgrowth include postoperative conditions (blind loops, enteroenterostomy, or gastrojejunocolic fistula), structural abnormalities (diverticula, strictures, or fistulas), motility disorders (diabetes mellitus, scleroderma, or pseudo-obstruction), achlorhydria (atrophic gastritis or gastric resections; achlorhydria is corrected with antibiotics), and impaired immunity. Two examples of impaired immunity are hypogammaglobulinemic sprue (in small-bowel biopsy specimens, no plasma cells are seen in the lamina propria and the villi are flat) and nodular lymphoid hyperplasia associated with IgA deficiency, which predisposes to *Giardia lamblia* infection.

- Deconjugated bile acids can be absorbed passively in the jejunum.

- Steatorrhea results from the intraluminal deficiency of bile acids.

- Diarrhea, vitamin B$_{12}$ deficiency with *normal or elevated* folate levels, postoperative or structural conditions, motility disorders, achlorhydria, and impaired immunity suggest bacterial overgrowth.

Noninvasive (Toxicogenic) Bacterial Diarrhea

Toxicogenic bacterial diarrhea, characterized by watery stools without fecal leukocytes, is caused by several organisms (Table 12.9).

Staphylococcus aureus

Diarrhea caused by *S aureus* is of rapid onset and lasts for 24 hours. There is no fever, vomiting, or cramps. The toxin is ingested with egg products, cream, and mayonnaise. Treatment is supportive.

Clostridium perfringens

The toxin of *C perfringens* (the "buffet pathogen") is ingested with precooked foods, usually beef and turkey, that have been kept warm under heating lamps in buffet lines. Heat-stable spores produce toxins. Although the bacteria are killed and the toxin is destroyed, the spores survive. When food is rewarmed, the spores germinate, producing toxin. The diarrhea is worse than the vomiting and is later in onset. It lasts 24 hours. Treatment is supportive.

Table 12.9 TOXICOGENIC CAUSES OF BACTERIAL DIARRHEA

ORGANISM	ONSET, H	MEDIATED BY CYCLIC AMP	FEVER	INTESTINAL SECRETION
Staphylococcus aureus	1–6	+	−	+
Clostridium perfringens	8–12	−	±	+
Escherichia coli	12	+	+	+
Vibrio cholerae	12	+	Due to dehydration	++++
Bacillus cereus	1–6	+	−	+

Abbreviations: −, absence of feature; +, presence of feature (++++, strong presence); ±, feature may be present or absent; AMP, adenosine monophosphate.

Escherichia coli

The toxin of *E coli*, which causes traveler's diarrhea, is ingested with water and salads. It is a plasmid-mediated enterotoxin. Treatment is rehydration with correction of electrolyte imbalance and administration of ciprofloxacin, norfloxacin, or trimethoprim-sulfamethoxazole. This pathogen may be important in epidemic diarrhea of the newborn.

Vibrio cholerae

The toxin of *V cholerae* is ingested with water. It is one of the few toxicogenic bacterial diarrhea illnesses in which antibiotics shorten the duration of the disease. Treatment is with tetracycline.

Bacillus cereus

Classically, the source of the *B cereus* toxin is fried rice in Asian restaurants. The toxin produces 2 syndromes: a rapid-onset syndrome that resembles *S aureus* infection and a slower-onset syndrome that resembles *C perfringens* infection. The diagnosis is typically made by clinical history but occasionally by isolating the organism from contaminated food. Treatment is supportive.

Other Toxicogenic Bacteria

Clostridium botulinum produces a neurotoxin that is ingested in improperly home-processed vegetables, fruits, and meats. It interferes with the release of acetylcholine from peripheral nerve endings. *Clostridiuim difficile* is discussed in the "Antibiotic Colitis" subsection of Chapter 9 ("Colon").

- Toxicogenic bacterial diarrhea: watery stools without fecal leukocytes.

- *Staphylococcus aureus*: rapid onset of diarrhea.

- *Clostridium perfringens*: "buffet pathogen" acquired from foods kept warm under heating lamps; delayed-onset diarrhea is the predominant symptom.

- *Escherichia coli*: traveler's diarrhea.

- *Vibrio cholerae*: one of the few toxicogenic diarrhea illnesses in which antibiotics shorten the duration of the disease; tetracycline is the treatment of choice.

- *Bacillus cereus*: source of toxin is fried rice in Asian restaurants.

Invasive Bacterial Diarrhea

Invasive bacterial diarrhea is characterized by fever, bloody stools, and fecal leukocytes. It is caused by several organisms (Table 12.10).

Shigella

Shigella infection is often acquired outside the United States. Bloody diarrhea is characteristic, and fever and bacteremia occur. Diagnosis is based on positive stool and blood cultures. Treatment is with ampicillin or a fluoroquinolone. Resistant strains are emerging for which chloramphenicol is an alternative. (Plasmids are responsible for antibiotic deactivation resistance.)

Salmonella (Non-Typhi)

In the United States, *Salmonella typhimurium* is the most common agent. The toxin is ingested with poultry. Fever and bloody diarrhea may be present. Diagnosis is based on a stool culture positive for *Salmonella*. Treatment is supportive. Severe symptoms should be treated with ciprofloxacin. Treating mild symptoms with other antibiotics may result in a prolonged carrier state.

Vibrio parahaemolyticus

The *V parahaemolyticus* toxin is ingested with undercooked shellfish. The infection is increasing in frequency in the United States (it is common in Japan). Fever and bloody diarrhea are the chief characteristics. Diagnosis is based on a stool culture positive for *Vibrio*. Antibiotics are of questionable value in treating this infection, but erythromycin may be most effective.

Escherichia coli

In the United States, enteroinvasive *E coli* is a rare cause of diarrhea. Enteroinvasive *E coli* involves the colon and causes abdominal pain with fever, bloody diarrhea, and profound toxicity (similar to *Shigella* infection). Shiga toxin–producing (also called enterohemorrhagic) *E coli* (serotype O157:H7) produces a cytotoxin that damages vascular endothelial cells. This serotype

Table 12.10 CAUSES OF INVASIVE BACTERIAL DIARRHEA

ORGANISM	FEVER	BLOODY DIARRHEA	BACTEREMIA	ANTIBIOTIC EFFECTIVENESS
Shigella	+	+	+	+
Salmonella	+	−	−	−
Vibrio parahaemolyticus	+	+	−	+[a]
Escherichia coli	+	+	−	−
Staphylococcus aureus (enterocolitis)	+	+	±	+
Yersinia enterocolitica	+	+	+	+
Campylobacter jejuni	+	+	±	+
Vibrio vulnificus	+	+	+	+

Abbreviations: −, absence of feature; +, presence of feature; ±, feature may be present or absent.

[a] Antibiotics are of questionable value, but erythromycin may be most effective.

can cause sporadic or epidemic illness from contaminated hamburger and raw milk. Enterohemorrhagic *E coli* infection should be suspected when bloody diarrhea occurs after eating hamburger and when bloody diarrhea is complicated by hemolytic uremic syndrome or thrombotic thrombocytopenic purpura. Antibiotic treatment has not been effective and is not recommended because it may increase the risk of development of hemolytic uremic syndrome or thrombotic thrombocytopenic purpura from the rapid release of toxin during bacterial death.

- Invasive bacterial diarrhea: fever, bloody stools, and fecal leukocytes.

- *Shigella*: bloody diarrhea.

- *Salmonella typhimurium*: bloody diarrhea may be present; treat with antibiotics only if blood cultures are positive.

- *Vibrio parahaemolyticus*: undercooked shellfish; bloody diarrhea.

- *Escherichia coli*: bloody stools, abdominal pain with fever; occurs after eating contaminated hamburger and may cause hemolytic uremic syndrome or thrombotic thrombocytopenic purpura.

Yersinia enterocolitica

The spectrum of disease caused by *Y enterocolitica* includes acute and chronic enteritis. Acute enteritis is similar to shigellosis and usually lasts 1 to 3 weeks. It is characterized by fever, diarrhea, leukocytosis, and fecal leukocytes. Chronic enteritis occurs especially in children with diarrhea, failure to thrive, hypoalbuminemia, and hypokalemia. Other features are acute abdominal pain (mesenteric adenitis), right lower quadrant pain, tenderness, nausea, and vomiting. The disease mimics appendicitis or Crohn disease. This gram-negative rod is hardy and can survive in cold temperatures. It grows on special cold-enriched medium. It is an invasive pathogen, with fecal-oral transmission in water and milk.

Extraintestinal manifestations are nonsuppurative arthritis and ankylosing spondylitis (associated with HLA-B27). Skin manifestations are erythema nodosum and erythema multiforme. Thyroid manifestations are Graves and Hashimoto diseases. Multiple liver abscesses and granulomata are present.

Treatment is with aminoglycosides or trimethoprim-sulfamethoxazole. The bacteria are variably sensitive to tetracycline and chloramphenicol. β-Lactamases are frequently produced, making penicillin resistance common.

- *Yersinia enterocolitica*: enteritis with acute abdominal pain (differential diagnosis includes appendicitis and Crohn disease).

- Fecal-oral transmission in water and milk.

- Manifestations include nonsuppurative arthritis and ankylosing spondylitis (associated with HLA-B27).

Campylobacter jejuni

The comma-shaped *C jejuni* organisms are motile, microaerophilic gram-negative bacilli. Transmission is linked to infected water, unpasteurized milk, poultry, sick dogs, and infected children. The incubation period is 2 to 4 days before invasion of the small bowel or colon. Infection results in the presence of blood and leukocytes in the stool. It may mimic granulomatous or idiopathic ulcerative colitis. It also may mimic small-bowel secretory diarrhea, with explosive, frequent watery diarrhea due to many *C jejuni* strains that produce a cholera-type toxin. The diarrhea usually lasts 3 to 5 days but may recur. Antibiotic treatment is with a macrolide antibiotic when severe, but treatment often is not needed. Postdiarrheal illnesses are hemolytic uremic syndrome and postinfectious arthritis.

- *Campylobacter jejuni*: transmission is linked to infected water, unpasteurized milk, poultry, sick dogs, and infected children.

- Infection may mimic granulomatous or idiopathic ulcerative colitis.
- Diarrhea usually lasts 3–5 days but may recur.

Vibrio vulnificus

Noncholera *V vulnificus* organisms are extremely invasive and produce necrotizing vasculitis, gangrene, and shock. They are routinely isolated from seawater, zooplankton, and shellfish along the Gulf of Mexico and both coasts of the United States, especially in the summer. The 2 clinical syndromes are 1) wound infection, cellulitis, fasciitis, or myositis after exposure to seawater or cleaning shellfish and 2) septicemia after the ingestion of raw shellfish (oysters). Patients at high risk of septicemia include those with liver disease, congestive heart failure, diabetes mellitus, renal failure, an immunosuppressive state, or hemochromatosis. Treatment is with tetracycline.

- *Vibrio vulnificus* is extremely invasive, producing necrotizing vasculitis, gangrene, and shock.
- Wound infection, cellulitis, fasciitis, or myositis occurs after exposure to seawater or cleaning shellfish.
- Septicemia occurs after the ingestion of raw shellfish (oysters).

Aeromonas hydrophila

Infection with *A hydrophila* is a frequent cause of diarrhea after a person has been swimming in fresh or brackish water. The organisms produce several toxins. Treatment is with trimethoprim-sulfamethoxazole and tetracycline.

MALABSORPTION DUE TO DISEASES OF THE SMALL INTESTINE

CELIAC DISEASE

Celiac disease (CD), also known as gluten-sensitive enteropathy, is a multisystem disorder affecting approximately 1% of the population. It may affect multiple organ systems and have protean manifestations. Iron deficiency anemia is the most common clinical manifestation of CD in adults. Gastrointestinal tract symptoms such as diarrhea are present in only approximately 50% of patients. Splenic atrophy may be a complication and cause an abnormal peripheral blood smear with Howell-Jolly bodies, which may be a clue to the diagnosis in 10% to 15% of patients. The pathognomonic skin manifestation is dermatitis herpetiformis. The measurement of serum IgA tissue transglutaminase antibodies is the test of choice for noninvasive screening. If the results are positive, a small-bowel biopsy should be performed. False-negative results can occur in the IgA-based tests because about 5% of patients with CD also have IgA deficiency. IgG-based testing or confirmation of normal total IgA levels should be performed with all sprue screening. If the result of the antibody testing is negative, another diagnosis should be considered. Small-bowel biopsy findings are not diagnostic. Diagnosis requires response to a gluten-free diet. If the patient has no response to the diet, the diet should be reviewed for inadvertent gluten ingestion. If symptoms recur after 10 to 15 years of successful dietary management, consider enteropathy-associated T-cell lymphoma, which is a characteristic complication of CD, especially if there is associated abdominal pain and weight loss.

- CD: iron deficiency anemia is the most common manifestation in adults.
- Splenic atrophy and an abnormal blood smear with Howell-Jolly bodies may be clues to the diagnosis in 10%-15% of patients.
- Enteropathy-associated T-cell lymphoma is a characteristic complication of CD.

TROPICAL SPRUE

In tropical sprue, diarrhea occurs 2 to 3 months after travel to the tropics. After 6 months, megaloblastic anemia develops because of folate deficiency and possible coexisting vitamin B_{12} deficiency. The pathogenesis is presumed to result from a type of bacterial overgrowth in the small bowel; however, the specific organism is somewhat controversial. Biopsies of the small bowel show villous atrophy, crypt hyperplasia, and an inflammatory infiltrate similar to findings in CD. Treatment is with tetracycline (250 mg 4 times daily) and folate with or without vitamin B_{12}.

- Tropical sprue: diarrhea and megaloblastic anemia after travel to the tropics.
- Cause: controversial.
- Treatment: tetracycline (250 mg 4 times daily) and folate with or without vitamin B_{12}.

WHIPPLE DISEASE

Whipple disease is a rare multisystem infectious disease that can involve the central nervous system (CNS), heart, kidneys, and small bowel. It occurs predominantly in middle-aged white men and is caused by chronic infection with the gram-positive bacillus *Tropheryma whipplei*. Diarrhea or steatorrhea is the most common presenting symptom. Arthritis is the most common extraintestinal symptom and affects the majority of patients. Whipple disease may involve the CNS, manifesting with oculomasticatory myorhythmia in 20% of patients. Oculomasticatory myorhythmia is pathognomonic and is characterized by continuous rhythmic jaw contractions that are synchronous with dissociated pendular vergence oscillations of the eyes. In the vast majority of patients with Whipple disease, the intestinal tract is involved regardless of the presence or absence of gastrointestinal tract symptoms.

Thus, the primary diagnostic approach to a patient with clinically suspected Whipple disease is upper endoscopy with mucosal biopsy. Intestinal biopsy specimens show the characteristic finding of macrophages with periodic acid-Schiff (PAS)-staining particles that represent *T whipplei* bacilli. Polymerase chain reaction assays may assist in detecting *T whipplei* DNA in the intestinal mucosa. Whipple disease should be suspected in patients who have recurrent arthritis, pigmentation, adenopathy, or CNS symptoms (dementia, myoclonus, ophthalmoplegia, visual disturbances, coma, or seizures). Treatment is with trimethoprim-sulfamethoxazole for 1 year.

- Suspect Whipple disease in patients who have recurrent arthritis, adenopathy, or CNS symptoms.

- Oculomasticatory myorhythmia is pathognomonic of Whipple disease.

- Small-bowel biopsy specimens show PAS-positive granules in macrophages.

- Treatment: trimethoprim-sulfamethoxazole for 1 year.

EOSINOPHILIC GASTROENTERITIS

Patients with eosinophilic gastroenteritis have a history of allergies (eg, asthma), food intolerances, and episodic symptoms of nausea, vomiting, abdominal pain, and diarrhea. Laboratory findings include peripheral eosinophilia, iron deficiency anemia, and steatorrhea or protein-losing enteropathy. Small-bowel radiographs show coarse folds and filling defects, and biopsy specimens show infiltration of the mucosa by eosinophils and, occasionally, the absence of villi. Parasitic infection should be ruled out. Treatment with corticosteroids produces a rapid response.

- Eosinophilic gastroenteritis: allergies, food intolerances, eosinophilia, and episodic intestinal symptoms.

- Rule out parasitic infection.

- Corticosteroids produce a rapid response.

SYSTEMIC MASTOCYTOSIS

Systemic mastocytosis is a clonal proliferation of mast cells with activating mutations in the *c-kit* gene. It is characterized by mast cell infiltration of tissues, including those in the bone marrow, spleen, liver, and gastrointestinal tract. The characteristic dermatologic finding is urticaria pigmentosa. Typical symptoms include pruritus, flushing, tachycardia, asthma, and headache caused by the release of histamine from mast cells. Gastrointestinal tract manifestations include diarrhea and peptic ulcer disease. Symptoms may be provoked by heat; hence, bath pruritus (ie, itching after a hot bath) is a clue to the diagnosis. Treatment includes histamine receptor blockers, anticholinergics, cromoglycate, and glucocorticoids.

Although the *c-kit* gene is mutated, the tyrosine kinase inhibitor, imatinib mesylate, is not an effective treatment.

- Systemic mastocytosis causes urticaria pigmentosa.

- Characteristic gastrointestinal tract manifestations include peptic ulcer disease and diarrhea.

- Bath pruritus is a clue to the diagnosis.

INTESTINAL LYMPHANGIECTASIA

Intestinal lymphangiectasia is caused by lymphatic obstruction that results in dilatation of intestinal lymphatic channels with subsequent lacteal rupture and leakage of chylomicrons and protein-rich fluid into the intestine. The clinical features are edema (often unilateral leg edema), chylous peritoneal or pleural effusions, and steatorrhea or protein-losing enteropathy. Laboratory findings include lymphocytopenia (average lymphocyte count, 0.6×10^9/L) due to enteric loss. Levels of all serum proteins, including immunoglobulins, are decreased. Small-bowel radiographs show edematous folds, and small-bowel biopsy specimens show dilated lacteals and lymphatics in the lamina propria that may contain lipid-laden macrophages. The same biopsy findings are seen in obstruction of mesenteric lymph nodes (lymphoma, Whipple disease, and Crohn disease) and obstruction of venous inflow to the heart (constrictive pericarditis and severe right heart failure). Diagnosis is based on abnormal small-bowel biopsy findings and enteric protein loss documented by finding increased α_1-antitrypsin levels in the stool. Treatment is with a low-fat diet and medium-chain triglycerides (they enter the portal blood rather than the lymphatics). Occasionally, surgical excision of the involved segment is useful if the lesion is localized.

- Intestinal lymphangiectasia: unilateral lymphedema of the leg and chylous peritoneal or pleural effusions.

- Lymphocytopenia is characteristic.

- Decreased levels of serum proteins.

- Biopsy specimens of the small intestine show dilated lymphatic channels.

- Treatment: low-fat diet and medium-chain triglycerides.

AMYLOIDOSIS

Amyloidosis is characterized by diffuse deposition of amorphous eosinophilic extracellular protein in the tissue. Gastrointestinal tract involvement can occur with AL amyloidosis, AA amyloidosis, and hereditary amyloidosis. The main sites of amyloid deposition are the walls of blood vessels and the mucous membranes and muscle layers of the intestine. Any portion of the gut may be involved. Amyloid damages tissues by infiltration (muscle and nerve infiltration causes motility disorders and malabsorption) and ischemia (obliteration of vessels causes ulceration and bleeding). Intestinal dysmotility can produce diarrhea, constipation, pseudo-obstruction, megacolon, and fecal incontinence. Clinical findings in amyloidosis include macroglossia, hepatomegaly, cardiomegaly, proteinuria, and peripheral neuropathy. Pinch (posttraumatic) purpura or periorbital purpura after proctoscopic examination may occur. Small-bowel radiography shows symmetrical, sharply demarcated thickening of the plicae circulares. Histologic examination of duodenal biopsy specimens shows amyloid deposits in up to 100% of patients. It is the diagnostic test of choice when amyloid is suspected as a cause of gastrointestinal tract symptoms. Amyloid deposits may not be seen on routine histologic stains; Congo red staining is required. Subcutaneous fat pad aspirate stained with Congo red can be used to make the diagnosis in 80% of patients.

MISCELLANEOUS SMALL-BOWEL DISORDERS

MECKEL DIVERTICULUM

A Meckel diverticulum results from persistence of the vitelline duct, which is the communication between the intestine and the yolk sac. It is the most frequent congenital abnormality of the small intestine and is an antimesenteric outpouching of the ileum usually occurring within 100 cm of the ileocecal valve. A Meckel diverticulum contains all layers of the intestinal wall and so is a true diverticulum. It may contain ectopic gastrointestinal tract mucosa, including gastric (most commonly), duodenal, biliary, colonic, or pancreatic tissue. The most common manifestation is painless, maroon stools, with peptic ulceration being the cause of bleeding secondary to acid production by the ectopic gastric mucosa within the Meckel diverticulum. Other manifestations include intestinal obstruction due to intussusception or volvulus around the band that fixes the diverticulum to the bowel wall. Diverticulitis of a Meckel diverticulum can occur and mimic acute appendicitis. The diagnostic test of choice is a Meckel scan (a technetium Tc 99m pertechnetate nuclear scan with mucous cells of gastric mucosa concentrating technetium), but false-positive and false-negative results can occur.

- Meckel diverticulum is the most common congenital abnormality of the small intestine.

- The most common manifestation is painless, maroon stools, and this diagnosis must be considered when young adults present with lower gastrointestinal tract bleeding.

AORTOENTERIC FISTULA

A history of gastrointestinal tract bleeding in a patient who has had a previous aortic graft demands immediate evaluation to rule out an aortoenteric fistula. If the patient presents with massive bleeding, do not attempt endoscopy or arteriography. Emergency surgery is indicated.

Management of a smaller bleeding episode is more controversial, and urgent computed tomography or extended upper endoscopy has been suggested as a possible alternative to surgical exploration. If the presence of a graft fistula is confirmed (by air in the vessel wall on computed tomography or erosion of a graft into the intestinal lumen on endoscopy), emergent surgery is indicated.

- If a patient presents with massive bleeding, do not attempt endoscopy or arteriography. Instead, emergency surgery is indicated.

CHRONIC INTESTINAL PSEUDO-OBSTRUCTION

Pseudo-obstruction is a syndrome characterized by the clinical findings of mechanical bowel obstruction but without occlusion of the lumen. The 2 types are primary and secondary.

The primary type, also called *idiopathic pseudo-obstruction*, is a visceral myopathy or neuropathy. It is associated with recurrent attacks of nausea, vomiting, cramping abdominal pain, distention, and constipation, which are of variable frequency and duration. If the cause is familial, the patient has a positive family history and the condition is present when the patient is young. Esophageal motility is abnormal (achalasia) in most patients; occasionally, urinary tract motility is abnormal. Diarrhea or steatorrhea results from bacterial overgrowth. Upper gastrointestinal tract and small-bowel radiographs show dilatation of the bowel and slow transit (not mechanical obstruction).

- Idiopathic pseudo-obstruction is due to a familial cause or to a sporadic visceral myopathy or neuropathy.

- Recurrent attacks have variable frequency and duration.

- Esophageal motility is abnormal in most patients.

- Steatorrhea is caused by bacterial overgrowth.

Secondary pseudo-obstruction occurs in the presence of underlying systemic disease or precipitating causes, including the following:

- Diseases involving the intestinal smooth muscle: amyloidosis, scleroderma, systemic lupus erythematosus, myotonic dystrophy, and muscular dystrophy.

- Neurologic diseases: Parkinson disease, Hirschsprung disease, Chagas disease, and familial autonomic dysfunction.

- Endocrine disorders: hypoparathyroidism.

- Drugs: antiparkinsonian medications (levodopa), phenothiazines, tricyclic antidepressants, ganglionic blockers, clonidine, and narcotics.

Approach to the Patient With Chronic Intestinal Pseudo-Obstruction

If a patient has chronic intestinal pseudo-obstruction, first rule out a mechanical cause for the obstruction. Second, look for an underlying precipitating cause such as metabolic abnormalities, medications, or an underlying associated disease. If a familial idiopathic cause is suspected, assess esophageal motility. Suspect scleroderma if intestinal radiography shows large-mouth diverticula of the small intestine. Suspect amyloidosis if the skin shows palpable purpura and if proteinuria and neuropathy are present.

- Secondary pseudo-obstruction is due to an underlying systemic disease or precipitating cause.
- Patients with scleroderma present with large-mouth diverticula of the intestine.
- Patients with amyloidosis present with palpable purpura, proteinuria, and neuropathy.

SUMMARY

- In osmotic diarrhea, stool volume is <1 L daily. Causes of osmotic diarrhea: lactase deficiency, sorbitol, and antacids.
- In secretory diarrhea, stool volume is >1 L daily. Causes of secretory diarrhea: bacterial toxins, neuroendocrine tumors, surreptitious ingestion of laxative, bile acid diarrhea, and fatty acid diarrhea.

- In exudative diarrhea, membrane permeability is abnormal and stool volume is typically small. Causes of exudative diarrhea: invasive bacterial pathogens and inflammatory bowel disease.
- Noninvasive (toxicogenic) bacterial diarrhea, characterized by watery stools without fecal leukocytes. Invasive bacterial diarrhea is characterized by fever, bloody stools, and fecal leukocytes.
- CD: iron deficiency anemia is the most common manifestation in adults.
- Tropical sprue: diarrhea and megaloblastic anemia after travel to the tropics.
- Suspect Whipple disease in patients who have recurrent arthritis, adenopathy, or CNS symptoms.
- Eosinophilic gastroenteritis: allergies, food intolerances, eosinophilia, and episodic intestinal symptoms. Rule out parasitic infection.
- Intestinal lymphangiectasia: unilateral lymphedema of the leg and chylous peritoneal or pleural effusions.

13.

LIVER AND BILIARY TRACT[a]

John J. Poterucha, MD

GOALS

- Interpret and evaluate abnormal liver function test results.

- Differentiate the various causes of liver disease: infectious, autoimmune, hereditary, and environmental.

- Understand the complications of end-stage liver disease.

- Understand the diagnosis and management of biliary tract disease.

INTERPRETATION OF ABNORMAL LIVER TEST RESULTS

The evaluation of patients who have abnormal liver test results includes many clinical factors: the patient's chief complaints, age, risk factors for liver disease, personal or family history of liver disease, medications, and physical examination findings. Designing a standard algorithm for the evaluation of abnormal liver test results has been challenging. Nevertheless, with some basic information, abnormalities can be evaluated in an efficient, cost-effective manner.

COMMONLY USED LIVER TESTS

AMINOTRANSFERASES

Aminotransferases are found in hepatocytes and are markers of liver cell injury or hepatocellular disease. Hepatocellular injury causes these enzymes to "leak" out of liver cells. Within a few hours after liver injury, increased levels of these enzymes can be detected in the serum. The aminotransferases are alanine aminotransferase (ALT) and aspartate aminotransferase (AST). ALT is more specific for liver injury than AST; however, markedly increased levels of muscle enzymes may be accompanied by increased levels of both AST and ALT. Because ALT has a longer half-life, improvements in ALT levels lag behind improvements in AST levels.

- Aminotransferases are markers of liver cell injury or hepatocellular disease.

ALKALINE PHOSPHATASE

Alkaline phosphatase is found on the hepatocyte membrane that borders the bile canaliculi (the smallest branches of the bile ducts). Because alkaline phosphatase is also found in bone and placenta, an isolated increase in the serum level of this enzyme should prompt further testing to determine whether the increase is from the liver or other tissues. One method of further testing is to determine alkaline phosphatase isoenzyme levels. Another method is to determine the level of γ-glutamyltransferase (GGT), an enzyme of intrahepatic biliary canaliculi that is more specific than alkaline phosphatase. Other than to confirm the hepatic origin of an increased level of alkaline phosphatase, GGT has little role in the diagnosis of diseases of the liver because its synthesis can be induced by many medications, thus reducing its specificity for clinically important liver disease.

- Isolated increase in the level of alkaline phosphatase should prompt further testing.

BILIRUBIN

Bilirubin is the water-insoluble product of heme metabolism that is taken up by the hepatocyte and conjugated with glucuronic acid to form monoglucuronides and diglucuronides. Conjugation makes bilirubin water soluble, allowing it to be excreted in the bile. Direct (conjugated) and indirect (unconjugated) fractions of bilirubin can be measured in the serum. Diseases characterized by overproduction of bilirubin, such

[a] Portions previously published in Poterucha JJ. Hepatitis. In: Bland KI, Büchler MW, Csendes A, Garden OJ, Sarr MG, Wong J, editors. General surgery: principles and international practice. 2nd ed. Vol. 1. London (UK): Springer-Verlag; ©2009. p. 921–32. Used with permission.

as hemolysis or resorption of a hematoma, are characterized by hyperbilirubinemia that is less than 20% conjugated. Hepatocyte dysfunction or impaired bile flow produces hyperbilirubinemia that is usually more than 50% conjugated bilirubin. Because conjugated bilirubin is water soluble and may be excreted in the urine, patients with liver disease and hyperbilirubinemia have dark urine. In these patients, the stools have a lighter color because of the absence of bilirubin pigments.

- Hyperbilirubinemia is usually <20% conjugated bilirubin in diseases characterized by overproduction of bilirubin.
- Hyperbilirubinemia is usually >50% conjugated bilirubin with hepatocyte dysfunction or impaired bile flow.

PROTHROMBIN TIME AND ALBUMIN

Prothrombin time (PT), expressed as the international normalized ratio (INR), and serum level of albumin are markers of liver synthetic function. Abnormalities of PT and albumin imply severe liver disease and should prompt an immediate evaluation. INR is a measure of the activity of coagulation factors II, V, VII, and X, all of which are synthesized in the liver. Because these factors are also dependent on vitamin K for synthesis, deficiencies of vitamin K also produce abnormalities of INR. Vitamin K deficiency can result from the use of antibiotics during a period of prolonged fasting, small-bowel mucosal disorders such as celiac disease, and severe cholestasis, with an inability to absorb fat-soluble vitamins. True hepatocellular dysfunction is characterized by an inability to synthesize clotting factors even when stores of vitamin K are adequate. A simple way to distinguish between vitamin K deficiency and liver dysfunction in a patient with a prolonged PT is to administer vitamin K. A 10-mg dose of oral vitamin K for 3 days or 10 mg of subcutaneous vitamin K normalizes the PT within 48 hours in a vitamin K–deficient patient, but it has no effect on the PT in a patient with decreased liver synthetic function.

Because albumin has a half-life of 21 days, serum levels do not decrease suddenly with liver dysfunction. However, the serum level of albumin can decrease relatively quickly in a severe systemic illness such as bacteremia. This rapid decrease most likely results from the release of cytokines and the accelerated metabolism of albumin. A chronic decrease of albumin in a patient without overt liver disease should prompt a search for albumin in the urine.

- PT and albumin are markers of liver synthetic function.

HEPATOCELLULAR DISORDERS

Hepatocellular disorders are diseases that primarily affect hepatocytes and are characterized predominantly by increases in aminotransferases. The disorders are best considered as acute (generally <3 months) or chronic. Acute hepatitis may be accompanied by malaise, anorexia, abdominal pain, and

Table 13.1 **COMMON CAUSES OF A MARKED ACUTE INCREASE IN ALT**

DISEASE	CLINICAL CLUE	DIAGNOSTIC TEST
Hepatitis A	Exposure history	IgM anti-HAV
Hepatitis B	Risk factors	HBsAg, IgM anti-HBc
Drug-induced hepatitis	Compatible medication or timing	Improvement after withdrawal of the agent
Alcoholic hepatitis	History of alcohol excess, AST:ALT >2, AST <400 U/L	Clinical improvement with abstinence
Hepatitic ischemia	History of hypotension & heart disease	Rapid improvement of aminotransferase levels
Acute biliary obstruction	Abdominal pain, fever	Cholangiography

Abbreviations: ALT, alanine aminotransferase; AST, aspartate aminotransferase; HAV, hepatitis A virus; anti-HBc, antibody to hepatitis B core antigen; HBsAg, hepatitis B surface antigen; U, units.

jaundice. ALT and AST levels are usually greater than 500 U/L. Common causes of a marked acute increase in ALT are listed in Table 13.1.

The level and pattern of aminotransferase elevation may be helpful in the differential diagnosis of acute hepatitis. Acute hepatitis due to viruses or drugs generally produces markedly elevated levels of aminotransferases, often in the thousands (units per liter). In general, the concentration of ALT is higher than that of AST. An ALT concentration greater than 5,000 U/L is usually caused by acetaminophen hepatotoxicity, hepatic ischemia ("shock liver"), or unusual viruses such as herpes simplex virus. Hepatic ischemia typically occurs in patients with preexisting cardiac disease after an episode of hypotension. Aminotransferase levels are very high but decrease considerably within a few days. Another cause of transient elevations of aminotransferase levels is transient bile duct obstruction, usually from a stone. These elevations can be as high as 1,000 U/L, but they decrease within 24 to 48 hours. In patients with pancreatitis, a transient increase in the AST or ALT concentration suggests gallstone pancreatitis. Alcoholic hepatitis is characterized by more modest increases in aminotransferase levels, which are always less than 400 U/L and, at times, near normal. In patients with alcoholic hepatitis, usually the AST:ALT ratio is greater than 2:1. Finally, patients with alcoholic hepatitis frequently have a markedly elevated level of bilirubin that is out of proportion to the aminotransferase elevations.

Diseases that produce a sustained (>3 months) increase in aminotransferase levels are in the category of chronic hepatitis. The increase (usually 2-fold to 5-fold) in aminotransferase levels is more modest than in acute hepatitis. Patients are usually asymptomatic but occasionally complain of fatigue and right upper quadrant pain. The differential diagnosis of

Table 13.2 COMMON CAUSES OF CHRONIC HEPATITIS

DISEASE	CLINICAL CLUE	DIAGNOSTIC TEST
Hepatitis C	Risk factors	Anti-HCV, HCV RNA
Hepatitis B	Risk factors	HBsAg
Nonalcoholic steatohepatitis	Obesity, diabetes mellitus, hyperlipidemia	Steatosis on liver imaging, liver biopsy
Alcoholic liver disease	History, AST:ALT >2	Clinical liver biopsy
Autoimmune hepatitis	ALT 200–1,500 U/L, usually female, other autoimmune disease	Strongly positive antinuclear or anti–smooth muscle antibody (or both), hypergammaglobulinemia, liver biopsy

Abbreviations: ALT, alanine aminotransferase; AST, aspartate aminotransferase; HBsAg, hepatitis B surface antigen; HCV, hepatitis C virus; U, units.

Table 13.3 COMMON CAUSES OF CHOLESTASIS

DISEASE	CLINICAL CLUE	DIAGNOSTIC TEST
Primary biliary cirrhosis	Middle-aged woman	Antimitochondrial antibody
Primary sclerosing cholangitis	Association with ulcerative colitis	Cholangiography (ERCP or MRCP)
Large bile duct obstruction	Jaundice or pain (or both)	Ultrasonography, ERCP, or MRCP
Drug-induced cholestasis	Compatible medication or timing	Improvement after withdrawal of the agent
Infiltrative disorder or malignancy	Other clinical features of malignancy, sarcoidosis, or amyloidosis	Ultrasonography, computed tomography, liver biopsy
Inflammation-associated cholestasis	Symptoms of underlying inflammatory state	Blood cultures, appropriate antibody tests

Abbreviations: ERCP, endoscopic retrograde cholangiopancreatography; MRCP, magnetic resonance cholangiopancreatography.

chronic hepatitis is relatively lengthy; the more important and common disorders are listed in Table 13.2.

- The level and pattern of aminotransferase elevation may be helpful in the differential diagnosis of hepatocellular disorders.

CHOLESTATIC DISORDERS

Diseases that predominantly affect the biliary system are called cholestatic diseases. They can affect the microscopic ducts (eg, primary biliary cirrhosis) or the large bile ducts (eg, pancreatic cancer causing obstruction of the common bile duct), or both (eg, primary sclerosing cholangitis). Generally, the predominant laboratory abnormality in these disorders is the alkaline phosphatase level. Although diseases that increase the bilirubin level are often referred to as cholestatic, severe hepatocellular injury (as in acute hepatitis) also produces hyperbilirubinemia because of hepatocellular dysfunction. The common causes of cholestasis are listed in Table 13.3.

JAUNDICE

Jaundice is visibly evident hyperbilirubinemia, which occurs when the serum bilirubin concentration exceeds 2.5 mg/dL. Evaluation of a patient with jaundice is an important diagnostic skill (Figure 13.1). It is important to differentiate conjugated from unconjugated hyperbilirubinemia. A common disorder that produces unconjugated hyperbilirubinemia is Gilbert syndrome, in which total bilirubin is generally less than 3.0 mg/dL and direct bilirubin is 0.3 mg/dL or less. The concentration of bilirubin is generally higher in the fasting state or in illness. A presumptive diagnosis of Gilbert syndrome can be made when an otherwise well person has unconjugated hyperbilirubinemia and normal levels of hemoglobin (which excludes hemolysis) and liver enzymes (which excludes liver disease).

Direct hyperbilirubinemia is a more common cause of jaundice than indirect hyperbilirubinemia. Patients with direct hyperbilirubinemia can be categorized as those with nonobstructive conditions and those with obstruction. Risk factors for viral hepatitis, a bilirubin concentration greater than 15 mg/dL, and persistently high aminotransferase levels suggest that the jaundice is from hepatocellular dysfunction. Abdominal pain, fever, or a palpable gallbladder (or a combination of these) suggests obstruction. A sensitive, specific, and noninvasive test to exclude obstructive causes of cholestasis is hepatic ultrasonography. With diseases characterized by obstruction of a large bile duct, generally ultrasonography demonstrates intrahepatic bile duct dilatation, especially if the bilirubin concentration is greater than 10 mg/dL and the patient has had jaundice for more than 2 weeks. Acute large bile duct obstruction, usually from a stone, may not allow time for the bile ducts to dilate. An important clue to the presence of an acute large duct obstruction is a marked but transient increase in the levels of aminotransferases. If the clinical suspicion for obstruction of the bile duct is still strong despite negative ultrasonographic results, magnetic resonance cholangiography should be considered. Uncomplicated gallbladder disease, such as cholelithiasis with or without cholecystitis, does not cause jaundice or abnormal liver test results unless a common bile duct stone or sepsis is present.

- In Gilbert syndrome, the total bilirubin is generally less than 3.0 mg/dL and direct bilirubin is 0.3 mg/dL or less.

- Uncomplicated gallbladder disease, such as cholelithiasis with or without cholecystitis, does not cause jaundice or abnormal liver test results unless a common bile duct stone or sepsis is present.

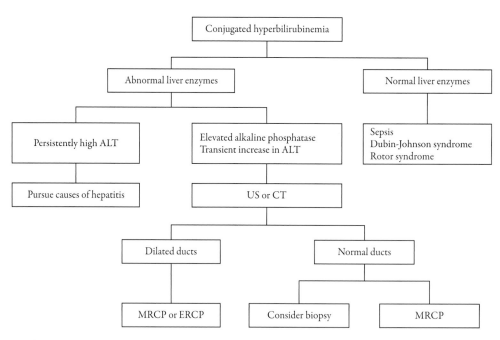

Figure 13.1 Evaluation of Conjugated Hyperbilirubinemia. ALT indicates alanine aminotransferase; CT, computed tomography; ERCP, endoscopic retrograde cholangiopancreatography; MRCP, magnetic resonance cholangiopancreatography; US, ultrasonography. (Adapted from Poterucha JJ. Approach to the patient with abnormal liver tests and fulminant liver failure. In: Hauser SC, editor. Mayo Clinic gastroenterology and hepatology board review. 3rd ed. Rochester [MN]: Mayo Clinic Scientific Press and Florence [KY]: Informa Healthcare USA; c2008. p. 283–92. Used with permission of Mayo Foundation for Medical Education and Research.)

ALGORITHMS FOR PATIENTS WITH ABNORMAL LIVER TEST RESULTS

Algorithms for patients with abnormal liver test results are at best only guidelines and at worst misleading. The patient's clinical presentation should be considered when interpreting abnormal results. In general, patients with abnormal liver test results that are less than 3 times the normal value can be observed unless the patient is symptomatic or the albumin level, INR, or bilirubin concentration is abnormal. Persistent abnormalities should be evaluated. Algorithms for the management of patients with increased levels of ALT or alkaline phosphatase are shown in Figures 13.2 and 13.3, respectively.

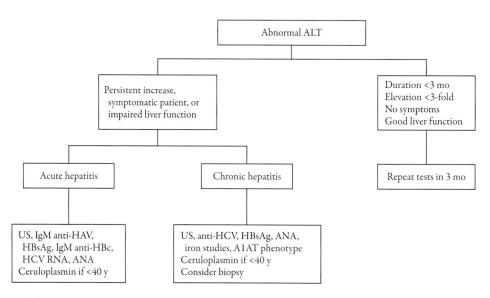

Figure 13.2 Evaluation of Abnormal Alanine Aminotransferase (ALT) Levels. A1AT indicates α_1-antitrypsin; ANA, antinuclear antibody; anti-HAV, hepatitis A virus antibody; anti-HBc, antibody to hepatitis B core antigen; anti-HCV, hepatitis C virus antibody; HBsAg, hepatitis B surface antigen; HCV, hepatis C virus; US, ultrasonography. (Adapted from Poterucha JJ. Approach to the patient with abnormal liver tests and fulminant liver failure. In: Hauser SC, editor. Mayo Clinic gastroenterology and hepatology board review. 3rd ed. Rochester [MN]: Mayo Clinic Scientific Press and Florence [KY]: Informa Healthcare USA; c2008. p. 283–92. Used with permission of Mayo Foundation for Medical Education and Research.)

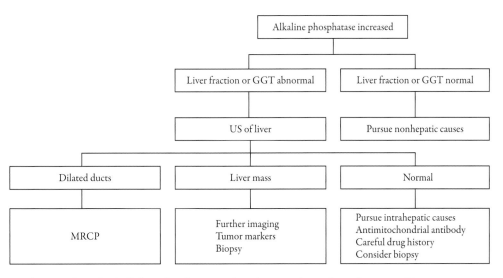

Figure 13.3 Evaluation of Increased Levels of Alkaline Phosphatase. GGT indicates γ-glutamyltransferase; MRCP, magnetic resonance cholangiopancreatography; US, ultrasonography. (Adapted from Poterucha JJ. Approach to the patient with abnormal liver tests and fulminant liver failure. In: Hauser SC, editor. Mayo Clinic gastroenterology and hepatology board review. 3rd ed. Rochester [MN]: Mayo Clinic Scientific Press and Florence [KY]: Informa Healthcare USA; c2008. p. 283–92. Used with permission of Mayo Foundation for Medical Education and Research.)

SPECIFIC LIVER DISEASES

VIRAL HEPATITIS

Hepatitis A

Owing to vaccination and improvements in food handling, hepatitis A virus (HAV) is becoming an unusual cause of acute hepatitis in the United States. The disease generally is transmitted by the fecal-oral route and has an incubation period of 15 to 50 days. Major routes of transmission of HAV are ingestion of contaminated food or water and contact with an infected person. Persons at highest risk of HAV infection are those living in or traveling to developing countries, children in day care centers, and homosexual men. Hepatitis caused by HAV is generally mild in children, who often have a subclinical or nonicteric illness. Infected adults are more ill and are usually icteric. The prognosis is excellent, although HAV can rarely cause acute liver failure. Chronic liver disease does not develop from HAV. Serum IgM anti-HAV is present during an acute illness and generally persists for 2 to 6 months. IgG anti-HAV appears slightly later, persists for life, and offers immunity from further infection.

- HAV is transmitted by ingestion of contaminated food or water or contact with an infected person.

- The incubation period is 15–50 days.

- IgM anti-HAV is present during the acute illness.

- The prognosis is excellent and chronic liver disease does not develop.

Hepatitis B

Hepatitis B virus (HBV) is a DNA virus that is transmitted by exposure to blood or contaminated body fluids. In high-prevalence areas (eg, certain areas of Asia and Africa), HBV is acquired perinatally or in early childhood. High-risk groups in the United States include persons born in an area where HBV is endemic (eg, parts of Asia and Africa), injection drug users, and persons with multiple sexual contacts. In the United States, most patients who have hepatitis B were born in Asia or sub-Saharan Africa. The clinical course of HBV infection varies. Many acute infections in adults are subclinical, and even when symptomatic, the disease resolves within 6 months with subsequent development of immunity. During acute hepatitis, symptoms (when present) are generally more severe than those of HAV infection. Jaundice rarely lasts longer than 4 weeks.

- HBV is transmitted by exposure to blood or contaminated body fluids.

- Infants may acquire infection from the mother.

- High-risk groups: persons born in an area where HBV is endemic, injection drug users, and persons with multiple sexual contacts.

- Most infections in adults are subclinical.

- Jaundice rarely lasts >4 weeks.

A brief guide to the interpretation of serologic markers of hepatitis B is shown in Table 13.4. Viral markers in the blood during a self-limited infection with HBV are shown in Figure 13.4. Note that IgM antibody to hepatitis B core antigen (anti-HBc) is nearly always present during acute hepatitis B.

Five percent of patients who acquire HBV as adults and 90% of those infected as neonates do not clear hepatitis B surface antigen (HBsAg) from the serum within 6 months and, thus, become chronically infected. The natural history of chronic infection is illustrated in Figure 13.5.

Table 13.4 HEPATITIS B SEROLOGIC MARKERS

TEST	INTERPRETATION OF POSITIVE RESULTS
Hepatitis B surface antigen (HBsAg)	Current infection
Antibody to hepatitis B surface (anti-HBs)	Immunity (immunization or resolved infection)
IgM antibody to hepatitis B core (IgM anti-HBc)	Usually recent infection; occasionally "reactivation" of chronic infection
IgG antibody to hepatitis B core (IgG anti-HBc)	Remote infection
Hepatitis B e antigen (HBeAg) or HBV DNA >10^4 IU/mL	Active viral replication
Antibody to hepatitis B e (anti-HBe)	Remote infection

Abbreviations: HBV, hepatitis B virus; IU, international units.

Adapted from Poterucha JJ. Chronic viral hepatitis. In: Hauser SC, editor. Mayo Clinic gastroenterology and hepatology board review. 4th ed. Rochester (MN): Mayo Clinic Scientific Press and New York (NY): Oxford University Press; c2011. p. 269–79. Used with permission of Mayo Foundation for Medical Education and Research.

Patients who are infected perinatally, typically those from Asia, generally go through an immune-tolerant phase that lasts until early adulthood. The immune tolerant phase is characterized by normal ALT, the presence of hepatitis B

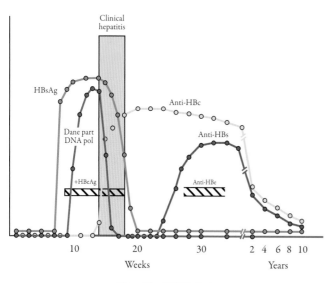

Figure 13.4 Viral Markers in Blood During Self-limited Hepatitis B Virus Infection. Anti-HBc indicates hepatitis B core antibody; anti-HBe, hepatitis B e antibody; anti-HBs, hepatitis B surface antibody; HBeAg, hepatitis B e antigen; HBsAg, hepatitis B surface antigen; part, particle; pol, polymerase. (Adapted from Robinson WS. Biology of human hepatitis viruses. In: Zakim D, Boyer TD, editors. Hepatology: a textbook of liver disease. Vol 2. 2nd ed. Philadelphia [PA]: WB Saunders Company; c1990. p. 890–945. Used with permission.)

e antigen (HBeAg), and very high HBV DNA levels. Liver histology shows "ground glass" hepatocytes but otherwise minimal changes. Treatment is not recommended. The immune-tolerant phase evolves under immune pressure into the HBeAg-positive chronic hepatitis B phase, characterized by elevated ALT, the presence of HBeAg, more than 10^4 IU/mL of HBV DNA, and active inflammation and often fibrosis on liver biopsy. This phase is generally considered to lead to progressive liver damage, including cirrhosis and an increased risk of hepatocellular carcinoma. At a rate of about 10% per year, patients mount an immune response that is sufficient to achieve a decrease in ALT, clearance of HBeAg, development of antibody to hepatitis B e antigen (anti-HBe) (seroconversion), and a decrease of HBV DNA levels to less than 2,000 IU/mL. This inactive carrier phase is generally not accompanied by progressive liver damage. Most patients remain in this phase for many years and have a better prognosis than patients with active liver inflammation and viral replication. Sixty percent of patients with chronic hepatitis B infection are in the inactive carrier phase.

About one-third of inactive carriers have a recurrence of chronic hepatitis characterized by an abnormal ALT level and an increased HBV DNA level. This may be associated with a recurrence of the HBeAg-positive state, although more commonly it is due to a precore or core promoter variant that produces HBeAg-negative chronic hepatitis B. This phase, similar to the HBeAg-positive phase, is associated with a progression of liver disease.

Patients with chronic hepatitis B and cirrhosis are at high risk of hepatocellular carcinoma, and liver ultrasonography should be performed every 6 to 12 months. After neonatal or early childhood acquisition of hepatitis B, hepatocellular carcinoma may develop even in the absence of cirrhosis, and surveillance is advised for the following patients: Asian men older than 40 years, Asian women older than 50 years, Africans older than 20 years, patients with a family history of hepatocellular carcinoma, and patients with persistent elevations of ALT and HBV DNA.

- IgM anti-HBc is nearly always present during acute hepatitis B.

- HBsAg is not cleared in 5% of patients acquiring HBV as adults and in 90% of those infected as neonates.

- Progressive liver injury occurs in chronically infected patients who have elevated ALT and HBV DNA levels >10^4 IU/mL.

- Certain patients with chronic hepatitis B are at high risk of hepatocellular carcinoma, and surveillance is advised.

Patients with chronic hepatitis B, an abnormal ALT level, and HBV DNA >10^4 IU/mL are candidates for therapy. Treatment options are compared and contrasted in Table 13.5. Treatment with peginterferon alfa results in a 30% response rate as measured by the loss of HBeAg, the suppression of HBV DNA, and the appearance of anti-HBe. Rarely, patients also clear HBsAg. Patients more likely to respond to peginterferon

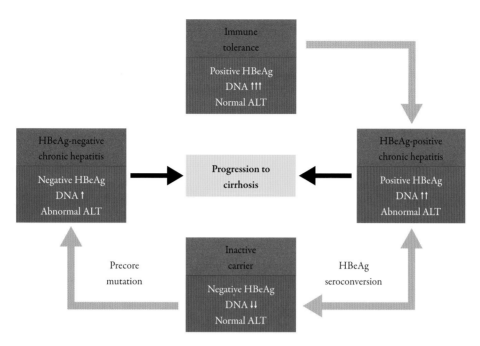

Figure 13.5 Phases of Chronic Hepatitis B Virus Infection. Black arrows represent histopathologic changes; gray arrows represent changes in serologic markers between phases; thin arrows represent an increase or decrease in DNA level (↑, low increase; ↑↑, moderate increase; ↓↓, moderate decrease; ↑↑↑, high increase). ALT indicates alanine aminotransferase; HBeAg, hepatitis B e antigen. (Adapted from Pungpapong S, Kim WR, Poterucha JJ. Natural history of hepatitis B virus infection: an update for clinicians. Mayo Clin Proc. 2007 Aug;82[8]:967–75. Used with permission of Mayo Foundation for Medical Education and Research.)

include those with high serum levels of aminotransferases, active hepatitis without evidence of cirrhosis on biopsy, and low serum levels of HBV DNA. Patients with HBV infection who have a response to peginterferon therapy may have a transient increase in aminotransferase levels after about 8 weeks of treatment. An acute hepatitis syndrome may be precipitated, and peginterferon is generally not given to patients with cirrhosis. Tenofovir, entecavir, lamivudine, adefovir, and telbivudine are oral agents that decrease HBV DNA levels and may result in clinical improvement, even in the presence of decompensation. The oral drugs are safer than peginterferon for patients with cirrhosis because flares of hepatitis and infectious complications are uncommon. Resistance is a concern with the oral agents; the highest rates of resistance occur with lamivudine, intermediate rates with adefovir and telbivudine, and low rates with entecavir and tenofovir. Because of their low resistance rates, entecavir and tenofovir are the preferred oral drugs of choice for the treatment of hepatitis B.

Hepatitis B immune globulin should be given to household and sexual contacts of patients with acute hepatitis B. Infants should receive hepatitis B vaccine. The marker of immunity is hepatitis B surface antibody (anti-HBs). Neonates often acquire hepatitis B perinatally if the mother is infected. Because infected neonates are at high risk of chronic infection, all pregnant women should be tested for HBsAg. If a pregnant woman is HBsAg-positive, the infant should receive both hepatitis B immunoglobulin and hepatitis B vaccine. This strategy may not be effective when HBV DNA is high in the mother, and some have advised administration of lamivudine or tenofovir during the third trimester in women who have an HBV DNA level of more than 10^7 U/mL.

Table 13.5 **AGENTS FOR TREATMENT OF HEPATITIS B VIRUS**

FEATURE	PEGINTERFERON	LAMIVUDINE	ADEFOVIR	ENTECAVIR	TELBIVUDINE	TENOFOVIR
Treatment duration	12 mo	Indefinite	Indefinite	Indefinite	Indefinite	Indefinite
Side effects	Many	Minimal	Rarely renal	Minimal	Minimal	Minimal
Monthly charge, $	1,700	385	1,013	932	816	771
Disease flare	Common	Rare	Rare	Rare	Rare	Rare
HBeAg seroconversion, %	27	20	12	21	22	20
Resistance	None	12%–15% yearly	1%–4% yearly	1%–2% yearly	22% at 2 y	None

Abbreviation: HBeAg, hepatitis B e antigen.

Patients who are HBsAg-positive and are receiving immunosuppressive therapy should also receive hepatitis B treatment, even if they do not meet the other recommendations for therapy. Treatment of those patients decreases the risk of hepatitis B flares that can be precipitated by immune suppression.

Hepatitis D

Hepatitis D virus (HDV), or delta agent, is a small RNA particle that requires the presence of HBsAg to cause infection. HDV infection can occur simultaneously with acute HBV infection (coinfection) or HDV may infect a patient with chronic hepatitis B (superinfection). Infection with HDV should be considered only for patients with HBsAg; it is diagnosed by anti-HDV seroconversion.

- HDV requires the presence of HBsAg to cause infection.

- HDV infection is diagnosed by anti-HDV seroconversion.

Hepatitis C

Hepatitis C virus (HCV), an RNA virus, is the most common chronic blood-borne infection in the United States. HCV has a role in 40% of all cases of chronic liver disease, and HCV infection is the most common indication for liver transplant. The most common risk factor is illicit drug use. Persons with a history of transfusion of blood products before 1990 (when routine testing of blood products for HCV was introduced) are also at considerable risk of infection with HCV. Sexual transmission of HCV occurs but seems to be inefficient. The risk of transmission of HCV to health care workers by percutaneous (needlestick) exposure is also low—approximately 2% for a needlestick exposure to an infected patient.

Antibodies to HCV (anti-HCV) indicate exposure to the virus and are not protective. The presence of anti-HCV can indicate either a current infection or a previous infection with subsequent clearance. The presence of anti-HCV in a patient with an abnormal ALT level and risk factors for hepatitis C acquisition is strongly suggestive of current HCV infection. The initial test used for anti-HCV determination is enzyme-linked immunosorbent assay (ELISA). Although this test is very sensitive (few false-negative results), false-positives occur. If the result for anti-HCV by ELISA is negative, the patient is unlikely to have hepatitis C. The specificity of ELISA is improved with the addition of the recombinant immunoblot assay (RIBA) for anti-HCV. A guide to the interpretation of anti-HCV test results is given in Table 13.6.

HCV infection is diagnosed by determining the presence of HCV RNA, which is sensitive and specific for the diagnosis of hepatitis C. Levels of HCV RNA do not correlate with disease severity and are mainly used to stratify the response to therapy. Similarly, hepatitis C genotypes do not affect disease severity but do affect treatment response.

- HCV is a parenterally transmitted virus and a common cause of chronic hepatitis.

Table 13.6 **INTERPRETATION OF ANTI-HCV RESULTS**

ANTI-HCV BY ELISA	ANTI-HCV BY RIBA	INTERPRETATION
Positive	Negative	False-positive ELISA; patient does not have true antibody
Positive	Positive	Patient has antibody[a]
Positive	Indeterminate	Uncertain antibody status

Abbreviations: ELISA, enzyme-linked immunosorbent assay; anti-HCV, antibodies to hepatitis C virus; RIBA, recombinant immunoblot assay.

[a] Anti-HCV does not necessarily indicate current hepatitis C infection (see text).

- Common modes of transmission are illicit drug use and transfusion of blood products before 1990.

- The presence of HCV RNA is used to diagnose HCV infection.

Patients with HCV infection rarely present with acute hepatitis. The natural history of hepatitis C is summarized in Figure 13.6. In about 60% to 85% of persons who acquire hepatitis C, a chronic infection develops; after chronic infection is established, subsequent spontaneous loss of the virus is rare. Consequently, most patients with hepatitis C present with chronic hepatitis with mild to moderate increases in ALT levels. Some patients have fatigue or vague right upper quadrant pain. Patients may also receive medical attention because of complications of end-stage liver disease or, rarely, extrahepatic complications such as cryoglobulinemia or porphyria cutanea tarda. Up to 30% of patients chronically infected with HCV have a persistently normal ALT level. Because the majority of patients with hepatitis C are asymptomatic, treatment is generally aimed at preventing future complications of the disease. Patients with cirrhosis due to HCV generally have had HCV infection for more than 20 years.

Most patients in the United States are infected with hepatitis C genotype 1. Combination therapy with peginterferon alfa, ribavirin, and either telaprevir or boceprevir is the current standard of care for patients with hepatitis C genotype 1 who are deemed candidates for treatment. This combination, given for 6 to 12 months (duration of treatment depends on histologic stage and rapidity of response), results in sustained clearance of HCV RNA from the serum in 70% of patients. Patients with genotype 2 or 3 who are treated with peginterferon and ribavirin have an 80% to 90% chance of having a sustained response to therapy. Pretreatment liver biopsy may be used to assess histologic stage but is not mandatory. Treatment is expensive and carries a risk of significant side effects; therefore, the decision to treat is individualized for each patient. Contraindications for hepatitis C therapy are decompensated cirrhosis, advanced age, major comorbid illnesses, severe autoimmune disease, severe psychiatric disease, and uncontrolled substance abuse. Patients who are not candidates for treatment should be evaluated annually with routine liver tests.

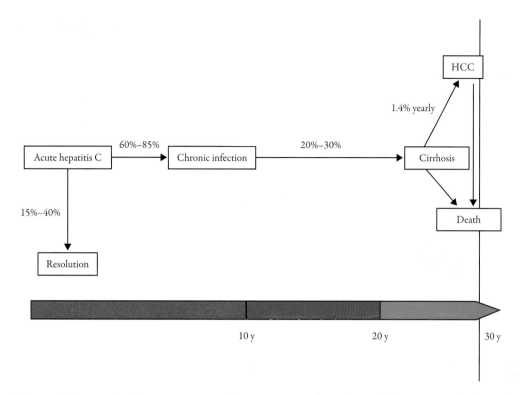

Figure 13.6 Natural History of Hepatitis C. Values are percentages of patients. HCC indicates hepatocellular carcinoma. (Adapted from Poterucha JJ. Chronic viral hepatitis. In: Hauser SC, editor. Mayo Clinic gastroenterology and hepatology board review. 4th ed. Rochester [MN]: Mayo Clinic Scientific Press and New York [NY]: Oxford University Press; c2011. p. 269–79. Used with permission of Mayo Foundation for Medical Education and Research.)

The risk of hepatocellular carcinoma complicating hepatitis C with cirrhosis is 1% to 4% per year. Surveillance with liver imaging every 6 to 12 months is advised for patients who are potential candidates for treatment with liver transplant, percutaneous ablation, transarterial chemoembolization, or radioembolization. Patients with HCV infection and decompensated cirrhosis should be considered for liver transplant.

- Symptomatic, clinically recognized acute hepatitis C is unusual.

- Of the patients who acquire HCV, 60%–85% remain chronically infected.

- Treatment of hepatitis C results in sustained clearance of HCV RNA in approximately 70%–90% of patients; response rates are highest in those infected with genotype 2 or 3.

- Patients with cirrhosis due to hepatitis C are at increased risk of hepatocellular carcinoma, particularly if they have a history of alcohol excess.

Hepatitis E

Hepatitis E virus is an enterically transmitted RNA virus that causes acute hepatitis primarily in patients who have lived or traveled in areas where the virus is endemic (India, Pakistan, Mexico, and Southeast Asia); however, hepatitis E is increasingly reported in patients who have not visited these areas. Clinically, hepatitis E resembles hepatitis A.

Other Viral Causes of Hepatitis

Epstein-Barr virus, cytomegalovirus, and herpesvirus may all cause hepatitis as part of a clinical syndrome. Infections with these agents are most serious in immunocompromised patients. Immunocompetent patients with infectious mononucleosis syndromes commonly have abnormal liver test results and mild increases in bilirubin levels, although clinically recognized jaundice is unusual. Herpes hepatitis generally occurs in immunosuppressed or pregnant patients and is characterized by fever, mental status changes, absence of jaundice, and AST and ALT levels greater than 5,000 U/L.

AUTOIMMUNE HEPATITIS

Autoimmune hepatitis was previously called autoimmune chronic active hepatitis because the diagnosis required 3 to 6 months of abnormal liver enzyme test results. However, 40% of patients with autoimmune hepatitis present with a clinical acute hepatitis. Autoimmune hepatitis can affect patients of any age, predominantly females. By definition, patients with autoimmune hepatitis should not have a history of drug-related hepatitis, HBV, HCV, or Wilson disease. Immunoserologic markers, such as antinuclear antibody (ANA), smooth muscle antibody, soluble liver antigen antibodies, or antibodies to liver-kidney microsomal

(LKM) antigens, are usually detected. Patients with autoimmune hepatitis may have other autoimmune diseases, including Hashimoto thyroiditis. Aminotransferase levels are generally 4 to 20 times the reference value, and most patients have an increased level of gamma globulin. Corticosteroids (30–60 mg daily) produce improvement in most patients, and the improvement in liver test results and gamma globulin levels is often dramatic. Azathioprine is often used to allow the use of lower doses of prednisone. Immunosuppressive doses should be decreased to control symptoms and to maintain the serum level of aminotransferases less than 5 times the reference value. Even after an excellent response to corticosteroids, relapse often occurs and the control of autoimmune hepatitis usually requires maintenance therapy.

- Autoimmune hepatitis is a chronic condition, but patients may present with acute hepatitis.

- Drug-related hepatitis, HBV, HCV, and Wilson disease should be excluded before making a diagnosis of autoimmune hepatitis.

- Immunoserologic markers are usually detected.

- Most patients have improvement with corticosteroid therapy, and the improvement in liver test results and gamma globulin levels is often dramatic.

- The control of autoimmune hepatitis usually requires maintenance therapy.

ALCOHOLIC LIVER DISEASE

Alcoholic Hepatitis

Long-term, excessive use of alcohol (>20 g daily for women and >40 g daily for men) can produce advanced liver disease. Alcoholic hepatitis is characterized histologically by fatty change, degeneration and necrosis of hepatocytes (with or without Mallory bodies), and an inflammatory infiltrate of neutrophils. Almost all patients have fibrosis, and they may have cirrhosis. Clinically, patients with alcoholic hepatitis may be asymptomatic or icteric and critically ill. Common symptoms include anorexia, nausea, vomiting, abdominal pain, and weight loss. The most common sign is hepatomegaly, which may be accompanied by ascites, jaundice, fever, splenomegaly, and encephalopathy. The level of AST is increased in 80% to 90% of patients, but it is almost always less than 400 U/L. The AST:ALT ratio is frequently greater than 2. Leukocytosis is commonly present, particularly in severely ill patients. Although the constellation of symptoms may mimic biliary disease, the clinical features are characteristic in an alcoholic patient. Because cholecystectomy carries a high morbidity among patients with alcoholic hepatitis, the clinical distinction is important.

- Alcoholic hepatitis is characterized by fatty change, degeneration and necrosis of hepatocytes (with or without Mallory bodies), and an inflammatory infiltrate of neutrophils.

- Common symptoms include anorexia, nausea, vomiting, abdominal pain, and weight loss.

- Common signs are hepatomegaly, ascites, jaundice, fever, splenomegaly, and encephalopathy.

- The level of AST is almost always <400 U/L in patients with alcoholic hepatitis.

- The AST:ALT ratio is frequently >2.

- Leukocytosis occurs in severely ill patients.

Poor prognostic markers of alcoholic hepatitis include encephalopathy, spider angiomata, ascites, renal failure, prolonged PT, and a bilirubin concentration greater than 20 mg/dL. Many patients have disease progression, particularly if alcohol intake is not curtailed. Corticosteroid therapy may be beneficial as an acute treatment of alcoholic hepatitis in patients with severe disease characterized by encephalopathy and a markedly prolonged PT. Pentoxifylline is a safe agent that has shown benefit in a single randomized controlled study. A *discriminant function* (DF) greater than 32 helps to identify patients with a poor prognosis:

$$DF = 4.6(PT_{patient} - PT_{control}) + bilirubin\ (mg/dL).$$

- Poor prognostic markers of alcoholic hepatitis: encephalopathy, ascites, renal failure, prolonged PT, and bilirubin >20 mg/dL.

- Corticosteroid therapy may be beneficial in severe disease.

Alcoholic Cirrhosis

Cirrhosis is defined histologically by septal fibrosis with nodular parenchymal regeneration. Only 60% of patients with alcoholic cirrhosis have signs or symptoms of liver disease, and most patients with alcoholic cirrhosis lack a clinical history of alcoholic hepatitis. Liver enzyme levels may be relatively normal in cirrhosis without alcoholic hepatitis. The prognosis of alcoholic cirrhosis depends on whether patients continue to consume alcohol and whether there are signs (jaundice, ascites, or gastrointestinal tract bleeding) of chronic liver disease. For patients who do not have ascites, jaundice, or variceal bleeding and who abstain from alcohol, the 5-year survival rate is 89%; for patients who have any of those complications and continue to consume alcohol, it is 34%. Liver transplant is an option for patients with end-stage alcoholic liver disease if they demonstrate that they can maintain abstinence from alcohol. The outcome of liver transplant for alcoholic liver disease is similar to that of transplant for other indications.

- Only 60% of patients with alcoholic cirrhosis have signs or symptoms of liver disease.

- Liver enzyme levels may be relatively normal.

- The 5-year survival for patients with alcoholic cirrhosis who abstain from alcohol is 89%.

- The 5-year survival for those who have signs and continue to consume alcohol is 34%.

- Liver transplant is an option for patients who can demonstrate a pattern of abstinence from alcohol.

NONALCOHOLIC FATTY LIVER DISEASE

Nonalcoholic fatty liver disease (NAFLD) is a common cause of abnormal levels of liver enzymes. A subset of NAFLD is nonalcoholic steatohepatitis (NASH), which is characterized histologically by fatty change and inflammation. Characteristically, patients with NAFLD have at least 1 of the following risk factors: obesity, hyperlipidemia, and diabetes. The aminotransferase levels are mildly abnormal, and the alkaline phosphatase level is increased in about one-third of patients. When advanced cirrhosis develops, fat may not be recognizable in liver tissue, and NASH most likely accounts for some cases of "cryptogenic" cirrhosis. The pathogenesis of NAFLD is unknown, and the effect of weight loss and control of hyperlipidemia and hyperglycemia is variable. In 10% of patients, NAFLD progresses to cirrhosis. The risk factors for more advanced disease are advanced age, marked obesity, and diabetes mellitus. Other than to control risk factors, there is no approved therapy for NAFLD. In patients with fat in the liver, it is important to rule out other diseases that result in steatosis, including hepatitis C, celiac disease, Wilson disease, and alcoholic liver disease.

Aggressive treatment of obesity, hyperlipidemia, and diabetes is indicated in patients with NAFLD. The weight loss that occurs after bariatric surgery improves the histologic features of NAFLD. Vitamin E has been shown to improve liver test results and histologic features in patients with NAFLD. Use of agents such as pioglitazone and rosiglitazone has resulted in biochemical and histologic improvement but also in weight gain. For treatment of hyperlipidemia, the statin drugs are safe in patients with NAFLD. For patients with NAFLD who are given potentially hepatotoxic medications, liver enzymes should be monitored regularly and use of the medications can continue as long as liver enzyme levels are less than 5-fold the reference value and liver function is preserved.

- There is no approved therapy for NAFLD other than risk factor control.

CHRONIC CHOLESTATIC LIVER DISEASES

Primary Biliary Cirrhosis

Primary biliary cirrhosis (PBC) is a chronic, progressive, cholestatic liver disease that primarily affects middle-aged women. Its cause is unknown but appears to involve an immunologic disturbance resulting in small bile duct destruction. In many patients, the disease is identified by an asymptomatic increase in alkaline phosphatase. Common early symptoms are pruritus and fatigue. Patients may have Hashimoto thyroiditis or sicca complex. Biochemical features include increased levels of alkaline phosphatase and IgM. When PBC is advanced, the concentration of bilirubin is high, the serum level of albumin is low, and PT is prolonged. Steatorrhea may occur because of progressive cholestasis. Fat-soluble vitamin deficiencies and metabolic bone disease are common.

Antimitochondrial antibodies are present in 90% to 95% of patients with PBC. The classic histologic lesion is granulomatous infiltration of septal bile ducts. Ursodiol treatment benefits patients who have this disease by improving survival and delaying the need for liver transplant. Cholestyramine and rifampin may be beneficial in the management of pruritus.

- PBC primarily affects middle-aged women.

- Common early symptoms: pruritus and fatigue.

- Alkaline phosphatase and IgM levels increase.

- Fat-soluble vitamin deficiencies and metabolic bone disease are common.

- Antimitochrondrial antibodies are present in 90%–95% of patients.

- Classic histologic lesion: granulomatous infiltration of septal bile ducts.

- Treatment: ursodiol.

Primary Sclerosing Cholangitis

Primary sclerosing cholangitis (PSC) is a chronic cholestatic liver disease characterized by obliterative inflammatory fibrosis of extrahepatic and intrahepatic bile ducts. An immune mechanism has been implicated. Patients may have an asymptomatic increase in the alkaline phosphatase level or progressive fatigue, pruritus, and jaundice. Bacterial cholangitis may occur in patients with dominant strictures or in whom instrumentation has been performed. Cholangiography, with either endoscopic retrograde cholangiopancreatography (ERCP) or magnetic resonance cholangiopancreatography (MRCP), establishes the diagnosis of PSC, showing short strictures of bile ducts with intervening segments of normal or slightly dilated ducts. This cholangiographic appearance may be mimicked by human immunodeficiency virus (HIV)-associated cholangiopathy (due to cytomegalovirus or *Cryptosporidium*), ischemic cholangiopathy after intra-arterial infusion of fluorodeoxyuridine, and IgG4-associated cholangitis.

- PSC: obliterative inflammatory fibrosis of extrahepatic and intrahepatic bile ducts.

- Asymptomatic increase in the alkaline phosphatase level.

- Cholangiography establishes the diagnosis.

- HIV-associated cholangiopathy mimics the cholangiographic appearance of PSC.

Seventy percent of patients with PSC have ulcerative colitis (UC), which may antedate, accompany, or even follow the diagnosis of PSC. Treatment of UC has no effect on the development or clinical course of PSC. Patients with PSC are at higher risk of cholangiocarcinoma; its development may be manifested by rapid clinical deterioration, jaundice, weight loss, and abdominal pain. There is no effective medical therapy for PSC. Treatment of PSC is generally supportive, and many patients have progressive liver disease and require liver transplant. Endoscopic balloon dilatation of bile duct strictures may offer palliation, especially in patients with recurrent cholangitis.

- UC occurs in 70% of patients with PSC.

- Treatment of UC has no effect on the development or clinical course of PSC.

- Patients with PSC are at higher risk of cholangiocarcinoma.

HEREDITARY LIVER DISEASES

Genetic Hemochromatosis

Genetic hemochromatosis is an autosomal recessively transmitted disorder characterized by iron overload. The physiologic defect appears to be an inappropriately high absorption of iron from the gastrointestinal tract. The *HFE* gene for genetic hemochromatosis has been identified. In the general population, the heterozygote frequency is 10%. Only homozygotes manifest progressive iron accumulation.

- Genetic hemochromatosis is a disorder of iron metabolism.

- Transmission is autosomal recessive.

- Only homozygotes have progressive iron accumulation.

Patients often present with end-stage disease, although an increased sensitivity to screening is aiding in earlier diagnosis. The peak incidence of clinical presentation is between the ages of 40 and 60 years. Iron overload is manifested more often and earlier in men than in women because women are protected by the iron losses of menstruation and pregnancy. Although hemochromatosis is now usually diagnosed from screening iron test results, clinical features include arthropathy, hepatomegaly, skin pigmentation, diabetes mellitus, cardiac dysfunction, and hypogonadism. Hemochromatosis should be considered in patients presenting with symptoms or diseases such as arthritis, diabetes, cardiac arrhythmias, or sexual dysfunction. Routine liver biochemistry studies generally show few abnormalities, and complications of portal hypertension are unusual. Transferrin saturation greater than 50% is the earliest biochemical iron abnormality in hemochromatosis. High serum levels of ferritin indicate tissue iron overload in patients with hemochromatosis. Increased levels of iron and ferritin may occur in other liver diseases, particularly advanced cirrhosis of any cause. Testing for mutations in the *HFE* gene is the standard method for diagnosing hemochromatosis. Of

the patients with hemochromatosis, 80% to 90% are homozygous for C282Y. Heterozygotes for C282Y generally do not have the disease. Patients who are C282Y heterozygote and H63D heterozygote (compound heterozygosity) may have iron overload.

Liver biopsy in patients with abnormal iron tests is done only if patients are negative for C282Y or if there is a concern about cirrhosis. The knowledge of cirrhosis is important because of the increased risk of hepatocellular carcinoma. Generally, hepatic iron levels in hemochromatosis are greater than 10,000 μg/g dry weight. A diagnostic algorithm is shown in Figure 13.7.

- Iron overload is more common in men.

- Clinical features: arthropathy, hepatomegaly, skin pigmentation, diabetes mellitus, cardiac dysfunction, and hypogonadism.

- Iron saturation and serum levels of ferritin are high.

- Standard tests for making the diagnosis: genetic testing and liver biopsy with quantification of hepatic iron concentration.

Patients with hemochromatosis should be treated with phlebotomy if the ferritin level is high. Those with C282Y homozygosity and a normal ferritin level can be observed every 2 to 3 years without treatment. The standard for phlebotomy is to remove 500 mL weekly to achieve a ferritin level less than 50 μg/L or iron saturation less than 50%. A maintenance program of 4 to 8 phlebotomies annually is then required. When initiated in the precirrhotic stage, removal of iron can render the liver normal and may improve cardiac function and control of diabetes. Treatment does not reverse arthropathy or hypogonadism, nor does it eliminate the increased risk (30%) of hepatocellular carcinoma if cirrhosis has already developed. All first-degree relatives of patients should be evaluated for hemochromatosis.

- Hemochromatosis is treated with repeated phlebotomies.

- Treatment does not reverse arthropathy or hypogonadism or eliminate the increased risk of hepatocellular carcinoma.

- First-degree relatives should be tested for hemochromatosis.

Wilson Disease

Wilson disease is an autosomal recessive disorder characterized by increased amounts of copper in tissues. The basic defect involves an inability of the liver to prepare copper for biliary excretion. The liver is chiefly involved in children and adolescents, whereas neuropsychiatric manifestations are more prominent in older patients. The Kayser-Fleischer ring is a brownish pigmented ring at the periphery of the cornea. It is not invariably present and is seen more commonly in patients with neurologic manifestations. Hepatic

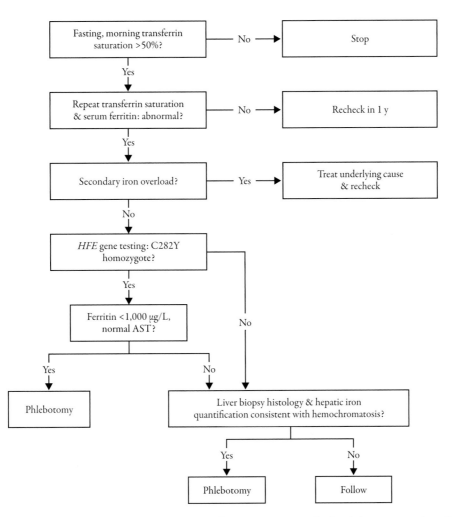

Figure 13.7 Diagnostic Algorithm for Genetic Hemochromatosis. Causes of secondary iron overload include anemias with ineffective erythropoiesis, multiple blood transfusions, and oral or parenteral iron supplementation. AST indicates aspartate aminotransferase. (Adapted from Brandhagen DJ, Fairbanks VF, Batts KP, Thibodeau SN. Update on hereditary hemochromatosis and the *HFE* gene. Mayo Clin Proc. 1999 Sep;74[9]:917–21. Used with permission of Mayo Foundation for Medical Education and Research.)

forms of Wilson disease include acute liver failure (often accompanied by hemolysis and renal failure), chronic hepatitis, steatohepatitis, and insidiously developing cirrhosis. The development of hepatocellular carcinoma is rare. Neurologic signs include tremor, rigidity, altered speech, and changes in personality. Fanconi syndrome and premature arthritis may occur.

- Wilson disease: an autosomal recessive disorder characterized by increased amounts of copper in tissues.

- Kayser-Fleischer ring is a brownish pigmented ring at the periphery of the cornea.

- Hepatocellular carcinoma is rare.

- Neurologic signs: tremor, rigidity, altered speech, and changes in personality.

Evidence of hemolysis (total bilirubin increased out of proportion to direct bilirubin), a low or normal level of alkaline phosphatase, and a low serum level of uric acid (due to uricosuria) suggest Wilson disease. The diagnosis is established on the basis of a low level of ceruloplasmin and an increased urinary or hepatic concentration of copper. Ceruloplasmin levels may be misleading—they may be increased by inflammation or biliary obstruction and decreased by liver failure of any cause. High concentrations of copper in the liver are found in Wilson disease, although similarly high values can also occur in cholestatic syndromes. Genetic testing for Wilson disease is developing but is currently most reliable for screening among first-degree relatives when a specific mutation in the proband has been identified. Standard treatments for Wilson disease are penicillamine, which chelates and increases the urinary excretion of copper, and trientine. Zinc inhibits absorption of copper by the gastrointestinal tract and can be used as adjunctive therapy. All siblings of patients should be evaluated for Wilson disease. Liver transplant corrects the metabolic defect of the disease.

- Diagnosis: low ceruloplasmin level and increased urinary or hepatic concentration of copper.

- Treatment: penicillamine or trientine; zinc.

- Liver transplant corrects the metabolic defect.

α_1-Antitrypsin Deficiency

α_1-Antitrypsin is synthesized in the liver. The gene is on chromosome 14. M is the common normal allele, and Z and S are abnormal alleles. Patients with the ZZ phenotype are at highest risk of liver disease. Inability to excrete the abnormally folded mutant protein results in intrahepatic accumulation of α_1-antitrypsin. Patients with α_1-antitrypsin deficiency may have a history of jaundice during the first 6 months of life. In later childhood or adulthood, cirrhosis may develop. Patients with α_1-antitrypsin–induced liver disease often lack clinically important lung disease, and infusions of α_1-antitrypsin do not protect against hepatic involvement. The prevalence of cirrhosis in patients with the MZ phenotype is likely increased, but the risk is small. Hepatocellular carcinoma may complicate α_1-antitrypsin deficiency when cirrhosis is present, especially in males. α_1-Antitrypsin deficiency is diagnosed by determining the α_1-antitrypsin phenotype or genotype. The serum levels of α_1-antitrypsin may vary and be unreliable. Liver transplant corrects the metabolic defect and changes the recipient's phenotype to that of the donor.

- Intrahepatic accumulation of α_1-antitrypsin causes liver disease.
- The diagnosis is made by determining the α_1-antitrypsin phenotype or genotype.
- Hepatocellular carcinoma can complicate α_1-antitrypsin deficiency, especially in males.
- Liver transplant corrects the metabolic defect.

ACUTE LIVER FAILURE

Acute liver failure is hepatic failure that includes encephalopathy developing less than 8 weeks after the onset of jaundice in patients with no history of liver disease. The common causes are listed in Box 13.1. Acute liver failure due to acetaminophen hepatotoxicity or hepatitis A carries a better prognosis than acute liver failure due to other causes. Poor prognostic markers include a drug-induced cause (other than acetaminophen), older age, grade 3 or 4 encephalopathy, acidosis, and INR greater than 3.5. Treatment is supportive, and patients should be transferred to a medical center where liver transplant is available.

- Acute liver failure is hepatic failure with encephalopathy developing <8 weeks after the onset of jaundice in patients with no history of liver disease.
- Poor prognostic markers include a drug-induced cause (other than acetaminophen), older age, grade 3 or 4 encephalopathy, and INR >3.5.

DRUG-INDUCED LIVER INJURY

Drugs cause toxic effects in the liver in different ways, often mimicking liver disease from other causes. With the notable exception of acetaminophen hepatotoxicity, most drug-induced liver disorders are idiosyncratic and not dose-related. Drug-induced liver injury accounts for 2% of the cases of jaundice in hospitalized patients and 50% of the cases of acute liver failure. Consequently, all drugs that have been used by a patient presenting with liver disease must be identified.

Acetaminophen toxicity is the most common cause of acute liver failure. Toxicity may occur at relatively low doses (eg, 3 g daily) in alcoholics because alcohol induces hepatic microsomal cytochrome P450 enzymes, which metabolize acetaminophen to its toxic metabolite. Acetaminophen hepatotoxicity is characterized by aminotransferase values greater than 5,000 U/L and often by renal failure. *N*-acetylcysteine should be given to any patient with acute liver failure in whom acetaminophen toxicity is suspected.

Valproic acid, tetracycline, and zidovudine may cause severe microvesicular steatosis associated with encephalopathy. Hepatotoxicity due to amiodarone may have histologic features that mimic those of alcoholic hepatitis or NAFLD. Antituberculous agents, including isoniazid, rifampin, and ethambutol, may cause acute hepatitis. Antibiotics are frequently associated with acute hepatitis. Amoxicillin-clavulanate is a relatively common cause of drug-induced liver injury and may result in prolonged cholestasis that can mimic large bile duct obstruction. Nitrofurantoin and minocycline can mimic autoimmune hepatitis. The chance of hepatotoxicity from lipid-lowering agents is extremely remote, even in patients with preexisting liver disease.

- Most drug-induced liver disorders are idiosyncratic, not dose-related.
- Drugs cause 2% of the cases of jaundice (in hospitalized patients) and 50% of the cases of acute liver failure.
- In alcoholics, acetaminophen toxicity may occur at lower doses than in nonalcoholics.

Box 13.1 **COMMON CAUSES OF ACUTE LIVER FAILURE**

Infective
  Hepatitis virus A, B, C (rare), D, and E
  Herpesvirus
Drug reactions and toxins
  Acetaminophen hepatotoxicity
  Idiosyncratic drug reaction
Vascular
  Ischemic hepatitis ("shock" liver)
  Acute Budd-Chiari syndrome
Metabolic
  Wilson disease
  Fatty liver of pregnancy
Miscellaneous
  Massive malignant infiltration
  Autoimmune hepatitis

- Antibiotics are a common cause of drug-induced liver injury.
- Amiodarone may cause hepatotoxicity that histologically mimics alcoholic hepatitis or NAFLD.
- Statins may cause mild liver test abnormalities but only rarely cause significant liver injury.

LIVER TUMORS

Hepatocellular Carcinoma

In the United States, 90% of hepatocellular carcinoma (HCC) cases occur in patients with cirrhosis. The level of α-fetoprotein is increased in only 50% of patients with HCC; however, a level of α-fetoprotein greater than 400 ng/mL in a cirrhotic patient with a liver mass is essentially diagnostic of HCC. A lesion that enhances on the hepatic arterial phase with "washout" on the portal venous phase on computed tomography (CT) or magnetic resonance imaging (MRI) in a patient with cirrhosis is very suggestive of HCC, and biopsy is often not necessary for diagnosis. Common metastatic sites are lymph nodes, lung, bone, and brain. Liver transplant is an option for patients with 3 or fewer lesions (largest <3 cm) or a single lesion smaller than 5 cm. Transplant is advised particularly for patients with cirrhosis who may not tolerate resection because of poor liver reserve. Transarterial chemoembolization, radioembolization, and percutaneous ablative techniques, such as alcohol injection or radiofrequency ablation, may be useful as primary or neo-adjuvant therapy.

- The α-fetoprotein level is increased in ≤50% of patients with HCC.
- Usually, imaging is characteristic and biopsy is not necessary for diagnosis.
- Common metastatic sites: lymph nodes, lung, bone, and brain.
- Treatment options: liver transplant, hepatic resection, transarterial chemoembolization, radioembolization, and percutaneous ablation.

Cholangiocarcinoma

The incidence of cholangiocarcinoma is increasing in the United States. Recognized risk factors are PSC, chronic biliary infection, and a history of choledochal cysts. Cholangiocarcinoma may be difficult to diagnose, especially in patients with PSC. For most patients, surgical resection is the treatment of choice, although resection is not possible in many patients. At some centers, liver transplant is considered in select patients with cholangiocarcinoma.

Adenoma

Adenomas are associated with the use of oral contraceptives or estrogen. Patients most commonly present with incidentally discovered liver mass lesions, although they can present with acute right upper quadrant pain and hemodynamic compromise because of bleeding. Avoidance of estrogens is advised for patients with hepatic adenomas.

Cavernous Hemangioma

Cavernous hemangioma is the most common benign tumor of the liver. CT or MRI with intravenous contrast is often diagnostic, demonstrating peripheral enhancement of the lesion. Cavernous hemangiomas generally require no treatment and are not estrogen dependent.

Focal Nodular Hyperplasia

Focal nodular hyperplasia (FNH) is a benign liver lesion that is probably a reaction to aberrant arterial flow to the liver. These lesions are typically discovered incidentally, although large lesions that stretch the liver capsule may cause abdominal pain. Diagnosis can usually be made with imaging; the characteristic findings are intense vascular enhancement on the hepatic arterial phase and a central scar. Bleeding from FNH is rare and malignant transformation does not occur; therefore, resection is not necessary. Similar to cavernous hemangioma, FNH is not estrogen dependent.

Metastases

Metastases are more common than primary tumors of the liver. Frequent primary sites are the colon, stomach, breast, lung, and pancreas. Surgical resection of isolated colon cancer metastases has a limited effect on long-term survival.

COMPLICATIONS OF END-STAGE LIVER DISEASE

Most of the complications of cirrhosis are due to the development of portal hypertension. The mechanism of portal hypertension is related to increases in both portal vein blood flow and intrahepatic resistance to flow. Increased flow is related to splanchnic vasodilatation. Increased resistance is related to sinusoidal narrowing from fibrous tissue and regenerative nodules as well as active vasoconstriction from alterations in production of endothelin and nitric oxide.

Ascites

The pathogenesis of ascites involves stimulation of the renin-angiotensin-aldosterone system, resulting in inappropriate renal sodium retention with expansion of plasma volume. Pleural effusion (hepatic hydrothorax) occurs in 6% of patients with cirrhosis and is right-sided in 67%. Edema usually follows ascites and is related to hypoalbuminemia and possibly to increased pressure on the inferior vena cava by the intra-abdominal fluid. The sudden onset of ascites should raise the possibility of hepatic venous outflow obstruction (Budd-Chiari syndrome).

Table 13.7 **USE OF THE SERUM-ASCITES ALBUMIN GRADIENT (SAAG) AND ASCITES PROTEIN TO DETERMINE THE CAUSE OF ASCITES**

SAAG, G/DL	ASCITES PROTEIN <2.5 G/DL	ASCITES PROTEIN ≥2.5 G/DL
≥1.1	Portal hypertension due to cirrhosis	Portal hypertension due to hepatic venous outflow obstruction (including right heart failure)
<1.1	Nephrotic syndrome	Malignancy, tuberculosis

Paracentesis is indicated at presentation to confirm the cause of ascites. Tests most useful for determining the cause of ascites are measurements of total protein and the serum-ascites albumin gradient (SAAG), which is calculated as

$$SAAG = [\text{serum albumin}] - [\text{ascitic fluid albumin}].$$

A SAAG of 1.1 g/dL or more indicates portal hypertension. Ascites due to portal hypertension induced by congestive heart failure can be distinguished from cirrhotic ascites because congestive heart failure (and other conditions associated with hepatic venous outflow obstruction such as Budd-Chiari syndrome) usually has an ascitic fluid protein level of 2.5 g/dL or more. Ascites from peritoneal carcinomatosis or tuberculosis generally has an ascitic fluid protein level of 2.5 g/dL or more and a SAAG of less than 1.1 g/dL (Table 13.7).

The treatment of ascites involves dietary sodium restriction and diuretics. Spironolactone (100–200 mg daily) and furosemide (20–40 mg daily) are usually used initially. The goal is to increase the concentration of urinary sodium and to allow the loss of 1 L of ascitic fluid (1 kg of body weight) per day. Paracentesis should be performed therapeutically in patients with tense ascites or with respiratory compromise from abdominal distention. Large-volume or even total paracentesis in combination with 6 to 8 g of albumin for each liter of ascitic fluid removed is safe and well tolerated. Refractory ascites is uncommon. Patients with cirrhotic ascites have a low concentration of urinary sodium (<10 mEq/mL on a random specimen) despite maximal diuretic therapy. Those who do not adhere to dietary sodium restriction excrete more than 80 mEq in 24 hours. For patients with refractory or resistant ascites, most physicians advocate therapeutic paracentesis as needed. A transjugular intrahepatic portosystemic shunt (TIPS) is effective in some patients with refractory ascites and is particularly useful for cirrhotic patients with pleural effusion as the main manifestation of fluid retention. Peritoneovenous shunts are complicated by disseminated intravascular coagulation and shunt malfunction and are rarely performed.

- The pathogenesis of ascites involves stimulation of the renin-angiotensin-aldosterone system, resulting in inappropriate renal sodium retention with expansion of plasma volume.

- Pleural effusion occurs in 6% of patients with cirrhosis and is right-sided in 67%.

- The sudden onset of ascites raises the possibility of hepatic venous outflow obstruction (Budd-Chiari syndrome).

- A SAAG ≥1.1 g/dL almost always indicates portal hypertension.

- Patients with cirrhotic ascites generally have a low concentration of urinary sodium.

- The mainstay of treatment is sodium restriction and diuretics; large-volume paracentesis is safe and well tolerated.

Spontaneous Bacterial Peritonitis

Spontaneous bacterial peritonitis (SBP) occurs in 10% to 20% of patients with cirrhosis who have ascites. SBP is a bacterial infection of ascitic fluid without an intra-abdominal source of infection. Fever, abdominal pain, and abdominal tenderness are classic symptoms; however, many patients have few or no symptoms. SBP should be considered in any patient with cirrhotic ascites, particularly if there has been clinical deterioration. For all patients presenting with ascites, diagnostic paracentesis is advisable as an initial step. Unless severe (INR >2.5 or platelets <10×10^9/mL), coagulopathy and thrombocytopenia are not contraindications for diagnostic paracentesis. A cell count and culture of ascitic fluid should be performed for all patients in whom SBP is being considered. Bedside inoculation of blood culture bottles with ascitic fluid increases the diagnostic yield of fluid cultures. SBP is more common in patients with large-volume ascites and in patients with a low ascitic fluid protein concentration (<1.0 g/dL). Also, blood from all patients with SBP should be cultured because almost 50% of these cultures are positive. Variants of SBP are listed in Table 13.8.

Table 13.8 **VARIANTS OF SPONTANEOUS BACTERIAL PERITONITIS**

CONDITION	ASCITIC FLUID Polymorpho-nuclear cells/mL	ASCITIC FLUID Culture Results	MANAGEMENT
Spontaneous bacterial peritonitis	>250	Positive	Antibiotics
Culture-negative neutrocytic ascites	>250	Negative	Antibiotics
Bacterascites	<250	Positive	Treat if symptoms of infection are present; otherwise, repeat paracentesis for cell count and cultures

SBP and culture-negative neutrocytic ascites should be treated, usually with a third-generation cephalosporin. Albumin should also be given (1.5 g/kg on day 1 and 1 g/kg on day 3). Polymicrobial infection of ascitic fluid should prompt a search for an intra-abdominal focus of infection; SBP nearly always involves only 1 organism. Patients with a prior episode of SBP are at high risk of recurrence, and daily prophylactic therapy (usually with norfloxacin) is recommended.

- SBP occurs in 10%–20% of patients with cirrhosis who have ascites.
- Classic symptoms: fever, abdominal pain, and abdominal tenderness.
- Many patients have few or no symptoms.
- Bedside inoculation of blood culture bottles with ascitic fluid increases the diagnostic yield.
- SBP is more common in patients with large-volume ascites and in patients with a low ascitic fluid protein concentration (<1.0 g/dL).
- Secondary prophylaxis is advised for patients with a previous episode of SBP.

Hepatorenal Syndrome

Hepatorenal syndrome is renal failure in the absence of underlying renal pathologic abnormalities in patients with portal hypertension. The differential diagnosis is given in Table 13.9. In cirrhotic patients presenting with renal insufficiency, hepatorenal syndrome is difficult to differentiate from prerenal azotemia; thus, a brief trial of volume expansion with albumin is indicated. Treatment is supportive, although vasoconstrictors such as midodrine or norepinephrine are used in patients with low blood pressure. After liver transplant, renal function usually improves, although this is confounded by the renal toxicity of the antirejection drugs tacrolimus and cyclosporine.

- Hepatorenal syndrome: renal failure with normal tubular function in a patient with portal hypertension.
- It is difficult to differentiate from prerenal azotemia.
- After liver transplant, renal function usually improves.

Portal Systemic Encephalopathy

Portal systemic encephalopathy is a reversible decrease in the level of consciousness of patients with severe liver disease. Disturbed consciousness, personality change, intellectual deterioration, and slowed speech are common manifestations. Patients often have asterixis (flapping tremor). The sudden development of portal systemic encephalopathy in patients with stable cirrhosis should prompt a search for bleeding, infection (especially SBP), or electrolyte disturbances; however, simple precipitating events are increased dietary protein, constipation, or sedatives. Serum and arterial levels of ammonia are usually increased but are not necessary for diagnosis. Lactulose decreases the nitrogenous compounds presented to the liver and is the first-line treatment for hepatic encephalopathy. Oral nonabsorbable antibiotics such as rifaximin or neomycin are given to patients who do not respond to or tolerate lactulose. Dietary protein restriction is advised only for patients with no response to medical therapy.

- Portal systemic encephalopathy: reversible decrease in the level of consciousness of patients with severe liver disease.
- Patients often have asterixis.
- If portal systemic encephalopathy develops suddenly, look for bleeding, infection, or electrolyte disturbances.
- Treatment: lactulose or nonabsorbable antibiotics.

Variceal Hemorrhage

Esophageal varices are collateral vessels that develop because of portal hypertension. Varices also can occur in other parts of the gut. Most patients with cirrhosis who have varices do not hemorrhage, but mortality among patients with a first hemorrhage is 10% to 20%. For patients who have cirrhosis but have not had bleeding, endoscopy to assess for the presence of varices is advised. Patients with moderate-sized or large varices, especially if there are red marks on the varices, should be treated with a nonselective β-blocker (nadolol or propranolol) to prevent bleeding. Endoscopic variceal ligation is an alternative to nonselective β-blockers. An algorithm for use of endoscopy to assess for esophageal varices is shown in Figure 13.8.

Table 13.9 **DIFFERENTIAL DIAGNOSIS FOR HEPATORENAL SYNDROME**

VARIABLE	PRERENAL AZOTEMIA	HEPATORENAL SYNDROME	ACUTE RENAL FAILURE
Urinary sodium concentration, mEq/L	<10	<10	>30
Urine to plasma creatinine ratio	>30:1	>30:1	<20:1
Urine osmolality	At least 100 mOsm > plasma osmolality	At least 100 mOsm > plasma osmolality	Equal to plasma osmolality
Urine sediment	Normal	Unremarkable	Casts, debris

Adapted from Arroyo V, Gines P, Guevara M, Rodes J. Renal dysfunction in cirrhosis: pathophysiology, clinical features and therapy. In: Boyer TD, Wright TL, Manns MP, Zakim D, editors. Zakim and Boyer's hepatology: a textbook of liver disease. 5th ed. Vol. 1. Philadelphia (PA): Saunders/Elsevier; c2006. p. 423–52. Used with permission.

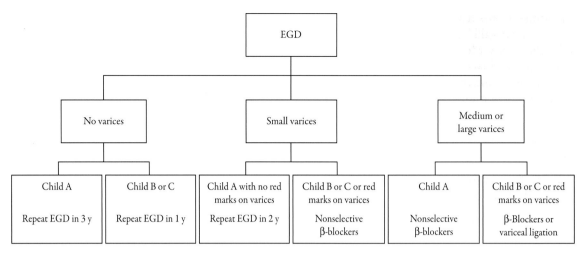

Figure 13.8 Prophylaxis of Esophageal Variceal Bleeding in Patients With Cirrhosis. Child indicates Child-Pugh class (A, B, or C, in order of increasing severity of cirrhosis); EGD, esophagogastroduodenoscopy.

Bleeding from esophageal varices is generally massive. For patients with acute bleeding, early endoscopy is indicated for diagnosis and treatment. Endoscopic therapy consists of band ligation or, less commonly, sclerotherapy. Octreotide decreases portal venous pressure and may also be given for acute variceal bleeding. All patients with cirrhosis who are hospitalized for gastrointestinal tract bleeding should receive prophylactic antibiotics.

- Bleeding from esophageal varices is generally massive.

- Esophageal varices are collateral vessels that result from portal hypertension.

- Most patients with cirrhosis who have varices do not hemorrhage.

- The first hemorrhage results in 10%–20% mortality.

- Early endoscopy is indicated for diagnosis and treatment.

Of patients who bleed from esophageal varices, 80% to 100% have recurrent bleeding within 2 years after the first episode; therefore, secondary prophylaxis is advised. Oral propranolol or nadolol may be used alone to prevent rebleeding in patients with preserved liver function, although most advocate serial endoscopic variceal ligation in combination with β-blockers until the varices have been obliterated. TIPS is effective in controlling refractory variceal bleeding. The incidence of portal systemic encephalopathy after TIPS is 10% to 40%, but this complication usually can be controlled with medical therapy. Patients bleeding from gastric varices are more likely to require TIPS than those bleeding from esophageal varices.

Patients with cirrhosis may also have gastrointestinal tract bleeding from portal hypertensive gastropathy. Bleeding from this lesion is usually gradual, and patients frequently present with iron deficiency anemia. Treatment is with nonselective β-blockers and administration of iron. Any patient with bleeding from varices or portal hypertensive gastropathy should be considered for liver transplant.

- Recurrent bleeding occurs in 80%–100% of patients.

- Patients with refractory bleeding are candidates for TIPS.

- The incidence of portal systemic encephalopathy after TIPS is 10%–40%.

BILIARY TRACT DISEASE

Gallstones and Cholecystitis

Gallstones can cause uncomplicated biliary pain, acute cholecystitis, common bile duct obstruction with cholangitis, and acute pancreatitis. Biliary pain is generally felt in the epigastrium or right upper quadrant and is usually severe and steady, lasting several hours. History is important; constant pain, food intolerance, and gaseousness are generally not features of biliary disease. Gallstones do not cause abnormal liver test results unless the common bile duct is obstructed or the patient has sepsis. Ultrasonography is 90% to 97% sensitive for detecting gallbladder stones. Cholecystitis may be suggested by gallbladder contraction, marked distention, surrounding fluid, or wall thickening. Ultrasonography also offers the opportunity to detect dilated bile ducts. If performed during an episode of pain, radionuclide biliary scanning is helpful in diagnosing cystic duct obstruction with cholecystitis. Positive test results are marked by nonvisualization of the gallbladder despite biliary excretion of radioisotope into the small intestine.

Asymptomatic patients with gallstones require no therapy, even in high-risk patients. Acalculous cholecystitis, probably precipitated by prolonged fasting and gallbladder ischemia, generally only occurs in patients hospitalized with critical illnesses. Clinical manifestations are fever and abdominal pain; liver test results may not be abnormal. Diagnosis is made with ultrasonography or radionuclide biliary scan. Patients with episodes of biliary colic or acute cholecystitis should have cholecystectomy. Patients with high surgical risk may undergo drainage with percutaneous cholecystostomy or an endoscopically placed nasocholecystic tube. Many patients without gallbladder stones have undergone cholecystectomy because of a decrease in gallbladder ejection fraction noted on radionuclide biliary scan. Most of these patients do not have resolution of pain, and therefore a decreased gallbladder ejection fraction should be interpreted with caution since often the patient's symptoms are unrelated to the finding.

- Ultrasonography is 90%–97% sensitive for detecting gallstones.
- Radionuclide biliary scanning helps diagnose cystic duct obstruction with cholecystitis.
- Asymptomatic patients with gallstones require no therapy.

Bile Duct Stones

Most bile duct stones originate in the gallbladder, although a few patients, such as those with preexisting biliary disease (eg, PSC), have primary duct stones. CT and ultrasonography are relatively insensitive for common bile duct stones, and diagnosis generally requires MRCP, ERCP, or endoscopic ultrasonography. ERCP also offers therapeutic potential for patients with bile duct stones and is the test of choice when clinical suspicion is high. Patients with bile duct stones can have minimal or no symptoms, or they can have life-threatening cholangitis with abdominal pain, fever, and jaundice. Common bile duct stones should be removed; in nearly all patients, this can be accomplished with ERCP. The urgency of the procedure depends on the clinical presentation. Patients with minimal symptoms can have elective ERCP, but those with cholangitis and fever unresponsive to antibiotics should have urgent endoscopic treatment. Patients with gallbladder stones who have a sphincterotomy and clearance of their duct stones have only a 10% chance of having additional problems with their gallbladder stones; thus, cholecystectomy can be avoided in patients who are at high risk of complications with surgery.

- Most bile duct stones originate in the gallbladder.
- Diagnosis of bile duct stones generally requires MRCP, ERCP, or endoscopic ultrasonography.
- Common bile duct stones should be removed.
- Urgent endoscopic treatment is needed if cholangitis and fever are unresponsive to antibiotics.

Malignant Biliary Obstruction

Malignant biliary obstruction is usually the result of carcinoma of the head of the pancreas, bile duct cancer, or metastatic malignancy to hilar nodes. If the disease is unresectable, palliative endoscopic stenting is as effective as surgical bypass. Patients with malignant biliary obstruction and impending duodenal obstruction are usually considered for palliative surgery, although endoscopic techniques can be attempted by expert endoscopists.

Gallbladder Carcinoma

Gallbladder carcinoma has a strong association with calcified gallbladder wall (porcelain gallbladder); therefore, prophylactic cholecystectomy is advised. Most patients with gallbladder carcinoma present at an advanced stage and have a poor prognosis.

SUMMARY

- Aminotransferases are markers of liver cell injury or hepatocellular disease.
- Hyperbilirubinemia is usually <20% conjugated bilirubin in diseases characterized by overproduction of bilirubin. Hyperbilirubinemia is usually >50% conjugated bilirubin with hepatocyte dysfunction or impaired bile flow.
- HAV is transmitted by ingestion of contaminated food or water or contact with an infected person. HBV is transmitted by exposure to blood or contaminated body fluids. HCV is a parenterally transmitted virus and a common cause of chronic hepatitis.
- Autoimmune hepatitis is a chronic condition, but patients may present with acute hepatitis. Drug-related hepatitis, HBV, HCV, and Wilson disease should be excluded before making a diagnosis of autoimmune hepatitis.
- Genetic hemochromatosis is a disorder of iron metabolism. Transmission is autosomal recessive.
- Wilson disease: an autosomal recessive disorder characterized by increased amounts of copper in tissues.
- Diagnosis of bile duct stones generally requires MRCP, ERCP, or endoscopic ultrasonography. Common bile duct stones should be removed.

PART III

PULMONARY DISEASES

14.

CRITICAL CARE MEDICINE

J. Christopher Farmer, MD

GOALS

- Understand how to identify and appropriately treat impending respiratory failure.

- Understand mechanical ventilation.

- Differentiate between types of shock.

- Summarize important concepts in the treatment of sepsis.

- Describe an approach to a patient in the intensive care unit (ICU) who has gastrointestinal tract (GI) hemorrhage.

INTRODUCTION

Critical care medicine is a multidisciplinary branch of medicine that focuses on intensive, broad-based support of patients who have life-threatening illnesses or a high risk of critical illness. The American Board of Internal Medicine does not include critical care medicine as a separate medical content area but rather includes this information as a cross-content area that comprises 10% of the total certification examination (14–18 questions) (http://www.abim.org/exam/certification/internal-medicine.aspx). Reflecting the examination's critical care content distribution, this chapter discusses, in rank order, the following critical care–specific content areas: 1) pulmonary (respiratory), 2) cardiology, 3) infectious diseases, 4) endocrinology, 5) gastroenterology, and 6) hematology. Refer to the content-specific chapters in this book for the other content areas, which are represented by 0 or 1 question on the examination.

RESPIRATORY CRITICAL CARE

AIRWAY MANAGEMENT

Compared with elective airway management in the operating room, emergent airway management in the ICU is associated with higher complication rates because of patient comorbidities, limited evaluation and planning time, and limited patient reserve. Internal medicine board examination questions typically focus on the following:

1. Recognition of impending respiratory failure and the patient's inability to properly maintain the airway

2. Assessment and recognition of the patient whose airway is difficult to maintain (including risk factors)

3. Various airway support techniques (use of oral airways, preoxygenation techniques, indications for intubation, etc)

Endotracheal intubation allows maximal control of the airway, enables delivery of specific inspired oxygen concentrations and positive pressure ventilation, and provides protection from aspiration. Indications for intubation include airway protection in cases of obstruction or loss of normal gag and cough reflexes, central nervous system injury or sedation with loss of normal control of ventilation, and any cause of respiratory failure requiring positive pressure–assisted ventilation. Complications of intubation include vomiting and aspiration, hypoxemia during the procedure, and inadvertent intubation of the esophagus.

Assessment and recognition of the risk factors for a patient with a potentially difficult airway—before attempting intubation—is imperative (Box 14.1). The widely used Mallampati classification (Figure 14.1) consists of classes I (easy intubation) to IV (difficult intubation):

1. Class I—entire tonsil is clearly visible

2. Class II—upper half of tonsil fossa is visible

3. Class III—soft palate and hard palate are clearly visible

4. Class IV—only hard palate is visible

Before intubation, the equipment, environment, and patient should be prepared. Proper preparation for unforeseen problems is of utmost importance (Box 14.2).

Pharmacotherapy to facilitate endotracheal intubation is generally not an expected knowledge area on the internal

PREDICTORS OF DIFFICULT MASK VENTILATION AND INTUBATION

Difficult mask ventilation
   Age >55 y
   BMI >26
   Edentulous
   Male
   Mallampati class IV
   Beard
   History of snoring
Difficult intubation
   Short thick neck
   Limited neck flexion or extension
   Thyromental distance <3 finger breadths
   Long upper incisors
   Presence of overbite
   Inability to jut mandibular incisors anterior to upper incisors
   Inability to open mouth >3 cm
   Mallampati class III or IV
   High arched palate

Abbreviation: BMI, body mass index (calculated as weight in kilograms divided by height in meters squared).

medicine certification examination. However, the risk of using a depolarizing muscle relaxant (eg, succinylcholine) in some patients can be substantial, and these risks should be known:

1. Risk of causing a precipitous, life-threatening hyperkalemia in patients with significant burn injuries, spinal cord injuries, demyelination syndromes, crush injuries, and renal failure

2. Risk of inducing a mechanical circumstance leading to an inability to intubate or ventilate (refractory upper airway obstruction)

- Recognition of impending respiratory failure is not always straightforward.

- Successful management is predicated on assessment of risk factors and proper preparation and planning.

- A backup method to direct laryngoscopy should be readily available.

- Use muscle relaxants with extreme caution.

RESPIRATORY FAILURE

Effective functioning of the respiratory system requires 1) normal central nervous system control, 2) intact neuromuscular transmission and bellows function, and 3) normal gas exchange at the alveolar-capillary level. Respiratory failure may result from physiologic impairment or disease at any of these levels. Respiratory failure is typically classified as hypoxemic or hypercapnic. Board examination questions typically focus on the following:

1. Ability to recognize impending respiratory failure: oxygenation, ventilation, and the work of breathing are no longer sustainable without mechanical intervention

2. Ability to discern the type of respiratory failure—hypoxemic or hypercapnic—and the specific type of support that is medically indicated.

3. Ability to calculate values for common physiologic perturbations that indicate the presence of respiratory failure, such as the alveolar-arterial (A-a) gradient

The determination of impending respiratory failure is based on clinical findings (arterial blood gas findings may be normal initially). Thus, it is important to assess the patient's breathing work (ie, effort), the presence or absence of worsening tachycardia and tachypnea, the presence or absence of altered

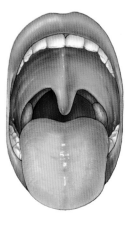

Class I

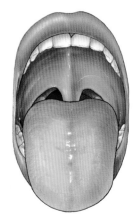

Class II

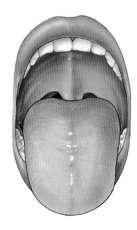

Class III

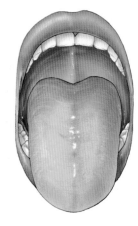

Class IV

Figure 14.1 Mallampati Classification. The Mallampati classification is based on the structures visualized with maximal mouth opening and tongue protrusion in the sitting position. (This test was originally described without phonation, but some have suggested that Mallampati Classification with or without phonation correlates with intubation difficulty: higher Mallampati scores are more likely to indicate greater intubation difficulty.)

sensorium not explained by other causes, and the amount of respiratory support needed to achieve an acceptable oxygen saturation as measured by pulse oximetry (SpO_2) (ie, the SpO_2 may still be >90%, but the patient's breathing effort and the required fraction of inspired oxygen [FIO_2] support may have significantly increased).

Hypoxemic Respiratory Failure

Hypoxemic respiratory failure is defined as severe or refractory hypoxemia that does not improve with the administration of supplemental oxygen and requires additional respiratory mechanical interventions. Effective gas exchange requires adequate alveolar ventilation for the elimination of carbon dioxide, oxygen uptake across the alveolar-capillary membrane, and the delivery of oxygen to tissues. Hypoxemia may result from the following:

1. Decrease in the inspired PO_2 (eg, at high altitude, including air travel, or with interruption of the oxygen supply)

2. Hypoventilation

3. Ventilation-perfusion ratio ($\dot{V}/\dot{Q}$) mismatch

4. Pulmonary shunt (diffusion barrier)

Hypoxemic respiratory failure proceeds along a continuum that begins with $\dot{V}/\dot{Q}$ mismatch and proceeds toward increased pulmonary shunt. For each step, calculation of the A-a gradient can be helpful when identifying and quantifying abnormal gas exchange. From arterial blood gas measurements, the A-a gradient is calculated as follows:

$$\text{A-a gradient} = [FIO_2 \times (P_{ATM} - P_{H_2O}) - (PaCO_2/0.8)] - PaO_2,$$

where sea level atmospheric pressure (P_{ATM}) = 760 torr and partial pressure of water vapor (P_{H_2O}) = 47 torr.

The A-a gradient = $PAO_2 - PaO_2$, where PAO_2 indicates partial pressure of oxygen in the alveoli. Normally, the A-a gradient is less than 10 torr in a young adult; it increases by 10 torr every decade thereafter.

Pulmonary shunt is defined as alveoli that are perfused but not ventilated. The absence of ventilation is caused by alveolar collapse (eg, atelectasis, loss of surfactant) or alveolar flooding (eg, alveolar capillary leak). Clinically, pulmonary shunt occurs when PaO_2 does not appropriately increase even with increased supplemental oxygen administration, as is common in patients with acute respiratory distress syndrome (ARDS) as discussed below.

Treatment of hypoxemic respiratory failure requires correction of hypoxia. For patients who have pulmonary shunting, this likely means the use of either invasive or noninvasive mechanical ventilation (discussed in the "Mechanical Ventilation" section). In addition to the use of mechanical ventilation, recognition and treatment of underlying causes, such as pneumonia and heart failure, is extremely important.

- The major causes of hypoxemia are low inspired PO_2, hypoventilation, $\dot{V}/\dot{Q}$ mismatch, and shunting.

Hypercapnic Respiratory Failure

Hypercarbic or hypercapnic respiratory failure is caused by inadequate alveolar ventilation that is generally the result of airway obstruction, increased pulmonary dead space, or failure of the respiratory "bellows" (eg, chest wall, diaphragm, or neural control). *Physiologic dead space* is the portion of a breath that does not participate in gas exchange (ie, in the hypopharynx, trachea, and conducting airways). The amount of dead space increases with several disease states, such as chronic lung disease (eg, chronic obstructive pulmonary disease [COPD] and asthma), ARDS, pulmonary embolism, pulmonary hypertension, and others.

Hypercapnia occurs when minute ventilation is not sufficient to compensate for the increased volume of lung dead space. As acute hypercapnia worsens, respiratory acidosis often follows, and the worsening of hypercapnic respiratory failure accelerates. This process is exacerbated in patients who have COPD and who also have abnormal diaphragmatic function and pathologically altered carbon dioxide central chemoreception.

The presence of an acute respiratory acidosis usually indicates impending or actual respiratory muscle fatigue. Therefore, unless the intrinsic work of breathing in real-time can be significantly decreased (eg, use of bronchodilators in patients with severe outflow obstruction), invasive or noninvasive mechanical ventilation support is typically required. If the respiratory musculature is fatigued and metabolic stores are depleted, a period of rest is required and the work of breathing must be relieved in some fashion.

- Major causes of hypercapnic respiratory failure include inadequate alveolar ventilation, increased pulmonary dead space, and failure of the respiratory "bellows."

Acute Respiratory Distress Syndrome

Board examination questions related to ARDS typically focus on 1) diagnosis of ARDS, 2) causes of ARDS, and 3) general principles of therapy. Board examinations must focus on "settled science," and there are many treatment areas related to ARDS that are still in flux and are therefore difficult to test.

Description

ARDS is diffuse lung injury that causes acute hypoxic respiratory failure. Acute lung injury (ALI) is a frequent primary cause of critical illness and may occur as a complication or as a coexisting feature of multisystem disease. ARDS is commonly defined as diffuse ALI with the following major features:

1. Diffuse (bilateral) pulmonary infiltrates—infiltration in 3 or 4 quadrants on the chest radiograph

2. Abnormal ratio of PaO_2 to FIO_2 (P/F ratio)—in ALI <300, and in ARDS <200

3. "Normal" volume status—pulmonary artery occlusion pressure <18 mm Hg, and lack of evidence of left atrial hypertension or volume overload (eg, on echocardiogram)

Several conditions are associated with ARDS (Table 14.1).

Mortality from ARDS has averaged about 50%. For the first 30 years after ARDS was described, no single therapy was shown to alter the outcome, although gradual improvement in overall mortality was attributed to multidisciplinary ICU management. Recently, in prospective controlled trials, a strategy of mechanical ventilation with reduced tidal volumes was associated with improved survival (discussed below).

Pathophysiology

The pathophysiology of ARDS is related to damage of alveolar-capillary units. Early changes include endothelial cell swelling and capillary leak, followed by interstitial edema and parenchymal inflammation. Mononuclear inflammation, loss of alveolar type I cells, and hyaline membrane formation typically develop within 2 or 3 days after an initial insult (eg, sepsis).

Fibrosis may subsequently develop within days to weeks after the initial insult that caused ARDS. Damage to type II alveolar cells leads to the loss of surfactant production. Ultimately, alveolar filling and alveolar collapse develop, and intrapulmonary shunting and $\dot{V}/\dot{Q}$ mismatch with hypoxemia are clinically apparent.

Treatment

Respiratory support for ARDS can be summarized as follows: *Excessive mechanical ventilation amplitude variation is bad.* After an initial insult, lung injury is exacerbated by high-pressure distention of alveoli and alveolar cycling (repeated opening and closing of alveolar sacs, leading to shear injury, also known as alveolar recruitment and derecruitment). Both processes (overdistention and alveolar cycling) further increase the proinflammatory cascade response in the lungs, which worsens the endothelial capillary leak and loss of surfactant and increases the rate of fibrosis. Treatment involves mechanical ventilation strategies (ie, lung-protective ventilatory strategies) that allow for lung healing. This concept is graphically depicted for an ARDS patient in Figure 14.2.

In 2000, a multicenter group of investigators affiliated with the ARDS Network showed improved survivorship among patients receiving a tidal volume of 6 mL/kg (based on ideal body weight) compared with a control group receiving a tidal volume of 12 mL/kg (based on ideal body weight). The smaller tidal volumes were used to maintain plateau airway

Table 14.1 **CONDITIONS ASSOCIATED WITH ACUTE RESPIRATORY DISTRESS SYNDROME (ARDS)[a]**

DISORDER OR TYPE OF DISORDER	CAUSE
Shock	Any cause
Sepsis	Lung infections, other bacteremic or endotoxic states
Trauma	Head injury, lung contusion, fat embolism
Aspiration	Gastric, near-drowning, tube feedings
Hematologic	*Transfusions,* leukoagglutinin, *disseminated intravascular coagulation,* thrombotic thrombocytopenic purpura
Metabolic	Pancreatitis, uremia
Drugs	Narcotics, barbiturates, aspirin
Toxic	Inhaled—oxygen, smoke Chemicals—paraquat Irritant gases—nitrogen dioxide, chlorine, sulfur dioxide, ammonia
Miscellaneous	Radiation, air embolism, altitude

[a] Italics indicate disorders and causes most commonly associated with ARDS.

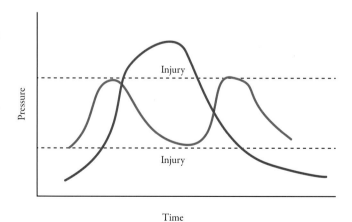

Figure 14.2 Lung-Protective Ventilatory Strategy for Patient With Acute Respiratory Distress Syndrome. Respiratory cycle tracing shows how mechanical ventilation (red line) keeps respiration out of the zones of injury (above the upper dashed line and below the lower dashed line). Blue line indicates respiration without mechanical ventilation.

pressures below 30 cm water. This is the only specific therapy for ARDS that has been shown to decrease mortality.

In patients treated with a lung-protective ventilatory strategy, the resulting level of alveolar ventilation may increase $PaCO_2$ (referred to as permissive hypercapnia) but does not appear to be harmful and may even decrease the degree of ventilator-induced lung injury. In other words, in patients who have ARDS or increased pulmonary dead space, the "pressure cost" required to achieve a normal PCO_2 often exceeds any benefit and may actually exacerbate ALI.

Finally, many clinicians use an open-lung ventilatory strategy, in which incremental positive end-expiratory pressure (PEEP) levels are used to maintain alveolar recruitment and to prevent alveolar cycling and derecruitment.

Patients with ARDS progress beyond simple $\dot{V}/\dot{Q}$ mismatch to pulmonary shunt. The clinical hallmark is that increasing the FIO_2 as a single maneuver does not improve oxygenation. PEEP is required to recruit alveoli; the goal is to improve oxygenation. A common board examination question asks what should be done next for a patient who has ARDS and inadequate oxygenation ($FIO_2 > 0.4–0.5$). PEEP is the first choice. In addition, patients with ARDS may have some alveoli (and lung segments) that are slow to open or recruit (the physiologic term is *prolonged alveolar time constant*). Besides providing PEEP for these patients, lengthening the duration of inspiration may be beneficial to allow for additional time for alveolar recruitment. How to improve alveolar recruitment is also a common ARDS subject area for board examination questions.

Because increased capillary permeability allows for larger volumes of intravascular fluid, a conservative fluid strategy to maintain adequate systemic perfusion is preferred and was recently validated in a large study. Supplemental nutrition (enteral feeding) is recommended throughout the course of critical illness if tolerated (both acute and chronic). Patient mobilization with ambulation and ventilator weaning are also initiated as early as possible for all patients with ARDS.

The role of corticosteroids in patients with ARDS remains controversial. Nitric oxide and other vasodilating agents in ARDS provide short-term improvement in oxygenation but no mortality benefit. Prone positioning has been used in an attempt to open flooded dependent alveoli and improve $\dot{V}/\dot{Q}$ matching and oxygenation; it has resulted in nonsustainable improvements in oxygenation with no effect on mortality and an increase in dislodgment and obstruction of endotracheal tubes.

- ARDS is defined as a P/F ratio <200 with bilateral pulmonary infiltrates and a normal volume status.

- A low–tidal volume strategy is the only ARDS treatment that has improved survival.

MECHANICAL VENTILATION

The goals of mechanical ventilation are 1) correct hypoxia, 2) support ventilation, 3) decrease the work of breathing, and 4) support lung injury healing. All modern forms of mechanical ventilation use positive pressure during inspiration. Inspiration is cycled to exhalation by either volume (ie, tidal volume delivery) or pressure (ie, pressure control).

Internal medicine board examination questions related to mechanical ventilation are basic and do not involve complex management decisions. As already mentioned, these examinations must focus on settled science, and there is much about mechanical ventilation that reflects individual and institutional preferences (eg, the use of synchronized intermittent mandatory ventilation [SIMV] or controlled mechanical ventilation [CMV]). Therefore, typical question content areas might include the following:

1. Recognition of complications caused by mechanical ventilation (eg, barotrauma or pneumothorax, auto-PEEP)

2. A plan for the next step (eg, if a patient with specified blood gas results is mechanically ventilated, what should be done next?)

3. Selection of noninvasive or invasive mechanical ventilation approaches for patients with specific conditions (eg, COPD, pneumonia, or ARDS)

4. Recognition of complications of mechanical ventilation (eg, barotrauma, high pressure ventilator alarm)

5. Indications for weaning a patient from mechanical ventilation

Mechanical ventilation is necessary for many patients who have loss of respiratory control, neuromuscular or respiratory pump failure, and severe disorders of gas exchange that do not respond to lesser levels of support. Patients who require mechanical ventilation usually meet the criteria for ventilator support listed in Table 14.2.

Table 14.2 **TYPICAL PHYSIOLOGIC CRITERIA FOR MECHANICAL VENTILATOR SUPPORT**

VARIABLE	VALUE
Respiratory rate, breaths/min	>25–30
Minute ventilation, L/min	>10–15
Maximal inspiratory pressure (force), cm water	<20
Vital capacity, mL/kg	<10
PaO_2, mm Hg	<60 when FIO_2 >0.60
PaO_2/FIO_2	<200
$PAO_2 – PaO_2$, mm Hg	>300 with FIO_2 =1.00
VD/VT	>0.60
pH	<7.20 (with a predominant respiratory component)

Abbreviations: FIO_2, fraction of inspired oxygen; $PAO_2 – PaO_2$, alveolar-arterial gradient in partial pressure of oxygen; VD, dead space volume; VT, tidal volume.

Modes of Mechanical Ventilation

Modes of mechanical ventilation refers to how a positive-pressure machine breath is delivered and its relation to the spontaneous breaths of the patient (eg, assist/control mode, intermittent mandatory ventilation [IMV], and pressure support ventilation). Table 14.3 outlines basic ventilator modes and basic initial invasive mechanical ventilation settings for a patient with respiratory failure.

Volume Preset Assist/Control Mode Ventilation

In this mode, a machine-assisted breath is delivered for every inspiratory effort by the patient. If no spontaneous breaths occur during a preset time interval, a controlled breath of predetermined volume is delivered by the ventilator. The backup rate determines the minimum minute ventilation the patient will receive.

The advantage of assist/control mode ventilation is that it allows maximal rest for the patient and maximal control of ventilation. The disadvantage is that hyperventilation or air trapping (or both) can occur in patients making rapid inspiratory efforts.

Pressure Support Ventilation

Pressure support ventilation may be used to assist spontaneously breathing patients, with or without IMV breaths. For each inspiratory effort by the patient, the ventilator delivers a high rate of flow of inspired gas, up to a preset pressure limit. This pressure support occurs only during the spontaneous inspiratory effort, so that the rate and pattern of respiration are determined by the patient.

Volume Preset IMV

Volume preset IMV allows a preset number of machine-assisted breaths of a given tidal volume. Between machine breaths, patients may breathe spontaneously. The IMV mode was developed as a weaning mode so that the number of mechanical breaths could be decreased gradually, allowing for increasing spontaneous ventilation. However, recent trials have shown that this mode of weaning is inferior to weaning with T-piece trials or pressure support ventilation.

Positive End-Expiratory Pressure

PEEP is intended to increase functional residual capacity, recruit partially collapsed alveoli, improve lung compliance, and improve $\dot{V}/\dot{Q}$ matching. It decreases atelectrauma (recruitment and derecruitment of alveoli). An adverse effect of PEEP is an excessive increase in intrathoracic pressure with decreased cardiac output. Overdistention of lung units may also worsen gas exchange because of ventilator-induced lung injury. At levels of PEEP greater than 10 to 15 cm water, barotrauma is of concern. The optimal PEEP may be defined as the lowest level of PEEP needed to achieve satisfactory oxygen delivery at a nontoxic FIO_2 (<0.60).

Complications of Mechanical Ventilation

Ventilator-Associated Pneumonia

Ventilator-associated pneumonia (VAP) is a serious preventable complication of mechanical ventilation. Mortality due to VAP can be decreased by prevention with use of a VAP bundle, as recommended by the Institute for Healthcare Improvement (IHI). The IHI Ventilator Bundle includes the following:

1. Elevation of the head of the bed

2. Daily sedation vacations and assessment of readiness to extubate

3. Peptic ulcer disease prophylaxis

4. Deep vein thrombosis prophylaxis

5. Daily oral care with chlorhexidine

- Implementing the IHI Ventilator Bundle can prevent VAP.

Intrinsic PEEP

Intrinsic PEEP, or *auto-PEEP*, is an important complication of positive pressure ventilation. Inadequate time during the expiratory phase of the respiratory cycle results in a new machine breath being delivered before the previous breath is completely exhaled. This may worsen hyperinflation, increase intrathoracic pressure, reduce venous return, and worsen associated complications (eg, barotrauma). Intrinsic PEEP may occur in spontaneously breathing patients with obstructive airway disease, but the effect is most important in mechanically ventilated patients. Treatment typically involves optimizing bronchodilator therapy and altering the ventilator cycle to allow maximal expiratory time.

- Auto-PEEP can be treated by allowing maximal expiratory time and by optimizing bronchodilator therapy.

Oxygen Toxicity

Pulmonary oxygen toxicity appears to be the result of direct exposure to high tensions of inspired oxygen or alveolar oxygen. For adults, oxygen toxicity is not believed to be of clinical concern if the FIO_2 is less than 0.40 to 0.50. Higher levels of inspired oxygen may be associated with acute tracheobronchitis (most likely an irritant effect). After several days of exposure, a syndrome of diffuse alveolar damage and lung injury may develop with pathologic features resembling those of ARDS.

- Oxygen toxicity is of concern with FIO_2 levels greater than 0.50.

Tracheostomy

Prolonged invasive mechanical ventilation increases the risk of tracheal injury and stenosis, bleeding, tracheoesophageal fistula, and, possibly, increased bronchial or pulmonary infections. For patients who require prolonged mechanical ventilation or airway support, the timing of tracheostomy is controversial. ARDS patients who receive a tracheostomy early in their clinical course have demonstrably improved

Table 14.3 BASIC VENTILATOR MODES AND SETTINGS

MODE	DESCRIPTION OR MECHANISM
Volume Control Modes	
A/C, also called CMV	• Active inhalation V_T is delivered up to a volume threshold & not a pressure threshold • Exhalation is passive; after the V_T is delivered, the machine releases & exhalation is driven by chest wall & lung elastance (recoil) • Patient initiates the respiratory cycle (unless apneic or paralyzed) • Machine senses inspiratory effort & then delivers machine-defined V_T for every breath • Does not allow patient to breathe spontaneously (ie, patient-defined V_T) • Machine rate (eg, CMV = 8/min) defines the minimum number of V_T breaths a patient will receive per minute • A patient who initiates more breaths per minute than the defined rate will receive those breaths at the machine-defined V_T
SIMV	• Active inhalation V_T is delivered up to a volume threshold & not a pressure threshold • Exhalation is passive; after the V_T is delivered, the machine releases & exhalation is driven by chest wall & lung elastance (recoil) • Patient initiates the respiratory cycle (unless apneic or paralyzed) • Machine senses inspiratory effort & then delivers machine-defined V_T for only the rate of machine breaths • Machine rate (eg, SIMV =8/min) defines the actual number of V_T breaths a patient will receive per minute • A patient who initiates more breaths per minute than the defined rate will receive those breaths at the patient-defined V_T (ie, the V_T of the spontaneous breaths can be different from the V_T of the machine breaths)
Pressure Control Modes	
PCV	• Can be used with either CMV or SIMV modes • Active inhalation V_T is delivered up to a pressure threshold & not a volume threshold • Exhalation is passive; after the V_T is delivered, the machine releases & exhalation is driven by chest wall & lung elastance (recoil) • Patient initiates the respiratory cycle (unless apneic or paralyzed)
Additional Support Modes	
CPAP	• This is a spontaneous breathing mode (ie, V_T & rate are not provided by the mechanical ventilator) • Continous positive pressure is delivered while a patient breathes spontaneously • This pressure is continuous, meaning that both inspiratory & expiratory phases of respiration are supplemented with positive pressure • CPAP may be delivered invasively (ie, through an endotracheal tube) or noninvasively (ie, with a tight-fitting mask or with high–gas flow nasal prongs)
PSV	• PSV augments spontaneous breaths with a machine-defined amount of positive pressure that is delivered only during inspiration • The purpose of PSV mode is to improve patient-machine synchrony (comfort) & to decrease the patient work of breathing; in some patients this may facilitate weaning from mechanical ventilation • PSV inspiratory positive flow continues while the patient inhales & then stops when the patient's flow decreases to less than a threshold value (usually <25% of the initial inspiratory flow rate) • Patients determine their spontaneous V_T during PSV breaths by controlling their flow rate. When they have had enough, they simply stop inspiring
Initial Invasive Mechanical Ventilation Settings	
Mode	• As indicated: CMV, SIMV, PSV, CPAP
Tidal volume	• Standard: 8–10 mL/kg ideal body weight (less is preferred) • ARDS: 6 mL/kg ideal body weight
Rate	• Titrate to desired V_M for P_{CO_2}, PEEP, & T_I
F_{IO_2}	• Maintain P_{O_2} > target value (usually 60 torr)
T_I	• Set to meet patient demand • Allow adequate time for exhalation
PEEP	• As indicated; maintain lower values unless needed for ARDS • Do not use as a prevention maneuver for atelectasis

Abbreviations: A/C, assist/control; ARDS, acute respiratory distress syndrome; CMV, controlled mechanical ventilation; CPAP, continuous positive airway pressure; F_{IO_2}, fraction of inspired oxygen; PCV, pressure control ventilation; PEEP, positive end-expiratory pressure; PSV, pressure support ventilation; SIMV, synchronized intermittent mandatory ventilation; T_I, inspiratory time; V_M, minute ventilation; V_T, tidal volume.

mortality. Tracheostomy has the advantages of decreased laryngeal injury, increased patient comfort, ease of suctioning, and, in certain patients, allowance for oral ingestion and speech. Tracheostomy is commonly considered for patients who have needed or are expected to need intubation and mechanical ventilation for more than 2 to 4 weeks.

- Tracheostomy is considered for patients requiring mechanical ventilation for >2–4 weeks.

Weaning (Liberation From Mechanical Ventilation)

Patients are candidates for weaning from mechanical ventilation when they are hemodynamically stable, underlying pathophysiologic processes (both pulmonary and nonpulmonary) are resolving, and they have adequately recovered from respiratory failure. It is important to identify these patients in order to decrease costs, ICU lengths of stay, and infectious and other complications of mechanical ventilation. The most effective and consistent way to wean patients is to use a protocol that involves a nurse or respiratory therapist. What seems to be most important is a daily spontaneous breathing trial after the patient seems ready for weaning, preceded by a daily interruption of sedation. This is typically done each morning with a T-piece system, or by using continuous positive airway pressure (CPAP) or pressure support ventilation (PSV) mode for 30 minutes to 2 hours. A weaning protocol is presented in Figure 14.3.

- Daily spontaneous breathing trials are helpful for patients who seem ready for weaning.

CARDIAC CRITICAL CARE

Cardiac-specific topics are largely covered in the "Cardiology" section of this book. Therefore, the present chapter focuses on chapter topics in which critical care and cardiology substantially overlap and are commonly included as board examination questions.

SHOCK

Shock is defined as the inadequate provision of oxygen and metabolic substrate to the tissues. Vital signs are typically not part of the definition; thus, hypotension is not necessary to establish a diagnosis of shock. Many patients present to critical care units with "undifferentiated shock" (ie, the cause may not be readily apparent). Initial assessment is aimed at determining the cause of shock. The following classification system is widely used (Table 14.4): 1) hypovolemic (hemorrhagic), 2) distributive, 3) cardiogenic, and 4) obstructive.

- Given systemic vascular resistance, cardiac output, and central venous pressure, be able to differentiate between different types of shock.

When patients present to an ICU or emergency department with undifferentiated shock and life-threatening hypoperfusion, time matters. Thus, instead of proceeding in a linear fashion (history first, and then examination, laboratory and imaging studies, and finally treatment), diagnosis and treatment must occur simultaneously. This is because failure to promptly restore perfusion status (within a few hours) results in secondary tissue damage from proinflammatory mediators (possibly leading to multiple organ failure). A typical sequence of events (amplification) is depicted in Figure 14.4.

In 2001, a landmark article was published on rapid resuscitation of patients who had shock caused by severe sepsis (Figure 14.5). There has been ongoing controversy about the end points of resuscitation and specific therapies used in that study. Nevertheless, the principles of the study are highly relevant: early recognition and treatment of hypoperfusion can decrease the ensuing inflammatory response to shock.

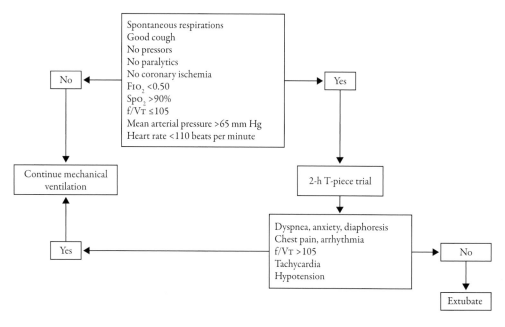

Figure 14.3 Ventilatory Weaning Protocol. FIO_2 indicates fraction of inspired oxygen; f/VT, respiratory frequency divided by tidal volume (rapid shallow breathing index); SpO_2, arterial oxygen saturation.

Table 14.4 CLASSIFICATION OF SHOCK[a]

SHOCK TYPE	PRELOAD (CENTRAL VENOUS PRESSURE)	WEDGE PRESSURE	SYSTEMIC VASCULAR RESISTANCE	CARDIAC OUTPUT	EXAMPLES OF CAUSES
Hypovolemic (hemorrhagic)	↓	↓	↑	↓	Bleeding Vomiting, diarrhea Diuretic use (excess) Diabetes mellitus Burns, exudative skin lesions Diabetes insipidus
Distributive	↔	↔	↓	↑	Sepsis Hyperthyroidism Liver disease Anaphylaxis Thiamine deficiency Spinal cord injury (neurogenic shock)
Cardiogenic	↑↔	↑	↑	↓	Pump failure (right or left) Acute coronary syndrome Acute mitral regurgitation
Tamponade (equalization of pressures)	↔	↔	↔	↔	Cardiac tamponade

[a] Arrows indicate increase (↑), decrease (↓), or no change (↔).

- Be familiar with the early goal-directed therapy algorithm.

ASSESSMENT OF HEMODYNAMIC STATUS (PERFORMANCE)

The use of pulmonary arterial catheters in ICU patients is disappearing, since it has been shown that harms exceed benefits. Thus, board examination questions about pulmonary arterial waveforms, wedge pressure, and other related topics are much less frequent. The use of bedside echocardiography and central venous pressure (CVP) monitoring has increased. The use of CVP monitoring has increased because early goal-directed therapy protocols for sepsis call for measuring central venous oxygen saturation. Examination questions therefore tend to

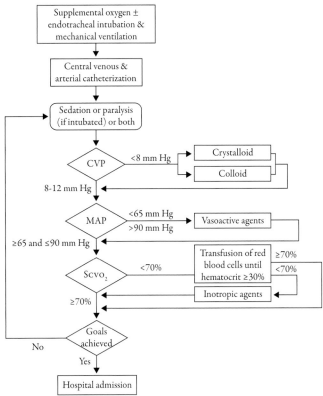

Figure 14.5 Protocol for Early Goal-Directed Therapy. CVP indicates central venous pressure; MAP, mean arterial pressure; Scvo₂, central venous oxygen saturation. (Adapted from Rivers E, Nguyen B, Havstad S, Ressler J, Muzzin A, Knoblich B, et al; Early Goal-Directed Therapy Collaborative Group. Early goal-directed therapy in the treatment of severe sepsis and septic shock. N Engl J Med. 2001 Nov 8;345[19]:1368–77. Used with permission.)

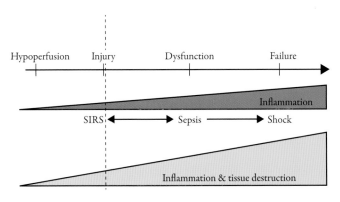

Figure 14.4 Shock: Time Matters. SIRS indicates systemic inflammatory response syndrome.

focus on the need to obtain additional hemodynamic monitoring data to sort out the type of shock and complications of these invasive procedures, or the examination provides hemodynamic results and then asks a question about next steps.

Peripheral veins are the preferred access sites in patients who require intravenous therapy. Indications for central venous access are lack of adequate peripheral veins, need for hypertonic or phlebitic medications or solutions, need for long-term access, need for measuring central pressures, and access for procedures (hemodialysis and cardiac pacing). The most common locations for central access are the internal jugular, subclavian, and femoral veins.

Relative contraindications include procedural inexperience of the practitioner, significant coagulopathy, inability to identify landmarks, infection or burn at the entry site, and thrombosis of the proposed central venous site. At most institutions today, central venous catheters are inserted with the help of direct ultrasonographic visualization.

Complications of central venous catheterization include bloodstream infections, cardiac arrhythmias, pneumothorax, air embolism, vascular injury, catheter or guidewire embolism, catheter knotting, bleeding, and other potential complications of needle or catheter misplacement.

The IHI has identified prevention of catheter-related bloodstream infections (CR-BSIs) with use of the IHI Central Line Bundle as a key element in improving patient outcomes and preventing morbidity. The key components of the Central Line Bundle are 1) hand hygiene; 2) maximal barrier precautions upon insertion; 3) chlorhexidine skin antisepsis; 4) optimal catheter site selection, with avoidance of the femoral vein for central venous access in adult patients; and 5) daily review of line necessity, with prompt removal of unnecessary lines. CR-BSIs are usually attributed to the migration of bacteria from the skin along the catheter tract. *CR-BSI* is usually defined as more than 15 colony-forming units per milliliter on semiquantitative culture of the catheter tip. *Catheter-related bacteremia* is defined as bacterial growth and blood cultures that are positive for the same organism as on the catheter tip. Risk factors include infected catheter site or cutaneous breakdown, multiple manipulations, the number of catheter lumens, and the duration of use of the same site (particularly after 3 or 4 days). Treatment of CR-BSIs should include catheter removal and replacement at another site if necessary.

- The Central Line Bundle is important in preventing CR-BSIs.

- Treatment of CR-BSIs includes prompt catheter removal.

INFECTIOUS DISEASES AND CRITICAL ILLNESS

Critical care–directed board examination questions typically focus on sepsis recognition and management, appropriate antibiotic selection for serious or life-threatening infections (see the "Infectious Diseases" section of this book), and infection control (eg, Central Line Bundle, VAP prevention).

Description

Sepsis is an exaggerated inflammatory response to a noxious (infectious) stimulus and is characterized by a severe catabolic reaction, widespread endothelial dysfunction, and release of innate inflammatory response components. To achieve a common terminology, *systemic inflammatory response syndrome* (*SIRS*) was introduced for findings of fever or hypothermia, tachycardia, hyperventilation, and leukocytosis or leukopenia regardless of cause. Not all SIRS is infection mediated. *Sepsis* is defined as SIRS with a known or presumed source of infection, and *severe sepsis* is defined as sepsis associated with organ system dysfunction and systemic effects, including hypotension, decreased urine output, or metabolic acidosis. *Septic shock* refers to persistent signs of organ hypoperfusion despite adequate fluid resuscitation.

The mortality of patients with sepsis and multiorgan failure may be greater than 70% to 90%. Adverse risk factors include age older than 65 years, continued systemic signs of sepsis, persistent deficit in oxygen delivery, and preexisting renal or liver failure. Physiologic scoring systems (eg, Acute Physiology and Chronic Health Evaluation [APACHE]) may predict outcome more accurately for subgroups of patients.

Complications

Multisystem organ failure, or *multiple-organ dysfunction syndrome* (*MODS*), is usually defined as acute dysfunction of 2 or more organ systems lasting more than 2 days. Sepsis is the most common cause. Corticosteroids have no known benefit and may cause adverse effects in patients with sepsis syndrome. The exception is patients who have a documented adrenal insufficiency and severe sepsis; they may benefit from low doses of hydrocortisone or methylprednisolone.

Treatment

The Surviving Sepsis Campaign is a group of organizations and professional societies that have created guidelines for the treatment of sepsis. These have been modified and updated at intervals. The use of activated protein C is no longer recommended. Primary therapies are described below.

Antibiotics
Use of antibiotics includes the following steps:

1. Collect samples for blood cultures before antibiotics are given

2. Obtain other cultures and imaging studies as indicated

3. Administer appropriate antibiotics within 1 hour of ICU admission (within 3 hours of emergency department admission)

4. Select specific antibiotics after 72 hours as appropriate and continue their use for 10 days

5. Control the source of the infection, and drain it if indicated

Resuscitation

Prompt resuscitation and correction of systemic hypoperfusion is critical (within 6 hours of initial presentation to the hospital). The most common error during resuscitation of medical patients with sepsis is inadequate administration of intravenous fluids during the first few hours after ICU admission. Use of blood products and inotropic support should also be considered as indicated. The early goal-directed therapy protocol (Figure 14.5) is not strictly endorsed as an absolute approach in this chapter because of lingering controversies (as mentioned above).

Corticosteroids

High-dose corticosteroids provide no benefit in sepsis and have been shown to cause harm. Various randomized controlled trials have suggested a mortality benefit from administration of low-dose hydrocortisone (100 mg intravenously every 6 hours) and fludrocortisone (50 mcg by mouth daily for 7 days) in patients who have sepsis and relative adrenal insufficiency. Their use, and the actual incidence of relative adrenal insufficiency, remains controversial. *Relative adrenal insufficiency* is defined as an increase in the serum cortisol level of less than 9 mg/dL in relation to baseline at 0, 30, and 60 minutes after intravenous administration of cosyntropin 250 mcg. The number needed to treat to save 1 life is 7. This test should not be used in patients who have received etomidate during endotracheal intubation (sedation) since it is a selective inhibitor of β-hydroxylase and could therefore blunt the cortisol response to corticotropin.

- Important concepts in sepsis include identification of the source of infection, early administration of antibiotics, and fluid resuscitation.

ENDOCRINOLOGY AND CRITICAL ILLNESS

Diabetic emergencies, acute thyroid conditions, and other endocrine emergencies are discussed in the "Endocrinology" section of this textbook. Board examination questions specifically related to critical care typically focus on glucose management in all ICU patients.

GLUCOSE MANAGEMENT

Two large randomized studies of intensive insulin therapy in surgical and medical ICUs in Belgium showed mortality benefit, but they raised questions of both internal and external validity and sparked debate in this area. It is generally agreed that allowing blood glucose levels to increase to 200 mg/dL or more is unacceptable. Conversely, maintaining strict normoglycemia (≤110 mg/dL) is associated with frequent episodes of hypoglycemia and may increase mortality. A blood glucose maintenance target of 140 to 180 mg/dL is currently encouraged, most recently in the multicenter Normoglycemia in

Intensive Care Evaluation–Survival Using Glucose Algorithm Regulation (NICE-SUGAR) trial.

- Intensive glucose management is associated with frequent hypoglycemia, and more lenient goals should be targeted.

GASTROENTEROLOGY AND CRITICAL ILLNESS

A review of gastroenterology, including acute conditions, is discussed in the "Gastroenterology and Hepatology" section of this textbook. Board examination questions specifically related to critical care typically focus on diagnosis and management of GI hemorrhage in ICU patients, fulminant hepatic failure, and conditions such as abdominal compartment syndrome.

GI HEMORRHAGE

Diagnosis

As with sepsis, underresuscitation for shock and hypoperfusion is a common shortfall in the management of ICU patients who have clinically significant GI hemorrhage. When significant GI blood loss is suspected, the focus should immediately shift to the assessment of perfusion status. Determine whether the patient has shock, either overt or cryptic. Do not exclusively use hemoglobin and hematocrit as quantification markers of blood loss and determinants of shock. As with other forms of shock, assess factors such as capillary refill time, urine output, presence or absence of altered sensorium, and lactate level and presence of metabolic acidosis. These are nonspecific but valuable indicators that help evaluate how sick the patient is and how aggressive the resuscitation must be. Table 14.5 correlates the amount of blood loss with clinical findings. Identification of the source of GI hemorrhage is important, but resuscitation has the highest priority.

For all patients with significant GI hemorrhage, the following considerations should be addressed on arrival because, by various mechanisms, they can directly influence the initial diagnosis and management of patients with GI hemorrhage and shock:

1. Presence of coagulopathy

2. Presence of shock

3. Presence of hypothermia

4. Use of medications that exacerbate GI bleeding or inhibit clotting

5. Active alcohol ingestion

6. Active non-GI comorbidities that worsen the outcome

7. Prior history of GI hemorrhage that required ICU admission

Table 14.5 Classification of Blood Loss

FEATURE	CLASS			
	I	II	III	IV
Blood loss, mL	<750	750–1,500	1,500–2,000	>2,000
Blood pressure	No change	Systolic: no change Diastolic: increased	Decreased	Hypotension (possibly severe)
Pulse, beats per minute	100	100–120	>120 (thready)	>120–140 (very thready)
Respiratory rate	Normal	Increased	Increased	Increased
Sensorium	Alert, thirsty	Anxious	Anxious or drowsy	Drowsy or obtunded
Urine output	Normal	Decreased	Oliguria	Oliguria or anuria

8. Presence of severe liver disease

9. Recent GI surgery that can be associated with GI bleeding

10. Prior history of conditions such as peptic disease, polyps, and diverticular disease

Management

The following are management priorities:

1. Administer necessary fluid and blood resuscitation

2. Correct coagulopathy

3. Reverse adverse medications if possible (eg, anticoagulants)

4. Notify the gastroenterology department about the patient and the possible need for emergent endoscopy

5. Notify the surgery department about the patient if transfusion requirements exceed 4 to 6 units of packed red blood cells

Upper endoscopy should be considered emergently for ICU patients who have the appropriate clinical history, hemodynamic instability, or persistent hematemesis or when coagulation variables cannot be effectively normalized and bleeding is ongoing. The goal of endoscopy is to identify the source of bleeding and, more importantly, to use interventional techniques to stop blood loss (eg, variceal banding, injection therapies of ulcers and varices, ablative therapies). Some patients receive a combination of these therapies. A very small number of patients with relentless variceal hemorrhage may require balloon tamponade therapy to staunch the bleeding. Empirical use of continuous infusion octreotide or vasopressin is not recommended for patients with upper GI hemorrhage unless 1) they have a proven prior history of significant variceal hemorrhage, 2) it is requested by the gastroenterologist before endoscopy, or 3) the patient has progressive hemodynamic instability. Vasopressin can exacerbate preexisting coronary ischemia and its use should be carefully considered before administration.

The treatment of acute lower GI hemorrhage is largely supportive. Resuscitate the patient, administer blood, correct coagulopathy, and involve other providers with the care plan early on (eg, gastroenterology department, surgery department). Identifying the source of bleeding can be difficult because active bleeding can be intermittent and elusive. Many patients presenting to an ICU with lower GI hemorrhage have had a previous episode. The role of emergent colonoscopy, especially in an unprepped patient, is not clearly defined. Various studies have reported widely disparate diagnostic yields with this test when performed under these circumstances. Other diagnostic adjuncts, such as arteriography or nuclear medicine scans, may be needed to more precisely identify the source of bleeding.

- Identify and treat shock in patients with GI hemorrhage.

- Notify and involve gastroenterology specialists early.

FULMINANT HEPATIC FAILURE

Patients with fulminant hepatic failure most typically present to the ICU without a prior history of liver disease. Their liver failure is typically manifest as overt hepatic synthetic failure with progressive coagulopathy and then worsening encephalopathy. These patients die of complications of hepatic failure, including infection or sepsis, multiorgan failure, and complications of cerebral edema (with or without central nervous system hemorrhage). ICU management and treatment is supportive, seeks possible reversible causes, and advances to orthotopic liver transplant quickly when the issues described above develop. Supportive ICU care includes the following:

1. Close surveillance for infections

2. Airway protection with endotracheal intubation earlier rather than later

3. Aggressive management of coagulopathy

4. Intracranial pressure monitoring and therapies when obtundation and evidence of intracranial pressure elevation are present

5. Maintenance of the perfusion status of other vital organs, such as the kidneys

- Seek reversible causes of fulminant hepatic failure and treat supportively.

ABDOMINAL COMPARTMENT SYNDROME

Primary abdominal compartment syndrome (ACS) is associated with abdominopelvic injury or disease that frequently requires early surgical or interventional radiologic intervention. Secondary ACS does not originate from the abdominopelvic region. Risk factors for ACS are severe penetrating and blunt abdominal trauma, ruptured abdominal aortic aneurysm, retroperitoneal hemorrhage, pneumoperitoneum, neoplasm, pancreatitis, massive ascites, liver transplant, abdominal wall burn eschar, abdominal surgery, high-volume fluid resuscitation (>3,500 mL in 24 hours), ileus, and pulmonary, renal, or liver dysfunction.

Normal intra-abdominal pressure (IAP) (ie, the pressure within the abdominal cavity) is approximately 5 to 7 mm Hg in critically ill adults. Intra-abdominal hypertension is defined by a sustained or repeated elevation of IAP (≥12 mm Hg) and is graded as follows:

- Grade I: IAP 12–15 mm Hg.
- Grade II: IAP 16–20 mm Hg.
- Grade III: IAP 21–25 mm Hg.
- Grade IV: IAP >25 mm Hg.

ACS is defined as a sustained IAP greater than 20 mm Hg (with or without abdominal perfusion pressure <60 mm Hg) that is associated with new organ dysfunction. If 2 or more risk factors for ACS are present, baseline IAP should be measured. Bladder pressure is the simplest accepted method of measuring IAP.

IAP levels greater than 15 mm Hg are associated with worsening total pulmonary compliance due to progressive elevation of the hemidiaphragms and basilar atelectasis, resulting in a progressive reduction in total lung capacity, functional residual capacity, and residual volume. This manifests clinically as bronchial breath sounds in both bases, elevated hemidiaphragms on chest radiography, and elevated peak and plateau pressures. Respiratory failure due to hypoventilation results from progressive elevation in IAP.

Further increases in intrathoracic pressure may worsen cardiac output through impaired venous return (due to elevated intrathoracic pressure and direct compression of the inferior vena cava and the portal vein by abdominal pressure) and diastolic heart failure (pressure applied to right and left ventricles results in stiff walls and impaired relaxation). These derangements result in reduced stroke volume that is only partly compensated for by increases in heart rate and contractility. The Starling curve is thus shifted down and to the right, and cardiac output continues to decrease with progressive elevation of IAP. These derangements are exacerbated by the frequent coexistence of hypovolemia or a systemic inflammatory condition, resulting in vasodilatation. Hence, diuresis is not appropriate since it would further reduce venous return and cardiac output. Decompression of the abdominal cavity results in nearly immediate reversal of respiratory failure.

- ACS is defined as IAP >20 mm Hg.
- Elevated intra-abdominal pressure causes both respiratory dysfunction and cardiac dysfunction.
- Decompression of the abdominal cavity is the treatment.

HEMATOLOGIC DISORDERS AND CRITICAL ILLNESS

Critical care–focused internal medicine board examination questions in this content domain typically focus on the following:

1. Most common causes of bleeding in ICU patients

2. Primary hematologic syndromes in the ICU with associated bleeding

3. ICU treatment of these disorders

ICU-RELATED BLEEDING DISORDERS

Diagnosis

Nearly all ICU-related bleeding disorders are acquired, and many of them are multifactorial. These disorders are most commonly associated with the following:

1. Medications that affect platelets or coagulation factors (or both)

2. Liver disease and loss of synthetic function

3. Drugs that bind with vitamin K

4. Thrombocytopenia (see item 1 in this list)

5. Other systemic disorders (eg, sepsis) that cause conditions such as disseminated intravascular coagulation

6. Dilutional coagulopathy

Thrombocytopenia is very common in ICU patients. It is often associated with various drugs, including heparin. In general, the causes are the same causes of thrombocytopenia in other care environments.

Similarly, coagulopathy develops in many ICU patients. Most commonly, prothrombin time is prolonged. In general the causes are the same causes of coagulopathy in other care environments.

Management

Treatment of bleeding disorders in the ICU is largely supportive and includes identifying and discontinuing the use of offending medications. Since discontinuation is not always possible, observation may be considered until either of the following indications develops:

1. Clinically significant bleeding develops

2. An invasive procedure, which may cause bleeding, is needed

- Drug-induced thrombocytopenia is very common in ICU patients; heparin is 1 of the most important causes.

SUMMARY

- Major causes of hypercapnic respiratory failure include inadequate alveolar ventilation, increased pulmonary dead space, and failure of the respiratory "bellows."

- ARDS is defined as a P/F ratio <200 with bilateral pulmonary infiltrates and a normal volume status.

- Tracheostomy is considered for patients requiring mechanical ventilation for >2–4 weeks.

- Types of shock: hypovolemic (hemorrhagic), distributive, cardiogenic, and obstructive.

- Important concepts in sepsis include identification of the source of infection, early administration of antibiotics, and fluid resuscitation.

- Identify and treat shock in patients with GI hemorrhage. Notify and involve gastroenterology specialists early.

15.

INTERSTITIAL LUNG DISEASES

Fabien Maldonado, MD, and Timothy R. Aksamit, MD

GOALS

- Understand the diagnostic approach to interstitial lung diseases.
- Identify key features and differentiating characteristics of interstitial lung diseases.

OVERVIEW

Interstitial lung diseases (ILDs), better described as diffuse parenchymal lung diseases, encompass a group of heterogeneous lung conditions characterized by various etiologies, clinical and radiologic manifestations, clinical courses, and responses to treatment. In this chapter, we use the American Board of Internal Medicine designation *ILDs*. Although more than 100 distinct entities have been described, the vast majority are rare enough to be considered clinical oddities. Prompt recognition of ILD and initiation of appropriate therapy can result in significant improvement of otherwise potentially life-threatening respiratory conditions.

Some ILDs are characterized by suggestive or even pathognomonic findings, but the majority are best diagnosed through a dynamic interaction between clinicians, radiologists, and pathologists. ILDs are thought to affect 1 in 3,000 to 1 in 4,000 persons in the general population and represent approximately 15% of all consultations for the general pulmonologist. Although there is no widely accepted definition for ILDs, they share the common feature of diffuse involvement of the lung parenchyma and may affect the pulmonary interstitium. By convention, infections, pulmonary edema, lung malignancies, and emphysema are excluded, but they should be carefully considered as part of the differential diagnosis (Box 15.1).

- Most ILDs need an integrated approach between clinicians, radiologists, and pathologists for accurate diagnosis.

There are 4 major categories of ILD:

1. ILDs of known cause (eg, drug-induced lung disease, connective tissue disease–related ILD [CTD-ILD])
2. Idiopathic interstitial pneumonias (Box 15.2)
3. Granulomatous ILDs (eg, sarcoidosis, hypersensitivity pneumonitis [HP])
4. Other ILDs (usually readily recognizable owing to characteristic findings)

The strategy for diagnosing ILD should follow a stepwise approach, including comprehensive history and thorough physical examination, pulmonary function tests (PFTs), radiologic studies (usually including high-resolution computed tomography [HRCT]), and, if needed, bronchoscopic or surgical (or both) lung biopsy (Figure 15.1). It is important to realize that for the majority of patients all tests are not necessary and the diagnosis may be achieved without histologic confirmation.

DIAGNOSIS

HISTORY

A detailed history is the most important step in the diagnosis of ILD (Table 15.1). Environmental (eg, pets, organic or mineral dust) or occupational exposures should be comprehensively investigated.

- The use of amiodarone, methotrexate, nitrofurantoin, chemotherapy, or radiotherapy should suggest iatrogenic lung disease.
- Insulation work or ship building should suggest asbestos-related disease; mining or sandblasting may be associated with silicosis.

Collagen vascular
   Dermatomyositis
   Rheumatoid arthritis
   Scleroderma
   Systemic lupus erythematosus
Drug-induced
   Chemotherapy
   Drug therapy
   Radiotherapy
Genetic
   Hermansky-Pudlak syndrome
   Metabolic storage disease
   Neurofibromatosis
   Tuberous sclerosis
Idiopathic
Infectious
   Chronic mycobacterial
   Chronic mycoses
Malignant
   Bronchoalveolar cell carcinoma
   Lymphangitic metastases
   Lymphoma
Occupational or inhalational
   Asbestosis
   Coal workers' pneumoconiosis
   Hypersensitivity
   Silicosis
   Toxic gas
Vasculitides
   Churg-Strauss syndrome
   Giant cell arteritis
   Wegener granulomatosis

- Idiopathic pulmonary fibrosis (IPF), desquamative interstitial pneumonia, and pulmonary Langerhans cell histiocytosis (PLCH) are more common in smokers; sarcoidosis and HP are more common in nonsmokers.

PHYSICAL EXAMINATION

Rales ("dry" or "Velcro crackles") suggest fibrosis, but they are nonspecific. Clubbing of the digits can be associated with IPF and asbestosis but is rare otherwise. Clubbing should raise concerns for alternative diagnoses (eg, lung or pleural malignancies, chronic suppurative lung diseases, right-to-left shunt, liver disease, inflammatory bowel diseases). Careful attention should be paid to extrapulmonary manifestations of systemic diseases such as musculoskeletal pain, sicca syndrome, esophageal dysmotility, and Raynaud phenomenon.

- Clubbing is rare in ILD aside from IPF and asbestosis.

PULMONARY FUNCTION STUDIES

The typical pattern is that of restriction, as evidenced by decreased lung volumes and preservation of flows. The

Idiopathic pulmonary fibrosis–usual interstitial pneumonia (IPF-UIP)
Nonspecific interstitial pneumonia (NSIP)
Sarcoidosis
Bronchiolitis obliterans with organizing pneumonia/cryptogenic organizing pneumonia (BOOP/COP)
Eosinophilic lung diseases
Lymphocytic interstitial pneumonia (LIP)
Alveolar microlithiasis
Lymphangioleiomyomatosis (LAM)
Langerhans cell histiocytosis/eosinophilic granulomatosis
Pulmonary alveolar proteinosis
Acute respiratory distress syndrome/acute lung injury
Others

diffusing capacity of lung for carbon monoxide (DLCO) is also reduced. When DLCO is reduced out of proportion to the rest of the PFTs, concurrent pulmonary hypertension or combined emphysema may be present. Some patients with ILD may present with mixed obstructive-restrictive disease, such as sarcoidosis, PLCH, lymphangioleiomyomatosis (LAM), HP, and chronic eosinophilic pneumonia.

IMAGING STUDIES

Although chest radiography (CXR) has been largely supplanted by HRCT, several characteristic findings are worth mentioning:

1. Alveolar opacities suggest potentially reversible diseases (caused by inflammation, edema, or alveolar hemorrhage) as opposed to reticular findings (more likely associated with irreversible fibrosis).

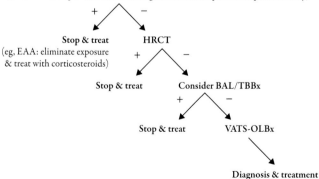

Figure 15.1 Strategy for Diagnosing Interstitial Lung Disease. BAL indicates bronchoalveolar lavage; CXR, chest radiography; EAA, extrinsic allergic alveolitis; HRCT, high-resolution computed tomography; OLBx, open lung biopsy; PFT, pulmonary function test; TBBx, transbronchial biopsy; VATS, video-assisted thoracoscopy; +, positive findings; –, negative findings.

Table 15.1 INTERSTITIAL LUNG DISEASES DISTINGUISHED BY HISTORY

EXPOSURE OR FEATURE	DISEASE
Amiodarone, methotrexate, nitrofurantoin, chemotherapy, radiotherapy	Drug-induced or iatrogenic lung disease
Insulation work, ship building, mining, sandblasting	Pneumoconioses
Birds, indoor hot tubs, moldy humidifiers	Hypersensitivity pneumonitis
Acute onset of disease	Acute eosinophilic pneumonia or organizing pneumonia Virtually rules out IPF and asbestosis (which evolve over months to years)
Current smoker	Desquamative interstitial pneumonia, IPF, pulmonary Langerhans cell histiocytosis
Former smoker, never smoker	Sarcoidosis, hypersensitivity pneumonitis

Abbreviation: IPF, idiopathic pulmonary fibrosis.

2. Distribution of the infiltrates may provide guidance. Use the mnemonic *CHAPS* to remember predominant upper lung opacities:

   a. *C*ystic fibrosis, *c*hronic eosinophilic pneumonia

   b. *H*P, *h*istiocytosis (PLCH)

   c. *A*llergic bronchopulmonary aspergillosis, *a*nkylosing spondylitis

   d. *P*neumoconioses

   e. *S*arcoidosis

3. Lower lung diseases include IPF, asbestosis, and aspiration.

4. Bilateral hilar lymphadenopathy should suggest sarcoidosis, silicosis, or, rarely, berylliosis (however, fungal or mycobacterial infections and lymphoma should be excluded).

5. Alveolar infiltrates in a "bat wing" distribution are typical of pulmonary alveolar proteinosis (PAP) (or cardiogenic pulmonary edema).

6. Peripheral opacities ("photographic negative of pulmonary edema") have been described in chronic eosinophilic pneumonia.

7. Pneumothorax may be the clinical manifestation of PLCH and LAM.

HRCT has revolutionized the diagnosis of ILD and often obviates the need for histopathologic examination. Several characteristic features should narrow the differential diagnosis. Alveolar opacities (consolidation or ground-glass infiltrates) suggest reversible disease, while reticular "fibrotic" infiltrates are less likely to resolve. Honeycombing, traction bronchiectases, and basal predominance are typical for usual interstitial pneumonia (UIP), a pattern necessary for the diagnosis of IPF (see section on IPF below). Thin-walled cysts suggest PLCH (upper lobe predominance) or LAM (diffuse lung involvement). A "crazy-paving" pattern (ground-glass infiltrates with septal thickening) is seen in PAP.

Micronodular infiltrates may be clustered around the bronchovascular bundles and subpleural areas (as in sarcoidosis and lymphangitic carcinomatosis) or randomly distributed (as in hematogenously spread diseases such as miliary tuberculosis). Centrilobular infiltrates (sparing subpleural spaces and bronchovascular bundles) may have a tree-and-bud pattern (fungal or mycobacterial infections) or they may not (HP and PLCH).

- Bilateral hilar lymphadenopathy is common in silicosis and sarcoidosis, but infections (fungal or mycobacterial) and lymphoma should be excluded.

- "Bat wing" distribution on CXR and "crazy-paving" pattern on HRCT are typical of PAP.

- A "photographic negative of pulmonary edema" is seen in chronic eosinophilic pneumonia.

- Thin-walled cysts are seen in PLCH and LAM.

LABORATORY STUDIES

Laboratory studies are rarely helpful in the diagnosis of ILD. Useful tests include a complete blood cell count with a differential blood count and liver and renal function tests. Subsequently, hepatitis and human immunodeficiency virus (HIV) serologies may be indicated. Other laboratory studies can be considered depending on the clinical picture:

1. Serologies for connective tissue disease are often obtained, particularly in the case of organizing pneumonia (OP) and nonspecific interstitial pneumonia (NSIP), the most common patterns seen in CTD-ILD.

2. Serum protein electrophoresis may be ordered if amyloidosis is a consideration.

3. HP antibody testing is usually limited to a few common offenders and is rarely helpful in practice.

4. The angiotensin-converting enzyme level, classically used to follow patients with sarcoidosis, is neither sensitive nor specific.

5. One notable exception is that of cytoplasmic antineutrophil cytoplasmic autoantibody (c-ANCA)–proteinase 3 antibodies, which are both sensitive and specific for Wegener granulomatosis.

- Laboratory studies are rarely helpful in ILD, except for the diagnosis of Wegener granulomatosis.

Bronchoscopic or surgical lung biopsy have limited roles. It is important to realize that the histopathologic diagnosis may only support a presumptive diagnosis without establishing it.

Bronchoscopy is relatively simple and safe. The main risks are pneumothorax (up to 5%) and bleeding (up to 2%). It is used primarily to exclude infection or malignancy; the biopsy samples are too small to establish a confident diagnosis in ILD. In selected cases, the findings can be diagnostic. For instance, a profusion of nonnecrotizing granulomas should suggest sarcoidosis (as opposed to necrotizing granulomas seen in fungal and mycobacterial infections and Wegener granulomatosis).

Bronchoalveolar lavage (BAL) can be done safely in nearly all patients (including anticoagulated patients) and can exclude infection. On occasion, it may offer some guidance:

1. A predominance of lymphocytes on the BAL is consistent with sarcoidosis (with a classically inverted CD4:CD8 ratio, typically >4) or HP (normal CD4:CD8 ratio).

2. Eosinophilic predominance is seen with acute and chronic eosinophilic pneumonia.

3. Hemosiderin-laden macrophages are seen in diffuse alveolar hemorrhage.

4. Lipid-laden macrophages are seen in aspiration pneumonia and, less commonly, in lipoid pneumonia.

5. A CD1a$^+$ (a marker of Langerhans histiocytes) cell count greater than 5% suggests PLCH as a possibility.

Surgical lung biopsy is still required in a minority of patients (approximately 30%). Although it usually allows for a confident diagnosis, the risks and benefits need to be weighed and discussed with the patient, since acute exacerbations of ILD have occurred postoperatively with dramatic consequences. For this reason, rapidly progressive ILD should be considered a relative contraindication to surgical lung biopsy.

- Bronchoscopy is safe and simple, but biopsy samples are generally too small for a definitive diagnosis, except for sarcoidosis.

- Lymphocytic predominance on BAL suggests sarcoidosis (high CD4:CD8 ratio) or HP (normal ratio).

- Hemosiderin-laden macrophages suggest alveolar hemorrhage; lipid-laden macrophages are associated with aspiration and lipoid pneumonia.

- PLCH can be diagnosed when more than 5% of BAL cells stain positive for CD1a.

ILDS OF KNOWN CAUSE

CONNECTIVE TISSUE DISEASE–RELATED INTERSTITIAL LUNG DISEASES

Virtually all connective tissue diseases may affect the lungs. CTD-ILDs are more common in females, with the exception of rheumatoid arthritis (RA), which is more common in men. The typical histopathologic patterns seen in CTD-ILD are NSIP and OP. In fact, these histopathologic diagnoses should suggest the possibility of a connective tissue disease limited to the lungs in otherwise asymptomatic patients.

- Treat the underlying cause. These ILDs tend to respond to treatment of the underlying inflammatory conditions with corticosteroids or other immunosuppressive agents as indicated.

RHEUMATOID ARTHRITIS

Differences between RA-ILD and other CTD-ILDs include the following:

- RA-ILD is more common in males.

- A UIP pattern is typically seen in RA-ILD, which is less responsive to treatment.

RA is commonly associated with pleural effusions, pulmonary nodules, and fibrosis (RA-ILD) but may affect any part of the respiratory system. Arytenoid arthritis may cause central airway obstruction, and in patients with RA, bronchiectases or constrictive bronchiolitis may develop. The possibility of drug-induced lung disease (sarcoidosis-like reaction with methotrexate; Goodpasture syndrome or constrictive bronchiolitis with penicillamine) should be considered.

SYSTEMIC LUPUS ERYTHEMATOSUS

Systemic lupus erythematosus typically causes NSIP or OP (or both). A life-threatening pulmonary complication is acute lupus pneumonitis, characterized by diffuse alveolar damage on lung biopsy, which is poorly responsive to treatment. Diaphragmatic weakness (myopathy) may result in "plate-like atelectasis" or, when severe, the classic "shrinking lung syndrome" characterized by low lung volumes in the absence of lung infiltrates.

INFLAMMATORY MYOPATHIES

Inflammatory myopathies (dermatomyositis and polymyositis) may cause NSIP and OP, respiratory muscle weakness, and recurrent aspiration. The antisynthetase syndrome is characterized by specific autoantibodies (anti-Jo1 being the most common) that are cytoplasmic and may not result in a positive antinuclear antibody. Clinical manifestations include lung fibrosis, arthritis, Raynaud phenomenon, and myositis. The finding of "mechanic's hands" in these patients is a clue to lung involvement (Figure 15.2).

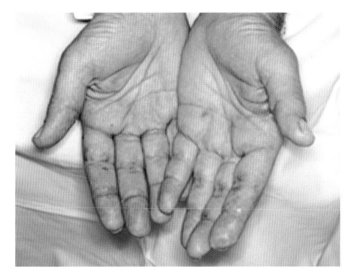

Figure 15.2 Dermatomyositis. "Mechanic's hands" are characterized by roughening and fissures of the skin on the lateral and palmar areas of the fingers. (Adapted from Khambatta S, Wittich CM. Amyopathic dermatomyositis. Mayo Clin Proc. 2010 Nov;85[11]:e82. Used with permission of Mayo Foundation for Medical Education and Research.)

SCLERODERMA

Scleroderma (systemic sclerosis) is associated with fibrosis (NSIP, OP, or less commonly UIP) and pulmonary hypertension (in up to 25% of the patients), particularly in limited scleroderma or CREST syndrome. Scleroderma may also cause recurrent aspiration due to esophageal dysmotility. Lymphocytic interstitial pneumonia (thought to represent a low-grade lymphoproliferative disorder) is a classic manifestation of Sjögren lung disease.

- RA-ILD affects more men than women and tends to have a UIP pattern.
- Acute lupus pneumonitis has a poor prognosis.
- Limited scleroderma is associated with pulmonary hypertension, while systemic sclerosis is associated with pulmonary fibrosis.

DRUG- AND THERAPY-INDUCED LUNG DISEASES

Various pharmacologic agents may cause drug-induced lung disease. Discontinuing use of the drug is mandatory and usually results in prompt clinical improvement. The use of corticosteroids is often recommended, but the evidence for this practice is anecdotal at best. The drugs discussed below should be presumed to be responsible for lung disease until proven otherwise.

Bleomycin Lung Toxicity

Bleomycin lung toxicity is the prototype of drug-induced lung disease. This antibiotic chemotherapeutic agent is used in various malignancies, primarily in Hodgkin disease. The toxicity is cumulative (and therefore subacute or chronic), resulting in progressive fibrosis that may be indistinguishable from IPF. Lung toxicity may be exacerbated by concurrent radiotherapy, renal failure, and high fractions of inspired oxygen. Rarely, the onset may be acute and associated with eosinophilia.

Methotrexate

Methotrexate may cause a hypersensitivity reaction that occurs early in the treatment. The typical manifestation is sarcoidosis-like, with bilateral hilar lymphadenopathy and diffuse lung infiltrates. Eosinophilia is present in 50% of the cases. Bronchoscopic lung biopsies may reveal ill-defined granulomas, and the cell count and differential count on BAL are similar to those in sarcoidosis with lymphocytic predominance. Sometimes the CD4:CD8 ratio is increased. Opportunistic infections should be excluded.

Nitrofurantoin

Nitrofurantoin is an antibiotic used to treat and prevent urinary tract infections. It may cause potentially life-threatening acute forms of lung toxicity (eosinophilic pneumonia) in 1 in 500 to 1 in 5,000 patients. A chronic form, similar in presentation to IPF, occurs in 1 in 50,000 patients. Discontinuing use of the drug is mandatory.

Amiodarone

Amiodarone, a drug commonly used in cardiovascular medicine, can cause lung toxicity, which is cumulative in the majority of cases after exposure to amiodarone at a dosage of more than 400 mg daily for 3 to 6 months. One particular radiologic characteristic of amiodarone lung toxicity is the presence of high-attenuation infiltrates on non-contrast HRCT, owing to the high iodine content of amiodarone. Treatment consists of discontinuing use of the drug, but because of its long half-life (2–3 months), clinical improvement may be delayed.

Illicit Substances

The use of illicit substances should be investigated. Opiate products cause pulmonary edema, and crack cocaine causes various lung manifestations, including eosinophilic pneumonia ("crack lung"), HP, bronchospasm, and diffuse alveolar hemorrhage.

Chemotherapy and Radiotherapy

A history of chemotherapy or radiotherapy (or both) should suggest the possibility of iatrogenic lung disease. Radiation pneumonitis typically occurs within 6 to 12 weeks of treatment and is usually limited to the field of radiation, but it may also affect other areas (including the contralateral lung, owing to OP). Treatment with corticosteroids may help, but progression toward chronic fibrosis may become evident months after treatment.

- Bleomycin toxicity is exacerbated by radiotherapy, uremia, and high fractions of inspired oxygen.

- Methotrexate lung disease resembles sarcoidosis.

- Lung infiltrates in females with recurrent urinary tract infections should suggest nitrofurantoin lung toxicity.

- High-attenuation lung infiltrates suggest amiodarone lung toxicity.

PNEUMOCONIOSES

Asbestos-Related Lung Diseases

Asbestos-related lung diseases should be suspected in patients with high-risk occupations (eg, insulation work, ship building, mining). Most pulmonary manifestations occur after a prolonged dormant period of 20 to 40 years, except for benign asbestos-related pleural effusion, which may occur within 10 years of exposure. Calcified pleural (or pericardial) plaques are a marker for asbestos exposure, but they do not generally cause symptoms. Other lung manifestations include the following:

- Asbestosis:

  a. An ILD with similarities to IPF, but asbestosis carries a better prognosis

  b. Treatment is supportive; corticosteroids are not indicated

- Rounded atelectasis:

  a. A focal subpleural opacity often confused with lung cancer

- Malignancy:

  a. Mesothelioma: a primary pleural malignancy with poor prognosis and few therapeutic options

  b. Bronchogenic carcinoma: although smoking is not a risk factor for mesothelioma, it acts synergistically with asbestos exposure and exponentially increases the risk of bronchogenic carcinoma

Silicosis

Silicosis occurs in patients exposed to silica (eg, mining, quarrying, sandblasting). The disease is distinct from asbestosis, and findings include bilateral hilar lymphadenopathy (occasionally eggshell calcifications) with clustered micronodular infiltrates that typically favor the apices of the lungs (as opposed to asbestosis which, like IPF, typically predominates in the bases). There are 3 characteristic associations:

1. Silicosis is a risk factor for tuberculosis, which should be excluded in patients whose respiratory condition worsens.

2. An association with connective tissue diseases has been described (Caplan syndrome).

3. Silicosis may be an independent risk factor for lung cancer, although to a much lesser extent than asbestos exposure.

- Asbestos exposure may result in pleural effusions, rounded atelectasis, fibrosis (asbestosis), mesothelioma, and bronchogenic carcinoma.

- Silicosis resembles sarcoidosis radiologically.

- Silicosis is associated with mycobacterial infections, connective tissue diseases, and lung cancer.

IDIOPATHIC INTERSTITIAL PNEUMONIAS

IDIOPATHIC PULMONARY FIBROSIS

IPF is the most common idiopathic interstitial pneumonia, and it affects males and females older than 50 years. The pathophysiology remains elusive but is thought to be secondary to poor wound healing of the lung characterized by exuberant fibrosis without underlying inflammation. No treatment has been effective; corticosteroids should not be used. Lung transplant is an option for selected patients.

UIP is a histopathologic diagnosis necessary for the diagnosis of IPF, but it may be seen in other diseases (eg, asbestosis, drug-induced lung disease, HP, CTD-ILD). Either a radiologic diagnosis (HRCT) or a histopathologic diagnosis of UIP is acceptable (ie, a surgical lung biopsy is not necessary if HRCT demonstrates typical IPF with honeycombing, traction bronchiectases, and basal predominance). Biopsy may precipitate an acute exacerbation, a life-threatening complication of IPF. Other complications include pulmonary hypertension and pneumothorax. The prognosis is poor; median survival is approximately 3 to 5 years. Other conditions associated with UIP should be excluded, since they may be more responsive to treatment.

- Corticosteroids are not useful in IPF and should not be used.

- A surgical lung biopsy is not needed to diagnose UIP when HRCT shows typical IPF; surgical lung biopsy may trigger an acute exacerbation.

NONSPECIFIC INTERSTITIAL PNEUMONIA

NSIP is the main differential diagnosis for IPF. Patients with NSIP present at a younger age (<50 years) and females predominate over males (2:1). The frequent presence of autoantibodies suggests that NSIP may be, at least in some cases, an autoimmune process. Radiologically, NSIP shows homogeneous involvement of the lungs, ground-glass opacities, and limited honeycombing and traction bronchiectases. NSIP is also a histopathologic diagnosis that may occur in other diseases (eg, CTD-ILD, HP, infections). Treatment with corticosteroids is usually effective, and the 5-year survival (about 80%) is much better than with IPF.

- NSIP responds to corticosteroids.

CRYPTOGENIC ORGANIZING PNEUMONIA

Cryptogenic organizing pneumonia (COP) was formerly known as idiopathic bronchiolitis obliterans with organizing pneumonia (BOOP). Typically, COP manifests as a recurrent flulike illness resistant to antibiotics with migratory infiltrates that progress over several months. Histopathologically, it is an alveolar-filling process (with intra-alveolar plugs of granulation tissue). The radiologic features include consolidation and ground-glass infiltrates (usually peripheral), and the pattern on PFTs is that of restriction rather than obstruction. Thus, BOOP is a misnomer (there is little bronchiolar involvement). COP is exquisitely responsive to treatment with corticosteroids, which should be administered for 3 to 6 months. Rebound after discontinuation is common, but COP generally responds to retreatment with corticosteroids. The absence of prompt improvement should suggest the possibility of secondary OP rather than COP. The most common underlying diagnoses are drug-induced lung disease, CTD-ILD, and hematologic malignancies.

- Persistent pneumonia with migratory infiltrates suggests COP.
- COP is exquisitely responsive to corticosteroids.
- Rebound is frequent after discontinuation of treatment.

Although not considered an idiopathic interstitial pneumonia, chronic eosinophilic pneumonia manifests much like COP, with recurrent flulike episodes and migratory, peripheral infiltrates (typically described as a "photographic negative of pulmonary edema"). It is also exquisitely responsive to corticosteroids and, like in COP, rebound is frequent after discontinuation of treatment. The main differences with COP are the upper lung predominance of the infiltrates and the eosinophilic infiltration of the lungs (peripheral eosinophilia is present in two-thirds of the cases).

- Chronic eosinophilic pneumonia resembles COP but affects the upper portions of the lungs and is characterized by pulmonary eosinophilia.

ACUTE INTERSTITIAL PNEUMONIA

Acute interstitial pneumonia (AIP), or Hamman-Rich syndrome, is characterized histologically by diffuse alveolar damage (presence of hyaline membranes), the histologic hallmark of acute respiratory distress syndrome (ARDS). In fact, the term *AIP* is equivalent to *idiopathic ARDS*. As with ARDS, the mortality is high (about 50%), but survivors have the potential for near-complete respiratory recovery.

ACUTE EOSINOPHILIC PNEUMONIA

Another rare type of idiopathic ARDS is acute eosinophilic pneumonia (not to be confused with chronic eosinophilic pneumonia); patients present with acute ARDS and eosinophilic infiltration of the lungs. The presentation is often dramatic and leads to acute respiratory failure and a need for mechanical ventilation. Affected persons are young; typically, they recently began smoking. The disease has affected military personnel returning from the Middle East. Acute eosinophilic pneumonia responds dramatically to corticosteroids without rebound after discontinued use. Treatment can be short (2 weeks). Pulmonary eosinophilia is common, but peripheral eosinophilia is rare.

- AIP, or Hamman-Rich syndrome, is idiopathic ARDS.
- Acute eosinophilic pneumonia is similar to AIP but is characterized by eosinophilic infiltration of the lungs and a dramatic response to corticosteroids.

DESQUAMATIVE INTERSTITIAL PNEUMONIA AND RESPIRATORY BRONCHIOLITIS– INTERSTITIAL LUNG DISEASE

Desquamative interstitial pneumonia (DIP) and respiratory bronchiolitis–interstitial lung disease (RB-ILD) are rare. Although classified as idiopathic, they are considered smoking-related lung diseases. They belong to the same spectrum of disease, with DIP on one end (primarily alveolar disease) and RB-ILD on the other (bronchiolar disease). Initially thought to be secondary to "desquamated" epithelial cells, the disease is now understood to result from the accumulation of pigment-laden macrophages in the airspaces (DIP) or around the bronchioles (RB-ILD) (or both). Smoking cessation is warranted and, if achieved, the prognosis is good.

- DIP and RB-ILD are smoking-related lung diseases, and smoking cessation is recommended.

GRANULOMATOUS ILDS

SARCOIDOSIS

Sarcoidosis is a granulomatous disease of unknown cause that typically affects patients younger than 50 years (African American females predominate). Patients may present with acute or gradual-onset lung disease, with possible progression toward end-stage diffuse fibrotic lung disease.

Sarcoidosis is one of the few lung diseases that predominantly affect nonsmokers and former nonsmokers (along with HP). Although the lungs (>90% of cases) and lymph nodes are the most commonly involved organs, the disease can affect virtually any organ, including the heart, liver, spleen, eye, bone, skin, bone marrow, parotid glands, pituitary, and reproductive organs, and the nervous system. Hypercalcemia, anemia, and increased liver enzyme levels may be noted. Familial clusters of sarcoidosis have been reported. The course of the disease is highly variable, from asymptomatic to life-threatening.

Imaging

Radiographic stage correlates with the severity of pulmonary disease and prognosis as follows:

- Stage 0: normal CXR.
- Stage I: hilar adenopathy.
- Stage II: hilar adenopathy with pulmonary infiltrates.
- Stage III: infiltrates without adenopathy.
- Stage IV: fibrotic lung disease.

CXR may also show characteristic bilateral hilar or mediastinal lymphadenopathy with occasional eggshell calcifications. Computed tomography of the chest may show clustered micronodules with a bronchovascular and subpleural distribution.

Diagnosis

In most cases, granulomatous histopathologic features need to be identified and other causes of granulomatous inflammation excluded (primarily fungal, mycobacterial, and other infections). If hilar adenopathy and parenchymal infiltrates are present, bronchoscopy with biopsy confirms granulomatous changes in more than 90% of cases. Thus, sarcoidosis must be considered a diagnosis of exclusion after other causes of granulomatous disease have been ruled out. The serum levels of angiotensin-converting enzyme are not sufficiently sensitive or specific to be of diagnostic value, but they may be helpful as a marker of disease activity.

Treatment

Corticosteroids are first-line therapy. However, whether immunosuppressive therapy, including corticosteroids, alters the natural course of the disease is debated. Other immunosuppressive regimens used as second-line therapy for pulmonary sarcoidosis have included methotrexate, azathioprine, pentoxifylline, and cyclosporine. Treatment is reserved for severe organ disease (including progressive lung disease). In up to 90% of patients with stage I pulmonary sarcoidosis, the disease is expected to remain stable or to resolve spontaneously with no treatment. Stage III pulmonary sarcoidosis is expected to spontaneously remit in only 10% of patients. Pulmonary sarcoidosis is expected to progress within 2 to 5 years after diagnosis, although increased disease activity can occur at any time.

- Sarcoidosis affects the lungs in 90% of cases and extrapulmonary organs in 30% of cases.
- Treatment with corticosteroids is indicated for only severe manifestations of the disease.

HYPERSENSITIVITY PNEUMONITIS

HP is an uncommon form of ILD. It is considered an allergic reaction to various organic antigens, including molds, grain dusts (farmer's lung), pets and birds (bird fancier's lung), and mycobacterial antigens (hot tub lung). Serum precipitins for specific antigens are inconsistently specific and have poor sensitivity for diagnostic purposes. The symptoms and clinical course are related temporally to antigen exposure. With acute disease, patients may have dyspnea, cough, fever, chest pain, headache, malaise, fatigue, and flulike illness. Chronic diffuse fibrotic lung disease may be indistinguishable from IPF.

The histopathologic features of HP show a range of bronchiolar-oriented, ill-defined, noncaseating granulomas with lymphocytic-predominant centrilobular infiltrates and varying degrees of fibrosis. A restrictive pattern is common on PFTs, although an airway component may also be present and result in an obstructive component. Bronchodilators may be needed to treat airflow obstruction. CXR generally shows reticulonodular changes, and HRCT often shows nonspecific nodules and ground-glass opacities predominantly in the upper lobes. Acute symptoms generally improve after the patient is no longer exposed to the antigen. Severe cases require treatment with corticosteroids.

- The granulomas in HP are poorly defined.
- Treatment consists of avoidance of allergens and, sometimes, administration of corticosteroids.

OTHER GRANULOMATOUS DISEASES

Other granulomatous diseases include infections such as fungal or mycobacterial infections. The granulomas are usually necrotizing, as opposed to those in sarcoidosis and HP. Wegener granulomatosis and Churg-Strauss syndrome should also be in the differential diagnosis. Response to intravenous injection of insoluble material, such as intravenous talcosis (as occurs in intravenous drug users), may result in diffuse lung granulomas centered on foreign bodies that are birefringent in polarized light.

OTHER ILDS

PULMONARY LANGERHANS CELL HISTIOCYTOSIS

PLCH is a rare cystic lung disease mostly affecting young white smokers. Spontaneous pneumothoraces are common (25% of cases). CXR shows diffuse interstitial infiltrates with classic cystic and micronodular changes, predominantly in the upper lobes. The distinctive nodular component and upper lobe predominance seen on HRCT differentiate PLCH from LAM (see below). Restriction is common, but a mixed pattern is also classically described. In the systemic variant of the disease (more common in children), there may be bone involvement and pituitary insufficiency (central diabetes insipidus). The combination of exophthalmos, diabetes insipidus, and lytic bone lesions (often in the skull) is known as Hand-Schüller-Christian disease. Aggregates of Langerhans cells interspersed with normal lung parenchyma are the characteristic histopathologic finding. An increase in the number of Langerhans cells can be detected by staining BAL specimens for CD1a (typically >5%), which is overexpressed in these cells. Absolute cessation of smoking is mandatory. The response to abstinence from all tobacco products varies, with stabilization or improvement noted in as many as two-thirds of patients. Langerhans cell histiocytosis increases the risk of bronchogenic cancer and lymphoma. The success of corticosteroid treatment and chemotherapy has been limited. Transplant is reserved for advanced, progressive disease.

- PLCH is another smoking-related lung disease, and cessation of smoking is mandatory.
- Pneumothorax is common in PLCH.
- Think of PLCH in a young smoker with pneumothoraces.

LYMPHANGIOLEIOMYOMATOSIS

LAM is a disease of women of childbearing age that may be associated with tuberous sclerosis (in up to 20% of cases). It is characterized clinically by a history of recurrent pneumothoraces (50%-80%), chylous pleural effusions (30%), diffuse infiltrates with hypoxemia, and airflow obstruction. Hemoptysis is common (25%). HRCT typically demonstrates well-defined cysts scattered homogeneously throughout the lungs, without nodules or interstitial fibrosis. Pregnancy or exogenous estrogens may worsen the course of the disease. The histopathologic features, similar to those of tuberous sclerosis, include a distinctive proliferation of atypical interstitial smooth muscle and thin-walled cysts within the lung. Extrapulmonary involvement may include uterine leiomyomas and renal angiomyolipomas. The response to treatment with hormonal manipulation has been limited. Currently, lung transplant is the definitive treatment. Sirolimus appears promising in the management of LAM.

- Cystic lung disease or recurrent pneumothoraces in young females suggest LAM.

- Pneumothorax, hemoptysis, chylous pleural effusions, and retroperitoneal pain or hemorrhage from ruptured angiomyolipomas are common.

PULMONARY ALVEOLAR PROTEINOSIS

PAP is a rare, idiopathic form of diffuse lung disease characterized by the filling of alveoli with proteinaceous material consisting mostly of phospholipoprotein (dipalmitoyl lecithin). A defect in the signaling of granulocyte-macrophage colony-stimulating factor (GM-CSF) is thought to contribute to the clinical manifestations. Most patients are smokers younger than 50 years, with a male predominance (male to female ratio, 3:1). Symptoms of dyspnea, cough, and low-grade fever are common. Many infectious, occupational, inflammatory, and environmental secondary causes of PAP-like presentations have been recognized. Increased predisposition to *Nocardia* infections has been reported. CXR may show an alveolar filling pattern infiltrate that resembles bat wings, mimicking pulmonary edema. A nonspecific but characteristic alveolar filling pattern seen with HRCT, described as a "crazy-paving" pattern with airspace consolidation and thickened interlobular septa, is suggestive of PAP. A milky white return of BAL fluid or lung biopsy findings usually indicate the diagnosis. In addition to smoking cessation, therapy has involved whole-lung lavage and, more recently, trials of GM-CSF.

- PAP is often due to a deficiency in GM-CSF or to autoantibodies directed against GM-CSF.
- Treatment with whole-lung lavage remains the standard of care for severe cases, although GM-CSF supplementation is sometimes effective.

SUMMARY

Diffuse lung disease includes a wide range of idiopathic and secondary lung disease processes that have various presentations and prognoses. A focused, complete medical history and physical examination in combination with judicious use of laboratory data, PFTs, chest imaging, bronchoscopy, and open lung biopsy when needed can narrow the differential diagnosis, provide important prognostic information, and guide therapeutic interventions.

16.

PULMONARY VASCULAR DISEASE, PULMONARY EMBOLISM, AND PULMONARY HYPERTENSION

Karen L. Swanson, DO

GOALS

- Characterize pulmonary vascular diseases, including pulmonary vasculitides.

- Describe the identification and management of patients with pulmonary embolism (PE) and pulmonary hypertension (PH).

PULMONARY VASCULAR DISEASE

Pulmonary vascular disease includes pulmonary vascular tumors, malformations, vasculitides, and lymphatic disorders.

PULMONARY VASCULAR TUMORS

Pulmonary vascular tumors are rare and usually metastatic at diagnosis. They may arise from the aorta, inferior vena cava, pulmonary arteries, or veins. Sarcomas and leiomyosarcomas are the most common tumors and may mimic pulmonary embolism. Breast, lung, prostate, pancreas, liver, and stomach cancers may metastasize to the pulmonary vasculature.

PULMONARY ARTERIOVENOUS MALFORMATION

Pulmonary arteriovenous malformations (PAVMs) directly communicate between pulmonary arteries and veins and bypass the pulmonary capillaries (Figure 16.1). Right-to-left shunting causes hypoxemia, brain abscesses, and stroke (through paradoxical embolism). PAVMs lack structural integrity and can rupture, leading to hemorrhagic complications including hemothorax.

PAVM may be idiopathic or acquired (from trauma, surgical procedures, or actinomycosis), or it may occur with hereditary hemorrhagic telangiectasia (HHT). PAVM occurs in 30% to 50% of cases of HHT, which is an autosomal dominant anomaly. Diagnostic criteria for HHT include telangiectasias (fingers, lips, and tongue), epistaxis (spontaneous and recurrent), visceral arteriovenous malformation (brain, lung, liver, and gastrointestinal tract), and family history.

Patients may report dyspnea and are often hypoxemic; both conditions worsen with exertion. Examination findings include clubbing and pulmonary bruit. Diagnosis is made with bubble echocardiography (to demonstrate intrapulmonary shunting) or through radionuclide or computed tomographic (CT) scanning. The mainstay of treatment is embolization through pulmonary angiography and, rarely, surgery.

- PAVM may be idiopathic or acquired, or it may occur with HHT.

- PAVM causes right-to-left shunting, leading to brain abscess, stroke, or hypoxemia.

- Think of PAVM in a young person with stroke.

HEPATOPULMONARY SYNDROME

Hepatopulmonary syndrome (HPS) is a complication of chronic liver disease. The diagnostic triad includes evidence of liver disease, intrapulmonary shunting, and hypoxemia. Hypoxemia is identified by an increased alveolar-arterial difference in Po_2—the $P(A-a)o_2$ gradient. The only treatment is liver transplant, which resolves hypoxemia and improves survival. HPS patients with Pao_2 less than 60 mm Hg receive exception points in the Model for End-Stage Liver Disease (MELD) scoring system and are given higher transplant priority because symptoms resolve with liver transplant.

- Liver transplant is the treatment of choice in HPS.

PULMONARY ARTERY ANEURYSM

Pulmonary artery aneurysms are usually asymptomatic and discovered on routine chest imaging. Many patients do not require treatment other than serial observation. Surgical indications include hemoptysis, continued growth, or refractory hypoxemia due to right-to-left shunting through the aneurysm.

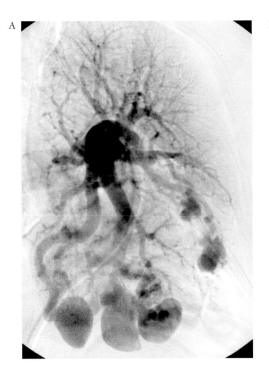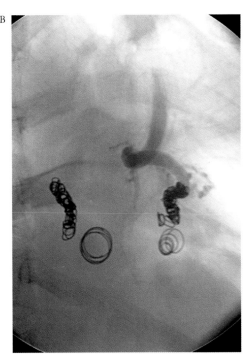

Figure 16.1 A, Pulmonary angiography documenting the presence of multiple, large pulmonary arteriovenous malformations. B, After coil embolization, there is complete lack of flow through the pulmonary arteriovenous malformations.

PULMONARY CAPILLARY HEMANGIOMATOSIS

Pulmonary capillary hemangiomatosis is a severe, idiopathic proliferation of pulmonary capillaries that is usually accompanied by PH. Symptoms include dyspnea, hemoptysis, and edema. CT scan shows a diffuse reticulonodular pattern with enlarged central pulmonary arteries. The diagnosis requires lung biopsy, which is usually not performed owing to excessive risk. There is no effective treatment. Median survival is 3 years without transplant.

PULMONARY VASCULITIDES

The pulmonary vasculitides are a heterogeneous group of disorders of unknown cause characterized by inflammation and necrosis of the arteries and sometimes veins. Signs and symptoms include fever, malaise, weight loss, palpable purpura, mononeuritis multiplex, arthralgias, and renal insufficiency. Specific pulmonary manifestations include hemoptysis, stridor, cough, and dyspnea.

GRANULOMATOSIS WITH POLYANGIITIS (WEGENER GRANULOMATOSIS)

Granulomatosis with polyangiitis (GPA) is a systemic vasculitis of small or medium-sized arteries and veins characterized by necrotizing granulomas of the upper and lower respiratory tract, glomerulonephritis, and small-vessel vasculitis. Most GPA (>90%) affects white persons. The male to female ratio is 2:1.

Affected organs include the ear, nose, and throat (rhinorrhea, purulent or bloody nasal discharge, nasal mucosal drying and crust formation, otitis media, and hearing loss), lungs (hemoptysis and alveolar hemorrhage), kidney (rapidly progressive glomerulonephritis), and skin (purpura and cutaneous nodules). Arthralgias and mononeuritis multiplex also occur. Two important signs of GPA are nasal septal perforation and ulceration of the vomer bone. The differential diagnosis of the saddle-nose deformity includes GPA, relapsing polychondritis, and leprosy. Massive alveolar hemorrhage is a life-threatening emergency. Clinical manifestations range from subacute to rapidly progressive respiratory failure.

- Major organs affected are represented by the mnemonic *ELKS* (*e*ar, nose, and throat; *l*ungs; *k*idney; and *s*kin).

- Important signs of GPA are nasal septal perforation and ulceration of the vomer bone.

- Differential diagnosis of saddle-nose deformity: GPA, relapsing polychondritis, and leprosy.

- Typical clinical scenario for GPA: The patient has systemic disease with major respiratory manifestations and renal involvement with focal segmental glomerulonephritis.

Laboratory tests may show a normocytic anemia, mild leukocytosis, mild thrombocytosis, positive rheumatoid factor, and a highly increased erythrocyte sedimentation rate (often >100 mm/h). Urinalysis may show hematuria, proteinuria, and red cell casts in 80% of patients.

Antineutrophil cytoplasmic autoantibodies (ANCAs) are used to corroborate the diagnosis of GPA. The 2 main patterns of ANCA are cytoplasmic (c-ANCA), which is directed to proteinase 3, and perinuclear (p-ANCA), which is targeted to myeloperoxidase (MPO). c-ANCA is highly specific and sensitive for GPA and is present in more than 90% of patients who have systemic disease. In active disease, the sensitivity is 91%, and the specificity is 98%; in inactive disease, the sensitivity is 63%, and the specificity is 99.5%.

- Positive c-ANCA without clinical evidence of disease does not establish the diagnosis.

- Some patients with active disease have negative c-ANCA.

- c-ANCA may be present in other diseases (eg, hepatitis C, microscopic polyangiitis, ulcerative colitis, sulfasalazine toxicity).

p-ANCA is positive in various diseases, including inflammatory bowel disease, autoimmune liver disease, rheumatoid arthritis, and other vasculitides. p-ANCA with specificity against MPO is closely associated with microscopic polyangiitis, leukocytoclastic vasculitis, pauci-immune necrotizing crescentic glomerulonephritis, and other vasculitides, including Churg-Strauss syndrome.

- Positive p-ANCA results occur in other vasculitides and collagen diseases.

- The presence of p-ANCA with specificity for MPO should suggest small-vessel vasculitis (microscopic polyangiitis).

The combination of corticosteroids and cyclophosphamide produces complete remission in more than 90% of patients with limited GPA. In severe GPA, intravenous corticosteroids and rituximab are recommended. Trimethoprim-sulfamethoxazole is effective in preventing disease relapse.

EOSINOPHILIC GRANULOMATOSIS WITH POLYANGIITIS (CHURG-STRAUSS SYNDROME)

Eosinophilic granulomatosis with polyangiitis is characterized by pulmonary and systemic vasculitis, extravascular granulomas, increased levels of IgE, and eosinophilia in patients with asthma or allergy. Allergic rhinitis, nasal polyps, nasal mucosal crusting, and septal perforation occur in more than 70% of patients. Almost all patients have refractory asthma. In more than 60% of patients, chest radiography (CXR) shows patchy and occasionally diffuse alveolar-interstitial infiltrates with a predilection for the upper two-thirds of the lungs. Pleural effusions develop in up to one-third. The response to systemic corticosteroids is dramatic.

- Features of eosinophilic granulomatosis with polyangiitis include refractory asthma, progressive respiratory distress, allergic rhinitis, nasal polyps, nasal mucosal crusting, septal perforation, tissue and blood eosinophilia, and increased levels of IgE.

GIANT CELL ARTERITIS

Giant cell arteritis, also known as temporal arteritis, cranial arteritis, and granulomatous arteritis, should be considered when older patients have a new cough or throat pain without an obvious cause. In fact, 10% of patients have prominent respiratory symptoms. Histopathology shows mononuclear infiltrates with giant cell formation in medium-sized and large pulmonary arteries. Pulmonary nodules, interstitial infiltrations, pulmonary artery occlusion, and aneurysms have been described. The response to corticosteroids is favorable.

- Respiratory symptoms are prominent in 10% of patients with giant cell arteritis.

- Cough, sore throat, and hoarseness occur in older persons without an obvious cause.

BEHÇET DISEASE

Behçet disease is a chronic, relapsing, multisystemic inflammatory disorder characterized by aphthous orogenital ulcerations (in >65% of patients), uveitis, cutaneous nodules or pustules, synovitis, and meningoencephalitis. Superficial venous thrombosis, deep vein thrombosis (DVT) of upper and lower extremities, and thrombosis of the inferior and superior venae cavae occur in 7% to 37% of patients. Pulmonary vascular involvement produces severe hemoptysis that is initially responsive to corticosteroids but which tends to recur; death is due to hemoptysis in 39% of patients. CXR may show lung infiltrates, pleural effusions, prominent pulmonary arteries, and pulmonary artery aneurysms. Aneurysms of the pulmonary artery communicating with the bronchial tree (bronchovascular anastomosis) should be considered in patients with Behçet disease and massive hemoptysis. Because of the high incidence of DVT, PE is common. Corticosteroids and chemotherapeutic agents have been used. The prognosis is poor if the patient experiences marked hemoptysis.

- Behçet disease: aphthous orogenital ulcerations, uveitis, cutaneous nodules, and meningoencephalitis.

- Severe hemoptysis is the cause of death in 39% of patients.

- A fistula between the airway and vascular structures is common.

- High incidence of DVT and PE.

TAKAYASU ARTERITIS

Takayasu arteritis, also known as pulseless disease, aortic arch syndrome, and reversed coarctation, is a chronic inflammatory disease of unknown cause affecting the aorta and its major branches, including the proximal coronary arteries, renal arteries, and the elastic pulmonary arteries. The pulmonary arteries are involved in more than 50% of patients, with lesions in medium-sized and large arteries. Perfusion lung scans show abnormalities in more than 75% of patients; pulmonary angiography shows arterial occlusion in 86%. Takayasu arteritis is most prevalent in East Asia and more common in women. Corticosteroids induce remission within days to weeks. Pulmonary involvement signifies a poor prognosis.

- Takayasu arteritis: pulmonary artery involvement occurs in >50% of patients and portends a poor prognosis.

ALVEOLAR HEMORRHAGE SYNDROMES

Diffuse hemorrhage into the alveolar spaces is called *alveolar hemorrhage syndrome*. Disruption of pulmonary capillaries (capillaritis) may result from any of the following: damage caused by different immunologic mechanisms (Goodpasture syndrome, renal-pulmonary syndromes, glomerulonephritis, and systemic lupus erythematosus), direct chemical or toxic injury (toxic or chemical inhalation, penicillamine, mitomycin, abciximab, all-*trans*-retinoic acid, trimellitic anhydride, and smoked crack cocaine), physical trauma (pulmonary contusion), and increased vascular pressure within the capillaries (mitral stenosis and severe left ventricular failure).

The severity of hemoptysis, anemia, and respiratory distress depends on the extent and rapidity of bleeding. Alveolar hemorrhage is present if hemosiderin-laden macrophages constitute more than 20% of the total alveolar macrophages recovered with bronchoalveolar lavage. The risk of alveolar hemorrhage increases with thrombocytopenia, abnormal coagulation variables, renal failure (creatinine ≥2.5 mg/dL), and heavy smoking. Treatment is with high-dose intravenous methylprednisolone or plasma exchange.

- Alveolar hemorrhage syndrome is caused by different mechanisms.
- Hemoptysis is not a consistent feature.
- Risk increases with thrombocytopenia, other coagulopathy, creatinine ≥2.5 mg/dL, and heavy smoking.
- Drugs that cause alveolar hemorrhage: penicillamine, abciximab, all-*trans*-retinoic acid, and mitomycin.

GOODPASTURE SYNDROME

Goodpasture syndrome is a classic example of a cytotoxic (type II) disease. The Goodpasture antigen (located in type IV collagen) is the primary target for the autoantibodies. The highest concentration of antigen is in the glomerular basement membrane (GBM). The alveolar basement membrane is affected by cross-reactivity with the GBM. Immunofluorescent microscopy shows linear deposition of IgG and complement along basement membranes. Anti-GBM antibody is positive in more than 90% of patients, but it is also present in persons exposed to influenza virus, hydrocarbons, or penicillamine and in some patients with systemic lupus erythematosus. The cause of Goodpasture syndrome is unknown.

- Goodpasture syndrome is a classic example of a cytotoxic (type II) disease.
- Anti-GBM antibody is positive in >90% of patients.
- Anti-GBM antibody is also present in persons exposed to influenza virus, hydrocarbons, or penicillamine and in some patients with systemic lupus erythematosus.

Patients with anti-GBM antibody–mediated nephritis demonstrate 2 principal patterns of disease: 1) young men presenting in their 20s with Goodpasture syndrome (glomerulonephritis and lung hemorrhage) and 2) elderly patients, especially women, presenting in their 60s with glomerulonephritis alone. In the classic form of Goodpasture syndrome (in younger patients), men are affected more often than women (male to female ratio, 7:1) and the average age at onset is approximately 27 years. Recurrent hemoptysis, pulmonary insufficiency, renal involvement with hematuria and renal failure, and anemia are the classic features. Pulmonary hemorrhage almost always precedes renal manifestations. Active cigarette smoking increases the risk of alveolar hemorrhage.

- Pulmonary hemorrhage almost always precedes renal manifestations.
- Active cigarette smoking increases the risk of alveolar hemorrhage.
- Typical clinical scenario for the classic form: A young man has glomerulonephritis and lung hemorrhage.
- Typical clinical scenario for the form in older patients: An elderly patient, especially a woman, has glomerulonephritis alone.

One-third of patients with anti-GBM disease test positive for p-ANCA–MPO; fulminant pulmonary hemorrhage is more likely to occur in p-ANCA–positive patients than in those who are p-ANCA–negative. Plasmapheresis is the treatment of choice. Although complete recovery can be expected in most patients treated with systemic corticosteroids, immunosuppressive agents, or plasmapheresis, relapse occurs in up to 7%.

- One-third of patients with anti-GBM disease test positive for p-ANCA–MPO.
- Patients with positive p-ANCA–MPO are more likely to have fulminant pulmonary hemorrhage.
- Plasmapheresis is the treatment of choice.

MICROSCOPIC POLYANGIITIS

Microscopic polyangiitis is distinct from classic polyarteritis nodosa, which typically affects medium-sized arteries. Pulmonary capillaritis is the most common lesion in microscopic polyangiitis but does not occur in classic polyarteritis nodosa. Microscopic polyangiitis is a systemic vasculitis associated with renal involvement in 80% of patients, characterized by rapidly progressive glomerulonephritis. Other features include weight loss (in 70% of patients), skin involvement (60%), fever (55%), mononeuritis multiplex (58%), arthralgias (50%), myalgias (48%), and hypertension (34%). Males are affected more frequently; median age at onset is 50 years. Alveolar hemorrhage is observed in 12% to 29% of patients and influences morbidity and mortality. ANCA (mostly p-ANCA–MPO) is detected in 75% of patients who have microscopic polyangiitis.

- Microscopic polyangiitis: progressive glomerulonephritis is a major feature.
- Pulmonary alveolar hemorrhage is observed in 12%-29% of patients.
- In 75% of patients, p-ANCA–MPO is positive.

IDIOPATHIC PULMONARY HEMOSIDEROSIS

Idiopathic pulmonary hemosiderosis (IPH) is a rare disorder of unknown cause and is a diagnosis of exclusion. Features include recurrent intra-alveolar hemorrhage, hemoptysis, transient infiltrates on CXR, and secondary iron deficiency anemia. IPH has been described in association with idiopathic thrombocytopenic purpura, autoimmune hemolytic anemia, and nontropical sprue (celiac disease).

Clinical features are chronic cough with intermittent hemoptysis, iron deficiency anemia, fever, weight loss, generalized lymphadenopathy (25% of patients), hepatosplenomegaly (20%), clubbing (15%), and eosinophilia (10%). The kidneys are not involved. Treatment is repeated blood transfusions, iron therapy, corticosteroids, and, possibly, cytotoxic agents. A 30% mortality rate within 5 years after disease onset has been reported.

- IPH is a diagnosis of exclusion.
- Generalized lymphadenopathy occurs in 25% of patients, hepatosplenomegaly in 20%, and clubbing in 15%.
- Kidneys are not involved.
- Eosinophilia occurs in 10% of patients.

PULMONARY LYMPHATIC DISORDERS

Pulmonary lymphatic disorders include lymphangioma, lymphangiomatosis, lymphangiectasis, and pulmonary lymphatic dysplastic syndromes. Pulmonary lymphatic dysplasia syndromes are a heterogeneous group of disorders. They include idiopathic lymphedema syndromes, idiopathic recurring chylous effusions, and yellow nail syndrome and are characterized by obstruction of proximal lymphatic channels with refractory accumulation of chyle. The immunoglobulin loss may result in immunodeficiency and the protein loss in malnutrition. Yellow nail syndrome consists of lymphedema, yellow dystrophic nails, and idiopathic pleural effusions or respiratory tract illness (or both) with bronchiectasis and recurrent pneumonias. The nails usually do not grow, and patients may wonder why the nails do not need to be trimmed.

- Pulmonary lymphatic disorders include lymphangioma, lymphangiomatosis, lymphangiectasis, and lymphatic dysplasia syndromes.

- Yellow nail syndrome consists of lymphedema, yellow dystrophic nails that do not grow, and idiopathic pleural effusions or recurrent lung infection (or both).

PULMONARY EMBOLISM

PE is the cause of death in 5% to 15% of hospitalized patients. Poor prognostic factors include age older than 70 years, cancer, congestive heart failure, chronic obstructive pulmonary disease, systolic arterial hypotension, tachypnea, and right ventricular hypokinesis. PE is detected in 25% to 30% of routine autopsies. Antemortem diagnosis is made in less than 30% owing to the variable and nonspecific presentation of patients with PE.

- PE is a common problem; consider PE in all patients who have lung symptoms.
- Antemortem diagnosis, made in <30% of cases, requires a high degree of awareness.
- The risk of death from untreated PE is 8%.

ETIOLOGY

The most common cause of PE is DVT of the lower extremities. In approximately 45% of patients with femoral and iliac DVT, emboli move to the lungs. Other sources of emboli include thrombi in the upper extremities, right ventricle, and indwelling catheters. The primary and secondary coagulation abnormalities that predispose to the development of DVT and PE are listed in Box 16.1. The incidence of DVT in various clinical circumstances is listed in Table 16.1. Idiopathic DVT, particularly when recurrent, may indicate the presence of neoplasm in 10% to 20% of patients. The presence of varicose veins does not increase the risk of DVT. Compression ultrasonography, the most commonly used noninvasive test, has a diagnostic accuracy of 90% to 95% in detecting iliac and femoral DVT. Serial compression ultrasonography is recommended for high-risk patients because of a 15% detection rate of DVT after an initial negative study. Magnetic resonance imaging has a high sensitivity and specificity for the diagnosis of pelvic DVT.

- DVT is detected in only 40% of cases of PE.
- Consider factor V Leiden mutation, the presence of lupus anticoagulant, and deficiencies of antithrombin III, protein S, and protein C among predisposing factors for DVT and PE.
- In idiopathic recurrent DVT, look for an occult neoplasm.

DIAGNOSTIC TESTS

Physical examination, electrocardiography, CXR, blood gas abnormalities, troponins, B-type natriuretic peptide (BNP), and increased plasma D-dimer level have low specificity and sensitivity for the diagnosis of PE but, when considered

Table 16.1 INCIDENCE OF DEEP VEIN THROMBOSIS (DVT) IN VARIOUS CLINICAL CIRCUMSTANCES

CLINICAL CIRCUMSTANCE	INCIDENCE OF DVT, %
Major abdominal surgery[a]	14–33
Thoracic surgery	25–60
Gynecologic surgery	
Patient age ≤40 y	<3
Patient age >40 y	10–40
Patient age >40 y with other risks	40–70
Urologic surgery	10–40
Hip surgery	50–75
Myocardial infarction	20–40
Congestive heart failure	70
Stroke with paralysis	50–70
Postpartum	3
Trauma	20–40

[a] Odds are 1:20 without prophylaxis and 1:50 with prophylaxis.

with high levels of BNP are at higher risk of in-hospital adverse events (odds ratio, 6.8) and 30-day all-cause mortality (odds ratio, 7.6). CXR findings may be normal and electrocardiographic findings nonspecific.

- CXR findings are normal in 30% of patients.
- The classic $S_1Q_3T_3$ pattern is seen in only 15% of patients.
- A negative D-dimer test excludes PE if there is low or intermediate pretest probability.

Both the PaO_2 and the $P(A-a)O_2$ gradient may be normal in 15% to 20% of patients. The $P(A-a)O_2$ gradient shows a linear correlation with the severity of PE. A normal $P(A-a)O_2$ gradient does not exclude PE. Most patients with acute PE are hypocapnic.

- The $P(A-a)O_2$ gradient correlates linearly with the severity of PE.
- A normal $P(A-a)O_2$ gradient does not exclude PE.

Ventilation-perfusion scanning is less commonly used in the diagnosis of acute PE and is generally reserved for patients with renal insufficiency or contrast allergy. A "high-probability" lung scan has a sensitivity of 41% and a specificity of 97% (90% probability of PE). A "low-probability" lung scan excludes the diagnosis of PE in more than 85% of patients. An "intermediate-probability" scan is associated with PE in 21% to 30%. Therefore, an intermediate-probability lung scan usually requires additional study. A negative or normal perfusion-only scan (excluding ventilation scan) rules out PE with a very high probability.

together, may be helpful. Plasma levels of D-dimer (a specific fibrin degradation product) are increased in DVT and PE. High levels have no positive predictive value for PE. A normal D-dimer level excludes PE in patients with low or intermediate pretest probability of PE. Age and pregnancy are associated with increased levels.

BNP and N-terminal proBNP (NT-proBNP) are specific markers of ventricular stress and have a strong correlation with right ventricular dysfunction in patients with PE. PE patients

- High-probability scan: 90% probability of PE.

- Intermediate-probability scan: 30% probability of PE.

- Low-probability scan: 15% probability of PE.

- Normal scan excludes PE in 100% of cases.

CT angiography permits ultrafast scanning of pulmonary arteries during contrast injection. Sensitivity and specificity rates greater than 95% have been reported. Spiral CT has the greatest sensitivity in the diagnosis of PE in the main, lobar, or segmental arteries. Ventilation-perfusion scanning is preferred for patients with possible chronic thromboembolic disease owing to the distal nature of the thrombotic material. Magnetic resonance imaging may have the advantage of detecting both DVT and PE. Dysfunction of the right ventricle (frequently seen in submassive, massive, and recurrent PE) can be detected with transthoracic Doppler echocardiography. Echocardiography is not necessary for all PE patients, especially those with normal BNP; however, it is extremely useful for the clinically unstable patient.

- Spiral CT has the greatest sensitivity in the diagnosis of acute PE.

- Ventilation-perfusion scan is helpful in assessing chronic thromboembolic disease.

Pulmonary angiography is the gold standard but has been largely replaced by CT angiography. It should be performed within 24 to 48 hours after the diagnosis has been considered. After pulmonary angiography, major complications occur in 1% of patients, and minor complications in 2%; mortality from the procedure is 0.5%.

TREATMENT

Goals of short-term treatment are to prevent recurrence of venous thromboembolism (extension and fatal PE) and to prevent long-term complications (late recurrence, post-thrombotic syndrome, chronic thromboembolic pulmonary hypertension). Therapy, including drug choice and duration, are discussed in detail in "Hematology: Thrombosis" (Chapter 36).

Thrombolytics

In massive PE or PE with hemodynamic instability, thrombolytic therapy is recommended. The use of thrombolytics in submassive, hemodynamically stable PE is controversial. Ideally, thrombolytic agents should be administered within 24 hours after PE. Heparin infusion is begun or resumed if the activated partial thromboplastin time is less than 80 seconds after thrombolytic therapy. The risk of intracranial bleeding in patients who have PE treated with thrombolytic drugs is about 1%.

- Thrombolytic agents should be administered within 24 hours after PE.

- Heparin therapy is necessary after thrombolytic therapy.

- Thrombolytic therapy: 1% risk of intracranial bleeding.

Inferior Vena Cava Interruption

Inferior vena cava interruption is indicated if anticoagulant therapy is contraindicated, complications result from anticoagulant therapy, anticoagulant therapy fails, a predisposition to bleeding is present, chronic recurrent PE and secondary pulmonary hypertension occur, or surgical pulmonary thromboendarterectomy has been performed or is intended to be performed. After the filter has been inserted, anticoagulant therapy is aimed at preventing DVT at the insertion site, inferior vena cava thrombosis, cephalad propagation of a clot from an occluded filter, and propagation or recurrence of lower extremity DVT. PE occurs in 2.5% of patients despite inferior vena cava interruption.

- Inferior vena cava interruption does not replace long-term anticoagulant therapy.

- PE occurs in 2.5% of patients despite inferior vena cava interruption.

PULMONARY HYPERTENSION

Elevation of pulmonary pressure (ie, PH) can be caused by an elevated pulmonary capillary wedge pressure, a high-flow state (increased cardiac output), or a true elevation in pulmonary vascular resistance (ie, pulmonary arterial hypertension [PAH]). PAH is present when the mean pulmonary arterial pressure (MPAP) is greater than 25 mm Hg at rest (or >35 mm Hg with exercise), the pulmonary capillary wedge pressure is less than 15 mm Hg, and the pulmonary vascular resistance is more than 3 Wood Units (>240 dynes·s·cm^{-5}). Pathologically, PAH is characterized by vasoconstriction, pulmonary vascular remodeling, and thrombosis in situ that leads to progressive increases in pulmonary vascular resistance, right-sided heart failure, and death. There are many causes of PH; a revised clinical classification categorizes the causes into 5 groups (Box 16.2).

- PH may be caused by an increased volume (elevated wedge pressure), a high-flow state (high cardiac output), or a true elevation in pulmonary vascular resistance (PAH).

- A revised clinical classification of PH defines 5 groups.

The clinical presentation of PH is nonspecific, and patients complain of progressive dyspnea, lower extremity edema, and fatigue. Blood testing, which may be helpful for identifying a cause for PH, includes connective tissue serologies, BNP, thyroid studies, liver enzymes, testing for human immunodeficiency virus, and a complete blood cell count. Full pulmonary function testing and overnight oximetry are essential to exclude pulmonary causes of PH. The diagnosis of PE needs to be excluded in all patients undergoing evaluation for PH.

- Blood tests and pulmonary evaluation are essential to determine the cause of PH.

- PE needs to be excluded in all patients with PH.

Typically, a diagnosis of PH is suggested by an increased right ventricular systolic pressure on transthoracic Doppler echocardiography and is confirmed with right-heart catheterization. Hemodynamic measurements at right-heart catheterization are important to exclude PH due to fluid overload or contributions from a high cardiac output (such as in liver disease, thyroid disease, or anemia). Patients who show vasoreactivity at right-heart catheterization (a decrease in MPAP or pulmonary vascular resistance by 20% with vasodilator challenge) may benefit from a trial of calcium channel blockers.

- Echocardiography is a good screening test; however, right-heart catheterization is imperative to define hemodynamic measurements.

- Rarely, patients with positive vasodilator response may respond to calcium channel blockers.

World Health Organization (WHO) functional class is a powerful predictor of survival. Patients in WHO functional class IV have a median survival of 6 months; in functional class III, 2.5 years; and in functional class I or II, 6 years. Extremes of age, decreased exercise capacity (6-minute walk distance), syncope, and signs of right ventricular failure carry a poor prognosis.

- WHO functional class is a powerful predictor of survival.

To date, no cure exists. However, several treatment options have been shown to improve quality of life, the hemodynamic profile, and survival. A meta-analysis of 23 randomized controlled trials involving PAH reported a 43% decrease in mortality and a 61% decrease in hospitalizations compared with placebo. Oxygen, diuretics, digoxin, and anticoagulation may be useful in the treatment of PAH. Other treatment options approved by the US Food and Drug Administration (FDA) for PAH patients in WHO functional class I include intravenous, subcutaneous, and inhaled prostanoids (epoprostenol, treprostinil, and iloprost); oral endothelin receptor antagonists (bosentan and ambrisentan); and oral phosphodiesterase type 5 inhibitors (sildenafil and tadalafil). Combination therapy has become the standard of care in PAH, although the long-term safety and efficacy data are not well defined. A stepwise approach appears beneficial. Drug-drug interactions are common.

- FDA-approved medications for PAH have all been shown to improve quality of life and the hemodynamic profile in randomized controlled trials.

- Combination therapy in PAH is common.

Balloon atrial septostomy confers a survival advantage for patients with Eisenmenger syndrome and PAH with patent foramen ovale. The creation of an interatrial right-to-left shunt can decompress the right heart chambers and increase left ventricular preload and cardiac output. Systemic oxygen therapy improves despite oxygen desaturation. Patients should be receiving optimal medical therapy before septostomy is considered, however, and this likely serves as a bridge to transplant.

Disease-specific therapy in PAH has reduced referral for lung transplant, but transplant is an important option for patients not responding to medical therapy. PAH patients with connective tissue disease have the worst prognosis; survival is better for PAH patients with congenital heart disease. The prognosis is poor for patients with pulmonary venoocclusive disease and pulmonary capillary hemangiomatosis due to the lack of effective medical therapy. Heart-lung and double-lung transplant have been performed.

- Consider the diagnosis of PH for patients with new-onset dyspnea.

- Transthoracic Doppler echocardiography can suggest the presence of PH; however, right-heart catheterization is diagnostic.

- Available treatment options for PAH may improve quality of life and survival.

SUMMARY

- The pulmonary vasculitides are a heterogeneous group of disorders. Patients may present with fever, malaise, weight loss, palpable purpura, mononeuritis multiplex, arthralgias, renal insufficiency, hemoptysis, stridor, cough, and dyspnea.

- Maintain a high degree of awareness for PE.

- Thorough evaluation, including pulmonary function tests and evaluation for PE, is indicated in the diagnostic workup of PH.

COMMON PULMONARY DISORDERS

John G. Park, MD

- Interpret chest radiographs and pulmonary function tests (PFTs).

- Manage obstructive airway diseases.

- Describe key features of cystic fibrosis (CF) and bronchiectasis.

- Characterize pleural fluid findings.

- Identify sleep-related breathing disorders.

SYMPTOMS AND SIGNS

COUGH

Cough is a common symptom that can be caused by lesions in the nose, pharynx, larynx, bronchi, lungs, pleura, or abdominal viscera. *Chronic cough* is cough that lasts 3 weeks or more. Most cases of chronic cough are caused by postnasal drip, asthma, gastroesophageal reflux (GERD), chronic obstructive pulmonary disease (COPD), or angiotensin-converting enzyme inhibitor (ACEI) use. In up to 90% of patients, chronic cough is due to more than 1 cause; initial treatment is usually empirical. Cough is often the presenting manifestation of asthma. ACEIs cause cough in 10% of patients who use ACEIs; there is a 10-fold decrease with use of angiotensin II receptor blocker. Bronchoscopy has a low diagnostic yield if chest radiographic (CXR) findings are normal. Complications of cough include cough syncope, rib fracture, and pneumothorax.

- Common causes of chronic cough are postnasal drip, asthma, GERD, COPD, and ACEI use.

HEMOPTYSIS

History, examination, and CXR findings are important in establishing the cause of hemoptysis. Bronchial arterial bleeding occurs in patients with chronic bronchitis, bronchiectasis, malignancies, or foreign bodies. Pulmonary arterial bleeding occurs in pulmonary arteriovenous malformations, fungus ball, tumors, vasculitis, pulmonary hypertension, and lung abscess. Pulmonary capillary bleeding occurs in mitral stenosis, left ventricular failure, pulmonary infarction, vasculitis, Goodpasture syndrome, and idiopathic pulmonary hemosiderosis. The most common cause of streaky hemoptysis is acute exacerbation of chronic bronchitis. The cause of death in massive hemoptysis is asphyxiation, not exsanguination.

- The most common cause of hemoptysis is an exacerbation of chronic bronchitis.

HISTORY AND EXAMINATION

An approach to the history and physical examination of patients with pulmonary disease is outlined in Box 17.1. Percussion and auscultation findings associated with various pulmonary conditions are listed in Table 17.1.

DIAGNOSTIC TESTS

PLAIN CHEST RADIOGRAPHY

The ability to identify normal radiographic anatomy is essential. A step-by-step method of CXR interpretation should be used so that subtle abnormalities are not missed (Table 17.2).

1. Initially, assess the CXR overall, without focusing on any specific area or abnormality.

    a. Note the extrapulmonary structures. For example, destructive shoulder arthritis may indicate rheumatoid arthritis and prompt a search for associated pulmonary manifestations. Absence of a breast shadow in a female patient should prompt evaluation for signs of pulmonary metastases of breast cancer. Visualization of a tracheostomy stoma or cannula may indicate previous laryngeal cancer, suggesting the possibility of complications such as aspiration pneumonia and lung metastases.

History
  Smoking
  Occupational exposure
  Exposure to infected persons or animals
  Hobbies & pets
  Family history of diseases of the lung & other organs
  Past malignancy
  Systemic (nonpulmonary) diseases
  Immune status (corticosteroid therapy, chemotherapy, cancer)
  History of trauma
  Previous chest radiography
Examination
  Inspection
    Respiratory rate, hoarseness of voice
    Respiratory rhythm (abnormal breathing pattern)
    Accessory muscles in action (FEV_1 <30%)
    Postural dyspnea (orthopnea, platypnea, trepopnea)
    Intercostal retraction
    Paradoxical motions of abdomen or diaphragm
    Cough (type, sputum, blood)
    Wheeze (audible with or without stethoscope)
    Pursed lip breathing or glottic wheeze (patients with COPD)
    Cyanosis (central vs peripheral)
    Conjunctival suffusion (CO_2 retention)
    Clubbing
    Thoracic cage (eg, anteroposterior diameter, kyphoscoliosis, pectus carinatum)
    Trachea, deviation
    Superior vena cava syndrome
  Asterixis, central nervous system status
  Cardiac impulse, jugular venous pressure, pedal edema (signs of cor pulmonale)
Palpation
  Clubbing
  Lymphadenopathy
  Tibial tenderness (hypertrophic pulmonary osteoarthropathy)
  Motion of thoracic cage (hand or tape measure)
  Chest wall tenderness (costochondritis, rib fracture, pulmonary embolism)
  Tracheal deviation, tenderness
  Tactile (vocal) fremitus
  Subcutaneous emphysema
  Succussion splash (effusion, air-fluid level in thorax)
Percussion
  Thoracic cage (dullness, resonance)
  Diaphragmatic motion (normal, 5–7 cm)
  Upper abdomen (liver)
Auscultation
  Tracheal auscultation
  Normal breath sounds
  Bronchial breath sounds
  Expiratory slowing
  Crackles
  Wheezes

Pleural rub
Mediastinal noises (mediastinal crunch)
Heart sounds
Miscellaneous (muscle tremor, etc)

Abbreviations: CO_2, carbon dioxide; COPD, chronic obstructive pulmonary disease; FEV_1, forced expiratory volume in the first second of expiration.

  b. Infradiaphragmatic abnormalities such as calcifications in the spleen, displacement of the gastric bubble and colon, and signs of upper abdominal surgery may indicate the cause of a pleuropulmonary process.

  c. Lateral CXRs are important in identifying retrocardiac and retrodiaphragmatic abnormalities.

• Initially look at the entire CXR.

• Look for extrapulmonary abnormalities before focusing on any obvious parenchymal findings.

2. View the skeletal thorax to exclude rib fracture, osteolytic and other lesions of the ribs, rib notching, missing ribs, and vertebral abnormalities. Changes due to previous thoracic surgical procedures (eg, coronary artery bypass, thoracotomy, lung resection, or esophageal surgery) may provide clues to the pulmonary disease.

3. Assess the intrathoracic but extrapulmonary structures such as the mediastinum (including the great vessels, esophagus, heart, lymph nodes, and thymus). A calcified mass in the region of the thyroid almost always indicates a goiter. An obliterated aortopulmonary window (a notch below the aortic knob on the left, just above the pulmonary artery) may indicate a tumor or lymphadenopathy. Right paratracheal and paramediastinal lymphadenopathy can be subtle. Hilar regions are difficult to interpret because lymphadenopathy, vascular prominence, or tumor may make the hila appear larger. The retrocardiac region may show hiatal hernia with an air-fluid level; this may be helpful in the diagnosis of reflux or aspiration.

• Note changes due to previous surgical procedures.

• Assess the mediastinal structures: esophagus, thyroid, thymus, and great vessels.

4. Examine the pleural regions for pleural effusion, pleural thickening (particularly in the apices), blunting of costophrenic angles, pleural plaques or masses, and pneumothorax. A lateral decubitus radiograph may be necessary to confirm the presence of free fluid in the pleural space. An air bronchogram depicting the major airways may indicate a large tumor (cut-off of air bronchogram) or consolidation from an infection.

5. Finally, evaluate the lung parenchyma. Notably, about 15% of the pulmonary parenchyma is located behind the heart and diaphragm; a lateral CXR is helpful in examining this region. It is important not to overinterpret increased interstitial lung markings. Generally, bronchovascular

Table 17.1 PERCUSSION AND AUSCULTATION FINDINGS IN PULMONARY CONDITIONS

CONDITION	CHEST EXPANSION	FREMITUS	RESONANCE	BREATH SOUNDS	EGOPHONY	BRONCHOPHONY
Pleural effusion[a]	Decreased	Decreased	Decreased	Decreased	Absent >> present	Absent >> present
Consolidation[b]	Decreased	Increased	Decreased	Bronchial	Present	Present
Atelectasis[c]	Decreased	Decreased	Decreased	Decreased	Absent > present	Absent > present
Pneumothorax	Variable	Decreased	Increased	Decreased	Absent	Absent

[a] The trachea is shifted contralaterally in effusion.

[b] Whispered pectoriloquy is present in consolidation.

[c] The trachea is shifted ipsilaterally in atelectasis.

markings should be visible throughout the lung parenchyma. The absence of any markings within the lung parenchyma suggests a bulla or an air-containing cyst. Apical areas should be evaluated carefully for the presence of pleural thickening, pneumothorax, small nodules, and subtle infiltrates.

- Examine the apices for thickening, pneumothorax, nodules, and subtle infiltrates.

- Examine the lung parenchyma behind the heart and diaphragm.

Common CXR abnormalities are depicted in Figures 17.1 through 17.26.

FLUOROSCOPY

Fluoroscopy is useful in localizing lesions during biopsy and aspiration procedures. It also is valuable in assessing

Table 17.2 **SYSTEMATIC APPROACH TO EVALUATION OF A CHEST RADIOGRAPH**

1. Check for patient identifier

2. Evaluate extrapulmonary structures
   Destructive arthritis
   Absence of breast shadow
   Evidence of previous surgery: sternal wires, valvular prosthesis, surgical staples demarcating previous lobectomy, etc
   Tracheostomy

3. Infradiaphragmatic abnormalities

4. Skeletal changes: rib fractures, notching, osteolytic lesions, etc

5. Intrathoracic, extrapulmonary structures: mediastinum, thyroid calcification, achalasia, aortopulmonary window, hilum, calcified adenopathy

6. Pleural region: blunting, calcification

7. Lung parenchyma: infiltrates, air bronchogram, nodules, cysts, abscess, pneumothorax

8. Lateral views to evaluate retrocardiac & retrodiaphragmatic spaces

diaphragmatic motion and in diagnosing diaphragmatic paralysis by the sniff test. Paradoxical motion of the diaphragm suggests diaphragmatic paralysis (but it is present in up to 6% of healthy subjects). Bilateral diaphragmatic paralysis diminishes the sensitivity of the test.

- Fluoroscopy is useful in diagnosing diaphragmatic paralysis through the sniff test.

COMPUTED TOMOGRAPHY

A high-resolution computed tomography (HRCT) scan can show characteristic features of pulmonary Langerhans cell granulomatosis, lymphangioleiomyomatosis, idiopathic pulmonary fibrosis, and lymphangitic pulmonary metastasis. Computed tomograpy (CT) is useful in staging lung cancer and in evaluating the presence of solitary pulmonary nodules, multiple lung nodules (metastatic), diffuse lung disease, pleural process, and calcification in nodules. Ultrafast CT with contrast media is used for diagnosing pulmonary embolism.

- HRCT is helpful in the diagnosis of intersitial lung disease.

MAGNETIC RESONANCE IMAGING

Magnetic resonance imaging (MRI) is recommended for the initial evaluation of a superior sulcus tumor (Pancoast tumor), lesions of the brachial plexus, and paraspinal masses that on CXR appear consistent with neurogenic tumors. MRI is superior to CT in evaluating chest wall masses and searching for small occult mediastinal neoplasms (eg, ectopic parathyroid adenoma).

- MRI is superior to CT in evaluating chest wall masses and searching for small occult mediastinal neoplasms.

OTHER IMAGING MODALITIES

Pulmonary angiography is useful in detecting pulmonary arteriovenous malformations, fistulas, and pulmonary embolisms. Peripheral or tiny pulmonary emboli, however, may not be

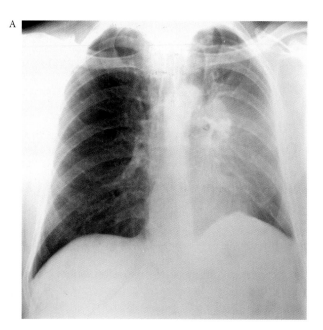
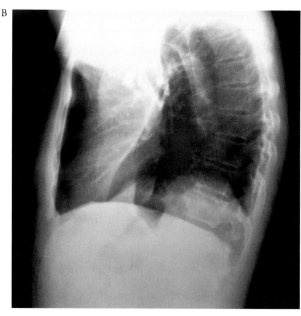

Figure 17.1 Collapsed Left Upper Lobe. A, Posteroanterior chest radiograph (CXR). B, Lateral CXR. The ground-glass haze over the left hemithorax is typical of a partially collapsed left upper lobe. In more than 50% of patients with collapsed lobes, loss of volume is evidenced by left hemidiaphragmatic elevation; the mediastinum is shifted to the left and the left hilum is pulled cranially. Also, the left main bronchus deviates cranially. Calcification in the left hilar mass represents an unrelated, old granulomatous infection. In panel B, the density from the left hilum down toward the anterior portion of the chest represents the partially collapsed left upper lobe. The radiolucency substernally is the right lung.

detected. Bronchial angiography is used for suspected bronchial arterial bleeding in massive hemoptysis. Radionuclide lung scans are used in the diagnosis of pulmonary embolism, although CT angiography is used increasingly more often. Quantitative radionuclide scans may be useful in assessing unilateral and regional pulmonary function in surgical candidates for lung resection.

- Pulmonary angiography, bronchial angiography, and radionuclide scans are useful in diagnosing lung pathology.

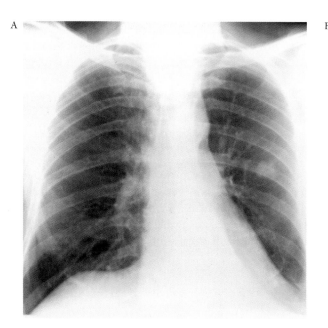
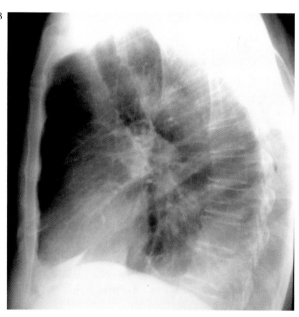

Figure 17.2 Collapsed Left Lower Lobe. A, Posteroanterior chest radiograph (CXR). B, Lateral CXR. Note nodule in left midlung field plus collapsed left lower lobe, seen as a density behind the heart. This entity represents 2 separate primary lung cancers: synchronous bronchogenic carcinomas. Do not stop with the first evident abnormality, such as the nodule in the midlung field, without looking carefully at all other areas. Panel B shows an increased density over the lower thoracic vertebrae without an obvious wedge-shaped infiltrate. Over the anterior portion of the hemidiaphragm, the small wedge-shaped infiltrate is not fluid in the left major fissure because the left major fissure is pulled away posteriorly. Instead, it is an incidental normal variant of fat pushed up into the right major fissure.

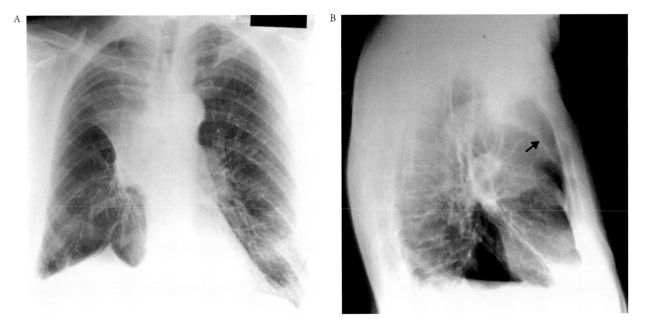

Figure 17.3 Collapsed Right Upper Lobe. A, Posteroanterior chest radiograph (CXR). B, Lateral CXR. Panel A shows classic "reversed *S*" mass in the right hilus with partial collapse of the right upper lobe. Loss of volume is evident with the elevation of the right hemidiaphragm. In panel B, the partially collapsed right upper lobe is faintly seen in the upper anterior portion of the hemithorax (arrow).

PULMONARY FUNCTION TESTS

The main indication for PFTs is dyspnea. Results of PFTs do not provide a diagnosis of lung disease, but they are useful in assessing the mechanical function of the respiratory system and quantifying lung function. PFTs can be used to distinguish obstruction, which indicates airflow limitation (eg, as in asthma, bronchitis, and emphysema), from restriction, which indicates limitation to full expansion of the lungs (eg, as in large pleural effusion or disease in the lung parenchyma, chest wall, or diaphragm). A combination of obstructive and restrictive patterns is also possible (eg, as in COPD with pulmonary fibrosis). An increase in flow rates (ie, >12% and 200 mL) after bronchodilator therapy suggests reversible component airway disease, although the absence of response does not preclude a clinical trial with inhaled bronchodilator medications.

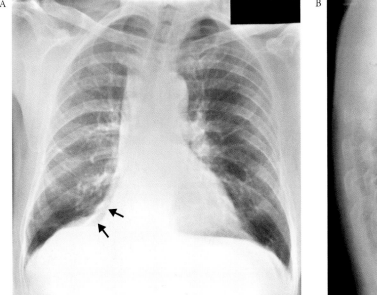
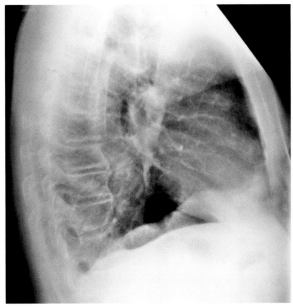

Figure 17.4 Collapsed Right Lower Lobe. A, Posteroanterior chest radiograph (CXR). B, Lateral CXR. This 75-year-old male smoker had hemoptysis for 1.5 years; his CXR had been read as "normal" on several occasions. In panel A, note the linear density (arrows) projecting downward and laterally along the right border of the heart. It projects below the diaphragm and is not a normal line. Also, the right hilum is not evident; it has been pulled centrally and downward because of carcinoma obstructing the bronchus of the right lower lobe. Note the very slight shift in the mediastinum to the right, indicative of a loss of volume. In panel B, in spite of a notable collapse of the right lower lobe, this collapse is represented by only a subtle increased density over the lower thoracic vertebrae.

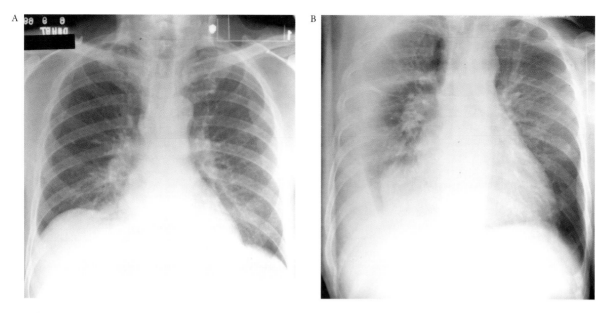

Figure 17.5 Effusion. A, Posteroanterior chest radiograph (CXR). B, Decubitus CXR. In panel A, an "elevated right hemidiaphragm" is actually an infrapulmonic (or subpulmonic) effusion, as seen in panel B. For unknown reasons, a meniscus is not formed in some people with infrapulmonic pleural effusion. Thus, a seemingly elevated hemidiaphragm should be examined with the suspicion that it could be infrapulmonic effusion. Subpulmonic effusion occurs more frequently in patients with nephrotic syndrome. Decubitus CXR or ultrasonography would disclose the free fluid.

- PFTs are useful in distinguishing between obstruction and restriction.

Provocation Inhalational Challenge

Provocation inhalational challenge with bronchospastic agents (eg, methacholine, exercise, etc) is useful when the diagnosis of asthma or hyperreactive airway disease is uncertain. A 20% decrease in forced expiratory volume in the first second

of expiration (FEV_1) from baseline is considered a positive test result, although up to 10% of healthy subjects show a positive response to an inhalational challenge. A negative test is helpful in ruling out hyperreactive airway disease. A false-positive test can result from airway hyperreactivity from recent infection or inflammation.

- A positive result with provocation is a 20% decrease in FEV_1 from baseline.

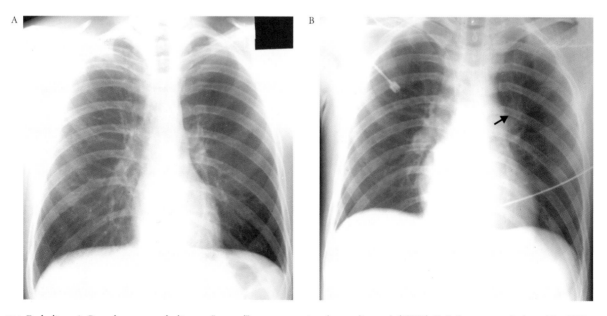

Figure 17.6 Embolism. A, Prepulmonary embolism on "normal" posteroanterior chest radiograph (CXR). B, Pulmonary embolism. The CXR is read as "normal" in up to 30% of patients with angiographically proven pulmonary embolism. In comparison with panel A, panel B shows a subtle elevation of the right hemidiaphragm. In panel A, the right and left hemidiaphragms are equal. In some series, an elevated hemidiaphragm is the most common finding with acute pulmonary embolism. Also, note the plumpness of the right pulmonary artery, prominent pulmonary outflow tract on the left (arrow in panel B), and subtle change in cardiac diameter. The patient was a 28-year-old man who was in shock from massive pulmonary emboli as a result of major soft tissue trauma produced by a motorcycle accident 7 days earlier.

A
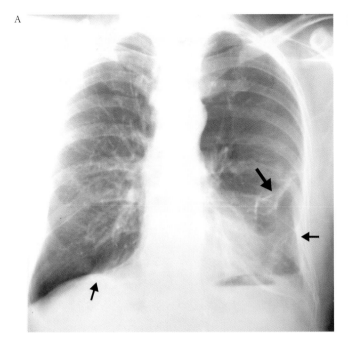

B
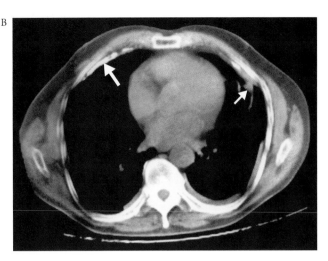

Figure 17.7 Asbestos Exposure. The patient was a 68-year-old asymptomatic man who smoked. A, Abnormal chest radiograph shows areas of pleural calcification (small arrows), particularly on the right hemidiaphragm. This is a tip-off to previous asbestos exposure. The process in the left midlung was worrisome (large arrow), perhaps indicating a new process such as bronchogenic carcinoma. B, Computed tomography disclosed rounded atelectasis (small arrow). The "comma" extending from this mass is characteristic of rounded atelectasis, which is the result of subacute to chronic pleural effusion resolving and trapping lung as it heals. Pleural calcification is apparent (large arrow).

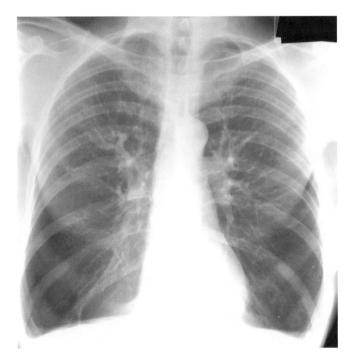

Figure 17.8 Panlobular Emphysema at the Bases Consistent With the Diagnosis of α_1-Antitrypsin Deficiency. Emphysema should not be read into a chest radiograph because all it usually represents is hyperinflation that can occur with severe asthma as well. However, there are diminished interstitial markings at the bases with radiolucency. Also, blood flow is increased to the upper lobes because that is where most of the viable lung tissue is.

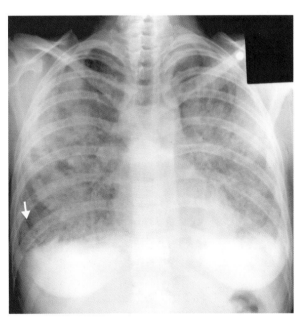

Figure 17.9 Lymphangitic Carcinoma in a 27-Year-Old Woman. This patient had a 6-week history of progressive dyspnea and weight loss. Because of her young age, neoplasm may not be considered initially. However, the chest radiographic features suggest it: bilateral pleural effusions, Kerley B lines as evident in the right base (arrow), and mediastinal and hilar lymphadenopathy in addition to diffuse parenchymal infiltrate.

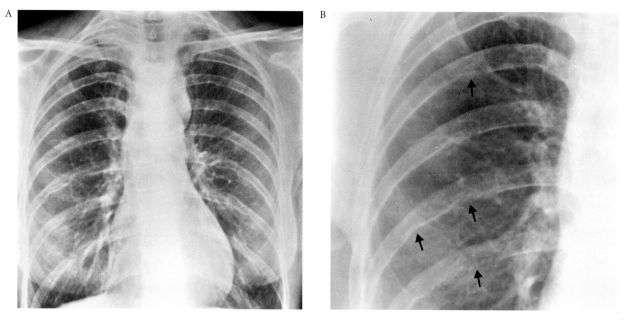

Figure 17.10 Coarctation. A and B, Posteroanterior chest radiographs showing coarctation with a tortuous aorta mimicking a mediastinal mass. This occurs in about one-third of patients with coarctation. Rib notching is indicated by the arrows in panel B.

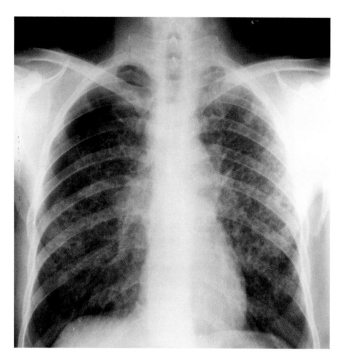

Figure 17.11 Histiocytosis X (or Eosinophilic Granuloma). Extensive change is predominantly in the upper two-thirds of the lung fields. Eventually 25% of the patients have pneumothorax, as seen on this chest radiograph (right side). The honeycombing, also described as microcysts, is characteristic of advanced histiocytosis X.

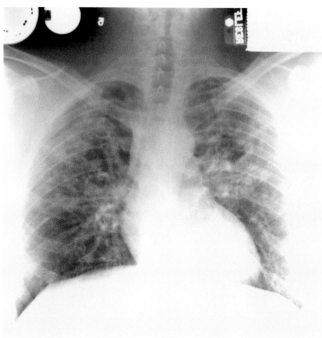

Figure 17.12 Sarcoidosis in a 35-Year-Old Patient. This chest radiograph shows the predominant parenchymal pattern seen in the upper two-thirds of the lungs in many patients with stage II or III sarcoidosis. The pattern can be interstitial, alveolar (which this one is predominantly), or a combination. There probably is some residual adenopathy in the hila and right paratracheal area.

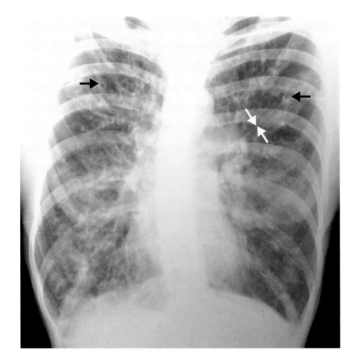

Figure 17.13 Advanced Cystic Fibrosis. This chest radiograph shows hyperinflation with low-lying hemidiaphragms, bronchiectasis (white arrows pointing to parallel lines), and microabscesses (black arrows) representing small areas of pneumonitis distal to the mucous plug that has been coughed out. Cystic fibrosis almost always begins in the upper lobes.

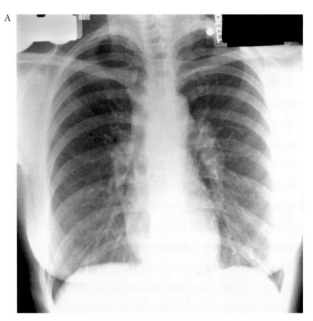

A

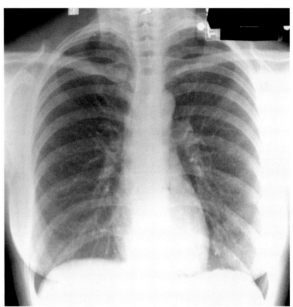

B

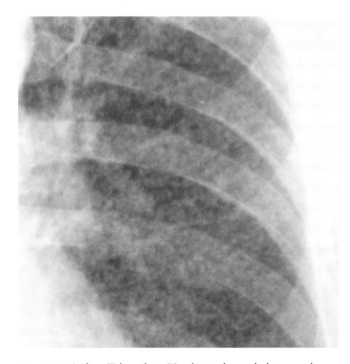

Figure 17.14 Miliary Tuberculosis. The chest radiograph shows a miliary pattern of relatively discrete micronodules, with little interstitial (linear or reticular) markings. Disseminated fungal disease has a similar appearance, as does bronchoalveolar cell carcinoma; however, the patients do not usually have the systemic manifestations of miliary tuberculosis. Other, less common differential diagnoses include lymphoma, lymphocytic interstitial pneumonitis, and pulmonary edema. *Pneumocystis jiroveci* pneumonia usually has a more interstitial reaction.

Figure 17.15 Pulmonary Sarcoidosis. A, Chest radiograph (CXR) of a 30-year-old woman who had stage I pulmonary sarcoidosis with subtle bilateral hilar and mediastinal adenopathy, particularly right paratracheal and left infra-aortic adenopathy. B, CXR 1 year later, after spontaneous regression of sarcoidosis.

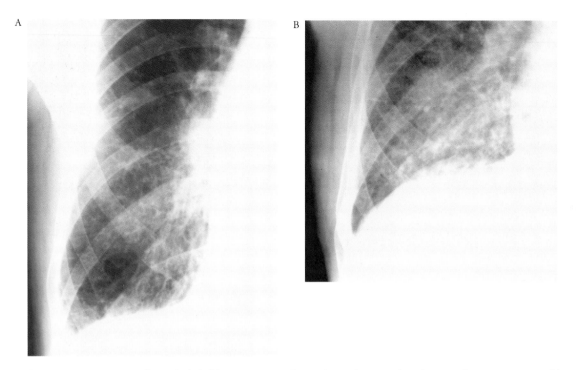

Figure 17.16 Kerley B Lines. These 2 examples can be helpful in interpreting chest radiographs. A, Kerley B lines are shown in a 75-year-old man with colon cancer. B, The Kerley B lines are from metastatic adenocarcinoma of the colon; they were a tip-off that the parenchymal process in this patient resulted from metastatic carcinoma and not from a primary pulmonary process such as pulmonary fibrosis, which was the working diagnosis.

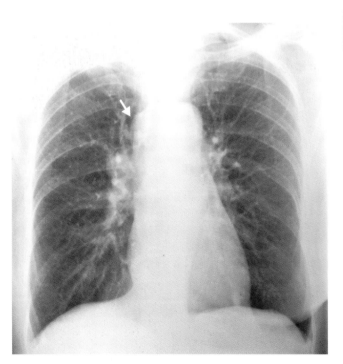

Figure 17.17 Metastatic Carcinoma of the Breast. This chest radiograph from a 55-year-old woman who had a right mastectomy for breast carcinoma now shows subtle but definite right paratracheal (arrow) and right hilar adenopathy from metastatic carcinoma of the breast.

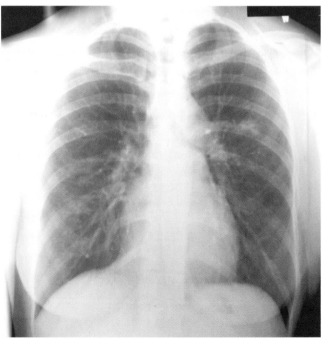

Figure 17.18 "Solitary Pulmonary Nodule." The nodule in the left midlung field is technically not a solitary pulmonary nodule because of another abnormality in the thorax that might be related to it, left infra-aortic adenopathy. The differential diagnosis would be bronchogenic carcinoma with hilar nodal metastasis or, as in this case, acute primary pulmonary histoplasmosis. Had this patient been in an area with coccidioidomycosis, that disease would also be included in the differential diagnosis.

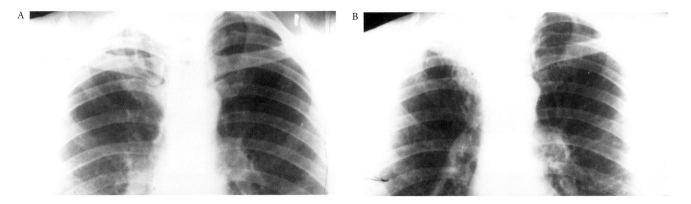

Figure 17.19 Pancoast Tumor. A, Subtle asymmetry at the apex of the right lung. The patient's symptoms at the time of the initial chest radiography were attributed to a cervical disk. B, The asymmetry was more obvious 3.5 years later when the Pancoast lesion (primary bronchogenic carcinoma) was diagnosed.

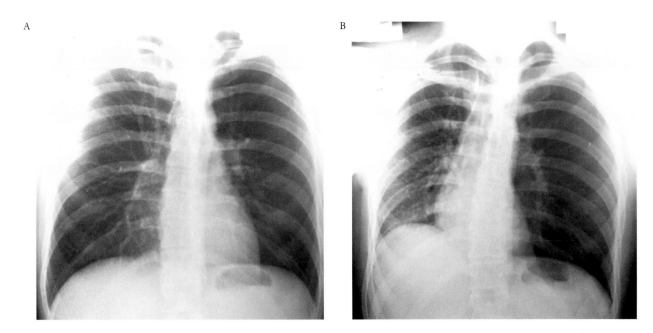

Figure 17.20 Bronchial Carcinoid. The adage that "not all that wheezes is asthma" should be remembered every time a patient with asthma is encountered and the condition does not seem to improve. A, In this patient, wheezes were predominant over the left hemithorax. B, The forced expiration film showed air trapping in the left lung. Bronchial carcinoid of the left main bronchus was diagnosed at bronchoscopy.

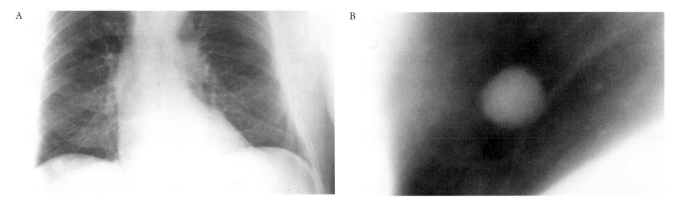

Figure 17.21 Adenocarcinoma. A, A solitary pulmonary nodule is evident below the right hemidiaphragm, where at least 15% of the lung is obscured. B, Tomography shows that the nodule has a discrete border but is noncalcified. It was not present 18 months earlier.

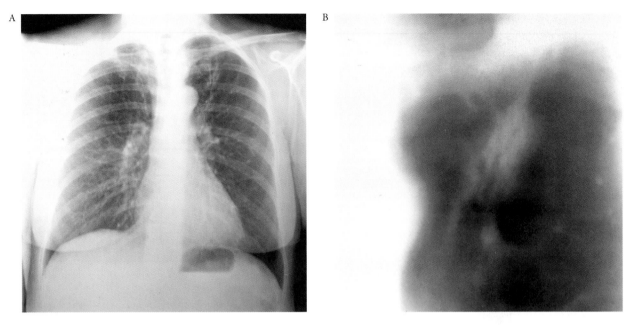

Figure 17.22 Infiltrate. A, Solitary infiltrate in the left upper lobe with air bronchogram, as evident on tomography or computed tomography. B, Air bronchogram should be considered a sign of bronchoalveolar cell carcinoma or lymphoma until proved otherwise.

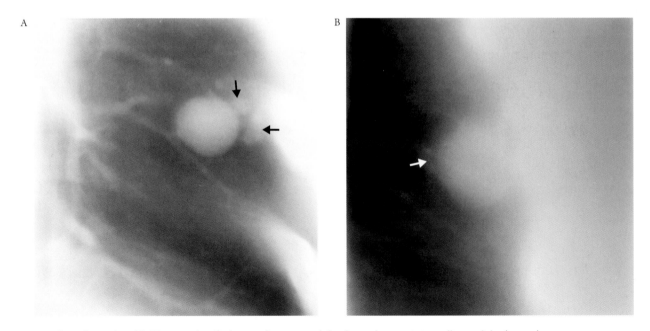

Figure 17.23 Granuloma. A and B, Tomography of solitary pulmonary nodules shows characteristic satellite nodules (arrows).

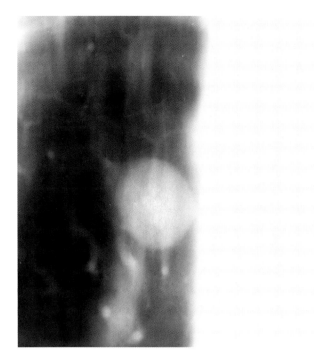

Figure 17.24 Popcorn Calcification of Hamartoma. This benign process can be seen also in granuloma.

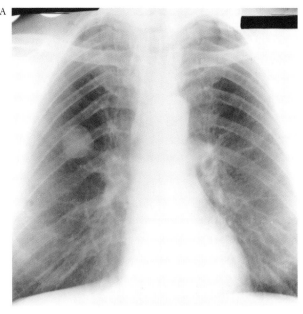

A

B

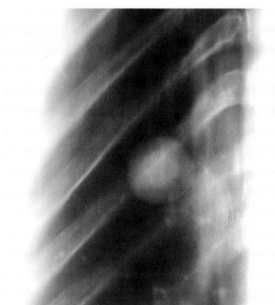

Figure 17.26 Bull's-Eye Calcification Characteristic of Granuloma in a Solitary Pulmonary Nodule. A and B, These nodules occasionally enlarge but almost never warrant removal.

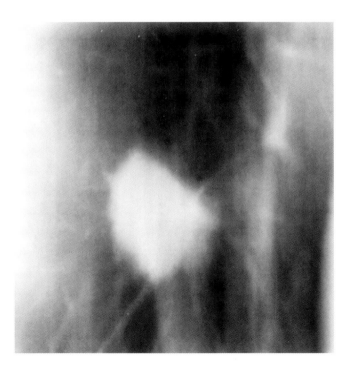

Figure 17.25 Primary Bronchogenic Carcinoma. Tomography of a solitary nodule shows the characteristic spiculation or sunburst effect. Spicules represent extension of the tumor into septa. Computed tomography showed a similar appearance.

Interpretation of PFT Results

The following is a simplified step-by-step approach to interpreting PFT results:

1. Evaluate volumes and flows separately.

2. Look at the flow-volume curve to see whether it suggests an obstructive ("scooped out" appearance) or a restrictive (high peak with narrow curve) pattern.

3. Look at the ratio of FEV_1 to forced vital capacity (FVC). An FEV_1/FVC ratio <70% suggests airflow obstruction. FEV_1 is used to classify the severity of airflow obstruction (Table 17.3).

4. If FEV_1/FVC is >70% but FEV_1 is reduced, look at total lung capacity (TLC). Reduced TLC suggests a restrictive defect (Table 17.3).

5. TLC, functional residual capacity (FRC), and residual volume (RV) indicate volumes. TLC = VC (vital capacity) + RV. Increases in TLC and RV suggest hyperinflation (asthma or COPD). If TLC and VC are decreased, consider restrictive lung disease (fibrosis) or loss of lung volume (surgery, diaphragmatic paralysis, or skeletal problems).

6. VC measured during a slow (not forced) expiration is not affected by airway collapse in COPD. FVC may be low with forced expiration because of airway collapse. In healthy subjects, VC = FVC.

7. FEV_1 and forced expiratory flow (FEF) of the midexpiratory phase ($FEF_{25\%-75\%}$) indicate flow rates. Flow rates are diminished in COPD, but smaller decreases can occur if lung volumes are low.

8. The maximal voluntary ventilation (MVV) test requires rapid inspiratory and expiratory maneuvers and, thus,

Table 17.3 **INTERPRETATION OF PULMONARY FUNCTION TESTING**

Obstruction is indicated by FEV_1/FVC <70%

FEV_1, Percentage of Predicted Value	Severity of Airflow Obstruction
>80	Borderline
<80 & >60	Mild
<60 & >40	Moderate
<40	Severe

Restriction is indicated by TLC <80% of predicted value (restrictive defect is only suggested by reduced vital capacity; TLC is needed for confirmation)

TLC, Percentage of Predicted Value	Severity of Restrictive Defect
<80 & >60	Mild
<60 & >50	Moderate
<50	Severe

Bronchodilator response requires both 12% & 200-mL improvement in FEV_1 after bronchodilator therapy

Methacholine challenge requires 20% decrease in FEV_1 after challenge to be considered positive

Abbreviations: FEV_1, forced expiratory volume in the first second of expiration; FVC, forced vital capacity; TLC, total lung capacity.

tests airflow through major airways and muscle strength. Disproportionately reduced MVV (MVV = FEV_1 × 35) may be from poor effort, variable extrathoracic obstruction, and respiratory muscle weakness. Respiratory muscle weakness can be assessed by maximum inspiratory pressure (PImax) and maximum expiratory pressure (PEmax). Clinical features should be correlated with the results of PFTs.

9. Diffusing capacity of lung for carbon monoxide (DLCO) is dependent on the thickness of the alveolocapillary membrane (T), the area of the alveolocapillary membrane (A), and the pressure difference between alveolar gas and venous blood (ΔPCO). Thus, DLCO is represented by the following:

$$DLCO = \frac{A \times \Delta P_{CO}}{T}$$

   a. Low DLCO

   1) Anatomical emphysema (decreased A)

   2) Anemia (effectively decreased A) (a decrease in hemoglobin by 1 g/dL diminishes DLCO by 7%)

   3) Restrictive lung diseases (decreased A or decreased T in pulmonary fibrosis or other interstitial lung diseases)

   4) Pneumonectomy (decreased A)

   5) Pulmonary hypertension (effectively decreased T)

   6) Recurrent pulmonary emboli (effectively decreased A)

   b. Increased DLCO

   1) Supine posture (increased A due to increased blood volume in upper lobes)

   2) Exercise (increased A due to increased blood volume)

   3) Polycythemia (increased A)

   4) Obesity (increased A due to increased blood volume)

   5) Left-to-right shunt (increased A)

   6) Some patients with asthma

   c. Isolated low DLCO (with normal PFT results)

   1) Pulmonary hypertension

   2) Multiple pulmonary emboli

   3) Combined diseases such as pulmonary fibrosis with COPD

   4) Anemia

10. Flow-volume curves are helpful to distinguish between intrathoracic and extrathoracic major airway obstructions. Flattening of the expiratory flow curve with

a normal inspiratory flow curve suggests intrathoracic airway obstruction. Flattening of the inspiratory flow curve alone suggests extrathoracic airway obstruction. Flattening of both flow curves suggests fixed airway obstruction, and the location cannot be determined.

Explanations for Table 17.4

Patient 1

The patient has typical features of emphysema. The FEV_1/FVC ratio indicates obstruction. The FEV_1 indicates that the obstruction is severe. The TLC indicates hyperinflation. The reduced $D_{L}CO$ suggests emphysema. The clinical diagnosis is severe obstructive disease with anatomical emphysema.

Patient 2

The PFT results suggest emphysema. In a young non-smoker, other causes of emphysema must be considered. The clinical diagnosis is severe emphysema caused by familial deficiency of α_1-antitrypsin.

Patient 3

Flow rates and lung volumes are decreased only slightly but are within normal limits. MVV is severely decreased. In this patient, $P_{I}max$ and $P_{E}max$ were severely decreased, suggesting muscle weakness. The clinical diagnosis is severe thyrotoxicosis with proximal muscle weakness (ie, thyrotoxic myopathy). This pattern of PFT results can also occur in neuromuscular diseases such as amyotrophic lateral sclerosis and myasthenia gravis.

Patient 4

As indicated by the FEV_1/FVC ratio and FEV_1, there is a moderately severe airflow obstruction. The normal TLC and residual volume suggest an absence of air trapping. The normal $D_{L}CO$ excludes anatomical emphysema or other parenchymal problems. Bronchodilator testing elicited improvement in lung volumes and flow rates. The clinical diagnosis is typical asthma.

Patient 5

This patient has normal lung volumes and flow rates (80%-120% of predicted normal). A former athlete, he recently noted cough and chest tightness after exertion. Previous PFT results were unavailable. The following are important points: 1) In a young, otherwise healthy patient, the lung volumes and flow rates are usually above normal and even higher in an athlete. 2) This patient may have had very high volumes and flow rates in the past, but without previous PFT results, no comparison can be made (if earlier PFT results were available, the new results might represent a severe decrease in pulmonary function). 3) The history suggests the possibility of exercise-induced asthma; spirometry after an exercise test showed a 28% reduction in flow rates 5 to 10 minutes after exercise ended. 4) Note the relatively high $D_{L}CO$, a phenomenon seen in patients with asthma. The clinical diagnosis is exercise-induced asthma.

Patient 6

This patient has a moderately severe decrease in lung volumes and normal flow rates. MVV is normal, but $D_{L}CO$ is severely diminished. These results suggest severe restrictive lung disease. The slightly diminished flow rates are the result of

Table 17.4 **TRY TO INTERPRET THESE RESULTS OF PULMONARY FUNCTION TESTS BEFORE READING THE EXPLANATIONS**

| | PATIENT | | | | | | | | |
FEATURE	*1*	*2*	*3*	*4*	*5*	*6*	*7*	*8*	*9*
Age, y/sex	73/M	43/M	53/F	43/M	20/M	58/F	40/M	28/F	44/M
Weight, kg	52	53	50	63	80	59	75	52	148
Tobacco, PY	63	NS	NS	NS	NS	NS	NS	NS	NS
Total lung capacity, %[a]	140	128	84	118	100	56	68	108	90
Vital capacity, %[a]	52	75	86	78	95	62	58	106	86
Residual volume, %[a]	160	140	90	110	90	65	80	98	90
FEV_1, %[a]	35	38	82	48	90	85	42	112	96
FEV_1/FVC, %	40	34	80	40	85	88	50	85	78
$FEF_{25\%-75\%}$, %[a]	18	14	80	35	88	82	24	102	88
Maximum voluntary ventilation, %[a]	62	48	40	60	120	108	62	88	90
$D_{L}CO$ (normal), mL/min/mm Hg	9 (22)	10 (28)	20 (20)	28 (28)	32 (34)	8 (26)	8 (28)	6 (32)	40 (28)

Abbreviations: $D_{L}CO$, diffusing capacity of lung for carbon monoxide; $FEF_{25\%-75\%}$, forced expiratory flow of the midexpiratory phase; FEV_1, forced expiratory volume in the first second of expiration; FVC, forced vital capacity; NS, nonsmoker; PY, pack-years of smoking.

[a] Percentage of the predicted value. Values of 80% to 120% are considered normal.

decreased lung volumes. The clinical diagnosis is biopsy-proven idiopathic pulmonary fibrosis. Patients who have had lung resection also have low lung volumes and decreased D_{LCO}.

Patient 7

The reduction in the FEV_1/FVC ratio suggests the presence of obstructive dysfunction. TLC is also decreased, which suggests additional restrictive lung disease. MVV is also reduced, and D_{LCO} is severely decreased. Compared with patient 6, this patient has obstructive disease plus severe restrictive lung disease. A very low D_{LCO} suggests parenchymal disease. CXR showed bilaterally diffuse nodular interstitial changes, especially in the upper two-thirds of the lungs. Biopsy specimens of the bronchial mucosa and lung showed extensive endobronchial sarcoidosis. The clinical diagnosis is severe restrictive lung disease from parenchymal sarcoidosis and obstructive dysfunction caused by endobronchial sarcoidosis.

Patient 8

This patient has normal lung volumes and flow rates. MVV is slightly decreased but within normal limits. D_{LCO} is very low. Pao_2 is 56 mm Hg. The clinical diagnosis is primary pulmonary hypertension.

Patient 9

This extremely obese patient has normal lung volumes and flow rates. D_{LCO} is abnormally high. Abnormally high D_{LCO} is reported to be a result of increased VC. The clinical diagnosis is obesity-related pulmonary dysfunction.

EXERCISE TESTING

Indications for cardiopulmonary exercise testing include unexplained dyspnea or effort intolerance, ability-disability evaluation, quantification of severity of pulmonary dysfunction, differentiation of cardiac from pulmonary causes of disability, evaluation of progression of a disease process, estimation of operative risks before cardiopulmonary surgery (lung resection or heart-lung or lung transplant), rehabilitation, and evaluation of need for supplemental oxygen.

- Cardiopulmonary exercise testing can help differentiate between cardiac and pulmonary causes of dyspnea.

INVASIVE TESTING

Bronchoscopy can be used for diagnostic and therapeutic purposes. It can be helpful in the evaluation of persistent cough, hemoptysis, lung nodule, atelectasis, diffuse lung disease, lung infections, suspected cancer, and staging of lung cancer. Therapeutic indications include atelectasis, retained secretions, tracheobronchial foreign bodies, airway stenosis, and obstructive lesions. Bronchoalveolar lavage is helpful in diagnosing opportunistic lung infections. Lung biopsy can be done through bronchoscopy, thoracoscopy, or thoracotomy.

- Bronchoscopy can be both diagnostic and therapeutic.

- Lung biopsy may be indicated in the evaluation of diffuse lung disease.

OBSTRUCTIVE LUNG DISEASES

Obstructive lung diseases include emphysema, bronchitis, asthma, bronchiectasis, CF, bronchiolitis, bullous lung disease, and airway stenosis. The 3 most prevalent obstructive lung diseases are emphysema, chronic bronchitis, and asthma.

Several features are useful for distinguishing these 3 diseases:

1. Age at onset—asthma: younger than 30 years; bronchitis: 50 or older; emphysema: 60 or older

2. Use of tobacco—asthma: no; bronchitis and emphysema: yes

3. Pattern—asthma: paroxysmal; bronchitis and emphysema: chronic and progressive

4. Sputum—asthma: absent or minimal; bronchitis: increased; emphysema: minimal or increased

5. CXR findings—asthma: usually normal; bronchitis: increased lung markings; emphysema: hyperinflation

6. $Paco_2$—asthma: normal or decreased during attack; bronchitis: increased; emphysema: normal or increased

7. Pao_2—asthma: normal or decreased during attack; bronchitis and emphysema: low

8. D_{LCO}—asthma: normal; bronchitis: normal or slightly decreased; emphysema: decreased

9. FEV_1—asthma: normal or decreased during attack; bronchitis and emphysema: decreased

10. Total lung capacity and residual volume—asthma: normal or increased during attack; bronchitis: normal or slightly increased; emphysema: increased greatly

11. Cor pulmonale—asthma and emphysema: rare; bronchitis: common

12. Hematocrit—asthma: normal; bronchitis and emphysema: normal or increased

The current working definition of COPD is a disease state characterized by airflow limitation that is not fully reversible. This definition implies that asthma, which is considered fully reversible (at least in its early stages), is separate from COPD. In some instances, however, the 2 diseases can coexist. A classification of the severity of COPD has been proposed and should guide management at various stages of the disease (Box 17.2). Note the difference in clinical staging of COPD from the classification of severity of airflow obstruction on the PFTs.

- The 3 most common obstructive lung diseases are emphysema, chronic bronchitis, and asthma.

- The severity of COPD guides management.

ETIOLOGY

Tobacco smoking is the major cause of COPD. Tobacco smokers have 10 times the risk of nonsmokers of dying of COPD, whereas pipe and cigar smokers have between 1.5 and 3 times the risk of nonsmokers. Smoking also increases the risk of COPD in persons who have α_1-antitrypsin deficiency. Occupational exposures, heredity (α_1-antitrypsin deficiency), infections, allergy (in asthma), and other factors are also involved in the etiology of COPD.

α_1-Antitrypsin is a secretory glycoprotein that inhibits proteolytic enzymes and, thus, protects the lungs from destructive emphysema. α_1-Antitrypsin deficiency is an autosomal recessive disease; the phenotypes are normal (PiMM), heterozygote (PiMZ), homozygote (PiZZ), and null (PiNull). Affected individuals often present in the third or fourth decade of life and have a family history of COPD. Hepatic cirrhosis develops in up to 3% of patients. Upper lobe centrilobular emphysema is the most common type of COPD in susceptible smokers. Lower lobe panlobular COPD is the usual pattern in patients with α_1-antitrypsin deficiency.

- In α_1-antitrypsin deficiency, smoking hastens the onset of emphysema.

- Tobacco smoke is most commonly associated with upper lobe centrilobular emphysema, while α_1-antitrypsin deficiency is associated with lower lobe panlobular COPD.

BULLOUS LUNG DISEASE

Bullous changes may be seen in Marfan and Ehlers-Danlos syndromes, burned-out sarcoidosis, and cadmium exposure, although small apical bullae are often present in healthy persons. Bullous lung disease is associated with an increased risk of lung cancer. Complications include pneumothorax, COPD, infection, formation of lung abscess, bleeding into a bulla, and compression of adjacent normal lung. Surgical therapy may improve lung function by 5% to 10% in 10% to 15% of patients.

ASTHMA

Asthma is discussed in Chapter 42 ("Asthma").

TREATMENT OF COPD

The therapeutic approach to COPD consists of reducing risk factors (eg, smoking cessation), identifying the severity of COPD, quantifying the pulmonary dysfunction and response to bronchodilator therapy, selecting appropriate bronchodilators, anticipating and appropriately treating complications, and educating the patient and family about long-term therapy. Proper inhalation technique is essential in optimal treatment. Practical aspects of managing COPD are outlined in Box 17.2.

Reducing Risk Factors

Because smoking is a major risk factor in the development and progression of COPD, smoking cessation should be discussed and programs offered to those who continue to smoke. Smoking cessation is discussed in Chapter 55 ("General Internal Medicine and Quality Improvement"). Decreased exposure to occupational dusts, gases, and fumes and other pollutants is also important in the management of COPD.

Bronchodilators

Bronchodilator drugs are administered to reverse bronchoconstriction (bronchospasm). They can be divided into β-adrenergic agonists (β_2-selective agonists), anticholinergics (ipratropium), antimuscarinics (tiotropium), adrenergic agonists (sympathomimetics), phosphodiesterase inhibitors (theophylline), mast cell inhibitors (cromolyn), leukotriene modifiers, antihistamines, anti-inflammatory agents (corticosteroids and methotrexate), and other agents (troleandomycin, γ-globulin, and mucolytics).

Short-Acting β-Adrenergic (β_2-Selective) Agonists

Short-acting β-adrenergic agonists are the most commonly used bronchodilators. They include albuterol, bitolterol, metaproterenol, pirbuterol, and terbutaline. In most patients, single doses of these agents produce clinically important bronchodilatation within 5 minutes (peak effect occurs 30–60 minutes after inhalation, with a beneficial effect lasting 3–4 hours). The dosage should be tailored on the basis of clinical features and potential side effects. Adverse effects include tremor, anxiety, restlessness, tachycardia, palpitations, increased blood pressure, and cardiac arrhythmias. Side effects are more likely in the presence of cardiovascular, liver, or neurologic disorders and in elderly patients. Rarely, paradoxical bronchospasm may result from tachyphylaxis (a rapidly decreasing response to a drug after a few doses) or from exposure to preservatives and propellants. A newer single-isomer β-agonist, levalbuterol, binds to β-adrenergic receptors with 100-fold greater affinity than albuterol. Metered dose inhalers are just as effective as nebulized medications, but the total dose of medication is higher in the nebulized formulation.

- Short-acting β-adrenergic agonists are widely used and provide immediate relief.

Long-Acting β-Adrenergic (β₂-Selective) Agonists

Long-acting β-adrenergic agonists include salmeterol and formoterol and are often used in moderate COPD. Salmeterol is highly lipophilic (albuterol is hydrophilic); hence, it has a depot effect in tissues. Salmeterol has a prolonged duration of action (10–12 hours) and inhibits the release of proinflammatory and spasmogenic mediators from respiratory cells. Salmeterol and formoterol are also effective in preventing exercise-induced asthma, methacholine-induced bronchospasm, and allergen challenge. Side effects are similar to those of other β-adrenergic agents. Salmeterol and other β-adrenergic bronchodilators may potentiate the actions of monoamine oxidase inhibitors and tricyclic antidepressants.

- Salmeterol and formoterol are an option for moderate COPD.

Anticholinergic Agents

Anticholinergic agents (eg, ipratropium and atropine) are useful in treating chronic bronchitis or asthmatic bronchitis. As a single agent, ipratropium is only modestly effective since it prevents bronchoconstriction caused by cholinergic agents, but it does not protect against bronchoconstriction produced by tobacco smoke, citric acid, sulfur dioxide, or carbon dust. Side effects include nervousness, headache, gastrointestinal tract upset, dry mouth, and cough. Ipratropium may aggravate narrow-angle glaucoma, prostatic hypertrophy, and bladder neck obstruction.

Tiotropium is a long-acting anticholinergic that improves bronchodilation in patients with COPD. It appears to be more effective than ipratropium in reducing the number of COPD exacerbations.

- Ipratropium may aggravate narrow-angle glaucoma, prostatic hypertrophy, and bladder neck obstruction.
- Tiotropium is a long-acting anticholinergic useful in COPD.

Phosphodiesterase Inhibitors

The use of phosphodiesterase inhibitors (eg, theophylline) has diminished with the increased use of β-agonists because phosphodiesterase inhibitors have a narrow therapeutic window, wide range of toxic effects (eg, cardiac arrhythmias and grand mal seizures), and interactions with other drugs. Nevertheless, theophylline increases the contractility of respiratory muscles in a dose-related fashion. The effects of various substances and circumstances on the clearance of theophylline are shown in Box 17.3.

- Theophylline use has substantially decreased owing to safety concerns.

Corticosteroids

Corticosteroids have no bronchodilating effect in patients with emphysema. Patients with bronchitis, however, may benefit from the anti-inflammatory action. A short course of systemic corticosteroid is useful in the treatment of acute COPD exacerbation since it reduces the duration and severity of the illness. Several large studies have suggested that the regular use of inhaled corticosteroids may be appropriate for patients who have a documented FEV_1 response to inhaled corticosteroids or for patients who have moderate to severe COPD and repeated exacerbations that require oral corticosteroid therapy. Inhaled corticosteroids can be given in conjunction with systemic (oral) corticosteroids, especially during the weaning period of long-term or high-dose systemic (oral) corticosteroids.

Box 17.3 AGENTS THAT AFFECT THEOPHYLLINE CLEARANCE

Agents that increase theophylline clearance
   β-Agonists
   Carbamazepine
   Dilantin
   Furosemide
   Hyperthyroidism
   Ketoconazole
   Marijuana
   Phenobarbital
   Rifampin
   Tobacco smoke
Agents that decrease theophylline clearance
   Allopurinol
   Antibiotics: macrolides, ciprofloxacin, norfloxacin, isoniazid
   β-Blocker: propranolol
   Caffeine
   Cirrhosis
   Congestive heart failure
   H_2-blocker: cimetidine
   Mexiletine
   Oral contraceptives
   Viral infection

- Oral corticosteroids are useful in acute COPD exacerbations.
- Inhaled corticosteroids may be indicated for selected patients with moderate to severe COPD.

Adjuvant Therapy

Antibiotic therapy is helpful for patients with symptoms suggestive of bacterial infection, especially during COPD exacerbations. Maintenance of good oral hydration, avoidance of tobacco smoking and other respiratory irritants, pneumococcal vaccination, annual influenza vaccination, and prompt treatment of respiratory infections are equally important.

Oxygen

Low-flow oxygen (<2 L/min) therapy is recommended when the PaO_2 is 55 mm Hg or less, arterial oxygen saturation (SaO_2) is 88% or less, or PaO_2 is 59 mm Hg or less if there is polycythemia or clinical evidence of cor pulmonale (ie, the presence of altered structure and function of the right ventricle due to pulmonary hypertension from a primary pulmonary disorder). The lack of carbon dioxide retention should be assured before recommending oxygen. The need for chronic or indefinite oxygen therapy should be reassessed after 3 months of treatment. Exercise therapy (ie, pulmonary rehabilitation) improves exercise tolerance and maximal oxygen uptake but does not improve PFT results.

- Indications for oxygen therapy: PaO_2 ≤55 mm Hg, SaO_2 ≤88%, or PaO_2 ≤59 mm Hg if the patient has polycythemia or cor pulmonale.

Surgery

Lung volume reduction surgery is beneficial in selected patients with COPD but is associated with increased mortality for patients with severe disease.

COMPLICATIONS AND CAUSES OF COPD EXACERBATIONS

The complications and causes of exacerbation of COPD include viral and bacterial respiratory infections (common agents are *Haemophilus influenzae*, *Moraxella catarrhalis*, and *Streptococcus pneumoniae*), cor pulmonale, myocardial infarction, cardiac arrhythmias, pneumothorax, pulmonary emboli, bronchogenic carcinoma, environmental exposure, oversedation, neglect of therapy, excessive oxygen use (suppression of hypoxemic drive and worsening ventilation-perfusion ratio [$\dot{V}/\dot{Q}$] mismatch), and excessive use of β_2-agonist (tachyphylaxis). Common findings in patients with emphysema include nocturnal oxygen desaturation, premature ventricular contractions, and episodic pulmonary hypertension. Severe weight loss (sometimes >50 kg) is noted in 30% of patients with severe COPD.

- The most common bacterial respiratory agents in COPD patients are *Haemophilus influenzae*, *Moraxella catarrhalis*, and *Streptococcus pneumoniae*.

CYSTIC FIBROSIS

CF is a common lethal autosomal recessive disease caused by a mutation of the gene that encodes for the CF transmembrane conductance regulator (CFTR), a protein that regulates epithelial cell chloride channels. All exocrine glands, except sweat glands, are affected, accounting for the majority of symptoms. Respiratory manifestations include persistent cough, sinusitis, nasal polyps, progressive cystic bronchiectasis, purulent sputum, atelectasis, hemoptysis, obstructive airway disease, and pneumothorax. Impaired mucociliary clearance leads to chronic infection, and bacteria such as *H influenzae*, *Staphylococcus aureus*, and *Pseudomonas aeruginosa* often colonize the airways. CF is the most common cause of COPD and pancreatic deficiency in the first 3 decades of life in the United States. Other common manifestations of CF are diabetes mellitus, acute or chronic pancreatitis, biliary disease, intussusception and fecal impaction, and male infertility due to defects in sperm transport (female infertility is also present in 20% of females with CF).

- CF is caused by a mutation in *CFTR*.
- CF affects all exocrine glands except sweat glands.
- Common manifestations of CF include sinusitis, nasal polyposis, bronchiectasis, obstructive airway disease, pancreatic insufficiency, biliary disease, and male infertility.

In 20% of patients, the diagnosis is not made until the adolescent years. Diagnosis in adults requires at least 3 of the following: clinical features of CF, positive family history, sweat chloride greater than 80 mEq/L, and pancreatic insufficiency. Quantitative pilocarpine iontophoresis (sweat chloride testing) is helpful in making the diagnosis; abnormal results on at least 2 tests are necessary for the diagnosis. This test must be performed with extreme care because inaccurate collection is a common source of misdiagnosis. Conditions associated with high levels of sodium and sweat chloride include smoking, chronic bronchitis, malnutrition, adrenal insufficiency, hypothyroidism, hypoparathyroidism, pancreatitis, hypogammaglobulinema, and ectodermal dysplasia. False-negative test results are common in edematous states and in persons receiving corticosteroids. The concentrations of sodium and sweat chloride increase with age.

- Diagnosis requires 3 of the following: CF clinical features, family history, pancreatic insufficiency, and sweat chloride >80 mEq/L.
- Numerous conditions can increase the sweat chloride levels in the absence of CF.

The average life span for persons with CF is approximately 37 years. Survival and quality of life are improved with aggressive chest physical therapy, prompt treatment of upper and lower respiratory tract infections, intensive nutritional support, and conditioning. Poor prognostic factors include female sex, residence in a non-Northern climate, pneumothorax, hemoptysis, recurrent bacterial infections, presence of *Burkholderia cepacia*, and systemic complications. Respiratory therapy for CF includes management of obstructive lung disease and respiratory infections, chest physiotherapy, postural drainage, immunization against influenza, hydration, and deoxyribonuclease therapy. Although systemic glucocorticoids are administered during acute exacerbations or to patients who have allergic bronchopulmonary aspergillosis, routine use has been associated with notable side effects and is not recommended. If patients with CF have decreased FEV_1 or evidence of chronic airway inflammation, and if sputum examination does not show nontuberculous mycobacteria, treatment with azithromycin (500 mg 3 times weekly) appears to improve FEV_1 and decrease the frequency of pulmonary exacerbations. The risk of death from CF is 38% to 56% within 2 years when FEV_1 has reached 20% to 30% of the predicted value. Bilateral lung transplant is an option for patients with declining lung function. The 5-year survival rate is between 40%-60%. The presence of *B cepacia*, however, is a contraindication for transplant.

- Due to improvement in treatments, the lifespan for patients with CF has increased.
- The 5-year survival rate after bilateral lung transplant is 40%-60%.

BRONCHIECTASIS

Bronchiectasis is ectasia, or dilatation, of the bronchi due to irreversible destruction of bronchial walls. Its clinical features are similar to those of COPD. Bronchiectasis is reversible in chronic bronchitis, acute pneumonia, and allergic bronchopulmonary aspergillosis. Bronchiectasis most commonly involves the lower lung fields; upper lobes are affected in CF and chronic mycotic and mycobacterial infections. Central (perihilar) involvement is suggestive of allergic bronchopulmonary aspergillosis.

- Bronchiectasis: similar clinical features as COPD.

Most cases of bronchiectasis are diagnosed clinically with chronic cough and expectoration of purulent sputum. Nonpulmonary symptoms include fetor oris, anorexia, weight loss, arthralgia, and clubbing. HRCT of the chest is the preferred test for definitive diagnosis. Findings include airway dilatation, dilated bronchi extending to periphery without tapering, bronchial wall thickening, bronchial obstruction due to inspissated purulent secretions, loss of volume, and air-fluid levels if cystic or saccular changes are present. PFT results usually indicate obstructive phenomena.

- Patients with bronchiectasis present with chronic cough and expectoration of purulent sputum.
- Diagnosis can be made clinically; HRCT is confirmatory.

In adults, many cases of bronchiectasis are related to adenoviral or bacterial infections (measles, influenza, adenovirus, or pertussis) in childhood. Various infections, including *Mycoplasma pneumoniae*, nontuberculous mycobacteria, and anaerobic organisms, have also been associated with bronchiectasis. Tuberculosis is a common cause of bronchiectasis, particularly in the upper lobes. Occasionally, chronic histoplasmosis and coccidioidomycosis cause bronchiectasis. In patients with chronic stable bronchiectasis, *P aeruginosa* is the predominant organism in respiratory secretions.

Ciliary dyskinesia is also associated with the development of bronchiectasis. Primary ciliary dyskinesia (PCD), which results from abnormal motion of cilia, causes many clinical problems, including nasal polyps, sinusitis, inner ear infection or deafness, and chronic bronchitis or bronchiectasis. Kartagener syndrome, an autosomal recessive disorder, is an example of PCD. Acquired ciliary defects occur in smokers, in patients with bronchitis, and in patients who have had viral infections. Both hypogammaglobulinemia and agammaglobulinemia are also associated with bronchiectasis. Central bronchiectasis is present in 85% of patients with allergic bronchopulmonary aspergillosis (ABPA) at the time of the initial diagnosis and has been used as a diagnostic criterion of the disease. Uncommon causes of bronchiectasis include yellow nail syndrome, α_1-antitrypsin deficiency, Felty syndrome, inflammatory bowel disease, toxic inhalation, and chronic tracheobronchial stenosis.

- Bronchiectasis is associated with viral and bacterial infections.
- Ciliary dyskinesia, hypogammaglobulinemia, agammaglobulinemia, and ABPA are common causes of bronchiectasis.

Complications of bronchiectasis include hemoptysis from bronchial (systemic) vessels (in 50% of patients), progressive respiratory failure with hypoxemia and cor pulmonale, and secondary infections due to fungi and noninfectious mycobacterioses. Routine culture of respiratory secretions is not warranted for all patients.

- The source of bleeding in bronchiectasis is the bronchial (systemic) circulation.

Treatment of bronchiectasis is aimed at controlling the symptoms and preventing complications. Predisposing conditions should be sought and treated aggressively (γ-globulin injections, removal of foreign body or tumor, control of aspiration, and treatment of infections of paranasal sinuses, gums, and teeth). Postural drainage, chest physiotherapy, humidification, bronchodilators, and cyclic antibiotic therapy are effective in many patients. Surgical treatment is reserved for patients with troublesome symptoms, localized disease, and severe hemoptysis. High-dose inhaled corticosteroid therapy (fluticasone) is reportedly effective in reducing the sputum inflammatory indices in bronchiectasis.

- Treatment of bronchiectasis consists of identifying and treating underlying conditions, controlling symptoms, and preventing complications.

PLEURAL EFFUSION

Excess pleural fluid collects in the pleural space when fluid accumulation exceeds removal mechanisms. Hydrostatic, oncotic, and intrapleural pressures regulate fluid movement in the pleural space. Any of the following mechanisms can produce pleural effusion:

1. Changes in capillary permeability (inflammation)

2. Increased hydrostatic pressure

3. Decreased plasma oncotic pressure

4. Impaired lymphatic drainage

5. Increased negative intrapleural pressure

6. Movement of fluid (through diaphragmatic pores and lymphatic vessels) from the peritoneum

The principal causes of pleural effusion are listed in Box 17.4. The diagnosis may be suggested by certain characteristics of the effusion. For example, obvious pus suggests empyema; an elevated salivary amylase level with pleural fluid acidosis suggests esophageal rupture; and a ratio of pleural fluid hematocrit to blood hematocrit greater than 0.5 suggests hemothorax. On the basis of clinical suspicion, testing of the effusion should be selective. Despite extensive testing of pleural fluid, the causes of up to one-third of pleural effusions remain unknown.

- Pleural effusion results when fluid accumulation exceeds the body's removal mechanisms.
- The causes of up to one-third of pleural effusions remain unknown, even after extensive testing.

DISTINGUISHING AN EXUDATE FROM A TRANSUDATE

Traditionally, an effusion with any *one* of the following is considered an exudate:

1. Ratio of pleural fluid protein to serum protein >0.5

2. Ratio of pleural fluid lactate dehydrogenase (LDH) to serum LDH >0.6

Box 17.4 PRINCIPAL CAUSES OF PLEURAL EFFUSION

Osmotic-hydraulic[a]
  Congestive heart failure
  Superior vena caval obstruction
  Constrictive pericarditis
  Cirrhosis with ascites
  Hypoalbuminemia
  Salt-retaining syndromes
  Peritoneal dialysis
  Hydronephrosis
  Nephrotic syndrome
Infections[b]
  Parapneumonic (bacterial) effusions
  Bacterial empyema
  Tuberculosis
  Fungi
  Parasites
  Viruses & mycoplasma
Neoplasms[b]
  Primary & metastatic lung tumors
  Lymphoma & leukemia
  Benign & malignant pleural tumors
  Intra-abdominal tumors with ascites
Vascular disease[b]
  Pulmonary embolism
  Wegener granulomatosis
Intra-abdominal diseases[b]
  Pancreatitis & pancreatic pseudocyst
  Subdiaphragmatic abscess
  Malignancy with ascites
  Meigs syndrome[a]
  Hepatic cirrhosis with ascites[a]
Trauma[b]
  Hemothorax
  Chylothorax
  Esophageal rupture
  Intra-abdominal surgery
Miscellaneous
  Drug-induced effusions[b]
  Uremic pleuritis[b]
  Myxedema[a]
  Yellow nail syndrome[b]
  Dressler syndrome[b]
  Familial Mediterranean fever[b]

[a] Usually a transudate.
[b] Usually an exudate.

---

3. Pleural fluid LDH greater than two-thirds of the upper limit of the reference range for serum LDH

A meta-analysis found that any *one* of the following findings can also be used to identify the fluid as an exudate:

1. Pleural fluid protein >2.9 g/dL

2. Pleural fluid cholesterol >45 mg/dL

3. Pleural fluid LDH >60% of the upper limit of the reference range for serum LDH

It is not necessary to perform all the above tests to differentiate a transudate from an exudate. Clinically, it is more useful to classify the cause by considering the source (organ system) of the fluid (Box 17.4). The most common cause of a transudate is congestive heart failure (pulmonary artery wedge pressure >25 mm Hg). The most common cause of an exudate is pneumonia (parapneumonic effusion).

- The most common cause of a transudate is congestive heart failure.

- The most common cause of an exudate is pneumonia.

Glucose and pH

The pleural fluid glucose concentration and pH usually change in tandem (ie, if the glucose concentration is low, the pH is low). Glucose levels are low (fluid glucose <60 mg/dL or ratio of fluid glucose to plasma glucose <0.5) in rheumatoid effusion, malignant mesothelioma, systemic lupus erythematosus, esophageal rupture, tuberculous pleurisy, and empyema. Pleural fluid pH is less than 7.30 in empyema, esophageal rupture, rheumatoid effusion, tuberculosis, malignancy, and trauma. A parapneumonic effusion with pH less than 7.20 likely represents empyema, and drainage with a chest tube should be considered. Empyema caused by *Proteus* species produces a pH greater than 7.8 (because of the production of ammonia).

Amylase

The concentration of amylase in the pleural fluid is increased in esophageal rupture because of leakage of salivary amylase. In any unexplained left-sided effusion, consider pancreatitis and measure the amylase level in the pleural fluid.

Chylous Effusion

Chylous effusion is suggested by a turbid or milky white appearance of the fluid. However, chylothorax is confirmed by the presence of chylomicrons. Supportive evidence includes a pleural fluid triglyceride concentration greater than 110 mg/dL. A concentration less than 50 mg/dL excludes chylothorax. A helpful mnemonic for causes of chylous effusion is *5 T's*: *t*horacic duct, *t*rauma, *t*umor (lymphoma), *t*uberculosis, and *t*uberous sclerosis (lymphangiomyomatosis). Lymphoma is the most common nontraumatic cause of chylothorax. Cholesterol effusions are not true chylous effusions but are known as pseudochylothorax and are seen with tuberculous or rheumatoid effusions.

Cell Counts

A hemorrhagic effusion (pleural fluid hematocrit >50% of serum hematocrit) is seen in trauma, tumor, asbestos effusion, pancreatitis, pulmonary embolism with infarctions, and other conditions. A bloody effusion in lung cancer usually denotes pleural metastasis, even if the cytologic results are negative. Pleural fluid eosinophilia (>10%) is nonspecific and occurs in trauma, pulmonary infarction, psittacosis, drug-induced effusion, pulmonary infiltrate with eosinophilia-associated effusions, benign asbestos pleural effusion, and malignancy. Pleural fluid lymphocytosis occurs in tuberculosis, chronic effusions, lymphoma, sarcoidosis, chylothorax, and some collagenoses (eg, yellow nail syndrome and chronic rheumatoid pleurisy).

Cytology

Cytologic examination is an important test in most adults with an "unknown" effusion. Positive fluid cytologic findings in primary lung carcinoma imply unresectability (stage IIIB disease).

Cultures

In tuberculosis, it is important to culture pleural biopsy specimens. Tuberculous effusions yield positive cultures in less than 15% of cases. Pleural biopsy has a higher (>75%) diagnostic yield in tuberculosis. The adenosine deaminase and interferon-γ levels are increased in tuberculous pleural effusion. Cultures have poor yields in viral infections.

Pleural Biopsy

Pleural biopsy is indicated if tuberculous pleural disease is suspected. Pleural biopsy through a thoracoscope improves the diagnostic yield of pleural effusions.

- If pH is <7.2 and clinical suspicion for infection is high, drainage for suspected empyema should be considered.

- Pleural fluid amylase is increased in esophageal rupture.

- A mnemonic for the causes of chylous effusions is *5 T's*: *t*horacic duct, *t*rauma, *t*umor (lymphoma), *t*uberculosis, and *t*uberous sclerosis (lymphangiomyomatosis).

- Pleural fluid lymphocytosis is often caused by tuberculosis, lymphoma, and chylothorax.

Complications of thoracentesis include pneumothorax (3%-20% of patients), hemothorax, pulmonary edema, intrapulmonary hemorrhage, hemoptysis, vagal inhibition, air embolism, subcutaneous emphysema, bronchopleural fistula, empyema, seeding of a needle tract with malignant cells, and puncture of the liver or spleen.

SLEEP-RELATED BREATHING DISORDERS

Sleep-related breathing disorders encompass various abnormal breathing patterns that occur during sleep. Complications include sleepiness and increased cardiovascular morbidity and mortality (Box 17.5).

OBSTRUCTIVE SLEEP APNEA–HYPOPNEA SYNDROME

Obstructive sleep apnea (OSA) is defined as periodic cessation of airflow (duration ≥10 seconds) due to obstruction of the upper airway during sleep with continued respiratory effort. Typically, the episode is terminated with a temporary arousal from sleep and return of normal upper airway patency. *Hypopnea* is defined as reduction in airflow for at least 10 seconds, usually with resultant desaturation of at least 4%. Hypopnea is also typically terminated by an arousal. Such periodic episodes of apnea and hypopnea usually result in fragmented sleep and periodic desaturations. OSA should be suspected in patients who are obese, have increased neck circumference, are known to snore, and complain of daytime sleepiness. An overnight polysomnogram is required to make the diagnosis of OSA, which is defined as having more than 5 episodes of apnea and hypopnea per hour of sleep. Although overnight oximetry may suggest the presence of OSA, it is neither sensitive enough to rule out the diagnosis nor specific enough to confirm it.

Box 17.5 SYSTEMIC DISORDERS THAT HAVE BEEN ASSOCIATED WITH SLEEP-RELATED BREATHING DISORDERS

Central nervous system
  Cerebrovascular accidents
  Cognitive impairments
  Excessive sleepiness
  Lower seizure threshold
  Recurrent headaches
Cardiovascular system
  Myocardial infarcts
  Hypertension
  Cardiac arrhythmia
  Acceleration of atherosclerosis
  Pulmonary hypertension
Endocrine system
  Insulin insensitivity
  Suppression of growth hormone release
  Alteration of progesterone & testosterone release
  Obesity
Gastrointestinal tract
  Gastroesophageal reflux disease
Respiratory system
  Hypercapnia
  Dyspnea
  Reduced exercise tolerance
Psychiatric
  Depression
  Insomnia
  Nocturnal panic disorders

OSA has been associated with multisystemic dysfunction (Box 17.5). Several studies suggest that there is an increase in postoperative complications and overall mortality among patients with untreated OSA.

- The diagnosis of OSA is made with overnight polysomnography.
- Overnight oximetry is neither sensitive nor specific for OSA.
- Untreated OSA is associated with increased postoperative complications and mortality.

CENTRAL SLEEP APNEA

Central sleep apnea (CSA) is defined as periodic cessation of airflow (duration ≥10 seconds) during sleep in the absence of upper airway obstruction, and presumably it is caused by lack of respiratory muscle stimulation. In contrast to OSA, airflow is gradually resumed and is not always associated with an arousal from sleep. CSA may occur in persons with neurologic abnormalities (eg, cerebrovascular accident, amyotrophic lateral sclerosis, and postpolio syndrome), endocrine dysfunctions (eg, acromegaly and hypothyroidism), congestive heart failure, or narcotic use, or it may be idiopathic. The respiratory pattern, which cycles between crescendo and decrescendo respirations followed by a pause, is known as *Cheyne-Stokes respiration* or *periodic respiration* and is often seen in persons with congestive heart failure (especially during acute exacerbation), at high altitude, and after a cerebrovascular event.

- CSA is periodic cessation of airflow without upper airway obstruction.
- Cheyne-Stokes respiration is associated with congestive heart failure, high altitude, and stroke.

SLEEP HYPOVENTILATION SYNDROME

Sleep hypoventilation syndrome is characterized by a reduction in minute ventilation, resulting in hypercapnia and usually hypoxemia during sleep. Features include daytime hypercapnia, pulmonary hypertension, and cor pulmonale. Most affected persons are obese (*obesity-hypoventilation syndrome*) or have severe respiratory or neurologic disease.

TREATMENT

Patients with these sleep disorders are treated with noninvasive positive pressure devices, such as continuous positive airway pressure (CPAP) and bilevel positive airway pressure (BiPAP) devices. Adequate titration can be achieved during a polysomnogram, but, in certain circumstances, an autotitrating CPAP device may be used. In severe cases, tracheostomy may be required. Treatment of CSA may require a special positive airway pressure device such as BiPAP or adaptive servo-ventilator. Weight loss is also helpful in the treatment of OSA and sleep hypoventilation syndrome in overweight and obese patients.

- Noninvasive positive pressure devices are used to treat these sleep disorders.
- Weight loss is recommended for overweight and obese patients with OSA and sleep hypoventilation syndrome.

SUMMARY

- PFTs are useful in distinguishing between obstruction and restriction.
- The therapeutic approach to COPD consists of reducing risk factors (eg, smoking cessation), identifying the severity of COPD, quantifying the pulmonary dysfunction and response to bronchodilator therapy, selecting appropriate bronchodilators, anticipating and appropriately treating complications, and educating the patient and family about long-term therapy.
- CF is caused by a mutation in *CFTR*. CF affects all exocrine glands except sweat glands. Common manifestations of CF include sinusitis, nasal polyposis, bronchiectasis, obstructive airway disease, pancreatic insufficiency, biliary disease, and male infertility.
- The most common cause of a transudate is congestive heart failure. The most common cause of an exudate is pneumonia.
- OSA is diagnosed with overnight polysomnography. Overnight oximetry is neither sensitive nor specific for OSA. Untreated OSA is associated with increased postoperative complications and mortality.
- CSA is periodic cessation of airflow without upper airway obstruction. Cheyne-Stokes respiration is associated with congestive heart failure, high altitude, and stroke.

PART IV

INFECTIOUS DISEASES

18.

INFECTIONS IN THE IMMUNOCOMPROMISED HOST, RECOGNITION AND MANAGEMENT OF BIOTERRORISM INFECTIONS, AND INFECTIOUS SYNDROMES CAUSED BY SPECIFIC MICROORGANISMS

Pritish K. Tosh, MD, M. Rizwan Sohail, MD, and Elie F. Berbari, MD

GOALS

- Recognize infections in the immunocompromised host.
- Describe bioterrorism agents.
- Review specific infectious syndromes.

INFECTIONS IN THE IMMUNOCOMPROMISED HOST

Infections in the immunocompromised host may occur in the setting of neutropenia, B-cell and T-cell deficiencies, immunoglobulin deficiencies, complement deficiencies, and macrophage dysfunction. Some patients have multiple defects due to both the underlying disease and its treatment.

FEBRILE NEUTROPENIA

Patients with neutropenia are at risk for infections with *Pseudomonas* species, gram-positive cocci, Enterobacteriaceae, and *Candida* and *Aspergillus* species. Patients who have neutropenia from the cytotoxic effects of chemotherapy, which breach normal mucosal and cutaneous barriers, are at the highest risk for infection. Fever in a patient with an absolute polymorphonuclear neutrophil count less than 0.5×10^9/L is usually due to translocation of bacteria from impaired mucosal surfaces. The oral mucosa and gingival crevices are rich sites for aerobic and anaerobic streptococci and the lower gastrointestinal tract, for enteric gram-negative organisms and anaerobes. With prolonged neutropenia, invasive fungal disease may occur. Because of the high risk for morbidity, patients with acute leukemia expected to have prolonged neutropenia are given antimicrobial prophylaxis with levofloxacin and a mold-active azole (posaconazole or voriconazole) during the period of neutropenia. Bacteremia occurs in about 20% of neutropenic fever episodes.

Because of the high risk for morbidity in patients presenting with febrile neutropenia, empiric antimicrobial therapy should be started (urgent indication). Initial empiric regimens include monotherapy with ceftazidime, cefepime, or an antipseudomonal carbapenem. All empiric antimicrobial treatments need to have activity against *Pseudomonas aeruginosa*. Alternative therapy with antipseudomonal penicillin plus an aminoglycoside is also acceptable. Vancomycin can be added to the initial regimen

- if a patient has severe mucositis
- when quinolone prophylaxis has been used
- when the patient is known to be colonized with methicillin-resistant *Staphylococcus aureus* or penicillin-resistant *Streptococcus pneumoniae*
- when an obvious catheter-related infection is present
- if the patient is hypotensive.

Empiric vancomycin therapy can be subsequently discontinued in this setting if cultures are negative for aerobic gram-positive organisms. If there is no response to therapy after 5 to 7 days and the patient remains neutropenic, empiric therapy with posaconazole or voriconazole should be considered.

Oral ulcerations and odynophagia are common with herpes simplex virus infections. The presence of ulcerating papules of ecthyma gangrenosum should suggest disseminated infections due to *Pseudomonas* or other gram-negative bacteria. Bloodstream infection with gram-positive organisms (*S aureus*, coagulase-negative staphylococci, enterococci, viridans streptococci, and *Corynebacterium jeikeium*) is often due to infected central venous catheters. *Streptococcus mitis* bacteremia may occur in the setting of mucositis and can be associated with sepsis and acute respiratory distress syndrome, especially in patients with leukemia.

Bacteremia due to anaerobic organisms is uncommon, except in cases of perirectal abscess, gingivitis, or neutropenic enterocolitis (typhlitis). Persistent fever and abdominal symptoms in the neutropenic host should raise this consideration. These infections are managed medically with antimicrobials that cover the anaerobic flora.

Disseminated fungal infections often arise in the setting of prolonged neutropenia and use of broad-spectrum antibiotics. *Candida* species should be considered in neutropenic persons with nodular or erythematous papular skin lesions, fluffy white chorioretinal exudates, and fever unresponsive to empiric antibacterial agents. In particular, the development of fever and an increased alkaline phosphatase level during recovery from neutropenia and the finding of microabscesses in the liver and spleen on computed tomography suggest the presence of disseminated candidiasis (hepatosplenic candidiasis). The therapy of hepatosplenic candidiasis requires months of antifungal therapy, usually with fluconazole. Nonresolving nodular or consolidative pulmonary infiltrates in the setting of prolonged antibacterial use and neutropenia suggest invasive aspergillosis. Affected patients may have an "air crescent" sign on computed tomography of the chest, and the diagnosis can be determined from a respiratory or tissue specimen or a positive result on serum *Aspergillus* galactomannan assay. The most effective agent for treatment of invasive aspergillosis is voriconazole. The presence of facial numbness, pain, or sinus disease in the setting of prolonged neutropenia raises suspicion for invasive mucormycosis (due most often to *Rhizopus* or *Mucor* species) and invasive aspergillosis. These conditions are diagnosed by examination of respiratory tract specimens or endoscopic biopsy and treated with débridement and intravenous liposomal amphotericin compounds.

- *Streptococcus mitis* bacteremia may occur in the setting of mucositis and can be associated with sepsis and acute respiratory distress syndrome, especially in patients with leukemia.

- The development of fever and an increased alkaline phosphatase level during recovery from neutropenia and the finding of microabscesses in the liver and spleen on computed tomography suggest the presence of disseminated candidiasis (hepatosplenic candidiasis).

- Nonresolving nodular or consolidative pulmonary infiltrates in the setting of prolonged antibacterial use and neutropenia suggest the possibility of invasive aspergillosis.

INFECTIONS IN TRANSPLANT RECIPIENTS

Recipients of hematopoietic stem cell transplants receive "conditioning" chemotherapy that often leads to prolonged neutropenia and mucositis in the early transplant period before engraftment. These patients have complications similar to those with febrile neutropenia. Additionally, those who receive allogeneic transplants are at risk for graft-vs-host disease augmenting the degree of immunosuppression.

In solid organ transplant recipients, the risk for specific infection can be classified according to the following:

Table 18.1 **OPPORTUNISTIC INFECTIONS IN SOLID ORGAN TRANSPLANT**

MONTH	TYPE OF INFECTION AFTER TRANSPLANT
1	Bacterial infections (related to wound, intravenous lines, urinary tract), herpes simplex virus, hepatitis B
1–4	Cytomegalovirus, *Pneumocystis carinii*, *Listeria monocytogenes*, *Mycobacterium tuberculosis*, *Aspergillus*, *Nocardia*, *Toxoplasma*, hepatitis B, *Legionella*
2–6	Epstein-Barr virus, varicella-zoster virus, hepatitis C, *Legionella*
>6	*Cryptococcus neoformans*, *Legionella*

posttransplant time course and serologic status of recipient and donor for certain infections (such as cytomegalovirus or toxoplasmosis). Most infections in the first month after transplant are common nosocomial infections such as wound infections, urinary tract infections, and line infections. Cytomegalovirus, a common infection after transplant, can present with fever, viremia, hepatitis, colitis, gastritis, retinitis, myocarditis, and pneumonitis. Cytomegalovirus-seronegative recipients of organs from a seropositive donor are at highest risk for cytomegalovirus disease. The time of occurrence of opportunistic infections after solid organ transplant is given in Table 18.1. Pathogens associated with various immunodeficiency states are listed in Table 18.2.

- The majority of infections in the first month after transplant are not opportunistic infections. Most infections are common nosocomial infections such as wound infections, urinary tract infections, and line infections.

- Cytomegalovirus is an important pathogen in patients who have had a transplant. Presentations can include febrile illness with viremia, hepatitis, colitis, gastritis, retinitis, myocarditis, and pneumonitis.

- Cytomegalovirus-seronegative recipients of organs from a seropositive donor are at highest risk for cytomegalovirus disease.

IMMUNOSUPPRESSIVE MEDICATIONS

Commonly used immunosuppressive agents such as cyclosporin, tacrolimus, sirolimus, mycophenolate mofetil, and azathioprine, often in combination with corticosteroids, are associated with several T-cell–mediated opportunistic infections, including *Pneumocystis jiroveci* pneumonia, nocardiosis (pulmonary, brain, and cutaneous), histoplasmosis, cryptococcosis, coccidioidomycosis, listeriosis, cytomegalovirus, varicella-zoster, and herpes simplex virus (Table 18.2). Alemtuzumab and fludarabine agents frequently used in chronic lymphocytic leukemia cause a prolonged impact on T cells and are associated with similar T-cell–mediated infections.

Table 18.2 PATHOGENS ASSOCIATED WITH IMMUNODEFICIENCY

IMMUNODEFICIENCY	USUAL CONDITIONS	PATHOGENS
Neutropenia ($<0.5 \times 10^9$/L)	Cancer chemotherapy, adverse drug reaction, leukemia	**Bacteria:** Aerobic gram-negative bacilli (coliforms & pseudomonads, *Staphylococcus aureus, viridans streptococci,* coagulase-negative *Staphylococcus*) **Fungi:** *Aspergillus, Candida* species
Cell-mediated immunity	Organ transplant, human immunodeficiency virus infection, lymphoma (especially Hodgkin disease), corticosteroid therapy	**Bacteria:** *Listeria, Salmonella, Nocardia, Mycobacterium (M tuberculosis & M avium), Legionella* **Viruses:** CMV, herpes simplex, varicella-zoster, JC virus **Parasites:** *Toxoplasma, Strongyloides stercoralis, Cryptosporidium* **Fungi:** *Candida, Cryptococcus, Histoplasma, Coccidioides, Pneumocystis jiroveci* (formerly *Pneumocystis carinii*)
Hypogammaglobulinemia or dysgammaglobulinemia	Multiple myeloma, congenital or acquired deficiency, chronic lymphocytic leukemia	**Bacteria:** *Streptococcus pneumoniae, Haemophilus influenzae* (type B) **Parasites:** *Giardia* **Viruses:** Enteroviruses
Complement deficiencies C2, 3 C5 C6–8 Alternative pathway	Congenital	**Bacteria:** *S pneumoniae, H influenzae, S aureus,* Enterobacteriaceae *Neisseria meningitidis, S pneumoniae, H influenzae, Salmonella*
Hyposplenism	Splenectomy, hemolytic anemia	*S pneumoniae, H influenzae, Capnocytophaga canimorsus* (formerly known as CDC group DF-2)
Defective chemotaxis	Diabetes, alcoholism, renal failure, lazy leukocyte syndrome, trauma, SLE	*S aureus,* streptococci, *Candida*
Defective neutrophilic killing	Chronic granulomatous disease, myeloperoxidase deficiency	**Catalase-positive bacteria:** *S aureus, Escherichia coli, Candida* species

Abbreviations: CMV, cytomegalovirus; SLE, systemic lupus erythematosus.

Adapted from Bartlett JG. Pocket book of infectious disease therapy. 9th ed. Baltimore (MD): Williams & Wilkins; c1998. p. 236. Used with permission.

Primary prophylaxis with trimethoprim-sulfamethoxazole to prevent *P jiroveci* pneumonia and acyclovir to prevent herpes simplex virus should be offered.

The tumor necrosis factor-α inhibitors infliximab (Remicade), adalimumab (Humira), and etanercept (Enbrel) are associated with impaired granuloma formation and infections due to mycobacteria and endemic fungi such as *Histoplasma*.

Natalizumab (Tysabri), an agent used for treatment of multiple sclerosis and Crohn disease, is associated with the development of progressive multifocal leukoencephalopathy.

- Prolonged use of high-dose corticosteroids may be associated with T-cell–mediated opportunistic infections, such as *P jiroveci* pneumonia.

- Tumor necrosis factor-α inhibitors infliximab (Remicade), adalimumab (Humira), and etanercept (Enbrel) are associated with mycobacteria and endemic fungi such as *Histoplasma*.

- Natalizumab (Tysabri), an agent used for treatment of multiple sclerosis and Crohn disease, is associated with the development of progressive multifocal leukoencephalopathy.

RECOGNITION AND MANAGEMENT OF BIOTERRORISM INFECTIONS

The Centers for Disease Control and Prevention classifies the following diseases as category A, high-priority diseases that pose a risk to national security: anthrax, tularemia, plague, botulism, smallpox, and viral hemorrhagic fevers.

The incubation period, lethality, chemotherapy, chemoprophylaxis, vaccine, and specimens that can be obtained for each agent are described in Table 18.3. The agents have high mortality rates, can be easily disseminated or transmitted from person to person, and have the potential to have a major public health impact.

ANTHRAX

In 2001, several cases of inhalational and cutaneous anthrax followed the deliberate dissemination of weaponized *Bacillus anthracis* spores through the mail. Inhalational anthrax is particularly deadly. It produces hemorrhagic mediastinitis, hemorrhagic meningitis, and bacteremia. A characteristic finding in inhalational anthrax is a widened mediastinum on chest radiography. Cutaneous anthrax usually manifests as a solitary papule that evolves into an eschar, typically with surrounding edema. Culture of blood, pleural fluid, cerebrospinal fluid, or

Table 18.3 TREATMENT FOR INFECTIONS POTENTIALLY CAUSED BY BIOTERRORISM

DISEASE

VARIABLE	Smallpox (Variola Major)	Anthrax (Bacillus Anthracis)	Botulism Toxin (Clostridium Botulinum)	Plague (Yersinia Pestis)	Tularemia (Francisella Tularensis)	Viral Hemorrhagic Fevers
Incubation period, d	7–17	1–14 (cutaneous); 1–42[a] (inhalational)	1–5	2–3	1–21	2–21
Lethality	High to moderate	Very high	High without respiratory support	High without treatment	Moderate if untreated	Variable
Chemotherapy[b]	Cidofovir (in vitro)	Cutaneous: Ciprofloxacin 500 mg PO every 12 h or Doxycycline 100 mg PO every 12 h Duration: 60 d Inhalational: Ciprofloxacin 500 mg IV every 12 h or Doxycycline 100 mg IV every 12 h Plus 1 or 2 antimicrobials with demonstrated susceptibility Duration: 60 d	CDC bivalent equine antitoxin for serotypes A, B (licensed) & monovalent for serotype E (investigational)	Streptomycin 1 g IM twice daily or Gentamicin 5 mg/kg IV once daily or Ciprofloxacin 400 mg IV every 12 h or 750 mg PO twice daily or Chloramphenicol 25 mg/kg IV 4 times daily or Doxycycline 100 mg IV twice daily Duration: 10 d	Streptomycin 1 g IM twice daily or Gentamicin 5 mg/kg daily IV or Ciprofloxacin 400 mg IV twice daily Duration: 10 d Doxycycline 100 mg IV twice daily or Chloramphenicol 15 mg/kg IV 4 times daily Duration: 14–21 d	Supportive care. Ribavirin (arena viruses or bunyaviruses) 30 mg/kg IV initial dose, then 16 mg/kg every 6 h × 4 d, then 8 mg/kg every 8 h for 6 d. Passive antibody for AHF, BHF, Lassa fever, & CCHF
Chemoprophylaxis	Vaccinia immune globulin 0.6 mL/kg IM (within 3 d of exposure)	Ciprofloxacin 500 mg PO twice daily or Doxycycline 100 mg PO twice daily Duration: 60 d[c]	NA	Doxycycline 100 mg PO twice daily or Ciprofloxacin 500 mg PO twice daily or Chloramphenicol 25 mg/kg PO 4 times daily Duration: 7 d	Doxycycline 100 mg PO twice daily or Ciprofloxacin 500 mg PO twice daily Duration: 14 d	NA
Vaccine	Calf lymph vaccinia vaccine: 1 dose by scarification	Anthrax vaccine: 0.5 mL SC at 0, 2, 4 wk, 6, 12, 18 mo, with annual boosters	DOD pentavalent toxoid for serotypes A-E (IND): 0.5 mL deep SC at 0, 2, 12 wk, then annual booster	Greer inactivated vaccine (FDA licensed) Not effective for aerosol exposure. No longer available	Live attenuated vaccine (IND). Recommended for laboratory personnel, not for postexposure prophylaxis	AHF candidate #1 vaccine (cross-protection for BHF) (IND). RVF inactivated vaccine (IND)

Specimen[d] Postexposure (0–24 h)	Nasal swab, sputum, induced sputum for culture & PCR	Nasal swab, sputum, induced sputum for culture, FA, & PCR	Nasal swabs, respiratory secretions for PCR & toxin assays. Serum for toxin assays	Nasal swab, sputum, induced sputum for culture, FA, & PCR	Nasal swab, sputum, induced sputum for culture, FA, & PCR	Nasal swabs & induced respiratory secretions for RT-PCR & viral culture
Clinical illness & convalescence	Serum for viral culture. Drainage from skin lesions, scrapings, tissue for microscopy, EM, viral culture, PCR	Blood for culture & PCR. CSF for Gram stain, culture, & PCR. Tissue for Gram stain, culture, IHC, & PCR. Acute & convalescent sera for toxin & antibody studies	Nasal swabs, respiratory secretion for PCR & toxin assays. Usually no IgM or IgG	Blood, sputum, & tissue for Gram stain, culture, FA, F-1 antigen assays, IHC, & PCR. Acute & convalescent sera for antibody assays	Blood for culture & PCR. Sputum & tissue for Gram stain, culture, FA, IHC, & PCR. Acute & convalescent sera for antibody assays	Serum for viral culture, acute & convalescent antibody assays. Tissue for microscopy, EM, IHC, PCR

Abbreviations: AHF, Argentine hemorrhagic fever (Junin virus); BHF, Bolivian hemorrhagic fever; CCHF, Congo-Crimean hemorrhagic fever; CDC, Centers for Disease Control & Prevention; CSF, cerebrospinal fluid; DOD, US Department of Defense; EM, electron microscopy; FA, fluorescent antibody; FDA, US Food & Drug Administration; IgG, immunoglobulin G; IgM, immunoglobulin M; IHC, immunohistochemistry; IM, intramuscularly; IND, investigational drug; IV, intravenously; NA, not applicable; PO, orally; PCR, polymerase chain reaction; RT-PCR, reverse transcription-polymerase chain reaction; RVF, Rift Valley fever; SC, subcutaneously.

[a] A human case of inhalational anthrax developed at 42 days after exposure to the accidental release of *B anthracis* in Sverdlosk, Russia. This long incubation period may have been due, in part, to the use of postexposure prophylaxis in that setting or to inaccuracies in information regarding the date of the release (or if there was more than 1). The incubation period for inhalational cases acquired outside this setting (millworkers & others) ranges from 1 to 7 days.

[b] Dosages are for adult patients only. See agent-specific recommendations for children & immunocompromised populations.

[c] Increased duration because of possibility of concomitant aerosol exposure.

[d] Should be obtained only in coordination with infection control, public health, & Laboratory Response Network.

Data from Woods CW, Ashford D. Identifying and managing casualties of biological terrorism. In: Rose BD, editor. UpToDate. Wellesley (MA): UpToDate; c2007. Available from: http://www.uptodate.com.

a skin lesion confirms the diagnosis of anthrax. Sputum rarely reveals the organism. Nasal swab culture is useful for epidemiologic purposes but is not sufficiently sensitive to diagnose individual exposures.

Bacillus anthracis organisms are usually susceptible to penicillins, tetracycline, clindamycin, vancomycin, rifampin, and the fluoroquinolones. Inhalational exposures should be treated with ciprofloxacin or doxycycline for at least 60 days. Combination therapy with multiple active drugs is preferred for inhalational anthrax.

- Widened mediastinum is a characteristic finding in inhalational anthrax.

- Inhalational anthrax requires prolonged therapy with multiple active drugs.

TULAREMIA

Francisella tularensis infection is spread by tick or deer fly bites, aerosol droplets, or direct contact with tissues of infected animals (eg, rabbits, muskrats, squirrels, and beavers). Typically, infection causes an eschar at the site of inoculation, regional lymphadenopathy, and high fevers. Pneumonia also can occur. Streptomycin and gentamicin are the most effective therapies. Tetracycline is also active, but its use is associated with a 10% relapse rate. *Francisella tularensis* bacteria have been identified as a potential bioterrorism agent.

- *Francisella tularensis* infection is spread by tick or deer fly bites, aerosol droplets, or direct contact with tissues of infected animals.

PLAGUE

From 1950 to 1991, there were 336 cases of plague in the United States. According to the Centers for Disease Control and Prevention, 10 to 15 human plague cases occur each year, mostly in rural areas. Plague is enzootic in the southwestern United States. New Mexico has 56% of cases, and 29% of cases are among American Indians. Rats and fleas are the vectors. There is concern that the organism *Yersinia pestis* could be used for bioterrorism. Clinical presentations include 1) regional lymphadenopathy with septicemia—the most common form—and 2) the pneumonic form (high case-fatality rate). Secondary cases of pneumonic plague can occur, and droplet isolation is recommended for hospitalized patients. Treatment is with streptomycin or tetracycline.

SMALLPOX

Because of global efforts at eradication, the last case of smallpox in the world was in 1977. However, the possibility remains for this virus to be used as a bioterrorism agent. The rash of this illness is classically described as being pustular, firm, and umbilicated. The lesions start in the throat and mouth and then progress to the face, trunk, and extremities. The lesions commonly affect the palms and soles. Secondary cases of this illness occur, and airborne isolation is needed for hospitalized patients. Treatment is supportive, and exposed persons should be given vaccination.

VIRAL HEMORRHAGIC FEVERS

Multiple viruses can cause hemorrhagic fever, such as Ebola, Marburg, Lassa, Crimean-Congo, and Rift Valley. The clinical presentation includes multiorgan involvement with fever, thrombocytopenia, and bleeding. Treatment is largely supportive, although intravenous ribavirin may be effective in Lassa fever. Secondary cases occur in viral hemorrhagic fevers, and airborne isolation precautions are recommended.

INFECTIOUS SYNDROMES CAUSED BY SPECIFIC MICROORGANISMS

BACTERIA

Actinomycetes

Actinomyces israelii, an anaerobic, gram-positive, branching, filamentous organism, is the most common cause of human actinomycosis. *Actinomyces israelii* is part of the normal flora of the mouth. Infections are associated with any condition that creates an anaerobic environment (such as trauma with tissue necrosis, pus). The pathologic characteristic is formation of "sulfur granules," which are clumps of filaments. Infection is not characterized by granuloma formation.

- The pathologic characteristic of actinomycosis is "sulfur granules" (clumps of filaments).

Lumpy jaw is caused by a perimandibular infection with *A israelii*. It is characterized by a chronic draining sinus and may follow a dental extraction. Pulmonary actinomycosis develops when aspirated material reaches an area of lung with decreased oxygenation (such as in atelectasis). This condition often occurs in association with poor dental hygiene. A chronic suppurative pneumonitis may develop and eventually result in a sinus tract draining through the chest wall. There may be subsequent perforation into the esophagus, pericardium, ribs, and vertebrae. Ileocecal perforation from focal actinomycosis has been reported. Appendicitis may be a predisposing factor.

- Lumpy jaw is caused by a perimandibular infection with *A israelii*. It is characterized by a chronic draining sinus and may follow a dental extraction.

Actinomyces israelii also may be found in culture of tubo-ovarian abscesses and other pelvic infections. It is especially associated with pelvic inflammatory disease developing in a woman with an intrauterine device.

- A prolonged course of penicillin is the preferred treatment of actinomycosis.

Bartonella Species

Bartonella bacilliformis, *Bartonella quintana*, and *Bartonella henselae* are the most common *Bartonella* species that cause human disease. Bartonellae are gram-negative bacteria that are commonly transmitted by various arthropods, such as lice, ticks, and fleas. *Bartonella henselae* (formerly *Rochalimaea henselae*) is the primary causative agent of cat-scratch disease. The disease is characterized by a papule or pustule at the site of inoculation, followed by tender enlargement of the regional lymph nodes. Low-grade fever and malaise also may be present. Exposure to domestic cats (especially kittens) is the main risk factor. About 10% of patients may have extranodal manifestations. Disseminated infection with any of the *Bartonella* species can occur in patients with AIDS. *Bartonella quintana* and *B henselae* infections in patients with human immunodeficiency virus (HIV) or AIDS or other immunocompromised patients can present with cutaneous and visceral involvement, particularly the liver. Cutaneous neovascular proliferation causes skin lesions called bacillary angiomatosis, which resembles an angioma and can be confused with Kaposi sarcoma. This infection presents in the bones as lytic lesions. *Bartonella henselae* and *B quintana* can cause bacteremia and endocarditis. *Bartonella henselae* is associated with cat exposure, and *B quintana* occurs more often in alcoholic, homeless persons without specific cat exposure. *Bartonella quintana* can be transmitted by the bite of infected cat fleas. *Bartonella* endocarditis usually presents subacutely and often requires surgical management.

Diagnosis of cat-scratch disease is based on the clinical picture and serologic evidence of antibodies to *B henselae* or other species. In biopsied tissue, the organisms can be seen with Warthin-Starry stain. Because cat-scratch disease is usually self-limited, treatment is indicated only for patients with significant symptoms or bothersome adenopathy. Azithromycin is the most effective antibiotic for treatment of cat-scratch disease. For bacteremia or endocarditis, prolonged treatment with erythromycin, azithromycin, or doxycycline is given. For endocarditis, an aminoglycoside may be added for the first 2 weeks of the 8- to 12-week therapy.

- *Bartonella henselae* and *B quintana* can cause bacteremia and endocarditis.

- *Bartonella henselae* is associated with cat exposure, and *B quintana* occurs more often in alcoholic, homeless persons without specific cat exposure.

Brucella

Most cases of brucellosis acquired in the United States occur in 4 states (Texas, California, Virginia, and Florida). Although rare (100–200 cases per year) in the United States, brucellosis may occur in meat handlers, persons exposed to livestock, or persons who consume unpasteurized milk or other unpasteurized dairy products. Brucellosis can also be acquired by microbiology technologists and should be considered when these persons present with an otherwise unexplained febrile illness.

Brucellosis should be suspected in recent immigrants with fever or travelers who become ill after returning from developing countries. Personnel in microbiology laboratories should be warned when cultures are sent for processing so as to allow special precautions to be taken. Brucellosis may cause a chronic granulomatous disease with caseating granulomas. Brucellosis (along with tuberculosis) is a cause of "sterile" pyuria. Chronic brucellosis is one of the infectious causes of fever of undetermined origin. Calcifications in the spleen may be an indication of the presence of infection (although histoplasmosis also causes splenic calcifications). Serologic testing, special blood cultures, and bone marrow cultures are helpful for making the diagnosis; results of blood cultures are usually positive in acute brucellosis. Treatment is with doxycycline along with streptomycin or rifampin. Trimethoprim-sulfamethoxazole may be effective.

- Brucellosis may cause fever of unknown origin and is associated with animal exposures.

Clostridium botulinum

Clostridium botulinum produces a heat-labile neurotoxin that inhibits acetylcholine release from cholinergic terminals at the motor end plate. Botulism usually is caused by the ingestion of contaminated food (home-canned products and improperly prepared or handled commercial foods). There is concern that the organism can be used as a bioterrorism agent. Wound botulism results from contaminated traumatic wounds. Neonatal botulism can result from consumption of contaminated honey.

The clinical symptoms of botulism include unexplained diplopia; fixed, dilated pupils; dry mouth; and descending flaccid paralysis with normal sensation. Patients are usually alert and oriented and have intact deep tendon reflexes. Fever is rare.

Treatment of botulism is primarily supportive. An equine antitoxin is available and helpful for preventing progression of the disease. In food-borne cases, purging the gut with cathartics, enemas, and emetics to remove unabsorbed toxin also may be of value. Antibiotic therapy does not affect the course of illness.

- Neurotoxin of *C botulinum* inhibits acetylcholine release from cholinergic terminals at the motor end plate.

- The clinical symptoms of botulism include unexplained diplopia; fixed, dilated pupils; dry mouth; and descending flaccid paralysis with normal sensation.

- Treatment of botulism is supportive. Antibiotic therapy is not indicated.

Clostridium tetani

Clostridium tetani is a strictly anaerobic gram-positive rod that produces a neurotoxin (tetanospasmin). This neurotoxin, when produced by organisms in infected wounds, is responsible for the clinical manifestations of tetanus. Although rare in the United States, 200 to 300 cases still occur annually, mostly in elderly persons who have never been immunized.

The first muscles affected by tetanus are controlled by cranial nerves, resulting in trismus. Eye muscles (cranial nerves III and IV) rarely are involved. As the disease progresses, other muscles become involved (generalized rigidity, spasms, and opisthotonos). Sympathetic overactivity is common (labile hypertension, hyperpyrexia, and arrhythmias). The diagnosis of tetanus is based on clinical findings, although a characteristic electromyogram is suggestive.

- The diagnosis of tetanus is based primarily on clinical findings, which are induced by a neurotoxin.

Treatment of tetanus includes supportive care, proper wound management, and administration of antiserum (human tetanus immune globulin). Penicillin G or metronidazole should be administered to eradicate vegetative organisms in the wound. Active tetanus does not induce protective immunity. Therefore, a primary tetanus immunization series should be given after an episode of tetanus.

- Active tetanus does not induce protective immunity to subsequent episodes of tetanus.

Corynebacterium diphtheriae

Diphtheria is a classic infectious disease that is easily prevented with vaccination. Epidemics of diphtheria recently occurred in states of the former Soviet Union. Diphtheria causes a focal infection of the respiratory tract (pharynx in 60%-70% of cases, larynx, nasal passages, or tracheobronchial tree). A tightly adherent, gray pseudomembrane is the hallmark of the disease, but disease can occur without pseudomembrane formation. Manifestations depend on the extent of involvement of the upper airway and the presence or absence of systemic complications due to toxin. Toxin-mediated complications include myocarditis (10%-25%), which causes congestive heart failure and arrhythmias, and polyneuritis (bulbar dysfunction followed by peripheral neuropathy). Respiratory muscles may be paralyzed.

- In diphtheria, toxin-mediated complications include myocarditis (10%-25%), which causes congestive heart failure and arrhythmias, and polyneuritis.

- Diphtheria may cause respiratory muscle paralysis.

The diagnosis of diphtheria is definitively established by culture with Löffler medium. Rapid diagnosis sometimes can be made with methylene blue stain or fluorescent antibody staining of pharyngeal swab specimens. Diphtheria is highly contagious. Equine antiserum is still the main therapy. Although there is no evidence that antimicrobial agents alter the course of disease, they may prevent transmission to susceptible hosts. Erythromycin and penicillin G are active against *C diphtheriae*. Nonimmune persons exposed to diphtheria should be evaluated and treated with erythromycin or penicillin G if culture results are positive. They should also be immunized with diphtheria-tetanus toxoid.

- Nonimmune persons exposed to diphtheria should be evaluated and treated with erythromycin or penicillin G if culture results are positive.

Cutaneous infection with *C diphtheriae* can occur in indigent persons and alcoholics. Preexisting dermatologic disease (most often in the lower extremities) is a risk factor. Lesions may appear "punched-out" and filled with a membrane, but they may be indistinguishable from other infected ulcers. Toxin-mediated complications (such as myocarditis and neuropathy) are uncommon. Diagnosis is established with methylene blue staining and culture of the lesion with Löffler medium.

- Cutaneous diphtheria is reported in indigent persons and alcoholics.

Nocardia

Nocardia organisms are aerobic, gram-positive, filamentous, and branching and are visualized with a modified acid-fast stain. *Nocardia asteroides* is the cause of most human infections in the United States (Figure 18.1). *Nocardia brasiliensis* and *Nocardia madurae* cause mycetomas. Infections are most often opportunistic, occurring in immunosuppressed patients, including those with HIV or AIDS, but infections can occur in normal hosts also.

- *Nocardia* infections are most often opportunistic, occurring in immunosuppressed patients.

The respiratory tract is the usual portal of entry for *Nocardia* infection. Chronic pneumonitis and lung abscess are the most common findings. Hematogenous spread to the brain is relatively common. Computed tomography or magnetic resonance imaging of the head is advised in immunocompromised patients with pulmonary nocardiosis. Spread

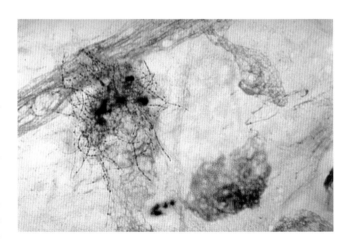

Figure 18.1 *Nocardia asteroides* (Modified Acid-Fast Stain, ×450).

also can occur to the skin (12%) and joints (3%). In patients with chronic pneumonia who have neurologic symptoms or signs, *Nocardia* brain abscess should be considered.

- In immunosuppressed patients with pulmonary nocardiosis, computed tomography of the head should be done to rule out concomitant brain abscess, even in the absence of symptoms.

Nocardiosis is not diagnosed until autopsy in up to 40% of cases. Antemortem diagnosis depends on obtaining appropriate stains and cultures (the organism will grow on fungal media). Because sputum culture is relatively insensitive, specimens obtained by bronchoscopy or open lung biopsy may be needed to confirm the diagnosis. The disease must be differentiated from other causes of chronic pneumonia (such as bacterial, actinomycotic, tubercular, fungal infections).

Therapy involves drainage of abscesses and high doses of sulfonamide drugs (trimethoprim-sulfamethoxazole is the current drug of choice). Some species of *Nocardia* show evidence of sulfonamide resistance. Other antimicrobial agents used for nocardiosis include imipenem, amikacin, minocycline, and cephalosporins. Therapy depends on antimicrobial susceptibility patterns. Newer drugs such as linezolid have activity against *Nocardia* species.

- Nocardiosis is diagnosed at autopsy in up to 40% of cases.
- Trimethoprim-sulfamethoxazole is the current treatment of choice.

SPIROCHETES

Leptospirosis

Leptospira interrogans infection is acquired by contact with urine from infected animals (eg, rats and dogs), and it causes a biphasic disease. Infections occur more often after a rainy season. The organism can enter directly through the skin from contaminated water that contains animal urine. Leptospirosis should be considered in the differential diagnosis of febrile travelers who were exposed to freshwater. The first phase, the leptospiremic phase, is characterized by abrupt-onset headache (98%), fever, chills, conjunctivitis, severe muscle aching, gastrointestinal symptoms (50%), changes in sensorium (25%), rash (7%), and hypotension. This phase lasts 3 to 7 days. Improvement in symptoms coincides with disappearance of *Leptospira* organisms from blood and cerebrospinal fluid. The second phase, the immune stage, occurs after a relatively asymptomatic period of 1 to 3 days, when fever and generalized symptoms recur. Meningeal symptoms often develop during this period. The second phase is characterized by the appearance of immunoglobulin M antibodies. Most patients recover after 1 to 3 days. However, in serious cases, hepatic dysfunction and renal failure may develop. Death in patients with leptospirosis usually occurs in the second phase as a result of hepatic and renal failure.

- *Leptospira interrogans* infection is acquired by contact with urine from infected animals (eg, rats and dogs).
- Leptospirosis is a biphasic disease.

The diagnosis of leptospirosis is established on the basis of clinical presentation and of cultures of blood and, rarely, cerebrospinal fluid in the first 7 to 10 days of infection. Urine cultures can remain positive in the second week of illness. Serologic testing by immunoglobulin M detection with enzyme-linked immunosorbent assay or microscopic agglutination test has a low sensitivity, especially in the acute phase, but it increases to 89% and 63% in the second phase of disease, respectively. The specificity of both tests is high (>94%) in all specimens. Treatment with penicillin G is effective only if given within the first 1 to 5 days from onset of symptoms. Oral amoxicillin or doxycycline can be used for mild-moderate illness.

- Treatment of leptospirosis with penicillin G is effective only if given within the first 1–5 days from onset of symptoms.

Lyme Disease

Epidemiology
Lyme disease is the most common vector-borne (*Ixodes* ticks) disease reported in the United States. The incidence of disease is highest in the spring and summer, when exposure to ticks is most common. Evidence suggests that ticks must be attached for more than 36 hours to transmit infection. Although Lyme disease has been reported in most states, it is most common in coastal New England and New York, the mid-Atlantic states, Oregon, northern California, and the Upper Midwest. The white-footed mouse and the white-tailed deer serve as zoonotic reservoirs for the etiologic agent *Borrelia burgdorferi*. Coinfections with *Babesia* or *Ehrlichia* species can occur in up to 15% of cases and may increase the severity of symptoms. Despite popular concern, the Infectious Diseases Society of America recognizes no chronic form of the disease.

- *Borrelia burgdorferi* is the etiologic agent of Lyme disease.

Clinical Syndromes
Stage 1 (early) occurs from 3 to 32 days after the tick bite. Erythema migrans (solitary or multiple lesions) is the hallmark of Lyme disease and occurs in 80% or more of infected persons. It can be associated with fever, lymphadenopathy, and meningismus. The rash of erythema migrans usually enlarges and resolves over 3 to 4 weeks. *Borrelia burgdorferi* disseminates hematogenously early in the course of the illness.

- Erythema migrans develops in ≥80% of patients with Lyme disease.

Stage 2 occurs weeks to months after stage 1. In 10% to 15% of cases, neurologic abnormalities develop (facial nerve palsy, lymphocytic meningitis, encephalitis, chorea, myelitis, radiculitis, and peripheral neuropathy). Carditis (reversible atrioventricular block) occurs in 5% to 10% of patients. Conduction abnormalities are mostly reversible, and permanent heart block is rare. Temporary pacing is necessary in approximately 30% of patients, but a permanent pacemaker is not indicated. Dilated cardiomyopathy has been reported, and conjunctivitis and iritis also occur.

- During stage 2 of Lyme disease, 10%-15% of patients have neurologic abnormalities.
- Carditis occurs in 5%-10% of patients with Lyme disease.

Stage 3, although uncommon, can develop months to years after initial infection. Monarticular or oligoarticular arthritis occurs in 50% of patients who do not receive effective therapy. It becomes chronic in 10% to 20%. Chronic arthritis is more common in those with HLA-DR2 and HLA-DR4. Other manifestations are acrodermatitis chronica atrophicans (primarily with European strains), progressive, chronic encephalitis, and dementia (rare). Most patients will have detectable serum antibodies against *B burgdorferi*. Magnetic resonance imaging may show demyelination.

Diagnosis
Anti-*B burgdorferi* antibodies can be detected by enzyme-linked immunosorbent assay after the first 2 to 6 weeks of illness. The Western blot test is the confirmatory serologic test for the diagnosis when the antibody response of screening enzyme-linked immunosorbent assay is positive. This 2-step test (endorsed by the Centers for Disease Control and Prevention) is both sensitive and specific for establishing the diagnosis of Lyme disease. Serologic tests should be ordered only in cases of a clinical syndrome compatible with Lyme disease. Serologic testing is likely to be negative in the early stage (ie, with the erythema migrans rash). Treatment without testing should be initiated in patients who reside in or visit endemic areas and have the characteristic skin lesion of erythema migrans. False-positive results occur with infectious mononucleosis, rheumatoid arthritis, systemic lupus erythematosus, echovirus infection, and other spirochetal disease.

Treatment
For stage 1 (early) Lyme disease in the absence of neurologic involvement or complete heart block, doxycycline (100 mg twice a day for 10–21 days), amoxicillin (500 mg 3 times a day for 10–21 days), and cefuroxime axetil (500 mg twice a day for 10–21 days) are effective therapeutic agents. Azithromycin, clarithromycin, and erythromycin are less effective than doxycycline and should generally be avoided. Because of the risk of vertical transmission, all pregnant women with active Lyme disease should be treated. Doxycycline is contraindicated in pregnant women and children younger than 8 years.

In Lyme carditis, the outcome is usually favorable. If first- or second-degree atrioventricular block is present, it should be treated with oral agents, whereas third-degree heart block should be treated with intravenous ceftriaxone, 2 g a day for 14

to 21 days, or intravenous penicillin G 20 million units a day for 14 to 21 days. Lyme meningitis, radiculopathy, or encephalitis should be treated parenterally.

- In Lyme carditis, the outcome is usually favorable.

The outcome in patients with facial palsy is also usually favorable. In one series, 105 of 122 affected patients completely recovered. Corticosteroids have no role. If only facial nerve palsy is present (no symptoms of meningitis or radiculoneuritis), oral therapy with doxycycline or amoxicillin is used. Patients with Lyme disease may have bilateral facial palsy. The therapy used if other neurologic manifestations are present is described below.

- The outcome in patients with facial palsy due to Lyme disease is usually favorable.

If Lyme meningitis is present, ceftriaxone, 2 g a day for 14 to 28 days, or intravenous penicillin G, 20 million units a day for 14 to 28 days, should be given. Radiculoneuritis and peripheral neuropathy may have a greater tendency for chronicity and often occur with meningitis. Treatment is the same as that for Lyme-associated meningitis. The regimens for encephalopathy and encephalomyelitis are identical to those for meningitis.

- Radiculoneuritis and peripheral neuropathy may have a greater tendency for chronicity and often occur with meningitis.

Optimal regimens for Lyme arthritis (oral vs intravenous) are not established. Intra-articular corticosteroids may cause treatment failures. Joint rest and aspiration of reaccumulated joint fluid are often needed. Response to antibiotics may be delayed. If no neurologic disease is present, doxycycline is given (100 mg orally twice a day for 28 days). An alternative regimen is amoxicillin and probenecid (500 mg each, 4 times a day for 28 days) or ceftriaxone (2 g per day intravenously for 14–28 days). Synovectomy may be necessary in the management of persistent monoarticular Lyme arthritis that has not responded to antimicrobial therapy.

Prevention
Prophylactic antibiotic therapy after a tick bite is not recommended. Use of single-dose doxycycline is recommended only if 1) the adult or nymphal *Ixodes scapularis* tick has been attached for 36 hours (as evidenced by engorgement of the tick or by certainty of time of exposure to tick), 2) prophylaxis can be started within 72 hours of tick removal, 3) the *B burgdorferi* prevalence rate is 20% among ticks within the region of the tick bite, and 4) doxycycline is not contraindicated. In the vast majority of tick bites, disease is not transmitted. Appropriate use of DEET (N,N-diethyl-3-methylbenzamide)- or picaridin-containing insect repellents and protective clothing are strongly recommended during outdoor activities.

- Prophylactic antibiotic therapy after a tick bite is not recommended, unless 1) the adult or nymphal *I scapularis* tick has been attached for 36 hours (as evidenced by engorgement of the tick or by certainty of time of exposure to tick), 2) prophylaxis can be started within 72 hours of tick removal, 3) *B burgdorferi* prevalence rate is 20% among ticks within the region of the tick bite, and 4) doxycycline is not contraindicated.

RICKETTSIAE

All rickettsial infections are transmitted by an insect vector, except Q fever (respiratory spread). All are associated with a rash, except Q fever and ehrlichiosis. The rash of Rocky Mountain spotted fever may be indistinguishable from that of meningococcemia. Rocky Mountain spotted fever rash begins on the extremities and moves centrally. The rash of typhus (both murine and endemic typhus) begins centrally and moves toward the extremities. Rocky Mountain spotted fever is most common in the mid-Atlantic states and Oklahoma, not the Rocky Mountain states. The pathophysiology of all rickettsial infections includes vasculitis and disseminated intravascular coagulation. Rickettsial pox is a common, although usually unrecognized, disease in urban areas of the United States. It is the only rickettsial disease characterized by vesicular rash. The mouse mite is the vector for rickettsial pox. A small eschar is present at the site of inoculation in 95% of patients.

- All rickettsial infections have an arthropod vector, except Q fever.

- All rickettsial infections are associated with a rash, except Q fever and ehrlichiosis.

- Rocky Mountain spotted fever rash begins on the extremities and moves centrally.

- Rocky Mountain spotted fever is most common in the mid-Atlantic states and Oklahoma, not the Rocky Mountain states.

Coxiella burnetii, the cause of Q fever, is acquired by inhalation of contaminated aerosol particles of dust, earth, or feces or after exposure to animal products, especially infected placentas. Sheep are common sources, but other animals, including cats, can harbor the disease (eg, a small outbreak occurred in a group of poker players after a cat gave birth beneath their card table). Disease manifests most commonly as an isolated febrile illness, and most such cases present with pneumonitis; 15% of patients have hepatitis (granulomatous), 1% have endocarditis, and some also present with central nervous system manifestations. Q fever is one of the causes of culture-negative endocarditis. It usually is diagnosed with serologic testing. Treatment is with tetracycline or fluoroquinolones.

- Among persons with Q fever, most have pneumonitis, and 15% have hepatitis.

- Q fever is one of the causes of culture-negative endocarditis.

Ehrlichia species are gram-negative intracellular bacteria that resemble rickettsial organisms and preferentially infect lymphocytes, monocytes, and neutrophils. The species that cause human ehrlichiosis are *Ehrlichia chaffeensis* (which infects monocytes), *Ehrlichia equi*, and *Anaplasma phagocytophilum* (formerly *phagocytophilia*) (which causes human granulocytic ehrlichiosis).

The disease is seasonal; the peak incidence is from May through July. The vectors are the common dog tick (*Dermacentor variabilis*), the lone star tick (*Amblyomma americanum*) for *E chaffeensis*, and *Ixodes* ticks (same vector as Lyme disease) for the agent of human granulocytic ehrlichiosis. The incubation period is approximately 7 days, followed by fever, chills, malaise, headache, and myalgia. Fewer than 50% of patients have a rash. Important laboratory features include leukopenia, thrombocytopenia, and increased levels of hepatic transaminases.

The severity of the disease is variable, but severe complications, including death, can occur. Coinfection with human granulocytic ehrlichiosis and *B burgdorferi* (Lyme disease) does occur and can be especially severe. Diagnosis depends on serologic analysis (indirect immunofluorescent assay) or detection by polymerase chain reaction amplification. Treatment is with doxycycline, 100 mg twice a day. Unlike the rickettsial diseases, chloramphenicol is often not effective against *Ehrlichia*.

FUNGI

Coccidioidomycosis

Coccidioides immitis is a dimorphic fungus: in tissue it exists as a spherule, and in culture at room temperature it is mycelial (filamentous). It forms arthrospores that are highly infectious. *Coccidioides immitis* is endemic in the southwestern United States, especially the San Joaquin Valley of California and central Arizona, and in Mexico. Disseminated disease is most likely to occur in males (especially Filipino and black), pregnant females, and immunocompromised hosts, including HIV-infected patients, regardless of sex. Nonpregnant white females seem to be more resistant to disseminated disease than white males.

- *Coccidioides immitis* is endemic in the southwestern United States and Mexico.

- Disseminated disease is most likely to occur in males (especially Filipino and black), pregnant females, and immunocompromised hosts, including HIV-infected patients.

Half to two-thirds of primary infections with *C immitis* are subclinical. The most common clinical manifestation is pneumonitis that is usually self-limited. Common manifestations are dry cough and fever (valley fever) that may resemble influenza. Associated findings include hilar adenopathy, pleural effusion (12%), thin-walled cavities (5%), and solid "coin" lesions. Disseminated infection predominantly affects the central nervous system, skin, bones, and joints.

- Primary infection with *C immitis* causes pneumonitis that is usually self-limited.

Coccidioidomycosis is one of the many infectious causes of erythema nodosum. When present, it usually indicates an active immune response that will control the infection. Erythema nodosum is more common in females and is often associated with arthralgias, especially of the knees and ankles.

- Coccidioidomycosis is one of the many infectious causes of erythema nodosum.

The diagnosis of coccidioidomycosis is based on detecting the organism by culture or biopsy with silver stains. A *C immitis* serologic (complement fixation) titer more than 1:4 is suggestive of infection. Skin testing is of epidemiologic value only. The diagnosis of coccidioidomycosis meningitis is usually established by detecting cerebrospinal fluid anticoccidioidal antibodies. A biopsy specimen may reveal a diagnostic *C immitis* spherule (Figure 18.2). Laboratory abnormalities may include eosinophilia and hypercalcemia.

Fluconazole, itraconazole, and amphotericin B are effective for therapy of coccidioidomycosis. The acute pulmonary form is usually self-limited, and observation may be adequate. However, therapy is indicated if a patient is pregnant, is immunocompromised (patients with AIDS or receiving immunosuppressive regimens for organ transplant or other medical reasons), or has worsening infection without therapy. Amphotericin B is the drug of choice for severe manifestations and for pregnant women with coccidioidomycosis. An alternative to fluconazole is itraconazole (200 mg twice daily). For meningitis, therapy with high-dose fluconazole is preferred and has largely replaced intrathecal amphotericin B. Because of the high relapse rate of *C immitis* meningitis, chronic suppressive therapy is necessary, usually with fluconazole. *Coccidioides* meningitis may be complicated by adhesive arachnoiditis. Newer antifungal medications such as voriconazole are active in vitro but clinical studies are not available, and caspofungin has limited in vitro activity against coccidioidomycosis. Because of their risk for teratogenicity, azole

antifungals such as fluconazole should be avoided during the first trimester of pregnancy.

- Fluconazole, itraconazole, and amphotericin B are effective for therapy of coccidioidomycosis.

- Therapy is indicated if a patient is pregnant, is immunocompromised, or has worsening infection without therapy.

Histoplasmosis

Histoplasma capsulatum is also a dimorphic fungus that grows as a small (3 mm in diameter) yeast in tissue. Culture at room temperature produces the mycelial form. Although present in many areas of the world, histoplasmosis is especially prevalent in the Ohio, Missouri, and Mississippi river valleys and parts of Mexico and Central America. Outbreaks have been associated with large construction projects and exposure to bird or bat droppings. Histoplasmosis is acquired by inhalation of spores and also can be transmitted by organ transplant from an infected donor. The risk of acquisition is increased with certain activities, including caving and bridge or other construction. Although healthy individuals may acquire histoplasmosis, patients with AIDS and those with cell-mediated immune deficiency are particularly susceptible to disseminated disease. *Histoplasma capsulatum* infection is one of the causes of caseating granulomata.

- Outbreaks of histoplasmosis have been associated with large construction projects and exposure to bird or bat droppings.

- Although healthy individuals may acquire histoplasmosis, patients with AIDS and those with cell-mediated immune deficiency are particularly susceptible to disseminated disease.

Primary (acute) histoplasmosis may be clinically indistinguishable from influenza or other upper respiratory tract infections. After resolution, multiple small, calcified granulomas may be seen on subsequent chest radiography. The progressive (disseminated) form of histoplasmosis is uncommon but serious. The disseminated form and reactivation of prior disease are most likely to occur in infants, elderly men, and immunosuppressed persons, including those with HIV or AIDS and those receiving therapy with tumor necrosis factor-α inhibitors such as etanercept and infliximab. Manifestations may resemble those of lymphoma, with weight loss, fever, anemia, increased erythrocyte sedimentation rate, and splenomegaly. Mucosal ulcers, which can occur throughout the gastrointestinal tract and mouth, are not infrequent. Disseminated histoplasmosis typically involves the reticuloendothelial system—bone marrow, spleen, lymph nodes, and liver. Bone marrow involvement may be associated with pancytopenia. As with tuberculosis, the adrenal glands may be infected, with resulting adrenal insufficiency. Chronic cavitary pulmonary disease due to *Histoplasma* may resemble tuberculosis and

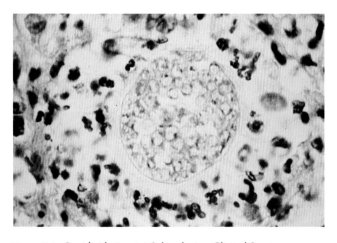

Figure 18.2 *Coccidioides immitis* Spherules in a Clinical Specimen (Grocott Methenamine-Silver Stain).

tends to occur in patients with preexistent pulmonary disease such as chronic obstructive pulmonary disease.

- Primary (acute) histoplasmosis may be indistinguishable from influenza or other upper respiratory tract infections.
- As with tuberculosis, the adrenal glands may be infected by *H capsulatum*, with resulting adrenal insufficiency.

The result of serologic testing—using complement fixation and immunodiffusion—if positive, is helpful for confirming the diagnosis of histoplasmosis, although the sensitivity may be decreased in immunosuppressed patients. Biopsy, silver staining, and cultures of infected tissues are the best means of diagnosis. Bone marrow stains and cultures and fungal blood cultures are frequently helpful. Biopsy specimens of mouth lesions can be diagnostic. Detection of *Histoplasma* antigen in urine, cerebrospinal fluid, or serum is sensitive and easily available as a diagnostic test, especially for the diagnosis and treatment of disseminated disease.

The mild, acute forms of histoplasmosis are usually self-limited and do not require therapy. Amphotericin B in a total dose of 35 mg/kg (given over time as 0.5–1 mg/kg per day) is the drug of choice for all severe, life-threatening cases. Itraconazole is effective for most nonmeningeal, non–life-threatening cases and has largely replaced ketoconazole. Itraconazole dosage is 200 to 400 mg per day (guided by serum drug concentrations) for 6 to 12 months. Patients with AIDS require chronic maintenance therapy.

Blastomycosis

Yet another dimorphic fungal pathogen is *Blastomyces dermatitidis*. In tissue, the yeast forms are thick-walled and have broad-based buds (±10 mm in diameter) (Figure 18.3). In culture at room temperature, a mycelial form is found. Blastomycosis is endemic in the southeastern and upper midwestern United States. Primary pulmonary blastomycosis may be asymptomatic and may disseminate hematogenously to bone, skin, or prostate. Granulomas occur, but calcification is less frequent than with histoplasmosis or tuberculosis.

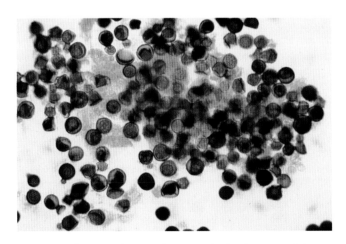

Figure 18.3 *Blastomyces dermatitidis* in Bronchoalveolar Lavage (Silver Stain, ×450).

Blastomycosis affects lung, skin, bone (especially the vertebrae), male genitalia (ie, prostate, epididymis, and testis), and the central nervous system. The pulmonary form has no characteristic findings: pleural effusion is rare, hilar adenopathy develops occasionally, and cavitation is infrequent. It often mimics carcinoma of the lung. Cutaneous involvement with blastomycosis is common. Lesions, especially on the face, are characteristically painless and nonpruritic and have a sharp, spreading border. Chronic crusty lesions may occur.

- Blastomycosis affects lungs, skin, bone (especially the vertebrae), and male genitalia (ie, prostate, epididymis, and testis).
- The most common clinical forms of blastomycosis are pulmonary and cutaneous.

The diagnosis of blastomycosis is based on the results of biopsy, stains, and cultures. Serologic and skin testing are rarely helpful.

Amphotericin B (total dose is 20–25 mg/kg) or itraconazole (200–400 mg per day for 6 months) is effective as therapy for blastomycosis. Amphotericin B is reserved primarily for life-threatening infections. Mild-to-moderate nonmeningeal blastomycosis can be treated with itraconazole (200–400 mg/day) for 6 months.

- Amphotericin B or itraconazole can be used to treat blastomycosis.

Sporotrichosis

Sporothrix schenckii, another dimorphic fungal pathogen, in tissue is a round, cigar-shaped yeast. In culture at room temperature it is mycelial. *Sporothrix schenckii* is most often found in soil, plants, plant products such as straw, wood, sphagnum moss, and thorny plants. Sporotrichosis is transmitted by cutaneous inoculation (rose-gardener's disease) and, rarely, through inhalation. It manifests as a suppurative and granulomatous reaction.

Cutaneous infection produces characteristic crusty lesions ascending the lymphatics of the extremities from the initial site of infection. Similar lesions may be produced by infection with *Mycobacterium marinum*, *Nocardia*, or cutaneous leishmaniasis. Septic arthritis can occasionally occur. Sporotrichosis occasionally may cause chronic pneumonitis (with cavitation and empyema) or meningitis.

- Cutaneous sporotrichosis produces characteristic crusty lesions ascending the lymphatics of the extremities from the initial site of infection.
- Sporotrichosis occasionally may cause chronic pneumonitis (with cavitation and empyema) or meningitis.

The diagnosis of sporotrichosis may be difficult and depends on clinical recognition of the cutaneous lesions in most instances. Biopsy, culture, or serologic testing may aid in the diagnosis.

For the lymphocutaneous or cutaneous form, itraconazole is the therapy of choice. An effective alternative is supersaturated solution of potassium iodide. Amphotericin B is recommended for disseminated disease (pulmonary, joint), although it may respond poorly to therapy.

Aspergillosis

Aspergillus is an opportunistic pathogen that causes infection in immunocompromised persons, particularly those with prolonged neutropenia or steroid use. Although any species of *Aspergillus* can cause disease, *Aspergillus fumigatus* is the most common pathogenic species. The organisms have large, septated hyphae (phycomycetes are nonseptated) branching at 45° angles (Figure 18.4). Especially in neutropenic hosts, they may invade blood vessels, producing a striking thrombotic angiitis similar to phycomycosis. Metastatic foci may cause suppurative abscess formation.

- *Aspergillus* organisms may invade blood vessels, producing a striking thrombotic angiitis.

The form of disease produced by aspergillosis primarily is determined by the nature of the immunologic deficit in the infected individual. Neutropenia predisposes to rapidly invasive bronchopulmonary disease with early dissemination to the brain and other tissues. The longer the duration of neutropenia, the higher the risk for invasive aspergillosis. Prompt therapy with high doses of amphotericin B and resolution of the neutropenia are necessary to control the disease. Diagnosis should be suspected when *Aspergillus* is isolated from any source in a susceptible individual.

T-cell deficiencies (primarily from corticosteroids) predispose to somewhat more indolent, though no less serious, forms of aspergillosis. Progressive pulmonary infiltrates, necrotic skin lesions, wound infections, and brain abscesses may result. Sinus infections with *Aspergillus* may be localized or invasive in patients with T-cell deficiencies.

Serologic testing is not helpful for diagnosing invasive *Aspergillus* in the compromised host.

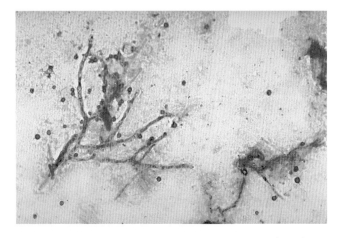

Figure 18.4 *Aspergillus fumigatus* in Bronchoalveolar Lavage (×450).

- Neutropenia predisposes to rapidly invasive bronchopulmonary disease with early dissemination to the brain and other tissues.

Aspergillus also can cause localized disease in persons with normal immunologic function. Chronic necrotizing pulmonary aspergillosis occurs in patients with pulmonary emphysema. The chronic, progressive infiltrates of this condition often require tissue sampling for diagnosis. Treatment with surgical resection and systemic antifungal therapy is sometimes curative.

Aspergillus may produce a "fungus ball" in preexisting lung bullae or cavities (such as from ankylosing spondylitis, previous tuberculosis, or emphysema). Hemoptysis is the main symptom. Surgical excision may be necessary to prevent lethal hemorrhage.

Localized colonization with *Aspergillus* is common and usually does not produce disease. However, otitis externa (swimmer's ear) and allergic bronchopulmonary aspergillosis are exceptions. The symptoms of allergic bronchopulmonary aspergillosis resemble those of asthma. It is characterized by migratory pulmonary infiltrates, thick, brown, tenacious mucous plugs in the sputum, eosinophilia, and high titers of anti-*Aspergillus* antibodies; it typically occurs in the setting of chronic asthma. Endophthalmitis due to *Aspergillus* may develop after ocular operation or trauma.

Aspergillus frequently colonizes the respiratory tract. Isolating the organism from the sputum of an immunocompetent host usually does not indicate disease and does not require treatment.

- Chronic necrotizing pulmonary aspergillosis occurs in patients with pulmonary emphysema.

- *Aspergillus* may produce a "fungus ball" in preexisting lung bullae or cavities (such as from ankylosing spondylitis, previous tuberculosis, or emphysema).

Aspergillus infections may respond poorly to currently available antifungal medications. Amphotericin B products are very effective, but they must be given in high doses. Lipid-based formulations of amphotericin B are advised for patients in whom nephrotoxicity develops with deoxycholate amphotericin B. Itraconazole was the first oral agent with substantial activity against *Aspergillus*. However, newer drugs such as voriconazole and caspofungin have potent in vitro and in vivo activity against *Aspergillus*. Intravenous voriconazole should be avoided in patients with severe kidney disease (glomerular filtration rate, <50 mL/min). Caspofungin is approved by the US Food and Drug Administration for refractory invasive aspergillosis. This has been used alone or in combination with amphotericin B products. Surgical débridement of infected tissues is often necessary for cure. Allergic bronchopulmonary aspergillosis responds to corticosteroid therapy, and itraconazole may be an important adjunctive therapy in decreasing or sparing the use of corticosteroids.

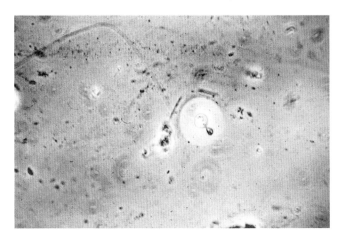

Figure 18.5 *Cryptococcus neoformans* in Cerebrospinal Fluid (×450).

Cryptococcosis

Cryptococcus neoformans is a yeast in both tissue and culture, is 4 to 7 mcm in diameter, and has thin-walled buds and a capsule (Figure 18.5). It is an opportunistic pathogen infecting persons with T-cell deficiency or dysfunction (eg, patients with Hodgkin disease, hematologic malignancy, organ transplant, exogenous corticosteroids, chronic liver disease, and AIDS). The respiratory tract is the usual portal of entry. Cryptococcosis does not incite much inflammatory reaction and calcification is rare.

- *Cryptococcus neoformans* is an opportunistic pathogen.

- *Cryptococcus* primarily infects persons with T-cell deficiencies or dysfunction (eg, Hodgkin disease, hematologic malignancy, organ transplant, exogenous corticosteroids, chronic liver disease, and AIDS).

Cryptococcus neoformans is acquired by inhalation. From the lungs it disseminates widely and easily crosses into the central nervous system. Pneumonia and meningitis are the most common forms of cryptococcosis. Meningitis may be insidious, with headache as the only symptom. Cranial nerve involvement may develop (including blindness with involvement of the optic nerve). Disseminated cryptococcosis also may cause an indolent form of cellulitis.

- Pneumonia and meningitis are the most common forms of *C neoformans* infection.

Cryptococcal infection can be diagnosed with fungal culture (eg, cerebrospinal fluid, blood, sputum, and urine), silver staining of biopsy tissue, or detection of *Cryptococcus* antigen in body fluids. The cryptococcal antigen test is the most helpful of all fungal serologic tests. It measures capsular antigen, whereas most other fungal serologic tests measure antibody response. Remember that *Cryptococcus* very commonly spreads to the central nervous system. Therefore, if *C neoformans* is isolated from any source (such as sputum, urine, and blood) in an immunosuppressed patient, a lumbar puncture should be done to rule out meningitis, even in the absence of symptoms.

The India ink preparation largely has been replaced by antigen detection assay.

Cryptococcal infections respond to treatment with amphotericin B or fluconazole. Choice of therapy depends on extent of disease and host immune function. Mild to moderate noncentral nervous system cryptococcosis can be treated with fluconazole for 6 to 12 months. However, severe presentation, immunocompromised hosts, and central nervous system involvement should be treated with amphotericin B. Combining oral flucytosine (100–150 mg/kg per day) with amphotericin B for 6 weeks allows a lower dose of amphotericin to be used. Unfortunately, relapse rates are high regardless of the treatment regimen given. In a recent study comparing fluconazole (200 mg per day) with amphotericin B for 10 weeks, fluconazole was as effective as amphotericin B ("effective" is defined as clinical improvement or resolution of symptoms with negative results for culture of cerebrospinal fluid). However, mortality in the first 2 weeks of therapy was higher with fluconazole (15% vs 8%).

Cryptococcosis in patients with AIDS is difficult to cure; however, the advent of highly active antiretroviral therapy has improved outcomes. The goal of therapy is to control the infection and then suppress it with long-term antifungal agents. A common approach is to initiate therapy with amphotericin B with flucytosine for at least 2 weeks. After 2 weeks of therapy with amphotericin B plus flucytosine, fluconazole therapy (400 mg per day) should be initiated for 8 weeks if the patient is clinically responding and has a negative result of cerebrospinal fluid fungal culture. Amphotericin therapy is continued until cerebrospinal fluid cultures are negative or there is unacceptable toxicity from the drug. Oral fluconazole therapy is continued indefinitely for patients with severe immunosuppression and poor immune reconstitution. Fluconazole therapy may be discontinued for patients who successfully complete a course of recommended therapy, remain asymptomatic, and have a sustained increase (ie, >6 months) in their CD4+ counts to more than 200 cells/mcL after antiretroviral therapy because studies show that the risk of recurrence is low. The newly approved caspofungin does not have any activity against *C neoformans*.

Candidiasis

Candida is a normal part of the human microflora. It grows as both yeast and hyphal forms simultaneously. Although *Candida albicans* is the most common species, numerous other species can cause human disease. *Candida* causes mucosal and cutaneous infections in both normal and immunocompromised hosts. Invasive disease primarily occurs in neutropenic hosts and as a nosocomial bloodstream infection.

Examples of candidiasis in the normal host include diaper rash and intertrigo, in which *Candida* growth on moist skin surfaces produces irritation. Vulvovaginal candidiasis is common, especially after a woman takes a course of antibiotics for an unrelated infection. Treatment with topical antifungal agents or a single dose of oral fluconazole is usually curative. Diabetes, corticosteroids, oral contraceptives, obesity, and HIV infection predispose to recurrent vulvovaginal candidiasis. Oral thrush may result from the same conditions.

Candida species cause 5% to 10% of nosocomial blood-stream infections. Candidemia most often occurs in critically ill patients receiving broad-spectrum antibiotics and parenteral nutrition. Neutropenia is another predisposing factor. Current blood culture techniques usually detect *Candida*, but culture results may be delayed. All intravenous catheters should always be removed or replaced when bloodstream infection with *Candida* is discovered. Metastatic abscesses can occur in any site after an episode of candidemia. *Candida* osteomyelitis or joint infections can occur as complications after an episode of line-related fungemia. Endophthalmitis may occur as long as 1 month after initial fungemia. For central venous catheter-related candidemias, catheter removal followed by amphotericin B (250–500 mg) or fluconazole is indicated.

Candida tropicalis, Candida parapsilosis, Candida glabrata, and multiple other species cause nosocomial illness, especially in immunocompromised patients. Note that these non-albicans species of *Candida* are more often resistant to fluconazole therapy, especially *C glabrata.*

Injection drug use is a risk factor for *Candida* endocarditis (and joint space infections, especially of the sternoclavicular joint). It is often caused by species other than *C albicans.*

- Fungemia develops from infected intravenous catheters, especially in the immunosuppressed host.

- Risk factors for *Candida* bloodstream infection include previous antibacterial therapy, cytotoxic or corticosteroid therapy, and parenteral nutrition.

- *Candida* endocarditis occurs most often in injection drug users.

- Diabetes, corticosteroids, oral contraceptives, obesity, and HIV infection predispose to recurrent vulvovaginal candidiasis.

Candida urinary tract infection is common in patients with urinary catheters and those receiving antibacterial drugs. Removal of the catheter is the primary therapy. If necessary, treatment with fluconazole or bladder irrigation with dilute amphotericin B may be curative, although recurrence is common.

Hepatosplenic candidiasis, also called chronic disseminated candidiasis, occurs during the recovery phase after prolonged neutropenia. Fever, abdominal pain, and increased alkaline phosphatase level suggest the diagnosis. Typical "bull's-eye" lesions can be seen with ultrasonography, computed tomography, or magnetic resonance imaging of the infected liver. Current guidelines (2004) of the Infectious Diseases Society of America recommend fluconazole (6 mg/kg per day) as the generally preferred antifungal in clinically stable patients. However, amphotericin B deoxycholate (0.6–0.7 mg/kg per day) or a lipid formulation of amphotericin B (3–5 mg/kg per day) is an option in ill patients or patients with refractory disease. Limited data suggest that caspofungin may be effective.

Candida esophagitis is a common cause of odynophagia in immunosuppressed patients, especially those with AIDS. Endoscopy is necessary to prove the diagnosis. *Candida* esophagitis is clinically indistinguishable from, and may coexist with, cytomegalovirus and herpes simplex virus esophagitis. Fluconazole is effective therapy for oral or esophageal candidiasis. Caspofungin is also active and is approved by the US Food and Drug Administration for treatment of candidemia or candidiasis caused by *Candida* species, including those that are resistant to azoles such as fluconazole. Caspofungin is available only as an intravenous drug.

- Hepatosplenic candidiasis typically develops as chemotherapy-induced neutropenia resolves.

- *Candida* esophagitis is clinically indistinguishable from, and may coexist with, cytomegalovirus and herpes simplex virus esophagitis.

Mucormycosis (*Rhizopus* Species, Zygomycetes)

Mucormycosis is a term used to describe infections caused by fungi of the order Mucorales. Older terms for this include phycomycosis and zygomycosis. There are many different fungi or Zygomycetes within this order that are pathogenic to humans. Of those, *Rhizopus* species are the most commonly isolated, followed by *Rhizomucor* and *Cunninghamella.* Mucormycosis is a disease of immunocompromised hosts. Pulmonary, nasal, and sinus infections are the most common. Facial pain, headache, and fever are common symptoms. Rhinocerebral mucormycosis results from direct extension into the brain. Diabetic ketoacidosis, neutropenia, renal failure, and deferoxamine therapy are all risk factors for this life-threatening infection. The diagnosis of mucormycosis depends on finding the typical black necrotic lesions (usually in the nose or on the palate) and is confirmed by biopsy. Treatment involves reversing the predisposing condition as much as possible, surgical débridement of necrotic tissue, and amphotericin B.

- The diagnosis of mucormycosis depends on finding the typical black necrotic lesions (usually in the nose or on the palate) and is confirmed by biopsy.

- Diabetic ketoacidosis, neutropenia, renal failure, and deferoxamine therapy are all risk factors for mucormycosis.

VIRUSES

Herpesviruses

There are now 8 known herpesviruses: herpes simplex virus (HSV) types 1 and 2, Epstein-Barr virus (EBV), cytomegalovirus (CMV), varicella-zoster virus (VZV), human herpesvirus 6 (HHV-6), HHV-7 (not yet known to be associated with clinical disease), and HHV-8. All herpesviruses are DNA viruses that share the characteristic of establishing latency after primary infection, whether or not symptomatic.

Serologic evidence of infection is common by adulthood: HSV 1, 87%; HSV 2, 20%; EBV, 95%; CMV, 50%; and VZV, 90%. The rate of infection increases in populations of lower socioeconomic status.

Herpes Simplex Virus

Primary infection with HSV results from exposure of skin or mucous membranes to intact viral particles. Latent infection is then established in sensory nerve ganglia. Genital HSV infection is caused by HSV type 2 in 80% of cases and by HSV type 1 in the remaining 20%. The reverse is true for oral HSV. Genital HSV is more likely to recur when caused by HSV type 2. Recurrence rates of oral and genital HSV can be decreased by 80% with chronic use of antiviral drugs. In normal hosts, this does not promote emergence of acyclovir-resistant strains.

Herpes simplex encephalitis is a nonseasonal, life-threatening illness usually caused by HSV type 1. Herpes simplex encephalitis causes confusion, fever, and, frequently, seizures. Simultaneous herpes labialis is present in 10% to 15% of cases. Antemortem diagnosis may be difficult. However, new techniques such as magnetic resonance imaging of the brain, showing characteristic temporal lobe involvement, and amplification of HSV DNA (polymerase chain reaction) from cerebrospinal fluid are extremely sensitive. Detecting periodic lateralized epileptiform discharges with electroencephalography is suggestive of herpes simplex encephalitis. Poor neurologic status, age older than 30 years, and encephalitis of more than 4 days in duration before initiation of therapy are associated with a poor outcome.

Neonatal HSV infection is acquired at the time of vaginal delivery. The mortality rate is high (20%) despite antiviral therapy. In neonates who survive, neurologic sequelae and recurrent HSV lesions are common. Cesarean section is recommended if a woman has active herpetic lesions at the time of delivery.

Acyclovir, famciclovir, valacyclovir, ganciclovir, foscarnet, and vidarabine inhibit replication of both HSV types 1 and 2. Acyclovir resistance may develop in patients with AIDS who are treated with multiple courses of acyclovir. Resistance usually is conferred by a mutation in the thymidine kinase gene, preventing phosphorylation of acyclovir to its active form.

- Recurrence rates of oral and genital HSV can be decreased by 80% with chronic suppressive therapy with acyclovir.

- Herpes simplex encephalitis can be diagnosed with magnetic resonance imaging and polymerase chain reaction amplification of HSV DNA from cerebrospinal fluid.

- Delivery by cesarean section is recommended if active genital lesions are present at the end of pregnancy.

HSV pneumonia is rare and usually occurs in immunosuppressed patients. When HSV is isolated from a respiratory source, it most commonly represents shedding from the oral mucosa rather than the lungs. HSV also is associated with visceral disease (such as esophagitis). Biopsy is required to reliably distinguish HSV from CMV or *Candida* esophagitis. Eczema herpeticum (Kaposi varicelliform eruption) occurs in areas of eczema. Large areas of skin are involved. Herpetic whitlow is a painful HSV infection of a finger, is most commonly acquired through contact with oral secretions (eg, in respiratory technicians, dentists, and anesthesiologists), and occasionally is acquired through needle stick. Herpetic whitlow can mimic a bacterial process, such as paronychia. Although nosocomial transmission of HSV is rare, recent reports stress the importance of mucous membrane precautions when treating all patients with HSV, particularly those with respiratory infection who undergo invasive procedures.

- Herpetic whitlow is a painful HSV infection of a finger, is most commonly acquired through contact with oral secretions, and occasionally is acquired through needle stick. It can mimic a bacterial process.

HSV can cause outbreaks among participants in contact sports (in wrestlers, it is called herpes gladiatorum). The infection is transmitted by skin-to-skin contact. Lesions appear on the head (78%), trunk (28%), and extremities (42%). The rash may be atypical. Large, ulcerative perianal lesions can develop in patients with AIDS. Some of the lesions are mistaken for decubitus ulcers.

- HSV can cause outbreaks among participants in contact sports.

- Large, ulcerative perianal lesions can develop in patients with AIDS.

Epstein-Barr Virus

Most acute EBV infections are asymptomatic. Symptomatic infectious mononucleosis causes the clinical triad of fever, pharyngitis (80%), and adenopathy. Splenomegaly occurs in 50% of cases. One of the most serious complications of mononucleosis is splenic rupture. Other complications include hemolytic anemia, airway obstruction, encephalitis, and transverse myelitis. Associated laboratory abnormalities include atypical lymphocytosis, thrombocytopenia, and mild increases in liver enzyme values. Corticosteroids may be beneficial for treatment of hemolytic anemia and acute airway obstruction. Ampicillin or amoxicillin given during infectious mononucleosis commonly causes a diffuse macular rash.

Table 18.4 differentiates EBV from other causes of mononucleosis. The diagnosis of infectious mononucleosis depends on detection of heterophile antibodies (monospot test) or specific EBV immunoglobulin M antibodies. False-negative results of the monospot test are more likely with increasing age.

- Infectious mononucleosis has the clinical triad of fever, pharyngitis, and adenopathy.

- Splenomegaly occurs in 50% of cases of infectious mononucleosis.

- One of the most serious complications is splenic rupture.

- If ampicillin is given during infectious mononucleosis, a rash often develops.

Table 18.4 INFECTIOUS MONONUCLEOSIS-LIKE SYNDROMES

DISEASE	PHARYNGITIS	ADENOPATHY	SPLENOMEGALY	ATYPICAL LYMPHOCYTES	HETEROPHILE	OTHER TEST
Infectious mononucleosis	++++	++++	+++	+++	+	Specific EBV antibody + (VCA IgM)
CMV	–	–	+++	++	–	CMV IgM
Toxoplasmosis	–	++++	+++	++		Toxoplasmosis serology
HIV	+	+++	–	++	–	HIV serology (will likely be negative) HIV viral load HIV p24 antigen

Abbreviations and symbols: CMV, cytomegalovirus; EBV, Epstein-Barr virus; HIV, human immunodeficiency virus; IgM, immunoglobulin M; VCA, viral capsid antigen; –, absent; +, ++, +++, and ++++, present to varying degrees.

Uncomplicated cases require symptomatic care only. The patient should not participate in contact sports for several months because of the risk for splenic rupture. Corticosteroids are not indicated for uncomplicated infection. Acyclovir and other antiviral drug therapy are not effective.

Chronic fatigue syndrome is a syndrome characterized by various nonspecific symptoms. EBV infection, however, does not cause chronic fatigue syndrome.

- No therapy is indicated for uncomplicated cases of infectious mononucleosis.

- EBV does not cause chronic fatigue syndrome.

EBV infection in males with X-linked lymphoproliferative syndrome is a rare disorder of young boys in whom fulminant EBV infections develop and is associated with a nearly 60% mortality rate. Complications include severe EBV hepatitis with liver failure and hemophagocytic syndrome with bleeding. In survivors, hypogammaglobulinemia, malignant lymphoma, aplastic anemia, and opportunistic infections develop. Acyclovir and corticosteroids do not seem to be beneficial.

In EBV-associated Burkitt lymphoma and nasopharyngeal carcinoma, patients have high titers of immunoglobulin A antibodies to EBV. Polyclonal and monoclonal B-cell lymphoproliferative syndromes have been associated with EBV in patients who have had organ transplant and in patients with AIDS. Oral hairy leukoplakia in patients with AIDS is associated with EBV infection and responds to acyclovir therapy. EBV recently has been associated with leiomyosarcomas in transplant recipients.

- Polyclonal and monoclonal B-cell lymphoproliferative syndromes have been associated with EBV.

Cytomegalovirus

Primary CMV infection is usually asymptomatic in immunocompetent patients, but it can cause a heterophile-negative mononucleosis syndrome. It is a significant cause of neonatal disease. Perinatal infection can occur in utero, intra partum, or post partum and can cause congenital malformations. Primary infection of the mother during pregnancy results in a 15% chance of fetal cytomegalic inclusion disease. Young children in day-care centers commonly shed CMV in their urine and saliva. Their parents are at risk of acquiring primary infection from an asymptomatic child. CMV can cause fever of unknown origin in healthy adults, especially in those with day-care–aged children.

CMV can be transmitted by leukocytes in blood transfusions. Use of leukocyte-poor packed red blood cells or blood from CMV-seronegative donors decreases the risk of transmission via this route. Symptomatic infection develops about 4 weeks after transfusion and manifests as fever with atypical lymphocytes in the peripheral blood smear. Serologic testing confirms the diagnosis. Viral cultures are rarely helpful in diagnosing CMV disease in the noncompromised patient.

- CMV can cause heterophile-negative mononucleosis syndrome.

- CMV can be transmitted by blood transfusion.

- Fever and infectious mononucleosis-like picture on peripheral smear are characteristics in postoperative patients who have received blood transfusions.

In persons with impaired cellular immunity (such as those with AIDS or organ and bone marrow transplant recipients), CMV causes serious infections (CMV syndrome, retinitis, pneumonia, gastrointestinal ulcerations, encephalitis, and adrenalitis). The diagnosis most often is established by isolation of CMV from blood or from culture, by histopathologic evidence of CMV infection in involved tissue (such as liver, lung, gastrointestinal tract), or from clinical findings alone (CMV retinitis).

- CMV causes serious infections (retinitis, pneumonia, gastrointestinal ulcerations, encephalitis, and adrenalitis) in patients who have AIDS or take immunosuppressive medications.

The manifestations of CMV disease in persons with advanced AIDS are protean. Disease is almost always caused by reactivation of latent infection in this setting. Finding CMV in the blood or urine of patients with AIDS is common and has a low predictive value for symptomatic CMV disease. CMV retinitis occurs in 20% to 30% of patients with advanced AIDS. Diagnosis is based on ophthalmologic examination. The relapse rate for CMV retinitis in AIDS is high, even with chronic antiviral therapy.

Solid organ and bone marrow transplant recipients are another group of patients at risk for CMV disease. It is the most common infection after solid organ transplant (occurring primarily in the first 6 months after transplant). Those at highest risk are CMV seronegative before transplant and receive an organ from a seropositive donor. Latent virus is present in almost all tissues and begins replicating shortly after transplant.

Symptomatic disease (CMV syndrome) usually develops in the first 4 to 8 weeks after a solid organ transplant and causes fever, leukopenia, increases in liver enzyme values, and end-organ involvement. CMV serum antigen testing or CMV detected in blood culture helps confirm the diagnosis. Patients who have had bone marrow transplant are especially at risk for CMV pneumonia. The mortality rate approaches 50% despite therapy. Prophylactic ganciclovir and, possibly, CMV immune globulin may decrease or delay posttransplant CMV disease.

- CMV retinitis occurs in 20%-30% of patients with advanced AIDS.
- CMV is the most common infectious complication of organ transplant.

Ganciclovir is the treatment of choice for most CMV infections in immunocompromised hosts. A randomized, placebo-controlled trial found that foscarnet and ganciclovir are equally efficacious for halting the progression of CMV retinitis in patients with AIDS but that patients taking foscarnet lived longer (12 vs 8 months). Both drugs are now approved for this indication. Full-dose induction therapy is given for 2 to 3 weeks, followed by chronic suppressive therapy indefinitely (usually as once-daily dosing). Oral valganciclovir has excellent bioavailability and can be used in select patients for suppression. Transplant recipients usually do not require suppressive medication after an episode of CMV disease. In patients with CMV pneumonia after bone marrow transplant, combining ganciclovir with intravenous immune globulin is more effective than ganciclovir alone. Nonimmunocompromised patients with CMV do not require treatment.

- Ganciclovir, valganciclovir, or foscarnet is the treatment of choice for most CMV infections.

Varicella-Zoster Virus
Primary infection with VZV usually occurs in childhood and causes chickenpox. Illness with chickenpox is more likely to be severe in adults and immunocompromised hosts. Varicella pneumonia occurs in 5% to 50% of cases. Pregnant women are especially vulnerable. They should be treated with high-dose acyclovir (10 mg/kg intravenously every 8 hours). Acyclovir is not associated with toxicity to the fetus. Pneumonia develops within 1 to 6 days after the onset of illness and usually recedes as the rash does. Encephalomyelitis is another serious complication of varicella infection, occurring predominantly in children. Onset is 3 to 14 days after the appearance of rash.

- Varicella pneumonia occurs in 5%-50% of adults with chickenpox.
- Pneumonia begins to improve with disappearance of rash.

After primary infection, VZV DNA persists in a latent state in sensory neuron ganglia. Reactivated infection causes zoster (shingles), which manifests as a painful vesicular rash in a dermatomal distribution. Involvement of the fifth cranial nerve, especially the ophthalmic branch, may be sight-threatening. In nonimmune persons exposed to zoster, primary VZV infection may develop. Neurologic complications of herpes zoster include motor paralysis (localized to the dermatomal distribution of rash), encephalitis, and myelitis.

- Herpes zoster infection often involves the fifth cranial nerve, especially the ophthalmic branch.

Varicella immune globulin can prevent primary VZV infection, especially when given within 96 hours of exposure. It is indicated for 1) VZV-seronegative immunocompromised hosts who have had close contact with a person with chickenpox and 2) newborns of mothers with varicella infection that occurs 5 days before or 2 days after delivery.

Ten percent of mothers with active varicella will transmit the infection to the fetus. Infection during the first trimester may result in limb hypoplasia, cortical atrophy, and chorioretinitis. During the third trimester, multiple visceral abnormalities can occur, including pneumonia. The fetal and neonatal mortality rate is about 30%.

- Among mothers with active varicella, 10% will transmit the infection to the fetus.

Treatment for varicella (primary varicella-zoster) infection is based on whether the patient is immunocompetent. Two randomized clinical trials showed that oral acyclovir (800 mg 5 times a day or equivalent) reduced the duration of skin lesions and viral shedding in adults and children. Its efficacy for reducing visceral complications (pneumonia) remains unknown. Early treatment (<24 hours) is necessary. The cost of therapy may limit its usefulness, but it is advocated by some to decrease the duration of illness. Acyclovir may reduce the risk of dissemination and of complications in immunocompromised patients. Treatment of zoster ophthalmicus reduces the incidence of uveitis and keratitis. For immunocompetent patients with zoster, 3 antiviral drugs (acyclovir, famciclovir, and valacyclovir) speed healing and reduce pain. Preliminary data suggest that the new antiviral agent famciclovir might decrease the duration of postherpetic neuralgia.

Corticosteroids do not prevent postherpetic neuralgia. For disseminated infections (encephalitis, cranial neuritis), a recent controlled trial showed that high-dose intravenous acyclovir decreases the duration of hospitalization. Acyclovir-resistant VZV infection (which can occur in patients with AIDS) can be treated with intravenous foscarnet or cidofovir.

Two effective live virus vaccines for VZV are available. One VZV vaccine (Varivax) is for primary prevention of varicella, and a new, different (higher attenuated varicella colony-forming units per milliliter) vaccine (Zostavax) is now available and recommended for prevention of herpes zoster (shingles) and postherpetic neuralgia in persons older than 60 years. VZV vaccine for primary prevention is recommended for children and VZV-seronegative adolescent and adult populations. It is contraindicated in pregnancy. Both live vaccines are contraindicated in patients with impaired cellular immunity such as AIDS, leukemias, lymphoma, chemotherapy, transplant, chronic corticosteroid therapy, or other cellular immunodeficiency states.

Human Herpesvirus 6

HHV-6 is a recently discovered lymphotropic virus. It causes the mild childhood infectious exanthem known as roseola infantum. Like CMV, reactivation of infection occurs after organ transplant. HHV-6 has been associated with pneumonitis after bone marrow transplant.

Human Herpesvirus 8

HHV-8 is also known as Kaposi sarcoma-associated virus. As the name implies, it is thought to be the causative agent of Kaposi sarcoma. It is related to EBV. Most recently, HHV-8 has been linked to body cavity-based lymphomas in patients with AIDS and Castleman disease.

Measles (Rubeola)

There was a substantial increase in measles cases in the late 1980s and early 1990s in unvaccinated preschool children and vaccinated high school and college students (1990: 27,786 cases). Prodromal upper respiratory tract symptoms are prominent. Oral lesions (Koplik spots) precede the rash. Both measles infection and measles vaccine cause temporary cutaneous anergy (false-negative purified protein derivative test). Infection may cause more significant immunologic suppression, as exemplified by cases of reactivated tuberculosis in persons with measles.

- In measles, oral Koplik spots precede the rash.
- Measles vaccine may cause temporary cutaneous anergy.

Complications of measles include encephalitis and pneumonia. Encephalitis is often severe. It usually occurs after a period of apparent improvement of measles infection. In primary measles pneumonia, large, multinucleated cells (Warthin-Finkeldey cells) are found on lung biopsy. Secondary bacterial infection is more common than primary measles pneumonia. *Staphylococcus aureus* and *Haemophilus influenzae* are the most common bacterial pathogens.

- Complications of measles include encephalitis.
- Secondary bacterial infection is more common than primary measles pneumonia.

Atypical measles occurs in patients vaccinated before 1968. After exposure to measles, atypical rash, fever, arthralgias, and headache (aseptic meningitis) may develop. The presence of a high titer of measles antibody in serum helps confirm the diagnosis.

Rubella

The prodromal symptoms of rubella are mild (unlike those of rubeola). Posterior cervical lymphadenopathy, arthralgia (70% in adults), transient erythematous rash, and fever are characteristic. Infection is subclinical in many cases. Central nervous system complications and thrombocytopenia are rare.

- The characteristics of rubella are posterior cervical lymphadenopathy, arthralgia (70% in adults), transient erythematous rash, and fever.

The greatest danger from rubella is to the fetus. When a pregnant female is exposed to rubella, rubella serologic testing should be done. If the titer indicates immunity, there is no danger and no further testing is indicated. If the titer indicates nonimmunity, the patient should be followed for evidence of clinical rubella. The serum titer should be checked again in 2 to 3 weeks to evaluate for evidence of asymptomatic infection. If the titer is not increased and there is no evidence of clinical rubella, then no intervention is indicated. If clinical rubella develops or seroconversion is demonstrated, there is a high risk of congenital abnormalities or spontaneous abortion. The risk varies from 40% to 60% if infection occurs during the first 2 months of gestation to 10% by the fourth month. Intravenous gamma globulin may mask symptoms of rubella, but it does not protect the fetus.

- Gamma globulin does not protect the fetus after exposure to rubella.

From 6% to 11% of young adults remain susceptible to rubella after receiving rubella vaccine. A pregnant female should not be given rubella vaccine because it can cause congenital abnormalities. Females of childbearing age should be warned not to become pregnant within 2 to 3 months from the time of immunization. Transient arthralgias develop in 25% of immunized women. Fever, rash, and lymphadenopathy also may develop. Symptoms may occur as long as 2 months after vaccination. They may be confused with other forms of arthritis.

Mumps

Mumps virus commonly affects glandular tissue. Parotitis, pancreatitis, and orchitis are characteristic manifestations. Orchitis occurs in 20% of males with mumps. It is unilateral in approximately 75%. Orchitis often is associated with recrudescence of malaise and chills, fever, headache, nausea, vomiting, and testicular pain. Sterility is uncommon, even after bilateral infection.

Although mumps cases are uncommon in the United States, in 2006 there was an outbreak of mumps. Approximately 5,000 cases were reported to the National Notifiable Diseases Surveillance System. Source of the initial cases was unknown. The median age of persons reported with mumps was 22 years, and the highest incidence was among the adults 18 to 24 years of age, many of whom were college students. Factors contributing to this outbreak included college campus environment, lack of a 2-dose measles-mumps-rubella college-entry requirement or lack of enforcement of a requirement, delayed recognition and diagnosis of mumps, mumps vaccine failure, vaccine that might be less effective in preventing asymptomatic infection or atypical mumps than in preventing parotitis, and waning immunity.

Clinical suspicion can be confirmed by serologic test (immunoglobulin M for mumps) within 5 days of illness onset or sending a parotid duct swab or other samples such as cerebrospinal fluid for viral cultures. If the initial immunoglobulin M antibody titer is negative, a second (convalescent) serum specimen for immunoglobulin M antibodies obtained 2 to 3 weeks after onset of the illness can be helpful for making the diagnosis. A 4-fold increase in immunoglobulin G antibodies compared with immunoglobulin G obtained initially can also help. Mumps virus can be transmitted by direct contact with respiratory droplets, saliva, or contaminated fomites. The incubation period is 16 to 18 days (range, 12–25 days) from exposure to onset of symptoms.

Mumps meningoencephalitis is one of the most common nonseasonal viral meningitides. It can cause low glucose values in the cerebrospinal fluid, mimicking bacterial meningitis. Deafness is a rare complication of mumps.

- Mumps meningoencephalitis is one of the most common nonseasonal viral meningitides.

Mumps polyarthritis is most common in men between the ages of 20 and 30 years. Joint symptoms begin 1 to 2 weeks after subsidence of parotitis, and large joints are involved. The condition lasts approximately 6 weeks, and complete recovery is usual. This condition may be confused with other forms of arthritis.

- Mumps polyarthritis is most common in men between the ages of 20 and 30 years.

Parvovirus B19

Parvovirus is a single-stranded DNA virus that infects the erythrocyte precursors in bone marrow, with resulting reticulocytopenia. It is the cause of erythema infectiosum (fifth disease) in children, transient arthritis in adults (which is symmetric, involves small joints, and can mimic rheumatoid arthritis), and aplastic crisis in persons with hemolytic

anemias. Infection during pregnancy results in a 5% chance of hydrops fetalis or fetal death. Serologic testing is the preferred diagnostic method in immunologically competent persons.

Parvovirus B19 infection may persist in immunosuppressed patients, resulting in red blood cell aplasia. Diagnosis is established by demonstration of giant pronormoblasts in bone marrow or identification of viral DNA in bone marrow or peripheral blood. Most patients respond to administration of commercial immune globulin infusions for 5 to 10 days. No treatment is recommended for parvovirus infections in the noncompromised host.

- Parvovirus B19 is the cause of erythema infectiosum (fifth disease) and transient, symmetric, small-joint arthritis.

- Parvovirus B19 virus can cause red blood cell aplasia in patients with AIDS.

Human T-Cell Lymphotropic Viruses

Human T-cell lymphotropic virus (HTLV)-I and -II are non-HIV human retroviruses. HTLV-I is endemic in parts of Japan, the Caribbean basin, South America, and Africa. It may be transmitted by sexual contact, infected cellular blood products (not clotting factor concentrates), and injection drug use. Vertical transmission (eg, breast-feeding and transplacental) also occurs. HTLV-I is associated with human T-cell leukemia/lymphoma and tropical spastic paraparesis (also known as HTLV-I–associated myelopathy). However, clinical disease never develops in 96% of persons infected with HTLV-I. HTLV-II causes no known clinical disease. The seroprevalence of HTLV-I or -II is as high as 18% in certain high-risk groups (injection drug users, patients attending sexually transmitted disease clinics) (HTLV-II is 2.5 times more prevalent than HTLV-I). Among voluntary blood donors, the seroprevalence in the United States is estimated at 0.016%. With current screening practices, the risk of transmission of HTLV-I or -II through blood transfusion is estimated to be 0.0014% (1/70,000 units).

- HTLV-I may be transmitted by sexual contact, infected blood products, and injection drug use.

- HTLV-I infection is usually asymptomatic but is associated with human T-cell leukemia and chronic myelopathy.

PARASITES

Helminths

Neurocysticercosis is an infection of the central nervous system with a larval stage of the pork tapeworm (*Taenia solium*). It is acquired by ingesting tapeworm eggs from fecally contaminated food (not from eating undercooked pork). It is endemic in Latin America, Asia, and Africa. Recent cases have been reported among household contacts of foreign-born persons (working as domestic employees). The infected persons had not traveled to an affected area. The most common presentation is seizures. Brain imaging reveals cystic or calcified brain lesions. Serum or cerebrospinal fluid serologic testing can aid in the diagnosis. Treatment with praziquantel or albendazole may be beneficial. Albendazole is considered superior for neurocysticercosis because of better central nervous system penetration. The coadministration of corticosteroids often is used to decrease cerebral inflammation associated with therapy.

- Neurocysticercosis is acquired by ingesting tapeworm eggs from fecally contaminated food.

- Seizures are the most common symptom of neurocysticercosis.

Strongyloides stercoralis is unique among the intestinal nematode infections. Unlike the other helminths, the larvae of this organism can mature in the human host (auto-infection). In immunocompromised hosts (neutropenia, steroids, AIDS, HTLV-I), a superinfection can develop with larval migration throughout the body. Gram-negative bacteremia is a common coinfection, resulting from disruption of the intestinal mucosa by the invasive larvae. Treatment is with ivermectin.

Trichinosis is acquired from eating undercooked meat, especially bear. Features include muscle pain (especially diaphragm, chest, and tongue), eosinophilia, and periorbital edema. Treatment is with mebendazole or albendazole.

Hookworm (*Necator americanus*) causes anemia. It is found mainly in tropical and subtropical regions. The larval form penetrates the skin. Walking barefoot is a risk factor. Treatment is with mebendazole or albendazole.

Ascariasis infection may cause intestinal obstruction or pancreatitis (worm migrates up the pancreatic duct). Treatment is with mebendazole or albendazole.

Schistosomiasis is a tropical disease that causes hepatic cirrhosis, hematuria, and carcinoma of the bladder. Transverse myelitis may develop as a result of schistosomiasis. It is acquired by direct penetration of the *Schistosoma cercariae* from contaminated water (lakes, rivers). Praziquantel is the drug of choice for schistosomiasis.

- Trichinosis is acquired from eating undercooked meat, especially bear.

- Transverse myelitis may develop as a result of schistosomiasis.

Protozoan Parasites

Acanthamoeba, a free-living ameba, causes amebic keratitis in persons swimming in fresh water while wearing soft contact lenses. The diagnosis is based on microscopic examination of scrapings of the cornea. Treatment is with topical antifungal agents. Patients often respond poorly to therapy and have progressive corneal destruction.

Symptomatic infection with *Entamoeba histolytica* (amebiasis) may cause diarrhea (often bloody), abdominal pain, and fever. Metronidazole, followed by a lumenocidal agent such as iodoquinol or paromomycin, is the preferred therapy (metronidazole does not kill amebae in the intestinal lumen).

Asymptomatic carriage of amebic cysts should be treated with one of the lumenocidal agents.

- Metronidazole, followed by a lumenocidal agent such as iodoquinol or paromomycin, is the preferred therapy for symptomatic amebiasis.

Invasive amebiasis may lead to distant abscesses (primarily the liver, but other organs can be involved). An amebic liver abscess usually is single and is commonly located in the posterior portion of the right lobe of the liver. The anatomical location, the fact that it is usually a single abscess, and the absence of other signs of bacterial infection help to distinguish amebic hepatic abscess from bacterial abscess. Serologic tests (complement fixation) are positive in more than 90% of patients with amebic abscess. Hepatic abscess may rupture through the diaphragm into the right pleural cavity.

- Amebic liver abscess may rupture through the diaphragm into the right pleural cavity.

Giardia lamblia is the parasite most frequently detected in state parasitology laboratories. Infection characteristically produces sudden onset of watery diarrhea with malabsorption, bloating, and flatulence. Prolonged disease that is refractory to standard therapy may occur in patients with immunoglobulin A deficiency. The organism may be detected in stool specimens. Stool *Giardia* antigen testing by enzyme-linked immunosorbent assay is very sensitive and may obviate duodenal aspirates for diagnosis. Metronidazole, tinidazole, or nitazoxanide are effective for treating giardiasis.

- *Giardia lamblia* is the parasite most frequently detected in state parasitology laboratories.

- Giardiasis causes sudden onset of watery diarrhea and malabsorption, bloating, and flatulence.

- Prolonged giardiasis is particularly common in patients with immunoglobulin A deficiency.

Toxoplasma gondii is acquired from eating undercooked meat or exposure to cat feces. Primary toxoplasmosis is usually asymptomatic. In immunocompetent persons it may cause a heterophile-negative mononucleosis-like syndrome. Toxoplasmosis causes brain and eye lesions and pneumonia in patients with AIDS. Immunocompromised patients with toxoplasmosis can be treated effectively with pyrimethamine in combination with either sulfadiazine or clindamycin. *Toxoplasma* chorioretinitis can occur in immunocompetent patients during primary infection. Patients may present with fever and blurry vision. On ophthalmologic examination, an acute retinochoroiditis causes marked vitreous reaction overlying the retinal infection, leading to the characteristic fundus picture of the optic nerve appearing as a "headlight in the fog."

- Toxoplasmosis is acquired from eating undercooked meat or exposure to cat feces.

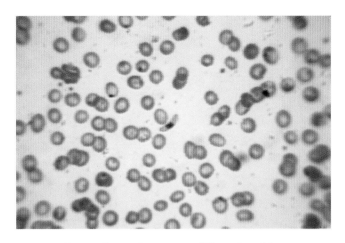

Figure 18.6 Banana-Shaped Gametocyte of *Plasmodium falciparum* in Thin Blood Smear.

- Toxoplasmosis may cause an infectious mononucleosis-like syndrome.

Malaria is endemic and spreading in many parts of the world. Spiking fevers, rigors, and headache are the hallmark of malaria. With falciparum malaria, the fevers may be irregular or continuous. *Plasmodium falciparum* is the most common cause of fever in a traveler returned from Africa. It is also more likely to cause malarial complications such as cerebral malaria, pulmonary edema, and death. *Plasmodium vivax* and *Plasmodium malariae* infections cause regular episodic fevers (malarial paroxysms). Recent reports indicate that, in Southeast Asia, a monkey plasmodium called *Plasmodium knowlesi* can cause clinical disease similar to that of *P falciparum*. Malaria is diagnosed by examination of thick and thin blood smears (Figure 18.6).

- Diagnosis of malaria is based on examination of thick and thin blood smears.

Prophylaxis for malaria is increasingly difficult because of drug-resistant *P falciparum*. Personal protection should always be used (such as mosquito nets, insect repellents containing DEET). For travelers to chloroquine-sensitive areas (Central America [north of Panama], Mexico, Haiti, the Dominican Republic, and the Middle East), chloroquine phosphate is still effective. In chloroquine-resistant areas, mefloquine, doxycycline, or an atovaquone-proguanil hydrochloride combination tablet (Malarone) is suggested. Sulfadoxine-pyrimethamine (Fansidar) or a combination of chloroquine with proguanil is not recommended for prophylaxis for chloroquine-resistant falciparum malaria. Travelers to the mefloquine-resistant areas of the Thai-Myanmar and Thai-Cambodian borders should use doxycycline or atovaquone-proguanil hydrochloride. Mefloquine should be avoided in patients with cardiac conduction abnormalities, depression or other psychiatric disorder, or seizure disorder. No regimen guarantees 100% prophylaxis. While receiving mefloquine, patients should be advised not to take halofantrine for a febrile illness because of the risk of fatal cardiac arrhythmias. All patients should be advised to seek medical attention if fever develops within 1 year after return from an endemic area.

Chloroquine is the preferred treatment of infection caused by *P vivax*, *P malariae*, and known chloroquine-susceptible strains of *P falciparum*. Chloroquine-resistant strains may respond to quinine and doxycycline, atovaquone-proguanil hydrochloride, mefloquine, or artemisinin derivatives (this agent is not freely [see below] available in the United States). For severe *P falciparum* infections, intravenous quinidine gluconate (intravenous quinine is not available in the United States) is effective. However, resistant cases of *P falciparum* might require treatment with doxycycline or clindamycin. Since July 2007, parenteral artesunate has been available in the United States for severe malaria treatment under an Investigational New Drug Protocol from the Centers for Disease Control and Prevention. This drug should be used in combination with another antimalarial agent for severe malaria in concordance with malaria treatment guidelines of the World Health Organization. Exchange transfusion may be beneficial for severely ill patients with parasitemia of more than 10%.

Primaquine is used to eradicate the exoerythrocytic phase of *Plasmodium ovale* and *P vivax* infections, preventing later relapses. Primaquine can cause hemolysis in persons with glucose-6-phosphate dehydrogenase deficiency.

Leishmaniasis is a protozoan disease transmitted by the sand fly bite. Visceral leishmaniasis (kala-azar, caused by *Leishmania donovani*) causes fever, hepatosplenomegaly, hypergammaglobulinemia, cachexia, and pancytopenia. It has been reported in patients with AIDS in Spain. Bone marrow examination (Giemsa stain) is often diagnostic. Cutaneous leishmaniasis (caused by *Leishmania tropica*, *Leishmania major*, *Leishmania braziliensis*, and *Leishmania mexicana*) occurs as a painless papule that progresses to an ulcer and may be self-limited. Cutaneous leishmaniasis has occurred in military personnel returning from Iraq (the "Baghdad boil") and Afghanistan. South and Central American forms of cutaneous leishmaniasis are often destructive and should be treated. Treatment is with antimony compounds or with amphotericin B or its liposomal formulations.

Babesia microti is a tick-borne illness transmitted by the same *Ixodes* tick that is responsible for Lyme disease and ehrlichiosis. It is a parasite that infects erythrocytes and causes fever, myalgias, and hemolytic anemia. Often asymptomatic in normal hosts, severe disease may develop in asplenic individuals. Babesiosis is endemic in the northeastern United States, especially around Nantucket, Martha's Vineyard, and Cape Cod. Cases of transfusion-transmitted babesiosis have been documented. The diagnosis is established by examination of peripheral blood smear or polymerase chain reaction amplification of *Babesia* DNA from peripheral blood. Treatment is with clindamycin and quinine or atovaquone plus azithromycin. Exchange transfusion has been needed in severely ill patients with high parasitemias. Simultaneous infection with babesiosis and Lyme disease may be especially severe.

- Babesiosis infects erythrocytes and causes fever, myalgias, and hemolytic anemia; asplenic patients may have a chronic, protracted illness.

19.

PULMONARY INFECTIONS AND MYCOBACTERIAL INFECTIONS

Pritish K. Tosh, MD, Elie F. Berbari, MD, and M. Rizwan Sohail, MD

GOALS

- Review viral pulmonary syndromes.

- Review the diagnosis and management of bacterial pneumonia.

- Understand the diagnosis and management of mycobacterial infections in immunocompetent and immunocompromised patients.

VIRAL INFECTIONS

VIRAL PNEUMONIA

Common causes of viral pneumonia are parainfluenza virus, adenovirus, and influenza viruses A and B. In adults, varicella (chickenpox) pneumonia is a severe illness, the resolution of which may be followed by nodular pulmonary calcification. In adults with chickenpox, cough (which occurs in 25% of patients), profuse rash, fever for more than 1 week, and age 35 years or older are the most important predictors of varicella pneumonia. Early therapy with intravenous acyclovir is recommended for patients at risk for pneumonia. Anecdotally, corticosteroids may be helpful in previously well patients with life-threatening varicella pneumonia; however, this intervention has not been tested in a large controlled trial. Herpes simplex virus may cause pneumonia in immunocompromised patients or in patients with extensive burns.

- Consider varicella pneumonia in adults who present with profuse rash, cough, and fever for more than 1 week; intravenous acyclovir is recommended for patients at risk.

Cytomegalovirus (CMV) pneumonia typically occurs in immunocompromised patients, such as those with AIDS who have CD4 counts less than 50/mcL, transplant recipients, and patients with hematologic malignancies. Diffuse, small nodular or hazy infiltrates are seen on chest radiography in 15%

of patients with pneumonia caused by CMV, but interstitial pneumonia due to CMV occurs in 50% of bone marrow graft recipients. Diagnosis of CMV pneumonia is made by finding characteristic inclusion bodies in affected cells, isolating the virus, or detecting CMV antigens or nucleic acids. Isolation of CMV from respiratory tract secretions does not always establish that infection is present.

- CMV infection is associated with immunocompromised patients, such as those with AIDS (CD4 count <50/mcL).

- Isolation of CMV from respiratory tract secretions does not always establish that infection is present.

AVIAN INFLUENZA A (H5N1) VIRUS

With birds serving as the original reservoir for avian influenza A, the first human infection was reported in 1997 in Hong Kong. Since then, the highly pathogenic avian influenza A (H5N1) virus, possessing genetic similarities to the virus linked to the 1918 influenza pandemic, has spread westward to infect poultry and rodents in central Europe. Bird-to-human transmission is the usual route of infection, but cases of human-to-human transmission through close contact have been suspected. By mid-2011, more than 500 cases of human infection had been documented, most in southern and eastern Asia, with a mortality rate of more than 50%. Infections characteristically occur in young, previously healthy persons who have come in contact with sick or dead birds. The illness manifests initially with pulmonary infiltrates and hypoxic respiratory failure consistent with acute respiratory distress syndrome followed by progression to multiorgan failure. Since avian influenza A (H5N1) is generally resistant to amantadine and rimantadine, the recommended first-line treatment is high-dose oseltamivir. Corticosteroids have been used adjunctively, but high-level studies have not been performed to confirm their efficacy. In 2007, the US Food and Drug Administration approved a vaccine for the national stockpile; it is not commercially available.

HANTAVIRUS PULMONARY SYNDROME

Hantavirus pulmonary syndrome, first recognized in the southwestern United States in 1993, is caused by an RNA virus (family, Bunyaviridae; genus, *Hantavirus*). The rodent reservoir for this virus is the deer mouse (*Peromyscus maniculatus*). Infection occurs by inhalation of rodent excreta. Epidemics have been related to environmental conditions that result in explosive growth of deer mouse populations. No human-to-human transmission has been documented. The syndrome is more common in the southwestern United States. Among persons with the syndrome, the median age is 32 years (range, 12–69 years), 52% are males, and 55% are Native Americans. The illness is characterized by a short prodrome of fever, myalgia, headache, abdominal pain, nausea or vomiting, and cough, followed by the abrupt onset of respiratory distress. Bilateral pulmonary infiltrates (noncardiogenic pulmonary edema) that occur within 48 hours after the onset of illness have been reported for all patients. Pleural effusions are common and can be transudative or exudative. Hemoconcentration, thrombocytopenia, and prolonged activated partial thromboplastin time are common; disseminated intravascular coagulation is rare. Early thrombocytopenia may provide a clue to the diagnosis of the infection. Myocardial suppression has been documented. Autopsy can show pleural effusions and edematous lungs, with interstitial mononuclear cells in the alveolar septa, alveolar edema, focal hyaline membranes, and occasional alveolar hemorrhage. *Hantavirus* antigens are detected with immunohistochemistry. Serologic (*Hantavirus*-specific immunoglobulin M or increasing titers of immunoglobulin G), polymerase chain reaction, and other studies are available. Treatment is supportive; the mortality rate is as high as 50%.

- The reservoir for *Hantavirus* is the deer mouse.

SEVERE ACUTE RESPIRATORY SYNDROME

Severe acute respiratory syndrome (SARS) is a viral respiratory infection caused by a novel coronavirus that previously had infected only animals. SARS is transmitted through aerosol and possibly fecal-oral routes. The majority of patients with SARS have been adults 25 to 70 years old who were previously healthy. Many of the cases have been reported in Asia, particularly Hong Kong, Taiwan, and the People's Republic of China; however, cases have been reported in other countries in Asia and in North America and Europe. Notably, no new cases have been documented since 2004. SARS has an incubation period of 2 to 10 days. The illness begins with fever (>38.0°C) and associated chills and rigors. Other frequent symptoms are headache, malaise, and myalgia. Within the first 7 days, a dry nonproductive cough and dyspnea develop, with hypoxemia. This worsens in 20% of patients, who require mechanical ventilation and treatment in an intensive care unit. Currently, the fatality rate is approximately 15%. Leukocyte counts generally have been normal or decreased, with more than 50% of patients having lymphopenia and thrombocytopenia. Increased levels of liver aminotransferases and creatine kinase have been noted. Treatment is primarily supportive, with no role for antivirals.

- SARS is caused by a coronavirus.

- No new cases have been documented since 2004.

INFLUENZA

Influenza causes annual, seasonal epidemics leading to tens of thousands of deaths each year in the United States. Two influenza A strains (H3N2 and H1N1) and one influenza B strain typically circulate during winter months and undergo minor antigenic mutations (antigenic drift) resulting in annual seasonal epidemics. Influenza pandemics occur more rarely (every 20–30 years) and are the result of major antigenic changes (antigenic shift) leading to large numbers of infections due to low levels of population immunity. During seasonal epidemics, 80% to 90% of deaths due to influenza occur in persons older than 65 years. Complications include 1) primary influenza pneumonia (interstitial desquamative pneumonia) and 2) secondary bacterial infection, which usually is caused by *S pneumoniae*, *Haemophilus*, or *S aureus*. Rare cases of toxic shock syndrome have been reported when *S aureus* pneumonia complicates influenza.

- About 80%-90% of deaths due to seasonal influenza occur in persons older than 65 years.

- Secondary infection usually is caused by *S pneumoniae* or *S aureus*.

Amantadine and rimantadine are effective against only influenza A viruses, not influenza B. Therapy is most beneficial if begun within 48 hours of onset of symptoms. Neuraminidase inhibitors (oseltamivir and zanamivir) are effective against disease caused by both influenza A and B. Both reduce the duration of symptoms by 1 day when given within 48 hours after onset of symptoms. Because of seasonal changes in antiviral resistance in circulating strains, recommendations for treatment from the Centers for Disease Control and Prevention should be consulted each year. When oseltamivir resistance is suspected, treatment with zanamivir or a combination of oseltamivir and rimantadine is recommended instead of oseltamivir alone.

Inactivated injectable influenza and live attenuated intranasal vaccines are used for the prevention of influenza. Target groups for vaccination with the inactivated vaccine are persons older than 50 years, residents of chronic care facilities, persons with cardiopulmonary disorders, healthy children between 6 and 23 months old, children 6 months to 18 years old receiving long-term aspirin therapy (to prevent Reye syndrome), health care personnel, employees of chronic care facilities, providers of home health care, and persons sharing the same household as high-risk persons. The live attenuated vaccine is approved only for healthy immunocompetent persons between the ages of 2 and 49 years. Adverse reactions to both vaccines include fever, myalgias, and hypersensitivity. For persons who did not receive the vaccine, amantadine, rimantadine, or oseltamivir can be used for influenza prevention and are effective for prophylactic use after exposure to a patient with influenza; amantadine and rimantadine are active against only influenza A. Amantadine is given at a dose of 200 mg per day; if the person is older than 65 years, only 100 mg per day is given to decrease the risk of adverse effects. The decreased dosage also is used for patients with impaired renal function or seizure disorders. Toxicity manifests as dizziness, restlessness, and insomnia. High-risk persons who have not received the vaccine during the influenza season should be considered for chemoprophylaxis.

- Target groups for influenza vaccine are persons older than 50 years, residents of chronic care facilities, persons with cardiopulmonary disorders, healthy children between 6 and 23 months old, children 6 months to 18 years old receiving long-term aspirin therapy (to prevent Reye syndrome), health care personnel, employees of chronic care facilities, providers of home health care, and household members of high-risk persons.

BACTERIAL INFECTIONS

COMMUNITY-ACQUIRED PNEUMONIA

There are more than 900,000 cases of community-acquired pneumonia (CAP) in persons older than 65 years in the United States each year. Despite the use of antimicrobials, mortality remains high. CAP and influenza combine to be the seventh leading cause of death in the United States. Common microbiologic causes of CAP are *Streptococcus pneumoniae*, *Mycoplasma pneumoniae*, *Haemophilus influenzae*, *Chlamydophila (Chlamydia) pneumoniae*, *Legionella* species, *Staphylococcus aureus*, and respiratory viruses (most commonly influenza and respiratory syncytial virus).

Where patients are treated for CAP is important because unnecessary hospitalizations for CAP increase costs. In addition, patients transferred to an intensive care unit for CAP care have worse outcomes than those who are directly admitted to an intensive care unit. Although not meant to supplant good clinical judgment, CAP risk stratification indices help clinicians decide the site-of-care for patients with CAP. The most validated index is the Pneumonia Severity Index, which calculates the risk of mortality using 20 demographic, comorbidity, physical examination, and laboratory risk factors. CURB-65, an alternative index, is validated and easier to use. In a patient suspected of having CAP, 1 point is given for each of the following: *C*onfusion, *U*remia (blood urea nitrogen >19 mg/dL), *R*espiratory rate (>30 breaths/min), *B*lood pressure (systolic <90 mm Hg or diastolic ≤60 mm Hg), and age ≥65 years. Patients with a CURB-65 score of 0 or 1 are at low risk and should be considered for outpatient therapy, a patient with a score of 2 should be considered for hospitalization or closely supervised outpatient treatment, a patient with a score of 3 should be hospitalized, and a patient with a score of 4 or 5 should be hospitalized and considered for care in an intensive care unit. Of the CURB-65 criteria, uremia is the only one that requires laboratory data. For patients suspected of having

CAP for whom laboratory data are not available, a modified index (CRB-65) can be used, in which the uremia risk factor is removed from the calculation. A patient with a CRB-65 score of 0 should be treated as an outpatient, a patient with a score of 1 or 2 should be considered for hospitalization, and a patient with a score of 3 or 4 should be hospitalized.

Chest imaging is a requirement for a diagnosis of CAP. Computed tomography is more sensitive, but chest radiography is usually sufficient. The usefulness of other diagnostic tests is more controversial because they are generally of low yield and infrequently affect clinical care. However, they can be helpful for individual patients and provide data for epidemiologic purposes. Other testing is optional for outpatients with CAP. Pretreatment culturing of blood and sputum should be performed on all patients hospitalized with CAP, and urinary antigen testing for *Legionella pneumophila* and *S pneumoniae* should be performed on patients requiring care in an intensive care unit. During influenza season, influenza testing should be performed on all patients with CAP who require hospitalization.

Empiric treatment of CAP should be directed toward the suspected pathogens on the basis of a patient's risk factors:

- For previously healthy patients who have not received antimicrobials in the prior 3 months, reside in locations with less than 25% macrolide resistance in *S pneumoniae*, and will be treated as outpatients, macrolide monotherapy (eg, erythromycin, azithromycin, or clarithromycin) is recommended, and doxycycline is recommended as an alternative.

- For patients with significant medical comorbidities who have received antimicrobials in the prior 3 months, have more than 25% macrolide resistance in *S pneumoniae*, and will be treated as outpatients, treatment options are as follows:

  a. A respiratory fluoroquinolone as monotherapy (eg, levofloxacin or moxifloxacin) *or*

  b. A β-lactam antibiotic *and* a macrolide *or* doxycycline as a single-agent alternative

- For patients with significant medical comorbidities or who have received antimicrobials in the prior 3 months and will be treated as inpatients, treatment options are as follows:

  a. A respiratory fluoroquinolone as monotherapy (eg, levofloxacin or moxifloxacin) *or*

  b. A β-lactam antibiotic *and* a macrolide *or* doxycycline as a single-agent alternative

- For patients who require management in an intensive care unit, recommended treatment is with a β-lactam antibiotic (eg, cefotaxime, ceftriaxone, or ampicillin-sulbactam) *and* azithromycin or a respiratory fluoroquinolone (eg, levofloxacin or moxifloxacin).

- Empiric treatment of methicillin-resistant *S aureus* with the addition of vancomycin or linezolid should be considered for patients with clinical risk factors such as end-stage renal disease, intravenous drug use, recent influenza infection, and prior use of antimicrobials, especially fluoroquinolones.

If the microbiologic cause of CAP is determined, antimicrobial therapy can be directed toward that pathogen. For hospitalized patients, intravenously administered antimicrobials can be switched to oral administration when the patient is hemodynamically stable, improving clinically, and able to take medications orally. The oral antimicrobial should be the same agent or of the same drug class as the intravenous antimicrobial. The duration of use of antimicrobials for CAP is variable but generally ranges between 7 and 10 days. Patients should be treated for a minimum of 5 days and until all but 1 of the following occurs before discontinuing use of antimicrobials: temperature 37.8°C or less, heart rate 100 beats per minute or less, respiratory rate 24 breaths per minute or less, systolic blood pressure 90 mm Hg or less, oxygen saturation 90% or more while breathing room air, ability to take oral medications, and normal mental status.

Streptococcus pneumoniae (pneumococcus) is a leading cause of community-acquired infections such as pneumonia, meningitis, otitis media, and sinusitis. Like many organisms, it is becoming increasingly resistant to traditional antibiotics. Potential complications of pneumococcal pneumonia include empyema and pericarditis from direct extension of infection. Empyema should be suspected when fever persists despite appropriate antibiotic therapy of pneumococcal pneumonia.

Asplenia predisposes to severe infections with *S pneumoniae* (and other encapsulated organisms). After splenectomy, fulminant (purpura fulminans) pneumococcal bacteremia with disseminated intravascular coagulation is more common and often fatal. Similarly, *S pneumoniae* infections are more frequent and unusually severe in smokers and patients with asthma, sickle cell disease, multiple myeloma, alcoholism, human immunodeficiency virus (HIV), or hypogammaglobulinemia.

Streptococcus pneumoniae is the leading cause of invasive bacterial respiratory disease in patients with HIV infection. Prophylaxis for *Pneumocystis jiroveci* pneumonia with trimethoprim-sulfamethoxazole may provide effective primary or secondary prophylaxis, but breakthrough infections with resistant organisms are not uncommon.

- Splenectomy predisposes to fulminant, often fatal, pneumococcal bacteremia with disseminated intravascular coagulation.

- *Streptococcus pneumoniae* infections are more frequent and unusually severe in smokers and patients with asthma, sickle cell disease, multiple myeloma, alcoholism, HIV, or hypogammaglobulinemia.

- *Streptococcus pneumoniae* is the leading cause of invasive bacterial respiratory disease in patients with HIV infection.

Infections due to *S pneumoniae* have traditionally been treated with penicillin. In January 2008, the Clinical and Laboratory Standards Institute published new *S pneumoniae* breakpoints and interpretations for penicillin (the preferred antimicrobial for susceptible *S pneumoniae* infections) for meningitis strains and nonmeningitis strains. Intermediate penicillin susceptibilities were removed from the meningitis strains, and breakpoints were increased substantially for nonmeningitis pneumococcal infections (Table 19.1).

With the new breakpoints, retrospective re-categorization of the isolates from 2006 to 2007 showed that 93% of the nonmeningitis isolates were penicillin-susceptible, 5.6% had intermediate susceptibility to penicillin, and 1% were fully penicillin-resistant. Among the meningitis isolates, 73% were penicillin-susceptible. Penicillin resistance among the meningitis isolates increased from 11% to 28%. These re-categorizations are important for decisions about empiric and specific pneumococcal therapy, depending on the syndrome. Penicillin resistance is conferred by an alteration of the penicillin-binding proteins, which results in a decreased affinity of these cell wall components for the penicillins. Penicillin-resistant strains are often resistant to other antibiotics such as the macrolides, trimethoprim-sulfamethoxazole, and, occasionally, cephalosporins. Risk factors for development of infection due to penicillin-resistant pneumococci include previous use of β-lactam antibiotics, nosocomial acquisition, and multiple previous hospitalizations.

Penicillin-resistant strains of *S pneumoniae* remain susceptible to vancomycin. High doses of cefotaxime, ceftriaxone, and imipenem also may be effective. Ciprofloxacin is not effective; however, the newer fluoroquinolones (levofloxacin, gatifloxacin, and moxifloxacin) are active against pneumococci. Resistance to levofloxacin is reported in about 1% of strains.

The pneumococcal vaccine is polyvalent, containing capsular polysaccharide from the 23 serotypes that most commonly cause pneumococcal infection. It is recommended for persons who are at an increased risk of invasive pneumococcal disease or complications. These include adults older than 65 years; patients of any age with chronic illness such as chronic cardiovascular disease (eg, congestive heart failure or cardiomyopathies), chronic pulmonary disease (eg, chronic obstructive pulmonary disease or emphysema), diabetes mellitus, alcoholism, asthma, chronic liver disease (cirrhosis), or asplenia; smokers; patients with cochlear implants; or patients with cerebrospinal fluid leaks. The vaccine can be given simultaneously with influenza virus vaccine. Pneumococcal vaccine booster is recommended 5 years after the initial dose in high-risk patients or in patients who received the first dose before age 65 years.

- Penicillin resistance is increasing in isolates of *Streptococcus*.

- Pneumococcal vaccine is recommended for patients at increased risk of invasive pneumococcal disease or complications.

Table 19.1 RECOMMENDATIONS FOR ANTIMICROBIAL THERAPY IN ADULTS WITH COMMUNITY-ACQUIRED BACTERIAL MENINGITIS

EMPIRIC THERAPY

Predisposing Factor	Common Bacterial Pathogens	Antimicrobial Therapy
Age, y		
16–50	*Neisseria meningitidis, Streptococcus pneumoniae*	Vancomycin plus a third-generation cephalosporin[a,b]
>50	*S pneumoniae, N meningitidis, Listeria monocytogenes,* aerobic gram-negative bacilli	Vancomycin plus a third-generation cephalosporin plus ampicillin[b,c]
With risk factor present[d]	*S pneumoniae, L monocytogenes, Haemophilus influenzae*	Vancomycin plus a third-generation cephalosporin plus ampicillin[b,c]

SPECIFIC ANTIMICROBIAL THERAPY

Microorganism, Susceptibility	Standard Therapy	Alternative Therapies
S pneumoniae		
Penicillin MIC		
<0.1 mg/L	Penicillin G or ampicillin	Third-generation cephalosporin,[b] chloramphenicol
0.1–1.0 mg/L	Third-generation cephalosporin[b]	Cefepime, meropenem
≥2.0 mg/L	Vancomycin plus a third-generation cephalosporin[b,c]	Fluoroquinolone[f]
Cefotaxime or ceftriaxone MIC		
≥1.0 mg/L	Vancomycin plus a third-generation cephalosporin[b,g]	Fluoroquinolone[f]
N meningitidis		
Penicillin MIC		
<0.1 mg/L	Penicillin G or ampicillin	Third-generation cephalosporin,[b] chloramphenicol
0.1–1.0 mg/L	Third-generation cephalosporin[b]	Chloramphenicol, fluoroquinolone, meropenem
L monocytogenes	Penicillin G or ampicillin[h]	Trimethoprim-sulfamethoxazole, meropenem
Group B streptococcus	Penicillin G or ampicillin[h]	Third-generation cephalosporin[b]
Specific Antimicrobial Therapy		
Escherichia coli & other Enterobacteriaceae	Third-generation cephalosporin[b]	Aztreonam, fluoroquinolone, meropenem, trimethoprim-sulfamethoxazole, ampicillin
Pseudomonas aeruginosa	Ceftazidime or cefepime[h]	Aztreonam,[h] ciprofloxacin,[h] meropenem[h]

H influenzae

β-Lactamase negative — Ampicillin — Third-generation cephalosporin,[b] cefepime, chloramphenicol, fluoroquinolone

β-Lactamase positive — Third-generation cephalosporin[b] — Cefepime, chloramphenicol, fluoroquinolone

Chemoprophylaxis[i]
N meningitidis — Rifampicin (rifampin), ceftriaxone, ciprofloxacin, azithromycin

Abbreviation: MIC, minimal inhibitory concentration.

[a] Only in areas with very low penicillin-resistance rates (<1%) should monotherapy with penicillin be considered, although many experts recommend combination therapy for all patients until results of in vitro susceptibility testing are known.

[b] Cefotaxime or ceftriaxone.

[c] Only in areas with very low penicillin-resistance & cephalosporin-resistance rates should combination therapy of amoxicillin (ampicillin) & a third-generation cephalosporin be considered.

[d] Alcoholism, altered immune status.

[e] Consider addition of rifampicin (rifampin) if dexamethasone is given.

[f] Gatifloxacin or moxifloxacin; no clinical data on use in patients with bacterial meningitis.

[g] Consider addition of rifampicin (rifampin) if the MIC of ceftriaxone is ≥2 mg/L.

[h] Consider addition of an aminoglycoside.

[i] Prophylaxis is indicated for close contacts (defined as those with intimate contact, which covers those eating & sleeping in the same dwelling & those having close social & kissing contacts) or health care workers who perform mouth-to-mouth resuscitation, endotracheal intubation, or endotracheal tube management. Patients with meningococcal meningitis who receive monotherapy with penicillin or amoxicillin (ampicillin) should also receive chemoprophylaxis, because carriage is not reliably eradicated by these drugs.

Note: The preferred intravenous doses in patients with normal renal & hepatic function: penicillin, 2 million units every 4 hours; amoxicillin or ampicillin, 2 g every 4 hours; vancomycin, 15 mg/kg every 8 to 12 hours; third-generation cephalosporin: ceftriaxone, 2 g every 12 hours, or cefotaxime, 2 g every 4 to 6 hours; cefepime, 2 g every 8 hours; ceftazidime, 2 g every 8 hours; meropenem, 2 g every 8 hours; chloramphenicol, 1 to 1.5 g every 6 hours; fluoroquinolone: gatifloxacin, 400 mg every 24 hours, or moxifloxacin, 400 mg every 24 hours, although no data on optimal dose is needed in patients with bacterial meningitis; trimethoprim-sulfamethoxazole, 5 mg/kg every 6 to 12 hours; aztreonam, 2 g every 6 to 8 hours; ciprofloxacin, 400 mg every 8 to 12 hours; rifampicin (rifampin), 600 mg every 12 to 24 hours; aminoglycoside: gentamicin, 1.7 mg/kg every 8 hours. The preferred dose for chemoprophylaxis: rifampicin (rifampin), 600 mg orally twice daily for 2 days; ceftriaxone, 250 mg intramuscularly; ciprofloxacin, 500 mg orally; azithromycin, 500 mg orally.

The duration of therapy for patients with bacterial meningitis has often been based more on tradition than on evidence-based data & needs to be individualized on the basis of the patient's response. In general, antimicrobial therapy is given for 7 days for meningitis caused by *Neisseria meningitidis* & *Haemophilus influenzae*, 10 to 14 days for *Streptococcus pneumoniae*, & at least 21 days for *Listeria monocytogenes*.

Adapted from van de Beek D, de Gans J, Tunkel AR, Wijdicks EFM. Community-acquired bacterial meningitis in adults. N Engl J Med. 2006 Jan 5;354(1):44–53. Used with permission.

LEGIONELLA

Legionellae organisms are fastidious gram-negative bacilli. *Legionella pneumophila* causes both CAP and nosocomial pneumonia, typically occurring in the summer months. Nosocomial legionellosis may be due to contaminated water supplies. Immunocompromised patients, especially those receiving long-term corticosteroid therapy, are especially susceptible to *Legionella* infections. Typical clinical features of legionellosis include weakness, malaise, fever, dry cough, diarrhea, pleuritic chest pain, relative bradycardia, diffuse rales bilaterally, and patchy bilateral pulmonary infiltrates.

Characteristic laboratory features of *Legionella* pneumonia may include decreased sodium and phosphorus values, increased leukocyte level, and increased liver enzyme values. Legionellae organisms will not grow on standard media. Diagnosis depends on results of special culture, finding organisms by direct fluorescent antibody staining, or detecting an increase in anti-*Legionella* antibody titers. Urine antigen detection is a more sensitive (>80%) and simple diagnostic test for *L pneumophila* infections, but only serogroup 1 is detected.

Legionellae organisms are intracellular parasites. As such, they are resistant to all β-lactam drugs and aminoglycosides in vivo. Effective agents for treating *Legionella* infection include macrolides, fluoroquinolones, and, to a lesser extent, doxycycline. Fluoroquinolones are considered drugs of choice for therapy. Some authorities recommend adding rifampin for severe infection.

- Immunocompromised patients, especially those receiving long-term corticosteroid therapy, are especially susceptible to *Legionella* infections.
- Diagnosis can be established by special *Legionella* culture, serologic tests, and urinary antigen detection.
- Therapy is with macrolides or fluoroquinolones.

MYCOPLASMA PNEUMONIAE

Mycoplasma pneumoniae organisms are one of the smallest microorganisms capable of extracellular replication. Because *Mycoplasma* organisms lack a cell wall, cell-wall–active antibiotics such as penicillins are ineffective in treating *Mycoplasma* infection. *Mycoplasma* infection is spread by droplet inhalation. It primarily infects young, previously healthy persons and presents with rapid onset of headache, dry cough, and fever. Results of physical examination are often unremarkable, with the possible exception of bullous myringitis. Chest radiography usually shows bilateral, patchy pneumonitis. The chest radiographic abnormalities are often out of proportion to the physical findings. Pleural effusion is present in 15% to 20% of cases. Neurologic complications include Guillain-Barré syndrome, cerebellar peripheral neuropathy, aseptic meningitis, and mononeuritis multiplex. Hemolytic anemia may occur late in the illness as a result of circulating cold hemagglutinins. Erythema multiforme may also occur. The diagnosis is established by specific complement fixation test. Cold agglutinins are nonspecific and unreliable for diagnosing *Mycoplasma*

infections. Fluoroquinolones, macrolides, and tetracyclines are effective therapies. Because immunity to *Mycoplasma* infection is transient, reinfection may occur. Clinical relapse of pneumonia occurs in up to 10% of cases of *Mycoplasma* pneumonia.

- *Mycoplasma pneumoniae* infection is spread by droplet inhalation.
- Chest radiography usually shows bilateral, patchy pneumonitis.
- Pleural effusion is present in 15%-20% of cases.
- Neurologic complications include Guillain-Barré syndrome, cerebellar peripheral neuropathy, aseptic meningitis, and mononeuritis multiplex.
- Cold hemagglutin hemolytic anemia and erythema multiforme may occur in patients with *Mycoplasma* pneumonia.

CHLAMYDOPHILA (CHLAMYDIA) PNEUMONIAE

Chlamydophila (Chlamydia) pneumoniae may also cause "atypical pneumonia." *Chlamydia trachomatis* and *Chlamydophila psittaci* are the other 2 chlamydial species that cause human disease. In young adults, *C pneumoniae* causes 10% of cases of pneumonia and 5% of cases of bronchitis. It has caused community outbreaks, and nosocomial transmission has occurred. Half of adults are seropositive for *C pneumoniae*. Birds are the source of infection with *C psittaci* (psittacosis), but there is no animal reservoir for *C pneumoniae*. Clinical manifestations of infection are usually mild and may resemble those caused by *M pneumoniae*. Pharyngitis occurs 1 to 3 weeks before the onset of pulmonary symptoms, and cough may last for weeks. The diagnosis is based on serologic testing. Treatment is with doxycycline or a macrolide. The newer fluoroquinolones such as levofloxacin and gatifloxacin have in vitro activity against *C pneumoniae*, but clinical efficacy studies are not available. Of note, trimethoprim-sulfamethoxazole and β-lactam antibiotics such as penicillins or cephalosporins are not active against chlamydial species.

- In young adults, *C pneumoniae* causes 10% of cases of pneumonia and 5% of cases of bronchitis.

MORAXELLA

Moraxella catarrhalis (formerly *Branhamella catarrhalis*) is a respiratory tract pathogen primarily causing bronchitis and pneumonia in persons with chronic obstructive pulmonary disease. It also may cause otitis media, sinusitis, meningitis, bacteremia, and endocarditis in immunosuppressed patients. Ampicillin resistance through β-lactamase production is common. Trimethoprim-sulfamethoxazole, the fluoroquinolones, and amoxicillin-clavulanate are effective for therapy.

BORDETELLA PERTUSSIS

The incidence of whooping cough is increasing as the protection afforded by immunization declines with age. Twelve percent of cases now occur in persons older than 15 years. *Bordetella pertussis* infection often results in persistent coughing in older children and adults. As many as 50 million adults are now susceptible to infection as a result of waning immunity. Whooping cough may cause severe lymphocytosis (>100 lymphocytes × 10^9/L). Diagnosis of *B pertussis* infection may be difficult. Molecular testing (polymerase chain reaction) of a nasopharyngeal aspirate is more sensitive, rapid, and reliable than cultures. Early treatment of pertussis with a macrolide (erythromycin, clarithromycin, or azithromycin) is recommended. The duration of treatment of pertussis is 14 days for the patient and 5 days for close contacts of affected patients for prevention, irrespective of age or vaccination status. Aerosolized bronchodilators or corticosteroids may alleviate the persistent coughing. A new pertussis-containing tetanus-diphtheria vaccine (Tdap) is now available for use in adults. It is given as a single booster to replace a dose of tetanus-diphtheria booster. This approach is particularly emphasized for adults who have close contact with infants (eg, parents, health care workers, and day care providers).

- *Bordetella pertussis* may cause severe lymphocytosis (>100 lymphocytes × 10^9/L).
- *Bordetella pertussis* can cause persistent cough in older children and adults.
- The treatment of choice is a macrolide antibiotic.

KLEBSIELLA, ENTEROBACTER, AND SERRATIA

Klebsiella pneumoniae is an important cause of both CAP and nosocomial pneumonia and often is associated with alcoholism, diabetes mellitus, and chronic obstructive pulmonary disease. Red currant jelly-colored sputum is characteristic. Lung abscess and empyema are more frequent with *K pneumoniae* than with other pneumonia-causing organisms, especially in alcoholics. Third-generation cephalosporins are the drugs of choice for treating most types of *Klebsiella*. Strains of *Klebsiella* resistant to ceftazidime have emerged. This resistance is caused by an extended-spectrum β-lactamase. Susceptibility testing results for such strains may erroneously report that they are susceptible to cefotaxime. If they are resistant to ceftazidime, consider them resistant to all cephalosporins. Resistance to carbapenem antibiotics through *K pneumoniae* carbapenemases has also emerged; treatment with antimicrobials such as colistin may be needed for these organisms.

- Lung abscess and empyema are more frequent with *K pneumoniae* than with other pneumonia-causing organisms, especially in alcoholics.

Enterobacter and *Serratia* are primarily associated with nosocomial infections. *Enterobacter* species such as *Enterobacter cloacae* or *Enterobacter aerogenes* often are resistant to third-

generation cephalosporins such as cefotaxime. Despite in vitro data suggesting susceptibility, β-lactamase production is induced when grown in the presence of cephalosporins. Carbapenems such as imipenem or meropenem, fluoroquinolones, cefepime, and trimethoprim-sulfamethoxazole are usually active against these strains.

- *Enterobacter* species often are resistant to third-generation cephalosporins such as cefotaxime, despite in vitro data suggesting susceptibility.

COXIELLA BURNETII

Coxiella burnetii, a rickettsia shed in the urine, feces, milk, and birth products of sheep, cattle, goats, and cats, is responsible for Q fever (named for the query associated with an outbreak in an Australian slaughterhouse in 1935). However, epidemiologic factors such as contact with cats or farm animals are identified for only 40% of patients. Humans are infected by inhalation of dried aerosolized material (eg, urine, feces, milk, or birth products of sheep, cattle, goats, or cats). The incubation period is 10 to 30 days. Clinical features include fever, myalgias, chills, chest pain, and cough (late in the course). The leukocyte count is normal, and the erythrocyte sedimentation rate is increased. Chest radiographic findings may be normal or show unilateral bronchopneumonia and small pleural effusions. Lobar consolidation is found in 25% of patients. Hepatitis and endocarditis can occur. Hyponatremia occurs in more than 25% of patients. Liver enzyme levels may increase. Indirect immunofluorescence is the diagnostic test of choice. Doxycycline is the treatment of choice, although prolonged duration of combination therapy with the addition of a macrolide or fluoroquinolone is often necessary for severe or complicated infections.

- *Coxiella burnetii* is a rickettsia that is responsible for Q fever.
- Humans are infected by inhalation of dried inoculum from urine, feces, milk, or birth products of sheep, cattle, goats, or cats.

FRANCISELLA TULARENSIS

Francisella tularensis is a gram-negative bacillus transmitted to humans from wild animals and from bites of ticks or deer flies. An analysis of an outbreak in Martha's Vineyard showed that the highest identifiable risk was associated with mowing grass and cutting brush. Aerosol inhalation can occur (eg, laboratory workers), and it is a potential bioterrorism agent. The incubation period for tularemia is 2 to 5 days. Cutaneous ulcer and lymphadenopathy are common features. Cough, fever, and chest pain are frequent, but many patients are asymptomatic. Chest radiography shows unilateral lower lobe patchy infiltrates (bilateral in 30% of patients) and pleural effusion (30% of patients). The leukocyte count can be normal; the organism is not seen with Gram staining of the sputum. Serologic testing (agglutinins) is considered diagnostic if it shows a fourfold increase in titer in paired samples 2 to 3 weeks apart or a single titer greater than 1:160. Intravenous streptomycin or gentamicin is the recommended antimicrobial regimen for *F tularensis* infection; ciprofloxacin or doxycycline given for 14 days is the recommended treatment for postexposure prophylaxis.

- Tularemia is transmitted to humans from wild animals and bites of ticks or deer flies. Mowing grass and cutting brush have also been identified as risk factors.

YERSINIA PESTIS

Yersinia pestis is a gram-negative bacillus that causes plague. It is more prevalent in New Mexico, Arizona, Colorado, and California than in other states. It is spread from wild rodents (occasionally cats), either directly or by fleas, usually in May to September. Because it is endemic to largely rural and uninhabited areas, the incidence of disease is low. The incubation period is 2 to 7 days. Clinical features include fever, headache, bubo (groin or axilla), cough, and tachypnea. Pneumonia occurs in 10% to 20% of patients. Pneumonic plague is the most serious and fulminant form of this disease. Chest radiography shows bilateral lower lobe alveolar infiltrates. Pleural effusion is common, and nodules and cavities can occur. The leukocyte count is higher than 15×10^9/L. The organism is seen with Giemsa or direct fluorescent antibody staining and in cultures of blood, lymph node, or sputum. Serologic testing gives positive results. Intravenous streptomycin or gentamicin is the recommended antimicrobial regimen for *Y pestis* infection; ciprofloxacin or doxycycline given for 7 days is the recommended treatment for postexposure prophylaxis.

- *Yersinia pestis* bacillus is most common in the southwestern United States.

BURKHOLDERIA PSEUDOMALLEI

Burkholderia pseudomallei is a gram-negative rod responsible for melioidosis. The disease is most prevalent in parts of Southeast Asia; sporadic cases have been reported in the United States. The organism is widely distributed in water and soil, and infection occurs after direct inoculation through the skin or, less commonly, by inhalation. Although the incubation period can be as short as 3 days, the disease remains latent and may become evident months to years later. Up to 2% of US Army personnel stationed in Vietnam were seropositive for *B pseudomallei*, even though the majority of them were free of clinical disease. Clinical features include acute community-acquired pneumonia, pleurisy, subacute presentation with upper lobe lesions (sometimes with cavitation), or chronic cavitary lung disease that resembles tuberculosis. Diagnosis is by positive findings on culture. Because *B pseudomallei* is often multidrug-resistant, definitive therapy is often dependent on antimicrobial susceptibility testing; empiric therapy with ceftazidime, meropenem, or imipenem should be considered if *B pseudomallei* infection is likely or while susceptibility tests are being performed.

- Melioidosis may resemble chronic cavitary tuberculosis.

NOCARDIA PNEUMONIA

Nocardia asteroides, *Nocardia brasiliensis*, and *Nocardia otitidiscaviarum* can cause pneumonia in susceptible persons. *N asteroides* is a weakly acid-fast saprophytic bacteria present in the soil, dust, plants, and water. Infection is more common in immunosuppressed patients and in those with pulmonary alveolar proteinosis. Primary infection leads to necrotizing pneumonia with abscess formation. No inflammatory response or granuloma formation occurs. Pulmonary nodules suggestive of cancer metastases and dense alveolar infiltrates are common chest radiographic findings. Infection may produce pleural effusion. Lymphohematogenous spread occurs in 20% of patients; in nearly all those patients, a brain abscess develops. The diagnosis is made at autopsy in 40% of cases. Isolation of the organism from the sputum of immunocompetent patients might represent colonization because the saprophytic state is well recognized; however, in an immunocompromised patient, this should be considered a true infection. Most *Nocardia* isolates are susceptible to trimethoprim-sulfamethoxazole, however initial combination therapy with the addition of imipenem, ceftriaxone, or amikacin should be considered in severe or complicated cases.

- Brain abscess is common in patients with disseminated *Nocardia* infection.

ASPIRATION PNEUMONIA

Aspiration pneumonia can be either acute or chronic. The acute type usually results from aspiration of a volume larger than 50 mL, with a pH less than 2.4. It produces classic aspiration pneumonia that is often sterile; the role of antibiotics in the absence of supporting cultures is unclear and controversial. Predisposing factors include nasogastric tube, anesthesia, coma, seizures, central nervous system problems, diaphragmatic hernia with reflux, and tracheoesophageal fistula. Nosocomial aspiration pneumonia is caused by *Escherichia coli*, *S aureus*, *K pneumoniae*, and *Pseudomonas aeruginosa*. Community-acquired aspiration pneumonias are caused by infections due to anaerobes (*Bacteroides melaninogenicus*, *Fusobacterium nucleatum*, and gram-positive cocci). Preventive measures are important. Chronic aspiration pneumonia results from recurrent aspiration of small volumes. Examples include patients with reflux aspiration who develop mineral oil granuloma. Symptoms include chronic cough, patchy lung infiltrates, and nocturnal wheeze.

- Acute aspiration pneumonia usually results from aspiration of a volume >50 mL, with a pH <2.4.

- Acute aspiration pneumonia is often sterile; the role of antibiotics in the absence of supporting cultures is unclear and controversial.

- Chronic aspiration pneumonia results from recurrent aspiration of small volumes.

LUNG ABSCESS

Lung abscess is a circumscribed collection of pus in the lung that leads to cavity formation; the cavity has an air-fluid level on chest radiography. Lung abscess usually is caused by bacteria, particularly anaerobic bacilli (30%-50% of cases), aerobic gram-positive cocci (25%), and aerobic gram-negative bacilli (5%-12%). Polymicrobial infections are most common. Suppuration leading to lung abscess can result from primary, opportunistic, and hematogenous lung infection. Primary lung abscess is caused by oral infection; aspiration accounts for up to 90% of all abscesses. Alcohol abuse and dental caries also contribute. Lung abscesses caused by opportunistic infections occur in elderly patients with a blood dyscrasia and in patients with cancer of the lung or oropharynx. In patients with advanced HIV infection, lung abscess can develop in association with a broad spectrum of pathogens, including opportunistic organisms. These patients have a poor prognosis. Hematogenous lung abscesses occur with septicemia, septic embolism, and sterile infarcts (3% of patients). A history of any of these conditions in association with fever, cough with purulent or bloody sputum, weight loss, and leukocytosis suggests the diagnosis. Chest radiography may show cavitated lesions. The abscess may rupture into the pleural space and cause empyema. Bronchoscopy may be necessary to obtain samples for culture, to drain the abscess, and to exclude obstructing lesions. High rates of morbidity and mortality (20%) are associated with lung abscess despite antibiotic therapy. The prognosis is worse for patients with a large abscess and for those infected with *S aureus*, *K pneumoniae*, and *P aeruginosa*. Treatment includes drainage (physiotherapy, postural, and bronchoscopic), antibiotics for 4 to 6 weeks, and surgical treatment if medical therapy fails.

- Hematogenous lung abscess occurs in septicemia and septic embolism.

- The cause is often polymicrobial, and prolonged antibiotic therapy is often needed.

MYCOBACTERIAL INFECTIONS

MYCOBACTERIUM TUBERCULOSIS

Mycobacterium tuberculosis causes the most common type of human-to-human chronic infection by mycobacteria worldwide. The most common mode of transmission is by inhalation of droplet nuclei from expectorated respiratory secretions. Of persons exposed to *M tuberculosis*, 30% become infected.

Among infected persons, active primary disease develops in less than 5% and active disease from reactivation develops in less than 5%. Active infection is diagnosed by documenting the presence of *M tuberculosis* in respiratory secretions or other body fluids or tissues. Sputum and gastric washings have an approximately 30% diagnostic yield. Bronchoscopy with bronchoalveolar lavage has an approximately 40% diagnostic yield, which increases to almost 95% if biopsy is performed. Culture of pleural fluid alone provides the diagnosis in less than 20% of cases, but culture of pleural biopsy specimens has a 70% diagnostic yield. Faster culture results are available with the use of broth culture systems (1.5–2 weeks) and nucleic acid amplification (8 hours). Culture-positive pulmonary tuberculosis with normal chest radiographic findings is not uncommon, and the incidence of this presentation is increasing. *Latent tuberculosis infection* is the current term for the condition in a person who does not have active tuberculosis but has a positive purified protein derivative (PPD) skin test. Such a person is infected with mycobacteria but does not have active disease.

- The PPD skin test indicates infection with mycobacteria and not active disease.

- Active infection should be confirmed by the growth of *M tuberculosis* in respiratory secretions or other body fluids or tissues.

- Bronchoscopically obtained specimens have a higher diagnostic yield.

- Chest radiographic findings can be normal in active tuberculosis.

A positive PPD tuberculin skin test is an example of a delayed (T-cell–mediated) hypersensitivity reaction. The test can be positive within 4 weeks after exposure to *M tuberculosis*. The PPD test is negative in 25% of patients with active tuberculosis. A false-negative PPD result can also occur in infections with viruses or bacteria, live virus vaccinations, chronic renal failure, nutritional deficiency, lymphoid malignancies, leukemias, corticosteroid and immunosuppressive drug therapy, newborn or elderly patients, recent or overwhelming infection with mycobacteria, and acute stress. The specificity of a positive PPD reaction is variable and is dependent on the prevalence of infection with nontuberculous mycobacteria. The annual risk of active tuberculosis for those who are PPD-positive depends on the underlying medical condition (annual risk in parentheses): HIV-positive (8%-10%), recent converters (2%-5%), abnormal chest radiograph (2%-4%), intravenous drug abuse (1%), end-stage renal disease (1%), and diabetes mellitus (0.3%). PPD skin testing should use a 5-tuberculin unit preparation; the widest induration is read at 48 and 72 hours. Prior vaccination with bacille Calmette-Guérin is not a contraindication for the PPD skin test. There is no reliable method to distinguish positive PPD results caused by bacille Calmette-Guérin vaccination from those caused by mycobacterial infections, although large reactions (≥20 mm) are not likely caused by bacille Calmette-Guérin.

The role of the serum interferon-γ release assay (QuantiFERON-TB Gold test, T-SPOT.*TB* test) continues to evolve and has the promise of increasing the specificity of testing to identify latent tuberculosis. The assay may help distinguish latent tuberculous infection from nontuberculous mycobacterial infection and bacille Calmette-Guérin vaccination because it measures interferon-γ production from a patient's blood sample incubated with *M tuberculosis*–specific antigens. Current Centers for Disease Control and Prevention guidelines suggest that the assay may be used in all circumstances in which the PPD skin test is used. Compared with the PPD skin test, the assay is probably less subject to reader bias and error, requires only a single health care visit, and is less likely to be positive after bacille Calmette-Guérin vaccine. Like the PPD skin test, the assay may be negative in patients who have active tuberculosis.

- The PPD reaction is a delayed type of hypersensitivity reaction.

- The PPD skin test can become positive within 4 weeks after exposure to *M tuberculosis*.

- The PPD skin test and interferon-γ release assay may be negative in a substantial proportion of patients with active tuberculosis.

- Compared with the PPD skin test, the interferon-γ release assay is probably less subject to reader bias and error, requires only a single health care visit, and is less likely to be positive after bacille Calmette-Guérin vaccine.

Targeted tuberculin testing for latent tuberculosis infection identifies persons at high risk for tuberculosis who would benefit from treatment of the infection. Indications for testing include persons with signs and symptoms suggestive of current tuberculosis infection, recent contacts with known or suspected cases of tuberculosis, abnormal chest radiographic findings compatible with past tuberculosis, patients with diseases that increase the risk of tuberculosis (silicosis, gastrectomy, diabetes mellitus, immune suppression, and HIV infection), and groups at high risk of recent infection with *M tuberculosis* (immigrants and long-time residents and workers in hospitals, nursing homes, or prisons). The following criteria apply to a positive PPD skin test:

1. Reaction 5 mm or more—persons with HIV infection, close contact with infectious cases, patients with organ transplants and other immunosuppressed patients (receiving the equivalent of 15 mg daily of prednisone for ≥1 month), and those with fibrotic lesions on chest radiography consistent with prior tuberculosis

2. Reaction 10 mm or more—immigrants within the past 5 years from high-prevalence countries; injection drug users; mycobacteriology laboratory workers; children younger than 4 years, or infants, children, and adolescents exposed to adults at high risk of tuberculosis; and employees and residents of high-risk congregate facilities including prisons, nursing homes, hospitals and other health care facilities, residential facilities for patients with AIDS, and homeless shelters; and patients with high-risk clinical conditions (eg, diabetes mellitus, silicosis, chronic renal failure, leukemias and lymphomas, carcinoma of the head or neck and lung, weight loss ≥10% of ideal body weight, gastrectomy, and jejunoileal bypass)

3. Reaction 15 mm or more—any person without a defined risk factor for tuberculosis

Pleural tuberculosis used to be more common in younger (<40 years) patients; now, it is more common among the elderly. In the United States, 4% of all tuberculous patients have pleural involvement, and pleural tuberculosis constitutes 23% of the cases with extrapulmonary tuberculosis. Effusions usually occur 3 to 6 months after the primary infection. Acute presentation (cough, fever, and pleuritic chest pain) is more common in younger patients. Bilateral exudative effusions occur in up to 8% of patients, and the PPD skin test is positive in more than 66%. The effusions typically have high protein levels (>5 g/dL), lymphocytosis (>50%), and low levels of glucose (<50 mg/dL). A low pleural fluid pH occurs in 20% of patients. Measurement of levels of the enzyme adenosine deaminase in the pleural fluid has a sensitivity of 70% to 90% for pleural tuberculosis, with a specificity that varies from less than 50% to 90%. The test is not diagnostic for pleural tuberculosis, and its main utility is to suggest tuberculosis infection if the adenosine deaminase level is very high or to rule out the diagnosis of pleural tuberculosis if the level is very low. Pleural biopsy specimens show caseous granulomas in up to 80% of patients, and cultures of biopsy specimens are positive in more than 75%. Cultures of pleural fluid are positive in only 20% to 40% of patients, and the sputum is positive in 40%. Bronchopleural fistula is a complication.

- Pleural tuberculosis is more common among the elderly.

- Effusion occurs 3–6 months after primary infection.

Miliary tuberculosis constitutes 10% of cases of extrapulmonary tuberculosis. It is characterized by the diffuse presence of small (<2 mm) nodules throughout the body. The spleen, liver, and lung are frequently involved. The disease can be acute and fatal or insidious in onset and slowly progressive. Chest radiography shows typical miliary lesions in more than 65% of patients. Sputum findings are negative in up to 80% of patients, and the PPD skin test is negative in approximately 50% of patients with miliary tuberculosis. Mortality is high (30%) even with therapy.

Tuberculous lymphadenitis (ie, scrofula) is the most common form of extrapulmonary tuberculosis. It is more common in children and young adults than in older persons. Cervical lymph nodes are affected most commonly; 1 or more nodes (painless, nontender, and rubbery) may be palpable. Abscess and sinus formation may occur.

Skeletal tuberculosis is becoming less common; when identified, it is more common in the young than in older adults. Any bone can be involved, but the vertebrae are involved in

50% of cases. Pott disease is *tuberculous spondylitis* and may produce severe kyphosis.

Tuberculous meningitis is the most common form of central nervous system involvement and is localized mainly to the base of the brain. It occurs more commonly in intravenous drug users who are HIV-positive and in immunocompromised patients. Tuberculous meningitis is often insidious in onset.

Abdominal tuberculosis frequently affects the peritoneum. *Ileocecal tuberculosis* can lead to ulcerative enteritis, strictures, and fistulas. *Genitourinary tuberculosis* is responsible for up to 13% of extrapulmonary disease. It is usually a late manifestation of the infection and is more common in older patients. The renal cortex is affected initially, and the infection can then spread to the renal pelvis, ureter, bladder, and genitalia. Sterile pyuria is an important feature.

Laryngeal tuberculosis is usually a complication of pulmonary tuberculosis.

Pericardial tuberculosis is usually due to hematogenous spread. Pericardial constriction may begin subacutely and become a chronic problem.

- Miliary tuberculosis is responsible for 10% of cases of extrapulmonary tuberculosis.
- Tuberculous lymphadenitis is the most common form of extrapulmonary tuberculosis.
- Tuberculous meningitis is often insidious in onset.

Tuberculosis is particularly prone to develop in HIV-positive persons. In these patients, a CD4 cell count less than 200/mcL and a PPD-positive status increase the risk. Furthermore, there is an increased rate of reactivation, increased rate of progressive primary infection, increased incidence of multidrug resistance, atypical clinical features, and increased progression of HIV disease. Among those who are HIV-positive and are exposed to *M tuberculosis*, nearly 40% develop primary tuberculosis, and the rate of reactivation is 8% to 10% per year. Tuberculous pleurisy and hilar and mediastinal lymphadenopathy are more common in patients with tuberculosis who have AIDS than in those who do not have AIDS. The diagnosis of tuberculosis in a patient with AIDS can be difficult owing to the varied manifestations. These patients may lack cavitation and granuloma formation and have negative sputum findings and negative PPD skin tests.

Treatment of tuberculosis in HIV-negative and HIV-positive patients is essentially identical with a few notable exceptions. Certain treatment schemes are contraindicated in HIV-infected patients because of a high rate of relapse due to resistant organisms or an increased risk of toxicity. Management of these patients is complex and requires expertise with both HIV and tuberculosis. Rifampin-containing regimens are effective in curing tuberculosis in HIV-positive patients. Initiation of HIV protease inhibitor therapy in patients who are HIV-positive or who have AIDS increases the symptoms and signs of the underlying mycobacterial infection. Rifampin accelerates the metabolism of protease inhibitors (decreased plasma levels) and leads to HIV resistance. Isoniazid prophylaxis for 12 months decreases the incidence of tuberculosis and increases the life expectancy for HIV-infected patients.

- Tuberculosis is particularly prone to develop in HIV-positive persons.
- The simultaneous presence of HIV and tuberculosis leads to increased severity of both infections.
- HIV protease inhibitor therapy may lead to worsening of the signs and symptoms of tuberculosis.

Definitive therapy is indicated for all patients with culture-positive tuberculosis. Treatment usually should include multidrug therapy (>2 drugs at a minimum; the use of 4 drugs is recommended) for all patients who have active tuberculosis (Tables 19.2 through 19.4; Figures 19.1 and 19.2). With rigidly administered 6-month regimens, more than 90% of patients are smear-negative after 2 months of therapy, more than 95% are cured, and less than 5% have relapse. A 9-month regimen provides a cure rate higher than 97% and a relapse rate less than 2%. All treatment programs should be recommended and preferably undertaken by physicians and health care workers experienced in the management of mycobacterial diseases. The most important impediment to lack of adequate therapy worldwide is the lack of adherence to the treatment.

Extrapulmonary tuberculosis can be treated effectively with either a 6- or 9-month regimen. However, miliary tuberculosis, bone and joint tuberculosis, and tuberculous meningitis in infants and children may require treatment for 12 or more months. Cavitary tuberculosis is often treated for 9 months. Systemic corticosteroid therapy may be useful in the prevention of pleural fibrosis, pericardial constriction, neurologic complications from tuberculous meningitis, tuberculous bronchial stenosis, and adrenal insufficiency caused by tuberculosis. Extrapulmonary tuberculosis confined to lymph nodes has no effect on obstetrical outcomes, but tuberculosis at other sites adversely affects the outcome of pregnancy.

- Miliary, skeletal, and meningeal tuberculosis may require >12 months of therapy.
- Corticosteroids are helpful for treating extrapulmonary tuberculosis.

Drug-resistant tuberculosis is an increasingly recognized problem. Drug resistance can develop against a single first-line drug. *Multidrug-resistant tuberculosis* (MDR-TB) refers to resistance that develops to at least both isoniazid and rifampin. *Extensively drug-resistant tuberculosis* (XDR-TB) is defined as resistance to at least both isoniazid and rifampin and resistance to fluoroquinolones or aminoglycosides. MDR-TB and XDR-TB are more likely in the following situations: nonadherence to treatment guidelines and treatment errors by physicians and health care workers, lack of adherence by patients, homelessness, drug addiction, and exposure to MDR-TB in high-prevalence countries with inadequate tuberculosis control programs. Multidrug resistance occurs rapidly in HIV-infected persons. The American Thoracic Society and the Centers for

Table 19.2 DRUG REGIMENS FOR CULTURE-POSITIVE PULMONARY TUBERCULOSIS CAUSED BY DRUG-SUSCEPTIBLE ORGANISMS

	INITIAL PHASE			CONTINUATION PHASE			RANGE OF TOTAL DOSES (MINIMAL DURATION)	RATING[a] (EVIDENCE)[b]	
								HIV Negative	HIV Positive
Regimen	Drugs	Interval & Doses[c] (Minimal Duration)	Regimen	Drugs	Interval & Doses[c,d] (Minimal Duration)				
1	INH RIF PZA EMB	7 d/wk for 56 doses (8 wk) *or* 5 d/wk for 40 doses (8 wk)[e]	1a	INH/RIF	7 d/wk for 126 doses (18 wk) *or* 5 d/wk for 90 doses (18 wk)[e]		182–130 (26 wk)	A (I)	A (II)
			1b	INH/RIF	Twice weekly for 36 doses (18 wk)		92–76 (26 wk)	A (I)	A (II)[f]
			1c[g]	INH/RPT	Once weekly for 18 doses (18 wk)		74–58 (26 wk)	B (I)	E (I)
2	INH RIF PZA EMB	7 d/wk for 14 doses (2 wk), *then* twice weekly for 12 doses (6 wk) *or* 5 d/wk for 10 doses (2 wk)[e], *then* twice weekly for 12 doses (6 wk)	2a	INH/RIF	Twice weekly for 36 doses (18 wk)		62–58 (26 wk)	A (II)	B (II)[f]
			2b[g]	INH/RPT	Once weekly for 18 doses (18 wk)		44–40 (26 wk)	B (I)	E (I)
3	INH RIF PZA EMB	3 times weekly for 24 doses (8 wk)	3a	INH/RIF	3 times weekly for 54 doses (18 wk)		78 (26 wk)	B (I)	B (II)
4	INH RIF EMB	7 d/wk for 56 doses (8 wk) *or* 5 d/wk for 40 doses (8 wk)[e]	4a	INH/RIF	7 d/wk for 217 doses (31 wk) *or* 5 d/wk for 155 doses (31 wk)[e]		273–195 (39 wk)	C (I)	C (II)
			4b	INH/RIF	Twice weekly for 62 doses (31 wk)		118–102 (39 wk)	C (I)	C (II)

Abbreviations: EMB, ethambutol; INH, isoniazid; PZA, pyrazinamide; RIF, rifampin; RPT, rifapentine.

[a] Definitions of ratings: A, preferred; B, acceptable alternative; C, offer when A and B cannot be given; E, should never be given.

[b] Definitions of evidence: I, randomized clinical trial; II, data from clinical trials that were not randomized or were conducted in other populations; III, expert opinion.

[c] When directly observed therapy is used, drugs may be given 5 days weekly & the necessary number of doses adjusted accordingly. Although there are no studies that compare 5 with 7 daily doses, extensive experience indicates this would be an effective practice.

[d] Patients with cavitation on initial chest radiograph & positive cultures at completion of 2 months of therapy should receive therapy for a 7-month (31 weeks; either 217 doses [daily] or 62 doses [twice weekly]) continuation phase.

[e] Drugs given for 5 days weekly are always given by directly observed therapy. Rating for these regimens is A (III).

[f] Not recommended for human immunodeficiency virus (HIV)-infected patients with CD4+ cell counts <100/mcL.

[g] Options 1c and 2b should be used only in HIV-negative patients who have negative sputum smears at the time of completion of 2 months of therapy & who do not have cavitation on the initial chest radiograph. For patients receiving this regimen & found to have a positive culture from the 2–month specimen, treatment should be extended an extra 3 months.

Adapted from Blumberg HM, Burman WJ, Chaisson RE, Daley CL, Etkind SC, Friedman LN, et al. American Thoracic Society/Centers for Disease Control and Prevention/Infectious Diseases Society of America: treatment of tuberculosis. Am J Respir Crit Care Med. 2003 Feb 15;167(4):603–62. Used with permission.

Disease Control and Prevention recommend an intensive phase of therapy with 4 drugs if the local rate of resistance to isoniazid is more than 4%. Even though the mortality from MDR-TB is high in HIV-positive and HIV-negative patients, appropriate treatment produces a favorable outcome (>80%). MDR-TB is often treated for 18 to 24 months.

• Drug-resistant tuberculosis may require multidrug (≥4 drugs) therapy.

To prevent drug resistance and to effectively decrease the number of cases of tuberculosis, many health care organizations recommend administration of antituberculous drugs by directly observed therapy (DOT) in which a health care provider monitors each patient as every dose of a 6-month regimen is taken. This approach makes a cure almost certain with drug-sensitive tuberculosis. The DOT regimen is particularly important for the homeless, chronic alcoholics, intravenous drug abusers, AIDS patients, and prison inmates. A fixed-dose combination should be considered in cases of newly diagnosed disease. Even though fixed-dose combinations of antituberculous drugs (isoniazid and rifampin; rifampin, isoniazid, and pyrazinamide) are available and have been strongly recommended by the World Health Organization, Centers for Disease Control and Prevention, American Thoracic Society, and the International Union Against Tuberculosis and Lung Disease, less than 25% of rifampin-containing therapies use the fixed-dose regimen. Treatment completion rates for

Table 19.3 **FIRST-LINE DRUGS FOR TUBERCULOSIS**[a,b]

DRUG	DOSE, MG/KG						ADVERSE REACTIONS	MONITORING
	Daily		2 Times Weekly[c]		3 Times Weekly[c]			
	Children[d]	Adults	Children[d]	Adults	Children[d]	Adults		
INH[e] (maximal dose, mg)	10–20 (300)	5 (300)	20–40 (900)	15 (900)	20–40 (900)	15 (900)	Liver enzyme elevation, hepatitis, peripheral neuropathy, mild effects on central nervous system, drug interactions	Baseline measurements of liver enzymes for adults / Repeat measurements if baseline results are abnormal, if patient is at high risk of adverse reactions, or if patient has symptoms of adverse reactions
RIF[f] (maximal dose, mg)	10–20 (600)	10 (600)	10–20 (600)	10 (600)	10–20 (600)	10 (600)	GI upset, drug interactions, hepatitis, bleeding problems, flulike symptoms, rash	Baseline measurements for adults: complete blood cell count, platelets, liver enzymes / Repeat measurements if baseline results are abnormal or if patient has symptoms of adverse reactions
PZA[g] (maximal dose, g)	15–30 (2)	15–30 (2)	50–70 (4)	50–70 (4)	50–70 (3)	50–70 (3)	Hepatitis, rash, GI upset, joint aches, hyperuricemia, gout (rare)	Baseline measurements for adults: uric acid, liver enzymes / Repeat measurements if baseline results are abnormal or if patient has symptoms of adverse reactions
EMB[h]	15–25	15–25	50	50	25–30	25–30	Optic neuritis	Baseline & monthly tests: visual acuity, color vision
SM[i] (maximal dose, g)	20–40 (1)	15 (1)	25–30 (1.5)	25–30 (1.5)	25–30 (1.5)	25–30 (1.5)	Ototoxicity (hearing loss or vestibular dysfunction), renal toxicity	Baseline & repeat as needed: hearing, kidney function

Abbreviations: EMB, ethambutol; GI, gastrointestinal tract; INH, isoniazid; PZA, pyrazinamide; RIF, rifampin; SM, streptomycin.

[a] Adjust weight-based dosages as weight changes.

[b] INH, RIF, PZA, & EMB are administered orally; SM is administered intramuscularly.

[c] Directly observed therapy should be used with all regimens administered 2 or 3 times weekly.

[d] Younger than 12 years.

[e] Hepatitis risk increases with age & alcohol consumption. Pyridoxine can prevent peripheral neuropathy.

[f] Severe interactions with methadone, oral contraceptives, & many other drugs. Drug colors body fluids orange & may permanently discolor soft contact lenses.

[g] Treat hyperuricemia only if patient has symptoms.

[h] Not recommended for children too young to be monitored for changes in vision unless tuberculosis is drug resistant.

[i] Avoid or decrease dose in adults older than 60 years.

Adapted from Centers for Disease Control and Prevention, Division of Tuberculosis. Elimination: core curriculum on tuberculosis. 3rd ed. c1994.

Table 19.4 TARGETED TUBERCULIN TESTING FOR LATENT TUBERCULOSIS INFECTION

PROPHYLACTIC GROUP DESCRIPTION	PPD SKIN TEST REACTION, MM
Persons with known or suspected HIV infection	≥5
Close contacts of person with infectious TB	≥5
Persons with chest radiographic findings suggestive of previous TB & inadequate or no treatment[a]	≥5
Persons who inject drugs & are known to be HIV-negative	≥10
Persons with certain medical conditions or factors Diabetes mellitus, silicosis, prolonged corticosteroid or other immunosuppressive therapy, cancer of the head & neck, hematologic & reticuloendothelial diseases (eg, leukemia & Hodgkin disease), end-stage renal disease, intestinal bypass or gastrectomy, chronic malabsorption syndromes, low body weight (≥10% below ideal)	≥10
Persons in whom PPD converted from negative to positive within the past 2 y	[b]

Age <35 y in the following high-prevalence groups:
  Persons born in areas of the world where TB is common (eg, Asia, Africa, Caribbean, & Latin America)
  Medically underserved, low-income populations including high-risk racial & ethnic groups (eg, Asians & Pacific Islanders, African Americans, Hispanics, & American Indians)
  Residents of long-term care facilities (eg, correctional facilities & nursing homes)
  Children <4 y
  Other groups identified locally as having an increased prevalence of TB (eg, migrant farm workers or homeless persons)
	≥10

Persons younger than 35 y with no known risk factors for TB	≥15
Occupational exposure to TB (eg, health care workers & staff of nursing homes, drug treatment centers, or correctional facilities)	[c]

Close contacts with an initial PPD skin test reaction <5 mm & normal findings on chest radiography
  Circumstances suggest a high probability of infection
  Evaluation of other contacts with a similar degree of exposure demonstrates a high prevalence of infection
  Child or adolescent
  Immunosuppressed (eg, HIV infection)
	<5

Abbreviations: HIV, human immunodeficiency virus; PPD, purified protein derivative of tubercle bacillus; TB, tuberculosis.

[a] Isolated calcified granulomas are excluded.

[b] Increase of ≥10 mm if person is younger than 35 years or is a health care worker; increase of ≥15 mm if person is 35 years or older.

[c] Appropriate cutoff for defining a positive reaction depends on the employee's individual risk factors for TB & on the prevelence of TB in the facility.

Adapted from Van Scoy RE, Wilkowske CJ. Antimicrobial therapy. Mayo Clin Proc. 1999 Oct;74(10):1038–48. Used with permission of Mayo Foundation for Medical Education and Research.

pulmonary tuberculosis are most likely to exceed 90% with DOT. However, DOT may not increase the cure rate in areas where the rate of cure is high (without DOT).

- DOT for 6 months is effective for preventing relapses and emergence of drug-resistant tuberculosis.
- DOT is also useful for the treatment of drug-resistant tuberculosis and tuberculosis in immunocompromised patients.
- A fixed-dose combination should be considered in cases of newly diagnosed disease.

Treatment of latent tuberculosis infection is indicated for persons with a positive PPD skin test who do not have active infection (Table 19.4). If an isoniazid-sensitive organism probably caused latent tuberculosis infection, the treatment options include isoniazid 300 mg daily or 900 mg biweekly.

Pyridoxine is usually added to prevent peripheral neuropathy, which is particularly common in patients with diabetes mellitus, alcohol abuse, or kidney disease. Rifampin (600 mg daily) is an alternative option. Previous combination therapy with rifampin and pyrazinamide is no longer routinely recommended because of the increased frequency of fatal hepatitis. Therapy with this combination should be supervised by a specialist. The recommended duration for therapy of latent tuberculosis infection is outlined below:

1. Isoniazid for HIV-positive adults and children: 12 months
2. Isoniazid for HIV-negative adults and children: 9 months
3. Rifampin, as an alternative to isoniazid: 4 months
4. Silicosis or old fibrotic lesion on chest radiography without active tuberculosis: 4-month therapy with isoniazid and rifampin, although 12 months of isoniazid alone is an acceptable alternative

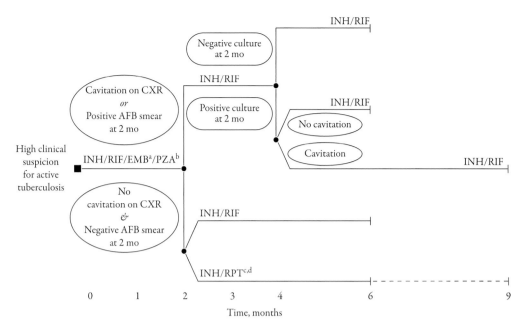

Figure 19.1 Treatment Algorithm for Tuberculosis. Patients in whom tuberculosis is proved or strongly suspected should have treatment initiated with isoniazid (INH), rifampin (RIF), pyrazinamide (PZA), and ethambutol (EMB) for the initial 2 months. Another acid-fast bacilli (AFB) smear and culture should be performed after 2 months of treatment. If cavities were seen on the initial chest radiograph (CXR) or the AFB smear is positive at completion of 2 months of treatment, the continuation phase of treatment should consist of INH and RIF daily or twice weekly for 4 months (total of 6 months of treatment). If cavitation was present on the initial CXR and if the culture at the completion of 2 months of therapy is positive, the continuation phase should be lengthened to 7 months (total of 9 months of treatment). If the patient has human immunodeficiency virus (HIV) infection and the CD4+ cell count is <100/mcL, the continuation phase should consist of daily or 3-times-weekly doses of INH and RIF. In patients without HIV infection who have no cavitation on CXR and negative AFB smears at completion of 2 months of treatment, the continuation phase may consist of either once-weekly doses of INH and rifapentine (RPT), or daily or twice-weekly doses of INH and RIF (total of 6 months) (bottom of figure). Patients receiving INH and RPT and whose 2-month cultures are positive should have treatment extended by an additional 3 months (total of 9 months). [a] Use of EMB may be discontinued when results of drug susceptibility testing indicate no drug resistance. [b] Use of PZA may be discontinued after it has been taken for 2 months (56 doses). [c] RPT should not be used in HIV-infected patients with tuberculosis or in patients with extrapulmonary tuberculosis. [d] Therapy should be extended to 9 months if the 2-month culture is positive. (Adapted from Blumberg HM, Burman WJ, Chiasson RE, Daley CL, Etkind SC, Friedman LN, et al. American Thoracic Society/Centers for Disease Control and Prevention/Infectious Diseases Society of America: treatment of tuberculosis. Am J Respir Crit Care Med. 2003 Feb 15;167[4]:603–62. Used with permission.)

In the United States, bacille Calmette-Guérin vaccine is recommended only for PPD-negative adults who are health care workers and live where the likelihood of transmission and subsequent infection with *M tuberculosis* strains resistant to isoniazid and rifampin is high, provided that comprehensive tuberculosis infection-control precautions have been implemented in the workplace and have not been successful. Bacille Calmette-Guérin vaccine is not recommended for HIV-positive children and adults.

NONTUBERCULOUS MYCOBACTERIA

Mycobacteria other than *M tuberculosis* and *Mycobacterium leprae* are commonly classified as *nontuberculous mycobacteria* (NTM) even though tubercle formation occurs. Most NTM have been isolated from natural water and soil. Human-to-human spread has not been documented. Natural waters are the source for most human infections caused by *Mycobacterium avium* complex; some cases are probably acquired from hospital tap water. Colonization or a saprophytic state of NTM is uncommon. NTM disease is not reportable in the United States.

- Human-to-human spread of NTM has not been documented.

- NTM disease is not reportable in the United States.

Chronic pulmonary disease is caused most frequently by *M avium* complex and *Mycobacterium kansasii*. Pulmonary disease is more common in older adults, those with underlying chronic obstructive pulmonary disease, smokers, alcohol abusers, and some children with cystic fibrosis. Pulmonary infection from *M avium* complex also develops in white women in their 60s who are HIV-negative and who do not have preexisting lung disease. Most of these patients (>90%) have bronchiectasis or small nodules without predilection for any lobe. High-resolution computed tomography may show associated multifocal bronchiectasis with small (<5 mm) nodular infiltrates. Bilateral nodular or interstitial lung disease (or both) or isolated disease in the right middle lobe or lingular disease is more predominant in elderly nonsmoking women. Hypersensitivity pneumonitis caused by exposure to *M avium* complex growing in a hot tub has been reported. *Mycobacterium avium* complex is responsible for 5% of the cases of mycobacterial lymphadenitis in adults and more than 90% of the cases in children. Lymphadenopathy is usually unilateral and nontender. Disseminated disease caused by NTM manifests as a fever of unknown origin in immunocompromised patients without AIDS.

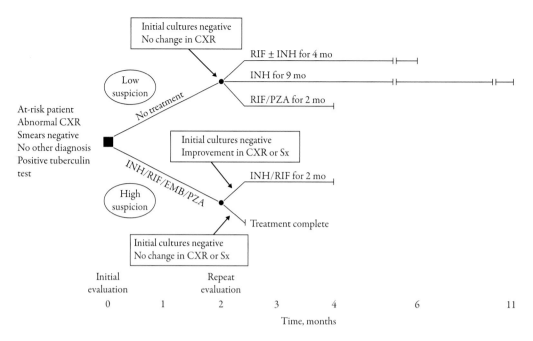

Figure 19.2 Treatment Algorithm for Active, Culture-Negative Pulmonary Tuberculosis (TB) and Inactive TB. The decision to begin treatment of a patient with sputum smears that are negative depends on the degree of suspicion that the patient has TB. If the clinical suspicion is high (bottom of figure), multidrug therapy should be initiated before acid-fast smear and culture results are known. If the diagnosis is confirmed by a positive culture, treatment can be continued to complete a standard course of therapy (see Figure 19.1). If initial cultures remain negative and treatment has consisted of multiple drugs for 2 months, there are 2 options depending on reevaluation at 2 months (bottom of figure): 1) If the patient demonstrates symptomatic or radiographic improvement without another apparent diagnosis, a diagnosis of culture-negative TB can be inferred. Treatment should be continued with isoniazid (INH) and rifampin (RIF) alone for an additional 2 months. 2) If the patient demonstrates neither symptomatic nor radiographic improvement, prior TB is unlikely and treatment is complete after treatment including at least 2 months of RIF and pyrazinamide (PZA) has been administered. In low-suspicion patients not initially receiving treatment (top of figure), if cultures remain negative, the patient has no symptoms, and the chest radiograph is unchanged at 2–3 months, the 3 treatment options are as follows: 1) INH for 9 months, 2) RIF with or without INH for 4 months, or 3) RIF and PZA for 2 months. The RIF/PZA 2-month regimen should be used only for patients who are not likely to complete a longer course of treatment and can be monitored closely. CXR indicates chest radiograph; EMB, ethambutol; Sx, signs and symptoms. (Adapted from Blumberg HM, Burman WJ, Chaisson RE, Daley CL, Etkind SC, Friedman LN, et al. American Thoracic Society/Centers for Disease Control and Prevention/Infectious Diseases Society of America: treatment of tuberculosis. Am J Respir Crit Care Med. 2003 Feb 15;167[4]:603–62. Used with permission.)

- *Mycobacterium avium* complex infection occurs in bronchiectasis.

HIV-infected persons are at high risk of NTM infections. More than 95% of NTM disease in HIV-infected persons is caused by *M avium* complex. In those with AIDS, disseminated infection occurs in up to 40% and localized infection in 5%; dissemination is more likely in those with a CD4 cell count less than 50/mcL. The risk of disseminated infection is 20% per year when the CD4 cell count is less than 100/mcL. High fever and sweats are common, as are anemia and increased alkaline phosphatase levels. Dissemination is usually documented with positive blood cultures (sensitivity, 90%).

- Disseminated *M avium* complex in AIDS is more likely when the CD4 count is <50/mcL.

- A single blood culture in disseminated *M avium* complex infection has a sensitivity of 90%.

Mycobacterium kansasii is the second most common cause of NTM pulmonary disease in the United States. It primarily affects adult white men. Approximately 90% of patients with *M kansasii* disease have cavitary infiltrates. *Mycobacterium*

kansasii infection can be clinically indistinguishable from tuberculosis; however, symptoms may be less severe and more chronic than with tuberculosis. In HIV-negative patients, common symptoms are cough (90%), purulent sputum (85%), weight loss (55%), and dyspnea (50%). In immunocompromised patients, including those with AIDS, the lung is most commonly involved and symptoms include fever, chills, night sweats, cough, weight loss, dyspnea, and chest pain. Disseminated *M kansasii* infection occurs in 20% of HIV-positive patients who have *M kansasii* pulmonary disease.

- Cavitation occurs in 90% of patients with *M kansasii* infection.

Specific skin tests are not available for the diagnosis of NTM. Routine cultures of sputum, blood, or stool are not recommended for asymptomatic patients. All specimens positive for acid-fast bacilli must be considered to indicate *M tuberculosis* until final culture results are available. Bronchoscopy or open lung biopsy is required for diagnosis in nearly half the cases. Therapy fails in half the patients. More than 80% of patients remain symptomatic, and 60% do not tolerate the initial multidrug regimen. Treatment of infections caused by NTM should be undertaken by a physician who specializes in infections caused by mycobacteria. The macrolides azithromycin and clarithromycin are important in the treatment of infections with *M avium* complex. Isoniazid is not used to treat infection with *M avium* complex. The current recommendation for treatment of pulmonary disease caused by *M kansasii* in adults is to use isoniazid, rifampin, and ethambutol. In patients who cannot tolerate 1 of these 3 drugs, clarithromycin can be substituted. Pyrazinamide is avoided because all isolates are resistant.

- Isoniazid is not used to treat infection with *M avium* complex.

- Macrolides are important in the therapy for infections with *M avium* complex, and isoniazid, rifampin, and ethambutol are clinically useful for *M kansasii*.

TOXICITY OF ANTITUBERCULOUS DRUGS

Isoniazid, rifampin, ethambutol, and pyrazinamide are considered first-line antituberculous medications. These 4 medications are the foundation of numerous treatment regimens for tuberculosis. Each has its own potential toxicity, and each can potentiate toxicity when used in combination. Hepatitis (aspartate aminotransferase usually >5 times the upper limit of the reference range) is the most common important adverse effect from antituberculous medications and is distinct from the mild increases in transaminases that occur in up to 20% of patients receiving these medications (aspartate aminotransferase usually >3 times the upper limit of the reference range). In adults receiving these medications, it is important to assess baseline liver function, creatinine level, complete blood cell count, and uric acid (if pyrazinamide is used) and to perform an ophthalmic examination (if ethambutol is used) before antituberculous therapy is begun. All patients should be evaluated periodically for adverse reactions to the drugs (Table 19.3).

Isoniazid

Clinically significant hepatitis occurs in less than 1% of patients receiving isoniazid, and the incidence increases with age. Middle-aged and black females are at higher risk. Hepatitis is more likely in patients who are "rapid acetylators," and peripheral neuropathy is more likely in those who are "slow acetylators." Isoniazid also causes rash, purpura, drug-induced systemic lupus erythematosus, seizures, optic neuritis, and arthritis. The addition of pyridoxine is recommended for patients with neuropathy (eg, patients with diabetes mellitus, uremia, alcoholism, or malnutrition), pregnancy, or seizure disorder. Before initiation of treatment of latent tuberculosis infection, baseline laboratory testing is indicated in patients with known liver disease or HIV infection, in pregnant women, in women in the immediate postpartum period (within 3 months after delivery), and in persons who drink alcohol regularly. Routine monitoring of liver function during treatment is recommended for patients with abnormal baseline liver function tests or those at risk of liver disease. Therapy should be stopped if the aspartate aminotransferase value is more than 5 times the upper limit of the reference range or 3 times more than the baseline value. Alcohol consumption should be avoided.

- The incidence of isoniazid-induced hepatitis increases with age.

- Isoniazid causes hepatitis and peripheral neuropathy.

- Stop therapy if aspartate aminotransferase is >5 times the upper limit of the reference range or 3 times more than the baseline value.

Rifampin

The overall incidence of serious adverse effects with rifampin is 1%. Gastrointestinal tract upset is the most common reaction. Larger or intermittent doses (>10 mg/kg) (or both) are associated with thrombocytopenia, flulike syndrome, hemolytic anemia, and cholestatic jaundice. Rash can occur, and use of the drug needs to be stopped for persistent rash. Hepatitis can also occur. Harmless orange discoloration of body secretions occurs. Rifampin induces liver microsomal enzymes, and it increases the metabolism of contraceptive pills, corticosteroids, warfarin, oral hypoglycemic agents, theophylline, anticonvulsant agents, ketoconazole, cyclosporine, methadone, and antiarrhythmic drugs (digitalis, quinidine, verapamil, and mexiletine); therefore, dosages of these drugs may have to be increased.

- Gastrointestinal tract upset is the most common adverse effect of rifampin.

- Rifampin induces liver microsomal enzymes.

Pyrazinamide

The most serious adverse reaction of pyrazinamide is liver damage. Hyperuricemia is common but gout is not, although arthralgias are reported occasionally. Rash and gastrointestinal tract upset are sometimes encountered.

- Liver damage is the most serious adverse reaction to pyrazinamide.

Ethambutol

Ethambutol in doses greater than 25 mg/kg causes retrobulbar neuritis in less than 3% of patients. Symptoms usually are observed 2 months after therapy has been initiated. Because ophthalmoscopic findings are normal in these patients, symptoms are important (blurred vision, central scotoma, and red-green color blindness). These symptoms precede changes in visual acuity. Optic neuritis is best prevented by giving a lower dose (15 mg/kg) during the maintenance phase of treatment. Renal failure prolongs the half-life of the drug and increases the frequency of ocular toxicity.

- Retrobulbar neuritis is a serious adverse effect of ethambutol.

- Renal failure prolongs the half-life of the drug and increases the frequency of ocular toxicity.

Streptomycin

Because streptomycin is excreted by the kidneys, the dosage should be decreased in renal insufficiency. The most common adverse effect is vestibular toxicity, which causes vertigo. Hearing loss may also occur. These effects are more likely in the elderly (>60 years). Ototoxicity and nephrotoxicity are related to both the cumulative dose and the peak serum concentration. Streptomycin should be avoided in pregnancy.

- Streptomycin-associated nephrotoxicity and vestibular toxicity are more common in persons >60 years.

- Streptomycin should be avoided in pregnancy.

PNEUMOCYSTIS JIROVECI INFECTION

Pneumocystis jiroveci (formerly *Pneumocystis carinii*) is a fungus with trophic and cyst forms. *Pneumocystis jiroveci* infections occur in immunosuppressed patients, especially those with AIDS (CD4 cell count ≤200/mcL) or malignancy, and after organ transplant. Infection causes alveolar and interstitial inflammation and edema with plasma cell infiltrates. Clinical features in patients with AIDS include the gradual onset of dyspnea, fever, tachypnea, and hypoxia. In patients without AIDS, the onset is more abrupt and progression to respiratory failure occurs quickly. Patients typically have relatively normal findings on lung examination and a patchy or diffuse interstitial or alveolar process on chest radiography. An upper lobe process is seen on the chest radiographs of patients receiving pentamidine aerosolized prophylaxis. The typical computed tomographic finding is ground-glass attenuation. However, this classic radiographic presentation is less frequent now and is being replaced by cystic lung disease, spontaneous pneumothorax, and an upper lobe distribution of parenchymal opacities. Routine laboratory data are unhelpful. The diagnosis can be made with induced sputum, bronchoalveolar lavage, or lung biopsy. Induced sputum or bronchoalveolar lavage is an excellent method for diagnosis, and the cyst stains best with methenamine silver nitrate. The number of organisms present in immunocompromised patients without AIDS is smaller and overall mortality is greater.

- An upper lobe process is seen on chest radiographs of patients receiving pentamidine aerosolized prophylaxis.

- A typical clinical scenario of *P jiroveci* infection is a patient with AIDS who has a CD4 cell count <200/mcL

and gradual onset of dyspnea, fever, tachypnea, hypoxia, cyanosis, cough; relatively normal findings on lung examination; and a patchy or diffuse interstitial or alveolar process on chest radiography.

PARASITIC DISEASES

Parasitic infections of the lung are less common in the United States than in other parts of the world. Travelers to regions where parasitic infestations are endemic may become infected and, when they return to the United States, present with difficult diagnostic problems. However, dirofilariasis is indigenous to the eastern and southeastern United States. Other parasitic infections, including helminthic infestations, also occur in the United States. The parasites most likely to cause pulmonary infections include *Paragonimus westermani* (paragonimiasis), *Echinococcus granulosus* (echinococcosis or hydatid disease), *Dirofilaria immitis* (dirofilariasis), *Schistosoma japonicum* and *Schistosoma mansoni* (schistosomiasis), and *Entamoeba histolytica* (amebiasis). Protozoal infections are more likely in patients whose cellular immunity is suppressed.

Dirofilariasis, caused by the heartworm that infects dogs, is transmitted to humans by mosquitoes. The disease is endemic to the Mississippi River Valley, the southeastern United States, and the Gulf Coast. Characteristically, the infection manifests as a well-defined solitary lung nodule or multiple lung nodules 1.5 to 2.5 cm in diameter. Eosinophilia occurs in less than 15% of patients. Serologic tests may aid in the diagnosis.

Echinococcosis has occurred in Alaska and the southwestern United States. When persons have lung disease, chest radiography shows well-defined round or oval cystic or solid lesions up to 15 cm in diameter. Rupture of the cysts can cause anaphylactic shock, hypersensitivity reactions, and seeding of adjacent anatomical areas. Liver involvement (in 40% with lung disease) and positive serologic findings are common.

Paragonimiasis is more likely in immigrants from Southeast Asia, but sporadic cases occur in the United States. It is transmitted typically through consumption of raw or undercooked crabs or crayfish. Respiratory features resemble those of chronic bronchitis, bronchiectasis, or tuberculosis. Profuse brown-colored sputum and hemoptysis can be seen. Pleural effusion is relatively common, and peripheral eosinophilia is common. Ova can be found in pleural fluid, bronchial wash, or sputum.

Schistosomiasis is not acquired in the United States. The infection leads to gradual development of secondary pulmonary hypertension caused by occlusion of the pulmonary arterial tree by the parasite. Cor pulmonale develops in 5% of patients.

Amebiasis may manifest as lobar pneumonia or lung abscess (pleuropulmonary complications are almost always right-sided). Rupture into the bronchial tree (hepatobronchial fistula) may be followed by expectoration of sputum that resembles anchovy paste or chocolate. Rupture of the liver abscess into the pleural space causes empyema along with respiratory distress in many patients. Pericardial involvement can also occur.

Strongyloidiasis involving the lungs may mimic asthma with eosinophilia. Risk factors include corticosteroid use, age older than 65 years, chronic lung disease, and chronic debilitating illness. Pulmonary signs and symptoms include cough, shortness of breath, wheezing, and hemoptysis in more than 90% of patients and pulmonary infiltrates in 90%. In a series of 20 patients with pulmonary strongyloidiasis, acute respiratory distress syndrome developed in 9 patients (45%). Preexisting chronic lung disease and the development of acute respiratory distress syndrome are important predictors of a poor prognosis.

- Typical clinical scenario of dirofilariasis is a patient from the Mississippi River Valley, southeastern United States, or Gulf Coast with a solitary lung nodule or multiple nodules. Dirofilariasis is transmitted by mosquitoes.

- Schistosomiasis can cause pulmonary hypertension.

- Amebiasis may result in pleuropulmonary complications that are almost always right-sided; rupture into the bronchial tree may occur, with sputum that resembles anchovy paste or chocolate.

- Strongyloidosis involving the lungs may mimic asthma with eosinophilia.

NONINFECTIOUS PULMONARY COMPLICATIONS IN AIDS

Infectious pulmonary complications in AIDS are discussed in Chapter 20 ("Pharyngitis, Sexually Transmitted Infections, Urinary Tract Infections, and Gastrointestinal Infections"). The noninfectious pulmonary complications in AIDS are discussed below (also see Chapter 21, "HIV Infection").

Nonspecific interstitial pneumonitis represents 30% to 40% of all episodes of lung infiltrates in patients with AIDS. Its incidence has decreased with the institution of highly active antiretroviral therapy. More than 25% of patients with this problem have concurrent Kaposi sarcoma, previous experimental treatments, or a history of *P jiroveci* pneumonia or drug abuse. The clinical features are similar to those of patients with *P jiroveci* pneumonia. Histologic examination of the lung may show various degrees of edema, fibrin deposition, and interstitial inflammation with lymphocytes and plasma cells. This condition is self-limited and often needs no therapy.

- Nonspecific interstitial pneumonitis occurs in up to 40% of patients with AIDS; *P jiroveci* pneumonia should be excluded.

Lymphocytic interstitial pneumonitis is caused by pulmonary infiltration with mature polyclonal B lymphocytes and plasma cells. It occurs most commonly in children and is diagnostic of AIDS when it occurs in a child younger than 13 years who is seropositive for HIV. Corticosteroid therapy may produce marked improvement. Pulmonary lymphoid hyperplasia has been reported in 40% of children with AIDS.

- Lymphocytic interstitial pneumonitis is diagnostic of AIDS when it occurs in a child <13 years who is seropositive for HIV.

Cystic lung disease is more common in patients with *P jiroveci* infections and in those receiving aerosolized pentamidine therapy. Cystic lesions are more common in the upper and mid lung zones. Chest computed tomography identifies these small or medium-size cystic lesions.

- Cystic lung disease is more common in patients with *P jiroveci* pneumonia and in those receiving aerosolized pentamidine therapy.

Bilateral synchronous pneumothorax occurs with increasing frequency in patients with *P jiroveci* pneumonia and in those receiving aerosolized pentamidine therapy. Other causes of pneumothorax include Kaposi sarcoma, tuberculosis, and other infections. Pneumothorax in patients with AIDS has a poor prognosis.

Pleural effusion is found in 25% of hospitalized patients with AIDS. Nearly one-third of the pleural effusions are due to noninfectious causes. Hypoalbuminemia is the leading cause of these effusions. Other important noninfectious causes include Kaposi sarcoma and atelectasis. Among the infectious causes, bacterial pneumonias, *P jiroveci* pneumonia, and *M tuberculosis* are important. Fungal infections can also produce pleural effusion. Large effusions are caused by tuberculosis and Kaposi sarcoma.

- Pleural effusion is caused by infections in two-thirds of hospitalized patients with AIDS.

- Kaposi sarcoma and tuberculosis cause large effusions.

Pulmonary hypertension has been found in patients with AIDS. It is more common in those with HLA-DR6 alleles. The mechanism is not clear, but HIV is thought to affect the endothelium directly and to cause vascular changes. The clinical, physiologic, and pathologic features are identical to those of primary pulmonary hypertension.

- Pulmonary hypertension is clinically identical to idiopathic pulmonary hypertension.

Kaposi sarcoma occurs with greater frequency among homosexuals with AIDS than among other patients with AIDS. It is believed to be caused by human herpesvirus 8. The incidence of its occurrence has diminished. Cutaneous lesions usually precede pulmonary Kaposi sarcoma. Previous or concurrent pulmonary opportunistic infections have been noted in more than 70% of patients with Kaposi sarcoma. Kaposi sarcoma occurs in the lungs of up to 35% of patients who have this tumor. The lung may be the only site in about 15% of patients. In most patients, the diagnosis of pulmonary Kaposi sarcoma is established only at autopsy. The diagnostic yield from bronchoscopy is 24% and from lung biopsy, 56%. Hemoptysis is an uncommon complication of Kaposi sarcoma, although endobronchial metastasis develops in 30% of patients. Multiple, discrete, raised, violaceous, or bright-red tracheobronchial lesions can be seen on bronchoscopy. Bronchoscopic biopsy is associated with a high incidence of considerable bleeding. Chest radiography may show typical nodular infiltrates in less than 10% of patients. Pleural effusion is present in more than two-thirds of patients with lung involvement with Kaposi sarcoma. Clinically, pulmonary Kaposi sarcoma is indistinguishable from *P jiroveci* pneumonia or opportunistic pneumonia.

- Pulmonary Kaposi sarcoma is usually preceded by cutaneous lesions.

- Lung involvement due to Kaposi sarcoma occurs in up to 35% of patients with this neoplasm.

- Clinically, pulmonary Kaposi sarcoma is indistinguishable from *P jiroveci* pneumonia or opportunistic pneumonia.

- Multiple, discrete, raised, violaceous, or bright-red tracheobronchial lesions can be seen on bronchoscopy.

Non-Hodgkin lymphoma involving the lungs occurs in less than 10% of patients with AIDS who have lymphoma.

The lymphoma in these patients is usually extranodal non-Hodgkin B-cell lymphoma. Lung involvement is a late occurrence. Nodules, masses, and infiltrates can be seen on chest radiography. A 6.5-fold increased incidence of primary lung cancer has been noted among patients with HIV infection and AIDS.

SUMMARY

- About 80%-90% of deaths due to seasonal influenza occur in persons ≥65 years.

- *Streptococcus pneumoniae* (pneumococcus) is a leading cause of community-acquired infections such as pneumonia, meningitis, otitis media, and sinusitis.

- Immunocompromised patients, especially those receiving long-term corticosteroid therapy, are susceptible to *Legionella* infections.

- The PPD skin test indicates infection with mycobacteria and not active disease.

20.

PHARYNGITIS, SEXUALLY TRANSMITTED INFECTIONS, URINARY TRACT INFECTIONS, AND GASTROINTESTINAL INFECTIONS

Pritish K. Tosh, MD, M. Rizwan Sohail, MD, and Elie F. Berbari, MD

GOALS

- Understand the epidemiology and management of sexually transmitted infections in patients with and without human immunodeficiency virus (HIV) infection.

- Distinguish differences in pathogenesis and management of urinary tract infections in men and women.

- Differentiate infectious diarrhea syndromes.

PHARYNGITIS

GROUP A β-HEMOLYTIC STREPTOCOCCI: *STREPTOCOCCUS PYOGENES*

Infections

Group A streptococci are responsible for several different clinical syndromes. *Streptococcus pyogenes* is the most common cause of bacterial pharyngitis. Although the pharyngitis is usually self-limited, antibiotic therapy (penicillin for 10 days or alternatives for patients with penicillin allergy) should be given to prevent acute rheumatic fever and suppurative complications. Penicillin also shortens the duration of symptoms if it is given within the first 24 hours of infection. Easily administered rapid antigen tests for streptococcal pharyngitis are specific, but they are not as sensitive (50%-70%) as a throat culture for detecting *S pyogenes*. The sensitivity of a rapid polymerase chain reaction test (LightCycler) for group A streptococci is 93%. Common complications of streptococcal pharyngitis include paratonsillar abscesses, otitis media, and sinusitis.

- Common complications of streptococcal pharyngitis include paratonsillar abscesses, otitis media, and sinusitis.

Nonsuppurative Complications

The nonsuppurative complications of group A streptococcal infection are acute rheumatic fever and acute glomerulonephritis. Treatment of group A streptococcal infection does not prevent poststreptococcal glomerulonephritis.

Rheumatic fever occurs only after streptococcal pharyngitis, never after skin infection. The diagnostic criteria for rheumatic fever are described in Box 20.1. Decreasing inflammation with aspirin (or corticosteroids) is the main therapy for acute rheumatic fever, although it will not prevent the development of chronic rheumatic heart disease.

- Treatment of group A streptococcal infection does not prevent poststreptococcal glomerulonephritis.

- Rheumatic fever occurs only after streptococcal pharyngitis, never after skin infection.

The risk for recurrent episodes of acute rheumatic fever with subsequent streptococcal infection is extremely high. Continuous antibiotic prophylaxis is effective for preventing these recurrences. Monthly injections of benzathine penicillin G or orally administered penicillin, sulfonamides, and erythromycin are effective for preventing recurrences of rheumatic fever. If there was no carditis with the initial rheumatic fever episode and no attack within the previous 5 years, prophylaxis may be discontinued after the age of 25 years. For patients who had significant carditis with residual valvular disease, lifelong prophylaxis may be necessary. Endocarditis prophylaxis is a separate issue. New recommendations do not advise prophylaxis for endocarditis to this group unless the patient has had a prior endocarditis or has a prosthetic valve. Acute glomerulonephritis may occur after infection with nephritogenic strains of *S pyogenes*. Both cutaneous infections and pharyngitis can result in acute glomerulonephritis.

- Continuous antibiotic prophylaxis is used to prevent recurrent acute rheumatic fever.

- Acute glomerulonephritis may occur after either streptococcal skin infections or pharyngitis.

SEXUALLY TRANSMITTED INFECTIONS

Sexually transmitted infections remain a major public health burden. About 19 million infections occur annually in the United States. Rates of sexually transmitted infections are higher in young African-American women and in men who have sex with men. The most common sexually transmitted infections are human papillomavirus, chlamydiosis, herpes simplex, and trichomoniasis. Although selected types of human papillomavirus are preventable with vaccination, other sexually transmitted infections require effective barriers to prevent transmission. These infections are characterized by their clinical presentations: 1) genital ulcers and lesions, 2) urethritis, 3) vulvovaginitis and cervicitis, 4) pelvic inflammatory disease, and 5) vaginal discharge.

GENITAL ULCERS AND LESIONS

Chancroid

In the United States, patients who present with genital ulcers usually have genital herpes, syphilis, or chancroid. These conditions are associated with an increased risk for HIV infection.

The combination of a painful genital ulcer and tender suppurative inguinal adenopathy is highly suggestive of chancroid, which is caused by *Haemophilus ducreyi*. Nevertheless, clinical inspection may not distinguish these 3 conditions, and all patients with genital ulcers should have syphilis serologic testing and herpes simplex virus (HSV) cell culture or polymerase chain reaction. In settings where chancroid is prevalent, such as in Africa and other tropical or subtropical regions, specialized culture for *H ducreyi* can be performed.

Chancroid is treated with azithromycin (1 g orally once), ceftriaxone (250 mg intramuscularly in a single dose), ciprofloxacin (500 mg orally twice a day for 3 days), or erythromycin base (500 mg orally 3 times a day for 7 days). Persons who have had sexual contact with an index patient during the 10 days preceding the patient's onset of symptoms should receive treatment.

Herpes Simplex Virus

At least 50 million persons in the United States are infected with HSV1 or HSV2. Most of them have not been diagnosed with genital herpes. Infected persons intermittently shed virus from the genital tract despite a lack of symptoms, leading to transmission. Isolation of HSV in cell culture or a type-specific polymerase chain reaction from genital lesions is the preferred virologic test. Herpes simplex may also be associated with erythema multiforme.

Antivirals can partially control the signs and symptoms of herpes episodes when they are used to treat first and recurrent episodes or when they are used as daily suppressive therapy. Recommended regimens for a first episode of genital HSV include acyclovir 400 mg orally 3 times a day for 7 to 10 days, acyclovir 200 mg orally 5 times a day for 7 to 10 days, famciclovir 250 mg orally 3 times a day for 7 to 10 days, or valacyclovir 1 g orally twice a day for 7 to 10 days.

Because recurrences are common, especially with HSV type 2, episodic or continuous suppressive antiviral therapy with acyclovir (400 mg orally twice a day), famciclovir (250 mg orally twice a day), valacyclovir (500 mg orally once a day), or valacyclovir (1 g orally once a day) are all effective in reducing the frequency of recurrences. Daily treatment with valacyclovir (500 mg daily) decreases the rate of HSV type 2 transmission in discordant, heterosexual couples in whom the source partner has a history of genital HSV type 2 infection.

HSV in Pregnancy

In the first trimester of pregnancy, the development of primary HSV infection may be associated with chorioretinitis, microcephaly, and skin lesions. The risk for transmission to the baby from an infected mother is 30% to 50% among women who acquire genital herpes near the time of delivery, 3% for women with a recurrence at delivery, and less than 1% among women with histories of recurrent herpes with no lesions at the time of delivery. Prevention of neonatal herpes relies on preventing acquisition of genital HSV late in pregnancy and avoiding exposure of the infant to herpetic lesions during delivery. Women without known genital herpes should be counseled to avoid intercourse during the third trimester with partners known to have or suspected of having genital herpes. Pregnant women without known orolabial herpes should be advised to avoid receptive oral sex during the third trimester with partners known to have or suspected to have orolabial herpes. At the onset of labor, all women should be questioned about symptoms of genital herpes, including prodromal symptoms, and examined carefully for herpetic lesions. Women without symptoms or signs of genital herpes or its prodrome can deliver vaginally. Acyclovir treatment late in pregnancy reduces the frequency of cesarean sections among women who have recurrent genital herpes by diminishing the frequency of recurrences at term. Women with recurrent genital herpetic lesions at the onset of labor should deliver by cesarean section to prevent neonatal herpes.

Syphilis

Syphilis is caused by the spirochete *Treponema pallidum*. The incidence of syphilis is highest in large cities among sexually active persons, particularly among inner city minority populations and men who have sex with men. Called the "great masquerader," syphilis may present with various manifestations, depending on the stage of disease, including a painless genital ulcer or chancre at the infection site; rash; mucocutaneous lesions; lymphadenopathy; cardiac, neurologic, and ophthalmic manifestations; auditory abnormalities; gummatous lesions; or simply a positive serologic test result. Because of the wide variety and transient nature of manifestations, syphilis is often overlooked.

Serologic tests for syphilis vary by laboratory. Some centers use the enzyme immunoassay for syphilis immunoglobulin M and G as a screening test, followed by a nontreponemal test, the rapid plasma reagin (RPR). Other centers use the RPR test initially and confirm the result with a more specific test such as the fluorescent treponemal antibody absorption test (FTA-ABS) (Table 20.1). Results of the FTA-ABS test are positive before VDRL testing (nontreponemal test), and thus they may be positive without a positive VDRL result in primary syphilis. VDRL results may be negative in 30% of patients with primary syphilis and can also be negative in late-latent infections.

Table 20.1 **LABORATORY DIAGNOSIS OF SYPHILIS**

SYPHILIS	TEST, % POSITIVE		
	VDRL	*FTA-ABS*	*MHA-TP*
Primary	70	85	50–60
Secondary	99	100	100
Tertiary	70	98	98

Abbreviations: FTA-ABS, fluorescent treponemal antibody absorption; MHA-TP, microhemagglutination assay for *Treponema pallidum*.

Adapted from Hook EW III. Syphilis. In: Goldman L, Ausiello D, editors. Cecil medicine. 23rd ed. Philadelphia (PA): Saunders Elsevier; c2008. p. 2280–8. Used with permission.

- The FTA-ABS test or other treponemal tests are the most sensitive serologic tests for the diagnosis of syphilis.

- The results of VDRL or RPR testing may be negative in 30% of patients with primary syphilis.

A chancre (clean, indurated ulcer) is the main manifestation of primary syphilis. It occurs at the site of inoculation and is usually painless. The incubation period is 3 to 90 days. It should be distinguished from HSV (painful) and chancroid (painful exudative ulcer). Diagnosis of primary syphilis can be made with dark-field examination of a specimen taken from the genital ulcer.

The manifestations of secondary syphilis result from hematogenous dissemination and usually occur 2 to 8 weeks after appearance of the chancre. Constitutional symptoms occur, in addition to rash, mucocutaneous lesions, alopecia, condylomata lata (ie, broad and flat verrucous syphilitic lesions located in warm, moist intertriginous areas, especially about the anus and genitals), lymphadenopathy, and various other symptoms and signs. The diagnosis is based on the clinical findings and results of serologic testing. The condition resolves spontaneously without treatment.

Latent syphilis is the asymptomatic stage after symptoms of secondary syphilis subside. Those that occur after 1 year are classified as late latent. The diagnosis is based on the results of serologic testing. For latent syphilis, a cerebrospinal fluid examination is indicated before treatment in patients with neurologic or ophthalmic abnormalities, in patients with other evidence of active tertiary syphilis (aortitis, gummas), before re-treatment of relapses, and in patients with HIV infection, especially those with a CD4 count less than 350 cells/mcL and a serum RPR result of more than 1:32.

Tertiary syphilis can involve all body systems (cardiovascular—aortitis involving the ascending aorta, which can cause aneurysms and aortic regurgitation; gummatous osteomyelitis; and hepatitis). However, neurosyphilis is the most common manifestation of tertiary syphilis in the United States. Neurosyphilis is often asymptomatic. Symptomatic disease is divided into several clinical syndromes that may overlap and occur at any time after primary infection. The diagnosis is made from cerebrospinal fluid examination; abnormalities include mononuclear pleocytosis and an increased protein value. VDRL testing of cerebrospinal fluid is only 30% to 70% sensitive. The FTA-ABS test on cerebrospinal fluid is highly sensitive but not specific. Any cerebrospinal fluid abnormality in a patient who is seropositive for syphilis must be investigated. Syndromes include meningovascular syphilis (occurs 4–7 years after infection and presents with focal central nervous system deficits such as stroke or cranial nerve abnormalities) and parenchymatous syphilis (general paresis or tabes dorsalis). Parenchymatous syphilis occurs decades after infection and may present as general paresis (chronic progressive dementia) or as tabes dorsalis (sensory ataxia, lightning pains, autonomic dysfunction, and optic atrophy).

- Neurosyphilis is the most common manifestation of tertiary disease in the United States.

- The diagnosis is made from cerebrospinal fluid examination.
- VDRL testing of cerebrospinal fluid is only 30%-70% sensitive.

Treatment of syphilis is based on whether the disease is early or late. For early syphilis (primary, secondary, or early latent [<1 year]), benzathine penicillin G 2.4 million units intramuscularly is used; follow-up serologic testing with RPR is done to ascertain response to therapy. Alternatives are doxycycline (100 mg twice daily for 14 days) or tetracycline (500 mg orally 4 times daily for 14 days). Erythromycin (500 mg orally 4 times daily) is the least effective. After treatment (especially in early syphilis), 10% to 25% of patients may experience a Jarisch-Herxheimer reaction, manifested by varying degrees of fever, chills, myalgias, headache, tachycardia, and hypotension. This reaction lasts for 12 to 24 hours and can be managed symptomatically.

Treatment for late disease (>1 year in duration, cardiovascular disease, gumma, late latent syphilis) is with benzathine penicillin 2.4 million units intramuscularly weekly for 3 weeks. Alternatives are doxycycline (100 mg orally twice daily) or tetracycline (500 mg orally 4 times daily) for 4 weeks.

Treatment of neurosyphilis is with aqueous penicillin G (12–24 million units intravenously per day) for 10 to 14 days or procaine penicillin (2.4 million units intramuscularly per day) plus probenecid (500 mg 4 times daily) for 10 to 14 days.

Pregnant patients should receive a penicillin-based regimen for treatment of all stages of syphilis. If a pregnant patient has a penicillin allergy, she should be desensitized to penicillin.

For early and secondary syphilis, follow-up clinical and serologic testing should be performed at 6 and 12 months. Re-treatment with 3 weekly injections of 2.4 million units of benzathine penicillin G should be given to patients with signs or symptoms that persist or whose VDRL result has a sustained 4-fold increase in titer. HIV testing should be performed if not done previously. If the VDRL titer does not decrease 4-fold by 6 months, consideration also should be given to re-treatment.

Patients with latent syphilis should have a follow-up examination at 6, 12, and 24 months. If the VDRL result increases 4-fold, if a high titer (>1:32) fails to decrease 4-fold within 12 to 24 months, or if signs or symptoms attributable to syphilis occur, a cerebrospinal fluid examination should be done to rule out the possibility of neurosyphilis and re-treatment should be done accordingly.

Follow-up in patients who receive treatment for neurosyphilis should include testing of cerebrospinal fluid every 6 months if cerebrospinal fluid pleocytosis was present initially; this testing is done until the results are normal. If the cell count is not decreased at 6 months or if the cerebrospinal fluid is not entirely normal at 2 years, re-treatment should be considered.

URETHRITIS SYNDROMES

The clinical syndrome of urethral pain and discharge is often associated with chlamydial infection, gonorrhea, and nongonococcal urethritis. A diagnosis is made on the basis of the following findings: the presence of mucopurulent or purulent discharge, a Gram stain of urethral secretions with 5 or more leukocytes per oil immersion field, or a positive result of leukocyte esterase test on first-void urine. The presence of gram-negative intracellular diplococci on a urethral smear is indicative of gonorrhea infection and is often accompanied by chlamydial infection. Nongonococcal urethritis is diagnosed when microscopy indicates inflammation without gram-negative intracellular diplococci. Urine or urethral exudates should be sent for testing for gonorrhea and *Chlamydia trachomatis*. *Chlamydia trachomatis* is a frequent cause of nongonococcal urethritis (15%-55% of cases); however, the prevalence varies by age group, with lower prevalence among older men. The etiologic agent of most cases of nonchlamydial nongonococcal urethritis is unknown; however, *Mycoplasma genitalium* is emerging as an increasingly recognized cause. Complications of nongonococcal urethritis among men infected with *C trachomatis* include epididymitis, prostatitis, and Reiter syndrome.

GONORRHEA

Neisseria gonorrhoeae is a gram-negative intracellular diplococcus. Rates of gonorrhea have remained stable, but resistance to therapy has increased. The disease often causes symptomatic urethritis and discharge in men, but it has few symptoms in women and may lead to cervicitis, infertility, ectopic pregnancy, and chronic pelvic pain. In women, concomitant proctitis is common (rectal cultures should be done in all women). Gonococcal pharyngitis is often asymptomatic. The diagnosis of gonorrhea may be made with a Gram stain of urethral exudate in men showing intracellular gram-negative diplococci or by using urine or urethral-cervical–based nucleic acid amplification tests.

- *Neisseria gonorrhoeae* commonly causes urethritis, cervicitis, pharyngitis, and proctitis.
- Asymptomatic carrier state occurs in both males and females, but it is more common in females.

Resistance to penicillin, tetracycline, and, most recently, fluoroquinolones has limited the treatment options to cephalosporins. Because concomitant chlamydial infection is often present, a second agent is often included in the treatment regimen. Primary treatment is ceftriaxone (125 mg intramuscularly) plus doxycycline (100 mg orally twice daily for 7 days) or azithromycin (a single 1-g dose) to also treat chlamydial infection. Cefixime (400 mg once daily) is available as a first-line oral option. Alternative therapies are limited for patients who are allergic to β-lactam. Spectinomycin is not available in the United States. Limited data suggest that high-dose azithromycin (2 g in 1 dose) might be an option. Pharyngeal infection is best treated with ceftriaxone. Therapy recommended for pregnant women includes ceftriaxone (125 mg intramuscularly) or cefixime (400 mg orally) plus azithromycin (1 g orally). Follow-up nucleic acid amplification tests 3 weeks after treatment are recommended for all pregnant women. All patients with sexually transmitted diseases should be tested for HIV. Sexual partners should be offered evaluation and treatment. Table 20.2 outlines the treatment of gonococcal infections.

Table 20.2 TREATMENT REGIMENS FOR GONOCOCCAL INFECTIONS AND ASSOCIATED CONDITIONS

INFECTION	RECOMMENDED REGIMEN	ALTERNATIVE REGIMEN
Cervix, urethra, rectum[a]	Ceftriaxone 125 mg IM in a single dose *Or* Cefixime[c] 400 mg PO in a single dose or 400 mg by suspension (200 mg/5 mL) *Plus* Treatment for *Chlamydia* infection if not ruled out	Spectinomycin[b] 2 g IM in a single dose *Or* Single-dose cephalosporin regimen
Pharynx[a]	Ceftriaxone 125 mg IM in a single dose *Plus* Treatment for *Chlamydia* infection if not ruled out	

Disseminated gonococcal infection[d]	Ceftriaxone 1 g IM or IV every 24 h	Cefotaxime 1 g IV every 8 h
		Or
		Ceftizoxime 1 g IV every 8 h
		Or
		Spectinomycin[b] 2 g IM every 12 h
		After 24–48 h of clinical improvement, switch:[e]
		  Cefixime 400 mg PO twice daily
		  Or
		  Cefixime[c] 400 mg by suspension (200 mg/5 mL)
		  Or
		  Cefpodoxime 400 mg PO twice daily

Pelvic inflammatory disease[f]	Parenteral A:
	  Cefotetan 2 g IV every 12 h
	  Or
	  Cefoxitin 2 g IV every 6 h
	  Plus
	  Doxycycline 100 mg PO or IV every 12 h
	Parenteral B:
	  Clindamycin 900 mg IV every 8 h
	  Plus
	  Gentamicin[g]
	Oral:[h]
	  Ceftriaxone 250 mg IM in a single dose
	  Plus
	  Doxycycline 100 mg PO twice daily for 14 d *with or without* metronidazole 500 mg PO twice daily for 14 d
	  Or
	  Cefoxitin 2 g IM in a single dose & probenecid 1 g PO concurrently in a single dose
	  Plus
	  Doxycycline 100 mg PO twice daily for 14 d *with or without* metronidazole 500 mg PO twice daily for 14 d
	  Or
	  Other parenteral third-generation cephalosporin[j]
	  Plus
	  Doxycycline 100 mg PO twice daily for 14 d *with or without* metronidazole 500 mg PO twice daily for 14 d
		Parenteral:
		  Ampicillin-sulbactam 3 g IV every 6 h
		  Plus
		  Doxycycline 100 mg PO or IV every 12 h
		
		Fluoroquinolones:[i] levofloxacin 500 mg PO once daily or ofloxacin 400 mg twice daily for 14 d *with or without* metronidazole 500 mg PO twice daily for 14 d

(continued)

INFECTION	RECOMMENDED REGIMEN	ALTERNATIVE REGIMEN
Epididymitis	Ceftriaxone 250 mg IM in a single dose *Plus* Doxycycline 100 mg PO twice daily for 10 d Ofloxacin[k] 300 mg PO twice daily for 10 d *Or* Levofloxacin 500 mg PO once daily for 10 d	

Abbreviations: IM, intramuscularly; IV, intravenously; PO, orally.

[a] These regimens are recommended for all adult & adolescent patients, regardless of travel history or sexual behavior.

[b] Spectinomycin is currently not available in the United States.

[c] The tablet formulation of cefixime is currently not available in the United States.

[d] A cephalosporin-based intravenous regimen is recommended for the initial treatment of disseminated gonococcal infection. This is particularly important when gonorrhea is detected at mucosal sites by nonculture tests.

[e] Switch to 1 of the following regimens to complete at least 1 week of antimicrobial therapy. Cefixime[c] 400 mg orally twice daily *or* cefixime 400 mg by suspension (200 mg/5 mL) twice daily *or* cefpodoxime 400 mg orally twice daily.

[f] Parenteral & oral therapy seem to have similar clinical efficacy for women with pelvic inflammatory disease of mild or moderate severity. Clinical experience should guide decisions regarding transition to oral therapy, which usually can be initiated within 24 hours of clinical improvement.

[g] Loading dose intravenously or intramuscularly (2 mg/kg of body weight), followed by maintenance dose (1.5 mg/kg) every 8 hours. Single daily dosing may be substituted.

[h] Oral therapy can be considered for women with mild to moderately severe acute pelvic inflammatory disease because the clinical outcomes with oral therapy are similar to those with parenteral therapy. Women who do not respond to oral therapy within 72 hours should be reevaluated to confirm the diagnosis & should be administered parenteral therapy on either an outpatient or an inpatient basis.

[i] If parenteral cephalosporin therapy is not feasible, use of fluoroquinolones with or without metronidazole may be considered if the community prevalence & individual risk of gonorrhea are low. Tests for gonorrhea must be performed before instituting therapy.

[j] Ceftizoxime or cefotaxime.

[k] For acute epididymitis most likely caused by enteric organisms or with negative gonococcal culture or nucleic acid amplification test.

Adapted from Workowski KA, Berman S; Centers for Diseases Control and Prevention (CDC). Sexually transmitted diseases treatment guidelines, 2010. MMWR Recomm Rep. 2010 Dec 17;59(RR-12):1-110. Erratum in: MMWR Recomm Rep. 2011 Jan 14;60(1):18. Dosage error in article text.

- Primary treatment of *N gonorrhoeae* includes ceftriaxone (125 mg intramuscularly) or cefixime (400 mg orally) plus doxycycline (100 mg orally twice daily for 7 days) or azithromycin (single 1-g dose).

- Fluoroquinolones are no longer recommended for empiric treatment of gonorrhea.

In 1% to 3% of patients, this infection may lead to disseminated gonococcal infection. Risk factors include complement deficiency, female sex, pharyngeal infection, pregnancy, and menstruation. It occurs most often in women during menstruation (when sloughing of endometrium allows access to blood supply, enhanced growth of gonococci due to necrotic tissue, and change in pH). There are 2 distinct phases. The bacteremic phase may manifest as tenosynovitis (around the wrists or ankles ["lovers heels"]); painful, distally distributed skin lesions (usually less than 30 in number, peripheral macular or pustular with a hemorrhagic component); and polyarthralgias involving the knees and elbows (the classic dermatitis arthritis syndrome). Rarely, a destructive form of infective endocarditis may develop, primarily affecting the aortic valve. Results of synovial fluid testing are usually negative. The nonbacteremic phase follows 1 week later and may present as monoarticular infectious arthritis of the knee, wrist, and ankle; results of joint culture are positive in about 50%. Culture specimens should be obtained from the urethra, cervix, rectum, and pharynx.

- Disseminated gonococcemia is most likely to occur during menstruation.

- A bacteremic phase may manifest as tenosynovitis, skin lesions, and arthralgias; joint cultures are usually negative.

- Rarely, a destructive form of infective endocarditis may develop, primarily affecting the aortic valve.

- A nonbacteremic phase may present as monoarticular arthritis of the knee, wrist, and ankle; results of joint cultures are positive in about 50%.

Treatment is with ceftriaxone (1 g intravenously daily for 7–10 days); alternatives include ceftriaxone for 3 or 4 days or until clinical improvement followed by oral cefixime (400 mg daily) to complete a course of 7 to 10 days. If the strain is tested and found to be penicillin-susceptible, treatment includes penicillin G (10 million units intravenously daily) for 7 to 10 days, or it is given for 3 or 4 days and then oral amoxicillin is used to finish a 7- to 10-day course. For meningitis, treatment includes ceftriaxone (1–2 g intravenously every 12 hours for at least 10–14 days). Alternative drugs are penicillin, if the strain is susceptible, and chloramphenicol. For endocarditis, ceftriaxone or penicillin is used for at least 28 days.

- Treatment of disseminated gonococcal infection is with ceftriaxone (1 g intravenously daily for 7–10 days).
- Chlamydial infections often coexist with gonococcal infection and should be treated empirically.

Nongonococcal Urethritis and Cervicitis

Chlamydia trachomatis genital infection is the most common reportable sexually transmitted infection. This organism causes urethritis in men and mucopurulent cervicitis, endometritis, and pelvic inflammatory disease in women. Its sequelae include tubal infertility, chronic pelvic pain, and ectopic pregnancy. Because this infection may be asymptomatic in half of affected men and three-fourths of affected women, screening for this infection is recommended for all sexually active women age 24 years or younger. The diagnosis is most often made from nucleic acid amplification tests or from urine or urethral-cervical specimens. Treatment of infected persons, whether symptomatic or not, reduces transmission. Two treatment regimens are highly effective, and the choice depends on patient compliance. Doxycycline (100 mg twice daily for 7 days) or azithromycin (a single 1-g oral dose) is standard treatment. Infected persons should abstain from sex until 1 week of treatment is completed. Women with *C trachomatis* cervicitis should be rescreened 3 to 4 months after treatment. *Ureaplasma urealyticum*, *Trichomonas vaginalis*, *M genitalium*, and HSV are less common causes of nongonococcal urethritis. If urethritis fails to resolve and reinfection or relapse of a chlamydial infection has been excluded, *Trichomonas* or tetracycline-resistant *Ureaplasma* infection should be considered. In this situation, empiric treatment consists of metronidazole (2 g orally in a single dose) plus erythromycin base (500 mg orally 4 times daily for 7 days) or erythromycin ethylsuccinate (800 mg orally 4 times daily for 7 days).

- Nongonococcal urethritis and cervicitis are most commonly caused by *C trachomatis*.

Epididymitis

This condition usually presents as a unilateral, painful scrotal swelling. In young, sexually active men (<35 years of age), *C trachomatis* and *N gonorrhoeae* are the common pathogens. Sexually transmitted acute epididymitis is usually accompanied by urethritis, which frequently is asymptomatic and is usually not accompanied by bacteriuria. In contrast, in older men, bacteriuria due to obstructive urinary disease is relatively common and is associated with urinary tract instrumentation, surgery, systemic disease, or immunosuppression. Aerobic gram-negative rods and enterococci predominate in this age group. Although epididymitis is principally a clinical diagnosis, color duplex Doppler ultrasonography has a sensitivity of 70% and a specificity of 88% for diagnosing acute epididymitis. The diagnostic evaluation of men in whom epididymitis is suspected should include a Gram stain of urethral secretions, a leukocyte esterase test on first-void urine, or a microscopic examination of first-void urine sediment (≥10 leukocytes per high-power field indicates pyuria).

Because empiric treatment may be needed before test results are available, ceftriaxone (250 mg intramuscularly) plus doxycycline (100 mg orally twice daily for 10 days) is the treatment of choice. In older men with test results that are negative tests for gonorrhea and *Chlamydia*, oral levofloxacin (500 mg daily for 10 days) or treatment based on the results of urine Gram stain, culture, and susceptibility test can be used.

- Epididymitis is usually unilateral.
- In young, sexually active men, *C trachomatis* and *N gonorrhoeae* are the common pathogens; in older men, the usual urinary tract pathogens are likely causes.

PELVIC INFLAMMATORY DISEASE

Pelvic inflammatory disease is the most frequent acute infection in nonpregnant, reproductive-age women. It is associated with considerable long-term sequelae, such as infertility, ectopic pregnancies, tubo-ovarian abscess, and chronic pelvic pain. The organisms responsible include *N gonorrhoeae*, *C trachomatis*, *Mycoplasma hominis*, and various aerobic gram-negative rods and anaerobes. Fitz-Hugh-Curtis syndrome is an acute perihepatitis caused by direct extension of *N gonorrhoeae* or *C trachomatis* to the liver capsule. Occasionally, a friction rub can be auscultated over the liver and "violin string" adhesions between the liver capsule and parietal peritoneum can be observed with laparoscopy. *Actinomyces* species can be a pathogen in patients with an intrauterine device. Pelvic inflammatory disease is usually diagnosed on the basis of clinical findings, including lower abdominal or adnexal tenderness, cervical motion tenderness, fever, abnormal cervical discharge, and evidence of *N gonorrhoeae* or *C trachomatis* infection. Early empiric therapy is recommended in women at risk. Sonography and laparoscopy are reserved for complicated cases.

- Pelvic inflammatory disease is a polymicrobial infection.
- Fitz-Hugh-Curtis syndrome is an acute perihepatitis caused by direct extension of *N gonorrhoeae* or *C trachomatis* to the liver capsule.
- The emphasis on early diagnosis is meant to decrease the incidence of infertility as a complication of pelvic inflammatory disease.

The goal of treatment is to prevent complications. Most women can receive treatment as outpatients and be reassessed within 1 to 3 days. Hospitalization is indicated when the outpatient therapy is precluded by severe nausea and vomiting, the diagnosis is uncertain, pelvic abscess or peritonitis is present, the patient is pregnant, the patient is an adolescent, or noncompliance is suspected. Table 20.2 outlines the treatment of pelvic inflammatory diseases.

Tubo-ovarian abscess may be characterized by an adnexal mass on physical examination or radiographic examination or by failure of antimicrobial therapy. Most abscesses 4 to 6 cm in diameter respond to medical therapy alone with the preferred regimen of ampicillin, gentamicin, and clindamycin. Large abscesses (>10 cm) often necessitate operation.

- Tubo-ovarian abscess is characterized by an adnexal mass on physical examination or radiographic examination or by failure of antimicrobial therapy.

VAGINITIS

Vaginitis is characterized by a vaginal discharge or vulvar itching, odor, or irritation. The 3 entities most frequently associated with vaginal discharge are bacterial vaginosis (a replacement of the normal vaginal flora by an overgrowth of anaerobic microorganisms, mycoplasmas, and *Gardnerella vaginalis*), trichomoniasis (*T vaginalis*), and candidiasis.

Bacterial Vaginosis

Bacterial vaginosis is the most common vaginal infection affecting women of childbearing age. Risk factors for bacterial vaginosis include multiple sex partners (increased incidence has also been reported among women who have sex with women), new partners, douching, and a lack of vaginal lactobacilli. Women with bacterial vaginosis are at increased risk for sexually transmitted infections, low-birth-weight infants, and a substantial reduction in their quality of life. Bacterial vaginosis is due to a change in local vaginal ecology from a flora of predominant lactobacilli to one of various anaerobic bacteria. Organisms associated with the syndrome include *Atopobium vaginae*, *Gardnerella*, *Prevotella*, *Mobiluncus* species, *M hominis*, *Megasphaera* species, and the Clostridiales bacteria (bacterial vaginosis–associated bacterium 1, 2, and 3).

Bacterial vaginosis can be diagnosed with clinical (Amsel) or microbiologic (Nugent) criteria. The Amsel clinical criteria require 3 of the following: a grayish white discharge that is homogeneous and coats the vaginal walls, "clue" cells on wet-mount examination, a vaginal fluid pH more than 4.5, and a "fishy" smell when secretion is mixed with 10% potassium hydroxide (positive "whiff" test). Rapid nucleic acid tests (eg, Affirm VPIII) can also be used.

Recommended treatment regimens include metronidazole (500 mg orally twice daily for 7 days), clindamycin (300 mg orally twice daily for 7 days) as an alternative, topical clindamycin cream (2% for 7 days), or metronidazole gel (0.75% intravaginal applicator nightly for 5 days) (the clindamycin cream appears less efficacious than the metronidazole regimens). Single-dose metronidazole therapy should not be used. Recurrence of bacterial vaginosis is common.

Treatment of recurrent disease should include re-treatment followed by a prolonged course of twice-weekly metronidazole gel. Bacterial vaginosis has been associated with adverse pregnancy outcomes. All symptomatic pregnant women should be treated. In pregnant patients, systemic therapy with metronidazole (500 mg twice daily for 7 days) or clindamycin (300 mg orally twice daily for 7 days) is recommended rather than topical therapy. Treatment of asymptomatic nonpregnant carriers is not recommended. Some experts recommend treatment of asymptomatic pregnant women at high risk for preterm delivery. Routine treatment of sex partners is not recommended.

- Bacterial vaginosis diagnosis is based on the presence of grayish white discharge that is homogeneous, the presence of "clue" cells on wet-mount examination, a vaginal fluid pH more than 4.5, and a "fishy" smell when secretion is mixed with 10% potassium hydroxide (positive "whiff" test).

- Therapy options are metronidazole (500 mg orally twice daily for 7 days) or clindamycin (300 mg orally twice daily for 7 days).

Trichomoniasis

Women with trichomoniasis may have a malodorous yellow-green vaginal discharge with vulvar irritation, dysuria, or dyspareunia. Petechial lesions may be noted on the cervix with colposcopy ("strawberry cervix"). Although sexual transmission is most common, trichomoniasis has been transmitted to health care workers via urine soaked sheets. The diagnosis is established from wet mount of vaginal secretions showing the motile organisms. The vaginal pH is usually more than 4.5. New rapid tests for trichomoniasis in women include the 10-minute dipstick assay (OSOM Trichomonas Rapid Test) and the 45-minute nucleic acid probe test (Affirm VPIII) that evaluates for *T vaginalis*, *G vaginalis*, and *Candida albicans*. Both of these tests are performed on vaginal secretions and have a sensitivity of more than 83% and a specificity of more than 97%; the rapid test for trichomoniasis is much more sensitive than the direct wet-mount examination.

Treatment is with metronidazole (2 g as a single dose) or tinidazole (2 g: 4 500-mg tablets as a single dose). A 7-day course of metronidazole (500 mg twice daily) is an alternative. Gastrointestinal tolerance may be better with tinidazole. All partners should be examined and treated. Although treatment in asymptomatic pregnant women is controversial, treatment in symptomatic pregnant women should be a one-time dose of 2 g of metronidazole.

- Infection with *T vaginalis* often is characterized by yellow-green, purulent discharge.

- Diagnosis is established with wet mount or a rapid test of vaginal secretions (the latter has increased sensitivity).

- Treatment of *T vaginalis* is with metronidazole or tinidazole orally.

Vulvovaginal Candidiasis

Vulvovaginal candidiasis is the second most common cause of vaginitis. The disease can be complicated or uncomplicated; in most cases it is uncomplicated. The majority of cases are due to *C albicans*, and a smaller number are due to *Candida glabrata*. The predominant symptoms of this condition are itching, soreness, burning, and dyspareunia, not discharge. Usually there is no odor, and discharge is scant, watery, and white. "Cottage cheese curds" may adhere to the vaginal wall. Microscopy using 10% potassium hydroxide to the discharge may show characteristic pseudohyphae, but it is insensitive for diagnosis, and culture may be needed. Complicated cases are recurrent (>4 per year), have severe symptoms, involve non-*albicans Candida*, or occur in the setting of immunosuppression, diabetes, pregnancy, or severe illness. In severe or recurrent cases, consider HIV infection. For uncomplicated vulvovaginal candidiasis, any of a number of topical antifungal azole agents used from 1 to 7 days or a single 150-mg oral dose of fluconazole may be used. Multiple-dose oral azole therapy is used for severe, refractory cases. In recurrent vulvovaginal candidiasis due to *C albicans*, fluconazole 150 mg every 3 days for 3 doses followed by 150 mg once weekly may be effective. In non-*albicans* cases, alternatives such as intravaginal boric acid capsules may be used.

- Vulvovaginal candidiasis is categorized as complicated or uncomplicated.

- In severe or recurrent cases, consider HIV infection.

URINARY TRACT INFECTIONS

IN FEMALES

Urinary tract infections (UTIs) are common in young women. Because urethritis or cystitis can occur with low colony counts of bacteria (10^3 colony-forming units), routine urine cultures in young women with dysuria are not recommended. Urinalysis should be done with or without a Gram stain. If pyuria and uncomplicated UTI are present, short-course treatment (3 days) should be initiated. Only if occult upper urinary tract disease, a complicated UTI, or sexually transmitted disease is suspected should appropriate culture and sensitivity testing be performed. Risk factors for occult infection and complications include emergency department presentation, low socioeconomic status, hospital-acquired infection, pregnancy, use of Foley catheter, recent instrumentation, known urologic abnormality, previous relapse, UTI at age younger than 12 years, acute pyelonephritis or 3 or more UTIs in 1 year, symptoms for more than 7 days, recent antibiotic use, diabetes mellitus, and immunosuppression. Causative organisms include *Escherichia coli* and *Staphylococcus saprophyticus*, *Proteus mirabilis*, or *Klebsiella pneumoniae*.

Staphylococcus saprophyticus is a unique species of coagulase-negative staphylococcus that is a common cause of urinary tract infections in young, sexually active women.

Coagulase-negative staphylococci are usually resistant to the β-lactam antibiotics. Unless in vitro susceptibility testing shows other active agents, serious infections due to coagulase-negative staphylococci should be treated with vancomycin. The fluoroquinolones may be active against some strains, but resistance may emerge rapidly. *Staphylococcus saprophyticus* and *Staphylococcus lugdunensis* are exceptions because they are usually susceptible to the penicillins, trimethoprim-sulfamethoxazole, and many other antibiotics.

- Routine urine cultures are not recommended in young women with dysuria.

- Organisms that commonly cause cystitis are *E coli* and *S saprophyticus*.

For the first episode of cystitis or urethritis, treatment is given but no investigation is needed. Short-course treatment (3 days) has fewer side effects than standard (7–10 days) therapy, and risk of relapse of infection is the same. Trimethoprim-sulfamethoxazole, nitrofurantoin, and fosfomycin are considered first-line antimicrobial options for uncomplicated urinary tract infections. In patients who fail to improve within 48 hours of treatment with first-line therapy, drug resistance should be suspected and an oral fluoroquinolone should be considered. Rates of trimethoprim-sulfamethoxazole resistance among *E coli* approach 20% in some communities. If recurrence develops after 3-day therapy, subclinical pyelonephritis or resistance should be considered. Urologic evaluation is usually not necessary. It should, however, be performed in patients with multiple relapses, painless hematuria, a history of childhood UTI, renal lithiasis, and recurrent pyelonephritis.

- For uncomplicated urinary tract infections, trimethoprim-sulfamethoxazole, nitrofurantoin, and fosfomycin are first-line agents.

- Short-course treatment (3 days) has fewer side effects than standard (7–10 days) therapy, and risk of relapse of infection is the same.

- Urologic evaluation should be pursued in patients with multiple relapses, painless hematuria, history of childhood UTI, renal lithiasis, and recurrent pyelonephritis.

Asymptomatic bacteriuria (>10^5 colony-forming units/mL) in a midstream urine specimen should be treated only in pregnant women and in patients undergoing urinary tract instrumentation. For acute uncomplicated pyelonephritis, levofloxacin 750 mg once daily for 5 days is equal in efficacy to 10 days of twice-daily therapy with ciprofloxacin. In patients sufficiently ill to require hospitalization, a third-generation cephalosporin or a fluoroquinolone can be used as empiric therapy over a course of 10 to 14 days. If enterococci are suspected on the basis of the Gram stain, ampicillin or piperacillin should be used. Cephalosporins and trimethoprim-sulfamethoxazole should not be used to treat enterococcal UTI. Oral regimens can be substituted quickly as the patient improves. A urine culture is recommended 1 to 2 weeks after completion of therapy only in pregnant women, children, and patients with recurrent pyelonephritis in whom suppressive therapy is being considered.

Recurrent UTIs are common in women. Prophylaxis may be offered to women who have 2 or more symptomatic UTIs within 6 months or 3 or more over 12 months. For these women, 3 options have all been shown to be effective: continuous prophylaxis, postcoital prophylaxis, or intermittent self-treatment. For postmenopausal women, vaginal estrogen supplementation is beneficial.

- Asymptomatic bacteriuria ($>10^5$ colony-forming units/mL) in a midstream urine specimen should be treated only in pregnant women and in patients undergoing urinary tract instrumentation.

- For acute uncomplicated pyelonephritis, 5 days of oral levofloxacin therapy is as effective as 10 days of twice-daily ciprofloxacin therapy.

- A follow-up urine culture is not usually recommended.

- Cephalosporins and trimethoprim-sulfamethoxazole should not be used to treat enterococcal UTI.

IN MALES

In men, UTI is less common, but it increases in frequency with age. Urologic abnormalities (such as benign prostatic hyperplasia) are common. Men with symptomatic dysuria should be investigated for sexually transmitted diseases and prostatism. When a UTI is suspected, urine culture and sensitivity testing should be done. Causative organisms include *E coli* in 50% of cases, other gram-negative organisms in 25%, enterococci in 20%, and others in 5%. If signs and symptoms of epididymitis, acute prostatitis, and pyelonephritis are present, treat accordingly. If uncomplicated lower UTI is present, treatment duration is 10 to 14 days. If symptoms persist or relapse, the urine culture should be repeated. If results are positive, treat for a minimum of 6 weeks. If culture results are negative, consider further evaluation for one of the chronic prostatitis-chronic pelvic pain syndromes.

- Causes of UTI in males include *E coli* in 50%, other gram-negative organisms in 25%, enterococci in 20%, and others in 5%.

- Men with UTI should not receive short-course therapy.

GASTROINTESTINAL INFECTIONS

BACTERIAL AND TOXIGENIC DIARRHEA

The principal causes of toxigenic diarrhea are listed in Table 20.3, and those of invasive diarrhea are listed in Table 20.4. Fecal leukocytes usually are absent in toxigenic diarrhea. In invasive diarrhea, fecal leukocytes may be present. The travel history is often important.

Campylobacter jejuni

Campylobacter jejuni is the most common cause of sporadic acute bacterial diarrhea. Outbreaks, although less common, are associated with consumption of unpasteurized dairy products and undercooked poultry. The incidence of disease peaks in summer and early fall. Diarrhea may be bloody. Fever usually is present. The diagnosis is established by isolation of the organism from stool culture. Treatment is usually symptomatic because the disease tends to be self-limited. Erythromycin (500 mg twice daily for 5 days) or azithromycin can be used when symptoms are prolonged or the host is immunocompromised.

- Outbreaks of bacterial diarrhea caused by *C jejuni* are associated with consumption of unpasteurized milk and undercooked poultry.

- Macrolide therapy is the therapy of choice for *Campylobacter*-associated diarrhea.

Staphylococcal Enterotoxin

Preformed enterotoxins produced by *Staphylococcus aureus* are a common cause of food poisoning in the United States.

Table 20.3 **CAUSES OF BACTERIAL DIARRHEA: TOXIGENIC**

ORGANISM	ONSET AFTER INGESTION, H	PREFORMED TOXIN	FEVER PRESENT	VOMITING PREDOMINATES
Staphylococcus aureus	2–6	Yes	No	Yes
Clostridium perfringens	8–16	No	No	No
Escherichia coli	12	No	No	No
Vibrio cholerae	12	No	Due to dehydration	No
Bacillus cereus				
a.	1–6	Yes	No	Yes
b.	8–16	No	No	No

Table 20.4 CAUSES OF BACTERIAL DIARRHEA: INVASIVE

ORGANISM	FEVER PRESENT	BLOODY DIARRHEA PRESENT	ANTIBIOTICS EFFECTIVE
Shigella species	Yes	Yes	Yes
Salmonella (non-*typhi*)	Yes	No	No
Vibrio parahaemolyticus	Yes	Yes (occasional)	No
Escherichia coli O157:H7	Yes	Yes	No
Campylobacter	Yes	Yes	Yes
Yersinia	Yes	Yes (occasional)	Sometimes

The toxin is heat stable and, therefore, is not destroyed by cooking contaminated foods. Preformed toxin by *S aureus* is ingested in contaminated food. It has a short incubation period of 4 to 6 hours. Onset is abrupt, with severe vomiting (often predominates), diarrhea, and abdominal cramps. The duration of infection is 8 to 24 hours. Diagnosis is based on rapid onset, absence of fever, and history. Treatment is supportive.

- Bacterial diarrhea due to *S aureus* is caused by ingestion of preformed toxin in contaminated food; it has a short incubation period (4–6 hours).

- Preformed enterotoxins produced by *S aureus* are not destroyed by cooking food.

- Diagnosis is based on rapid onset, absence of fever, and history.

Clostridium perfringens

Bacterial diarrhea caused by *C perfringens* is associated with ingestion of bacteria that produce toxin in vivo, often in improperly prepared or stored precooked foods (meat and poultry products). Food is precooked and toxin is destroyed but spores survive; when food is rewarmed, spores germinate. When food is ingested, toxin is produced. Diarrhea is more severe than vomiting, and abdominal cramping is prominent. Onset of symptoms is later than with *S aureus* infection. Duration of illness is 24 hours. The diagnosis is based on the later onset of symptoms, a typical history. Treatment is supportive.

- In diarrhea caused by *C perfringens*, ingested bacteria produce toxin in vivo in precooked food.

- Diarrhea is more severe than vomiting; abdominal cramping is prominent.

Bacillus cereus Toxin

Two types of food poisoning are associated with *B cereus* infection. Profuse vomiting follows a short incubation period (1–6 hours); this is associated with the ingestion of a preformed toxin (usually in fried rice). A disease with a longer incubation occurs 8 to 16 hours after consumption; profound

diarrhea develops and usually is associated with eating meat or vegetables. The diagnosis is confirmed by isolation of the organism from contaminated food. The illness is self-limited and treatment is supportive.

Escherichia coli

Diarrhea caused by *E coli* can be either enterotoxigenic or enterohemorrhagic. Enterotoxigenic *E coli* is the most common etiologic agent of traveler's diarrhea. Treatment consists of fluid and electrolyte replacement along with loperamide plus a fluoroquinolone or rifaximin. Medical evaluation should be sought if fever and bloody diarrhea occur. For prophylaxis, travelers should use food and water precautions. Routine prophylactic use of trimethoprim-sulfamethoxazole, ciprofloxacin, and doxycycline is not recommended. The use of bismuth subsalicylate as primary prophylaxis in travelers reduces the incidence of enterotoxigenic *E coli*-associated diarrhea by up to 60%.

- Enterotoxigenic *E coli* is the most common etiologic agent in traveler's diarrhea.

- Treatment consists of fluid and electrolyte replacement along with loperamide plus a fluoroquinolone or rifaximin.

Escherichia coli O157:H7 causes an uncommon form of bloody diarrhea. This agent has been identified as the cause of waterborne illness, outbreaks in nursing homes and child care centers, and sporadic cases. It also has been transmitted by eating undercooked beef and other contaminated food products. Bloody diarrhea, severe abdominal cramps, fever, and profound toxicity characterize this enterohemorrhagic illness. It may mimic ischemic colitis. At extremes of age (old and young), the infection may produce hemolytic uremic syndrome and death. This organism should be considered in all patients with hemolytic uremic syndrome. Antibiotics are not known to be effective and may increase the likelihood of hemolytic uremic syndrome.

- *Escherichia coli* O157:H7 has been identified as the cause of waterborne illness, outbreaks in nursing homes and child care centers, and sporadic cases.

- Eating undercooked beef also transmits *E coli* O157:H7.

- Bloody diarrhea, severe abdominal cramps, and profound toxicity characterize *E coli* O157:H7 infection; it may resemble ischemic colitis.

- Infection should be considered in all patients with hemolytic uremic syndrome.

- Antibiotic therapy is not recommended.

Shigella

Diarrhea caused by *Shigella* species is often acquired outside the United States. It often is spread from person to person or consumption of contaminated food or water. Bloody diarrhea is characteristic, bacteremia may occur, and fever is present. The diagnosis is confirmed by stool culture and blood culture (occasionally positive). Treatment is with ampicillin, trimethoprim-sulfamethoxazole, norfloxacin, ciprofloxacin, or azithromycin. Resistance to ampicillin, trimethoprim-sulfamethoxazole, fluoroquinolone, or azithromycin has been reported. The illness may precede the onset of spondyloarthropathy (reactive arthritis) in persons with HLA-B2 and group B *Shigella flexneri*.

- Diarrhea caused by *Shigella* species is associated with person-to-person transmission and the consumption of contaminated food or water.

- Bloody diarrhea is characteristic, bacteremia may occur, and fever is present.

- The illness may precede the onset of spondyloarthropathy (reactive arthritis) in persons with HLA-B2 and group B *S flexneri*.

Salmonella

Salmonella (non-*typhi*)-associated illness most commonly is caused by *Salmonella enteritidis* and *Salmonella typhimurium* in the United States. It is associated with consumption of contaminated foods or with exposure to reptiles and snakes, pet turtles, ducklings, and iguanas. Large outbreaks have been associated with produce and even contaminated peanut butter, food sources that were previously not associated with this infection. *Salmonella* infection is a common cause of severe diarrhea and may cause septicemia in patients with sickle cell anemia or AIDS. *Salmonella* bacteremia can lead to hematogenous seeding of abdominal aortic plaques resulting in mycotic aneurysms. In *Salmonella* enteritis, fever is usually present, and bloody diarrhea is often absent (a characteristic distinguishing it from *Shigella* infection). The diagnosis is based on stool culture. Treatment is supportive. Antibiotics may prolong the carrier state and do not affect the course of the disease. Antibiotics are used if results of blood culture are positive. Reactive arthritis may be a complication of this illness.

- Large outbreaks of *Salmonella* gastroenteritis have recently been associated with produce and peanut butter, food sources that were not previously associated with this infection.

- *Salmonella* infection may cause septicemia in patients with sickle cell anemia or AIDS.

- Bloody diarrhea is often absent (a feature distinguishing it from *Shigella* infection).

- *Salmonella* bacteremia can lead to hematogenous seeding of abdominal aortic plaques resulting in mycotic aneurysms.

- In nonbacteremic patients with *Salmonella*-associated diarrhea, antibiotics may prolong the carrier state and do not affect the course of the disease.

Salmonella serotype *typhi* is rare in the United States; often, it is found in travelers returning from endemic regions who present with fever. Patients with typhoid fever have relative bradycardia and rose spots (50%). The leukocyte count may be decreased. Blood cultures usually are positive within approximately 10 days of symptom onset, whereas stool cultures become positive later.

There are many nontyphoidal *Salmonella* species. *Salmonella typhimurium* and *S enteritidis* produce gastroenteritis and occasionally bacteremia. Nontyphoidal *Salmonella* species can cause chronic bacteremia and infections of atherosclerotic aortic aneurysms. Urinary tract infections caused by *Salmonella* particularly occur in patients who are coinfected with *Schistosoma haematobium*. Antimicrobial resistance is increasingly common with *Salmonella* serotype *typhi*. Most cases of *Salmonella* gastroenteritis resolve without therapy. Serious or invasive infections should be treated with a third-generation cephalosporin or fluoroquinolone pending susceptibility data.

- *Salmonella* serotype *typhi* is rare in the United States and often found encountered in travelers returning from endemic regions who present with fever.

- Urinary tract infections caused by *Salmonella* particularly occur in patients who are coinfected with *S haematobium*.

LISTERIA MONOCYTOGENES

Listeria monocytogenes is a gram-positive rod, often mistaken for a diphtheroid in clinical cultures. Most often recognized as a cause of meningitis, it can be associated with food-borne diarrhea, typically acquired from processed deli meats, paté, or hot dogs consumed in the summer. The incubation period ranges from 6 hours to 90 days. The mean onset is about 24 hours (range, 6–240 hours). In most persons, febrile gastroenteritis is self-limited over 2 or 3 days. Infection can be severe and disseminate to involve multiple organs and cause meningitis in patients with cellular immune defects (those with a transplant or HIV, those taking immunosuppressive medications). In pregnant women, it may present as a flulike illness and can lead to fetal death or premature birth. Neonatal infection, also called "granulomatosis infantiseptica," may result from transplacental transmission of *Listeria*. Diagnosis is made by stool or blood culture. Severe listerial infections are usually treated with ampicillin plus gentamicin.

- *Listeria monocytogenes* enteritis is typically acquired from processed deli meats, paté, or hot dogs.

- Infection can be severe and disseminate to involve multiple organs in patients with cellular immune defects.

- In pregnant women, *L monocytogenes* infection may present as a flulike illness and can lead to fetal death or premature birth.

VIBRIO SPECIES

Vibrio cholerae causes a toxigenic bacterial diarrhea. In the United States, consumption of raw or undercooked shellfish such as oysters is the most common source of infection with pathogenic vibrios (eg, *Vibrio parahaemolyticus*, *Vibrio vulnificus*). Disease usually manifests as self-limited enteritis. Cholera, caused by *V cholerae*, continues to cause periodic pandemics, the most recent affecting South and Central America. Cholera is rare in the United States and Canada, even in travelers. Epidemics of cholera continue in many countries around the world, with a recent widespread outbreak in Haiti. Antibiotics (tetracycline) shorten the duration of illness. Fluid replacement therapy is the mainstay of management.

- Epidemics of cholera continue in many countries around the world, including a recent widespread outbreak in Haiti.

- Consumption of raw or undercooked shellfish such as oysters is the most common source of infection with pathogenic vibrios (eg, *V parahaemolyticus*, *V vulnificus*).

Vibrio parahaemolyticus infection is acquired by eating undercooked shellfish. It is a common bacterial cause of acute food-borne illness in Japan and is appearing with increasing frequency in the United States (along the Atlantic Gulf Coast and on cruise ships). Acute onset of explosive, watery diarrhea and fever are characteristic. The diagnosis is determined with stool culture. Antibiotic therapy is not required.

- Antibiotic therapy is not required for *V parahaemolyticus* infection.

YERSINIA ENTEROCOLITICA

Yersinia enterocolitica is the etiologic agent of several major clinical syndromes: enterocolitis, mesenteric adenitis, erythema nodosum, polyarthritis, Reiter syndrome, and bacteremia associated with contaminated blood products. Approximately 20% of infected patients have sore throat. Infection with *Y enterocolitica* causing mesenteric adenitis can mimic acute appendicitis. Acquisition of infection is thought to be associated with eating contaminated food products. The organism has been cultured from chocolate milk, meat, mussels, poultry, oysters, and cheese.

- In adults with *Y enterocolitica* infection, erythema nodosum, polyarthritis, and Reiter syndrome can develop.

- Infection with *Y enterocolitica* causing mesenteric adenitis can mimic acute appendicitis.

CLOSTRIDIUM DIFFICILE

Clostridium difficile infection should be distinguished from other forms of antibiotic-associated diarrhea (ie, watery stools, no systemic symptoms, and negative tests for *C difficile* toxin). Symptoms often occur after exposure to antibiotics and health care settings. Antibiotics with high biliary concentrations and broad aerobic and anaerobic activity are associated with *C difficile* infection. It occurs more commonly in the elderly, and is associated with an increased morbidity. The disease spectrum ranges from mild diarrhea to severe, life-threatening colitis. Typical features are profuse, watery stools; crampy abdominal pain; constitutional illness; unexplained leukocytosis; the presence of fecal leukocytes; and a positive result of *C difficile* toxin assay. In patients with a negative result of toxin assay in whom suspicion for the disease is high, proctoscopy or flexible sigmoidoscopy can be used to look for pseudomembranes. Disease can be localized to the cecum (postoperative patient with ileus) and can present as fever of unknown origin. A new toxigenic strain (North America pulsed-field type 1, NAP-1) associated with a binary toxin has become epidemic and is associated with fluoroquinolone resistance and more severe disease. Treatment of mild-moderate disease consists of metronidazole (500 mg orally 3 times daily for 10 days) or vancomycin (125 mg orally 4 times daily for 7–10 days). Oral vancomycin is preferred in cases of severe disease. If a patient is unable to take drugs orally, intravenous metronidazole (not vancomycin) or vancomycin enemas can be used. Relapse is frequent (>15% of cases) and necessitates re-treatment. Repeat stool testing after treatment is not recommended. Total colectomy may be lifesaving in severe cases.

- Colitis caused by *C difficile* often occurs in the setting of recent antibiotic use.

- Features of colitis caused by *C difficile* are profuse, watery stools; crampy abdominal pain; constitutional illness; fecal leukocytes; and leukocytosis.

- Treatment of *C difficile* infection is with metronidazole (500 mg orally 3 times daily for 10 days) or vancomycin (125 mg orally 4 times daily for 7–10 days).

- Oral vancomycin is preferred in severe cases.

- Relapse occurs in at least 15% of cases.

VIRAL DIARRHEA

Many types of viral diarrhea can be defined by their seasonal epidemiology. Rotavirus infection is the most common cause of sporadic mild diarrhea in children. It may be spread from children to adults. It usually occurs during the winter.

Vomiting is a more common early manifestation than watery diarrhea. Hospitalization for dehydration is common in young children. Diagnosis is made by detection of antigen in stool. Treatment is symptomatic.

Noroviruses are a common cause of epidemic diarrhea and "winter vomiting disease" in older children and adults and have high secondary attack rates. Outbreaks have been reported from day-care facilities, nursing homes, hospitals, family gatherings, and cruise ships. Various contaminated foods such as shellfish, undercooked fish, cake frosting, salads, and water have been implicated. The illness is an explosive, self-limited (36 hours) condition with severe nausea, vomiting, watery diarrhea, and dehydration. Treatment is symptomatic.

- Outbreaks of norovirus are associated with eating shellfish, undercooked fish, cake frosting, and salads and with drinking contaminated water.

- Numerous outbreaks of noroviruses have occurred on cruise ships.

- Illness, although potentially severe and dominated by vomiting, is self-limited.

PARASITIC DIARRHEA

The travel and exposure histories are critical to determining which agents should be sought. The parasitic conditions that are most common in the United States are giardiasis, amebiasis, and cryptosporidiosis. Giardiasis may present with abdominal bloating, weight loss, and flatulence. Hosts at risk are homosexual men, hikers with exposures to streams, day-care contacts, and persons with immunoglobulin A deficiency or HIV. A wet preparation examination of stool or a *Giardia* antigen test may establish the diagnosis. Treatment is with metronidazole or tinidazole.

Entamoeba histolytica infection is acquired through ingestion of contaminated water or food containing cysts from an infected carrier. The disease may be more common in immigrants from regions with high endemic rates of amebiasis such as Central and South America. Infected persons most commonly present with a subacute onset of colitis or liver abscess. The diagnosis can be made by stool testing or serum antibody tests. Treatment is with metronidazole (750 mg 3 times daily for 7–10 days). After treatment, the intestinal carrier state is eradicated with paromomycin or iodoquinol.

Cryptosporidium parvum is an important cause of diarrhea, especially in persons with AIDS, who may have a chronic, debilitating illness. Cryptosporidiosis is also a cause of self-limited diarrhea in otherwise healthy persons. Waterborne outbreaks have been reported in Georgia and Wisconsin. They occur most often in late summer or fall. The organism is resistant to chlorination and can best be eliminated from water sources by microfiltration. Thirty-five percent of patients have a coinfection, most commonly with *Giardia*.

The stool *Cryptosporidium* enzyme-linked immunosorbent assay–based antigen test has sensitivity of 87%, specificity 99%, and positive predictive value 98%. It has to be ordered specifically if cryptosporidiosis is in the differential diagnosis.

There is no effective therapy for *Cryptosporidium*. Paromomycin and nitazoxanide, a new drug, show some efficacy. Nitazoxanide has efficacy of 56% to 88% in immunocompetent patients.

- Cryptosporidiosis is an important cause of diarrhea in patients with AIDS.

- Waterborne outbreaks have been reported.

- The diagnosis may be missed on standard stool examination for ova and parasites.

Cyclospora cayetanensis is a protozoan that can cause persistent diarrhea, fever, and profound fatigue. First described in travelers to tropical areas of the world, disease due to *Cyclospora* also has been linked to consumption of contaminated food shipped to the United States (eg, raspberries from Guatemala). Like *Cryptosporidium*, the organism may not be detected on routine stool examinations; therefore, testing specific to the organism should be ordered. The illness can be effectively treated with trimethoprim-sulfamethoxazole.

- Infection with *C cayetanensis* causes persistent diarrhea, fever, and profound fatigue.

- Disease due to *Cyclospora* has been linked to consumption of contaminated food shipped to the United States (raspberries from Guatemala).

INTRA-ABDOMINAL ABSCESSES

Intra-abdominal abscesses may arise from a hematogenous, contiguous, traumatic, or operative route. Hepatic abscesses are among the most common and may be bacterial or nonbacterial in origin. Nonbacterial organisms are *Candida* and *E histolytica* (amebic abscess). However, most hepatic abscesses are bacterial in origin as a result of portal vein bacteremia from an intestinal source such as appendicitis or diverticulitis; bacteremia from a primary focus elsewhere; biliary tract origin, as in obstruction or ascending cholangitis; direct extension (subphrenic abscess); or trauma. Most often, patients present with the insidious onset of symptoms of malaise and anorexia followed by right upper abdominal pain and fever. Computed tomography is the best test for diagnosis of intra-abdominal and hepatic abscesses. The microbiologic nature is variable, depending on the origin. Biliary-source infections are usually due to enteric gram-negative bacteria such as *E coli* or *Enterobacter* species, whereas intestinal sources are often polymicrobial (Enterobacteriacae, *Streptococcus anginosus* group, and *Bacteroides*). The initial evaluation of a hepatic abscess should include blood cultures and amebic serologic tests. If the amebic serologic results are negative, aspiration should be performed and antibiotics directed according to culture results. Pyogenic abscesses are best managed by percutaneous drainage and antimicrobial therapy. Empiric options include ampicillin plus gentamicin, a fluoroquinolone plus metronidazole, or a third-generation cephalosporin plus metronidazole, a β-lactam/β-lactamase inhibitor combination, or a carbapenem. If a hematogenous route is suspected, an agent that is active against staphylococci should be used in the regimen.

Splenic abscesses are much less common but occur in a few specific settings: infective endocarditis, malignancies, trauma, and sickle cell disease. Patients may present with fever, vague abdominal pain, or left-sided pleuritic pain. Unexplained thrombocytosis in the setting of fever should raise the concern for splenic abscess. Because of the predominance of endocarditis as the source, streptococci are found most often. Small abscesses (<3 cm) can be managed with percutaneous drainage and directed antimicrobial therapy. Large abscesses usually require splenectomy.

Perinephric abscesses are rare; they usually arise in the setting of complicated upper urinary tract infections. The presence of upper tract instrumentation or infected stones may be risk factors. The microbes are usually those associated with upper urinary tract infection (*E coli*, *Proteus*, *Klebsiella*, and *Candida*). Hematogenous renal abscesses may occur with candidemia or *S aureus* bacteremias.

Psoas abscesses arise in the setting of contiguous spread from infections involving the retroperitoneum. They may be of perivertebral, genitourinary, or gastrointestinal (eg, Crohn disease, diverticulitis) origin. Hematogenous spread occurs with *S aureus* infection. The psoas muscle is also a site of tuberculous abscesses. Management is percutaneous drainage and directed antimicrobial therapy.

Pancreatic abscesses are rare and occur several weeks following a prolonged bout of pancreatitis with infected pancreatic necrosis. These infections are often polymicrobial and reflect the biliary and intestinal flora and staphylococci. Treatment is percutaneous drainage and directed antimicrobial therapy.

- Surgery is rarely needed for intra-abdominal abscesses if percutaneous drainage is accessible.

- Splenic abscesses are much less common but occur in a few specific settings: infective endocarditis, malignancies, trauma, and sickle cell disease.

- Psoas abscesses arise in the setting of contiguous spread from infections involving the retroperitoneum. They may be of perivertebral, genitourinary, or gastrointestinal (eg, Crohn disease, diverticulitis) origin.

21.

HIV INFECTION[a]

Mary J. Kasten, MD, and Zelalem Temesgen, MD

GOALS

- Identify how human immunodeficiency virus (HIV) is transmitted and what behaviors and conditions affect the risk of transmission.

- Review the natural history of HIV infection and AIDS, including AIDS-defining conditions.

- Recognize when treatment for HIV is indicated and understand the basic principles of antiretroviral treatment.

- Recognize when prophylaxis is indicated for opportunistic infection in HIV-infected patients and for which infections it should be given.

AIDS was first reported in 1981, when gay men presented with *Pneumocystis* pneumonia or Kaposi sarcoma. HIV was identified as the cause of AIDS in 1984. Testing for HIV became available in the United States in 1985. Considerable gains in the understanding and treatment of HIV have been made during the past 30 years.

There are 2 types of HIV: HIV-1 and HIV-2. Most reported cases of HIV disease around the world are caused by HIV-1. HIV-2 occurs predominantly in western Africa. Although HIV-1 and HIV-2 are clinically indistinguishable and have identical modes of transmission, HIV-2 is less easily transmitted than HIV-1 and slower to progress to AIDS.

- There are 2 types of HIV: HIV-1 and HIV-2.

- Most reported cases of HIV disease are caused by HIV-1.

EPIDEMIOLOGY

An estimated 33.3 million people in the world are living with HIV. Approximately 2.6 million people were infected with the virus in 2009. More than 25 million people have died of AIDS, 1.8 million in 2009 alone. More than 90% of the people living with HIV reside in developing countries where resources for diagnosis, prevention, and management of HIV are scarce. In the United States, an estimated 1.2 million persons are living with HIV; about one-fifth of these do not know they are infected. Persons with undiagnosed infection are thought to be responsible for a substantial proportion of new infections in the United States.

Nearly half of all persons with newly diagnosed HIV in the United States are African Americans even though they make up only 13% of the general population. One-fourth of newly diagnosed cases in the United States are in women. Globally, half of HIV-infected persons are women.

- Persons with undiagnosed HIV infection are responsible for a substantial proportion of HIV transmission.

- Globally, half of HIV-infected persons are women.

TRANSMISSION

HIV is transmitted sexually, perinatally, by parenteral inoculation (eg, intravenous drug injection, occupational exposure), through blood products, and, less commonly, through donated organs or semen. Sexual transmission is the most common means of infection. Conditions that may increase the risk of sexually acquiring HIV infection include traumatic intercourse (ie, receptive anal), ulcerative genital infections (including syphilis, herpes simplex, and chancroid), and lack of circumcision. The proper use of latex condoms substantially reduces the risk of HIV transmission. Nonoxynol spermicide increases the risk of HIV transmission; therefore, condoms that do not contain spermicide are preferred for HIV prevention. Perinatal transmission can occur in utero, at the time of birth, and through breast milk.

a Portions previously published in Warnke D, Barreto J, Temesgen Z. Antiretroviral drugs. J Clin Pharmacol. 2007 Dec;47(12):1570–9. Used with permission; treatment guidelines for opportunistic infections based on Benson CA, Kaplan JE, Masur H, Pau A, Holmes KK; CDC; National Institutes of Health; Infectious Diseases Society of America. Treating opportunistic infections among HIV-infected adults and adolescents: recommendations from CDC, the National Institutes of Health, and the HIV Medicine Association/Infectious Diseases Society of America. MMWR Recomm Rep. 2004 Dec 17;53(RR-15):1–112. Erratum in: MMWR Morb Mortal Wkly Rep. 2005 Apr 1;54(12):311.

Table 21.1 RISK OF ACQUIRING HIV, BY TYPE OF EXPOSURE

TYPE OF EXPOSURE	RISK, %
Transfusion of HIV-positive blood	>90
Percutaneous needlestick	0.3
Receptive anal intercourse	0.5
Receptive penile-vaginal intercourse	0.1
Insertive intercourse	0.05–0.07
Oral intercourse	0.005–0.01
Blood to mucous membranes	0.09
Blood to nonintact skin	<0.1

Abbreviation: HIV, human immunodeficiency virus.

The mode of transmission of HIV infection varies from region to region. In North America, men who have sex with men make up the largest population of those living with HIV and those with a new diagnosis. In sub-Saharan Africa, heterosexual intercourse is the primary mode of transmission of HIV. In eastern Europe and central Asia, more than half of new HIV infections are due to the use of nonsterile equipment used for injecting drugs.

In the United States, all blood donations have been routinely tested for HIV-1 antibody since early 1985. This practice has virtually eliminated the transmission of HIV through blood products in the United States.

- The risk of acquiring HIV varies greatly depending on the exposure (Table 21.1).

- The risk of sexually acquiring HIV varies greatly: receptive anal intercourse > receptive vaginal intercourse > insertive intercourse >>> oral intercourse.

- Circumcision decreases the risk of acquiring HIV infection.

- Proper use of latex condoms decreases HIV transmission during sex.

LABORATORY DIAGNOSIS

The enzyme-linked immunosorbent assays (ELISAs) and enzyme immunoassays (EIAs) are the most common assays used as a screening test for HIV-1 infection. They detect HIV-specific antibodies. They have high (>99%) sensitivity and specificity but low positive predictive values in low-prevalence populations. For this reason, positive results require confirmation with an additional test. False-positive results can occur for several reasons. These include the presence of cross-reacting antibodies in certain patients (eg, multiparous women and persons who have received

multiple transfusions) and participation in HIV vaccine studies. Causes of false-negative results include testing during the pre-seroconversion (window) period, bone marrow transplant, agammaglobulinemia, seroreversion in late-stage disease, and infection with HIV-2 or unusual HIV subtypes (eg, subtypes O and N). Technical or laboratory error can be a cause of both false-positive and false-negative results. Rapid tests for HIV with high sensitivity and specificity similar to conventional HIV screening tests have been approved by the US Food and Drug Administration (FDA); positive results of these tests also require confirmatory testing.

Individuals with positive results of ELISA, EIA, or a rapid test should undergo confirmatory testing, usually Western blot (WB) antibody testing. The guidelines of the Centers for Disease Control and Prevention (CDC) for interpretation of the WB test are as follows: the presence of antibody against any 2 of the 3 major viral gene products (p24, gp41, or gp120/gp160) is classified as positive; an HIV WB result is classified as negative if no major or minor bands are present; results that cannot be classified as positive or negative on the basis of these criteria are categorized as indeterminate. If results are indeterminate, the clinician should assess the risk of HIV infection in the patient and retest in 1 to 3 months. HIV RNA assays may be of additional help in these cases, particularly if a patient is at high risk for HIV infection. The risk of HIV infection is extremely low in patients with repeatedly indeterminate WB results.

- An HIV ELISA, EIA, or an FDA-approved rapid test should be used to screen people for chronic HIV infection.

- HIV WB testing is used to confirm positive results of screening tests for HIV.

The CDC recommends that screening for HIV infection be performed routinely for all patients 13 to 64 years old. An opt-out approach, similar to what has been used successfully for many years with pregnant women, is recommended. With the opt-out approach, testing is performed after the patient is notified, unless the patient declines. Neither separate written consent nor prevention counseling is required; general consent for medical care is considered sufficient to encompass consent for HIV testing. It is hoped that routine screening will lead to earlier diagnosis and earlier treatment of HIV and thus improved health, extended lifespan, decrease in HIV transmission, and decrease in the stigma of testing. Studies have shown that most people, once HIV is diagnosed, change their behavior to decrease risk of transmission to others.

Patients who engage in behaviors that place them at risk of being infected with HIV should be screened on a regular basis. All pregnant women should be screened for HIV infection even if the results of previous screening have been negative. Chronic HIV infection should be considered in patients with many different presentations; some of the more common clues are listed in Box 21.1.

NATURAL HISTORY OF HIV DISEASE

ACUTE HIV INFECTION

Days to weeks after exposure to HIV, most infected persons present with a brief illness that may last from a few days to a few weeks. This period of illness is associated with an enormous amount of circulating virus, a rapid decline in the CD4 cell count, and a vigorous immune response. Occasionally, CD4 counts decrease to levels at which patients can present with opportunistic illness. Patients often present with a mononucleosis-like illness, but the clinical manifestations of acute HIV infection are extremely varied (Table 21.2). Severe acute infections have been associated with more rapid progression of HIV disease. One should consider acute HIV infection in patients with any unusual febrile illness or viral-like syndrome. Results of ELISA are usually negative (window period), and the results of WB testing should be negative or indeterminate. However, p24 antigen, HIV culture, and polymerase chain reaction results may be positive. During acute symptomatic infection, the viral load (HIV RNA level) is high, generally more than 100,000 copies/mL, and patients are highly infectious.

- Acute HIV infection occurs within days to weeks after exposure to HIV.

- Acute HIV often presents with a mononucleosis-type illness.

- Acute HIV can imitate many other illnesses and syndromes.

- Results of WB testing should be negative or indeterminate for HIV with acute infection.

Table 21.2 FREQUENCY OF SYMPTOMS AND FINDINGS ASSOCIATED WITH ACUTE HIV-1 INFECTION

SYMPTOM OR FINDING	PERCENTAGE OF PATIENTS
Fever	>80–90
Fatigue	>70–90
Rash	>40–80
Headache	32–70
Lymphadenopathy	40–70
Pharyngitis	50–70
Myalgia or arthralgia	50–70
Nausea, vomiting, or diarrhea	30–60
Night sweats	50
Aseptic meningitis	24
Oral ulcers	10–20
Genital ulcers	5–15
Thrombocytopenia	45
Leukopenia	40
Elevated hepatic-enzyme levels	21

Abbreviation: HIV, human immunodeficiency virus.

Adapted from Kahn JO, Walker BD. Acute human immunodeficiency virus type 1 infection. N Engl J Med. 1998 Jul 2;339(1):33–9. Used with permission.

- The viral load is usually very high during acute HIV.

CHRONIC HIV INFECTION

After acute HIV infection, CD4 counts rebound, although not always to baseline, and the viral load decreases to a set point that often stays stable for years. Over time, most patients have a gradual loss of CD4 cells. Some patients remain asymptomatic with relatively preserved CD4 counts for more than a decade; other patients progress to AIDS in 2 to 3 years. The loss of CD4 cells eventually places the individual at risk for opportunistic infections and other complications of HIV. The CDC defines AIDS as known HIV infection with a CD4 count less than 200 cells/mcL or HIV infection associated with an AIDS-defining illness (Box 21.2).

- Gradual loss of CD4 cells is the hallmark of HIV infection.

- The rate of progression to AIDS is variable.

The illnesses and conditions associated with HIV infection vary greatly depending on an individual's CD4 count and other behaviors. Figure 21.1 illustrates the natural history of HIV infection and the stages at which conditions that are commonly associated with HIV infection occur.

Box 21.2 **AIDS-DEFINING CONDITIONS IN ADULTS**

Candidiasis of bronchi, trachea, or lungs

Candidiasis, esophageal

Cervical cancer, invasive

Coccidioidomycosis, disseminated or extrapulmonary

Cryptococcosis, extrapulmonary

Cryptosporidiosis, chronic intestinal (>1 mo duration)

Cytomegalovirus disease (other than liver, spleen, or nodes)

Cytomegalovirus retinitis (with loss of vision)

Encephalopathy, HIV-related

Herpes simplex: chronic ulcer(s) (>1 mo duration) or bronchitis, pneumonitis, or esophagitis

Histoplasmosis, disseminated or extrapulmonary

Isosporiasis, chronic intestinal (>1 mo duration)

Kaposi sarcoma

Lymphoma, Burkitt (or equivalent term)

Lymphoma, immunoblastic (or equivalent term)

Lymphoma, primary, of brain

Mycobacterium avium complex or *Mycobacterium kansasii*, disseminated or extrapulmonary

Mycobacterium tuberculosis, any site

Mycobacterium, other species or unidentified species, disseminated or extrapulmonary

Pneumocystis jiroveci pneumonia

Pneumonia, recurrent

Progressive multifocal leukoencephalopathy

Salmonella septicemia, recurrent

Toxoplasmosis of brain

Wasting syndrome due to HIV

Abbreviation: HIV, human immunodeficiency virus.

Adapted from Schneider E, Whitmore S, Glynn MK, Dominguez K, Mitsch A, McKenna MT. Revised surveillance case definitions for HIV infection among adults, adolescents, and children aged <18 months and for HIV infection and AIDS among children aged 18 months to <13 years—United States, 2008. MMWR Morb Mortal Wkly Rep. 2008 Dec 5;57(RR10):1–8.

PRIMARY CARE AND HIV INFECTION

IMMUNIZATIONS

Patients with HIV infection should have routine immunizations, but live virus vaccines should be given cautiously and generally avoided in patients with CD4 counts less than 200 cells/mcL. One should consider deferring vaccination for patients with low CD4 cell counts and immunizing them once their immune system has improved. Alternatively, immunizations can be given and potentially repeated after immune recovery.

All patients with HIV infection who are not immune to or infected with hepatitis B should receive the hepatitis B series. Antibody response to the vaccination should be verified after the series is completed.

Hepatitis A vaccine is recommended for all patients who are at risk, including men who have sex with men, travelers to developing countries, and patients with hepatitis B or C or other liver disease.

Pneumovax should be given to all HIV-infected patients with CD4 counts more than 200 cells/mcL. A one-time revaccination 5 years after initial immunization is recommended. Pneumococcal vaccination should also be considered for patients with CD4 counts less than 200 cells/mcL who are not responding immunologically to antiretroviral medication.

All HIV-infected patients should receive annual inactivated influenza vaccine.

- A CD4 count <200 cells/mcL is associated with adverse effects of live virus vaccines.

- A CD4 count <200 cells/mcL is associated with a poorer response to immunization.

PROPHYLAXIS AGAINST OPPORTUNISTIC INFECTIONS

HIV-infected persons are susceptible to many unusual infections depending on their CD4 count. A few can be prevented with immunization or appropriate prophylaxis. Recommendations and indications for primary prevention of *Pneumocystis* pneumonia (PCP), *Mycobacterium avium* complex (MAC) infection, and toxoplasmosis are listed in Table 21.3. Primary prophylaxis against other infections is not routinely recommended. Primary prophylaxis against PCP and toxoplasmosis can be discontinued when the CD4 count is 200 cells/mcL or more for 3 months or more. Primary prophylaxis against MAC can be discontinued when the CD4 count is 100 cells/mcL or more for 3 months or more.

- A CD4 count <200 cells/mcL or thrush is an indication for PCP prophylaxis.

- A CD4 count <100 cells/mcL with a positive immunoglobulin G serologic result to toxoplasmosis is an indication for toxoplasmosis prophylaxis.

- A CD4 count <50 cells/mcL is an indication for MAC prophylaxis.

SUBSTANCE ABUSE

Many patients with HIV have healthy lifestyles, but others use illicit drugs, drink alcohol to excess, or smoke. It is imperative to address these issues with HIV-infected patients, and this should be done in a nonjudgmental way that helps patients move toward healthier behaviors. Illicit drug use is not a contraindication to antiretroviral medication, and many drug users are compliant with use of HIV medications. The provider needs to be aware of what substances are being used to ensure there are no worrisome drug interactions between prescribed and nonprescribed substances. Many patients with HIV smoke; as HIV-infected patients live longer and do well with HIV, illness related to tobacco use is increasing, including an increased risk of lung cancer and heart disease.

- Lifestyles and habits of patients with HIV need to be addressed because they may affect treatment and outcome.

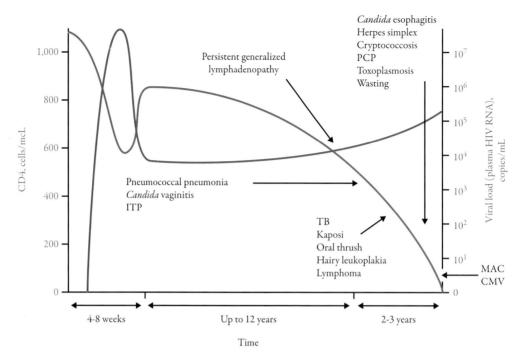

Figure 21.1 Natural History of Human Immunodeficiency Virus (HIV) Infection: CD4 Counts, Viral Load, and Clinical Manifestations. CMV indicates cytomegalovirus; ITP, idiopathic thrombocytopenic purpura; MAC, *Mycobacterium avium* complex; PCP, *Pneumocystis* pneumonia; TB, tuberculosis.

CANCER SCREENING

Three malignancies (Kaposi sarcoma, non-Hodgkin lymphoma, and invasive cervical cancer) have been designated as AIDS-defining cancers. Several other malignancies, although not classified as AIDS-defining, seem to be more common among people infected with HIV. HIV-infected patients who are generally well whether or not they are receiving antiretroviral treatment should have routine cancer screening as recommended for uninfected persons, with the exception of the need for more frequent Papanicolaou (Pap) smears. HIV-infected women should have a Pap smear at the time of diagnosis. If the result is normal, the Pap smear should be repeated in 6 months

Table 21.3 **PRIMARY PROPHYLAXIS FOR PCP, TOXOPLASMOSIS, AND MAC**

PATHOGEN/DISEASE	INDICATION	FIRST-CHOICE THERAPY	ALTERNATIVE THERAPY
Pneumocystis jiroveci pneumonia (PCP)	CD4 <200 cells/mcL or oropharyngeal candidiasis	TMP-SMX DS or TMP-SMX SS 1 tablet PO daily	TMP-SMX DS PO 3 times weekly *or* dapsone 100 mg or 50 mg PO bid *or* dapsone 50 mg PO daily + pyrimethamine 50 mg PO weekly + leucovorin 25 mg PO weekly *or* aerosolized pentamidine 300 mg monthly *or* atovaquone 1,500 mg PO daily
Toxoplasma gondii encephalitis	*Toxoplasma* IgG-positive with CD4 <100 cells/mcL	TMP-SMX DS 1 tablet PO daily	TMP-SMX DS 1 tablet PO 3 times weekly *or* TMP-SMX SS 1 tablet PO daily *or* dapsone 50 mg 1 tablet PO daily + pyrimethamine 50 mg & leucovorin 25 mg PO weekly *or* dapsone 200 mg + pyrimethamine 75 mg + leucovorin 25 mg weekly *or* atovaquone 1,500 mg + pyrimethamine 25 mg + leucovorin 10 mg PO daily
MAC disease	CD4 <50 cells/mcL after ruling out active MAC infection	Azithromycin 1,200 mg PO once weekly *or* clarithromycin 500 mg PO twice weekly *or* azithromycin 600 mg PO twice weekly	Rifabutin 300 mg PO daily (adjust based on interactions with antiretroviral therapy)

Abbreviations: bid, twice daily; DS, double strength; Ig, immunoglobulin; MAC, *Mycobacterium avium* complex; PCP, *Pneumocystis* pneumonia; PO, orally; SS, single strength; TMP-SMX, trimethoprim-sulfamethoxazole.

Adapted from Kaplan JE, Benson C, Holmes KK, Brooks JT, Pau A, Masur H. Guidelines for prevention and treatment of opportunistic infections in HIV-infected adults and adolescents: recommendations from CDC, the National Institutes of Health, and the HIV Medicine Association of the Infectious Diseases Society of America. MMWR Morb Mortal Wkly Rep. 2009 Apr 10;58(RR04):1–198.

and then annually. HIV-infected women with abnormal results of Pap smears should be followed by a practitioner with expertise in preventing cervical cancer in HIV-infected women. An anal Pap smear should be considered for men and women who have a history of receptive anal intercourse because of the increased incidence of human papillomavirus–related anal cell cancer, but it is not yet routinely recommended.

SELECTED INFECTIONS AND CONDITIONS ASSOCIATED WITH HIV INFECTION

PNEUMOCYSTIS PNEUMONIA

One of the most common opportunistic infections in patients with AIDS is PCP. It typically occurs in patients with CD4 counts less than 200 cells/mcL. Other risk factors include CD4 percentage less than 15%, oral thrush, recurrent bacterial pneumonia, high HIV-1 RNA level, unintentional weight loss, and previous episodes of PCP. The onset of illness is usually insidious, with several days to weeks of fever, exertional dyspnea, chest discomfort, weight loss, malaise, and night sweats. Chest radiography typically shows bilateral interstitial pulmonary infiltrates; a lobar distribution and spontaneous pneumothoraces may also occur. Patients with early disease can have a normal chest radiograph. Pleural effusion is uncommon. Thin-section computed tomography usually shows patchy ground-glass infiltrates. Arterial blood gas analysis usually shows hypoxemia and respiratory alkalosis. Increased lactate dehydrogenase level is common but not specific for PCP.

Several methods are used for the diagnosis of PCP. In HIV-infected persons, staining for *Pneumocystis* organisms in hypertonic saline-induced expectorated sputum is 55% to 90% sensitive, and bronchoalveolar lavage is 90% to 97% sensitive. Transbronchial lung biopsy increases the sensitivity of

staining for *Pneumocystis* to about 100%. Open lung biopsy is rarely required for the diagnosis of PCP in HIV-infected patients. Extrapulmonary *Pneumocystis* disease is uncommon but can be present in any organ.

- Staining for *Pneumocystis* organisms in induced sputum is a sensitive and noninvasive method for diagnosing PCP in patients with HIV infection.

The treatment of choice for PCP is trimethoprim-sulfamethoxazole (TMP-SMX). The usual recommended dosage is 15 mg/kg per day (trimethoprim component) in 3 or 4 equally divided doses for 21 days. If there is no improvement 4 to 8 days after treatment is begun, switching to another drug should be considered. Alternative treatment options are listed in Table 21.4. Controlled studies have shown that adjunctive corticosteroid therapy increases survival in patients with moderate to severe disease, defined as room air Po_2 less than 70 mm Hg or an alveolar-arterial Po_2 difference (A-a gradient) more than 35 mm Hg. When indicated, adjunctive corticosteroid therapy should be started immediately; a delay may compromise its effectiveness. The recommended corticosteroid program for severe PCP is prednisone 40 mg twice daily for 5 days followed by 40 mg daily for 5 days followed by 20 mg daily until treatment is completed.

- The treatment of choice for PCP is TMP-SMX.
- Adjunctive corticosteroid therapy increases survival in patients with moderate to severe disease.

Primary prophylaxis for PCP is reviewed in Table 21.3. Secondary prophylaxis (prevention of PCP after an episode of PCP) is also with TMP-SMX and should generally be discontinued if patients have sustained a CD4 count of more than

Table 21.4 DRUG THERAPY FOR *PNEUMOCYSTIS* PNEUMONIA

PREFERRED THERAPY, DURATION OF THERAPY	ALTERNATIVE THERAPY
For moderate to severe PCP TMP-SMX: 15–20 mg TMP & 75–100 mg SMX/kg daily IV administered every 6 to 8 h, may switch to PO after clinical improvement Duration: 21 d	For moderate to severe PCP Pentamidine 4 mg/kg IV daily infused over ≥60 minutes; certain specialists reduce dose to 3 mg/kg IV daily because of toxicities *Or* Primaquine 15–30 mg (base) PO daily plus clindamycin 600–900 mg IV every 6 to every 8 h or clindamycin 300–450 mg PO every 6 to 8 h
For mild to moderate PCP Same daily dose of TMP-SMX as above, administered PO in 3 divided doses; *or* TMP-SMX (160 mg/800 mg or DS) 2 tablets tid Duration: 21 d	For mild to moderate PCP Dapsone 100 mg PO daily & TMP 15 mg/kg PO daily (3 divided doses) *Or* Primaquine 15–30 mg (base) PO daily + clindamycin 300–450 mg PO every 6 to every 8 h *Or* Atovaquone 750 mg PO bid with food

Abbreviations: bid, twice daily; DS, double strength; IV, intravenously; PCP, *Pneumocystis* pneumonia; PO, orally; tid, 3 times daily; TMP-SMX, trimethoprim-sulfamethoxazole.

Adapted from Kaplan JE, Benson C, Holmes KK, Brooks JT, Pau A, Masur H. Guidelines for prevention and treatment of opportunistic infections in HIV-infected adults and adolescents: recommendations from CDC, the National Institutes of Health, and the HIV Medicine Association of the Infectious Diseases Society of America. MMWR Morb Mortal Wkly Rep. 2009 Apr 10;58(RR04):1–198.

200 cells/mcL for at least 3 months as a result of antiretroviral therapy. Rarely, PCP occurs at higher CD4 counts, and secondary prophylaxis should then be continued longer.

TUBERCULOSIS

Tuberculosis (TB) is the most common HIV-associated opportunistic infection globally. TB is a preventable disease; all patients with HIV infection should be screened with either a tuberculin skin test or an interferon-γ release assay. All HIV-infected patients with a positive test result (≥5 mm for the skin test), a past history of a positive test result, or recent exposure to a person with active TB should be treated for latent TB provided they have no symptoms or signs to suggest active infection and have not been previously treated. Box 21.3 reviews effective treatment programs for latent TB. TB occurs among HIV-infected persons at all CD4 counts. However, clinical manifestations generally differ depending on the degree of immunosuppression. When TB occurs late in the course of HIV infection, it tends to have atypical features, such as extrapulmonary disease, disseminated disease, and unusual chest radiographic appearance (lower lung zone lesions, intrathoracic adenopathy, diffuse infiltrations, and lower frequency of cavitation). Patients with low CD4 counts and TB have a high mortality rate (70%) and often have a fulminant course leading to death in 2 to 3 months. When TB occurs early in the course of HIV infection (CD4 count >350 cells/mcL), it tends to manifest with the classic presentation of upper lobe fibronodular infiltrates with cavitation.

- TB can occur at all CD4 counts in HIV infection.
- TB that occurs late in HIV infection tends to have atypical features and a more aggressive course.
- A tuberculin skin test result of ≥5 mm is interpreted as positive in HIV-infected patients.
- All HIV-infected patients with latent TB should be treated.

The diagnosis of TB requires evaluation with a chest radiograph, sputum samples for acid-fast bacillus smear and culture, and aspiration or tissue biopsy if extrapulmonary disease is suspected. Mycobacterial blood cultures are useful in cases of disseminated disease. In patients with relatively intact immune function, the yield of sputum smear and culture is similar to that in HIV-negative patients.

The management of HIV-infected patients taking antiretroviral agents and undergoing treatment for active TB is complex. Protease inhibitors and nonnucleoside analogue reverse transcriptase inhibitors (NNRTIs) have significant interactions with the rifamycins (rifampin, rifabutin, and rifapentine) used to treat mycobacterial infections. Compared with rifampin, rifabutin has substantially less activity as an inducer of cytochrome P450. Substitution of rifabutin for rifampin in treatment regimens for TB is a practical choice for patients who are also undergoing therapy with protease inhibitors or with NNRTIs. TB in HIV-infected persons that is susceptible to all first-line antituberculosis drugs may be treated with the standard 6-month drug program. Clinicians should consider factors that increase a person's risk for a poor clinical outcome (eg, lack of adherence to TB therapy, delayed conversion of *Mycobacterium tuberculosis* sputum cultures from positive to negative, and delayed clinical response) when deciding the total duration of TB therapy. Directly observed therapy is recommended. Patients who have successfully completed a regimen of treatment for TB do not require secondary prophylaxis or chronic maintenance therapy. Patients with multiple drug-resistant TB are at high risk for relapse and treatment failure. Treatment regimens for these patients are complex and require expertise in management of both TB and HIV infection.

- Antituberculosis drugs, particularly the rifamycins, interact with many anti-HIV drugs.
- A 6-month course of treatment may be used for pulmonary TB that is susceptible to all first-line antituberculosis drugs.

Paradoxical reactions have been reported with the concurrent administration of antiretroviral and antituberculosis therapy. These reactions, termed *immune reconstitution inflammatory syndrome*, are attributed to the recovery of the patient's delayed hypersensitivity response and include hectic fevers, lymphadenopathy, worsening of chest radiographic manifestations of TB (eg, miliary infiltrates, pleural effusions), and worsening of original tuberculous lesions (eg, expanding central nervous system lesions). Changes in antituberculosis or antiretroviral therapy are rarely needed. If the symptoms are severe, a short course of steroids to suppress the enhanced immune response can be attempted while continuing with antituberculosis and antiretroviral therapy. Patients with both active TB and HIV benefit from prompt antiretroviral treatment of HIV in addition to treatment of TB despite the risk of immune reconstitution inflammatory syndrome.

Box 21.3 PREFERRED REGIMENS FOR THE TREATMENT OF LATENT TUBERCULOSIS INFECTION

Isoniazid 300 mg PO daily + pyridoxine 50 mg PO daily for 9 mo

Isoniazid 900 mg twice weekly + pyridoxine 50 mg PO twice weekly for 9 mo

Rifampin 600 mg PO daily for 4 mo

Abbreviation: PO, orally.

MYCOBACTERIUM AVIUM COMPLEX INFECTION

Organisms of the *Mycobacterium avium* complex (MAC) are ubiquitous in the environment and include *M avium* and *Mycobacterium intracellulare*. They cause disseminated infection in HIV-infected persons, especially when immunosuppression is severe (CD4 count <50 cells/mcL). Disseminated MAC infection is a common systemic bacterial infection in patients with AIDS and very low CD4 counts. Common presentations include low-grade fever, night sweats, weight loss, fatigue, abdominal pain, and diarrhea. Hepatomegaly, splenomegaly, and lymphadenopathy may be present. Common laboratory abnormalities include anemia and increased alkaline phosphatase levels. Blood cultures are usually positive; however, organisms can also be isolated from stool, respiratory tract secretions, bone marrow, liver, and other biopsy specimens.

- MAC causes infection when immunosuppression is severe (CD4 count <50 cells/mcL).

- MAC is the most common systemic bacterial infection in HIV-infected patients with AIDS.

The organisms of MAC are resistant to conventional antimycobacterial agents. The current recommended treatment regimen includes one of the newer macrolides (eg, clarithromycin, azithromycin), ethambutol, and 1 or 2 additional drugs with activity against MAC. These include rifabutin, rifampin, ciprofloxacin, amikacin, and clofazimine. Rifabutin is thought to be the best option for a third agent; in randomized clinical trials, it has been shown to improve survival and to reduce the emergence of drug resistance. Similar to the paradoxical reactions with TB, an immune reconstitution and inflammatory syndrome of focal lymphadenitis and fever without bacteremia has been noted. Treatment for MAC can be discontinued in patients who have completed more than 12 months of treatment, are asymptomatic, and have a sustained increase in their CD4 counts to more than 100 cells/mcL for at least 6 months. However, therapy (not prophylaxis with a single drug) will need to be resumed if CD4 counts decrease to less than 100 cells/mcL.

- MAC is resistant to conventional antimycobacterial drugs.

- Lifelong maintenance therapy is needed in HIV-infected persons with a history of MAC disease if they do not have sustained immune reconstitution.

For patients with AIDS whose CD4 count is less than 50 cells/mcL, prophylaxis with azithromycin 1,200 mg weekly or clarithromycin 500 mg twice daily is recommended. Rifabutin 300 mg daily is an alternative if these drugs are not tolerated. The detection of MAC organisms in the respiratory or gastrointestinal tract when a blood culture is negative is not, in itself, an indication for prophylaxis or treatment. Primary prophylaxis may be discontinued in patients with CD4 counts of more than 100 cells/mcL and a sustained suppression of HIV plasma RNA for more than 3 to 6 months.

- Prophylaxis for MAC is indicated for patients with AIDS whose CD4 count is <50 cells/mcL.

CRYPTOCOCCUS NEOFORMANS DISEASE

Cryptococcus neoformans is a yeast that is acquired by inhaling it into the lungs, where it can cause symptomatic pneumonia, particularly in immunocompromised persons or in persons with lung disease. The organism has a strong propensity for dissemination to the central nervous system. The most common manifestation of *C neoformans* disease in HIV-infected patients is cryptococcal meningitis, which usually occurs when the CD4 count is less than 50 cells/mcL. The onset is insidious; symptoms are nonspecific (eg, fever, headache, malaise) and may have a waxing and waning course. Classic meningeal symptoms (eg, neck stiffness or photophobia) are present in only one-fourth to one-third of patients. Brain imaging findings are nonspecific; cerebral atrophy and ventricular enlargement are the most common findings. Cerebrospinal fluid findings may be minimal but frequently include an increased opening pressure, mild mononuclear pleocytosis, and increased protein value. Glucose levels may be normal or slightly low. The India ink preparation is positive in more than 70% of cases. The serum and cerebrospinal fluid cryptococcal antigen test has a sensitivity of 93% to 99% for cryptococcal meningitis. Cultures of cerebrospinal fluid are usually positive. Blood cultures are positive for *C neoformans* in up to 75% of HIV-infected persons with cryptococcal meningititis.

Adverse prognostic factors include altered mental status on presentation and high fungal burden (positive result of India ink test, high antigen titers, and extraneural disease). Increased intracranial pressure is common and may be associated with headache, confusion, or cranial nerve palsies. Aggressive management of intracranial pressure with daily lumbar puncture or placement of lumbar drains significantly minimizes morbidity and mortality from this illness.

- The organism *C neoformans* has a strong propensity for dissemination to the central nervous system.

- The most common manifestation of *C neoformans* disease in patients with HIV is cryptococcal meningitis.

- Cryptococcal antigen testing of cerebrospinal fluid is the most sensitive test for cryptococcal meningitis.

- Increased intracranial pressure is associated with increased mortality and should be managed aggressively with repeated lumbar punctures.

Initial therapy should include amphotericin B with flucytosine for 2 weeks; this is followed by fluconazole 400 mg daily for a total of 10 weeks. This initial therapy is followed by fluconazole (200 mg daily) for chronic maintenance therapy. Chronic maintenance therapy can be discontinued if the patient remains asymptomatic and has a sustained increase in CD4 count to more than 200 cells/mcL for 6 months. However, chronic suppression or maintenance therapy needs to be reinitiated if the CD4 count decreases to less than 200 cells/mcL. Although fluconazole and itraconazole can reduce the frequency of cryptococcal disease, routine primary prophylaxis is not recommended for several reasons. These include cost, the relative infrequency of cryptococcosis, the possibility of drug interactions, and the potential for development of drug resistance.

- Initial therapy for *C neoformans* infection in HIV includes amphotericin B with flucytosine followed by fluconazole.

- Routine primary prophylaxis for *C neoformans* disease is not recommended.

Immune reconstitution disease related to *Cryptococcus* may occur in patients with excellent virologic and immunologic response to HIV treatment. Generally, this occurs within 1 to 6 weeks of initiating antiretroviral treatment. Presentation is often with headache and more severe meningismus and inflammation in the cerebrospinal fluid than were seen at the time of the original diagnosis of meningitis. Cultures are usually sterile. Increased opening pressure should be managed with drainage.

CYTOMEGALOVIRUS

Cytomegalovirus (CMV) disease usually affects persons with advanced HIV disease (CD4 count <50 cells/mcL). Other risk factors include previous opportunistic infections and high plasma HIV-1 RNA level (>100,000 copies/mL). Chorioretinitis is the most common clinical manifestation of CMV in patients with HIV infection. The usual symptoms are floaters, visual field deficits, and painless loss of vision. Funduscopic examination reveals yellowish or white retinal infiltrates with or without intraretinal hemorrhage. In CMV gastrointestinal disease, the esophagus and colon are most commonly involved, and the disease manifests with dysphagia, abdominal pain, and bloody diarrhea. Hepatitis, pneumonitis, sclerosing cholangitis, encephalitis, adrenalitis, polyradiculopathy, and myelopathy can also be caused by CMV.

Agents used for the treatment of CMV disease and their general characteristics are listed in Table 21.5. The preferred therapy for sight-threatening lesions is immediate placement of a ganciclovir intraocular implant plus valganciclovir

900 mg orally twice daily for 14 to 21 days followed by valganciclovir once daily until immune recovery. For gastrointestinal disease, maintenance therapy can be deferred until relapse is actually demonstrated. Immune recovery uveitis, characterized by inflammation in the anterior chamber or vitreous, can occur in patients who experience a substantial increase in the CD4 count 4 to 12 weeks after antiretroviral therapy is started. Chronic maintenance therapy can be discontinued if patients remain asymptomatic and have a sustained increase in the CD4 count to more than 100 cells/mcL for 3 to 6 months. All patients whose maintenance therapy is discontinued should undergo regular ophthalmologic monitoring for detection of relapse and immune recovery uveitis. Chronic maintenance therapy will need to be reinitiated if there is ophthalmologic evidence of relapse or the CD4 counts decrease to less than 100 cells/mcL.

All patients with AIDS should undergo annual funduscopic examination to screen for CMV retinitis and other HIV-related eye disease and should have prompt evaluation of visual complaints. Routine prophylaxis against CMV is not recommended because of concerns regarding treatment-induced toxicities (such as neutropenia and anemia), conflicting reports of efficacy, lack of proven survival benefit, and cost.

- CMV disease usually affects persons with advanced HIV.

- CMV can cause chorioretinitis, gastrointestinal disease, hepatitis, and other organ involvement.

- CMV retinitis is painless and can lead to blindness.

SYPHILIS

Sexually transmitted diseases, including syphilis, that cause genital ulceration may be cofactors for acquiring HIV infection. In general, the clinical manifestations of syphilis are similar to those among non–HIV-infected persons. However, atypical presentations may occur. For example, in primary syphilis, multiple or atypical chancres can

Table 21.5 DRUGS USED FOR TREATMENT OF CYTOMEGALOVIRUS DISEASE

DRUG	DOSAGE	MAJOR ADVERSE EFFECT
Systemic		
Ganciclovir IV	5 mg/kg twice daily	Bone marrow suppression
Valganciclovir	900 mg PO twice daily	Bone marrow suppression
Foscarnet IV	60 mg/kg 3 times daily or 90 mg/kg twice daily	Renal toxicity
Cidofovir IV[a]	5 mg/kg weekly for 2 wk, followed by 5 mg/kg every 2 wk	Renal toxicity
Local anti-CMV therapy for retinitis		
Ganciclovir intraocular-release device (Vitrasert)[b]	Every 6 mo	Retinal detachment
Ganciclovir intravitreal injection[b]	2,000 mcg in 0.05–0.1 mL	Bone marrow suppression
Foscarnet intravitreal injection[b]	1.2–2.4 mg in 0.1 mL	Renal toxicity

Abbreviations: CMV, cytomegalovirus; IV, intravenously; PO, orally.

[a] Vigorous hydration and coadministration of probenecid are required to limit renal toxicity.

[b] Local anti-cytomegalovirus therapy should be accompanied by systemic therapy, such as oral ganciclovir, to avoid the risk of development of extraocular diseases.

occur. Neurosyphilis has been reported to occur earlier and more frequently and to progress more rapidly in patients with AIDS than in HIV-negative patients. Concomitant uveitis and meningitis also may be more common among HIV-1–infected patients with syphilis. There are reports of false-negative and false-positive serologic tests for syphilis in patients with HIV. However, serologic response to infection seems to be similar in HIV-positive and HIV-negative persons, and there are no specific clinical manifestations of syphilis that are unique to HIV.

Management of HIV-1–infected patients with syphilis is similar to the management of non–HIV-infected persons. A few points deserve emphasis regarding HIV infection and syphilis:

- Close follow-up is necessary to detect potential treatment failures and disease progression.

- Lumbar puncture is recommended for all HIV-infected patients with late latent syphilis or latent syphilis of unknown duration.

- Penicillin-based treatment is recommended, whenever possible, for all stages of syphilis in HIV-infected persons.

TOXOPLASMOSIS

Toxoplasma gondii, a protozoan, is the most common cause of focal central nervous system lesions in patients with AIDS. The most common symptoms of *Toxoplasma* encephalitis include headache and confusion; fever may be absent. Focal neurologic deficits occur in 69% of cases. The median CD4 count at diagnosis is 50 cells/mcL. Multiple ring-enhancing lesions with associated edema are usually noted on brain imaging studies. Magnetic resonance imaging is more sensitive than computed tomography for identifying lesions. The differential diagnosis of central nervous system mass lesions in patients with AIDS includes not only toxoplasmosis but also lymphoma and other infections, such as TB, cryptococcosis, histoplasmosis, bacterial abscess, and progressive multifocal leukoencephalitis.

- The organism *T gondii* is the most common cause of focal central nervous system lesions in patients with AIDS.

- Multiple ring-enhancing lesions usually are noted on brain imaging studies.

Empiric antitoxoplasmosis therapy is indicated in patients with AIDS and positive *Toxoplasma* serologic testing who present with multiple intracranial lesions. The absence of anti-toxoplasma immunoglobulin (Ig) G antibody makes a diagnosis of toxoplasmosis unlikely. Effective treatment should result not only in amelioration of symptoms but also in a reduction of the number, size, and contrast enhancement of the brain lesions. If the patient is seronegative for *Toxoplasma*, has a single mass lesion on both computed tomography and magnetic resonance imaging, or did not achieve the desired response after an empiric course of antitoxoplasmosis therapy for 10 to

---

Box 21.4 **TREATMENT OF HIV-ASSOCIATED TOXOPLASMOSIS**

Preferred treatment
Pyrimethamine 200 mg PO loading dose followed by 50–75 mg PO daily + leucovorin 10–25 mg PO daily + sulfadiazine 1,000–1,500 mg PO every 6 h

Alternative treatments
Pyrimethamine (leucovorin)[a] + clindamycin 600 mg IV or PO every 6 h

TMP-SMX 5 mg/kg (trimethoprim component) IV or PO every 12 h

Pyrimethamine (leucovorin)[a] + atovaquone 1,500 mg PO twice daily

Pyrimethamine (leucovorin)[a] + azithromycin 900–1,200 mg PO daily

Atovaquone 1,500 mg PO twice daily

Atovaquone 1,500 mg PO twice daily + sulfadiazine 1,000–1,500 mg PO every 6 h

Abbreviations: HIV, human immunodeficiency virus; IV, intravenously; PO, orally; TMP-SMX, trimethoprim-sulfamethoxazole.

[a] All pyrimethamine regimens should include leucovorin 10 to 25 mg orally daily to prevent drug-induced hematologic toxicity.

---

14 days, the diagnosis of *Toxoplasma* encephalitis should be questioned and a diagnostic brain biopsy considered.

Drugs used for the treatment of HIV-associated toxoplasmosis are listed in Box 21.4. The initial regimen of choice is the combination of pyrimethamine plus sulfadiazine plus leucovorin. The preferred alternative regimen for patients unable to tolerate or who fail to respond to first-line therapy is pyrimethamine plus clindamycin plus leucovorin. Acute therapy should be continued for at least 6 weeks if there is clinical and radiologic improvement. Suppressive therapy (secondary prophylaxis), with the same agents used for acute therapy but at a reduced dose, is necessary to prevent relapse. Secondary prophylaxis can be discontinued in patients who successfully complete initial therapy, remain asymptomatic with respect to signs and symptoms of toxoplasmosis, and have a sustained (ie, >6 months) increase in their CD4 counts to more than 200 cells/mcL with antiretroviral therapy. Secondary prophylaxis should be started again if the CD4 count decreases to less than 200 cells/mcL. All HIV-infected persons with a CD4 count of less than 100 cells/mcL who are seropositive for *Toxoplasma* should receive primary prophylaxis against *Toxoplasma* encephalitis, as reviewed in Table 21.3.

- Pyrimethamine plus sulfadiazine plus leucovorin is the preferred treatment regimen for toxoplasmosis in patients with AIDS.

- The agent of choice for primary prophylaxis against *Toxoplasma* encephalitis is TMP-SMX.

HIV-infected patients should be tested for IgG antibody to *Toxoplasma* as part of their initial work-up; if the result is negative, they should be counseled about the various potential sources of *Toxoplasma* infection, such as raw or undercooked meat and handling of cat litter.

PROGRESSIVE MULTIFOCAL LEUKOENCEPHALOPATHY

Progressive multifocal leukoencephalopathy is a demyelinating disease caused by the JC virus, a polyomavirus. Symptoms and signs are progressive, variable, and usually chronic or subacute. Symptoms include cognitive dysfunction, dementia, seizures, ataxia, aphasia, cranial nerve deficits, and focal deficits such as hemiparesis and visual field cuts. Fever is usually absent. Occasionally, symptoms present rapidly and progress in a few weeks to dementia or coma.

Diagnosis is based on clinical findings and magnetic resonance imaging, which shows characteristic white matter changes (bright areas on T2-weighted images) without contrast enhancement or mass effect. Routine cerebrospinal fluid studies are generally nondiagnostic, but identification of JC virus DNA in the cerebrospinal fluid by polymerase chain reaction may confirm the diagnosis. Absence of JC virus DNA does not rule out progressive multifocal leukoencephalopathy.

There is no established specific therapy for progressive multifocal leukoencephalopathy. The prognosis has considerably improved with antiretroviral treatment, and approximately half of patients with a good response to antiretroviral treatment have long-term remission. Thus, all patients with progressive multifocal leukoencephalopathy should be receiving effective antiretroviral therapy.

- Progressive multifocal leukoencephalopathy is caused by the JC virus.

- The diagnosis is based on clinical findings and on white matter changes on magnetic resonance imaging.

- All patients with HIV and progressive multifocal leukoencephalopathy should be receiving effective antiretroviral therapy.

MUCOCUTANEOUS CANDIDIASIS

Mucocutaneous disease, such as oral thrush, recurrent vaginitis, and candidal esophagitis, is common. Candidal esophagitis is an AIDS-defining condition. Systemic candidal infection, including candidemia, is rare unless additional risk factors for disseminated fungal infection such as severe neutropenia or indwelling catheters are present.

Mucocutaneous disease can often be successfully treated with clotrimazole troches or nystatin suspension or pastilles. Fluconazole is used for the treatment of candidal esophagitis and topical treatment failures. Amphotericin B or caspofungin can be used for azole failures.

Diagnosis of oropharyngeal candidiasis is usually clinical and is based on the appearance of lesions. Visualization of the organisms by microscopic examination of scrapings provides supportive diagnostic information.

The diagnosis of esophageal candidiasis is usually made presumptively on clinical grounds (retrosternal burning pain or odynophagia in a patient with a low CD4 count or oral candidiasis). A diagnostic trial of antifungal therapy is recommended before endoscopy is used for identifying the cause of the disease. Fluconazole 100 to 400 mg daily by mouth is usually used for 14 to 21 days to treat esophageal candidiasis.

Chronic maintenance therapy for recurrent oropharyngeal or vulvovaginal candidiasis is not recommended unless recurrences are frequent or severe. Fluconazole 100 to 200 mg daily can be used to prevent esophageal candidiasis or other problematic candidiasis.

ENTERIC DISEASE

A wide variety of organisms (protozoa, bacteria, fungal and viral organisms, including HIV itself) can cause diarrhea in patients with HIV. The CD4 count as a surrogate for the level of immunosuppression is an important guide when considering the differential diagnosis. For example, diarrhea due to MAC or CMV does not usually occur with CD4 counts of more than 100/mcL. Initial evaluation of patients with HIV infection who have considerable diarrhea, with or without abdominal pain or weight loss, after exclusion of dietary and medication causes, should include stool cultures for bacteria, 3 separate stool specimens for ova and parasites and acid-fast bacilli, testing for *Clostridium difficile*, and specific examination for cryptosporidiosis, isosporiasis, microsporidiosis, and cyclosporiasis. If no cause is found, sigmoidoscopy with biopsies should be done to look for CMV in patients with low CD4 counts. If this result is also negative, upper endoscopy or colonoscopy with biopsy of the terminal ileum can sometimes recover treatable pathogens in the small bowel.

SALMONELLA INFECTION

In contrast to immunocompetent persons, HIV-infected persons are more likely to have *Salmonella* infection that is severe, invasive, and widespread. Bacteremia is common and constitutes an AIDS-defining diagnosis. The source for *Salmonella* infection is usually ingestion of contaminated food, particularly undercooked poultry and eggs. Salmonellosis can present in 3 ways in HIV infection: a self-limited gastroenteritis; a more severe and prolonged diarrheal disease associated with fever, bloody diarrhea, and weight loss; and septicemia, with or without gastrointestinal symptoms. In the United States, the majority of cases of *Salmonella* septicemia are caused by nontyphoidal strains, in particular *Salmonella enteritidis* and *Salmonella typhimurium*. Bacteremia can occur with each of these syndromes and has a propensity for relapse.

Ciprofloxacin is the preferred agent for treatment. The treatment duration for mild gastroenteritis without bacteremia is 10 to 14 days. However, for patients with advanced HIV-1 disease (CD4 count <200 cells/mcL) or for those who have *Salmonella* bacteremia, treatment for 4 to 6 weeks is recommended. Alternatives to the fluoroquinolone antibiotics include TMP-SMX or third-generation cephalosporins (eg, ceftriaxone or cefotaxime).

- HIV-infected persons are more likely to have *Salmonella* infection that is severe, invasive, and widespread.

- Ciprofloxacin is the preferred antibiotic for the treatment of *Salmonella* infection.

CRYPTOSPORIDIOSIS, ISOSPORIASIS, MICROSPORIDIOSIS, AND *CYCLOSPORA* INFECTION

Cryptosporidium parvum, Isospora belli, Cyclospora cayetanensis, and several species of Microsporidia, including *Enterocytozoon bieneusi* and *Encephalitozoon intestinalis*, are all causative agents of generally self-limited diarrheal infections in immunocompetent patients. In HIV-infected patients with low CD4 cell counts, chronic diarrhea (often with malabsorption) can develop from all of these organisms. *Cryptosporidium* can also involve the gallbladder or biliary tract. Diarrhea due to all of these organisms resolves with antiretroviral therapy and immune recovery. Isosporiasis and *Cyclospora* infections can be effectively treated with TMP-SMX DS (160 mg of TMP and 800 mg of SMX) 4 times daily for 10 days. Suppressive treatment with TMP-SMX until immune recovery occurs is recommended after treatment. There is no specific, consistently effective pharmacologic or immunologic therapy for cryptosporidiosis or microsporidiosis. Cryptosporidiosis can be identified when specimens are stained with either a modified acid-fast procedure or a fluorescent assay (immunofluorescent assay or enzyme immunoassay) that uses monoclonal antibodies to *Cryptosporidium* antigens. Isosporiasis can also usually be identified with a modified acid-fast stain of stool or biopsy specimens. Microsporidiosis and *Cyclospora* infections require special selective stains or electron microscopy for definitive diagnosis.

- *Cryptosporidium parvum, Isopora belli*, several species of Microsporidia, and *Cyclospora cayetanensis* can all cause profuse, watery diarrhea, crampy abdominal pain, anorexia, flatulence, and malaise in patients infected with HIV.

- Isosporiasis and *Cyclospora* infections can both be treated with high-dose TMP-SMX.

- Antiretroviral therapy and immune recovery are the most effective treatments for cryptosporidiosis, isosporiasis, microsporidiosis, and *Cyclospora* infections.

BACILLARY ANGIOMATOSIS

Bacillary angiomatosis caused by *Bartonella quintana* and *Bartonella henselae* is characterized by vascular proliferative lesions that can involve any organ in the body. The most commonly involved site is the skin, where it may present as nodules or plaques that are sometimes difficult to differentiate from those of Kaposi sarcoma. Other sites include bone, lymph nodes, brain, respiratory tract, and gastrointestinal tract. Characteristic fluid-filled spaces occasionally are noted in the liver and spleen and are called peliosis hepatis or peliosis splenis. Patients with bacillary angiomatosis usually have CD4 counts less than 100 cells/mcL. *Bartonella* infection is a common cause of fever in late-stage AIDS. Chills, malaise, anorexia, and weight loss can also occur. Definitive diagnosis by culture of the organism can be challenging, and the diagnosis is often made by a combination of characteristic pathologic findings, demonstration of the organism on Warthin-Starry stain, polymerase chain reaction testing, and serologic testing. Treatment is with erythromycin or doxycycline for at least 3 months.

- Bacillary angiomatosis is characterized by vascular proliferative lesions in skin and other organs.

- The differential diagnosis of skin lesions includes Kaposi sarcoma.

- Treatment of bacillary angiomatosis is with erythromycin or doxycycline.

AIDS-ASSOCIATED MALIGNANCIES

KAPOSI SARCOMA

Kaposi sarcoma, a vascular tumor, is an AIDS-defining illness and is most common in men who have sex with men. Human herpesvirus 8 (HHV-8), also known as Kaposi sarcoma–associated herpesvirus, has been established as the etiologic agent of Kaposi sarcoma. HHV-8 appears to be sexually transmitted, and with HIV it synergistically acts to induce changes of Kaposi sarcoma. Histologically, whorls of spindle-shaped cells and abnormal proliferation of small blood vessels are seen. Skin, lung, and the gastrointestinal tract are the commonly affected organs. Early on, skin lesions are often mistaken for benign vascular lesions. Treatment options include local therapy (eg, radiotherapy, intralesional chemotherapy, and cryotherapy) and systemic therapy (eg, chemotherapy and interferon-alfa). Liposome-encapsulated anthracycline chemotherapeutic agents enable delivery of high doses of effective drug with fewer adverse effects. Antiretroviral therapy has resulted in a substantial reduction in the incidence of Kaposi sarcoma and has been associated with a reduction in tumor burden and disease progression. Therefore, antiretroviral therapy is recommended for all HIV-infected patients with Kaposi sarcoma.

- Kaposi sarcoma is most common among men who have sex with men.

- Kaposi sarcoma is related to HHV-8 infection.

- Antiretroviral treatment and immune recovery are important aspects of treatment of Kaposi sarcoma.

NON-HODGKIN LYMPHOMA

Non-Hodgkin lymphoma is much more common (as high as 200-fold increased risk) among HIV-infected patients than in the general population. It is a heterogeneous group of malignancies with varying biologic behavior and occurs in patients with widely ranging levels of immune function. The vast majority of non-Hodgkin lymphomas in patients with HIV are of B-cell origin. Intermediate- or high-grade B-cell non-Hodgkin lymphoma is a CDC-defined AIDS diagnosis. As patients with AIDS live longer, this complication is likely to become more frequent. It commonly presents with constitutional symptoms (fever, night sweats, and weight loss), lymphadenopathy, and involvement of extranodal sites such as the central nervous system, bone marrow, gastrointestinal tract, and liver. Involvement of the brain can manifest as an isolated disease (primary central nervous system lymphoma) or as leptomeningeal involvement in the context of spread of lymphoma elsewhere. The optimal treatment of HIV-associated non-Hodgkin lymphoma has not been well defined. Current recommendations suggest that most patients should receive standard-dose chemotherapy, PCP prophylaxis (regardless of CD4 count), and growth factor support. Additionally, highly active antiretroviral therapy should be a component of the strategy.

- The vast majority of non-Hodgkin lymphomas in patients with HIV are of B-cell origin.

- Non-Hodgkin lymphoma in HIV commonly presents with constitutional symptoms (eg, fever, night sweats, and weight loss), lymphadenopathy, and involvement of extranodal sites.

PRIMARY CENTRAL NERVOUS SYSTEM LYMPHOMA

The incidence of primary central nervous system lymphoma (PCNSL) in HIV-infected individuals is 1,000-fold higher than that in the general population. It occurs most often in the advanced stages of AIDS at a median CD4 count of less than 50 cells/mcL and is almost always associated with Epstein-Barr virus. The result of polymerase chain reaction testing of cerebrospinal fluid for Epstein-Barr virus is usually positive in patients with HIV and PCNSL but rarely positive in patients with toxoplasmosis or other causes of central nervous system brain lesions. The clinical presentation includes headache, confusion, lethargy, personality changes, memory loss, focal neurologic deficits, and seizure. Brain imaging studies show single or multiple contrast-enhancing lesions, which may be difficult to distinguish from those of toxoplasmosis. Biopsy is required for definitive diagnosis. Whole-brain radiation has been the primary treatment of PCNSL. Despite good initial radiographic response rates, the survival rate is poor with median survival times of 2 to 5 months. Since the advent of potent combination antiretroviral therapy, the incidence of PCNSL has declined, and antiretroviral therapy in combination with radiation has been associated with an improved prognosis compared with brain radiation alone.

- PCNSL is associated with Epstein-Barr virus infection.

- PCNSL usually occurs in patients with advanced AIDS.

- Lesions of PCNSL found on imaging studies may be difficult to distinguish from those of toxoplasmosis.

ANTIRETROVIRAL AGENTS

THE REPLICATION CYCLE OF HIV

A working knowledge of the HIV replication cycle is essential for understanding the mechanism of action of antiretroviral agents. Figure 21.2 reviews the interaction between the virus and the host cell that leads to production of infectious virions.

Currently, 25 individual antiretroviral drugs and 6 coformulated products categorized in 6 classes have been approved by the FDA for the treatment of HIV. The 6 classes of antiretroviral drugs are nucleoside and nucleotide analogue reverse transcriptase inhibitors (NRTI), nonnucleoside analogue reverse transcriptase inhibitors (NNRTI), protease inhibitors, fusion inhibitors, integrase inhibitors, and chemokine coreceptor antagonists.

NUCLEOSIDE AND NUCLEOTIDE ANALOGUE REVERSE TRANSCRIPTASE INHIBITORS

The NRTIs were the first agents to be developed as antiretrovirals. These agents are structurally similar to nucleic acids (the building blocks of RNA and DNA). They block HIV reverse

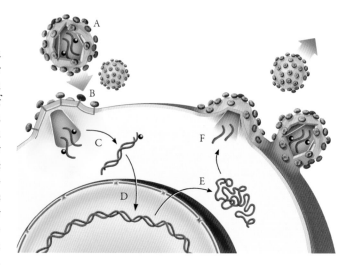

Figure 21.2 Life Cycle of Human Immunodeficiency Virus. A, The virus is an enveloped virus that contains viral genomic RNA and various Gag and Pol protein products. B, The interaction between the envelope proteins of the virus and CD4 receptor and other receptors of the host cell leads to the binding of the viral envelope and the host cytoplasmic membrane. C, The viral reverse transcriptase enzyme catalyzes the conversion of viral RNA into DNA. D, The viral DNA enters the nucleus and becomes inserted into the chromosomal DNA of the host cell. E, Expression of the viral genes leads to production of viral RNA and proteins. F, These viral proteins, as well as viral RNA, are assembled at the cell surface into new viral particles and leave the host cell by a process called budding. During the process of budding, they acquire the outer layer and envelope. At this stage, the protease enzyme cleaves the precursor Gag and Gag-Pol proteins into their mature products.

transcriptase activity by competing with nucleic acids and acting as chain terminators in the synthesis of proviral DNA.

- NRTIs are structurally similar to nucleic acids.

- NRTIs block HIV reverse transcriptase activity and prevent synthesis of proviral DNA.

- Currently, 8 individual NRTIs are licensed for clinical use in the United States. Zalcitabine (ddC), because of its low potency, high pill burden, and adverse events, is no longer used in clinical practice, and its production has been discontinued. In addition to these individual drugs, there are 5 coformulated products that contain 2 or 3 reverse transcriptase inhibitors in a single pill. General characteristics of currently available NRTIs are described in Table 21.6.

Resistance to NRTIs is associated with mutations in the *Pol* gene that codes for the enzyme reverse transcriptase. Specific mutations that confer resistance to individual agents have been identified, whereas other mutations confer cross-resistance to several agents.

The most serious toxicity of NRTIs is an unusual and potentially fatal syndrome consisting of severe hepatomegaly with steatosis and lactic acidosis in the absence of hypoxemia. Mitochondrial DNA depletion induced by NRTIs is responsible for this clinical syndrome. This syndrome is a class-wide toxicity. However, stavudine (d4T), didanosine (ddI), and zalcitabine (ddC) are the drugs most frequently associated with it. Stavudine and didanosine should not be used together because of the high risk for development of symptomatic lactic acidosis. Lamivudine (3TC), abacavir (ABC), tenofovir (TDF), and emtricitabine (FTC) are considered to have low mitochondrial toxicity potential.

Clinically, this syndrome usually has an insidious onset with initial gastrointestinal symptoms (nausea, anorexia, abdominal pain, vomiting), but it can progress rapidly and cause tachycardia, tachypnea, hyperventilation, jaundice, muscular weakness, and mental status changes. Occasional patients present with multiorgan failure. Associated laboratory abnormalities include an increased lactate level, low arterial pH, increased anion gap, increased liver enzyme values, and an increased bilirubin level. Lactate levels should be obtained only when patients' complaints are consistent with the presentation of this syndrome. Routine monitoring of the lactic acid level is not recommended. Once the presence of this syndrome is highly suspected, use of all antiretrovirals should be discontinued and symptomatic support with hydration instituted. Once lactate levels have returned

Table 21.6 GENERAL CHARACTERISTICS OF NUCLEOSIDE ANALOGUE REVERSE TRANSCRIPTASE INHIBITORS

DRUG NAME (ALIAS)	DOSING & ADJUSTMENTS	METABOLISM	TOXIC/ADVERSE EFFECTS
Abacavir (ABC)	300 mg twice daily or 600 mg once daily No food effect No adjustment needed for renal insufficiency Dose adjustment for hepatic impairment required	Hepatic by alcohol dehydrogenase & glucuronyl transferase	Diarrhea, anorexia, nausea, vomiting, headache, fatigue, hypersensitivity reaction
Didanosine (ddI)	Body weight ≥60 kg: 400 mg once daily Body weight <60 kg: 250 mg once daily Take 1/2 h before or 2 h after a meal Dose adjustment for renal insufficiency required	Unknown	Rash, abdominal pain, diarrhea, nausea, vomiting, asthenia, headache, fever, pancreatitis, peripheral neuropathy
Emtricitabine (FTC)	200-mg capsule once daily or 240 mg (24 mL) oral solution once daily Take without regard to meals Dose adjustment for renal insufficiency required	Limited, oxidation & conjugation	Hyperpigmentation of skin, rash, diarrhea, nausea, vomiting, headache
Lamivudine (3TC)	150 mg twice daily or 300 mg once daily Take without regard to meals Dose adjustment for renal insufficiency required	5.6% to transsulfoxide metabolite	Decrease in appetite, nausea, vomiting, headache, fatigue, pancreatitis in children
Stavudine (d4T)	Body weight ≥60 kg: 40 mg twice daily Body weight <60 kg: 30 mg twice daily Take without regard to meals Dose adjustment for renal insufficiency required	Intracellular phosphorylation to active metabolite	Rash, diarrhea, nausea, vomiting, headache, lipoatrophy, hyperlipidemia, peripheral neuropathy, muscle weakness
Tenofovir (TDF)	300 mg once daily Take without regard to meals Dose adjustment for renal insufficiency required	Intracellular hydrolysis	Diarrhea, flatulence, nausea, vomiting, osteopenia, renal impairment
Zidovudine (ZDV)	300 mg twice daily or 200 mg 3 times daily Take without regard to meals Dose adjustment for renal insufficiency required	Hepatic glucuronidation	Headache, nausea, anorexia, vomiting, anemia, leukopenia, myopathy, lipoatrophy, hyperlipidemia

Adapted from Panel on Antiretroviral Guidelines for Adults and Adolescents: Guidelines for the use of antiretroviral agents in HIV-1-infected adults and adolescents. Department of Health and Human Services. December 1, 2009; 1–161. [cited 2011 Nov 23]. Available from: http://www.aidsinfo.nih.gov/ContentFiles/AdultandAdolescentGL.pdf.

to normal, antiretroviral drug therapy can be reintroduced with NRTIs that have low potential for mitochondria toxicity ([cited 2011 Nov 23]. Available from: http://www.aidsinfo.nih.gov/ContentFiles/AdultandAdolescentGL.pdf).

- A rare and potentially fatal syndrome of lactic acidosis in the absence of hypoxemia can occur with NRTIs.

- Symptomatic lactic acidosis is most common with stavudine, didanosine, and zalcitabine.

- Use of stavudine and didanosine together is contraindicated.

Hypersensitivity reactions have been reported in approximately 5% of patients receiving abacavir. Symptoms consist of rash accompanied by systemic signs and symptoms such as fever, fatigue, nausea, vomiting, diarrhea, or abdominal pain. These symptoms usually appear within the first 6 weeks of treatment. The rash is usually maculopapular but can be variable in appearance. Hypersensitivity reactions also may occur without a rash. Symptoms usually resolve rapidly when use of the drug is discontinued. Once use of abacavir has been discontinued because of adverse effects, it should not be reintroduced. More severe symptoms, including death, have been reported when use of abacavir is reinstituted. A genetic marker, HLA-B*5701, has been associated with an increased risk for development of a hypersensitivity reaction to abacavir and is more common

in whites. HLA-B*5701 testing is now recommended before starting therapy with abacavir; other drugs should be chosen if a patient is positive for HLA-B*5701.

- Patients in whom abacavir therapy is being considered should be tested for HLA-B*5701.

- Abacavir should not be reintroduced once its use has been discontinued because of adverse effects.

NONNUCLEOSIDE ANALOGUE REVERSE TRANSCRIPTASE INHIBITORS

The NNRTIs bind directly and noncompetitively to the enzyme reverse transcriptase. They block DNA polymerase activity by causing conformational change and disrupting the catalytic site of the enzyme. Unlike nucleoside analogues, NNRTIs are not incorporated into viral DNA. They have no activity against HIV-2.

- NNRTIs bind directly and noncompetitively to the enzyme reverse transcriptase.

- NNRTIs are not active against HIV-2.

Five NNRTIs have been approved for the treatment of HIV: delavirdine, efavirenz, etravirine, nevirapine, and rilpivirine (Table 21.7). When first-generation NNRTIs

Table 21.7 GENERAL CHARACTERISTICS OF NONNUCLEOSIDE REVERSE TRANSCRIPTASE INHIBITORS

DRUG NAME (ALIAS)	DOSING & ADJUSTMENTS	METABOLISM	TOXIC/ADVERSE EFFECTS
Delavirdine (DLV)	400 mg 3 times daily Take without regard to meals No adjustment for renal insufficiency	CYP substrate, CYP3A4 inhibitor	Rash, hepatotoxicity, headache
Efavirenz (EFV)	600 mg once daily at or before bedtime Take on an empty stomach to reduce adverse effects No adjustment for renal insufficiency	CYP3A4 & 2B6 substrate, mixed CYP3A4 inducer or inhibitor	Rash, central nervous system symptoms (dizziness, light-headedness, abnormal dreams, difficulty with concentration), hepatotoxicity
Etravirine (ETR)	200 mg twice daily Take after a meal No adjustment for renal insufficiency	CYP3A4, 2C9, & 2C19 substrate 3A4 inducer; 2C9 & 2C19 inhibitor	Rash, hypersensitivity reaction
Nevirapine (NVP)	200 mg once daily for 14 days (lead-in period); thereafter, 200 mg twice daily Take without regard to meals No adjustment for renal insufficiency	CYP3A4 substrate, CYP3A4 inducer	Rash, hepatotoxicity, including symptomatic hepatitis & fatal hepatic necrosis
Rilpivirine (RPV)	25 mg once daily Take with a meal No adjustment for renal insufficiency	CYP3A substrate, CYP3A4 inhibitors (protease inhibitors, macrolides, azole antifungals) can increase levels of RPV, highly protein-bound, requires stomach acid for absorption (PPIs contraindicated, avoid H2RAs, take RPV 2 h before or 4 h after antacids)	Headache, insomnia, depression, transient rash, increased transaminase levels, increased total and LDL cholesterol levels. May prolong QT interval—use caution or avoid QT-interval–prolonging drugs

Abbreviations: CYP, cytochrome P450; H2RA, histamine$_2$-receptor antagonist; LDL, low-density lipoprotein; PPI, proton pump inhibitor.

Adapted from Panel on Antiretroviral Guidelines for Adults and Adolescents: Guidelines for the use of antiretroviral agents in HIV-1-infected adults and adolescents. Department of Health and Human Services. December 1, 2009; 1–161. [cited 2011 Nov 23]. Available from: http://www.aidsinfo.nih.gov/ContentFiles/AdultandAdolescentGL.pdf.

(nevirapine, delavirdine, efavirenz) and rilpivirine are administered as a single agent or as a part of an inadequately suppressive treatment regimen, resistance emerges rapidly. Mutations conferring resistance to one drug generally confer cross-resistance to the other first-generation NNRTIs. Cross-resistance to nucleoside analogues or protease inhibitors has not been observed. Patients in whom an RPV-based regimen fails are more likely to have failure with genotypic resistance to other NNRTIs, including etravirine.

Nevirapine, efavirenz, and etravirine all interact with the hepatic cytochrome P450 system. NNRTIs may change the metabolism of and thus lower the plasma levels of coadministered drugs that are metabolized by the cytochrome P450 system. Similarly, drugs that induce or inhibit cytochrome P450 activity may have an effect on the plasma concentrations of NNRTIs. Rash is a common adverse effect associated with NNRTIs. Malformations of the fetus have been noted in primates and humans exposed to efavirenz. Therefore, efavirenz is contraindicated in pregnant women.

- Mutations conferring resistance to one first-generation NNRTI generally confer cross-resistance to the other first-generation NNRTIs.

- Etravirine, a second-generation NNRTI, has a different resistance profile than the first-generation NNRTIs.

- Efavirenz is contraindicated in pregnant women because of the risk of fetal malformations.

PROTEASE INHIBITORS

Protease inhibitors (PIs) exert their antiviral effect by inhibiting HIV-1 protease. HIV-1 protease is a complex enzyme responsible for the cleavage of the large viral Gag and Gag-Pol polypeptide chains into smaller, functional proteins. This process takes place in the final stages of the HIV life cycle. Inhibition of the protease enzyme results in the release of structurally disorganized and noninfectious viral particles. PIs have antiviral activity in both acutely and chronically infected cells. They are metabolized by the cytochrome P450 system and are themselves, to varying degrees, inhibitors of this system. This leads to a considerable number of interactions with drugs that are inducers, inhibitors, or substrates of this system.

Currently, 9 PIs are approved for the treatment of HIV (Table 21.8).

- PIs exert their antiviral effect by inhibiting HIV-1 protease.

- PIs have considerable interactions with drugs that are metabolized through the P450 system.

The PIs have shown potent antiretroviral, immunologic, and clinical benefits in HIV-infected persons, but their long-term efficacy and safety have not been completely elucidated. Metabolic complications of these drugs have included hyperglycemia, diabetes mellitus, and abnormalities of lipid metabolism. Of note, similar metabolic abnormalities have been reported in patients taking antiretroviral regimens that do not contain PIs.

- Metabolic complications of PIs have included hyperglycemia, frank diabetes mellitus, and abnormalities of lipid metabolism.

The issue of resistance among PIs is complex and incompletely understood. Mutations that confer drug resistance have been identified in protease genes. Several of these mutations have been found to be key for individual PIs. Nevertheless, accumulation of several mutations is usually necessary for high-level resistance to occur, and cross-resistance is common among the various PIs.

The inhibitory effect of PIs on each other's metabolism has led to the common clinical practice of prescribing PIs with low-dose (100–400 mg daily) ritonavir. This enhances the pharmacokinetic profile of the PIs, allowing for decreased pill burden, more convenience (no food requirement), and less frequent dosing regimens.

FUSION INHIBITORS

Enfuvirtide (T-20) is the only fusion inhibitor that is currently approved by the FDA (Table 21.9). It binds a region of the HIV envelope glycoprotein gp41 and prevents viral fusion with the target cell membrane. The current indication for enfuvirtide is for treatment in patients who have experienced multiple regimen failures. Three noteworthy toxicities have been reported in clinical trials of enfuvirtide. Almost everyone experiences injection-site reactions that are typically erythematous nodules, are mild to moderate in severity, and rarely cause discontinuation of use of the drug. Much less frequent are hypersensitivity reactions. Bacterial pneumonia was noted at a higher frequency in enfuvirtide-treated patients than patients in the comparator arms.

INTEGRASE INHIBITORS

Raltegravir is the only currently approved integrase inhibitor (Table 21.10). HIV-1 integrase is essential for viral replication, and loss of integrase activity prevents viral DNA from becoming integrated into the cellular genome. Raltegravir has very potent anti–HIV-1 activity. Raltegravir is generally well tolerated. It has been used successfully in both treatment-naïve patients and in salvage programs.

CHEMOKINE CORECEPTOR ANTAGONISTS

Maraviroc is the only currently FDA-approved chemokine coreceptor (CCR5) antagonist (Table 21.11). HIV enters CD4 cells via the cluster of differentiation 4 (CD4) receptor and a coreceptor, either CCR5 or C-X-C chemokine receptor 4 (CXCR4). Virus strains in patients with early disease usually use CCR5 and are called R5 viruses. In later-stage HIV, both receptors or purely CXCR4 may be used; these viruses are called dual-mixed tropism viruses or X4 viruses, respectively. Maraviroc is effective against only R5 virus, and

Table 21.8 GENERAL CHARACTERISTICS OF PROTEASE INHIBITORS

DRUG NAME (ALIAS)	DOSING & ADJUSTMENTS	METABOLISM	TOXIC/ADVERSE EFFECTS
Atazanavir (ATZ)	ATZ 300 mg + RTV 100 mg once daily Take with food No adjustment for renal insufficiency Dose adjustment for hepatic impairment required	CYP3A4 substrate & inhibitor	Indirect hyperbilirubinemia; prolonged PR interval, including symptomatic first-degree AV block; nephrolithiasis; hyperglycemia; fat maldistribution; possible increased bleeding episodes in patients with hemophilia
Darunavir (DRV)	DRV 800 mg + RTV 100 mg once daily (for treatment-naïve) Antiretroviral-experienced: DRV 600 mg + RTV 100 mg twice daily Take with food No dose adjustment for renal insufficiency required	CYP3A4 substrate & inhibitor	Rash, hepatotoxicity, diarrhea, nausea, headache, hyperlipidemia, transaminase increased, hyperglycemia, fat maldistribution, possible increased bleeding episodes in patients with hemophilia
Fosamprenavir (FPV)	FPV 1,400 mg twice daily or FPV 1,400 mg + RTV 100–200 mg once daily (not recommended for treatment-experienced) FPV 700 mg + RTV 100 mg twice daily Take without regard to meals No dose adjustment for renal insufficiency required Dose adjustment for hepatic impairment required	CYP3A4 substrate, inhibitor, & inducer	Rash, diarrhea, nausea, vomiting, headache, hyperlipidemia, transaminase increased, nephrolithiasis, hyperglycemia, fat maldistribution, possible increased bleeding episodes in patients with hemophilia
Indinavir (IDV)	IDV 800 mg + RTV 100–200 mg twice daily Take without regard to meals No dose adjustment for renal insufficiency required Dose adjustment for hepatic impairment required	CYP3A4 substrate & inhibitor	Nephrolithiasis, GI intolerance, nausea, indirect hyperbilirubinemia, hyperlipidemia, headache, asthenia, blurred vision, dizziness, rash, metallic taste, thrombocytopenia, alopecia, hemolytic anemia, hyperglycemia, fat maldistribution, possible increased bleeding episodes in patients with hemophilia
Lopinavir/ ritonavir (LPV/r)	LPV/r 400 mg/100 mg twice daily or LPV/r 800 mg/200 mg once daily (once daily not recommended for treatment-experienced or pregnant women) Take without regard to meals No dose adjustment for renal insufficiency required	CYP3A4 substrate & inhibitor	GI intolerance, nausea, vomiting, diarrhea, asthenia, hyperlipidemia (especially hypertriglyceridemia), increased serum transaminases, hyperglycemia, fat maldistribution, possible increased bleeding episodes in patients with hemophilia
Nelfinavir (NFV)	1,250 mg twice daily or 750 mg 3 times daily Take with food No dose adjustment for renal insufficiency required	CYP 2C19 & 3A4 substrate & inhibitor Has an active metabolite	Diarrhea, hyperlipidemia, hyperglycemia, fat maldistribution, possible increased bleeding episodes in patients with hemophilia, increased serum transaminase
Ritonavir (RTV)	Current use only as a pharmacokinetic enhancer for other PIs: 100–400 mg per day in 1 dose or 2 divided doses Take with food No dose adjustment for renal insufficiency required	CYP3A4 & 2D6 substrate & inhibitor	GI intolerance, nausea, vomiting, diarrhea, paresthesias (circumoral & extremities), hyperlipidemia (especially hypertriglyceridemia), hepatitis, asthenia, taste perversion, hyperglycemia, fat maldistribution, possible increased bleeding episodes in patients with hemophilia
Saquinavir (SQV)	SQV 1,000 mg + RTV 100 mg twice daily Take within 2 h after a meal No dose adjustment for renal insufficiency required	CYP3A4 substrate & inhibitor	GI intolerance, nausea, diarrhea, headache, increased transaminase enzymes, hyperlipidemia, hyperglycemia, fat maldistribution, possible increased bleeding episodes in patients with hemophilia
Tipranavir (TPV)	TPV 500 mg + RTV 200 mg twice daily Take without regard to meals No dose adjustment for renal insufficiency required	CYP3A4 substrate & inducer (but when combined with RTV, the net effect is inhibition)	Hepatotoxicity (including clinical hepatitis), rash, intracranial hemorrhages, hyperlipidemia (especially hypertriglyceridemia), hyperglycemia, fat maldistribution, possible increased bleeding episodes in patients with hemophilia

Abbreviations: AV, atrioventricular; CYP, cytochrome P450; GI, gastrointestinal; PI, protease inhibitor.

Adapted from Panel on Antiretroviral Guidelines for Adults and Adolescents: Guidelines for the use of antiretroviral agents in HIV-1-infected adults and adolescents. Department of Health and Human Services. December 1, 2009; 1–161. [cited 2011 Nov 23]. Available from: http://www.aidsinfo.nih.gov/ContentFiles/AdultandAdolescentGL.pdf.

Table 21.9 GENERAL CHARACTERISTICS OF FUSION INHIBITORS

DRUG NAME (ALIAS)	DOSING & ADJUSTMENTS	METABOLISM	TOXIC/ADVERSE EFFECTS
Enfuvirtide (T-20)	90 mg (1 mL) subcutaneously twice daily No adjustment for renal insufficiency	Catabolism to its constituent amino acids	Local injection site reactions, increased bacterial pneumonia, hypersensitivity reaction

Adapted from Panel on Antiretroviral Guidelines for Adults and Adolescents: Guidelines for the use of antiretroviral agents in HIV-1-infected adults and adolescents. Department of Health and Human Services. December 1, 2009; 1–161. [cited 2011 Nov 23]. Available from: http://www.aidsinfo.nih.gov/ContentFiles/AdultandAdolescentGL.pdf.

therefore a tropism assay to ensure that R5 virus is present is recommended before starting treatment with maraviroc.

- Maraviroc is a pure CCR5 antagonist.

- A tropism assay should be done before initiating treatment with maraviroc.

GUIDELINES FOR USE OF ANTIRETROVIRAL THERAPY FOR HIV INFECTION

Guidelines addressing the issue of antiretroviral therapy in different populations and situations have been developed and are updated regularly electronically as new information becomes available (http://www.aidsinfo.nih.gov/). There is broad agreement that antiretroviral therapy should be initiated in adults with symptoms ascribed to HIV infection regardless of the CD4 cell count. The optimal time to start antiretroviral therapy in asymptomatic patients is less clear. Current guidelines recommend initiating antiretroviral therapy in asymptomatic patients with less than 350 CD4 cells/mcL. Treatment has been proved to decrease morbidity and mortality related to HIV and to improve quality of life. Treatment is also recommended for patients with a CD4 cell count between 350 and 500 cells/mcL, but the strength of this recommendation is less than that for patients with lower CD4 cell counts. Initiating antiretroviral therapy for asymptomatic HIV-infected persons who have CD4 cell counts of more than 500 cells/mcL remains controversial. Benefits of early treatment include prevention of potentially irreversible damage to the immune system, decreased risk of HIV-associated complications, and decreased risk of transmission of HIV to others. Table 21.12 reviews the current recommendations for antiretroviral treatment in treatment-naïve patients.

Antiretroviral therapy is recommended for 3 conditions, regardless of CD4 cell counts: 1) pregnancy, 2) HIV-associated nephropathy, and 3) hepatitis B virus coinfection in which treatment for hepatitis B virus is indicated.

Perinatal transmission of HIV has dramatically decreased in the United States since the 1990s. This decrease is a result of recommendations from the US Public Health Service for universal prenatal HIV counseling and HIV testing of all pregnant women, in addition to antiretroviral therapy for reduction of perinatal HIV transmission. Zidovudine administered to the mother during the antepartum and intrapartum periods and to the newborn for the first 6 weeks of life reduces the perinatal transmission of HIV by two-thirds. Antiretroviral therapy should be offered to all HIV-1 infected women during pregnancy. Treatment is recommended to prevent transmission of HIV to the child and for the long-term health of the mother. The regimen should be a potent 3-drug program; efavirenz should be avoided because of the risk of fetal malformation. Ideally, zidovudine is incorporated into the antiretroviral regimen. Zidovudine should also be given to the newborn for the first 6 weeks of life. The currently preferred antiretroviral treatment regimen for pregnant women is lopinavir/ritonavir (coformulated as Kaletra) twice daily with zidovudine and lamivudine (coformulated as Combivir). Cesarean section has also been shown to substantially decrease the risk of transmission of HIV to the infant at the time of delivery. Elective cesarean section is recommended for women with viral loads of more than 1,000 copies/mL. Women in developed countries with access to clean water and formula should avoid breast-feeding, which can transmit HIV to the infant.

Patients coinfected with hepatitis B who need treatment for hepatitis B should also be treated for HIV with a program that includes drugs active against both HIV and hepatitis B. Thus, the combination of tenofovir and emtricitabine or tenofovir and lamivudine should be used as the nucleoside backbone of the regimen.

- All patients with symptomatic HIV infection should be offered antiretroviral treatment.

Table 21.10 GENERAL CHARACTERISTICS OF INTEGRASE INHIBITORS

DRUG NAME (ALIAS)	DOSING & ADJUSTMENTS	METABOLISM	TOXIC/ADVERSE EFFECTS
Raltegravir (RAL)	400 mg twice daily Take without regard to food No adjustment for renal insufficiency	Uridine diphosphoglucuronosyl-transferase 1A1-mediated glucuronidation	Nausea, headache, diarrhea, fever, increased creatine kinase

Adapted from Panel on Antiretroviral Guidelines for Adults and Adolescents: Guidelines for the use of antiretroviral agents in HIV-1-infected adults and adolescents. Department of Health and Human Services. December 1, 2009; 1–161. [cited 2011 Nov 23]. Available from: http://www.aidsinfo.nih.gov/ContentFiles/AdultandAdolescentGL.pdf.

Table 21.11 GENERAL CHARACTERISTICS OF CHEMOKINE CORECEPTOR (CCR5) ANTAGONISTS

DRUG NAME (ALIAS)	DOSING & ADJUSTMENTS	METABOLISM	TOXIC/ADVERSE EFFECTS
Maraviroc (MVC)	300 mg twice daily with drugs that are not strong CYP3A inhibitors 150 mg twice daily with drugs that are strong CYP3A inhibitors 600 mg twice daily with drugs that are CYP3A inducers Take without regard to food No adjustment for renal insufficiency	CYP3A4 substrate	Abdominal pain, cough, dizziness, musculoskeletal symptoms, pyrexia, rash, upper respiratory tract infections, hepatotoxicity, orthostatic hypotension

Abbreviation: CYP, cytochrome P450.

Adapted from Panel on Antiretroviral Guidelines for Adults and Adolescents: Guidelines for the use of antiretroviral agents in HIV-1-infected adults and adolescents. Department of Health and Human Services. December 1, 2009; 1–161. [cited 2011 Nov 23]. Available from: http://www.aidsinfo.nih.gov/ContentFiles/AdultandAdolescentGL.pdf.

- Antiretroviral treatment should be considered for all asymptomatic HIV-infected individuals with CD4 cell count of less than 500 cells/mcL.

- All pregnant women should receive antiretroviral treatment.

RECOMMENDATIONS FOR POSTEXPOSURE PROPHYLAXIS

Numerous studies have estimated that the average risk for HIV transmission is approximately 0.3% after percutaneous exposure to HIV-infected blood and more than 90% with transfusion of HIV-infected blood (Table 21.1). A retrospective case-control study of health care workers found that the use of zidovudine was associated with a 79% decrease in the risk for HIV transmission. Results of that study, results from studies in animals, and data from the Pediatric AIDS Clinical Trials Group on the efficacy of zidovudine for preventing perinatal transmission of HIV prompted the US Public Health Service to issue recommendations for prophylaxis in health care workers after occupational exposure to HIV. Systems of care, including written protocols, should be in place to prompt reporting and to facilitate management of exposed health care workers.

- In health care workers, the use of zidovudine is associated with a 79% decrease in the risk for HIV transmission.

The risk of infection after exposure is a function of the type of exposure and the infectivity of the exposure source. Infectivity is related to viral load. An undetectable viral load is associated with a very small chance of infectivity, but it does not lower the risk to zero. Exposure to a hollow needle, a deep puncture wound, or an exposure with visible blood on the device or needle is considered a high-risk exposure in the health care setting. Receptive anal intercourse with a partner known to be HIV-infected and with a high viral load is a high-risk sexual exposure. For most HIV exposures, a 4-week regimen of 2 or 3 antiretroviral drugs is recommended. The preferred 2-drug combinations are 1) zidovudine plus lamivudine (or emtricitabine) or 2) tenofovir plus lamivudine (or emtricitabine). The addition of a PI is recommended for

Table 21.12 ANTIRETROVIRAL THERAPY RECOMMENDATIONS FOR TREATMENT-NAÏVE PATIENTS WITH NO RESISTANCE: 2 NRTIS + (1 PI, 1 NNRTI, OR RALTEGRAVIR[a])

AGENT	PREFERRED	ALTERNATIVE
NRTI combination	Coformulated tenofovir + emtricitabine (Truvada)	Coformulated zidovudine + lamivudine (Epzicom) *or* coformulated zidovudine + lamivudine (Combivir) Emcitrabine & lamivudine can be interchanged when not used in a coformulation
PI	Atazanavir + ritonavir once daily *or* Darunavir + ritonavir once daily	Fosamprenavir + ritonavir *or* coformulated lopinavir + ritonavir (Kaletra) *or* saquinavir + ritonavir twice daily
NNRTI	Efavirenz[b]	Nevirapine
Raltegravir[a]		

Abbreviations: NNRTI, nonnucleoside reverse transcriptase inhibitor; NRTI, nucleoside reverse transcriptase inhibitor; PI, protease inhibitor.

[a] Raltegravir is the preferred and only currently available integrase inhibitor.

[b] Unless pregnancy likely.

Adapted from Panel on Antiretroviral Guidelines for Adults and Adolescents: Guidelines for the use of antiretroviral agents in HIV-1-infected adults and adolescents. Department of Health and Human Services. December 1, 2009; 1–161. [cited 2011 Nov 23]. Available from: http://www.aidsinfo.nih.gov/ContentFiles/AdultandAdolescentGL.pdf.

exposures with an increased risk of transmission or when resistance to one of the recommended drugs is known or suspected. The sooner postexposure prophylaxis is started, the more likely it is to be effective. Postexposure prophylaxis is not generally recommended if more than 72 hours have elapsed since the exposure. Individual clinicians may prefer other antiretroviral drugs or combinations because of local knowledge and experience.

- The risk of HIV infection is a function of the type of exposure and the infectivity of the exposing source.

- Postexposure prophylaxis should be started as soon as possible and no later than 72 hours after exposure.

VIRAL LOAD AND RESISTANCE TESTING

The goal of antiretroviral treatment is maximal viral suppression for as long as possible with a gradual improvement in the CD4 cell counts and immune recovery. Response to treatment is evaluated by monitoring plasma HIV RNA (viral load) levels. HIV-1 RNA testing should be performed at baseline and repeated every 3 to 4 months during therapy or at more frequent intervals if the situation warrants. A minimal change in plasma viremia is considered a 3-fold or $0.5\text{-}\log_{10}$ increase or decrease. A substantial decrease in the CD4 cell count is a decrease of more than 30% from baseline for absolute cell numbers and a decrease of more than 3% from baseline in percentages of cells.

- A $0.5\text{-}\log_{10}$ change in viral load is considered potentially significant.

In cases of therapy failures, a new regimen consisting of at least 2 new agents, without cross-resistance to the drugs in the failed regimen, should be substituted. Resistance testing (genotyping or phenotyping) has been found to be useful for making the appropriate drug selection for incorporation into a salvage treatment regimen.

Resistance testing (genotyping) is now recommended at the time of initial diagnosis of HIV infection to identify transmitted primary HIV drug resistance, which has been associated with suboptimal response to initial antiretroviral therapy. Resistance testing should be done even if the patient is not ready to start treatment because the dominant virus population of a patient often reverts to wild-type virus with time. If the decision to initiate antiretroviral therapy is made, then repeat resistance testing at the time treatment is started should be performed because it is possible for a patient to acquire drug-resistant virus in the interval between the initial resistance testing and the initiation of antiretroviral therapy ([cited 2011 Nov 23]. Available from: http://www.aidsinfo.nih.gov/ContentFiles/PerinatalGL.pdf).

SUMMARY

- The goal of antiretroviral treatment is maximal viral suppression with improvement in the CD4 cell counts and immune recovery.

- Resistance testing (genotyping) is recommended at the time of initial diagnosis of HIV infection to identify transmitted primary HIV drug resistance.

22.

HEALTH CARE–ASSOCIATED INFECTIONS, INFECTIONS OF THE CENTRAL NERVOUS SYSTEM, INFECTIVE ENDOCARDITIS, SKIN AND SOFT TISSUE INFECTIONS, AND BONE AND JOINT INFECTIONS

Pritish K. Tosh, MD, M. Rizwan Sohail, MD, and Elie F. Berbari, MD

GOALS

- Review the diagnosis and management of health care–associated pneumonias.

- Review the diagnosis and management of bone and joint infections and central nervous system infections.

- Review the prevention and treatment of infective endocarditis.

- Review the diagnosis and management of common skin and soft tissue infections.

HEALTH CARE–ASSOCIATED INFECTIONS

HOSPITAL-ACQUIRED PNEUMONIA, VENTILATOR-ASSOCIATED PNEUMONIA, AND HEALTH CARE–ASSOCIATED PNEUMONIA

Hospital-acquired pneumonia (HAP), ventilator-associated pneumonia (VAP), and health care–associated pneumonia (HCAP) cause 25% of all infections in the intensive care unit and are the basis for 50% of all antimicrobials prescribed in the hospital. These are generally bacterial infections. They are associated with high morbidity and mortality. However, those occurring before the fifth day of hospitalization are generally caused by organisms that are more susceptible to antimicrobials and have a better prognosis than those occurring on or after the fifth hospital day. The diagnostic and therapeutic approaches to HAP, VAP, and HCAP are similar.

HAP is pneumonia that develops in a non-intubated patient more than 48 hours after hospital admission. VAP is pneumonia that develops in a patient more than 48 hours after intubation. HCAP is pneumonia that develops within

90 days of hospitalization that has lasted for 2 days or more, within 90 days of residence in a nursing home or long-term care facility, within 90 days of attending a clinic in a hospital or hemodialysis center, or within 30 days of receiving antimicrobials, chemotherapy, or wound care.

The microbiologic causes of HAP, VAP, and HCAP include aerobic gram-negative bacteria (such as *Escherichia coli*, *Klebsiella*, *Serratia*, *Proteus*, *Citrobacter*, *Enterobacter*, *Pseudomonas*, and *Acinetobacter*) and *Staphylococcus aureus*, including methicillin-resistant, or multiple drug-resistant, *S aureus* (MRSA). The basic principles of treatment include 1) treating early, because morbidity and mortality increase with delays in antimicrobial treatment; 2) knowing regional bacteriology and susceptibility; 3) stewarding antimicrobials to reduce unnecessary antimicrobial use and selection pressure for resistant organisms; and 4) applying prevention strategies.

HAP, VAP, and HCAP should be suspected when there is a new infiltrate and clinical signs of lower respiratory tract infection such as fever, purulent sputum, leukocytosis, and decline in oxygenation. A blood culture and culture of lower respiratory tract secretions (eg, obtained with bronchoalveolar lavage) should be performed before starting or changing therapy with antimicrobials, but they should not delay the initiation of therapy with new antimicrobials. If a patient has clinical improvement 48 to 72 hours after HAP, VAP, or HCAP is suspected and tracheal aspirate cultures are negative, use of antimicrobials can safely be stopped.

Empiric antimicrobial therapy should be based on local microbiologic and susceptibility data. In general, initial empiric therapy should include an anti-pseudomonal β-lactam (eg, cefepime, ceftazadime, imipenem, meropenem, doripenem, or piperacillin-tazobactam) *plus* an anti-pseudomonal aminoglycoside or fluoroquinolone (eg, amikacin, gentamicin, tobramycin, ciprofloxacin, or levofloxacin) *plus* vancomycin or linezolid for coverage of MRSA. In patients with recent antimicrobial exposure, antimicrobials of a different drug class should be used for empiric therapy. Antimicrobial therapy can be narrowed once the cause and antimicrobial susceptibilities are known. If started early, antimicrobial therapy can be stopped after 7 days, with the exception of infections caused by *Pseudomonas*, for which 14 or more days are often needed.

The following are recommended strategies for the prevention of HAP, VAP, and HCAP:

General
    Staff education and hand hygiene
    Surveillance of infections in the intensive care unit, including susceptibility
Aspiration precautions
    Semirecumbent position (30°-45°) rather than supine
    Preference of enteral feeding over parenteral nutrition
Intubation and mechanical ventilation
    Avoid reintubation
    Noninvasive ventilation should be used when possible in select patients
    Orotracheal and orogastric tubes are preferred over nasotracheal and nasogastric tubes
    Continuous aspiration of subglottic secretions should be used
    Endotracheal tube cuff pressure should be maintained >20 cm H_2O
    Contaminated condensate should be carefully removed from ventilator circuits
    Protocols to reduce sedation and accelerate weaning should be enacted

CATHETER-RELATED BLOODSTREAM INFECTION

Approximately 5 million central venous catheters are placed in the United States annually. About 1 in 20 of these catheters get infected. Indeed, catheter-related bloodstream infection (CR-BSI) is the most common cause of health care–associated bacteremia in the United States. CR-BSI is associated with substantial cost (about $28,000 per survivor), increased length of stay (average 6.5 days), and substantial mortality (10%-25%).

Catheter infection may present with local manifestations (port, tunnel, or exit site infection) or CR-BSI. Local infections are easy to recognize and always necessitate removal of the infected catheter. However, CR-BSI may present without any inflammatory signs or drainage from the exit site or tunnel. In these situations, blood should be simultaneously drawn from the catheter and a peripheral site. If cultures of blood drawn from the catheter have positive results 2 hours before the cultures from the peripheral site (differential time to positivity), this finding has high correlation (>80%) with catheter infection. If the catheter is urgently removed (eg, because of absence of an alternative source of infection), the catheter tip should be submitted for culture. Growth of more than 15 colony-forming units (per milliliter) of bacteria is highly suggestive of the catheter being the source of bloodstream infection.

- Differential time to culture positivity (cultures of blood drawn from the catheter are positive 2 hours before those

from the peripheral site) or a catheter tip with growth >15 colony-forming units per milliliter suggests the catheter as the source of bloodstream infection.

Removal of the infected catheter is always the preferred method of treating CR-BSI. Antibiotic lock therapy, in combination with systemic antimicrobial agents, is a key ingredient of catheter salvage attempts. A clinically unstable patient, presence of local or systemic complications, and infection with virulent organisms (such as *S aureus*, *Candida*, or gram-negative bacteria) warrant removal of an infected catheter.

COMMON NOSOCOMIAL PATHOGENS

S aureus

Staphylococcus aureus is a common cause of nosocomial infections, including surgical site infections, CR-BSI, and VAP. In cases in which nosocomial *S aureus* bacteremia is caused by a removable focus of infection (such as an intravenous catheter), a 2-week course of therapy may be sufficient if the infected catheter is quickly removed; such an approach leads to rapid resolution of fever and bacteremia. However, most cases of community-acquired *S aureus* bacteremia should be treated for 4 to 6 weeks with parenteral antibiotics because of the potential for metastatic abscesses and infective endocarditis. Some experts recommend using transesophageal echocardiography in all cases of *S aureus* bacteremia to screen for endocarditis. Urine cultures positive for *S aureus* should raise concern for *S aureus* bacteremia with secondary seeding of the urinary tract.

- Cases of community-acquired *S aureus* bacteremia should be treated for 4–6 weeks with parenteral antibiotics.

Most *S aureus* strains produce β-lactamase (a penicillinase) and thus are resistant to penicillin G or amoxicillin but are susceptible to β-lactam–β-lactamase inhibitor combination drugs such as amoxicillin-clavulanic acid. The semisynthetic penicillins (nafcillin, oxacillin) and first-generation cephalosporins remain active and are drugs of choice against methicillin-sensitive *S aureus* (MSSA) strains. Strains of *S aureus* with resistance to the β-lactam antibiotics have spread worldwide. This resistance is caused by an alteration of the penicillin-binding proteins in the cell wall. These strains, referred to as MRSA, are resistant to all β-lactam antibiotics, and often to other classes of antibiotics, but remain susceptible to drugs such as vancomycin, linezolid, or daptomycin. Strains of MRSA with decreased susceptibility to vancomycin have also emerged. Vancomycin intermediately resistant *S aureus* (VISA) has a minimum inhibitory concentration (MIC) of 4 to 8 mcg/mL, whereas vancomycin-resistant *S aureus* (VRSA) has an MIC of 16 or more mcg/mL.

If *S aureus* is penicillin susceptible (<5% of clinical isolates), penicillin G is the most active agent. For penicillin-allergic patients, effective alternatives include cefazolin and vancomycin. If the isolate is methicillin-susceptible, then nafcillin, oxacillin, or cephalosporins (first-generation) have better efficacy than vancomycin. Vancomycin is the most reliable and well-studied drug for treating serious infections caused by MRSA. Linezolid, dalfopristin/quinupristin, daptomycin, and tigecycline are newer drugs that are also active against MRSA. Some strains of MRSA may retain susceptibility to trimethoprim-sulfamethoxazole, minocycline, or the macrolides. However, these antibiotics are mostly used for treatment of non–life-threatening infections such as skin and soft tissue infections or chronic suppression of hardware-associated *S aureus* infections after completion of a parenteral antibiotic course for acute infection.

Staphylococcus aureus organisms frequently colonize the nares, which may predispose to invasive infections. Subclinical nasal colonization can result in nosocomial transmission of MRSA. Topical mupirocin ointment or other therapies (such as trimethoprim-sulfamethoxazole with or without rifampin) may temporarily eradicate the nasal colonization and have been successful for reducing the rate of postoperative wound infection. However, recolonization after a short interval is frequent.

- Vancomycin is the most reliably active drug for treating serious infections caused by MRSA.

Coagulase-Negative Staphylococci

Staphylococcus epidermidis is the most common of the coagulase-negative staphylococci, although many other staphylococcal species are included in this group. For clinical purposes, they are mostly interchangeable, except *Staphylococcus lugdunensis*, which is more aggressive and clinically behaves like *S aureus*. Coagulase-negative staphylococci are normal skin flora. They are opportunistic pathogens that commonly cause infections associated with medical devices. They rarely cause disease in otherwise healthy persons.

Coagulase-negative staphylococci are frequently associated with intravascular device–related bacteremias, infections associated with cardiac devices (ie, pacemakers, defibrillators), prosthetic valve endocarditis, osteomyelitis (usually after joint arthroplasty or other prosthetic implantations), meningitis after neurosurgical procedures, and infections of ventriculoperitoneal shunts and atrioventricular shunts. Treatment usually requires removal of the foreign body and administration of appropriate antibiotics. Coagulase-negative staphylococci have also been associated with peritonitis in patients undergoing chronic ambulatory peritoneal dialysis.

Determining the significance of blood cultures growing coagulase-negative staphylococci can be difficult. True infections generally result in systemic symptoms with multiple positive blood cultures, whereas a single positive blood culture is generally a contaminant.

Treatment duration for bacteremia due to coagulase-negative staphylococci is variable. Although a catheter-related bacteremia can be adequately treated with antibiotics administered for 1 to 2 weeks, prosthetic valve endocarditis due to coagulase-negative staphylococci warrants a 6-week regimen of vancomycin plus rifampin, with gentamicin added for the first 2 weeks. Moreover, valve replacement surgery may be necessary in recalcitrant cases.

- Unless in vitro susceptibility testing shows alternative active agents, serious infections due to coagulase-negative staphylococci should be treated with vancomycin.

- Removal of infected hardware usually is necessary to cure infections due to coagulase-negative staphylococci.

Pseudomonas aeruginosa

Pseudomonas aeruginosa is typically associated with nosocomial infection and is frequently resistant to common antibiotics. *Pseudomonas aeruginosa* and *S aureus* are the most frequent causes of infections complicating severe burn injuries. Other infections caused by *P aeruginosa* include folliculitis associated with hot tub use, osteomyelitis (particularly in injection drug users), malignant otitis externa in patients with diabetes mellitus, complicated urinary tract infections, ventilator-associated pneumonias, and pulmonary infections in patients with cystic fibrosis. Patients with neutropenia are also at high risk for *Pseudomonas* infection, especially bacteremia. Hence, the febrile neutropenic patient should be treated empirically with antipseudomonal antibiotics while culture results are pending. Ecthyma gangrenosum, a necrotizing skin lesion, may develop in neutropenic patients with bacteremia due to *P aeruginosa*.

- *Pseudomonas aeruginosa* and *S aureus* are the most frequent causes of infections complicating massive burns.

- Patients with neutropenic fever should receive empiric antipseudomonal coverage while culture results are pending.

Agents active against most *P aeruginosa* organisms include the extended-spectrum penicillins (piperacillin, ticarcillin), aminoglycosides, ceftazidime and cefepime (the only cephalosporins reliably active against this organism), aztreonam, meropenem, imipenem, doripenem, and ciprofloxacin. Ertapenem, unlike the other carbapenems, does not have activity against *P aeruginosa*. Administering 2 active drugs, usually a β-lactam and an aminoglycoside, is recommended when treating serious infections caused by *P aeruginosa*, especially endocarditis. Antibiotic resistance frequently emerges during and after treatment.

- Use 2 active agents against *P aeruginosa* for all serious infections until susceptibility data are available.

Stenotrophomonas (Xanthomonas) maltophilia

Stenotrophomonas maltophilia infection usually occurs in nosocomial settings. Its most notable trait is its resistance to imipenem and meropenem and also the aminoglycosides, quinolones, except occasionally levofloxacin, and most β-lactam drugs. *Stenotrophomonas maltophilia* is usually susceptible to trimethoprim-sulfamethoxazole and ticarcillin-clavulanate.

- *Stenotrophomonas maltophilia* is resistant to imipenem and meropenem.

INFECTIONS OF THE CENTRAL NERVOUS SYSTEM

BACTERIAL MENINGITIS

Infectious causes of meningitis can be categorized as acute or chronic and as bacterial or non-bacterial. Acute bacterial meningitis is an infectious disease emergency that all internists should be able to recognize and promptly treat. The incidence of bacterial meningitis is estimated to be 3.0 cases per 100,000 person-years, and its overall case fatality rate is 25% in adults. Common predisposing conditions for community-acquired meningitis include acute otitis media, altered immune states, alcoholism, pneumonia, diabetes mellitus, sinusitis, and a cerebrospinal fluid leak. Risk factors for death among adults with community-acquired meningitis include age 60 years or older, altered mental status at presentation, pneumococcal cause, and occurrence of seizures within 24 hours of symptom onset. In two-thirds of patients, classic features of fever and nuchal rigidity are present.

The epidemiology of community-acquired bacterial meningitis has shifted as a consequence of effective vaccination for *Haemophilus influenzae* type B and likely will further evolve with widespread use of the 7-valent vaccine for *Streptococcus pneumoniae* and the meningococcal conjugate vaccine. Currently, the organisms most commonly causing community-acquired meningitis in adults are *S pneumoniae* (38%), *Neisseria meningitidis* (14%), *Listeria monocytogenes* (11%), streptococci (7%), *S aureus* (5%), *H influenzae* (4%), and gram-negative bacilli (4%).

Patients who are at risk for central nervous system mass lesions or have signs of increased intracranial pressure should undergo noncontrast computed tomography of the head before undergoing lumbar puncture. Indications for computed tomography before lumbar puncture include age older than 60 years, immunocompromised host, new-onset seizures, papilledema, altered consciousness, or focal neurologic deficits. Treatment with empiric antibiotics should not be delayed if computed tomgraphy is necessary and could be started once blood for culture has been drawn.

Typical cerebrospinal fluid characteristics in bacterial meningitis include a cell count of 1,000 to 5,000/mcL (range, <100–10,000) and a glucose value less than 40 mg/dL or a cerebrospinal fluid–serum glucose ratio less than 0.4. The differential cell count is more likely to show a predominance of neutrophils. The Gram stain is positive in 60% to 90% of the cases. Countercurrent immunoelectrophoresis or latex agglutination tests may provide results in 15 minutes and are useful for the detection of *H influenzae* type B; *S pneumoniae*; *N meningitidis* types A, B, C, and Y; *E coli* K1; and group B streptococci in the absence of a positive Gram stain. Cerebrospinal fluid cultures are positive in 70% to 85% of cases. Blood cultures also may be positive and should be routinely performed in all cases of suspected bacterial meningitis. Polymerase chain reaction methods are being increasingly used to diagnose meningitis due to *S pneumoniae*, *H influenzae* type B, *Streptococcus agalactiae*, *L monocytogenes*, and *N meningitidis*.

Management of suspected community-acquired bacterial meningitis is outlined in Figure 22.1, and recommendations for antimicrobial therapy are listed in Table 22.1.

Recent guidelines from Infectious Diseases Society of America suggest a role for the use of dexamethasone in the early treatment of suspected pneumococcal meningitis in adults and *H influenzae* type B meningitis in children. There is inadequate evidence to support dexamethasone use for other pathogens responsible for bacterial meningitis. It is important to remember that corticosteroids are beneficial when they are administered either concurrently or before antimicrobial therapy. The optimal approach is to obtain a cerebrospinal fluid sample and administer dexamethasone and then the appropriate empiric antibiotic. Dexamethasone 0.15 mg/kg should be given 10 to 20 minutes *before* the first dose of antibiotics and the dose repeated every 6 hours for the first 2 to 4 days. If it is subsequently determined that the patient does not have pneumococcal meningitis, dexamethasone therapy should be discontinued.

- Risk factors for death in bacterial meningitis are age ≥60 years decreased mental status at admission, seizures within 24 hours of symptom onset, and pneumococcal cause.

- Gram stains of cerebrospinal fluid are positive in 60%-90% of cases.

- Organisms most commonly causing community-acquired infection in adults are *S pneumoniae*, *N meningitidis*, *L monocytogenes*, and *H influenzae*.

The causative organisms, affected age groups, and predisposing factors in bacterial meningitis are listed in Table 22.2, and empiric treatment in various age and patient groups is outlined in Table 22.3.

Immunocompromised hosts, pregnant women, and elderly patients should receive an empiric antibiotic regimen that includes coverage for *L monocytogenes*. High-dose ampicillin is the treatment of choice. An aminoglycoside can be added to treatment with ampicillin if *L monocytogenes* meningitis is confirmed. High-dose intravenous trimethoprim-sulfamethoxazole is an alternative for patients with penicillin allergy. *Listeria monocytogenes* can be mistakenly reported as a diphtheroid on cerebrospinal fluid culture and labeled a contaminant.

- Immunocompromised hosts, pregnant women, and the elderly should receive an empiric antibiotic regimen that includes high-dose ampicillin as coverage for *L monocytogenes*.

MENINGOCOCCAL MENINGITIS

Neisseria meningitidis is a gram-negative diplococcus that is carried in the nasopharynx of otherwise healthy persons. It initiates invasion by penetrating the airway epithelial layer. Because of widespread use of *H influenzae* vaccination in children, *N meningitidis* has emerged as a leading cause of bacterial meningitis in children and young adults. Most

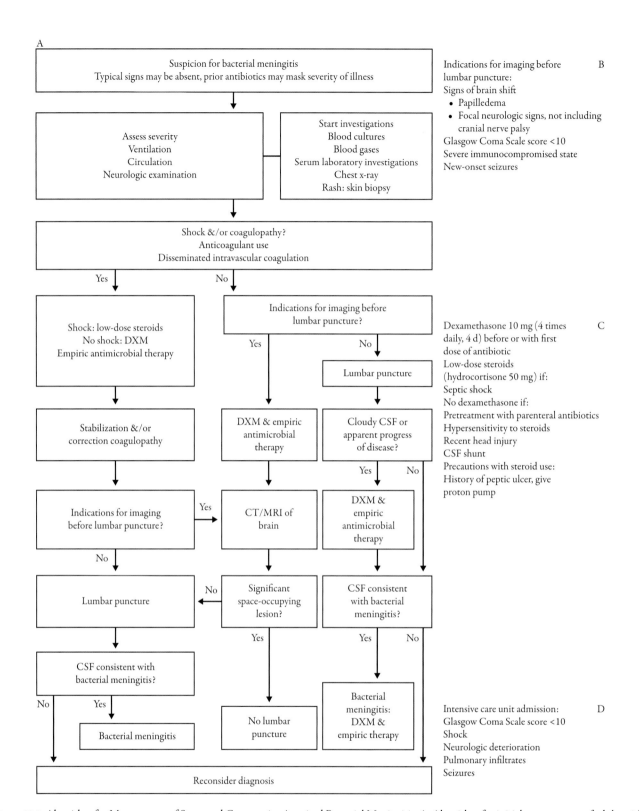

Figure 22.1 Algorithm for Management of Suspected Community-Acquired Bacterial Meningitis. A, Algorithm for initial management of adults with bacterial meningitis. B, Indications for performing imaging before lumbar puncture. C, Recommendations for adjunctive dexamethasone therapy in adults with bacterial meningitis. D, Criteria for admission of patients with bacterial meningitis to the intensive care unit. CSF indicates cerebrospinal fluid; CT, computed tomography; DXM, dexamethasone; MRI, magnetic resonance imaging. (Adapted from van de Beek D, de Gans J, Tunkel AR, Wijdicks EFM. Community-acquired bacterial meningitis in adults. N Engl J Med. 2006 Jan 5;[Suppl Appendix]354[1]:44–53. Used with permission.)

Table 22.1 RECOMMENDATIONS FOR ANTIMICROBIAL THERAPY IN ADULTS WITH COMMUNITY-ACQUIRED BACTERIAL MENINGITIS

EMPIRIC THERAPY

Predisposing Factor	Common Bacterial Pathogens	Antimicrobial Therapy
Age, y		
16–50	*Neisseria meningitidis, Streptococcus pneumoniae*	Vancomycin plus a third-generation cephalosporin[a,b]
>50	*S pneumoniae, N meningitidis, Listeria monocytogenes,* aerobic gram-negative bacilli	Vancomycin plus a third-generation cephalosporin plus ampicillin[b,c]
With risk factor present[d]	*S pneumoniae, L monocytogenes, Haemophilus influenzae*	Vancomycin plus a third-generation cephalosporin plus ampicillin[b,c]

SPECIFIC ANTIMICROBIAL THERAPY

Microorganism, Susceptibility	Standard Therapy	Alternative Therapies
S pneumoniae		
Penicillin MIC		
<0.1 mg/L	Penicillin G or ampicillin	Third-generation cephalosporin,[b] chloramphenicol
0.1–1.0 mg/L	Third-generation cephalosporin[b]	Cefepime, meropenem
≥2.0 mg/L	Vancomycin plus a third-generation cephalosporin[b,c]	Fluoroquinolone[f]
Cefotaxime or ceftriaxone MIC		
≥1.0 mg/L	Vancomycin plus a third-generation cephalosporin[b,g]	Fluoroquinolone[f]
N meningitidis		
Penicillin MIC		
<0.1 mg/L	Penicillin G or ampicillin	Third-generation cephalosporin,[b] chloramphenicol
0.1–1.0 mg/L	Third-generation cephalosporin[b]	Chloramphenicol, fluoroquinolone, meropenem
L monocytogenes	Penicillin G or ampicillin[h]	Trimethoprim-sulfamethoxazole, meropenem
Group B streptococcus	Penicillin G or ampicillin[h]	Third-generation cephalosporin[b]
Escherichia coli & other Enterobacteriaceae	Third-generation cephalosporin[b]	Aztreonam, fluoroquinolone, meropenem, trimethoprim-sulfamethoxazole, ampicillin
Pseudomonas aeruginosa	Ceftazidime or cefepime[h]	Aztreonam,[h] ciprofloxacin,[h] meropenem[h]

(*continued*)

EMPIRIC THERAPY

H influenzae	
β-Lactamase negative	Ampicillin
β-Lactamase positive	Third-generation cephalosporin,[b] cefepime, chloramphenicol, fluoroquinolone
	Cefepime, chloramphenicol, fluoroquinolone
Chemoprophylaxis[i]	
N meningitidis	Third-generation cephalosporin[b]
	Rifampicin (rifampin), ceftriaxone, ciprofloxacin, azithromycin

Abbreviation: MIC, minimal inhibitory concentration.

[a] Only in areas with very low penicillin-resistance rates (<1%) should monotherapy with penicillin be considered, although many experts recommend combination therapy for all patients until results of in vitro susceptibility testing are known.

[b] Cefotaxime or ceftriaxone.

[c] Only in areas with very low penicillin-resistance & cephalosporin-resistance rates should combination therapy of amoxicillin (ampicillin) & a third-generation cephalosporin be considered.

[d] Alcoholism, altered immune status.

[e] Consider addition of rifampicin (rifampin) if dexamethasone is given.

[f] Gatifloxacin or moxifloxacin; no clinical data on use in patients with bacterial meningitis.

[g] Consider addition of rifampicin (rifampin) if the MIC of ceftriaxone is ≥2 mg/L.

[h] Consider addition of an aminoglycoside.

[i] Prophylaxis is indicated for close contacts (defined as those with intimate contact, which covers those eating & sleeping in the same dwelling & those having close social & kissing contacts) or health care workers who perform mouth-to-mouth resuscitation, endotracheal intubation, or endotracheal tube management. Patients with meningococcal meningitis who receive monotherapy with penicillin or amoxicillin (ampicillin) should also receive chemoprophylaxis, because carriage is not reliably eradicated by these drugs.

Note: The preferred intravenous doses in patients with normal renal & hepatic function: penicillin, 2 million units every 4 hours; amoxicillin or ampicillin, 2 g every 4 hours; vancomycin, 15 mg/kg every 8 to 12 hours; third-generation cephalosporin: ceftriaxone, 2 g every 12 hours, or cefotaxime, 2 g every 4 to 6 hours; cefepime, 2 g every 8 hours; ceftazidime, 2 g every 8 hours; meropenem, 2 g every 8 hours; chloramphenicol, 1 to 1.5 g every 6 hours; fluoroquinolone: gatifloxacin, 400 mg every 24 hours, or moxifloxacin, 400 mg every 24 hours, although no data on optimal dose is needed in patients with bacterial meningitis; trimethoprim-sulfamethoxazole, 5 mg/kg every 6 to 12 hours; aztreonam, 2 g every 6 to 8 hours; ciprofloxacin, 400 mg every 8 to 12 hours; rifampicin (rifampin), 600 mg every 12 to 24 hours; aminoglycoside: gentamicin, 1.7 mg/kg every 8 hours. The preferred dose for chemoprophylaxis: rifampicin (rifampin), 600 mg orally twice daily for 2 days; ceftriaxone, 250 mg intramuscularly; ciprofloxacin, 500 mg orally; azithromycin, 500 mg orally.

The duration of therapy for patients with bacterial meningitis has often been based more on tradition than on evidence-based data & needs to be individualized on the basis of the patient's response. In general, antimicrobial therapy is given for 7 days for meningitis caused by *Neisseria meningitidis* & *Haemophilus influenzae*, 10 to 14 days for *Streptococcus pneumoniae*, & at least 21 days for *Listeria monocytogenes*.

Adapted from van de Beek D, de Gans J, Tunkel AR, Wijdicks EFM. Community-acquired bacterial meningitis in adults. N Engl J Med. 2006 Jan 5;354(1):44–53. Used with permission.

Table 22.2 ORGANISMS INVOLVED, AFFECTED AGE GROUPS, AND PREDISPOSING FACTORS IN BACTERIAL MENINGITIS

ORGANISM	AGE GROUP	COMMENT	PREDISPOSING FACTORS
Streptococcus pneumoniae	Any age, but often elderly	Most common cause of recurrent meningitis in adults	Cerebrospinal fluid leak, alcoholism, splenectomy, functional asplenia, multiple myeloma, hypogammaglobuline-mia, Hodgkin disease, HIV
Neisseria meningitidis	Infants to 40 y	Petechial rash is common Epidemics occur in closed populations	Terminal component complement deficiency
Haemophilus influenzae, type B	>Neonate to 6 y	Significant decrease in incidence since licensure of *H influenzae* B vaccine	Hypogammaglobulinemia in adults, HIV, splenectomy, functional asplenia
Escherichia coli, group B streptococci	Neonates		Maternal colonization
Gram-negative bacilli	Any age	*Staphylococcus aureus* & coagulase-negative staphylococci also common after neurosurgical procedure	Neurosurgical procedures, bacteremia due to urinary tract infection, pneumonia, etc, *Strongyloides* hyperinfection syndrome
Listeria monocytogenes	Neonates; immunosuppressed		

Abbreviation: HIV, human immunodeficiency virus.

sporadic cases (95%-97%) are caused by serogroups B, C, and Y, whereas A and C strains are usually observed in epidemics. Risk factors for meningococcal infection include host and environmental factors. Host defects include terminal complement component (C5-C9) deficiencies, which increase attack rates but are associated with low mortality, and properdin defects, which increase the risk of invasive disease. The organism is spread via airborne droplets from asymptomatic pharyngeal carriers. Environmental factors include a preceding viral respiratory infection; household, barracks, or dormitory crowding; chronic medical illnesses; corticosteroid use; and active or passive smoking. Travel to the "meningitis belt" of north central Africa or to the Haj in

Saudi Arabia is a risk factor for meningococcal meningitis, and vaccination is required.

Neisseria meningitidis infection often begins with a mild upper respiratory tract illness that may then disseminate into the bloodstream, leading to the development of a petechial rash that often occurs around the same time as the development of fever and meningeal signs. The diagnosis can be made by visualizing the small Gram-negative diplococci on a cerebrospinal fluid Gram stain. Treatment is with penicillin G if the MIC concentration is less than 0.1 mcg/mL, otherwise high-dose ceftriaxone or cefotaxime is preferred.

Close contacts of the index case (hospital workers with direct exposure to respiratory secretions during intubation or

Table 22.3 EMPIRIC THERAPY FOR BACTERIAL MENINGITIS

AGE GROUP/PATIENT GROUP	COMMON PATHOGENS	ANTIMICROBIAL THERAPY
Age		
0–4 wk	Group B streptococci, *Escherichia coli*, *Listeria monocytogenes*, *Klebsiella pneumoniae*, *Enterococcus* spp, *Salmonella* spp	Ampicillin plus cefotaxime or ampicillin plus an aminoglycoside
1–23 mo	Group B streptococci, *E coli*, *L monocytogenes*, *Haemophilus influenzae*, *Streptococcus pneumoniae*, *Neisseria meningitidis*	Vancomycin plus cefotaxime or ceftriaxone
2–50 y	*N meningitidis*, *S pneumoniae*	Vancomycin plus cefotaxime or ceftriaxone
>50 y	*S pneumoniae*, *L monocytogenes*, aerobic gram-negative bacilli	Vancomycin plus either cefotaxime or ceftriaxone plus ampicillin (cephalosporins have NO activity vs *Listeria*)
Basilar skull fracture	*S pneumoniae*, *H influenzae*, group A β-hemolytic streptococci	Vancomycin plus cefotaxime or ceftriaxone
Post-neurosurgery	Coagulase-negative staphylococci, *Staphylococcus aureus*, aerobic gram-negative bacilli (including *P aeruginosa*)	Vancomycin plus cefepime or ceftazidime or meropenem

Adapted from Tunkel AR, Hartman BJ, Kaplan SL, Kaufman BA, Roos KL, Scheld WM, et al. Practice guidelines for the management of bacterial meningitis. Clin Infect Dis. 2004 Nov 1;39(9):1267–84. Epub 2004 Oct 6. Used with permission.

mouth-to-mouth resuscitation, roommates, household contacts, day-care center members, persons exposed to patients' oral secretions) should be offered chemoprophylaxis within 24 hours of exposure. For adults, ceftriaxone (250 mg intramuscularly), rifampin (600 mg twice daily for 2 days), or ciprofloxacin (use only in patients 18 years or older, 500 mg for 1 dose) has been used. Cases of ciprofloxacin-resistant *N meningitidis* have been reported recently in Minnesota and North Dakota (in these cases, ceftriaxone, rifampin, or azithromycin is an alternative). Because the carrier state is not eliminated by penicillin, the index patient may require one of these prophylaxis regimens for eradication of carriage. Immunization of certain populations (eg, military recruits, college students living in dormitories, Haj pilgrims, patients with terminal complement component deficiencies or asplenia) is also recommended. Two meningococcal vaccines are currently available for serogroups A, C, Y, and W-135: the older polysaccharide vaccine (Menomune) and a newer conjugate vaccine (Menactra, MCV4) that offers longer protection. The MCV4 vaccine is now recommended at entry to high school.

- Terminal component complement deficiencies can predispose patients to repeated episodes of meningococcal meningitis.

- If the risk for the carrier state is high (household contacts), rifampin, ceftriaxone, or ciprofloxacin should be given for prophylaxis within 24 hours of index case.

PNEUMOCOCCAL MENINGITIS

Streptococcus pneumoniae is the most common cause of bacterial meningitis in adults (Figure 22.2), including those with recurrent meningitis due to cerebrospinal fluid leaks. Meningitis due to susceptible strain of *S pneumoniae* can still be treated successfully with high-dose penicillin G. However, given the spread of penicillin-resistant strains, bacterial meningitis should be empirically treated with high-dose cefotaxime or ceftriaxone, in combination with vancomycin, while awaiting the susceptibility results. Adjunctive treatment with dexamethasone has been shown to be beneficial if started at the same time or before the first dose of antibiotic.

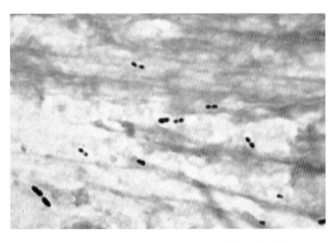

Figure 22.2 *Streptococcus pneumoniae* in Sputum (Gram Stain).

- The most common cause of bacterial meningitis in adults is *S pneumoniae*.

- Consider the possibility of a cerebrospinal fluid leak in patients with recurrent *S pneumoniae* meningitis.

Haemophilus influenzae

Widespread use of the vaccine against *H influenzae* B has dramatically reduced the incidence of invasive disease in children. Non-typeable strains of *H influenzae* more frequently cause disease in adults (primarily respiratory infection). Infections caused by *H influenzae* include pneumonia, meningitis, epiglottitis, and primary bacteremia. The organism is associated with infectious exacerbations of chronic obstructive pulmonary disease and with sinusitis and otitis media. Chronic lung disease, pregnancy, human immunodeficiency virus infection, hypogammaglobulinemia, splenectomy, and malignancy are risk factors for invasive disease.

- Chronic lung disease, pregnancy, human immunodeficiency virus infection, splenectomy, and malignancy are risk factors for invasive disease due to *H influenzae*.

Up to 40% of *H influenzae* organisms recovered from adults with invasive disease are resistant to ampicillin by virtue of β-lactamase production. Nonmeningeal infections with *H influenzae* can be treated with trimethoprim-sulfamethoazole, third-generation cephalosporins, fluoroquinolones, or a β-lactam–β-lactamase inhibitor combination such as ampicillin-sulbactam.

- Approximately 40% of *H influenzae* clinical isolates are resistant to ampicillin.

Infection with *H influenzae* is now an uncommon cause of meningitis in adults, although it can occur with hypogammaglobulinemia, asplenia, or cerebrospinal fluid leak. Third-generation cephalosporins (cefotaxime or ceftriaxone) are the drugs of choice for *H influenzae* meningitis.

LISTERIOSIS

Listeria monocytogenes is a small, motile, gram-positive, rod-shaped organism. Meningitis and bacteremia are the most common clinical manifestations of infection. *Listeria* organisms may be difficult to visualize on Gram stain of spinal fluid. The elderly, neonates, pregnant women, and persons taking corticosteroids are at highest risk for invasive disease due to *Listeria*. Epidemics have been associated with consumption of contaminated dairy products and some ready-to-eat foods such as hot dogs and luncheon meats. Diarrhea is usually a feature of epidemic listeriosis.

Penicillin and ampicillin are the most effective agents against *Listeria*. Antimicrobial coverage for *Listeria* (with ampicillin or trimethoprim-sulfamethoxazole) should always be included for bacterial meningitis in patients who are older than 50 years or are immunosuppressed. Combination therapy with an aminoglycoside is often recommended for treatment of severe disease. *Listeria* is always resistant to the cephalosporins. Trimethoprim-sulfamethoxazole is an effective alternative for the penicillin-allergic patient. Treatment should be continued for 2 to 4 weeks to prevent relapse of disease.

- The elderly, neonates, pregnant women, and persons taking corticosteroids are at highest risk for disease due to *Listeria*.
- Epidemics mainly are associated with consumption of contaminated dairy products and some ready-to-eat foods such as hot dogs and luncheon meats.
- Diarrhea may be a feature of epidemic listeriosis.

GROUP B β-HEMOLYTIC STREPTOCOCCI: STREPTOCOCCUS AGALACTIAE

This organism, a frequent part of the normal flora of the genital and gastrointestinal tracts, is an important cause of postpartum maternal and neonatal infections. It is also an important cause of bacteremia and metastatic infection in elderly adults, especially nursing home residents or those with chronic underlying diseases such as diabetes. In this population, mortality is as high as 38%. The penicillins are the treatment of choice for infections caused by *S agalactiae*. Meningitis, which most commonly occurs in neonates, is best treated with penicillin (or ampicillin) plus gentamicin. Prepartum vaginal culture for group B streptococcus may identify persons at highest risk for infection and allow eradication of the organism before delivery.

ASEPTIC MENINGITIS AND ENCEPHALITIS

The aseptic meningitis syndrome is characterized by an acute onset of meningeal symptoms, fever, cerebrospinal fluid pleocytosis (usually lymphocytic), and negative results of bacterial cultures from the cerebrospinal fluid. Noninfectious causes include medications, such as nonsteroidal anti-inflammatory drugs and trimethoprim-sulfamethoxazole; chemical meningitis; and neoplastic meningitis. Often, this syndrome is a meningoencephalitis due to viruses, which can be differentiated by an accurate exposure history and seasonality (Table 22.4).

In managing a patient with meningoencephalitis, an attempt should be made to establish an etiologic diagnosis. Cerebrospinal fluid analysis should always be performed. Cultures for bacteria and fungus and polymerase chain reaction assays for herpes simplex virus, Epstein-Barr virus, varicella-zoster virus, the enteroviruses, and *Mycobacterium tuberculosis* may be helpful. Cerebrospinal fluid and serum antigen tests for *Cryptococcus neoformans* and urine antigen tests for histoplasmosis or blastomycosis may be useful in the appropriate setting. *Treponema pallidum* (syphilis) and *Borrelia burgdorferi* (Lyme disease) infections can be detected with the cerebrospinal fluid VDRL test and *B burgdorferi*-specific antibody test in the cerebrospinal fluid and serum, respectively. For patients in whom there is a clinical suspicion of herpes simplex virus encephalitis but negative results on initial cerebrospinal fluid polymerase chain reaction, repeat testing in 1 to 3 days may yield positive results.

Besides cerebrospinal fluid investigations, blood tests may be helpful for establishing a cause for the encephalitis. Serologic testing for human immunodeficiency virus, Epstein-Barr virus, and *Mycoplasma pneumoniae* may be useful. Depending on epidemiologic exposure, additional serologic tests on serum samples may be indicated (Table 22.4).

Imaging may be helpful for establishing a cause of encephalitis. Magnetic resonance imaging may be helpful for localizing findings in specific infections such as herpes simplex virus encephalitis (which localizes to the temporal lobes) or for excluding conditions such as acute disseminated encephalomyelitis, which requires high-dose corticosteroids rather than anti-infective therapy. Electroencephalography can be helpful for identifying patients with nonconvulsive seizure activity who are confused, obtunded, or comatose. Electroencephalography shows characteristic periodic lateralized epileptiform discharges in herpes simplex virus encephalitis.

Table 22.4 EPIDEMIOLOGIC CLUES TO INFECTIOUS CAUSES OF ACUTE ASEPTIC MENINGITIS AND MENINGOENCEPHALITIS

SEASON, EXPOSURE, & RISK FACTORS	PATHOGEN
Late summer or fall	Enteroviruses
Winter	Mumps
Rodent urine	Lymphocytic choriomeningitis virus
Mosquito bites	Eastern and Western Equine viruses, West Nile virus, St. Louis virus, La Crosse virus
Ticks	Lyme disease, *Ehrlichia* or *Anaplasma* infection, Rocky Mountain spotted fever
Risk factors for sexually transmitted infections	Herpes simplex virus or human immunodeficiency virus
Immunocompromised patient	*Cryptococcus neoformans*
Travel to endemic area	Histoplasmosis, blastomycosis, coccidioidomycosis, Japanese encephalitis virus, yellow fever, rabies, tickborne encephalitis

Empiric therapy for encephalitis should always include intravenous high-dose acyclovir and antibiotics (to cover the possibility of bacterial meningitis), including doxycycline if risk factors for *Rickettsia* or *Ehrlichia* infections are present. Once an etiologic agent is identified, therapy should be targeted to that pathogen and use of other antimicrobial agents should be discontinued.

- Characteristic features of aseptic meningitis are fever, neck stiffness, cerebrospinal fluid pleocytosis (usually lymphocytic), and negative results of bacterial cultures.

- Empiric therapy for meningoencephalitis should include acyclovir until herpes simplex virus-1 infection is excluded by polymerase chain reaction test of cerebrospinal fluid.

CHRONIC MENINGITIS SYNDROME

Signs and symptoms of meningeal inflammation are more subtle in chronic meningitis and evolve over weeks to months. Chronic meningitis may be due to either infectious or noninfectious causes. Delayed presentation with apathy or altered mentation can occur. The cerebrospinal fluid profile shows inflammatory changes. The infection is most often due to organisms such as *Brucella*, *Nocardia*, spirochetes (syphilis, Lyme disease), fungi (*Cryptococcus*, *Coccidioides*, *Histoplasma*, *Blastomyces*), mycobacteria, and parasites.

OTHER CAUSES OF CENTRAL NERVOUS SYSTEM INFECTIONS

Poliovirus

Although wild-type polio has been eliminated from the Western Hemisphere, it remains endemic in parts of Asia and Africa. Disease still can be imported from these areas. Notably, a recent outbreak in the Netherlands occurred among members of religious groups that were not vaccinated. Polio is most often an asymptomatic infection. The virus affects the nuclei of cranial nerves and anterior motor neurons of the spinal cord, causing a flaccid paralysis. When paralysis develops, it is usually asymmetric. Vaccine-related polio, although rare, can occur with the live oral polio vaccine (OPV). In July 2000, a vaccine-strain polio outbreak occurred in the Dominican Republic and Haiti. Patients traveling to these countries are advised to receive an injectable inactivated polio vaccine booster. A polio-like illness in the United States, without travel or exposure, should also raise suspicion for West Nile virus.

Rabies

A high index of suspicion is a requisite for antemortem diagnosis of rabies. Cardinal clinical manifestations are hydrophobia and copious salivation. Rabies should be considered in any case of encephalitis or myelitis of unknown cause, especially in persons who have recently traveled outside the United States. The virus spreads along peripheral nerves to the central nervous system. The most common sources of exposure are dogs, cats, skunks, foxes, raccoons (Florida, Connecticut), wolves, and bats. Spread by other animals is very rare. Rodents rarely, if ever, transmit rabies.

Rabies acquisition in the United States is predominantly related to bat bites, which may not be apparent, especially if they occur during sleep. Aerosol spread is possible, and it is most often due to exposure to bats during spelunking or in medical laboratories. Annually, 1 or 2 cases of rabies are reported in the United States. From 1995 to 2006, 7 of 37 cases in the United States were due to exposure to rabid animals outside the country, whereas the majority of the rest (28, including 4 transplant recipients from a donor with rabies) were from exposure to bats in the United States. Rabies also has been reported to occur in patients after corneal transplant. The risk for nosocomial transmission is low.

Definitive diagnosis of rabies encephalitis is established by finding Negri bodies on biopsy of the hippocampus. Serum and cerebrospinal fluid can be tested for rabies antibodies when trying to diagnose the disease. Direct fluorescent antibody testing of a skin biopsy specimen from the nape of the neck can be used to detect rabies antigen.

- Rabies should be considered in any case of encephalitis or myelitis of unknown cause.

- Most common sources of exposure are dogs, cats, skunks, foxes, raccoons, wolves, and bats, but rarely rodents.

Any bite by bats or other animals suspected of carrying rabies should be taken very seriously. Post-bite management includes observing the animal, if possible, immediate soap and water washing of the wound, administering rabies immunoglobulin (injected into the bite site), and starting the postexposure rabies vaccine schedule. Human diploid vaccine is more effective and less toxic than the older duck embryo vaccine. Human rabies immunoglobulin is now widely available, mitigating the need to use horse serum immunoglobulin. However, rabies immunoglobulin and vaccine are not of benefit after the onset of clinical disease. Pre-exposure rabies vaccination is advised for patients likely to be in situations that put them at high risk for rabies, such as occupational exposure in veterinary medicine, spelunking, and prolonged stay in rabies-endemic countries. Pre-exposure vaccination mitigates the need for rabies immunoglobulin and decreases the postexposure doses to only 2 (days 0 and 3 after the bite).

SLOW VIRUSES AND PRION-ASSOCIATED CENTRAL NERVOUS SYSTEM DISEASES

Progressive Multifocal Leukoencephalopathy

Progressive multifocal leukoencephalopathy is caused by a papovavirus (JC virus) and usually occurs in immunocompromised patients, such as those with AIDS, leukemia, lymphoma, and immunosuppression for organ transplant. It can cause either diffuse or focal central nervous system abnormalities. Despite its name, progressive multifocal leukoencephalopathy usually causes solitary brain lesions, as seen on computed tomography or magnetic resonance imaging. Results of spinal fluid analysis are normal in most cases, and the diagnosis is based on brain biopsy. Detection of JC virus DNA by polymerase chain reaction testing of cerebrospinal fluid, in appropriate clinical context, confirms the diagnosis. However, the sensitivity of this test is low. There is no effective therapy directed at the JC virus. However, antiretroviral drugs in AIDS cases and reduction of immunosuppression in transplant patients lead to improvement.

- Progressive multifocal leukoencephalopathy is associated with AIDS, leukemia, lymphoma, and immunosuppression for organ transplant.

- JC virus is the causative pathogen for progressive multifocal leukoencephalopathy.

Subacute Sclerosing Panencephalitis (Inclusion Body Encephalitis)

This is a progressively fatal disease of children and adolescents. It is thought to be due to rubeola (measles) virus. Patients are younger than 11 years in 80% of cases. Onset is insidious, with progressive mental deterioration. Later, myoclonic jerks and diffuse abnormalities occur. Measles antibody levels in sera and cerebrospinal fluid are markedly increased. Brain biopsy is necessary to confirm the diagnosis (inclusion body encephalitis). Unfortunately, there is no proven treatment, and the disease is uniformly fatal.

Creutzfeldt-Jakob Disease

This is a rare, degenerative, and fatal disease of the central nervous system. It occurs equally in both sexes, usually at older ages. There are both familial and sporadic forms of the disease. It usually presents as rapidly evolving dementia with myoclonic seizures. Prions (small proteinaceous infectious particles without nucleic acid) have been proposed as the cause of this disease. Nosocomial transmission of Creutzfeldt-Jakob disease can occur via corneal transplant recipients and exposure to cerebrospinal fluid. Several cases in Great Britain in the recent past were linked to consumption of beef from cattle that had bovine spongiform encephalopathy. There is no treatment for Creutzfeldt-Jakob disease.

- Creutzfeldt-Jakob disease presents as rapidly evolving dementia with myoclonic seizures.

INFECTIVE ENDOCARDITIS

Infective endocarditis is universally fatal without treatment. The hallmark of endocarditis is formation of vegetations (a mass of fibrin, platelets, microcolonies of organisms, and scant inflammatory cells) on cardiac valves. Endocarditis can be broadly categorized into native and prosthetic valve endocarditis.

NATIVE VALVE ENDOCARDITIS

Native valve infective endocarditis is more common in men and patients older than 65 years. The age- and sex-adjusted incidence rate of infective endocarditis is 5 to 7 cases per 100,000 person-years. Mitral valve prolapse, bicuspid aortic valves, and aortic sclerosis are the principal predisposing valvular lesions in the absence of prosthetic materials. Increasingly, cases are associated with health care exposures such as hemodialysis and prolonged intravenous therapy.

Infective endocarditis may present acutely or subacutely, depending on the virulence of the infecting organism. In 75% of patients with native valve endocarditis, clinical features include fever, malaise, weight loss, and skin lesions. Heart murmurs are described in 85% of cases, and up to one-third may have a new murmur. Atypical presentation is more frequent in the elderly, especially with low-virulence organisms such as enterococci.

The diagnosis of infective endocarditis is based on the modified Duke criteria, which include pathologic, clinical, microbiologic, and echocardiographic findings (Boxes 22.1 and 22.2 and Figure 22.3). Clinical criteria are subdivided into major and minor criteria. Duke criteria have been validated in multiple studies and have a very high specificity and negative predictive value for endocarditis.

The microbiologic cause of endocarditis partly depends on whether the infection was acquired in the community or health care setting. Most cases of community-acquired native

---

Box 22.1 MODIFIED DUKE CRITERIA FOR THE DIAGNOSIS OF INFECTIVE ENDOCARDITIS

Definite infective endocarditis
  Pathologic criteria
    Microorganisms on culture or histologic examination of a vegetation, a vegetation that has embolized, or an intracardiac abscess specimen, *or*
    Pathologic lesions; vegetation or intracardiac abscess confirmed by histologic examination showing active endocarditis
  Clinical criteria[a]
    2 major criteria, *or*
    1 major criterion & 3 minor criteria, *or*
    5 minor criteria
Possible infective endocarditis
    1 major criterion & 1 minor criterion, *or*
    3 minor criteria
Rejected
    Firm alternative diagnosis explaining evidence of infective endocarditis, *or*
    Resolution of infective endocarditis syndrome with antibiotic therapy for ≤4 days, *or*
    No pathologic evidence of infective endocarditis at surgery or autopsy, with antibiotic therapy for ≤4 days, *or*
    Does not meet criteria for possible infective endocarditis, as above

[a] See Box 22.2 for definitions of major & minor criteria.

Adapted from Li JS, Sexton DJ, Mick N, Nettles R, Fowler VG Jr, Ryan T, et al. Proposed modifications to the Duke criteria for the diagnosis of infective endocarditis. Clin Infect Dis. 2000 Apr;30(4):633–8. Epub 2000 Apr 3. Used with permission.

valve endocarditis are due to viridans group streptococci (ie, *Streptococcus sanguis*, *Streptococcus mutans*, and *Streptococcus mitis*), *S aureus*, and enterococci. Less common causes include *Streptococcus bovis* (associated with gastrointestinal malignancy), *S pneumoniae*, coagulase-negative staphylococci (*Staphylococcus lugdunensis* has a behavior similar to that of *S aureus*), gram-negative bacilli, and fungi. In injection drug users, *S aureus* (60%), streptococci (16%), gram-negative bacilli (13.5%), polymicrobial infection (8.1%), group JK *Corynebacterium* (1.4%), and *Candida* species may be culprits. Tricuspid valve involvement is common in injection drug users and patients with health care–associated endocarditis due to central venous catheters or cardiac devices.

Empiric antibiotic therapy before obtaining blood for culture is the most common cause of culture-negative endocarditis. Other reasons for culture-negative endocarditis include infection with fastidious organisms that are difficult to cultivate in blood cultures, such as *Bartonella* species, *Chlamydia* species, *Tropheryma whippelii*, fungi, and *Coxiella burnetii*. The most frequent causes of culture-negative endocarditis are listed in Box 22.3. Several of these can be diagnosed with serologic tests or molecular assays. The HACEK group (*Haemophilus* species, *Actinobacillus actinomycetemcomitans*, *Cardiobacterium hominis*, *Eikenella* species, and *Kingella kingae*) has become a less frequent cause of culture-negative endocarditis because the organisms are more easily detected with contemporary blood culturing systems.

Treatment guidelines for native valve infective endocarditis are listed in Table 22.5.

Native valve endocarditis may be complicated by invasion and destruction of the valve or endocardium or by distant embolization. Large vegetations, more than 15 mm, increase the risk for embolization. The risk for embolization is greatest before the receipt of appropriate antimicrobials and decreases after the first week of therapy. Large vegetations may be associated with prolonged, yet unrecognized infection or specific microorganisms such as group B streptococci, HACEK, and fungi. Embolization may lead to strokes, mycotic aneurysms, and splenic, hepatic, and renal abscesses. Abscesses due to native valve infective endocarditis need to be drained before valve replacement.

The indications for surgical treatment of native valve infective endocarditis are listed in Box 22.4.

- Congestive heart failure, refractory to medical management, is the most common indication for valve replacement surgery in native valve endocarditis.

PROSTHETIC VALVE ENDOCARDITIS

Prosthetic valve endocarditis accounts for 1% to 5% of all endocarditis cases. However, the increasing number of patients with prosthetic valves and pacemakers is increasing the population at risk. Prosthetic valve endocarditis can be broadly categorized into early and late onset. Early-onset prosthetic valve endocarditis is an infection occurring within 2 months after valve replacement surgery, whereas late-onset prosthetic valve endocarditis occurs more than 2 months postoperatively.

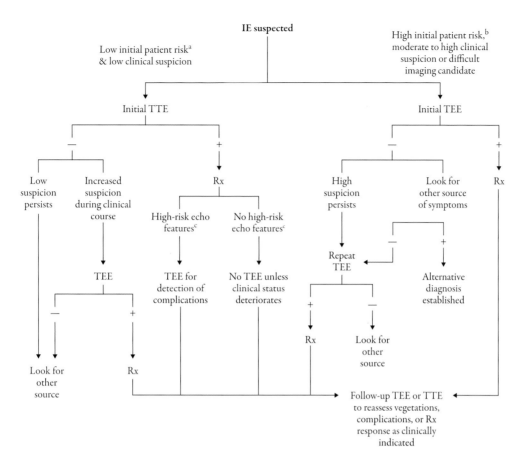

Figure 22.3 An Approach to the Use of Echocardiography (Echo) for the Diagnosis of Infective Endocarditis (IE). [a]For example, a patient with fever and a previously known heart murmur and no other stigmata of IE. [b]High initial patient risks include prosthetic heart valves, many congenital heart diseases, previous endocarditis, new murmur, heart failure, or other stigmata of endocarditis. [c]High-risk echocardiographic features include large or mobile vegetations, valvular insufficiency, suggestion of perivalvular extension, or secondary ventricular dysfunction. Rx indicates antibiotic treatment for endocarditis; TEE, transesophageal echocardiography; TTE, transthoracic echocardiography. (Adapted from Bayer AS, Bolger AF, Taubert KA, Wilson W, Steckelberg J, Karchmer AW, et al. Diagnosis and management of infective endocarditis and its complications. Circulation. 1998 Dec 22–29;98[25]:2936–48. Used with permission.)

Box 22.3 CAUSES OF CULTURE-NEGATIVE ENDOCARDITIS

Previous use of antibiotics
HACEK organisms
   Haemophilus spp
   Actinobacillus actinomycetemcomitans
   Cardiobacterium hominis
   Eikenella spp
   Kingella kingae
Nutritionally variant streptococci (*Abiotrophia* spp)
Neisseria spp
Listeria monocytogenes
Brucella spp
Fungi
Mycobacteria
Legionella spp
Coxiella burnetii
Chlamydia spp
Mycoplasma spp
Nocardia spp
Rothia dentocariosa
Bartonella spp

Staphylococci are the leading cause of prosthetic valve endocarditis. Some studies suggest that the aortic valve is affected more often than the mitral valve. Most early-onset cases often are due to infections introduced in the perioperative setting, such as coagulase-negative staphylococci and *S aureus*. In contrast, late-onset cases are frequently due to hematogenous seeding of prosthetic valves from a distant focus of infection. Therefore, the microbiologic nature of late-onset prosthetic valve endocarditis has certain similarities to that of community-acquired native valve endocarditis. The microorganisms that cause prosthetic valve endocarditis are outlined in Table 22.6. Persistent bacteremia, congestive heart failure, abscess formation, and stroke are predictors of higher mortality in patients with prosthetic valve endocarditis.

Treatment regimens for prosthetic valve endocarditis are summarized in Table 22.7.

SPECIFIC PATHOGENS CAUSING ENDOCARDITIS

Staphylococcus aureus

See the section "Health Care–Associated Infections."

Table 22.5 TREATMENT OF NATIVE VALVE INFECTIVE ENDOCARDITIS

MICROORGANISMS	THERAPY[a]	ALTERNATIVE THERAPY[a]
Penicillin-sensitive viridans group streptococci and *Streptococcus bovis* (MIC, ≤0.1 mcg/mL)	Aqueous crystalline penicillin G, 12–18 × 10^6 U/24 h IV either continuously or in 6 equally divided doses for 4 wk Or Ceftriaxone sodium 2 g IV or IM for 4 wk[c] Or Aqueous penicillin G, 12–18 × 10^6 U/24 h IV either continuously or in 6 equally divided doses for 2 wk *Plus* Gentamicin sulfate,[d] 1 mg/kg IV or IM every 8 h for 2 wk	Vancomycin,[b] 30 mg/kg IV in 2 equally divided doses, not to exceed 2 g/24 h unless serum levels are monitored for 4 wk Vancomycin therapy is recommended for patients allergic to β-lactams (immediate-type hypersensitivity); serum concentration of vancomycin should be obtained 1 h after completion of the infusion & should be in the range of 30–45 mcg/mL for twice-daily dosing
Relatively penicillin-resistant viridans group streptococci (MIC, >0.1 mcg/mL & <0.5 mcg/mL)	Aqueous crystalline penicillin G, 24 × 10^6 U/24 h IV either continuously or in 4–6 equally divided doses for 4 wk *Plus* Gentamicin sulfate,[d] 1 mg/kg IV or IM every 8 h for 2 wk	Vancomycin,[b] 30 mg/kg IV in 2 equally divided doses, not to exceed 2 g/24 h unless serum levels are monitored for 4 wk Vancomycin therapy is recommended for patients allergic to β-lactams (immediate-type hypersensitivity); serum concentration of vancomycin should be obtained 1 h after completion of the infusion & should be in the range of 30–45 mcg/mL for twice-daily dosing
Enterococci (gentamicin- or vancomycin-susceptible) or viridans group streptococci with MIC ≥0.5 mcg/mL or nutritionally variant streptococci (All enterococci causing endocarditis must be tested for antimicrobial susceptibility in order to select optimal therapy)	Aqueous crystalline penicillin G, 18–30 × 10^6 U/24 h IV either continuously or in 6 equally divided doses for 4–6 wk Or Ampicillin sodium 12 g/24 h IV either continuously or in 6 equally divided doses *Plus* Gentamicin sulfate,[d] 1 mg/kg IV or IM every 8 h for 4–6 wk (4-wk therapy recommended for patients with symptoms ≤3 mo in duration; 6-wk therapy recommended for patients with symptoms >3 mo in duration)	Vancomycin,[b] 30 mg/kg IV in 2 equally divided doses, not to exceed 2 g/24 h unless serum levels are monitored for 4–6 wk *Plus* Gentamicin,[d] 1 mg/kg IV or IM every 8 h for 4–6 wk Vancomycin therapy is recommended for patients allergic to β-lactams (immediate-type hypersensitivity); serum concentration of vancomycin should be obtained 1 h after completion of the infusion & should be in the range of 30–45 mcg/mL for twice-daily dosing Cephalosporins are not acceptable alternatives for patients allergic to penicillin
High-level aminoglycoside-resistant *Enterococcus faecalis*: ceftriaxone 2 g IV every 12 h *plus* ampicillin 2 g IV every 4 h for 4–6 wk	Linezolid, 1,200 mg/24 h IV or PO in 2 divided doses for ≥8 wk Or Dalfopristin/quinupristin, 22.5 mg/kg per 24 h IV in 3 divided doses for ≥8 wk	Patients with endocarditis caused by these strains should be treated in consultation with an infectious diseases specialist Cardiac valve replacement may be necessary for bacteriologic cure Cure with antimicrobial therapy alone may be <50% Severe, usually reversible thrombocytopenia may occur with use of linezolid, especially after 2 wk of therapy Dalfopristin/quinupristin only effective against *E faecium* & can cause severe myalgias, which may require discontinuation of therapy Only small number of patients have reportedly been treated with imipenem/cilastatin-ampicillin or ceftriaxone + ampicillin

Organism		
Enterococcus faecalis	Ampicillin sodium, 12 g/24 h IV in 6 divided doses for ≥8 wk — Or — Ceftriaxone sodium, 2 g/24 h IV or IM in 1 dose for ≥8 wk — Plus — Ampicillin sodium, 12 g/24 h IV in 6 divided doses for ≥8 wk — *Pediatric dose* (should not exceed that of a normal adult): linezolid 30 mg/kg per 24 h IV or PO in 3 divided doses; dalfopristin/quinupristin 22.5 mg/kg per 24 h IV in 3 divided doses; imipenem/cilastatin 60–100 mg/kg per 24 h IV in 4 divided doses; ampicillin 300 mg/kg per 24 h IV in 4–6 divided doses; ceftriaxone 100 mg/kg per 24 h IV or IM once daily	Imipenem/cilastatin, 2 g/24 h IV in 4 equally divided doses for ≥8 wk — Plus — Ampicillin sodium, 12 g/24 h IV in 6 divided doses for ≥8 wk — Or — Ceftriaxone sodium, 2 g/24 h IV or IM in 1 dose for ≥8 wk — Plus — Ampicillin sodium, 12 g/24 h IV in 6 divided doses for ≥8 wk
Staphylococcus aureus[e] Methicillin-sensitive	Nafcillin sodium or oxacillin sodium, 2.0 g IV every 4 h for 4–6 wk — Plus — Gentamicin sulfate (optional),[d] 1 mg/kg every 8 h IV or IM for first 3–5 d — Benefit of additional aminoglycoside has not been established	Cefazolin (or other first-generation cephalosporins in equivalent dosages), 2 g IV every 8 h for 4–6 wk — Plus — Gentamicin (optional),[d] 1 mg/kg every 8 h IV or IM for first 3–5 d — Cephalosporins should be avoided in patients with immediate-type hypersensitivity to penicillin — Vancomycin,[b] 30 mg/kg IV in 2 equally divided doses, not to exceed 2 g/24 h unless serum levels are monitored for 4–6 wk — Vancomycin therapy is recommended for patients allergic to β-lactams (immediate-type hypersensitivity); serum concentration of vancomycin should be obtained 1 h after completion of the infusion & should be in the range of 30–45 mcg/mL for twice-daily dosing — Daptomycin 6 mg/kg once daily may be used as an alternative in right-sided endocarditis due to MSSA or MRSA
Methicillin-resistant	Vancomycin,[b] 30 mg/kg IV in 2 equally divided doses, not to exceed 2 g/24 h unless serum levels are monitored for 4–6 wk	Consult infectious diseases specialist — Daptomycin 6 mg/kg once daily may be used as an alternative in right-sided endocarditis due to MSSA or MRSA
HACEK group	Ceftriaxone sodium, 2 g IV or IM for 4 wk[c] — Or — Ampicillin[f]-sulbactam 12 g/24 h IV in 4 divided doses for 4 wk — Or — Ciprofloxacin 1,000 mg/24 h PO or 800 mg/24 h IV in 2 divided doses if unable to tolerate alternatives — Cefotaxime sodium or other third-generation cephalosporins may be substituted	Consult infectious diseases specialist
Neisseria gonorrhoeae	Ceftriaxone, 1–2 g every 24 h for ≥4 wk	Aqueous crystalline penicillin G, 20×10^6 U/24 h IV either continuously or in 6 equally divided doses for 4 wk, for penicillin-susceptible isolates
Gram-negative bacilli	Most effective single drug or combination of drugs IV for 4–6 wk	

(*continued*)

Table 22.5 TREATMENT OF NATIVE VALVE INFECTIVE ENDOCARDITIS (CONTINUED)

MICROORGANISMS	THERAPY[a]	ALTERNATIVE THERAPY[a]
Urgent empiric treatment for culture-negative endocarditis	Vancomycin,[b] 30 mg/kg IV in 2 equally divided doses, not to exceed 2 g/24 h unless serum levels are monitored for 6 wk *Plus* Gentamicin sulfate,[d] 1.0 mg/kg IV every 8 h for 6 wk	
Fungal endocarditis	Amphotericin B *Plus* Flucytosine (optional) *Plus* Cardiac valve replacement (flucytosine levels should be monitored)	
Suspected *Bartonella*, culture negative	Ceftriaxone sodium, 2 g/24 h IV or IM in 1 dose for 6 wk *Plus* Gentamicin sulfate, 3 mg/kg per 24 h IV or IM in 3 divided doses for 2 wk *With or without* Doxycycline 200 mg/kg per 24 h IV or PO in 2 divided doses for 6 wk	Consult infectious diseases specialist

Abbreviations: HACEK, *Haemophilus* spp, *Actinobacillus actinomycetemcomitans*, *Cardiobacterium hominis*, *Eikenella* spp, and *Kingella kingae*; IM, intramuscularly; IV, intravenously; MIC, minimal inhibitory concentration; MRSA, methicillin-resistant *Staphylococcus aureus*; MSSA, methicillin-sensitive *Staphylococcus aureus*; PO, orally.

[a] Dosages recommended are for patients with normal renal function.

[b] Vancomycin dosage should be reduced in patients with impaired renal function. Vancomycin given on an mg/kg basis produces higher serum concentrations in obese patients than in lean patients. Therefore, in obese patients, dosing should be based on ideal body weight. Each dose of vancomycin should be infused over at least 1 hour to reduce the risk of the histamine-release "red man" syndrome.

[c] Patients should be notified that IM injection of ceftriaxone is painful.

[d] Dosing of gentamicin on an mg/kg basis produces higher serum concentrations in obese patients than in lean patients. Therefore, in obese patients, dosing should be based on ideal body weight. (Ideal body weight for men is 50 kg + 2.3 kg per inch over 5 feet, and ideal body weight for women is 45.5 kg + 2.3 kg per inch over 5 feet.) Relative contraindications to the use of gentamicin are age older than 65 years, renal impairment, or impairment of the eighth nerve. Other potentially nephrotoxic agents (such as nonsteroidal anti-inflammatory drugs) should be used cautiously in patients receiving gentamicin.

[e] For treatment of endocarditis due to penicillin-susceptible staphylococci (MIC, <0.1 mcg/mL), aqueous crystalline penicillin G, 12–18 × 10⁶ U/24 h IV either continuously or in 6 equally divided doses for 4 to 6 weeks, can be used instead of nafcillin or oxacillin. Shorter antibiotic courses have been effective in some injection drug users with right-sided endocarditis due to *Staphylococcus aureus*. The routine use of rifampin is not recommended for the treatment of native valve staphylococcal endocarditis.

[f] Ampicillin should not be used if laboratory tests show β-lactamase production.

Data from Wilson WR, Karchmer AW, Dajani AS, Taubert KA, Bayer A, Kaye D, et al; American Heart Association. Antibiotic treatment of adults with infective endocarditis due to streptococci, enterococci, staphylococci, and HACEK microorganisms. JAMA. 1995 Dec 6;274(21):1706–13; adapted from Steckelberg JM, Guiliani ER, Wilson WR. Infective endocarditis. In: Giuliani ER, Fuster V, Gersh BJ, McGoon MD, McGoon DC, editors. Cardiology: fundamentals and practice. 2ⁿᵈ ed. Vol 2. St. Louis (MO): Mosby Year Book; c1991, p. 1739–72. Used with permission of Mayo Foundation for Medical Education and Research; and adapted from Baddour LM, Wilson WR, Bayer AS, Fowler VG Jr, Bolger AF, Levison ME, et al. Infective endocarditis: diagnosis, antimicrobial therapy, and management of complications: a statement for healthcare professionals from the Committee on Rheumatic Fever, Endocarditis, and Kawasaki Disease, Council on Cardiovascular Disease in the Young, and the Councils on Clinical Cardiology, Stroke, and Cardiovascular Surgery and Anesthesia, American Heart Association: executive summary. Circulation. 2005 Jun 14;111(23):3167–84. Used with permission.

Viridans Group Streptococci

Several species of non-Lancefield typeable streptococci are referred to as the viridans group of streptococci. These are part of normal oral and enteric flora. This group of organisms is a common cause of subacute bacterial endocarditis, which should be suspected when viridans group of streptococci are found in blood cultures. Like the pneumococci, these organisms are increasingly likely to display variable resistance to penicillin.

- Viridans group of streptococci are part of normal oral and enteric flora and are usually associated with subacute native valve endocarditis.

Enterococci

Enterococci are an increasingly important cause of bacterial endocarditis. Enterococci are resistant to many antimicrobial agents, including all of the cephalosporins. This resistance allows the organisms to proliferate and cause infections in the hospital setting. Even in susceptible strains, penicillin or vancomycin monotherapy only inhibits bacterial growth but is not bactericidal. Moreover, strains that are resistant to both the penicillins and vancomycin (vancomycin-resistant enterococci) are spreading worldwide. Linezolid, dalfopristin/quinupristin, and daptomycin are used in cases of vancomycin-resistant enterococci infection. However, these agents are also bacteriostatic and not bactericidal. Of note, dalfopristin/quinupristin is active against only *Enterococcus faecium* and not against *E faecalis*.

To achieve the bactericidal activity necessary to cure endocarditis due to enterococci, a combination of penicillin (or ampicillin) plus gentamicin (or streptomycin) is required. The choice of aminoglycoside depends on the results of susceptibility testing. The duration of therapy depends on how long the patient has been ill with endocarditis. Four weeks of therapy is adequate for native valve endocarditis that has been present for less than 3 months and is uncomplicated. When a patient is symptomatic for longer than 3 months, has a prosthetic valve, or is allergic to penicillin, in which case vancomycin needs to be used, there is an unacceptable failure rate

with the 4-week regimen. Therefore, 6 weeks of therapy is recommended. Vancomycin is considered less effective than penicillin and therefore should be used only in cases of penicillin resistance or if a patient is allergic to penicillin. Optimal regimens for isolates resistant to both gentamicin and streptomycin are unknown. A valve replacement procedure may increase the chance for successfully treating subacute bacterial endocarditis due to drug-resistant enterococci.

- Enterococcal endocarditis is best treated with a combination of penicillin (or ampicillin) plus gentamicin (or streptomycin).

Haemophilus Species Other Than *influenzae*

Haemophilus parainfluenzae, H aphrophilus, and *H paraphrophilus* are part of normal oral flora. When these or other members of the HACEK (*Haemophilus* species; *Actinobacillus actinomycetemcomitans; Cardiobacterium hominis; Eikenella corrodens;* and *Kingella* species) group of organisms are recovered from blood cultures, infective endocarditis should be suspected. Large valvular vegetations with systemic emboli are frequent with HACEK endocarditis. Usual treatment is with ceftriaxone or ampicillin-sulbactam (if the organism is susceptible) for 4 weeks.

ADDITIONAL FACTS ABOUT INFECTIVE ENDOCARDITIS

Transesophageal echocardiography is superior to transthoracic echocardiography for the diagnosis and assessment of complications of infective endocarditis. The sensitivity of transthoracic echocardiography for diagnosing endocarditis is less than 50% in most series, whereas it is more than 95% with transesophageal echocardiography. Transesophageal echocardiography is especially useful for detection of cardiac abscesses or mycotic aneurysms, visualization of vegetations less than 5 mm in size, pulmonic valve infection, and vegetation attached to prosthetic valves or cardiac device leads.

Daptomycin 6 mg/kg daily has an efficacy similar to that of standard therapy in *S aureus* bacteremia and endocarditis and causes less nephrotoxicity than β-lactam– or vancomycin-based regimens. However, longer use of daptomycin is associated with more frequent increases in the creatine kinase level.

Short-course combination therapy, which includes an aminoglycoside in *S aureus* endocarditis, may be associated with increased nephrotoxicity. Combination therapy with rifampin should be used only in cases of prosthetic valve endocarditis due to staphylococci. Use of rifampin in uncomplicated cases of *S aureus* bacteremia and native valve endocarditis has been associated with prolonging the duration of bacteremia and increased mortality.

There is a well-recognized association between *Streptococcus bovis* bacteremia and carcinoma of the colon or other colonic disease. The *S bovis* organisms are clinically similar to the viridans group of streptococci and are generally susceptible to penicillin and the cephalosporins.

Table 22.6 CAUSATIVE ORGANISMS FOR PROSTHETIC VALVE ENDOCARDITIS (PVE) IN 556 PATIENTS

CAUSATIVE ORGANISM	TOTAL, NO. (%) (N=556)	EARLY PVE, NO. (%) (n=53)	LATE PVE, NO. (%) (n=331)
Staphylococcus aureus	128 (23.0)	19 (35.9)	61 (18.4)
Methicillin-sensitive *S aureus*	82 (14.7)	8 (15.1)	43 (13.0)
Methicillin-resistant *S aureus*	36 (6.5)	10 (18.9)	11 (3.3)
Coagulase-negative staphylococci	94 (16.9)	9 (17.0)	66 (19.9)
Enterococcus spp	71 (12.8)	4 (7.5)	42 (12.7)
Viridans streptococci	67 (12.1)	1 (1.9)	34 (10.3)
Culture negative	62 (11.2)	9 (17.0)	41 (12.4)
Streptococcus bovis	29 (5.2)	1 (1.9)	22 (6.7)
Fungal	23 (4.1)	5 (9.4)	11 (3.3)
Polymicrobial	10 (1.8)	0	6 (1.8)
HACEK spp	8 (1.4)	0	7 (2.1)
Escherichia coli	7 (1.3)	1 (1.9)	3 (0.9)
Streptococcus agalactiae	5 (0.9)	0	3 (0.9)
Propionibacterium acnes	4 (0.7)	0	3 (0.9)
Streptococcus group G	4 (0.7)	0	3 (0.9)
Propionibacterium NOS	3 (0.5)	0	2 (0.6)
Pseudomonas aeruginosa	3 (0.5)	1 (1.9)	1 (0.3)
Streptococcus anginosus	3 (0.5)	0	2 (0.6)
Streptococcus NOS	3 (0.5)	0	2 (0.6)
Streptococcus pneumoniae	3 (0.5)	0	3 (0.9)
Listeria monocytogenes	2 (0.4)	0	2 (0.6)
Micromonas micros	2 (0.4)	0	2 (0.6)
Mycobacterium spp	2 (0.4)	0	1 (0.3)
Serratia marcescens	2 (0.4)	1 (1.9)	0
Streptococcus gallolyticus	2 (0.4)	0	0
Streptococcus group B	2 (0.4)	0	0
Streptococcus group C	2 (0.4)	0	1 (0.3)

Abbreviations: HACEK, *Haemophilus* spp, *Actinobacillus actinomycetemcomitans*, *Cardiobacterium hominis*, *Eikenella* spp, and *Kingella kingae*; NOS, not otherwise speciated.

Adapted from Wang A, Athan E, Pappas PA, Fowler VG Jr, Olaison L, Paré C, et al. Contemporary clinical profile and outcome of prosthetic valve endocarditis. JAMA. 2007 Mar 28;297(12):1354–61. Used with permission.

INFECTIONS OF CARDIOVASCULAR IMPLANTABLE ELECTRONIC DEVICES

Permanent pacemakers, implantable cardioverter-defibrillators, and other cardiac devices are being increasingly used and are associated with infectious complications. Infections associated with these devices may present as localized generator pocket infection or systemic infection associated with bacteremia or lead endocarditis. Staphylococci (*S aureus* and coagulase-negative staphylococcus) account for two-thirds of the cases. Regardless of the infecting pathogen and clinical presentation, complete removal of the infected device (including generator and transvenous leads) is a requisite for curing these infections.

Box 22.5 and Figure 22.4 summarize Mayo Clinic guidelines for the diagnosis and management of cardiac devices. American Heart Association endorsed these guidelines in the updated Scientific Statement published in 2010.

Table 22.7 TREATMENT OF PROSTHETIC VALVE INFECTIVE ENDOCARDITIS

ORGANISM	THERAPY[a]	ALTERNATIVE THERAPY/COMMENTS[a]
Staphylococcus aureus or coagulase-negative staphylococci: methicillin-resistant	Vancomycin,[b] 30 mg/kg IV in 2 equally divided doses, not to exceed 2 g/24 h unless serum levels are monitored for ≥6 wk *Plus* Rifampin,[c] 300 mg PO every 8 h for ≥6 wk *Plus* Gentamicin sulfate,[d] 1 mg/kg IV or IM every 8 h for first 2 wk of therapy. (If organism is not susceptible to gentamicin, ciprofloxacin may be substituted if the organism is susceptible in vitro)	Rifampin increases the amount of warfarin sodium required for antithrombotic therapy
Staphylococcus aureus or coagulase-negative staphylococci: methicillin-susceptible	Nafcillin sodium or oxacillin sodium, 2 g IV every 4 h for ≥6 wk *Plus* Rifampin,[c] 300 mg orally every 8 h for ≥6 wk *Plus* Gentamicin sulfate,[d] 1 mg/kg IV or IM every 8 h for first 2 wk of therapy. (If organism is not susceptible to gentamicin, ciprofloxacin may be substituted if the organism is susceptible in vitro)	Rifampin increases the amount of warfarin sodium required for antithrombotic therapy First-generation cephalosporins or vancomycin should be used in patients allergic to β-lactams Cephalosporins should be avoided in patients with immediate-type hypersensitivity to penicillin or to methicillin-resistant staphylococci
Enterococci (gentamicin- or vancomycin-susceptible) or viridans group streptococci or nutritionally variant streptococci or *Streptococcus bovis* (All streptococci causing endocarditis must be tested for antimicrobial susceptibility in order to select optimal therapy)	Aqueous crystalline penicillin G, 18–30 × 10⁶ U/24 h IV either continuously or in 6 equally divided doses for 6 wk *Or* Ampicillin sodium, 12 g/24 h IV either continuously or in 6 equally divided doses *Plus* Gentamicin sulfate,[d] 1 mg/kg IV or IM every 8 h for 6 wk	Vancomycin,[b] 30 mg/kg IV in 2 equally divided doses, not to exceed 2 g/24 h unless serum levels are monitored for 4–6 wk *Plus* Gentamicin sulfate,[d] 1 mg/kg IV or IM every 8 h for 4–6 wk Vancomycin therapy is recommended for patients allergic to β-lactams (immediate-type hypersensitivity); serum concentration of vancomycin should be obtained 1 h after completion of the infusion & should be in the range of 30–45 mcg/mL for twice-daily dosing Cephalosporins are not acceptable alternatives for patients allergic to penicillin
Enterococcus faecium	Linezolid, 1,200 mg/24 h IV or PO in 2 divided doses for ≥8 wk *Or* Dalfopristin/quinupristin, 22.5 mg/kg per 24 h IV in 3 divided doses for ≥8 wk	Patients with endocarditis caused by these strains should be treated in consultation with an infectious diseases specialist Cardiac valve replacement may be necessary for bacteriologic cure Cure with antimicrobial therapy alone may be <50% Severe, usually reversible thrombocytopenia may occur with use of linezolid, especially after 2 wk of therapy Dalfopristin/quinupristin only effective against *E faecium* & can cause severe myalgias, which may require discontinuation of therapy Only small number of patients have reportedly been treated with imipenem/cilastatin-ampicillin or ceftriaxone + ampicillin

(continued)

Table 22.7 TREATMENT OF PROSTHETIC VALVE INFECTIVE ENDOCARDITIS (CONTINUED)

ORGANISM	THERAPY[a]	ALTERNATIVE THERAPY/COMMENTS[a]
Enterococcus faecalis	Imipenem/cilastatin, 2 g/24 h IV in 4 equally divided doses for ≥8 wk *Plus* Ampicillin sodium, 12 g/24 h IV in 6 divided doses for ≥8 wk *Or* Ceftriaxone sodium, 2 g/24 h IV or IM in 1 dose for ≥8 wk *Plus* Ampicillin sodium, 12 g/24 h IV in 6 divided doses for ≥8 wk *Pediatric dose* (should not exceed that of a normal adult): linezolid 30 mg/kg per 24 h IV or PO in 3 divided doses; dalfopristin/quinupristin 22.5 mg/kg per 24 h IV in 3 divided doses; imipenem/cilastatin 60–100 mg/kg per 24 h IV in 4 divided doses; ampicillin 300 mg/kg per 24 h IV in 4–6 divided doses; ceftriaxone 100 mg/kg per 24 h IV or IM once daily	

Abbreviations: IM, intramuscularly; IV, intravenously; PO, orally.

[a] Dosages recommended are for patients with normal renal function.

[b] Vancomycin dosage should be reduced in patients with impaired renal function. Vancomycin given on an mg/kg basis produces higher serum concentrations in obese patients than in lean patients. Therefore, in obese patients, dosing should be based on ideal body weight. Each dose of vancomycin should be infused over at least 1 hour to reduce the risk of the histamine-release "red man" syndrome.

[c] Rifampin plays a unique role in the eradication of staphylococcal infection involving prosthetic material; combination therapy is essential to prevent emergence of rifampin resistance.

[d] Dosing of gentamicin on an mg/kg basis produces higher serum concentrations in obese patients than in lean patients. Therefore, in obese patients, dosing should be based on ideal body weight. (Ideal body weight for men is 50 kg + 2.3 kg per inch over 5 feet, and ideal body weight for women is 45.5 kg + 2.3 kg per inch over 5 feet.) Relative contraindications to the use of gentamicin are age older than 65 years, renal impairment, or impairment of the eighth nerve. Other potentially nephrotoxic agents (such as nonsteroidal anti-inflammatory drugs) should be used cautiously in patients receiving gentamicin.

Data from Wilson WR, Karchmer AW, Dajani AS, Taubert KA, Bayer A, Kaye D, et al; American Heart Association. Antibiotic treatment of adults with infective endocarditis due to streptococci, enterococci, staphylococci, and HACEK microorganisms. JAMA. 1995 Dec 6;274(21):1706–13; and adapted from Baddour LM, Wilson WR, Bayer AS, Fowler VG Jr, Bolger AF, Levison ME, et al. Infective endocarditis: diagnosis, antimicrobial therapy, and management of complications: a statement for healthcare professionals from the Committee on Rheumatic Fever, Endocarditis, and Kawasaki Disease, Council on Cardiovascular Disease in the Young, and the Councils on Clinical Cardiology, Stroke, and Cardiovascular Surgery and Anesthesia, American Heart Association: executive summary. Circulation. 2005 Jun 14;111(23):3167–84. Used with permission.

Box 22.5 **GUIDELINES FOR THE DIAGNOSIS AND MANAGEMENT OF CARDIAC DEVICE INFECTIONS**

All patients should have at least 2 blood specimens drawn for culture at initial evaluation

Generator tissue should be obtained for Gram stain & culture, & lead tip tissue should be obtained for culture

Patients who either have positive blood cultures or have negative blood cultures but had recently received antibiotics before blood cultures were done should have TEE to assess for device-related endocarditis

Sensitivity of TTE is low & is not recommended to evaluate for device-related endocarditis

Patients with negative blood cultures & recent prior use of antibiotics & valve vegetations on TEE should be managed in consultation with an infectious diseases expert

All patients with device infection should undergo complete device removal, regardless of clinical presentation

A large (>1 cm) lead vegetation is not a stand-alone indication for surgical lead removal

Blood cultures should be repeated in all patients after device explantation. Patients with persistently positive blood cultures should have treatment for at least 4 weeks with antimicrobials even if TEE is negative for vegetations or other evidence of infection

Duration of antimicrobial therapy should also be extended to ≥4 wk in patients with complicated infection (endocarditis, septic venous thrombosis, osteomyelitis, metastatic seeding)

Adequate débridement & control of infection should be achieved at all sites before reimplantation of a new device

Reevaluation for continued need of the device should be performed before new device placement

If an infected cardiac device cannot be removed, then long-term suppressive antibiotic therapy should be administered after completing an initial course of treatment & securing a clinical response to therapy. Opinion of an infectious diseases expert should be sought

Abbreviations: TEE, transesophageal echocardiography; TTE, transthoracic echocardiography.

Adapted from Sohail MR, Uslan DZ, Khan AH, Friedman PA, Hayes DL, Wilson WR, et al. Management and outcome of permanent pacemaker and implantable cardioverter-defibrillator infections. J Am Coll Cardiol. 2007 May 8;49(18):1851–9. Epub 2007 Apr 23. Used with permission.

PREVENTION OF BACTERIAL ENDOCARDITIS

Recommendations for the prevention of bacterial endocarditis were revised and simplified in 2007. Endocarditis prophylaxis is no longer recommended before genitourinary or gastrointestinal procedures regardless of the cardiac lesions. Prophylaxis for infective endocarditis is now recommended only in patients with high-risk cardiac lesions: those with prosthetic heart valves, previous history of infective endocarditis, or congenital heart disease and in recipients of a cardiac transplant who develop valvulopathy of their transplanted heart (Box 22.6). For these high-risk patients, prophylaxis is indicated before dental procedures that involve manipulation of the gingival tissue or periapical region of the teeth or perforation of the oral mucosa. Current recommendations for antibiotic prophylaxis before a dental procedure are summarized in Table 22.8.

- Antibiotic prophylaxis for infective endocarditis is no longer recommended for genitourinary or gastrointestinal procedures.
- Prophylaxis for infective endocarditis is recommended only for patients with prosthetic cardiac valves, previous infective endocarditis, or congenital heart disease and cardiac transplant recipients with valvulopathy who are undergoing dental procedures.

SKIN AND SOFT TISSUE INFECTIONS

Specific skin and soft tissue infections can be characterized by their visual appearance, including vesicles, bullae, folliculitis, crusted lesions, papular lesions, ulcerations, and cellulitis.

Cellulitis is an acute, spreading infection of the dermis and subcutaneous tissue. Cellulitis is most common in tissue damaged by trauma and in extremities with impaired venous or lymphatic drainage (eg, the arm after mastectomy or the leg after saphenous vein harvest for coronary artery bypass grafting). Minor inflammation or disruption of skin integrity from tinea pedis may serve as a portal of entry for β-hemolytic streptococci (Figure 22.5). The involved area, usually on the lower extremity, is tender, warm, erythematous, and swollen. It lacks sharp demarcation from uninvolved skin. Recurrent cellulitis may develop in patients with a history of dermatitis or malignancy or a prior history of ipsilateral limb cellulitis. Severe group A streptococcal infection can complicate dermatomal varicella infection.

Erysipelas is a superficial cellulitis with prominent lymphatic involvement, presenting with an indurated peau d'orange appearance with a raised border that is well demarcated from normal skin. This infection is painful and most often occurs in the elderly. Recent reports have associated erysipelas with "toxic strep" syndrome.

It is important to exclude animal or human bites, hot tub folliculitis, necrotizing fasciitis, fish tank or water exposures, and mixed infections in diabetics. In most cases, cellulitis is due to β-hemolytic streptococci. A first-generation oral or parenteral cephalosporin (cephalexin or cefazolin) is the usual initial choice if MRSA is not suspected.

Impetigo describes a superficial skin infection. Historically, *Streptococcus pyogenes* was the most common cause of impetigo. Since the 1980s, however, most cases of impetigo have been caused by *S aureus* or mixed infections with both *S aureus* and β-hemolytic streptococci.

The approach to treatment of cellulitis is guided by the type of skin and soft tissue infection and the severity of clinical presentation. Empiric antibiotic therapy should include MRSA coverage if it is suspected on the basis of local epidemiologic factors. If a patient presents with a purulent lesion, it should

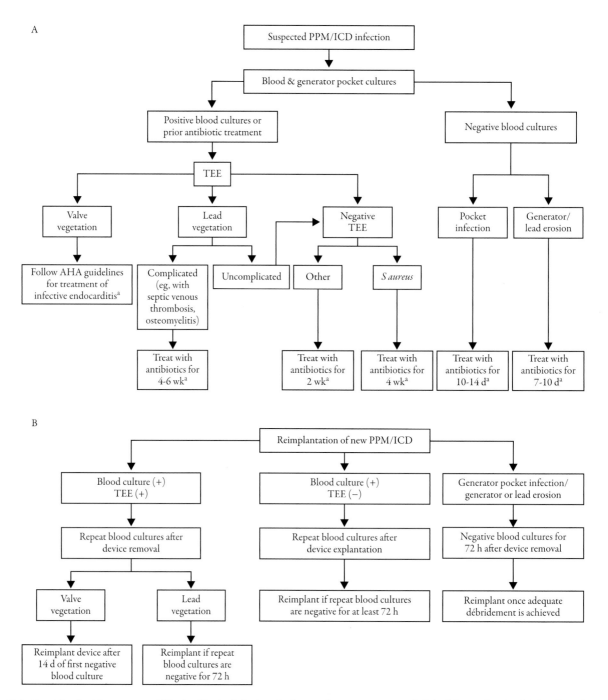

Figure 22.4 Algorithm for Management of Cardiac Device Infection. A, Approach to management of adults (also see Box 22.6). This algorithm applies only to patients with complete device explantation. B, Guidelines for reimplantation of new device (also see Box 22.5). [a]Duration of antibiotic treatment should be counted from the day of device explantation. AHA indicates American Heart Association; ICD, implantable cardioverter-defibrillator; PPM, permanent pacemaker; *S aureus*, *Staphylococcus aureus*; TEE, transesophageal echocardiography; +, positive; −, negative. (Adapted from Sohail MR, Uslan DZ, Khan AH, Friedman PA, Hayes DL, Wilson WR, et al. Management and outcome of permanent pacemaker and implantable cardioverter-defibrillator infections. J Am Coll Cardiol. 2007 May 8;49[18]:1851–9. Epub 2007 Apr 23. Used with permission.)

be drained and sent for Gram stain and bacterial culture to exclude community-acquired MRSA.

Unusual causes of soft tissue infection are *Eikenella corrodens* and oral anaerobes after human bites (knuckles cellulitis after fist fight), *Pasteurella multocida* after cat or dog bites, *Capnocytophaga canimorsus* after dog bites, *Aeromonas hydrophila* after freshwater exposure or exposure to leeches, *Vibrio vulnificus* after saltwater exposure, *Erysipelothrix rhusiopathiae* and *Streptococcus iniae* after fish exposure, and *P aeruginosa* after hot tub exposure.

Several severe complications can occur with soft tissue infections. These include necrotizing fasciitis (usually due to a polymicrobial infection or a toxin-producing group A *Streptococcus*) and pyomyositis (usually due to *S aureus*).

Necrotizing infections are best managed with surgery and directed antimicrobials, including a protein synthesis inhibitor such as clindamycin and a β-lactam antibiotic for invasive group A streptococcal syndromes (Figure 22.5).

The mortality rate associated with streptococcal necrotizing fasciitis is 30%, even in previously healthy patients and with appropriate treatment. Most patients require débridement or amputation of affected tissues. Effective treatment requires early recognition of the illness with prompt initiation of antibiotic treatment, along with early and aggressive surgical débridement of devitalized tissue when indicated.

Unlike many other pathogens, group A streptococci remain susceptible to the penicillins. The cephalosporins (first-generation) and vancomycin are effective alternative drugs. Erythromycin-resistant strains are reported but are so far uncommon in the United States. There is mounting evidence that clindamycin in combination with penicillin is the most effective antibiotic for treating streptococcal necrotizing fasciitis.

- Clindamycin in combination with penicillin is the most effective antibiotic for treating streptococcal necrotizing fasciitis.

- Effective treatment of necrotizing fasciitis requires early recognition with prompt initiation of antibiotic treatment, along with early surgical débridement of devitalized tissue.

Table 22.8 **REGIMENS FOR A DENTAL PROCEDURE**

SITUATION	AGENT	REGIMEN: SINGLE DOSE 30 TO 60 MIN BEFORE PROCEDURE	
		Adults	*Children*
Oral	Amoxicillin	2 g	50 mg/kg
Unable to take oral medication	Ampicillin *Or*	2 g IM or IV	50 mg/kg IM or IV
	Cefazolin or ceftriaxone	1 g IM or IV	50 mg/kg IM or IV
Allergic to penicillins or ampicillin—oral	Cephalexin[a,b] *Or*	2 g	50 mg/kg
	Clindamycin *Or*	600 mg	20 mg/kg
	Azithromycin or clarithromycin	500 mg	15 mg/kg
Allergic to penicillins or ampicillin & unable to take oral medication	Cefazolin or ceftriaxone[b] *Or*	1 g IM or IV	50 mg/kg IM or IV
	Clindamycin	600 mg IM or IV	20 mg/kg IM or IV

Abbreviations: IM, intramuscularly; IV, intravenously.

[a] Or other first- or second-generation oral cephalosporin in equivalent adult or pediatric dosage.

[b] Cephalosporins should not be used in an individual with a history of anaphylaxis, angioedema, or urticaria with penicillins or ampicillin.

Adapted from Wilson W, Taubert KA, Gewitz M, Lockhart PB, Baddour LM, Levison M, et al. Prevention of infective endocarditis: guidelines from the American Heart Association: a guideline from the American Heart Association Rheumatic Fever, Endocarditis, and Kawasaki Disease Committee, Council on Cardiovascular Disease in the Young, and the Council on Clinical Cardiology, Council on Cardiovascular Surgery and Anesthesia, and the Quality of Care and Outcomes Research Interdisciplinary Working Group. Circulation. 2007 Oct 9;116(15):1736–54. Epub 2007 Apr 19. Used with permission.

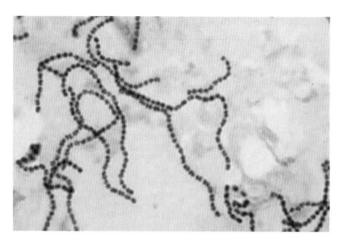

Figure 22.5 Chaining of β-Hemolytic Streptococcus in a Blood Culture (Gram Stain).

TOXIC SHOCK SYNDROME

Group A streptococci produce many disease-causing exotoxins. Scarlet fever may develop in persons with no previous immunity to erythrogenic toxin. Production of hyaluronidase causes the rapidly advancing margins characteristic of cellulitis due to β-hemolytic streptococci. Streptococcal exotoxin A is similar to the toxin produced by *S aureus*, which causes toxic shock syndrome.

Streptococcal toxic shock syndrome is similar to staphylococcal toxic shock syndrome (see below). Patients have invasive group A streptococcal infections with associated hypotension and 2 of the following: renal impairment, coagulopathy, liver impairment, adult respiratory distress syndrome, rash (may desquamate), or soft tissue necrosis. Symptoms are caused by production of streptococcal toxin (pyrogenic exotoxin A). Most patients have skin or soft tissue infection, are younger than 50 years, and are otherwise healthy compared with patients with invasive group A streptococcal infections without the streptococcal toxic shock syndrome. They may present only with severe limb pain without skin lesions. Most patients are bacteremic (in contrast to toxic shock syndrome due to *S aureus*). Treatment includes early administration of antibiotics, supportive care, and surgical débridement if needed. The case-fatality rate is 30%. Although there is no reported resistance to penicillin, clindamycin plus high-dose penicillin G is the preferred regimen because clindamycin may suppress exotoxin and M-protein production in addition to its activity against group A streptococci. In severe cases, consideration should be given to the use of early intravenous immunoglobulin therapy.

- Symptoms of toxic streptococcal syndrome are caused by production of streptococcal toxin.

- Most patients are bacteremic (different from toxic shock syndrome due to *S aureus*).

- Clindamycin plus high-dose penicillin G is the preferred antibiotic regimen.

Staphylococcal toxic shock syndrome is caused by the establishment or growth of a toxin-producing strain of *S aureus* in a nonimmune person. Clinical scenarios associated with this syndrome include prolonged, continuous use of tampons in young menstruating women, postoperative and nonoperative wound infections, localized abscesses, and *S aureus* pneumonia developing after influenza. It is a multisystem disease. Clinical criteria include fever, hypotension, erythroderma (often leads to desquamation, particularly on palms and soles), and involvement in 3 or more organ systems. Onset is acute; blood culture results are usually negative. The condition is caused by production of staphylococcal toxin (toxic shock syndrome toxin 1, TSST-1). Treatment is supportive; subsequent episodes are treated with a β-lactam antibiotic, which decreases the frequency and severity of subsequent attacks. The relapse rate may be as high as 30% to 40% (menstruation-related disease). The mortality rate is 5% to 10%.

- Toxic shock syndrome is caused by a toxin-producing strain of *S aureus* in a nonimmune person.

- Toxic shock syndrome is a multisystem disease: fever, hypotension, and erythroderma (often leads to desquamation, particularly on palms and soles).

- The onset of toxic shock syndrome is acute; results of blood culture are usually negative.

- Toxic shock syndrome is caused by production of staphylococcal toxin (TSST-1).

SKIN AND SOFT TISSUE INFECTION DUE TO UNUSUAL ORGANISMS

Community-Acquired Methicillin-Resistant *S aureus* (CA-MRSA)

CA-MRSA should be suspected 1) in patients with recurrent furunculosis, 2) in patients with cellulitis who have a prior personal history or a family member or close contact with a case of CA-MRSA, and 3) in patients who fail to respond to antimicrobial coverage for methicillin-sensitive *S aureus* (MSSA) and streptococci. Options for treatment in these cases include trimethoprim-sulfamethoxazole, clindamycin, or doxycycline with or without rifampin. The use of vancomycin, daptomycin, or linezolid should be strongly considered in patients who fail to respond to initial therapy, who are quite ill at initial presentation, and in whom multidrug-resistant *S aureus* is suspected.

Pasteurella multocida

Pasteurella multocida is a common cause of acute cutaneous infection after a cat or dog bite. Soft tissue infection after a dog or cat bite should be treated with amoxicillin-clavulanate or a combination of fluoroquinolone and clindamycin to cover oral flora pathogens of the biting animal and skin flora of the infected person.

- *Pasteurella multocida* is a common cause of cutaneous infection after a cat or dog bite.
- Soft tissue infection after a dog or cat bite should be treated with amoxicillin-clavulanate.

Capnocytophaga canimorsus (Formerly DF-2)

This organism may cause rapidly progressive soft tissue infection, bacteremia, and fulminant sepsis in splenectomized patients who are bitten by domestic animals such as dogs. Treatment is with penicillins or cephalosporins.

- *Capnocytophaga* can cause acute soft tissue infection and fulminant sepsis in splenectomized persons after a dog bite.
- Treatment with penicillins or cephalosporins is effective.

Vibrio vulnificus

Vibrio vulnificus can cause a severe bullous soft tissue infection in patients with underlying cirrhosis or hemochromatosis. Disease is usually acquired by the ingestion of raw oysters or through injury sustained in warm salt water. Chronic liver disease predisposes to infection. After the abrupt onset of fever and hypotension, multiple hemorrhagic bullae develop. Clinical syndromes associated with *V vulnificus* include bacteremia, gastroenteritis, and cellulitis. Even with prompt therapy, mortality exceeds 30%. Bacteremia or cellulitis is treated with tetracycline, cefotaxime, or ciprofloxacin. *Vibrio vulnificus* is not uniformly susceptible to the aminoglycosides.

- *Vibrio vulnificus* infection is usually acquired by the ingestion of raw oysters or through injury sustained in warm salt water.
- *Vibrio vulnificus* may cause a severe bullous soft tissue infection, especially in persons with underlying cirrhosis or hemochromatosis.

BONE AND JOINT INFECTIONS

ACUTE BACTERIAL ARTHRITIS (NONGONOCOCCAL)

Acute bacterial arthritis is most commonly due to hematogenous seeding (usually in the setting of trauma, injection drug use, and hemodialysis) in a patient with underlying crystalline or rheumatoid arthritis. The hip and knee joints are the 2 most commonly involved joints. These infections are commonly due to *S aureus* (most common) and β-hemolytic streptococci. *Salmonella* infection may occur in patients with sickle cell disease. Gram-negative aerobic bacilli cause 20% of septic arthritis cases; *P aeruginosa* infection is associated with injection drug use. Clinical features include fever, joint pain, and swelling.

All suspected septic joints should be aspirated. Infected synovial fluid is usually turbid, and the leukocyte count generally exceeds $40 \times 10^9/L$ (about 75% polymorphonuclear neutrophils). This condition may overlap and be confused with other inflammatory arthropathies. Gram stain is positive in 50% of cases. Joint culture results are typically positive. Radiographs are not helpful in routine cases because destructive changes may take more than 2 weeks to occur. The duration of therapy is for 2 to 4 weeks. Empiric therapy should include agents directed against *S aureus* and gram-negative bacilli. Drainage is essential. Percutaneous, arthroscopic, or open procedures are used. Hip, shoulder, and sternoclavicular joint involvement, development of loculations, and persistently positive culture results are the indications for arthroscopy or open débridement.

- Acute bacterial arthritis (nongonococcal) is most commonly due to hematogenous spread of bacteria.
- Bacteria most commonly involved are gram-positive aerobic cocci; *S aureus* is most common.
- Fever, pain, and swelling are frequent.
- Synovial fluid is turbid; the leukocyte count generally exceeds $40 \times 10^9/L$.
- Blood culture results are often positive.
- Drainage is essential.

VIRAL ARTHRITIS

Viral arthritis often presents as transient, self-limited polyarthritis. It may be caused by rubella (also may occur after vaccination), hepatitis B, mumps, coxsackievirus, adenovirus, parvovirus B19, human immunodeficiency virus, Ross River virus, and chikungunya virus infections in travelers. Parvovirus can cause a chronic symmetric, small joint arthritis that mimics rheumatoid arthritis, especially in women.

CHRONIC MONOARTICULAR ARTHRITIS

Tuberculosis and nontuberculous mycobacteria and fungi should be considered in patients presenting with insidious-onset arthritis and chronic arthritis. Exposure to fish tank or brackish water should raise the possibility of *Mycobacterium marinum* septic arthritis typically involving the small hand joints. A history of travel to the southwestern United States or being a gardener should raise the possibility of *Coccidioides immitis* and *Sporothrix schenckii*, respectively. In patients with chronic monoarticular arthritis of the knee and a history of tick exposure, positive serologic results, or erythema migrans, chronic Lyme arthritis should be considered.

OSTEOMYELITIS

Osteomyelitis can occur as a result of hematogenous seeding, contiguous spread of infection to bone from adjacent soft tissues and joints, or direct inoculation of infection into the bone as a result of trauma or surgery.

Hematogenous osteomyelitis is usually monomicrobial, whereas osteomyelitis due to contiguous spread or direct inoculation is usually polymicrobial. Acute hematogenous osteomyelitis is more common in children, but it can occur in adults in the setting of prolonged bacteremias, intravenous drug use, dialysis, and sickle cell disease. *Staphylococcus aureus*, coagulase-negative staphylococci, and aerobic gram-negative bacilli are the most common organisms. In long bone involvement, the acute onset of pain and fever is typical. In vertebral infection, pain may be the sole feature. Compatible radiographic changes and bone biopsy for culture and pathologic examination are used to establish the diagnosis. Results of blood culture may be positive. Specific parenteral antibiotic therapy is used for 3 to 6 weeks on the basis of culture and sensitivity test results. Débridement is usually not necessary unless a sequestrum is present.

- *Staphylococcus aureus* is a common organism in acute hematogenous osteomyelitis.

- Acute onset of pain and fever is typical.

Chronic, contiguous osteomyelitis more commonly occurs in adults, particularly in the setting of traumatic wounds, vascular insufficiency, and diabetic foot ulcers. The infections are usually mixed, but *S aureus* is the single most commonly isolated organism. In the presence of foreign bodies (such as plate or screws), coagulase-negative staphylococci is often the culprit. Local pain, tenderness, erythema, and draining sinuses are common. Fever is atypical unless there is concurrent cellulitis. Compatible radiographic changes (often vague) and bone biopsy for culture and pathologic examination are used to establish the diagnosis. Blood culture results are rarely positive. Adequate débridement, removal of dead space, soft tissue coverage, and fixation of infected fractures are essential. Specific parenteral antibiotic therapy is given for 4 to 6 weeks. If a foreign body is retained in patients with staphylococcal osteomyelitis, a rifampin-based therapy such as the combination of fluoroquinolones and rifampin is warranted.

- *Staphylococcus aureus* is the most common causative organism in chronic osteomyelitis.

- Coagulase-negative staphylococci are common pathogens if a foreign body is present.

- Local pain, tenderness, erythema, and draining sinuses are common.

- Antibiotic therapy is given for 4–6 weeks.

DISKITIS AND VERTEBRAL INFECTIONS

Infection of the intervertebral disk and the adjacent vertebrae may occur with or without associated epidural or psoas abscesses. These infections most often arise from hematogenous dissemination of infection from the skin and soft

tissues, genitourinary tract, infective endocarditis, infected intravenous sites, injection drug use, or respiratory tract infection. The incidence is greatest among males, peaks in the fifth decade of life, and is increasing, particularly among the elderly. Risk factors for spine infections include advanced age, immunocompromise, diabetes, intravenous drug use, renal failure, bacteremia, cancer, chronic corticosteroid use, intravascular devices, and recent instrumentation or spine surgery.

The clinical presentation of vertebral osteomyelitis includes localized insidious pain and tenderness in the spine area in 90% of patients. Most commonly affected is the lumbar or lumbosacral region; cervical disease may occur in patients with head and neck infections or in injection drug users. Fever is present in less than half of cases. Because of the clinical uncertainty, a delay in diagnosis by weeks to months occurs, which can lead to motor and sensory deficits in 15% of patients. The erythrocyte sedimentation rate is increased in more than 90% of cases, and the leukocyte count is increased in less than 50%.

Plain radiography may show vertebral end-plate irregularity 2 to 8 weeks after the onset of symptoms, but it is neither sensitive nor specific. Gadolinium-enhanced magnetic resonance imaging is the most useful test for diagnosis because of its high sensitivity (96%) and specificity (94%). In patients who cannot undergo magnetic resonance imaging, computed tomography or nuclear scanning may help establish the diagnosis. The best nuclear study for imaging disk space infections is technetium combined with gallium citrate scanning. Computed tomography-guided percutaneous aspiration or biopsy is often used to identify the causative organism. If the initial result is negative, the test should be repeated before proceeding to an open biopsy procedure.

Staphylococcus aureus and coagulase-negative staphylococci are the most common microorganisms cultured in vertebral osteomyelitis. *Mycobacterium tuberculosis* and *Brucella* are common in regions endemic for these organisms. Most patients can be managed conservatively with antimicrobials. Antibiotics should be given parenterally for a minimum of 4 to 6 weeks or longer if there is extensive vertebral destruction or undrained collections. Surgical interventions are limited to patients with progressive neurologic deterioration, spinal instability, progressive epidural abscess, or failed medical therapy.

SUMMARY

- Differential time to culture positivity (cultures of blood drawn from the catheter are positive 2 hours before those from the peripheral site) or a catheter tip with growth >15 colony-forming units per milliliter suggests the catheter as the source of bloodstream infection.

- Vancomycin is the most reliably active drug for treating serious infections caused by MRSA.

- Organisms most commonly causing community-acquired infection in adults are *S pneumoniae*, *N meningitidis*, *L monocytogenes*, and *H influenzae*.

- Characteristic features of aseptic meningitis are fever, neck stiffness, cerebrospinal fluid pleocytosis (usually lymphocytic), and negative results of bacterial cultures.

- Antibiotic prophylaxis for infective endocarditis is no longer recommended for genitourinary or gastrointestinal procedures.

- Toxic shock syndrome is a multisystem disease: fever, hypotension, and erythroderma (often leads to desquamation, particularly on palms and soles).

- *Staphylococcus aureus* is the most common causative organism in chronic osteomyelitis.

PART V

RHEUMATOLOGY

23.

NONARTICULAR RHEUMATISM

Kevin G. Moder, MD

- Review the diagnosis of common rheumatologic disorders: fibromyalgia, low back pain, and bursitis.

- Differentiate the various vasculitic syndromes using clinical data and laboratory testing.

- Understand treatment options for and toxic effects of treatments of vasculitis.

FIBROMYALGIA

Fibromyalgia is a condition characterized by chronic widespread musculoskeletal pain. Older terms used to describe this condition include fibrositis, tension myalgias, and psychogenic rheumatism. The 1990 American College of Rheumatology classification critieria for fibromyalgia state that the pain should be present for at least 3 months and should involve areas on both sides of the body above and below the waist and some part of the axial skeleton. Symptoms should not be explained by coexisting diseases or conditions. To meet classification criteria for fibromyalgia, 11 of 18 tender points must be present (Box 23.1). Fibromyalgia affects 2% to 10% of populations studied. It accounts for 15% of all visits to general internists in the United States; 75% to 95% of all patients are women. It is unusual for the diagnosis to be made in a person younger than 12 years or after age 65 years. Of the patients (or their parents), 60% recall childhood growing pains (leg pains). Fibromyalgia is often associated with psychosocial stress.

- Fibromyalgia is characterized by chronic widespread musculoskeletal pain.

- Fibromyalgia affects 2%-10% of populations studied; 75%-95% of patients are women.

There are new preliminary 2010 diagnostic criteria for fibromyalgia. The new criteria include a widespread pain index, in which the body is divided into 19 areas, and 1 point is given for each painful area. There is also a symptom severity score involving fatigue, waking unrefreshed, cognitive symptoms, and somatic symptoms. The usefulness of these criteria are being assessed.

SYMPTOMS

Patients with fibromyalgia report pain all over the body and describe their pain differently than do patients with rheumatoid arthritis. Patients with fibromyalgia poorly localize their pain, referring it to muscle attachment sites or muscles. The discomfort may be worse late in the day after activity. Some patients report morning stiffness; it is usually not as long or as severe as in patients with inflammatory arthritis, in whom the duration of stiffness often exceeds 1 hour. Physical activity or changes in the weather typically aggravate the symptoms. Most patients describe nonrestorative, nonrestful sleep. Psychosocial stress, anxiety, and depression frequently are present. Other patient complaints can include subjective joint swelling (without objective synovitis on examination), arthralgias, headaches, and paresthesias. About a third of patients have multiple somatic visceral symptoms, including urinary irritability, pelvic pain, temporomandibular joint symptoms, and irritable bowel syndrome.

- Patients with fibromyalgia typically describe pain all over the body.

- Physical activity or weather changes typically aggravate the symptoms.

- Multiple somatic symptoms, including headaches, paresthesias, numbness, and irritable bowel symptoms, are common.

- Widespread chronic musculoskeletal pain can be associated with psychosocial stress.

DIAGNOSIS

A detailed history and physical examination exclude most rheumatologic and neurologic diseases. The finding of painful

Box 23.1
1990 CLASSIFICATION CRITERIA FOR FIBROMYALGIA

Widespread pain
    Above & below the waist
    Right & left sides of the body
    Axial pain
Pain in at least 11 of 18 tender points (bilateral)
    Occiput
    Low cervical area
    Trapezius
    Supraspinatus
    Second rib
    Lateral epicondyle
    Gluteus
    Greater trochanter
    Knee
Symptoms present for at least 3 months

points at muscle attachment sites supports the diagnosis of fibromyalgia. No laboratory test confirms the diagnosis of fibromyalgia. Laboratory tests are used to rule out other conditions and usually are unrevealing. Vitamin D levels have been reported to be low in some patients with chronic pain syndromes, including fibromyalgia. Response to vitamin D replacement, however, is variable. Radiographs of specific, particularly problematic, joints may be helpful for identifying coexisting conditions. For example, patients with fibromyalgia may also have degenerative joint disease of a particular joint that contributes to their pain. If sleep disturbance is prominent, a sleep study may be helpful.

- Chronic widespread musculoskeletal pain not explained by physical findings of a rheumatic disease supports the diagnosis of fibromyalgia.
- No laboratory test confirms the diagnosis of fibromyalgia.

NATURAL HISTORY

Fibromyalgia is a chronic waxing and waning condition. Patients have periods of pain and dysfunction alternating with periods of feeling reasonably well. Over a period of years, a patient's symptoms and concerns can shift considerably from musculoskeletal concerns to fatigue or other associated symptoms. There is no increased physical disability in patients who have had fibromyalgia for longer periods in comparison with those for whom the diagnosis is recent.

TREATMENT

Treatment includes reassurance and education, addressing sleep problems, and establishing an exercise program. Nonsteroidal anti-inflammatory drugs, simple analgesics, and medications to help with sleep (such as tricyclic antidepressants) have a role in some patients. Comprehensive

fibromyalgia treatment programs may benefit some patients. Chronic pain management techniques may also be helpful for patients with impaired life skills.

Several controlled trials have shown that the antidepressant agent duloxetine is efficacious for patients with fibromyalgia with or without depression. This agent seems to be efficacious in female patients but less so in males with fibromyalgia. Pregabalin, which is used for treatment of peripheral neuropathy, has also been shown to be beneficial in some patients with fibromyalgia. Pramipexole has been shown to be beneficial in a subset of patients with fibromyalgia.

- In fibromyalgia, symptoms wax and wane.
- Several thereapeutic approaches, including medications, may provide symptomatic relief.

LOW BACK PAIN

One-third of all people older than 50 years have episodes of acute low back pain. Chronic low back pain is the most common compensable work-related injury. The vast majority of episodes of acute low back pain cannot be explained on a structural basis. Only 3% of patients presenting with acute low back pain have an identifiable cause that is not apparent after the initial interview and physical examination. More than 90% of patients have resolution with or without the help of a medical practitioner within the first 6 weeks after symptoms occur.

- Only 3% of patients presenting with acute low back pain have an identifiable cause that is not apparent after the initial interview and physical examination.
- More than 90% of episodes of acute low back pain resolve with or without the help of a medical practitioner within the first 6 weeks after symptoms occur.

DIAGNOSIS

During the initial evaluation of acute low back pain, it is important to look for signs, symptoms, and findings suggestive of radiculopathy, myelopathy, or cauda equina. In the absence of evidence for acute spinal cord compromise, spinal infection, or neoplastic involvement, immediate pursuit of a cause for the acute back pain is usually unrevealing. Objective leg weakness or bladder or bowel dysfunction is an indication for more extensive examination and possible surgical decompression. Involuntary weight loss and pain that increase with recumbency suggest a neoplastic or infectious process. Pain that worsens with coughing, straining, or sneezing suggests irritation of the dura mater. Radiating pain, weakness, or numbness in an extremity implicates irritation of a spinal nerve root.

Exertional calf or thigh cramping but normal peripheral pulses suggest the pseudoclaudication of spinal stenosis. Pseudoclaudication symptoms improve with leaning forward on a shopping cart while walking or with sitting (not standing still). Typically, pseudoclaudication also begins in the back or buttock and gradually radiates down the thigh into the leg. This is in contrast to claudication, which usually begins distally and then gradually spreads proximally.

Referred pain from the hips, abdomen, and pelvis can sometimes be interpreted as low back pain. An insidious onset with prominent morning stiffness suggests an inflammatory axial arthropathy.

- Objective leg weakness or bladder or bowel dysfunction in patients with low back pain is an indication for more extensive examination.

- Involuntary weight loss and pain that interferes with sleep suggest a neoplastic or infectious process.

- Exertional calf or thigh cramping but normal peripheral pulses suggest pseudoclaudication.

- An insidious onset with prominent morning stiffness suggests an inflammatory axial arthropathy.

In the absence of specific historical or physical examination findings, laboratory or plain radiographic findings often are unrevealing. The radiographic findings of spondylosis, disk degeneration, facet osteoarthritis, transitional lumbosacral segments, Schmorl nodes, spina bifida occulta, or mild scoliosis are often incidental findings not relevant to a patient's complaints of acute back pain. Bone scanning, electromyography, computed tomography, or magnetic resonance imaging are usually not necessary to evaluate acute low back pain. The indications for spinal radiography in patients with acute low back pain are listed in Box 23.2.

TREATMENT

The treatment of acute nonspecific low back pain begins with reassuring the patient, because 90% of all patients with acute low back pain have considerable improvement in 6 weeks. Temporary modification of activities may lessen symptoms. Bed rest should never be prescribed for more than 3 days to treat acute nonspecific low back pain. Longer bed rest has not been shown to be beneficial and may prolong disability. Short-term use of narcotic analgesics or tramadol can supplement the use

---

Box 23.2 **INDICATIONS FOR SPINAL RADIOGRAPHY IN PATIENTS WITH ACUTE LOW BACK PAIN**

First episode of acute back pain is after age 50 y
History of back disease
History of back surgery
History of neoplasm
Acute history of direct trauma to the back
Fever
Weight loss
Severe pain unrelieved in any position
Neurologic symptoms or signs

---

of acetaminophen, nonsteroidal anti-inflammatory drugs, and muscle relaxants such as cyclobenzaprine. Physical therapy measures include local heat and ice massage. Pelvic traction and transcutaneous electrical nerve stimulation add little to the management of acute nonspecific low back pain. Epidural glucocorticosteroid injections are best suited to acute disk herniation, although their role is controversial. Injections into the facets are helpful occasionally, particularly if the patient describes a locking or catching as part of the pain syndrome.

- In 90% of patients, acute low back pain (local or sciatic presentations) remits within 6 weeks.

- Pelvic traction and transcutaneous electrical nerve stimulation add little to the management of acute nonspecific low back pain.

BURSITIS

A bursa is a fluid-filled sac lined with a membrane. Bursae are present in the areas where tendons and muscles move over bony prominences. Additional bursae can form in response to irritative stimuli. Trauma or overuse, crystalline disease, chronic inflammatory arthritis, and infection cause bursitis. Common locations of bursitis include the olecranon and the greater trochanter.

Treatment of aseptic bursitis may involve immobilization, ice compresses, nonsteroidal anti-inflammatory drugs, bursal aspiration, corticosteroid injections, and, occasionally, physical therapy.

- Always consider infection or crystalline disease in the differential diagnosis of acute bursitis.

Septic bursitis may result from puncture wounds or cellulitis, or it can occur after a local injection. In many cases of septic bursitis, no clear portal of entry for infection is apparent. The organisms frequently responsible for infection are staphylococci and streptococci. Patients with septic superficial bursitis present with localized pain and swelling. Warmth about the area of the superficial bursa should raise the possibility of a septic bursa. If there is doubt, the bursa should be aspirated with strict aseptic technique. The needle should enter from the side through uninvolved skin—not at the point of maximal fluctuance—to avoid creating a chronic draining fistula.

When infection is suspected, empiric treatment with antistaphylococcal and antistreptococcal antibiotics should be given pending the microbiologic results. Gram stains are positive in only 40% to 60% of patients. The number of leukocytes in infected bursal fluid can be low compared with that in infected joint fluid. This difference may be due to the modest blood supply of the bursae compared with that of joints. Patients with more severe infections or with associated cellulitis frequently do not respond to outpatient management. Repeated aspirations or even surgical débridement is necessary in some cases.

- Septic bursitis frequently occurs without evidence of a portal of entry.

- Bursal warmth is the best predictor of infection.

- Gram stains are positive in only 40%-60% of patients.

- The number of leukocytes in infected bursal fluid can be low.

- Patients with more severe infections should be hospitalized.

POLYMYALGIA RHEUMATICA

Polymyalgia rheumatica is a clinical syndrome characterized by the onset of aching and morning stiffness in the proximal musculature (hip and shoulder girdles). It is more common in females than males and usually occurs in patients older than 60 years. Patients usually have an increased erythrocyte sedimentation rate; autoantibody results, including rheumatoid factor, cyclic citrullinated peptide antibodies, and antinuclear antibody, are usually negative or normal. Many patients have a mild normochromic anemia. A small number of patients may have a normal sedimentation rate; the C-reactive protein value is usually increased in these cases. In patients in whom the acute-phase reactants are normal and there is uncertainty about the diagnosis, radionucleotide joint scanning can be done. In patients with active polymyalgia rheumatica, radionuclide joint scanning confirms hip and shoulder synovitis, a finding supporting synovitis as the cause of the symptoms. The presence of other specific diseases such as rheumatoid arthritis, chronic infection, inflammatory myositis, or malignancy should be excluded. Patients with polymyalgia rheumatica have prompt (within 24–72 hours) response to small doses of prednisone (10–20 mg daily).

- A patient with polymyalgia rheumatica typically is elderly and presents with aching and morning stiffness in the proximal musculature and increased erythrocyte sedimentation rate.

FEATURES AND DIFFERENTIAL DIAGNOSIS

Patients with polymyalgia rheumatica complain of stiffness and pain that are most prominent in the mornings and after prolonged sitting. Because of these symptoms, they have difficulty getting comfortable at night to sleep. They occasionally have mild constitutional symptoms, including sweats, fevers, anorexia, and weight loss. Very prominent constitutional features and markedly increased erythrocyte sedimentation rate could suggest associated giant cell arteritis. Extremity edema or oligoarticular synovitis can occur, particularly at the knees, wrists, and shoulders. Polyarticular small joint arthritis is not a feature. Box 23.3 summarizes the rheumatic syndromes and other diseases that occasionally present with a polymyalgia rheumatica-like syndrome. Clinical evaluation and screening laboratory tests usually distinguish polymyalgia rheumatica from these other conditions. A variant known as the RS3PE syndrome (remitting symmetric seronegative synovitis with

---

Box 23.3 SYSTEMIC ILLNESSES PRESENTING WITH A POLYMYALGIA-LIKE SYNDROME

RHEUMATIC SYNDROMES	OTHER SYSTEMIC ILLNESSES
Systemic vasculitis	Paraneoplastic syndromes
Myositis	Systemic amyloidosis
Systemic lupus erythematosus	Infectious endocarditis
Seronegative rheumatoid arthritis	Hyperthyroidism
Polyarticular osteoarthritis	Hypothyroidism
Fibromyalgia	Hyperparathyroidism
Remitting seronegative, symmetric synovitis & peripheral edema	Osteomalacia
	Depression

---

pitting edema) can occur, primarily in older men. Patients with this syndrome present with symptoms of polymyalgia rheumatica but also synovitis and marked edema in the hands or feet.

- In polymyalgia rheumatica, stiffness is more prolonged in the mornings, and patients describe gelling (ie, stiffening again after prolonged inactivity).

- Prominent constitutional features and markedly increased erythrocyte sedimentation rate could suggest associated giant cell arteritis.

- Extremity edema or oligoarticular synovitis can occur.

PATHOGENESIS AND RELATIONSHIP TO GIANT CELL ARTERITIS

Polymyalgia rheumatica can begin before, appear simultaneously with, or develop after the symptoms of giant cell arteritis. The pathogenesis of polymyalgia rheumatica is unknown. Clinicians appreciate the close relationship between giant cell arteritis and polymyalgia rheumatica. Up to 15% of patients with polymyalgia rheumatica also have giant cell arteritis. Familial aggregation and increased incidence in patients of northern European background suggest a genetic predisposition. HLA-DR4 is associated with these conditions more commonly than would be expected by chance. Among patients with giant cell arteritis, 40% have symptoms of polymyalgia rheumatica during the course of their disease.

- Up to 15% of patients with polymyalgia rheumatica also have giant cell arteritis.

- Among patients with active giant cell arteritis, 40% have symptoms of polymyalgia rheumatica.

- Polymyalgia rheumatica can begin before, appear simultaneously with, or develop after the symptoms of giant cell arteritis.

TREATMENT

All patients with polymyalgia rheumatica should have a considerable response within 4 days of treatment with low-dose prednisone (10-20 mg/day). Sometimes, split-dose prednisone (5 mg 3 times per day) is more effective than the same single daily dose (15 mg once per day). Patients should be followed clinically, and usually the erythrocyte sedimentation rate should be measured monthly to monitor for disease activity. Polymyalgia rheumatica is thought to be a self-limited disease, but relapses can occur. Prednisone is discontinued in more than half of patients within 2 years. A minority of patients may be at risk of later appearance of giant cell arteritis. Patients with polymyalgia rheumatica that does not respond promptly to corticosteroids or those who have severe symptoms suggestive of giant cell arteritis (head, jaw, and arm claudication; visual loss; significantly different blood pressures for the right and left arms) should have a temporal artery biopsy. Occasionally, a patient presents with polymyalgia rheumatica and over time the condition evolves into true rheumatoid arthritis.

- All patients with polymyalgia rheumatica should have a considerable response within 4 days of treatment with prednisone.

- Polymyalgia rheumatica is usually a self-limited disease, although relapses occur, and a minority of patients may be at risk of late appearance of giant cell arteritis.

VASCULITIC SYNDROMES

Vasculitis, or angiitis, is an inflammatory disease of blood vessels. Damage to the vessel wall and stenosis or occlusion of the vessel lumen by thrombosis and progressive intimal proliferation of the vessel result in the clinical manifestations of the illness. The distribution of the vascular lesions and the size of the blood vessels involved vary considerably in different vasculitic syndromes and in different patients with the same syndrome. Vasculitis can be transient, chronic, self-limited, or progressive. It can be the primary abnormality or due to another systemic process. Histopathologic classification does not distinguish local from systemic illness or secondary from primary insult. The key clinical features suggestive of vasculitis are listed in Box 23.4. Vasculitis "look-alikes," or simulators, are listed in Box 23.5. These diseases and conditions should be considered whenever a patient's condition suggests vasculitis. Common test abnormalities found in patients with vasculitis are listed in Box 23.6. The ability to recognize characteristic clinical patterns of involvement is very helpful for making the diagnosis of systemic necrotizing vasculitis.

- Vasculitic symptoms reflect the nonspecific systemic features of inflammation (constitutional features) and the ischemic consequences of vascular occlusion.

SPECIFIC VASCULITIC SYNDROMES

Giant Cell Arteritis

Giant cell arteritis, also known as temporal arteritis, predominantly affects persons of northern European ancestry

---

Box 23.4 COMMON CLINICAL FEATURES IN PATIENTS WITH VASCULITIS

Constitutional features
  Fever
  Weight loss
  Fatigue
  Anorexia
Cutaneous manifestations
  Palpable purpura
  Necrotic ulcers
  Livedo reticularis
  Urticarial lesions
  Digital infarcts
Musculoskeletal features
  Arthralgia
  Arthritis
  Myalgia
  Claudication
Neurologic features
  Peripheral neuropathy
  Mononeuritis multiplex
  Cerebrovascular accidents
  Headache
Other
  Cough
  Hemoptysis
  Edema
  Hypertension
  Abdominal pain

---

older than 50 years. Three-quarters of patients are women. The prevalence exceeds 223 cases per 100,000 persons older than 50 years. Polymyalgia rheumatica symptoms may develop in 40% to 50% of all patients with giant cell arteritis. Up to 15% of patients with polymyalgia rheumatica have temporal artery biopsy findings positive for giant cell arteritis. There is considerable morbidity with this disease; however, the

---

Box 23.5 SYNDROMES THAT MIMIC VASCULITIS

Cardiac myxoma with embolization
Infective endocarditis
Thrombotic thrombocytopenic purpura
Atheroembolism: cholesterol or calcium emboli
Ergotism
Pseudoxanthoma elasticum
Ehlers-Danlos type 4
Neurovasculopathy secondary to antiphospholipid syndrome
Arterial coarctation or dysplasia
Infectious angiitis
  Lyme disease
  Rickettsial infection
  HIV infection

Abbreviation: HIV, human immunodeficiency virus.

Box 23.6 LABORATORY AND RADIOGRAPHIC
ABNORMALITIES IN VASCULITIS

Anemia
Increased values of acute phase reactants (CRP or ESR)
Increased values on liver function tests
Increased creatinine value
Active urine sediment
Proteinuria
Abnormal results on chest radiography
   Nodules
   Alveolar hemorrhage
   Pulmonary infiltrates

Abbreviations: CRP, C-reactive protein; ESR, erythrocyte sedimentation rate.

Box 23.7 CLASSIC CLINICAL FEATURES OF GIANT
CELL ARTERITIS

Fever, weight loss, fatigue
Polymyalgia rheumatica symptoms
Temporal headache
Jaw or tongue claudication
Ocular symptoms
   Blindness
   Diplopia
   Ptosis
   Scalp tenderness
   Dry cough
   Peripheral large vessel vasculitis (10%)

rate of blindness is declining. Affected patients are at higher subsequent risk of aortic aneurysms. The mortality rate for patients with giant cell arteritis is similar to that for the general population.

- Giant cell arteritis is most common in persons of northern European ancestry.

- Polymyalgia rheumatica may develop in 40%-50% of patients with giant cell arteritis.

- Up to 15% of patients with polymyalgia rheumatica have temporal artery biopsy findings positive for giant cell arteritis.

Pathology

Giant cell arteritis involves the primary and secondary branches of the aorta in a segmental or patchy fashion. However, any artery, and occasionally veins, can be affected. It is unusual for intracranial arteries to be involved. Histopathologically, all layers of the vessel wall are extensively disrupted, with intimal thickening and a prominent mononuclear and histiocytic infiltrate. Multinucleated giant cells infiltrate the vessel wall in 50% of cases. Fragmentation and disintegration of the internal elastic membrane, the other characteristic features, are closely associated with the accumulation of giant cells and vascular occlusive symptoms.

- Giant cell arteritis affects primary and secondary branches of the aorta in a segmental or patchy fashion.

Clinical Features

Early clinical features of giant cell arteritis include temporal headache, polymyalgia rheumatica symptoms, fatigue, and fever. The classic features of this disease are listed in Box 23.7. Arteritis of the branches of the ophthalmic or posterior ciliary arteries causes ischemia of the optic nerve (ischemic optic neuritis) and blindness. Less often, retinal arterioles are occluded. Blindness occurs in fewer than 15% of untreated patients. Large peripheral artery involvement in giant cell arteritis occurs in about 10% of patients. Extremity claudication, Raynaud phenomenon, aortic dissection, decreased pulses, and vascular bruits suggest large

peripheral artery involvement. Patients with large peripheral artery involvement do not differ from those with more classic giant cell arteritis, either histologically or with regard to laboratory findings. Patients who have had giant cell arteritis are at increased risk for the development of aneurysms.

- A patient with giant cell arteritis typically is 60 years old and presents with temporal headache, polymyalgia rheumatica-like symptoms, fatigue, and fever. The sedimentation rate is markedly increased. Physical examination shows scalp tenderness.

- Blindness occurs in <15% of untreated patients.

Diagnosis

The necessary length of an adequate temporal artery biopsy specimen is controversial. However, because of patchy involvement and skin lesions, a length of at least 1 cm is recommended. In 15% of patients, the biopsy is positive on the opposite side if that on the initial side is negative. Typical laboratory abnormalities in acute active giant cell arteritis include a markedly increased erythrocyte sedimentation rate, moderate normochromic anemia, and thrombocytosis. A mild increase in liver enzyme values, most typically alkaline phosphatase, occurs in one-third of patients because of granulomatous hepatitis. The erythrocyte sedimentation rate is rarely normal in patients with active giant cell arteritis.

- The temporal artery biopsy specimen needed to test for giant cell arteritis should be at least 1 cm long to compensate for patchy involvement.

- In 15% of patients with giant cell arteritis, the biopsy is positive on the opposite side if that on the initial side is negative.

- Typical laboratory abnormalities in giant cell arteritis are markedly increased erythrocyte sedimentation rate, moderate normochromic anemia, and thrombocytosis.

Treatment

Treatment is initiated with corticosteroids when the diagnosis of giant cell arteritis is considered and the biopsy

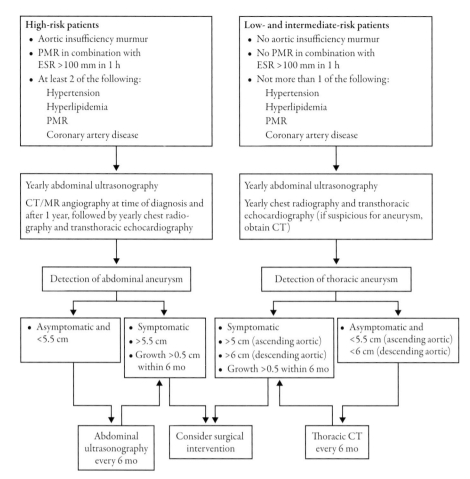

High-risk patients
- Aortic insufficiency murmur
- PMR in combination with ESR >100 mm in 1 h
- At least 2 of the following:
  Hypertension
  Hyperlipidemia
  PMR
  Coronary artery disease

Low- and intermediate-risk patients
- No aortic insufficiency murmur
- No PMR in combination with ESR >100 mm in 1 h
- Not more than 1 of the following:
  Hypertension
  Hyperlipidemia
  PMR
  Coronary artery disease

Yearly abdominal ultrasonography

CT/MR angiography at time of diagnosis and after 1 year, followed by yearly chest radiography and transthoracic echocardiography

Yearly abdominal ultrasonography

Yearly chest radiography and transthoracic echocardiography (if suspicious for aneurysm, obtain CT)

Detection of abdominal aneurysm

Detection of thoracic aneurysm

- Asymptomatic and <5.5 cm

- Symptomatic
- >5.5 cm
- Growth >0.5 cm within 6 mo

- Symptomatic
- >5 cm (ascending aortic)
- >6 cm (descending aortic)
- Growth >0.5 within 6 mo

- Asymptomatic and <5.5 cm (ascending aortic) <6 cm (descending aortic)

Abdominal ultrasonography every 6 mo

Consider surgical intervention

Thoracic CT every 6 mo

Figure 23.1 Suggested Diagnostic Algorithm for Early Detection of Aortic Aneurysms in Giant Cell Arteritis. Screening should be considered only in patients without major factors for adverse outcome from thoracic or abdominal aneurysm repair. CT indicates computed tomography; ESR, erythrocyte sedimentation rate; MR, magnetic resonance; PMR, polymyalgia rheumatica. (Adapted from Bongartz T, Matteson EL. Large-vessel involvement in giant cell arteritis. Curr Opin Rheumatol. 2006 Jan;18[1]:10–7. Used with permission.)

is requested. A temporal artery biopsy specimen remains positive for disease even after several weeks of corticosteroid treatment. Initial treatment includes prednisone, typically 40 to 60 mg/day. A higher dose of corticosteroids can be given parenterally in cases of visual or life-threatening symptoms. A recent study suggested parenteral corticosteroids initially may lessen the total duration and cumulative dose needed. Most symptoms of giant cell arteritis begin to respond within 24 hours after corticosteroid therapy is initiated. Visual changes that are present for more than a few hours are often irreversible. Alternate-day administration of corticosteroids does not control symptoms in at least half of patients.

- Treatment is initiated with corticosteroids when the diagnosis of giant cell arteritis is considered and the biopsy is requested.

- Initial treatment of giant cell arteritis includes prednisone, typically 40–60 mg/day.

- Alternate-day administration of corticosteroids does not initially control symptoms in at least half of patients.

Outcome

Giant cell arteritis typically has a self-limited course. In 24 months, half of patients are able to discontinue treatment with corticosteroids. An effective steroid-sparing agent has not

been identified, but methotrexate or azathioprine has been used in some patients. The diagnosis of giant cell arteritis does not influence mortality rates. Relapse may occur in a third of patients, and a thoracic or abdominal aneurysm develops in a third. Screening guidelines for aortic aneurysms are shown in Figure 23.1.

- Giant cell arteritis typically has a self-limited course over about 2 years, although relapses and late consequences, including aortic aneurysms, occur.

- Patients with a history of giant cell arteritis are at increased risk for the development of aneurysms.

Takayasu Arteritis

Takayasu arteritis is also known as aortic arch syndrome or pulseless disease. Each year, about 2.6 new cases per 1,000,000 population occur. Most patients are between the ages of 15 and 40 years. At least 80% of them are female. This disease is more common in Asia, Latin America, and Eastern Europe. Its histopathologic features cannot be distinguished from those of giant cell arteritis. Takayasu arteritis affects the aorta and its primary branches. The arterial wall is irregularly thickened, and luminal narrowing, dilatations, aneurysms, and distortions are present. The aortic valve and coronary ostia can be involved.

Classification criteria for Takyasu arteritis are listed in Box 23.8.

- Among patients with Takayasu arteritis, most are female and between the ages of 15 and 40 years.

- The aorta and its primary branches are most commonly affected.

Clinical and Laboratory Features

The constitutional features of fever, weight loss, fatigue, and arthralgia can precede symptoms of ischemia to the brain or claudication of the extremities. Renovascular hypertension, pulmonary hypertension, and coronary artery insufficiency can complicate Takayasu arteritis. Cutaneous vasculitis, erythema nodosum, and synovitis occasionally occur in cases of active Takayasu arteritis. Compromise of the cerebral vasculature can lead to dizziness, blurry or fading vision, syncope, and, occasionally, stroke. Physical examination findings confirm vascular bruits, absence of peripheral pulses, and, occasionally, fever. When the disease is active, results of laboratory studies usually show increased erythrocyte sedimentation rate, normochromic anemia, and thrombocytosis. However, in some cases of active disease, the erythrocyte sedimentation rate is normal. The diagnosis can be confirmed with conventional angiography, although magnetic resonance angiography may become the imaging method of choice.

- Renovascular hypertension, pulmonary hypertension, and coronary artery insufficiency can complicate Takayasu arteritis.

- Patients with active Takayasu arteritis can have a normal erythrocyte sedimentation rate, although this finding is rare.

- A patient with Takayasu arteritis typically is young and presents with fever, weight loss, fatigue, and arthralgia. Physical examination shows carotid bruits and absence of peripheral pulses. On laboratory testing, there is a mild normochromic anemia, and the erythrocyte sedimentation rate is increased.

Treatment and Outcome

Corticosteroid therapy alone is usually adequate for controlling the inflammation. Methotrexate or cyclophosphamide treatment is indicated in resistant cases. On average, patients receive corticosteroids for about 2 years. Late stenotic complications are amenable to vascular operation and bypass grafting. Survival is more than 90% at 10 years. Congestive heart failure from previous coronary artery involvement and cerebrovascular accidents are major causes of mortality.

- Survival in patients with Takayasu arteritis is >90% at 10 years.

Classic Polyarteritis Nodosa and Microscopic Polyangiitis

Systemic necrotizing vasculitis occurs alone or in association with several diseases (secondary). When it occurs as a primary vasculitis, it is most commonly a small vessel antineutrophil cytoplasmic antibody (ANCA)–associated disease of Wegener granulomatosis or microscopic polyangiitis. Medium-vessel polyarteritis nodosa, frequently associated with hepatitis B, is far less common. A secondary necrotizing vasculitis can occur in association with rheumatoid arthritis, systemic lupus erythematosus, other connective tissue diseases, cryoglobulinemia, hepatitis C infection, hairy cell leukemia, and other malignant conditions.

- Systemic necrotizing vasculitis occurs alone or in association with several diseases.

- ANCA-associated vasculitis disorders of Wegener granulomatosis and microscopic polyangiitis are more common than classic polyarteritis nodosa.

Pathology

These diseases are characterized by transmural inflammation and necrosis of blood vessels. Classic polyarteritis nodosa affects medium-sized muscular arteries. ANCA-associated vasculitis affects arterioles, venules, and capillaries. The size of the affected vessels plays a large part in determining the clinical manifestations of the syndromes.

- Systemic vasculitis may affect a spectrum of vessel sizes.

Clinical Features

Systemic vasculitis usually is associated with prominent constitutional features, including fever, fatigue, weight loss, and, occasionally, myalgia or arthralgia, along with manifestations of multisystem organ involvement. Virtually any organ can be affected eventually. Rarely, vasculitis is limited to a single organ or found incidentally associated with cancer at the time of operation and cured by surgical removal. Other cases are limited to isolated involvement of the skin (cutaneous vasculitis) or peripheral nerves.

Classic polyarteritis nodosa is a necrotizing vasculitis of small and medium-sized arteries and is associated with vascular nephropathy (usually without glomerulonephritis), causing multiple renal infarctions, hypertension, and renal failure.

Hypertension develops as a result of angiographically demonstrable renal artery compromise or, less commonly, glomerular involvement. Lung involvement is very uncommon. Patients with classic polyarteritis nodosa are usually ANCA-negative.

Microscopic polyangiitis is distinguished from polyarteritis nodosa as a necrotizing vasculitis that affects capillaries, venules, and arterioles and most frequently presents with pauci-immune and sometimes rapidly progressive necrotizing glomerulonephritis. Proteinuria is common, and, rarely, a nephritic syndrome may develop. There is an active urinary sediment, with red blood cells and red cell casts characteristic of glomerular involvement. Renal insufficiency is frequently noted at presentation, and glomerulonephritis causes oliguric renal failure in one-third of all patients. Renal angiography in microscopic polyangiitis is usually normal. Hypertension is uncommon. Lung involvement, including pulmonary capillaritis and hemorrhage, eventually may affect up to a third of patients with microscopic polyangiitis.

Systemic vasculitis may be a manifestation or complication of other diseases. This secondary vasculitis complicates hepatitis C infection, rheumatoid arthritis, Sjögren syndrome, mixed cryoglobulinemia, hairy cell leukemia, myelodysplastic syndrome, and other hematologic malignancies. Some forms of secondary vasculitis have more favorable clinical presentations. For example, systemic rheumatoid vasculitis most commonly manifests with constitutional symptoms, skin lesions, and neuropathy. It rarely causes a necrotizing glomerulonephritis or pulmonary hemorrhage.

- Systemic vasculitis is associated with prominent constitutional features, including fever, fatigue, weight loss, and, occasionally, myalgia or arthralgia, along with manifestations of multisystem organ involvement.

- Secondary vasculitis may be a complication of other diseases.

- Classic polyarteritis nodosa usually does not affect the lungs.

Diagnosis

Abnormal laboratory findings include normocytic anemia, increased erythrocyte sedimentation rate, and thrombocytosis. Microscopic polyangiitis presents with a myeloperoxidase-specific perinuclear (p-) ANCA in 90% of cases. Hypocomplementemia is not common in patients with active vasculitis. However, low complement may be evident if immune complexes such as cryoglobulins are part of the pathogenesis of secondary vasculitis or if vasculitis occurs in association with systemic lupus erythematosus. Hepatitis B infection occurs in a small proportion of patients with ANCA-negative (classic) polyarteritis nodosa and should always be sought, because treatment is directed against the infection. Hepatitis C is associated with mixed cryoglobulinemia, and vasculitis may occur in patients with cryoglobulinemia.

Evaluation should document the extent and severity of the condition. The confirmatory test typically is angiography or biopsy of involved tissue showing vasculitis. The biopsy

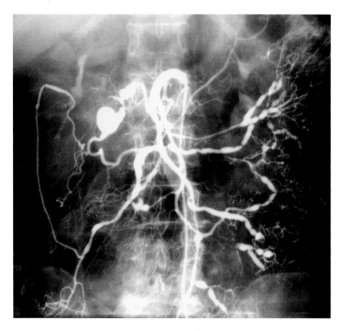

Figure 23.2 Visceral Polyarteritis Nodosa. Angiography shows the classic features of smooth tapers followed by normal or dilated vessels. Note the large saccular aneurysm in the hepatic artery. (Adapted from Audiovisual Aids Subcommittee of the Education Committee of the American College of Rheumatology. Syllabus: revised clinical slide collection on the rheumatic diseases and 1985, 1988, and 1989 slide supplements. Atlanta [GA]: American College of Rheumatology. Used with permission.)

should be of accessible symptomatic tissue. If medium-sized vessel polyarteritis nodosa is suspected, visceral angiography, including views of the renal and mesenteric arteries, shows saccular or fusiform aneurysm formation coupled with smooth, tapered stenosis alternating with normal or dilated blood vessels (Figure 23.2). In some cases, other imaging methods such as ultrasonography and magnetic resonance angiography may be helpful and less invasive than conventional angiography.

- Microscopic polyangiitis often presents with positive myeloperoxidase-specific p-ANCA.

- Hepatitis B infection occurs in a small proportion of patients with ANCA-negative (classic) polyarteritis nodosa.

- Confirmatory diagnostic tests include angiography or biopsy of involved tissue showing vasculitis.

- Visceral angiography often shows saccular or fusiform aneurysm formation coupled with smooth, tapered stenosis in patients with classic polyarteritis nodosa.

Treatment

The cornerstone of treatment is early diagnosis and corticosteroid therapy. Cytotoxic or antimetabolite drugs such as cyclophosphamide, methotrexate, mycophenolate mofetil, and azathioprine are often used in combination with corticosteroids. The choice of the second agent is usually determined by the severity and type of organ involvement and patient comorbid conditions. Five factors have been identified that are associated with increased mortality in patients with polyarteritis nodosa (Box 23.9). In patients with 1 or more of these factors, strong consideration should be given to using cyclophosphamide.

A new treatment that has shown promise in some patients with systemic vasculitis, especially those with Wegener granulomatosis, is rituximab. When a patient's condition deteriorates in the face of potent treatment, consider possible progression of disease, superimposed infection, or noninflammatory, proliferative, occlusive vasculopathy.

- Cyclophosphamide, mycophenolate mofetil, methotrexate, and azathioprine are often used in conjuction with corticosteroids for the treatment of systemic vasculitis.

- Rituximab is a new therapy that has shown promise in some cases of ANCA-associated vasculitis.

Outcome

In the first year after diagnosis of systemic vasculitis, deaths are related to the extent of disease activity, particularly gastrointestinal tract ischemia and renal insufficiency. Distinguishing classic polyarteritis nodosa from microscopic polyangiitis and type of organ involvement may influence treatment, complications, relapse rate, and mortality (Table 23.1).

After 1 year, complications of treatment, including infections in the immunocompromised patient, contribute most to mortality rates. With treatment, survival at 7 years is about

Table 23.1 FEATURES OF POLYARTERITIS NODOSA AND MICROSCOPIC POLYANGIITIS

CHARACTERISTIC	POLYARTERITIS NODOSA	MICROSCOPIC POLYANGIITIS
Vessels involved	Small & medium-sized	Capillaries, venules, arterioles
ANCA	Often negative	Usually p-ANCA (MPO)-positive
Renal involvement	Ischemic nephropathy	Often glomerulonephritis
Pulmonary involvement	Seldom	Alveolar hemorrhage in 1/3

Abbreviations: ANCA, antineutrophil cytoplasmic antibody; MPO, myeloperoxide; p-ANCA, perinuclear ANCA.

70% for microscopic polyangiitis and about 80% for classic polyarteritis nodosa.

- In the first year after diagnosis, deaths are related to the extent of disease activity, particularly gastrointestinal tract ischemia and renal insufficiency.

- Complications from treatment affect long-term mortality.

- A patient with systemic vasculitis typically presents with fever, fatigue, weight loss, arthralgia, mononeuritis multiplex, and renal failure. Laboratory testing shows increased sedimentation rate and anemia.

Churg-Strauss Vasculitis

Churg-Strauss vasculitis, or Churg-Strauss syndrome, is similar to microscopic angiitis and Wegener granulomatosis in that it involves small vessels and may be associated with ANCA antibodies. The median age at onset is about 38 years (range, 15–69 years). Churg-Strauss vasculitis is defined by 1) a history of, or current symptoms of, asthma, 2) peripheral eosinophilia ($>1.5\times10^9$ eosinophils/L), and 3) systemic vasculitis of at least 2 extrapulmonary organs. There is a slight male predominance. The histopathologic features of the disease include eosinophilic extravascular granulomas and granulomatous or nongranulomatous small vessel necrotizing vasculitis. It typically involves the small arteries, veins, arterioles, and venules.

- Churg-Strauss vasculitis is defined by asthma, eosinophilia, and systemic vasculitis involving at least 2 extrapulmonary systems.

- It involves small arteries, veins, arterioles, and venules.

Clinical Features

Churg-Strauss syndrome is thought to evolve in 3 stages. Patients need not progress in an orderly manner from 1 stage to another. There usually is a prodrome of allergic rhinitis, nasal polyposis, or asthma. In the second stage, peripheral blood and tissue eosinophilia develops, suggesting Löffler syndrome. Chronic eosinophilic pneumonia and gastroenteritis may remit or recur over years. The third stage is life-threatening vasculitis. Transient, patchy pulmonary infiltrates or nodules, pleural effusions, pulmonary angiitis and cardiomegaly, eosinophilic gastroenteritis, extravascular necrotizing granulomata of the skin, mononeuritis multiplex, and polyarthritis can complicate Churg-Strauss syndrome. A Churg-Strauss–like syndrome has been reported in some patients treated with the asthma medication zafirlukast. Less than half of patients with Churg-Strauss vasculitis are ANCA-positive. If they are positive, the ANCA-staining pattern is usually perinuclear and the antibodies are usually directed against myeloperoxidase (p-ANCA with myeloperoxidase).

- Churg-Strauss syndrome involves a prodrome of allergic rhinitis, nasal polyposis, or asthma.

- Peripheral blood and tissue eosinophilia develops.
- Transient, patchy pulmonary infiltrates, extravascular necrotizing granulomata of the skin, and mononeuritis multiplex can complicate Churg-Strauss syndrome.

Treatment and Outcome

The 1-year survival with treated Churg-Strauss syndrome is similar to that with microscopic polyangiitis. There is more cardiac involvement but fewer renal deaths than in polyarteritis nodosa. Treatment includes corticosteroids with or without the addition of cytotoxic agents. The eosinophilia resolves with treatment.

- In Churg-Strauss syndrome, there is more cardiac involvement but fewer renal deaths than in polyarteritis nodosa.
- A patient with Churg-Strauss syndrome typically presents with a history of bronchial asthma with recent worsening of pulmonary symptoms and development of mononeuritis multiplex. There is a history of nasal polyposis. Palpable purpura is noted on physical evaluation. On laboratory testing, the eosinophil count is markedly increased.

Buerger Disease

Buerger disease, or thromboangiitis obliterans, occurs almost exclusively in young adult smokers. There is a male predominance. Patients usually present with ischemic injury to fingers or, less commonly, toes. Buerger disease affects the small and medium-sized arteries and veins of the extremities. Acute vasculitis in Buerger disease is accompanied by characteristic intraluminal thrombus that contains microabscesses. Usually, the disease is arrested when smoking is stopped. In contrast to other forms of vasculitis, Buerger disease is best thought of as a vasculopathy in that it does not require immunosuppressive therapy.

- Buerger disease occurs almost exclusively in young adult smokers.
- Patients present with ischemic injury to fingers or toes.
- The disease is arrested when smoking is stopped.

Wegener Granulomatosis

Clinical Features

Wegener granulomatosis is a well-recognized pathologic triad of upper and lower respiratory tract necrotizing granulomatous inflammation and focal segmental necrotizing glomerulonephritis. Wegener granulomatosis occurs in less than 1 person annually per 100,000 population. The peak incidence of the disease occurs in the fourth and fifth decades of life. There is a slight male predominance. Eighty-five percent of patients have generalized disease, including glomerulonephritis; 15% can present with local inflammation involving only the upper respiratory tract or kidneys. The clinical features of this disease are summarized by the mnemonic ELKS: involvement of ear/nose/throat, lung, kidney, and skin. Lung involvement most commonly includes thick-walled, centrally cavitating pulmonary nodules. Alveolitis and pulmonary hemorrhage occur in up to 20% of patients. Biopsy in patients with renal involvement usually does not show changes that are specific for Wegener granulomatosis. Renal biopsy often shows focal segmental necrotizing glomerulonephritis and, occasionally, granulomatous vasculitis. Skin involvement may include urticaria, petechiae, papules, vesicles, ulcers, pyoderma, and livedo reticularis. Inflammatory arthritis is usually oligoarticular and transient, occurring early in the clinical presentation. Central nervous system involvement includes distal sensory neuropathy, mononeuritis multiplex, and cranial nerve palsies. Conjunctivitis, uveitis, and proptosis are not unusual. Neurosensory hearing loss has been described together with serous otitis and inner ear vasculitis. Wegener granulomatosis–associated subglottic tracheal stenosis due to chondritis should be distinguished from primary polychondritis. On laboratory testing, cytoplasmic (c-) ANCA test with antibodies directed against PR3 is positive.

- In a typical case of Wegener granulomatosis, a 50-year-old patient presents with the triad of upper and lower respiratory tract necrotizing granulomatous inflammation and focal segmental necrotizing glomerulonephritis. On laboratory testing, the c-ANCA test is positive.
- The clinical features of Wegener granulomatosis are summarized by the mnemonic ELKS: involvement of ear/nose/throat, lung, kidney, and skin.
- Alveolitis and pulmonary hemorrhage occur in up to 20% of patients.
- Central nervous system involvement includes distal sensory neuropathy, mononeuritis multiplex, and cranial nerve palsies.

Pathologic Diagnosis

The diagnosis of Wegener granulomatosis may require finding characteristic pathologic features in biopsy specimens. Biopsy of the upper respiratory tract suggests the diagnosis in 55% of patients, but only 20% have granulomata or vasculitis associated with necrosis. An open lung biopsy has a higher diagnostic yield than transbronchial biopsy. As mentioned previously, renal biopsy usually does not show changes specific for Wegener granulomatosis. Relevant laboratory findings in active Wegener granulomatosis include nonspecific increases in the erythrocyte sedimentation rate and platelet count, normocytic anemia, and low levels of albumin. A positive result of c-ANCA directed against proteinase 3 test in a patient with the clinical features of Wegener granulomatosis may be sufficient for diagnosis, especially if tissue is not easily obtained.

- Laboratory findings in Wegener granulomatosis include nonspecific increases in erythrocyte sedimentation rate and platelet count and normocytic anemia.

- The diagnosis of Wegener granulomatosis is established with a positive result of c-ANCA directed against proteinase 3 and granulomatous inflammation on biopsy.

ANCA

c-ANCA is directed against proteinase 3, a serine protease from azurophilic granules. c-ANCA occurs in more than 90% of active cases of generalized Wegener granulomatosis. Occasionally, it is found in idiopathic crescentic glomerulonephritis, microscopic polyarteritis nodosa, and Churg-Strauss syndrome. The antibody titer tends to correlate with disease activity in an individual patient.

p-ANCA is directed against myeloperoxidase and other neutrophil cytoplasmic constituents. p-ANCA (anti-myeloperoxidase–specific) is found in idiopathic crescentic glomerulonephritis, microscopic polyarteritis nodosa, Churg-Strauss syndrome, in occasional cases of Wegener granulomatosis, and other connective tissue diseases. Therefore, a positive p-ANCA result with antibodies directed against myeloperoxidase can be suggestive of vasculitis. However, p-ANCA directed against other antigens is much less specific. It can occur in patients with inflammatory bowel disease, autoimmune liver disease, other connective tissue diseases, malignancies, and even drug-induced syndromes.

- Proteinase 3, c-ANCA occurs in >90% of active cases of Wegener granulomatosis.
- Non–myeloperoxidase p-ANCA is found in many different conditions.

Treatment and Outcome

If untreated, generalized Wegener granulomatosis is associated with a mean survival of 5 months and 95% mortality in 1 year. More than 95% of patients eventually have clinical remission with oral cyclophosphamide treatment. Corticosteroids are useful initially, and the dose can be tapered quickly after the disease is controlled. Mortality in the first year of disease is related primarily to the inflammatory process, with pulmonary hemorrhage or renal failure. In subsequent years, drug toxicity may dominate, with opportunistic infection and increasing risk of neoplasm and hemorrhagic cystitis related to the use of cyclophosphamide. Relapses even years after treatment are not uncommon.

Recent studies have suggested that rituximab may be efficacious in the treatment of patients with Wegener granulomatosis. Studies are currently under way to better define the optimal patients and regimens for use of this agent in ANCA-associated vasculitis, including Wegener granulomatosis.

There is also a role for use of trimethoprim-sulfamethoxazole. It may be efficacious in limited Wegener disease and also may be useful as an adjuvant to other therapy. This is in addition to its use for prophylaxis of *Pneumocystis* pneumonia.

- If untreated, generalized Wegener granulomatosis is associated with a mean survival of 5 months.

- Cyclophosphamide has revolutionized the treatment of Wegener granulomatosis and dramatically altered the natural history.
- Corticosteroids are useful initially, and the dose can be tapered quickly after the disease is controlled.
- Rituximab is a potential new therapy for Wegener granulomatosis and other ANCA-associated vasculitides.

In recent years there has been an initiative to change the nomenclature and no longer use the term *Wegener granulomatosis*. There is a proposal to instead use the term *granulomatosis with polyangitis*. This would be one type of vasculitis under the more general heading of "ANCA-associated vasculitis."

Small Vessel Vasculitis and Cutaneous Vasculitis

Clinical Features

Small vessel vasculitis occurs by itself or complicates many infectious, neoplastic, and connective tissue diseases. The most common cause of isolated cutaneous vasculitis is drugs. It manifests with urticaria, palpable purpura, livedo reticularis, or skin ulceration. Small vessel vasculitis occurs with many illnesses; a partial listing is given in Box 23.10.

- The most common cause of isolated cutaneous vasculitis is a medication reaction.
- Isolated cutaneous vasculitis manifests with urticaria, palpable purpura, livedo reticularis, or skin ulceration.

Box 23.10 CONDITIONS WITH SMALL VESSEL VASCULITIS

Systemic small vessel vasculitis
  Systemic vasculitis
    Wegener granulomatosis
    Polyarteritis (primary & secondary)
    Churg-Strauss vasculitis
    Takayasu arteritis
    Schönlein-Henoch purpura/vasculitis
  Serum sickness
  Goodpasture syndrome
Nonsystemic small vessel vasculitis
  Hypocomplementemic urticarial vasculitis
  Leukocytoclastic vasculitis related to:
    Rheumatoid arthritis
    Sjögren syndrome
    Systemic lupus erythematosus
    Other connective tissue diseases
  Drug-induced & postinfectious angiitis
  Mixed cryoglobulinemia
  Malignancy-associated vasculitis
  Inflammatory bowel disease
  Organ transplant-associated vasculitis
  Hypergammaglobulinemic purpura of Waldenström

- It can complicate most types of primary and secondary systemic vasculitis.

Histopathology

A neutrophilic- or (uncommonly) lymphocytic-predominant infiltrate surrounds small arteries, veins, arterioles, or venules. The histopathologic picture called "leukocytoclastic vasculitis" includes immune complexes deposited in vessel walls, along with fibrin deposition, endothelial cell swelling and necrosis, and a polymorphonuclear leukocytoclasis with scattering of nuclear fragment or nuclear dust. A classic clinical correlate of leukocytoclastic vasculitis is palpable purpura. This is a pathologic diagnosis and not a specific clinical condition.

- A classic clinical correlate of leukocytoclastic vasculitis is palpable purpura.

Diagnosis

The clinician must interpret small vessel or cutaneous vasculitis as a clinical finding and not a diagnosis. These various conditions are distinguished clinically and pathologically. For instance, Schönlein-Henoch vasculitis is suggested by the clinical features of abdominal pain or gastrointestinal hemorrhage in addition to the classic picture of lower extremity purpura, arthritis, and hematuria. Schönlein-Henoch vasculitis has immunoglobulin A deposition in vessel walls and normal complement levels. Mixed cryoglobulinemia has circulating cryoglobulins and evidence of complement consumption. Complement levels, especially C4, may be low transiently in hypersensitivity vasculitis. Hypersensitivity vasculitis is almost always a nonsystemic small vessel vasculitis temporally related to infection, ingestion of drugs, or, less commonly, malignancy. The results of other laboratory studies are nonspecific. The leukocyte count and platelet count may be increased. Eosinophilia may be present. The erythrocyte sedimentation rate usually is increased.

- Complement levels may be low in mixed cryoglobulinemia and hypersensitivity vasculitis.
- Schönlein-Henoch vasculitis has 4 classic clinical features: lower extremity purpura, arthritis, gastrointestinal hemorrhage, and nephritis. Immunoglobulin A is noted on biopsy.

Treatment and Outcome

The outcome of nonsystemic small vessel vasculitis depends on the underlying condition. Control of the infection or discontinuing use of the offending drug may be all that is required. In other cases, corticosteroids or nonsteroidal anti-inflammatory drugs are beneficial. Hypersensitivity vasculitis is usually self-limited, but it may recur with repeated exposure to the antigen or drug.

- The outcome is good in nonsystemic small vessel vasculitis.
- Hypersensitivity vasculitis may recur with repeated exposure to the antigen or drug.

Cryoglobulinemia

Cryoglobulins are immunoglobulins that reversibly precipitate at reduced temperatures. They are grouped into 2 major categories. Type I cryoglobulins are aggregates of a single monoclonal immunoglobulin and generally are associated with multiple myeloma, Waldenström macroglobulinemia, and lymphomas. They usually are found in high concentrations (1–5 g/dL). Patients with type I cryoglobulins are often asymptomatic. Symptoms of type I cryoglobulinemia are usually related to increased viscosity and include headaches, visual disturbances, nosebleeds, Raynaud phenomenon, and ischemic ulceration from occlusion of arterioles and venules by precipitated immune complexes. Vasculitis is rare.

- Type I cryoglobulins are aggregates of a single monoclonal immunoglobulin.
- Patients with type I cryoglobulins are often asymptomatic.
- Symptoms of type I cryoglobulinemia are usually related to increased viscosity.
- Vasculitis is rare in type I cryoglobulinemia.

Type II and type III cryoglobulins consist of more than 1 class of immunoglobulin (mixed cryoglobulinemia) and can occur alone (essential, primary) or be due to another disease. Type II cryoglobulinemia involves a monoclonal immunoglobulin (usually immunoglobulin M) with anti-immunoglobulin specificity. Affected patients often have a positive rheumatoid factor. Type III cryoglobulinemia involves polyclonal immunoglobulins (usually immunoglobulin M) directed against other polyclonal immunoglobulins (usually immunoglobulin G). Other components of the immune complexes formed in mixed cryoglobulinemia include hepatitis C antigen, other infectious agents, cellular/nuclear antigens, and complement. These immune complexes precipitate slowly and are present in smaller quantities (50–500 mg/dL) than type I cryoglobulins.

Type II cryoglobulins frequently are associated with chronic infections (most commonly hepatitis C), autoimmune disorders, and, occasionally, lymphoma. The immune complexes that form precipitate on endothelial cells in peripheral blood vessels and fix complement, promoting vasculitic inflammation. The size of immune complexes, ability to fix complement, persistent immunoglobulin M production, and many other factors may influence the clinical presentation of mixed cryoglobulinemia. The typical presentation is that of nonsystemic small vessel vasculitis with palpable purpura, urticaria, and cutaneous ulceration. Peripheral neuropathy, arthralgia, and arthritis are common. Less commonly, mixed cryoglobulinemia is complicated by hepatosplenomegaly, pneumonitis or pulmonary hemorrhage, focal segmental necrotizing glomerulonephritis, serositis (pleurisy, pericarditis), and thyroiditis.

- Type II cryoglobulins frequently are associated with chronic infections (most often hepatitis C) and immune disorders.

- The typical presentation of type II cryoglobulinemia is nonsystemic small vessel vasculitis with palpable purpura, urticaria, and cutaneous ulceration.

- Peripheral neuropathy, arthralgia, and arthritis are common in type II cryoglobulinemia.

Laboratory Studies

Patients with type II cryoglobulinemia and small vessel vasculitis usually have an increased erythrocyte sedimentation rate, increased immunoglobulin levels, positive rheumatoid factor, and low levels of complement. Evidence of chronic hepatitis infection (particularly hepatitis C) frequently is identified. For cryoglobulin testing, it is important to draw blood into a warmed syringe and to keep it warm until transferred to a cryocrit tube. Cooled specimens must be kept for up to 3 days to identify type II cryoglobulins. Serum protein electrophoresis, immunoelectrophoresis, and quantitative immunoglobulin determinations can be helpful in some cases.

- In type II cryoglobulinemia, immunoglobulin levels and the erythrocyte sedimentation rate are increased, rheumatoid factor is positive, and complement levels are low.

- Evidence of chronic hepatitis infection (particularly hepatitis C) frequently is identified in type II cryoglobulinemia.

Outcome

The clinical course depends on the underlying associated conditions and on the organs involved. Progressive renal disease is the most common systemic complication. Pulmonary hemorrhage can be life-threatening.

- Outcome depends on associated conditions and organs involved.

- Progressive renal disease is the most common systemic complication.

Box 23.11 PALPABLE PURPURA: DIFFERENTIAL DIAGNOSIS

Polyarteritis
Churg-Strauss syndrome
Wegener granulomatosis
Schönlein-Henoch purpura/vasculitis
Cryoglobulinemic vasculitis
Connective tissue disease-associated vasculitis (rheumatoid arthritis, Sjögren syndrome, systemic lupus erythematosus)
Hypersensitivity vasculitis
  Drugs, infection, malignancy

Skin Lesions Associated With Vasculitis

Palpable purpura suggests leukocytoclastic vasculitis, but this pathologic diagnosis does not define the clinical syndrome. Box 23.11 outlines the differential diagnosis of palpable purpura. Nodules or papules diagnosed as necrotizing granuloma on biopsy occur in Churg-Strauss syndrome, Wegener granulomatosis, rheumatoid arthritis, and, occasionally, systemic lupus erythematosus. Other nodules or papules without necrotizing granulomata can be the sign of angiocentric lymphoproliferative disorders or sarcoidosis or they may be related to inflammatory bowel disease. Urticarial or pustular lesions complicate hypocomplementemic vasculitis, inflammatory bowel arthritis syndrome, and Behçet syndrome. Livedo reticularis, which is associated with proliferative endarteropathy, occurs in connective tissue diseases and antiphospholipid antibody syndrome and in association with cholesterol emboli and many systemic necrotizing vasculitides.

- Urticarial or pustular lesions complicate hypocomplementemic vasculitis, inflammatory bowel arthritis syndrome, and Behçet syndrome.

- Livedo reticularis occurs in connective tissue diseases and antiphospholipid antibody syndrome.

24.

INFLAMMATORY AND NONINFLAMMATORY ARTHRITIS

Clement J. Michet, MD

GOALS

- Review the diagnosis, clinical features, complications, and treatment of rheumatoid arthritis and other rheumatoid disorders.

- Review the diagnosis, clinical features, and treatment of osteoarthritis and its clinical subsets.

RHEUMATOID ARTHRITIS

Rheumatoid arthritis is a chronic systemic inflammatory disease characterized by joint destruction. It affects 0.03% to 1.5% of the population worldwide. Women are affected 3 times more frequently than men. Its incidence peaks between the ages of 35 and 45 years; however, the age-related prevalence of the disease increases even after age 65. The presentation of an unknown antigen to genetically susceptible persons is believed to trigger rheumatoid arthritis. Recently, cigarette smoking has been identified as a risk factor for seropositive rheumatoid arthritis.

There is an immunogenetic predisposition to the development of rheumatoid arthritis. Class II major histocompatibility complex molecules on the surface of antigen-presenting cells are responsible for initiating cellular immune responses and for stimulating the differentiation of B lymphocytes into plasma cells that produce antibody. Most white patients with rheumatoid arthritis have class II major histocompatibility complex type HLA-DR4 or HLA-DR1 or both. HLA-DR4 can be divided into 5 subtypes, 2 of which independently promote susceptibility to rheumatoid arthritis ("shared epitope"). The relative risk of rheumatoid arthritis is increased 3 to 5 times in white Americans with HLA-DR4. The concordance of rheumatoid factor–positive rheumatoid arthritis is increased 6 times among dizygotic twins. The risk of rheumatoid arthritis in a monozygotic twin is increased 30 times when a sibling has the disease.

- Rheumatoid arthritis affects 0.03%-1.5% of the population.

- Most white Americans with rheumatoid arthritis have class II major histocompatibility complex type HLA-DR4 or HLA-DR1 or both.

- The concordance of rheumatoid factor–positive rheumatoid arthritis is increased 6 times among dizygotic twins.

- The risk of rheumatoid arthritis in a monozygotic twin is increased 30 times when a sibling has the disease.

NATURAL HISTORY OF RHEUMATOID ARTHRITIS

In the majority of patients, the onset of the joint disease is insidious, occurring over weeks to months. However, in a third of patients, the onset is rapid, occurring over days or weeks. Early in the course of the disease, most patients have oligoarthritis. Their disease becomes polyarticular with time. Ten percent to 20% of patients have relentlessly progressive arthritis, and 70% to 90% have persistent, chronic, and progressive arthritis. The course may be slow, fluctuating, or rapid, but the end point is the same: disabling and destructive arthritis. Seventy percent of patients experience polycyclic disease, with repeated flares interrupted by partial or complete remissions. Spontaneous remissions in the polycyclic or progressive group almost never occur after 2 years of disease. Patients who experience a persisting polyarthritis with increased acute-phase reactants and a positive rheumatoid factor or anti–cyclic citrullinated peptide (CCP) antibody are at high risk for early erosive disease within 1 to 2 years of symptom onset and early disability. The relationship between disease duration and inability to work is nearly linear. After 15 years of rheumatoid arthritis, 15% of patients are completely disabled. Life expectancy in seropositive rheumatoid arthritis is shortened, but it may be improving with more aggressive early intervention in the illness. Age, disease severity, comorbid cardiovascular disease, and functional status predict mortality. Educational level and socioeconomic factors also influence mortality.

- In a third of patients, the onset of rheumatoid arthritis is rapid (days or weeks).

- Among patients with rheumatoid arthritis, 70%-90% have persistent, chronic, progressive arthritis.

- Joint damage occurs early in patients with seropositive disease.

- The relationship between disease duration and inability to work is nearly linear.

PATHOGENESIS OF RHEUMATOID ARTHRITIS

The immune reaction begins in the synovial lining of the joints in a genetically predisposed person. The earliest pathologic changes in the disease are microvascular injury that increases vascular permeability and the accumulation of inflammatory cells (CD4+ lymphocytes, polymorphonuclear leukocytes, and plasma cells) in the perivascular space. Proinflammatory cytokines are released. Mediators of inflammation promote synovial angiogenesis and synovial cell proliferation, the accumulation of neutrophils in synovial fluid, and the maturation of B cells into plasma cells. Plasma cells in the joint locally synthesize rheumatoid factor and other antibodies that promote inflammation. Immune complexes activate the complement system, releasing chemotactic factors and promoting vascular permeability and opsonization. Phagocytosis releases lysosomal enzymes and fosters the digestion of collagen, cartilage matrix, and elastic tissues. The release of oxygen-free radicals injures cells. Damaged cell membranes set free phospholipids that fuel the arachidonic acid cascade.

The local inflammatory response becomes self-perpetuating. Cytokines continue to play an important role, including tumor necrosis factor-α, interleukin-1, and interleukin-6. Proliferating synovium of activated macrophages and fibroblasts polarizes into a centripetally invasive pannus, destroying the weakened cartilage and subchondral bone. Chondrocytes, stimulated in the inflammatory milieu, release their own proteases and collagenases.

Patients have swelling, pain, and joint stiffness with the onset of vascular injury of the synovial lining, angiogenesis, and cellular proliferation. Joint warmth, swelling, pain, and limitation of motion worsen as the synovial membrane proliferates and the inflammatory reaction builds. In studies of early arthritis, histologic and radiographic evidence of rheumatoid synovitis is found in clinically unaffected joints, an indication that the disease is present before clinical manifestations appear.

Rheumatoid factor is an immunoglobulin (Ig) directed against the Fc portion of IgG. It is not specific for rheumatoid arthritis, and the prevalence of rheumatoid factor increases with aging in healthy persons. Rheumatoid factor may be detected in other inflammatory diseases such as primary Sjögren syndrome, systemic lupus erythematosus, mixed cryoglobulinemia, hepatitis C, and systemic vasculitis.

Anti-CCP antibodies are detected in the majority of patients with seropositive rheumatoid arthritis. These target antigens are found in peptides containing citrulline, an amino acid resulting from posttranslational enzyme modification of arginine. Unlike rheumatoid factor, these antibodies are specific for rheumatoid arthritis. They are present at the onset of disease, and in a high titer they are associated with progressive erosive disease.

- Swelling, pain, and joint stiffness occur with the onset of immune-mediated vascular injury of the synovial lining, angiogenesis, and cellular proliferation.

- Anti-CCP antibodies are equally sensitive and more specific than rheumatoid factor for the diagnosis of early, erosive rheumatoid arthritis.

- Cytokines, in particular tumor necrosis factor-α, and immune complexes, including rheumatoid factor, are important components of the joint inflammatory reaction in rheumatoid arthritis.

CLINICAL FEATURES OF RHEUMATOID ARTHRITIS

The joints most commonly involved in early rheumatoid arthritis are the metacarpophalangeal, proximal interphalangeal, wrist, and metatarsophalangeal joints (more than 85% of patients) (Figure 24.1). The distal interphalangeal joints are typically spared. The distribution of involvement is symmetric and polyarticular (5 or more joints); predominantly, small joints are involved. Ultimately, multiple other joints may be involved, including the knees, ankles, elbows, shoulders, and the cricoarytenoid and C1–2 articulations. Joints affected with rheumatoid arthritis are warm and swollen. The joint enlargement feels spongy and occurs with the thickening of the synovium. An associated joint effusion may make the joint feel fluctuant. Patients describe deep aching and soreness in the involved joints, which are aggravated by use and can be present at rest.

- The joints most commonly involved in early rheumatoid arthritis are the metacarpophalangeal, proximal interphalangeal, wrist, and metatarsophalangeal joints.

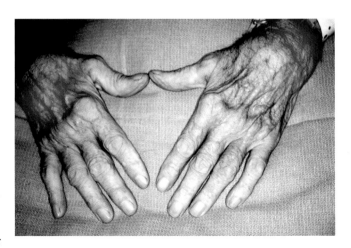

Figure 24.1 Moderately Active Seropositive Rheumatoid Arthritis. The patient has soft tissue swelling across the entire row of metatarsophalangeal joints and proximal interphalangeal joints bilaterally and soft tissue swelling mounding up over the wrists. Note the nearly complete lack of change at the distal interphalangeal joints.

- The distribution of involvement in rheumatoid arthritis is symmetric and polyarticular; predominantly, small joints are involved.
- Hallmarks of joint inflammation in rheumatoid arthritis are stiffness, heat, redness, soft tissue swelling, pain, and dysfunction.

CONSTITUTIONAL FEATURES OF RHEUMATOID ARTHRITIS

Morning stiffness of more than 1 hour, "gelling" throughout the body, and recurrence of the stiffness after resting are some of the many constitutional features that complicate rheumatoid arthritis. Fatigue, weight loss, muscle pain, excessive sweating, or low-grade fever may be reported by patients presenting with rheumatoid arthritis. Adult seropositive rheumatoid arthritis is not a cause of fever of unknown origin because temperatures greater than 38.3°C cannot be attributed to the disease.

MUSCULOSKELETAL COMPLICATIONS OF RHEUMATOID ARTHRITIS

The musculoskeletal complications of rheumatoid arthritis are listed in Box 24.1.

Cervical Spine

Half of all patients with chronic rheumatoid arthritis have radiographic involvement of the atlantoaxial joint. It is diagnosed from cervical flexion and extension radiographs showing subluxation. Alternatively, some patients have subaxial subluxations, typically at 2 or more levels. The cervical instability is usually asymptomatic; however, patients may have pain and

---

Box 24.1 MUSCULOSKELETAL COMPLICATIONS OF RHEUMATOID ARTHRITIS

Characteristic deformities
Boutonnière deformity of the finger, with hyperextension of the distal interphalangeal joint & flexion of the proximal interphalangeal joint
Swan-neck deformity of the finger, with hyperextension at the proximal interphalangeal joint & flexion of the distal interphalangeal joint
Ulnar deviation of the metacarpophalangeal joints; it can progress to complete volar subluxation of the proximal phalanx from the metacarpophalangeal head
Compression of the carpal bones & radial deviation at the carpus
Subluxation at the wrist
Valgus of the ankle & hindfoot
Pes planus
Forefoot varus & hallux valgus
Cock-up toes from subluxation at the metatarsophalangeal joints

---

stiffness in the neck and occipital region. Patients may present dramatically with drop attacks or tetraplegia, but more commonly progression can be slow and subtle with symptoms of hand weakness or paresthesias or signs of cervical myelopathy. Interference with blood flow by ischemic compression of the anterior spinal artery or vertebral arteries (vertebrobasilar insufficiency) causes the neurologic symptoms. All patients with destructive rheumatoid arthritis should be managed with intubation precautions and the assumption that cervical instability is present. New neurologic symptoms mandate urgent neurologic evaluation, including magnetic resonance imaging of the cervical spine and consideration of surgical intervention. Indications for surgical treatment include neurologic or vascular compromise and intractable pain. In active patients, prophylactic cervical spine stabilization is recommended when there is evidence of extreme (>8 mm) subluxation of C1 over C2. The probability of cervical involvement is predicted by the severity and chronicity of peripheral arthritis.

- Half of all patients with chronic rheumatoid arthritis have radiographic involvement of the atlantoaxial joint.
- Patients with cervical spine involvement by rheumatoid arthritis may present with occipital pain, signs of myelopathy, weakness and paresthesias of the hands, or drop attacks.
- Indications for surgical treatment in rheumatoid arthritis are neurologic or vascular compromise or intractable pain.
- The probability of cervical involvement is predicted by the severity and chronicity of peripheral arthritis.

Popliteal Cyst

Flexion of the knee markedly increases the intra-articular pressure of a swollen joint. This pressure produces an out-pouching of the posterior components of the joint space, termed a popliteal or a Baker cyst. Ultrasonographic examination of the popliteal space confirms the diagnosis. A popliteal cyst should be distinguished from a popliteal artery aneurysm, lymphadenopathy, phlebitis, and (more rarely) a benign or malignant tumor. The cyst can rupture down into the calf or, rarely, superiorly into the posterior aspect of the thigh. Rupture of the popliteal cyst with dissection into the calf may resemble acute thrombophlebitis and is called pseudothrombophlebitis. Fever, leukocytosis, and ecchymosis around the ankle (crescent sign) can occur with the rupture. Treatment of an acute cyst rupture includes bed rest, elevation of the leg, ice massage or cryocompression, and an intra-articular injection of corticosteroid. Treatment of the popliteal cyst requires improvement in the knee arthritis.

- Popliteal cyst is also called Baker cyst.
- Rupture of a popliteal cyst may resemble acute thrombophlebitis (pseudothrombophlebitis).
- Ultrasonography can distinguish a cyst from a popliteal artery aneurysm, lymphadenopathy, phlebitis, and tumor.

Tenosynovitis

Tenosynovitis of the finger flexor and extensor tendon sheaths is common. It presents with diffuse swelling between the joints and a palpable grating within the flexor tendon sheaths in the palm with passive movement of the digit. Other tenosynovial syndromes in rheumatoid arthritis include de Quervain and wrist tenosynovitis. Persistent inflammation can produce stenosing tenosynovitis, loss of function, and, ultimately, rupture of tendons. Treatment of acute tenosynovitis includes immobilization, warm soaks, nonsteroidal anti-inflammatory drugs, and local injections of corticosteroid in the tendon sheath.

- Tenosynovitis of the finger flexor and extensor tendon sheaths is common and can lead to tendon rupture.

Carpal Tunnel Syndrome

Rheumatoid arthritis is a common cause of carpal tunnel syndrome. The sudden appearance of bilateral carpal tunnel syndrome should raise the question of an early inflammatory arthritis. This syndrome is associated with paresthesias of the hand in a typical median nerve distribution. Discomfort may radiate up the forearm or into the upper arm. The symptoms worsen with prolonged flexion of the wrist and at night. Late complications include thenar muscle weakness and atrophy and permanent sensory loss. Treatment includes resting splints, control of inflammation, and local injection of glucocorticosteroid. Surgical release is recommended for persistent symptoms.

- Rheumatoid arthritis is a common cause of carpal tunnel syndrome.

- Carpal tunnel syndrome is associated with paresthesias of the hand in a typical median nerve distribution.

EXTRA-ARTICULAR COMPLICATIONS OF RHEUMATOID ARTHRITIS

Extra-articular complications of rheumatoid arthritis occur almost exclusively in patients who have high titers of rheumatoid factor. In general, the number and severity of the extra-articular features vary with the duration and severity of disease. Many of the classical extra-articular manifestations of rheumatoid arthritis have become less common with the advent of more aggressive treatment of early disease.

Rheumatoid Nodules

Rheumatoid nodules are the most common extra-articular manifestation of seropositive rheumatoid arthritis. More than 20% of patients have rheumatoid nodules, which occur over extensor surfaces and at pressure points. They are rare in the lungs, heart, sclera, and dura mater. The nodules have characteristic histopathologic features. A collagenous capsule and a perivascular collection of chronic inflammatory cells surround a central area of necrosis encircled by palisading fibroblasts. Breakdown of the skin over rheumatoid nodules, with ulcers and infection, can be a major source of morbidity. The infection can spread to local bursae, infect bone, or spread hematogenously to joints.

- Extra-articular complications in rheumatoid arthritis occur almost exclusively in seropositive rheumatoid arthritis.

- Rheumatoid nodules are the most common extra-articular complication.

- Rheumatoid nodules occur over extensor surfaces and at pressure points and are prone to ulceration and infection.

Rheumatoid Vasculitis

Rheumatoid vasculitis usually occurs in persons with severe, deforming arthritis and a high titer of rheumatoid factor. The vasculitis is mediated by the deposition of circulating immune complexes on the blood vessel wall. At its most benign, it occurs as rheumatoid nodules, with small infarcts over the nodules and at the cuticles. Proliferation of the vascular intima and media causes this obliterative endarteropathy, which has little associated inflammation. It is best managed by controlling the underlying arthritis. Leukocytoclastic or small vessel vasculitis produces palpable purpura or cutaneous ulceration, particularly over the malleoli of the lower extremities.

This vasculitis can cause pyoderma gangrenosum or peripheral sensory neuropathy. Secondary polyarteritis, which is clinically and histopathologically identical to polyarteritis nodosa, results in mononeuritis multiplex. Occasionally, the vasculitis occurs after the joint disease appears "burned out."

- Rheumatoid vasculitis usually occurs in the setting of severe, deforming arthritis and a high titer of rheumatoid factor.

- Rheumatoid vasculitis is mediated by the deposition of circulating immune complexes on the blood vessel wall.

- Rheumatoid vasculitis comprises a spectrum of vascular disease, including rheumatoid nodules and obliterative endarteropathy, leukocytoclastic or small vessel vasculitis, and secondary polyarteritis (systemic necrotizing vasculitis).

Neurologic Manifestations

Neurologic manifestations of rheumatoid arthritis include mild peripheral sensory neuropathy. Painful sensory-motor neuropathy (mononeuropathy) suggests vasculitis or nerve entrapment (eg, carpal tunnel syndrome). Cervical vertebral subluxation can cause myelopathy. Erosive changes may promote basilar invagination of the odontoid process of C2 into the underside of the brain, causing spinal cord compression and death.

Pulmonary Manifestations

Pleural disease has been noted in more than 40% of autopsies in cases of rheumatoid arthritis, but clinically significant pleural disease is less frequent. Characteristically, rheumatoid pleural effusions are asymptomatic until they become large enough to interfere mechanically with respiration. The pleural fluid is an exudate with a concentration of glucose that is low (10–50 mg/dL) because of impaired transport of glucose into the pleural space. Pulmonary nodules appear singly or in clusters. Single nodules have the appearance of a coin lesion. Nodules typically are pleural-based and may cavitate and create a bronchopleural fistula. Pneumoconiosis complicating rheumatoid lung disease, or Caplan syndrome, results in a violent fibroblastic reaction and large nodules.

Acute interstitial pneumonitis is a rare complication that may begin as alveolitis and progress to respiratory insufficiency and death. Interstitial fibrosis is a chronic, slowly progressive process. It has physical findings of diffuse dry crackles on lung auscultation and a reticular nodular radiographic pattern affecting both lung fields, initially in the lung bases. A decrease in the diffusing capacity for carbon dioxide and a restrictive pattern are characteristic pulmonary function test findings. Interstitial disease is highly associated with smoking. Bronchiolitis obliterans with or without cryptogenic organizing pneumonia may occur with rheumatoid arthritis or its treatment. It produces an obstructive picture on pulmonary function testing and typically responds to corticosteroid treatment. High-resolution computed tomography is useful for distinguishing these different interstitial rheumatoid lung syndromes and predicting treatment response. Methotrexate treatment causes a hypersensitivity lung reaction in 1% to 3% of patients. It can present insidiously with a dry cough or with life-threatening pneumonitis.

- Rheumatoid pleural disease is common but asymptomatic until pleural effusions interfere with respiration.
- The exudative pleural fluid is remarkable for low levels of glucose.
- High-resolution computed tomography helps to distinguish among rheumatoid-associated interstitial lung diseases, including interstitial pneumonitis, interstitial fibrosis, and bronchiolitis obliterans with or without cryptogenic organizing pneumonia.
- Methotrexate hypersensitivity pneumonitis may be a life-threatening complication of therapy.

Cardiac Complications

Pericarditis has been noted in 50% of autopsies in cases of rheumatoid arthritis. However, patients rarely present with acute pericardial symptoms or cardiac tamponade. Recurrent effusive pericarditis without symptoms may evolve to chronic constrictive pericarditis. Signs of unexplained edema or ascites may be the presenting manifestations. Untreated constrictive pericarditis has a very high 1-year mortality of 70%. It will not respond to medical therapies. Surgical pericardiectomy is necessary.

- Patients rarely present with acute pericardial symptoms despite frequent serous pericarditis.
- Rheumatoid pericardial disease frequently presents with edema or ascites due to occult constrictive disease.
- Chronic constrictive pericarditis necessitates surgical treatment.

Liver Abnormalities

Patients with rheumatoid arthritis can have increased levels of liver enzymes, particularly alkaline phosphatase. Increased levels of aspartate aminotransferase, γ-glutamyltransferase, and acute-phase proteins and hypoalbuminemia also occur in active rheumatoid arthritis. Liver biopsy shows nonspecific changes of inflammation. Nodular regenerative hyperplasia is rare and causes portal hypertension and hypersplenism. Many medications used to treat rheumatoid arthritis may cause increased levels of the transaminases.

- Increased levels of liver enzymes, particularly alkaline phosphatase, may occur in rheumatoid arthritis.
- Nodular hyperplasia of the liver can rarely complicate rheumatoid arthritis and lead to portal hypertension and hypersplenism.
- Many medications used to treat rheumatoid arthritis increase the levels of transaminases.

Ophthalmic Abnormalities

Keratoconjunctivitis sicca, or secondary Sjögren syndrome, is the most common ophthalmic complication in rheumatoid arthritis. Episcleritis and scleritis also occur independently of the joint inflammation and are usually treated topically. Severe scleritis progressing to scleromalacia perforans causes blindness. Infrequent ocular complications of rheumatoid arthritis include episcleral nodules, palsy of the superior oblique muscle caused by tenosynovitis of its tendon sheath (Brown syndrome), and uveitis. Retinopathy is an infrequent complication of antimalarial drug treatment.

- Keratoconjunctivitis sicca, or secondary Sjögren syndrome, is the most common ophthalmic complication in rheumatoid arthritis.
- Severe scleritis progressing to scleromalacia perforans causes blindness.

LABORATORY FINDINGS IN RHEUMATOID ARTHRITIS

Nonspecific alterations in many laboratory values are common. In very active disease, normocytic anemia (hemoglobin value about 10 g/dL), leukocytosis, thrombocytosis, hypoalbuminemia, and hypergammaglobulinemia are common. Rheumatoid factor (IgM) occurs in 90% of patients, but its presence may not be detected for months after the initial joint symptoms occur. A positive rheumatoid factor is not specific for rheumatoid arthritis. Diseases in boldface type in Box 24.2 are most likely to have high titers of rheumatoid factor. Five percent of the general population has a low titer of rheumatoid factor. Anti-CCP antibodies are more specific for rheumatoid arthritis and may be present when rheumatoid factor is absent. Antinuclear antibodies are common in seropositive rheumatoid disease. C-reactive protein correlates with disease activity, but it is not more helpful than the erythrocyte sedimentation rate. Active rheumatoid arthritis is associated with low iron-binding capacity, low plasma levels of iron, and an increased ferritin value, unless the patient is iron-deficient.

- Normocytic anemia, leukocytosis, thrombocytosis, and hypoalbuminemia are common in active rheumatoid arthritis.

- Rheumatoid factor is not specific for the diagnosis of rheumatoid arthritis.

- Anti-CCP antibodies may be present when rheumatoid factor is absent. They are not present in the other diseases associated with a factor.

Synovial fluid is cloudy and light yellow, has poor viscosity, and typically contains 10,000 to 75,000 leukocytes/mL, predominantly neutrophils.

RADIOGRAPHIC FINDINGS OF RHEUMATOID ARTHRITIS

The radiographic findings in early rheumatoid arthritis are normal or show soft tissue swelling and periarticular osteopenia. Later, the characteristic changes of periarticular osteoporosis, symmetric narrowing of the joint space, and marginal bony erosions become obvious. These signs are most common in radiographs of the hands and forefeet. Radiographic changes at end-stage rheumatoid arthritis include subluxation and other deformities, joint destruction, fibrous ankylosis, and, rarely, bony ankylosis.

- The characteristic radiologic changes in rheumatoid arthritis include periarticular osteoporosis, symmetric narrowing of the joint space, and bony erosions of the joint margin. These occur earliest in the hands and metatarsal phalangeal joints.

DIAGNOSIS OF RHEUMATOID ARTHRITIS

Adult rheumatoid arthritis should be considered in a person older than 16 years with inflammatory joint symptoms lasting for more than 6 weeks. The time criterion is important because there are viral arthropathies, such as parvovirus B19 infection, that mimic acute rheumatoid arthritis. Morning stiffness lasting for more than 30 minutes, small joint involvement in the metatarsophalangeal joints (morning metatarsalgia), metacarpophalangeal joints with tenderness and swelling, and more than 3 joints affected are clues to an early rheumatoid arthritis presentation. Of the 7 criteria of the American Rheumatism Association, listed in Box 24.3, 4 are used to classify cases as definite rheumatoid arthritis for research studies, but the vast majority of patients with early rheumatoid arthritis do not meet these criteria. The detection of CCP antibody has allowed rheumatologists to identify rheumatoid arthritis very early in the clinical evolution of the disease before patients would meet these classification criteria.

TREATMENT OF RHEUMATOID ARTHRITIS

The management of patients with rheumatoid arthritis requires making the correct diagnosis, determining the functional status of the patient, and selecting the goals of management with the patient. Goals of management include relieving inflammation and pain and maintaining function.

The principles emphasized by *physical medicine* include bed rest or rest periods, improving nonrestorative sleep, and joint protection (including modification of activities of daily life, range-of-motion exercises, orthotics, and splints, if they help the pain). Exercise should begin with range of motion and stretching to overcome contracture. Strengthening and conditioning exercises should be prescribed carefully, depending on the activity of the patient's disease.

The primary goal of rheumatoid arthritis therapy is to begin treatment as soon as the diagnosis is made. Using nonsteroidal anti-inflammatory drugs alone for rheumatoid arthritis is not recommended. Treatment should be managed and advanced with the goal of achieving low disease activity based on a targeted disease activity score.

The choice of first *disease-modifying antirheumatic drug* (DMARD) is determined by the potential for early joint damage. Therefore, in seropositive patients, methotrexate is the drug of choice. In seronegative polyarthritis, sulfasalazine, hydroxychloroquine, or minocycline may be options. Uninterrupted treatment with a disease-modifying agent for 3 to 6 months is usually necessary to assess its effect. Traditionally, DMARDs have been used sequentially, although recent studies have shown an enhanced benefit with early combination DMARD treatments that include methotrexate. Tapered oral corticosteroid therapy is another option in some protocols for early rheumatoid arthritis. Evidence supporting the pivotal pro-inflammatory role of tumor necrosis factor α in rheumatoid arthritis has been exploited clinically with the development of several effective tumor necrosis factor α antagonists. These generally are reserved for patients not responding to trials of more traditional and less expensive DMARDs, although evidence is accumulating that early use of these agents may result in better disease control. Abatacept (a T-cell costimulatory inhibitor), tocilizumab (an interleukin-6 inhibitor), and rituximab (an anti-CD20 B-cell–depleting agent) are options in treatment failures.

- Goals of management of rheumatoid arthritis include relieving inflammation and pain and maintaining function.
- A disease-modifying regimen is started when rheumatoid arthritis is diagnosed, and treatment should be guided by targeting improvement to a low level of disease activity. Methotrexate is the DMARD of choice in early seropositive rheumatoid arthritis.

- Low-dose or tapered prednisone may be necessary to preserve function and diminish joint damage during the initiation of DMARD therapy.
- With disease-modifying agents, uninterrupted treatment for 3–6 months is needed to assess efficacy. Combination DMARD therapy has become more common.

An *orthopedic surgical procedure* for resistant rheumatoid arthritis remains the most important therapeutic option for preserving or enhancing function. Synovectomy of the wrist and nearby tendon sheaths is beneficial when medication alone fails to control the synovitis. The operation preserves joint function and prevents the lysis of extensor tendons that can result in a loss of function. Synovectomy of the knee, either open or through an arthroscope, can delay the progression of rheumatoid arthritis from 6 months to 3 years. Removal of nodules and treatment for local nerve entrapment syndromes are also important surgical treatments for rheumatoid arthritis. Arthroplasty is reserved for patients in whom medical management has failed and in whom intractable pain or compromise in function developed because of a destroyed joint. Arthroplasty, arthrodesis (wrist), and synovectomy are important components of well-balanced rheumatology treatment programs. Total joint arthroplasty has a slightly poorer long-term outcome in rheumatoid arthritis than in osteoarthritis. Nevertheless, joint replacement has had a major impact on reducing patient disability.

- Orthopedic surgery is the most important advance in the treatment of medically resistant rheumatoid arthritis.
- Total joint arthroplasty has a slightly poorer long-term outcome in rheumatoid arthritis than in osteoarthritis.

CONDITIONS RELATED TO RHEUMATOID ARTHRITIS

Seronegative Rheumatoid Arthritis

Rheumatoid factor–negative (seronegative) rheumatoid arthritis is not associated with extra-articular manifestations. However, the arthritis usually is destructive, deforming, and otherwise indistinguishable from seropositive rheumatoid arthritis.

- Seronegative rheumatoid arthritis is not associated with extra-articular manifestations.

Seronegative Rheumatoid Arthritis of the Elderly

A subgroup of patients older than 60 years with seronegative rheumatoid arthritis may have milder arthritis. In this subgroup, polyarticular inflammation suddenly develops and is controlled best with low doses of prednisone. The presence of anti-CCP antibodies may help to distinguish this condition from polymyalgia rheumatica. Minimal destructive changes and deformity occur. Some elderly patients with seronegative arthritis, such as men in their 70s, present with acute polyarthritis and pitting edema of the hands and feet, so-called RS3PE (remitting symmetric seronegative synovitis with pitting edema). They have a prompt and gratifying response to low doses of prednisone. RS3PE typically runs a course similar to that of polymyalgia rheumatica. Rheumatoid arthritis may develop in some patients. Some cases are found to be a paraneoplastic disorder.

- In a patient older than 60 years, if rheumatoid factor–negative polyarticular arthritis suddenly develops, it is best controlled initially with low doses of prednisone.

Adult-Onset Still Disease

Systemic juvenile rheumatoid arthritis is known as Still disease. It has quotidian (fever spike with return to normal all in 1 day) high-spiking fevers, arthralgia, arthritis, seronegativity (negative rheumatoid factor and antinuclear antibody), leukocytosis, macular evanescent rash, serositis, lymphadenopathy, splenomegaly, and hepatomegaly. Fever, rash, and arthritis are the classic triad of Still disease.

Adult-onset Still disease has a slight female predominance. Its onset typically occurs between ages 16 and 35 years. Temperature more than 39°C occurs in a quotidian or double quotidian pattern in 96% of patients. The rash has a typical appearance: a macular salmon-colored eruption on the trunk and extremities. The transient rash is usually noticed at the time of increased temperature. Arthritis occurs in 95% of these patients. In one-third of patients, the joint disease is progressive and destructive. Adult-onset Still disease has a predilection for the wrists, shoulders, hips, and knees. Sixty percent of patients complain of a sore throat at onset, which can confuse the diagnosis with rheumatic fever; however, the course is much more prolonged than that of acute rheumatic fever. Weight loss is common. Lymphadenopathy occurs in two-thirds of patients and hepatosplenomegaly in about half. Pleurisy, pneumonitis, and abdominal pain occur in less than a third of patients. The serum ferritin level is markedly increased.

Treatment of adult-onset Still disease includes high doses of aspirin or indomethacin. Corticosteroids may be needed to control the systemic symptoms. Half of patients require methotrexate to control the systemic and articular features. Interleukin-1 inhibitor therapy may be useful for managing resistant cases.

- Fever, rash, and arthritis are the classic triad of Still disease.

- Rheumatoid factor and antinuclear antibodies are absent in Still disease.

- There is a predilection for the wrists, shoulders, hips, and knees.

- Sore throat occurs at onset in 60% of patients.

Felty Syndrome

Felty syndrome has the classic triad of rheumatoid arthritis, leukopenia, and splenomegaly. Classic Felty syndrome usually

---

Box 24.4 FEATURES OF FELTY SYNDROME

Classic triad
    Rheumatoid arthritis
    Leukopenia
    Splenomegaly
Other features
    Recurrent fevers with & without infection
    Weight loss
    Lymphadenopathy
    Skin hyperpigmentation
    Lower extremity ulcers
    Vasculitis
    Neuropathy
    Keratoconjunctivitis sicca
    Xerostomia
    Other cytopenias

---

occurs after 12 years or more of rheumatoid arthritis. It occurs in less than 1% of patients with seropositive rheumatoid arthritis. Splenomegaly either may not be clinically apparent or may manifest only after the arthritis and leukopenia have been present for some time. Other features of Felty syndrome are listed in Box 24.4. Patients with this syndrome frequently have bacterial infections, particularly of the skin and lungs. Infection related to the cytopenia is the major cause of mortality. High titers of rheumatoid factor are the rule, and a positive antinuclear antibody occurs in two-thirds of patients. Hypocomplementemia often occurs with active vasculitis. Patients often die of sepsis despite vigorous antibacterial treatment. Treatment can include corticosteroids, methotrexate, granulocyte colony-stimulating factor, and splenectomy. Differential diagnosis includes the large granular lymphocyte syndrome.

- Felty syndrome occurs in <1% of patients with seropositive rheumatoid arthritis.

- Felty syndrome has the classic triad of rheumatoid arthritis, leukopenia, and splenomegaly.

- High titers of rheumatoid factor are the rule in Felty syndrome.

- Patients with Felty syndrome frequently die of infection.

Sjögren Syndrome

Sjögren syndrome has a triad of clinical features: keratoconjunctivitis sicca (with or without lacrimal gland enlargement), xerostomia (with or without salivary gland enlargement), and connective tissue disease (usually rheumatoid arthritis). Histologically, CD4 lymphocytic infiltration and destruction of lacrimal salivary glands characterize it. Clinically, it manifests with dry eyes and dry mouth. Primary Sjögren syndrome is diagnosed predominantly in middle-aged women. Additional features of primary Sjögren syndrome are listed in Box 24.5. Most patients have a polyclonal hypergammaglobulinemia.

Classic triad
    Arthritis: typically episodic polyarthritis
    Dry eyes
    Dry mouth (& other dry mucous membranes)
Other features
    Constitutional features: fatigue, malaise, myalgia
    Raynaud phenomenon
    Cutaneous vasculitis
    CNS abnormalities
        Cerebritis, CNS vasculitis
        Stroke
        Multiple sclerosis-like illness
    Peripheral neuropathy
        Sensory
        Autonomic
        Interstitial lung disease
        Pleurisy

Abbreviation: CNS, central nervous system.

Autoantibodies typically are present, including rheumatoid factor, antinuclear antibodies, and antibodies to extractable nuclear antigens (SSA and SSB).

Patients can present with primary Sjögren syndrome without any additional connective tissue disease. The primary syndrome typically has episodic and nondeforming arthritis. More commonly, rheumatoid arthritis, systemic lupus erythematosus, scleroderma, polyarteritis nodosa, or polymyositis accompanies Sjögren syndrome. There is no perfect definition for Sjögren syndrome, and no test is completely diagnostic. Simple dry eyes of the elderly, benign sicca syndrome, is distinguished from Sjögren syndrome by the absence of SSA antibodies. Patients with Sjögren syndrome, but not the rheumatoid factor–negative, SSA antibody–negative sicca syndrome, have an increased risk for development of non-Hodgkin lymphoma.

Treatment of primary Sjögren syndrome is mainly symptomatic. Pilocarpine, 5 mg orally 4 times daily, improves salivary and lacrimal gland function in the majority of the patients. Adverse effects, including flushing and sweating, limit its usefulness. In addition to hydration, systemic therapy is indicated if there is evidence of systemic inflammation.

A Sjögren-like syndrome has been described in patients with human immunodeficiency virus (HIV) infection and hepatitis C. Other infiltrative diseases of the parotid glands should also be considered, including sarcoidosis, lymphoma, or an Ig-G4–related inflammatory syndrome.

- Sjögren syndrome presents with dry eyes, dry mouth, and a connective tissue disorder (usually rheumatoid arthritis).

- Sjögren syndrome can exist by itself or with another formal connective tissue disease such as rheumatoid arthritis, systemic lupus erythematosus, scleroderma, or myositis.

- Treatment focuses on control of inflammation and symptoms of dryness.

- A Sjögren-like syndrome has been described in patients with HIV infection and hepatitis C.

OSTEOARTHRITIS

Osteoarthritis is the failure of articular cartilage and subsequent degenerative changes in subchondral bone, bony joint margins, synovium, and para-articular fibrous and muscular structures. Osteoarthritis is the most common rheumatic disease; 80% of patients have some limitation of their activities, and 25% are unable to perform major activities of daily living. The prevalence of osteoarthritis is strongly associated with aging. Joints most commonly affected include the knee, hand, spine, metatarsophalangeal, and hip. Radiologic evidence of the disease greatly exceeds the prevalence of symptomatic cases.

- Osteoarthritis is the most common chronic rheumatic disease.

PATHOGENESIS OF OSTEOARTHRITIS

Two principal changes associated with osteoarthritis are the progressive focal degeneration of articular cartilage and the formation of new bone in the floor of the cartilage lesion at the joint margins (osteophytes). Not all the mechanisms causing osteoarthritis have been identified. Current theories include 1) mechanical process: cartilage injury, particularly after impact loading, and 2) biochemical process: failure of cartilage repair processes to adequately compensate for injury. A combination of mechanical and biochemical processes likely contributes in most cases of osteoarthritis. It must be emphasized that osteoarthritis is not just the consequence of "wear and tear."

- Osteoarthritis is associated with progressive focal degeneration of articular cartilage and subsequent degeneration of surrounding soft tissues and proliferation (osteophytosis) of bone.

- Osteoarthritis is not the consequence of normal use ("wear and tear").

CLINICAL FEATURES OF OSTEOARTHRITIS

The pain of an osteoarthritic joint is usually described as a deep ache. Subchondral bone edema contributes to the pain. The pain occurs with use of the joint and is relieved with rest and cessation of weight bearing. As the disease progresses, the involved joint may be symptomatic with minimal activity or even at rest. The pain originates in the structures around the disintegrating cartilage (there are no nerves in cartilage). There may be stiffness in the joint with initial use, but this initial stiffness is not prolonged as it is in inflammatory arthritis, such as rheumatoid arthritis. Although the symptoms are related predominantly to mechanical failure and motion limits, joint debris and the associated repair process promote mild inflammation, accumulation of synovial fluid, and mild hypertrophy of the synovial membrane. Acute inflammation can transiently occur at Heberden nodes (distal interphalangeal joints with prominent osteophytes as a consequence of osteoarthritis) or at the knee with tearing of a degenerative meniscal cartilage.

- Osteoarthritic pain is usually described as a deep ache with joint use and is improved with rest.
- Stiffness with initial use of the joint is not prolonged in osteoarthritis as it is in inflammatory arthritis (rheumatoid arthritis).

Physical examination documents joint margin tenderness, fine crepitus, limits to motion, and enlargement of the joint. The enlargement is usually bony (proliferation of cartilage and bone to form osteophytes), but it can include effusions and mild synovial thickening. Deformity is a late consequence of the osteoarthritis and is associated with atrophy or derangement of the local soft tissues, ligaments, and muscles. Radiographic or physical examination evidence of the severity of osteoarthritis does not reliably predict a patient's symptoms.

CLINICAL SUBSETS OF OSTEOARTHRITIS

Primary Osteoarthritis

Primary osteoarthritis is cartilage failure without a known cause that would predispose to osteoarthritis. It almost never affects the shoulders, elbows, ankles, metacarpophalangeal joints, or ulnar side of the wrist. It is divided into several clinical patterns, as described below.

Generalized osteoarthritis involves the distal interphalangeal joints, proximal interphalangeal joints, first carpometacarpal joints, hips, knees, and spine (Figure 24.2). It occurs most frequently in middle-aged postmenopausal women.

Isolated nodal osteoarthritis is primary osteoarthritis that affects only the distal interphalangeal joints. It occurs predominantly in women and has a familial predisposition.

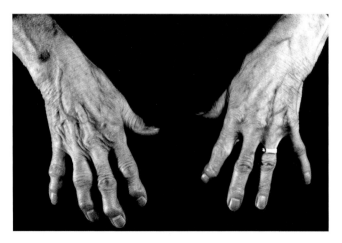

Figure 24.2 Generalized Osteoarthritis. Note prominent bony swelling at the proximal (Bouchard nodes) and distal (Heberden nodes) interphalangeal joints. The metacarpophalangeal joints are spared. Early hypertrophic changes are seen on profile at the first carpometacarpal joint, giving a slight squaring of the hand deformity, appreciated best on the left.

Isolated hip osteoarthritis is more common in men than in women. It has no clear association with obesity or activity. Many cases are now thought to be related to mild bony structural abnormalities such as femoral acetabular impingement.

Erosive osteoarthritis affects only the distal and proximal interphalangeal joints. Patients with erosive osteoarthritis have episodes of local inflammation. Mucous cyst formation at the distal interphalangeal joint is common. Painful flare-up of the disease recurs for years. Symptoms usually begin about the time of menopause. Bony erosions and collapse of the subchondral plate—features not usually seen in primary osteoarthritis—with osteophytes are markers of erosive osteoarthritis. Joint deformity can be severe. In many cases, bony ankylosis develops. Ankylosis is usually associated with relief of pain. The synovium is intensely infiltrated with mononuclear cells. This condition may be confused with rheumatoid arthritis.

Diffuse idiopathic skeletal hyperostosis (DISH), also known as Forestier disease, is a variant of primary osteoarthritis and occurs chiefly in men older than 50 years. The diagnosis requires finding characteristic exuberant, flowing osteophytosis that connects 4 or more vertebrae with preservation of the disk space. DISH must be distinguished from typical osteoarthritis of the spine with degenerative disk disease and from ankylosing spondylitis. Extraspinal sites of disease involvement include calcification of the pelvic ligaments, exuberant osteophytosis at the site of peripheral osteoarthritis, well-calcified bony spurs at the calcaneus, and heterotopic bone formation after total joint arthroplasty. Patients with DISH are often obese, and 60% have diabetes mellitus or glucose intolerance. Symptoms include mild back stiffness and, occasionally, back pain. Pathologically and radiologically, DISH is distinct from other forms of primary osteoarthritis.

- Primary osteoarthritis almost never affects the shoulders, elbows, ankles, metacarpophalangeal joints, or the ulnar side of the wrist.
- Generalized osteoarthritis involves the distal interphalangeal joints, proximal interphalangeal joints, first carpometacarpal joints, hips, knees, and spine.
- Isolated nodal osteoarthritis is primary osteoarthritis affecting only the distal interphalangeal joints.
- Isolated hip osteoarthritis is more common in men than in women.
- Erosive osteoarthritis affects only the distal and proximal interphalangeal joints.
- DISH is a variant of primary osteoarthritis and should be distinguished from ankylosing spondylitis.

Secondary Osteoarthritis

Secondary osteoarthritis is cartilage failure caused by some known disorder, trauma, or abnormality. Any patient with an unusual distribution of osteoarthritis or widespread chondrocalcinosis should be considered to have secondary

Table 24.1 INHERITED DISORDERS OF CONNECTIVE TISSUE

CONDITION	GENE DEFECT	CHARACTERISTICS
Marfan syndrome (autosomal dominant)	Fibrillin gene	Hypermobile joints: osteoarthritis, arachnodactyly, kyphoscoliosis Lax skin, striae, ectopic ocular lens Aortic root dilatation (aortic insufficiency), mitral valve prolapse, aneurysms, & aortic dissection
Ehlers-Danlos syndrome (10 subtypes)	Type I & type III collagen gene defects	Joint hypermobility, friable skin, osteoarthritis Type III collagen defects associated with vascular aneurysms
Osteogenesis imperfecta (autosomal dominant & recessive variations; the most common heritable disorder of connective tissue: 1:20,000; 4 subtypes)	Type I collagen gene defects	Brittle bones, blue sclerae, otosclerosis & deafness, joint hypermobility, & tooth malformation
Type II collagenopathies: Achondrogenesis type II Hypochondrogenesis Spondyloepiphyseal dysplasia Spondyloepimetaphyseal dysplasia Kniest dysplasia Stickler syndrome Familial precocious osteoarthropathy	Type II collagen gene defects	Spectrum from lethal (achondrogenesis) to premature osteoarthritis (Stickler syndrome)
Achondroplasia (autosomal dominant)	Fibroblast growth factor III receptor gene defect	Dwarfism, premature osteoarthritis
Pseudoachondroplasia	Cartilage oligomeric matrix protein (COMP) gene defect	Short stature, premature osteoarthritis
Multiple epiphyseal dysplasia (autosomal dominant)		

osteoarthritis. Secondary osteoarthritis frequently complicates trauma and the damage caused by inflammatory arthritis. Inherited disorders of connective tissue and several metabolic abnormalities, including ochronosis, hemochromatosis, Wilson disease, and acromegaly, are complicated by secondary osteoarthritis. Paget disease of bone, involving the femur or pelvis about the hip joint, can predispose to osteoarthritis.

- Osteoarthritis involving the shoulder, metacarpophalangeal joints, or isolated large joints or with chondrocalcinosis should prompt physicians to consider secondary causes of osteoarthritis.

Trauma or injury to joint and supporting periarticular tissues predisposes persons to the most common type of secondary osteoarthritis. Stress from repeated impact loading could weaken subchondral bone. Internal joint derangement with ligamentous laxity or meniscal damage alters the normal mechanical alignment of the joint. Isolated large joint involvement is a clue to posttraumatic osteoarthritis. Chronic rotator cuff tear with subsequent loss of shoulder joint cartilage (cuff arthropathy) and knee osteoarthritis that develops years after meniscal cartilage damage are examples of secondary osteoarthritis.

Congenital malformations of joints, such as congenital hip dysplasia and epiphyseal dysplasia, lead to premature osteoarthritis. Other developmental abnormalities, including slipped capital femoral epiphysis and Legg-Calvé-Perthes disease (idiopathic avascular necrosis of the femoral head), first present as premature osteoarthritis years after they occur. Inherited disorders of connective tissue frequently predispose the affected person to premature osteoarthritis. Table 24.1 describes several inherited disorders, including their gene defects and characteristics.

- Injury to joint or supporting periarticular tissues can predispose to osteoarthritis.

- Posttraumatic osteoarthritis is the most common form of secondary osteoarthritis.

- Isolated large joint involvement is a clue to posttraumatic osteoarthritis.

Hemochromatosis

Hemochromatosis was formerly considered an unusual autosomal recessive disorder of white males. It is now considered the commonest inherited disease. The full clinical spectrum of hemochromatosis includes hepatomegaly, bronze skin pigmentation, diabetes mellitus, the consequences of pituitary insufficiency, and degenerative arthritis. The arthropathy affects up to 50% of patients with hemochromatosis and generally resembles osteoarthritis; however, it involves the metacarpophalangeal joints and shoulders, joints not typically affected by generalized primary osteoarthritis. Attacks of acute pseudogout arthritis may occur in relation to deposition of calcium pyrophosphate dihydrate crystals. Chondrocalcinosis is commonly superimposed on chronic osteoarthritic change in hemochromatosis. The pathogenesis of joint degeneration in hemochromatosis is not clear.

- Arthropathy affects up to 50% of patients with hemochromatosis.

- The arthropathy of hemochromatosis involves the metacarpophalangeal joints and shoulders.

Wilson Disease

Wilson disease is a rare autosomal recessive disorder. Arthropathy occurs in 50% of adults with Wilson disease. This disease is suspected in anyone younger than 40 years with unexplained hepatitis, cirrhosis, or movement disorder. The diagnosis is suggested when the serum level of ceruloplasmin is less than 200 mg/L. Arthropathy is unusual in children with the disease. The radiologic appearance varies somewhat from that of primary osteoarthritis; there are more subchondral cysts, sclerosis, cortical irregularities, and radiodense lesions, which occur centrally and at the joint margins. Focal areas of bone fragmentation occur, but they are not related to neuropathy. Although chondrocalcinosis occurs, calcium pyrophosphate dihydrate crystals have not been observed in the synovial fluid.

- Arthropathy occurs in 50% of adults with Wilson disease.

- Arthropathy is unusual in children with Wilson disease.

Apatite Microcrystals

Apatite microcrystals are associated with degenerative arthritis and are found in patients with hypothyroidism, hyperparathyroidism, and acromegaly. They occur without an associated endocrinopathy. The role of microcrystalline disease in the progression of osteoarthritis is unclear, especially in the absence of acute recurrent flares of pseudogout.

Neuropathic Arthropathy (Charcot Joint)

Neuropathic arthropathy (Charcot joint) commonly affects patients with diabetes mellitus. Men and women are equally affected. Patients with diabetic neuroarthropathy have had diabetes an average of 16 years. Frequently, the diabetes is poorly controlled. Diabetic peripheral neuropathy causes blunted pain perception and poor proprioception. Repeated microtrauma, overt trauma, small vessel occlusive disease (diabetes), and neuropathic dystrophic effects on bone contribute to neuroarthropathy.

Patients may present with an acute arthritic condition that includes swelling, erythema, and warmth. The foot, particularly the tarsometatarsal joint, is involved most commonly in patients with diabetes. Patients usually describe milder pain than suggested by the clinical condition and radiographic appearances. They walk with an antalgic limp. Callus formation occurs over the weight-bearing site of bony damage, and the callus subsequently blisters and ulcerates. Infection can spread from skin ulcers to the bone. Osteomyelitis frequently complicates diabetic neuroarthropathy and should be suspected when an affected patient with diabetes has sudden worsening of his or her glucose control. Radiography shows disorganized normal joint architecture. Bone and cartilage fragments later coalesce to form characteristic sclerotic loose bodies. There is an attempt at reconstruction with new bone formation. This periosteal new bone is inhibited by small vessel ischemic change in some patients with diabetes. Diabetic osteopathy is a second form of neuroarthropathy. Osteopenia of para-articular areas, particularly the distal metacarpals and proximal phalanges, results in rapidly progressive osteolysis and juxta-articular cortical defects. This can be associated with osteomyelitis.

Initial treatment in patients with diabetes includes good local foot care, treatment of infection, and protected weight bearing. Involvement of the knee, lumbar spine, and upper extremity is uncommon. Classically, hip and spinal neuroarthropathy is caused by tertiary syphilis, and shoulder neuroarthropathy is associated with cervical syringomyelia.

- Neuropathic arthropathy (Charcot joint) most commonly affects the feet and ankles of patients with diabetes mellitus.

- Neuropathic arthropathy is a consequence of peripheral neuropathy and local injury.

- Osteomyelitis is caused by skin ulcers extending to the bone and should be suspected when an affected patient with diabetes has sudden worsening of his or her glucose control.

Avascular Necrosis

Avascular necrosis of bone, also known as osteonecrosis of bone, may lead to collapse of the articular surface and subsequent osteoarthritis. It usually occurs in the hip after femoral neck fracture. Systemic corticosteroid therapy increases the risk of this disorder. Avascular necrosis of the bone has other causes, including alcoholism, sickle cell disease, and systemic lupus erythematosus (Box 24.6). No underlying cause can be identified in 10% to 25% of patients.

Box 24.6 **MNEMONIC DEVICE FOR CAUSES OF ASEPTIC NECROSIS OF BONE**

A	Alcohol, atherosclerotic vascular disease
S	Steroids, sickle cell anemia, storage disease (Gaucher disease)
E	Emboli (fat, cholesterol)
P	Postradiation necrosis
T	Trauma
I	Idiopathic
C	Connective tissue disease (especially SLE), caisson disease

Abbreviation: SLE, systemic lupus erythematosus.

Avascular necrosis of bone usually affects the hips, shoulders, knees, or ankles. Treatment is conservative, including reduced weight bearing and analgesics. Some investigators have treated patients successfully with vascularized bone grafts in the bed of necrotic trabecular bone, although controlled studies are not available. Core decompression may help with pain but does not influence progression to osteoarthritis. When there is evidence of cortical bone collapse, progression to advanced osteoarthritis is inevitable. The most sensitive test for avascular necrosis is magnetic resonance imaging. Plain radiography is insensitive to early aseptic necrosis.

- Avascular necrosis usually occurs in the hip after femoral neck fracture and may lead to osteoarthritis.

- Alcoholism and corticosteroid use are other common causes of avascular necrosis.

Hypertrophic Osteoarthropathy

Hypertrophic osteoarthropathy is characterized by clubbing of the fingernails and painful distal long bone periostitis. The patient may have a noninflammatory arthritis at the ankles, knees, or wrists. This condition complicates primary and metastatic pulmonary malignancies, chronic pulmonary infections, cystic fibrosis, and hypoxic congenital heart disease. Treatment is usually symptomatic.

Hemophilic arthropathy, a type of progressive degenerative arthropathy, is more destructive than primary osteoarthritis. Patients with hemophilia and recurrent hemarthroses are at risk for hemophilic arthropathy. Widening of the intercondylar notch of the knees is an early radiographic feature suggesting the diagnosis of this condition.

RADIOGRAPHIC FEATURES OF OSTEOARTHRITIS

The radiographic features of osteoarthritis do not always predict the extent of symptoms. With aging, radiographic osteoarthritis is far more prevalent than the clinical illness. Common radiographic features include osteophyte formation, asymmetric joint-space narrowing, subchondral bony sclerosis, and subchondral cysts. Later bony changes include malalignment and deformity (Figure 24.3). In the spine, the radiographic finding called spondylosis includes anterolateral spinous osteophytes, degenerative disk disease with disk-space narrowing, and facet sclerosis. A defect in the bony structure of the posterior neural arch produces spondylolysis. With bilateral spondylolysis, subluxation of one vertebra on another may occur, a condition called spondylolisthesis. The causes of spondylolisthesis are trauma, osteoarthritis, and congenital. No laboratory studies of blood are useful in the diagnosis of osteoarthritis.

- Common radiographic features of osteoarthritis include osteophyte formation, asymmetric joint-space narrowing, subchondral bony sclerosis, subchondral cysts, and buttressing of angle joints.

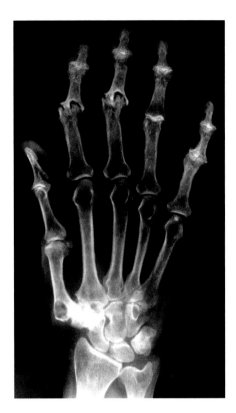

Figure 24.3 Severe Osteoarthritis. Hypertrophic changes, asymmetric joint-space narrowing, and subchondral sclerosis are prominent at the interphalangeal joints and at the first carpometacarpal joint. Note that the metacarpophalangeal joints are completely spared, distinguishing this arthritis from rheumatoid arthritis. Also, there is joint-space narrowing and sclerosis at the base of the thumb at the first carpometacarpal joint and between the trapezium and the scaphoid. Osteoarthritis does not affect the entire wrist compartment equally. The involvement seen here is the most common. An additional interesting feature seen here is central erosions at the second and third proximal interphalangeal joints. This variant occasionally has been called erosive osteoarthritis.

- No laboratory studies of blood are useful in the diagnosis of osteoarthritis.

THERAPY FOR OSTEOARTHRITIS

Therapeutic goals include relieving pain, preserving joint motion and function, and preventing further injury and wear of cartilage. Weight loss (especially in knee osteoarthritis), use of canes or crutches, correction of postural abnormalities, and proper shoe support are helpful measures. Isometric or isotonic range-of-motion exercises and muscle strengthening provide para-articular structures with extra support and help reduce symptoms. Relief of muscle spasm with local application of heat or cold to decrease pain can help. Addressing the patient's ability to cope with the illness may be more helpful than medication therapy alone.

Initial drug therapy should be analgesics, such as acetaminophen (1 g 4 times daily as needed). Nonsteroidal anti-inflammatory drugs are beneficial for inflammatory flares of osteoarthritis and usually do not need to be taken in anti-inflammatory doses every day. Selective use of opioid analgesics can be considered for disabling pain, especially in persons who are not surgical candidates. Intra-articular corticosteroids offer some temporary relief but should be used only if there is a symptomatic effusion or synovitis. Hyaluronic acid injections have small symptomatic benefit in selected patients with osteoarthritis of the knee.

Joint arthroplasty relieves pain, stabilizes joints, and improves function. Total joint arthroplasty is very successful at the knee, shoulder, or hip. Box 24.7 describes the indications for total joint arthroplasty. Arthroscopy removes loose bodies and trims torn menisci to correct lockup or giving way of the joint. In patients with established osteoarthritis of the knee, arthroscopic procedures have very limited or no lasting benefit. Herniated disks or spinal stenosis with radicular symptoms may require decompression.

- Simple analgesics such as acetaminophen are the first choice for treating osteoarthritis.

ARTHRITIS IN CHRONIC RENAL FAILURE

Up to 75% of patients undergoing chronic renal dialysis have musculoskeletal complaints after 4 years of dialysis. Renal failure arthritis affects the interphalangeal joints, metacarpophalangeal joints, wrists, shoulders, and knees. Symmetric joint-space narrowing and para-articular osteoporosis, subchondral cysts, and erosions have been described. There is no osteophytosis to confuse this condition with osteoarthritis. The synovial fluid is noninflammatory, and the synovitis on biopsy is nonspecific. Possible causes of this arthritis include apatite microcrystal deposition, hyperparathyroidism, and renal failure amyloidosis. Aseptic necrosis occasionally affects large joints.

After 10 years of hemodialysis, 65% of patients have pathologic or radiologic evidence of amyloid deposition (renal failure amyloid arthropathy). The amyloid is composed of β_2-microglobulin, is arthrotropic, and results in complete joint-space loss that occurs over a 3- to 12-month period. Shoulder pain and stiffness syndrome and carpal tunnel syndrome are strongly related to this amyloid deposition. Currently, treatment is aimed at relieving the symptoms.

- Up to 75% of patients undergoing chronic renal dialysis have musculoskeletal complaints after 4 years of dialysis.

- Destructive arthritis, shoulder pain and stiffness syndrome, and carpal tunnel syndrome are strongly related to amyloid deposition.

SUMMARY

RHEUMATOID ARTHRITIS

- Joint damage occurs early in patients with seropositive disease.

- Anti-CCP antibodies are equally sensitive and more specific than rheumatoid factor for the diagnosis of early, erosive rheumatoid arthritis.

- The distribution of involvement in rheumatoid arthritis is symmetric and polyarticular; predominantly, small joints are involved.

- A disease-modifying regimen is started when rheumatoid arthritis is diagnosed, and treatment should be guided by targeting improvement to a low level of disease activity. Methotrexate is the DMARD of choice in early seropositive rheumatoid arthritis.

- Low-dose or tapered prednisone may be necessary to preserve function and diminish joint damage during the initiation of DMARD therapy.

- With disease-modifying agents, uninterrupted treatment for 3–6 months is needed to assess efficacy. Combination DMARD therapy has become more common.

OSTEOARTHRITIS

- Osteoarthritis is the most common chronic rheumatic disease.

- Osteoarthritic pain is usually described as a deep ache with joint use and is improved with rest.

- Primary osteoarthritis almost never affects the shoulders, elbows, ankles, metacarpophalangeal joints, or the ulnar side of the wrist.

- Generalized osteoarthritis involves the distal interphalangeal joints, proximal interphalangeal joints, first carpometacarpal joints, hips, knees, and spine.

25.

GOUT AND SPONDYLOARTHROPATHIES

William W. Ginsburg, MD

GOALS

- To be able to diagnose gout and pseudogout.
- List the indications and adverse effects of medications used to treat gout and pseudogout.
- Recognize the characteristic findings of the spondyloarthropathies.
- Understand the indications for and treatment of the spondyloarthropathies.

CRYSTALLINE ARTHROPATHIES

HYPERURICEMIA AND GOUT

Hyperuricemia occurs in 2% to 18% of normal populations. It is associated with hypertension, renal insufficiency, obesity, and arteriosclerotic heart disease. The prevalence of clinical gouty arthritis ranges from 0.1% to 0.4%. There is a family history of gout in 20% of patients with gouty arthritis. Ninety percent of patients with gout have underexcretion of uric acid.

- Hyperuricemia is associated with hypertension, renal insufficiency, obesity, and arteriosclerotic heart disease.
- There is a family history of gout in 20% of patients with gouty arthritis.

Important Enzyme Abnormalities in the Uric Acid Pathway

Abnormalities of the uric acid pathway lead to several conditions (Figure 25.1).

Lesch-Nyhan syndrome is a complete deficiency of hypoxanthine-guanine phosphoribosyltransferase. It is an X-linked recessive disease. Therefore, it typically affects boys; clinical features include hyperuricemia, self-mutilation, choreoathetosis, spasticity, growth retardation, and severe gouty arthritis.

Overactivity of 5-phosphoribosyl-1-pyrophosphate synthetase is associated with hyperuricemia, X-linked genetic inheritance, and gouty arthritis.

Adenosine deaminase deficiency is inherited in an autosomal recessive pattern. It causes a combined immunodeficiency state with severe T-cell and mild B-cell dysfunction. Features of the disorder are hypouricemia, recurrent infection, and chondro-osseous dysplasia. Treatment for the disorder is with irradiated frozen red blood cells or marrow transplant.

Xanthine oxidase deficiency is also inherited in an autosomal recessive pattern. It is characterized by hypouricemia, xanthinuria with xanthine stones, and myopathy associated with deposits of xanthine and hypoxanthine.

Causes of Secondary Hyperuricemia

Secondary hyperuricemia can be attributed to overproduction or underexcretion of uric acid (Box 25.1). Important causes of overproduction of uric acid include cancer, psoriasis, and sickle cell anemia. Important causes of underexcretion of uric acid include chronic renal insufficiency, lead nephropathy, alcohol, diabetic ketoacidosis, and drugs, notably thiazide diuretics, nicotinic acid, and cyclosporine.

Factors Predisposing to Gout and Pseudogout

Factors that precipitate gout and pseudogout include trauma, surgery, alcohol use, and acidosis.

Clinical Manifestations of Acute Gout

In 50% of patients with gout, the metatarsophalangeal joint of the great toe is involved initially (podagra). Rapid joint swelling is associated with extreme tenderness. Uric acid crystals, which are needle-shaped and strongly negatively birefringent under polarized light, are found in the joint during an acute

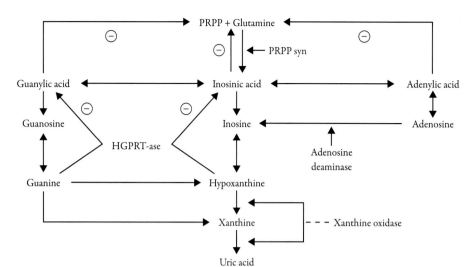

Figure 25.1 Purine Metabolism. HGPRT-ase indicates hypoxanthine-guanine phosphoribosyltransferase; PRPP, phosphoribosylpyrophosphate; PRPP syn, phosphoribosylpyrophosphate synthetase; –, feedback inhibition.

Box 25.1 CAUSES OF SECONDARY HYPERURICEMIA

Overproduction of uric acid
  Myeloproliferative disorders
    Polycythemia, primary or secondary
    Myeloid metaplasia
    Chronic myelocytic leukemia
  Lymphoproliferative disorders
    Chronic lymphocytic leukemia
  Plasma cell proliferative disorders
    Multiple myeloma
  Disseminated carcinoma & sarcoma
  Sickle cell anemia, thalassemia, & other forms of chronic hemolytic anemia
  Psoriasis
  Cytotoxic drugs
  Infectious mononucleosis
  Obesity
  Increased purine ingestion
Underexcretion of uric acid
  Intrinsic renal disease
    Chronic renal insufficiency of diverse cause
    Saturine gout (lead nephropathy)
  Drug-induced
    Thiazide diuretics, furosemide, ethacrynic acid, ethambutol, pyrazinamide, low-dose aspirin, cyclosporine, nicotinic acid, laxative abuse, levodopa, rasburicase
  Endocrine conditions
    Adrenal insufficiency, nephrogenic diabetes insipidus, hyperparathyroidism, hypoparathyroidism, pseudohypoparathyroidism, hypothyroidism
  Metabolic conditions
    Diabetic ketoacidosis, lactic acidosis, starvation, ethanolism, glycogen storage disease type I, Bartter syndrome
  Other
    Sarcoidosis
    Down syndrome
    Beryllium disease

---

attack. The diagnosis of gout is established by the demonstration of uric acid crystals in the joint aspirate. The joint fluid is inflammatory, and the polymorphonuclear neutrophil count is between 5 and 75×10^9/L.

Gout occurs most commonly in middle-aged men, but, after menopause, the incidence of gout in women increases. Although gout is usually monarticular and usually involves the joints in the lower extremity, attacks may become polyarticular over time.

- Podagra is the initial presentation of gout in 50% of cases.

- Uric acid crystals are strongly negatively birefringent under polarized light microscopy.

- Gout is usually monarticular and most often involves the joints in the lower extremities.

Treatment of Acute Gouty Arthritis

Nonsteroidal anti-inflammatory drugs (NSAIDs) are the drugs of choice for the treatment of acute gouty arthritis and should be used for a 7- to 10-day course. These drugs are relatively contraindicated in patients with congestive heart failure, active peptic ulcer disease, or renal insufficiency. NSAIDs should not be used in patients with nasal polyps and aspirin sensitivity because they may cause bronchospasm.

- NSAIDs are the drugs of choice for an acute attack of gouty arthritis.

- NSAIDs should be avoided in patients with congestive heart failure, peptic ulcer disease, or renal insufficiency.

- Intra-articular or oral corticosteroids and subcutaneous adrenocorticotropic hormone are other treatments, especially in patients who have contraindications to NSAIDs.

- Allopurinol, febuxostat, or probenecid therapy should not be initiated until the acute attack completely subsides. If patients are already receiving these medications, their use should be continued.

- Because of severe gastrointestinal adverse effects, high-dose oral colchicine is rarely used for an acute attack.

Treatment During Intercritical Period

Oral colchicine, 0.6 mg twice daily, should be given prophylactically with probenecid, allopurinol, and febuxostat for 6 to 12 months to prevent exacerbation of acute gout. Long-term use of low-dose colchicine can be associated with a myopathy and neuropathy, especially in patients with renal insufficiency. A myoneuropathy may appear in patients taking medications that affect colchicine metabolism via the cytochrome P450 system. These include cyclosporine, simvastatin, lovastatin, atorvastatin, diltiazem, cimetidine, verapamil, and amiodarone. If a statin is needed in conjunction with colchicine in a patient with renal insufficiency, fluvastatin and pravastatin are preferred because they are not handled by the cytochrome P450 system.

Probenecid inhibits tubular reabsorption of filtered and secreted urate. Probenecid should not be used if the patient has a creatinine clearance less than 50 mL/minute or a history of kidney stones or if 24-hour uric acid value is more than 1,000 mg. Notably, probenecid delays renal excretion of indomethacin and may increase the risk of methotrexate toxicity.

- Colchine should be used with caution in patients with renal impairment.

Allopurinol is a xanthine oxidase inhibitor and can precipitate gout. Its use should not be started during an acute attack. Allopurinol can cause a severe toxicity syndrome: eosinophilia, fever, hepatitis, decreased renal function, and erythematous desquamative rash. It should be given in the lowest dose possible to keep the uric acid value less than 6 mg/dL. In patients with chronic renal disease, the starting dose should always be low (50–100 mg) and increased slowly. If allopurinol is used in conjunction with 6-mercaptopurine or azathioprine, the dose of 6-mercaptopurine or azathioprine needs to be reduced at least 25% or bone marrow toxicity can occur.

- Allopurinol use should not be initiated during an acute attack.

Febuxostat is a recently approved non–purine xanthine oxidase inhibitor. It can be used in patients who are intolerant of allopurinol or who have mild to moderate renal insufficiency.

Pegloticase (uricase) converts uric acid to allantoin. It was recently approved for chronic gout refractory to conventional therapy. In patients with tophaceous deposits it promotes resolution.

Miscellaneous Points of Importance

1. Renal function is not necessarily adversely affected by an increased serum urate concentration.

2. Correction of hyperuricemia has no apparent effect on renal function.

3. Most rheumatologists do not treat asymptomatic hyperuricemia.

4. 30% of patients with chronic tophaceous gout are positive for rheumatoid factor (usually weakly positive).

5. 10% of patients with acute gout are positive for rheumatoid factor (usually weakly positive).

6. 5%–10% of patients will have a gout and a pseudogout attack simultaneously.

7. 50% of synovial fluids aspirated from first metatarsophalangeal joints of asymptomatic patients with gout have crystals of monosodium urate.

8. Up to 33% of patients with acute gout have a normal level of serum uric acid at the time of the acute attack.

9. Gout in a premenopausal female is very unusual.

10. There are reports of superimposed gout occurring in Heberden and Bouchard nodes in older women taking thiazide diuretics.

11. A septic joint can trigger a gout or pseudogout attack in a predisposed person. Synovial fluid should always be analyzed for crystals, Gram stain, and culture.

12. The frequency of gout in patients who have had cardiac transplant is high (25%). (Both cyclosporine and diuretics cause hyperuricemia.)

CALCIUM PYROPHOSPHATE DEPOSITION DISEASE

Etiologic Classification

Diseases associated with calcium pyrophosphate deposition disease (CPPD) include hyperparathyroidism, hemochromatosis-hemosiderosis, hypothyroidism, and hypomagnesemia.

Pseudogout

When CPPD causes an acute inflammatory arthritis, the term *pseudogout* is applied. CPPD pseudogout is an acute inflammatory arthritis caused by CPPD. CPPD crystals are weakly positively birefringent under polarized light microscopy. Pseudogout most commonly affects the knees, but the wrists, elbows, ankles, and intervertebral disks can be affected. It usually occurs in older individuals. Chondrocalcinosis is found on radiographs in most patients with pseudogout.

- Pseudogout is an acute inflammatory arthritis caused by CPPD.

- Knees are most commonly affected.

Treatment of Pseudogout

For treatment of acute attacks of pseudogout, NSAIDs or an injection of steroid preparation can be used. Prophylactic oral colchicine can lead to a decrease in the frequency and severity of attacks.

BASIC CALCIUM PHOSPHATE DISEASE (HYDROXYAPATITE DEPOSITION DISEASE)

Presentation

Clinical presentations of basic calcium phosphate disease include 1) acute inflammation, including calcific tendinitis, osteoarthritis with inflammatory episodes, periarthritis or arthritis dialysis syndrome, and calcinotic deposits in scleroderma and 2) chronic inflammation, including severe osteoarthritis and Milwaukee shoulder or knee (advanced glenohumeral and knee osteoarthritis, rotator cuff tear, noninflammatory paste-like joint fluid containing hydroxyapatite).

- Basic calcium phosphate disease can present as acute or chronic inflammation.

Diagnosis and Treatment

Individual crystals cannot be seen on routine polarization microscopy (Table 25.1). Small, round (shiny coin) bodies 0.5 to 100 mcm are seen. On electron microscopy, these represent lumps of needle-shaped crystals. Positive identification requires transmission electron microscopy or elemental analysis. Alizarin red stain showing calcium staining provides a presumptive diagnosis (if CPPD is excluded). Treatment involves NSAIDs and intra-articular steroids.

- In basic calcium phosphate disease, individual crystals are not seen on polarization microscopy.
- Positive identification requires transmission electron microscopy.

CALCIUM OXALATE ARTHROPATHY

Calcium oxalate arthropathy occurs in patients with primary oxalosis and in patients undergoing chronic hemodialysis. It can cause acute inflammatory arthritis. Crystals are large, bipyramidal, and birefringent. Calcium oxalate can cause chondrocalcinosis.

- Calcium oxalate arthropathy occurs in patients with primary oxalosis and patients undergoing chronic hemodialysis.

OTHER CRYSTALS IMPLICATED IN JOINT DISEASE

Cholesterol crystals are a nonspecific finding and have been found in the synovial fluid of patients with various types of chronic inflammatory arthritis. Cryoglobulin crystals are found in essential cryoglobulinemia and paraproteinemia. Corticosteroid crystals are found in an arthritis flare after a corticosteroid injection, and Charcot-Leyden crystals have been found in hypereosinophilic syndromes. In patients undergoing hemodialysis, aluminum phosphate crystals can develop.

SPONDYLOARTHROPATHIES

Conditions that form the spondyloarthropathies include ankylosing spondylitis, reactive arthritis, enteropathic spondylitis, and psoriatic arthritis.

Spondyloarthropathies are characterized by the following: involvement of the sacroiliac joints (uncommon in rheumatoid arthritis), peripheral arthritis that is usually asymmetric and oligoarticular, absence of rheumatoid factor, acute anterior uveitis, association with HLA-B27, and enthesopathy (disorder of muscle or tendinous attachment to bones).

The HLA region of chromosome 6 contains genes of the human histocompatibility complex. Every person has 2 of

Table 25.1 **DIFFERENTIAL DIAGNOSIS OF BASIC CALCIUM PHOSPHATE DISEASE ACCORDING TO RESULTS OF SYNOVIAL FLUID ANALYSIS**

DIAGNOSIS	LEUKOCYTE COUNT, ×10⁹/L	DIFFERENTIAL	POLARIZATION MICROSCOPY
Degenerative joint disease	<1	Mononuclear cells	Negative
Rheumatoid arthritis	5–50	PMNs	Negative
Gout	5–100	PMNs	Monosodium urate
Pseudogout	5–100	PMNs	CPPD
Hydroxyapatite	5–100	PMNs	Negative
Septic arthritis	≥100	PMNs	Negative

Abbreviations: CPPD, calcium pyrophosphate deposition disease; PMNs, polymorphonuclear leukocytes.

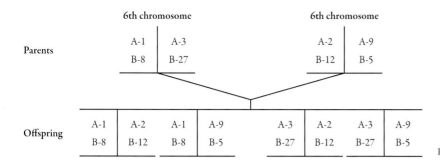

	6th chromosome				6th chromosome		
Parents	A-1 B-8	A-3 B-27			A-2 B-12	A-9 B-5	

Offspring	A-1 B-8	A-2 B-12	A-1 B-8	A-9 B-5	A-3 B-27	A-2 B-12	A-3 B-27	A-9 B-5

Figure 25.2 Inheritance of HLA Antigens.

chromosome 6, 1 inherited from each parent. On each of these there is an HLA-A and HLA-B allele. Therefore, everyone has 2 HLA-A types and 2 HLA-B types. With regard to inheritance, an offspring has a 50% chance of acquiring a specific HLA-A or HLA-B antigen from a parent (Figure 25.2). Siblings have a 25% chance of being identical for all 4 HLA-A and HLA-B alleles.

The frequency of HLA-B27 in control populations is as follows: whites (United States), 8%; African Americans, 2% to 4%; Asians, 1%; Haida (North American Indian), 50%. In randomly selected persons with HLA-B27, the chance of the disease developing is 2%. In B27-positive relatives of B27-positive patients with ankylosing spondylitis, the risk of the disease developing is 20%.

The rheumatic diseases associated with HLA-B27 are

1. Ankylosing spondylitis (HLA-B27 in >90%)

2. Reactive arthritis (>80%)

3. Enteropathic spondylitis (approximately 75%)

4. Psoriatic spondylitis (approximately 50%)

ANKYLOSING SPONDYLITIS

Ankylosing spondylitis is a chronic systemic inflammatory disease that affects the sacroiliac joints, the spine, and the peripheral joints. Sacroiliitis and low back pain define this disease.

Features

Characteristic features of low back pain in ankylosing spondylitis are the following: age at onset usually between 15 and 40 years, insidious onset, duration of more than 3 months, morning stiffness, improvement with exercise, family history, and diffuse radiation of back pain.

Findings of ankylosing spondylitis on physical examination are listed in Table 25.2. Other physical findings in ankylosing spondylitis are listed in Table 25.3. Radiographic findings in ankylosing spondylitis include sacroiliac sclerosis and possible erosions, spine involvement with squaring of the vertebral bodies, syndesmophytes, and bamboo spine. In patients with

early disease, magnetic resonance imaging can detect inflammation in the sacroiliac joints even when radiographs of the sacroiliac joints are normal.

Laboratory Findings

The erythrocyte sedimentation rate may be increased, there may be an anemia of chronic disease, rheumatoid factor is absent, and 95% of white patients are positive for HLA-B27.

Extraspinal Involvement

Enthesopathic involvement is characteristic of ankylosing spondylitis and the other spondyloarthropathies and includes plantar fasciitis, Achilles tendinitis, and costochondritis. Hip and shoulder involvement are common (up to 50%), but peripheral joints can be affected, usually with asymmetric involvement of the lower extremities.

Extraskeletal Involvement

Other findings in active disease include 1) fatigue, 2) weight loss, 3) low-grade fever, and 4) uveitis. Uveitis is an important clue to the diagnosis of spondyloarthropathies and is not found in adults with rheumatoid arthritis. Uveitis typically flares at a time the arthritis is inactive. Osteoporosis is a common complication of ankylosing spondylitis and can occur in early stages of the disease. Late complications can include traumatic spinal fracture leading to cord compression, cauda

Table 25.2 **FINDINGS IN ANKYLOSING SPONDYLITIS**

CHARACTERISTIC	FINDING
Scoliosis	Absent
Decreased range of movement	Symmetric
Tenderness	Diffuse
Hip flexion with straight-leg raising	Normal
Pain with sciatic nerve stretch	Absent
Hip involvement	Frequently present
Neurodeficit	Absent

Table 25.3 RESULTS OF TESTING IN ANKYLOSING SPONDYLITIS

TEST	METHOD	RESULTS
Schober	Make a mark on the spine at level of L5 & 1 at 10 cm directly above with the patient standing erect. Patient then bends forward maximally & the distance between the 2 marks is measured	An increase of <5 cm indicates early lumbar involvement
Chest expansion	Measure maximal chest expansion at nipple line	Chest expansion of <5 cm is clue to early costovertebral involvement
Sacroiliac compression	Exert direct compression over sacroiliac joints	Tenderness or pain suggests sacroiliac involvement

equina syndrome (symptoms include neurogenic bladder, fecal incontinence, and radicular leg pain), fibrotic changes in upper lung fields, aortic insufficiency, complete heart block, or secondary amyloidosis.

Differential Diagnosis

The differential diagnosis includes diffuse idiopathic skeletal hyperostosis, osteitis condensans ilii, fusion of sacroiliac joint seen in paraplegia, osteitis pubis, infection, and degenerative joint disease. The clinical symptoms of diffuse idiopathic skeletal hyperostosis are "stiffness" of spine and relatively good preservation of spine motion. It generally affects middle-aged and elderly men. Patients with diffuse idiopathic skeletal hyperostosis can have dysphagia related to cervical osteophytes. Criteria for the condition are "flowing" ossification along the anterolateral aspect of at least 4 contiguous vertebral bodies, preservation of disk height, absence of apophyseal joint involvement, absence of sacroiliac joint involvement, and extraspinal ossifications, including ligamentous calcifications.

Osteitis condensans ilii usually affects young to middle-aged females with normal sacroiliac joints. Radiography shows sclerosis on the iliac side of the sacroiliac joint only. The sacroiliac joint also can be involved with 1) tuberculosis, 2) metastatic disease, 3) gout, 4) Paget disease, or 5) other infections (eg, *Brucella, Serratia, Staphylococcus*).

Treatment

Treatment involves physical therapy (upright posture is very important), exercise (swimming), cessation of smoking, genetic counseling, and drug therapy with NSAIDs. Tumor necrosis factor inhibitors can provide benefit for spinal and peripheral joint symptoms. Adalimumab is more effective than etanercept for preventing recurrent uveitis.

REACTIVE ARTHRITIS

Reactive arthritis is an aseptic arthritis induced by a host response to an infectious agent rather than direct infection. HLA-B27 is associated in 80% of cases. Reactive arthritis develops after infections with *Salmonella, Shigella flexneri, Yersinia enterocolitica, Campylobacter jejuni, Clostridium*

difficile, and *Chlamydia trachomatis*. Inflammatory eye disease (conjunctivitis or uveitis) and mucocutaneous disease (balanitis, oral ulcerations, or keratoderma) can occur. Keratoderma blennorrhagicum is a characteristic skin disease on the palms and soles that is indistinguishable histologically from psoriasis. Joint predilection is for the toes and asymmetric large joints in the lower extremities. It can cause "sausage" toe, as can psoriatic arthritis. Cardiac conduction disturbances and aortitis can develop. Long-term studies indicate that the disease remains episodically active in 75% of patients and that disability is a frequent outcome.

Treatment is with NSAIDs. Sulfasalazine and methotrexate are used in patients with chronic disease. Treatment with tetracycline or erythromycin-type antibiotics may decrease the duration and severity of illness in some cases of *Chlamydia*-triggered reactive arthritis.

ARTHRITIS ASSOCIATED WITH INFLAMMATORY BOWEL DISEASE

Two distinct types of arthritis are associated with chronic inflammatory bowel disease:

1. Oligoarthritis of the peripheral joints tending to correlate with the activity of the bowel disease

2. Enteropathic spondylitis that is not a complication of the bowel disease. It may be diagnosed many years before the onset of bowel symptoms, and its subsequent progress bears little relationship to the bowel disease. Approximately 75% of patients with enteropathic spondylitis and inflammatory bowel disease are HLA-B27–positive.

In patients with arthritis, NSAIDs must be used with caution because they may flare the bowel disease. Infliximab or adalimumab are the drugs of choice to treat both spondylitis and Crohn disease. Etanercept is not beneficial for Crohn disease.

PSORIATIC ARTHRITIS

Psoriatic arthritis develops in approximately 25% of patients with psoriasis. Pitting of nails is strongly associated with joint disease. "Sausage" finger or toe is characteristic of psoriatic arthritis. "Pencil-in-cup" deformity of the distal and proximal interphalangeal joints is found on radiography.

There are 5 clinical groups of psoriatic arthritis: 1) predominantly distal interphalangeal joint involvement, 2) asymmetric oligoarthritis, 3) symmetric polyarthritis-like rheumatoid arthritis but negative for rheumatoid factor, 4) arthritis mutilans, and 5) psoriatic spondylitis. Treatment is with NSAIDs, methotrexate, and tumor necrosis factor inhibitors.

UVEITIS AND RHEUMATOLOGIC DISEASES

Various rheumatologic diseases are associated with uveitis, particularly the spondyloarthropathies. Uveitis is uncommon in rheumatoid arthritis and systemic lupus erythematosus. Nongranulomatous uveitis without any other associated symptoms may be associated with HLA-B27 in almost 50% of patients. Other causes of uveitis include sarcoid, Behçet syndrome, polychondritis, and juvenile idiopathic arthritis, especially in young females who are antinuclear antibody–positive.

BEHÇET SYNDROME

The common manifestations of Behçet syndrome include oral and genital ulcers and uveitis. Behçet syndrome is most common in Middle Eastern countries and Japan. HLA-B51 is associated with the syndrome. Uveitis, synovitis, cutaneous vasculitis, and meningoencephalitis may be present. Treatment is with corticosteroids, although more aggressive immunosuppression often is required.

OSTEOID OSTEOMA

Osteoid osteoma is a benign bone tumor. Bone pain at night is relieved by aspirin or another NSAID.

BYPASS ARTHRITIS

Bypass arthritis occurs in patients who have had intestinal bypass operations. The most commonly affected joints are metacarpophalangeal, proximal interphalangeal, wrists, knees, and ankles. Bypass arthritis is commonly associated with dermatitis. Circulating immune complexes composed of bacterial antigens are thought to be the cause of this disorder. Treatment consists of NSAIDs and antibiotics such as tetracycline, but reanastomosis may be necessary for complete resolution of symptoms.

SUMMARY

- Spondyloarthropathies are characterized by sacroiliitis, uveitis, peripheral arthritis, enthesopathic involvement, and an association with HLA-B27.

- Dactylitis ("sausage" finger or toe) is characteristic of psoriatic arthritis and reactive arthritis.

- Gout and pseudogout are diagnosed from synovial fluid analysis demonstrating characteristic crystals.

- The treatment of acute gout and pseudogout is with NSAIDs unless contraindicated.

- A uric acid value <6 mg/dL is the goal of therapy with probenecid, allopurinol, or febuxostat.

26.

SYSTEMIC LUPUS ERYTHEMATOSUS AND INFECTIONS[a]

William W. Ginsburg, MD

GOALS

- To diagnose and treat lupus and other connective tissue diseases.

- To interpret results of autoimmune tests.

- To recognize adverse effects of medications used to treat lupus and other connective tissue diseases.

- To recognize rheumatologic manifestations of various infections.

SYSTEMIC LUPUS ERYTHEMATOSUS

Systemic lupus erythematosus (SLE) is a chronic inflammatory disease of unknown cause with a wide spectrum of clinical manifestations and variable course characterized by exacerbations and remissions. Antibodies that react with nuclear antigens commonly are found in patients with the disease. Genetic, hormonal, and environmental factors seem to be important in the cause.

DIAGNOSIS

Findings in patients with SLE are listed in Box 26.1. At least 4 of the findings are needed for the diagnosis of SLE.

EPIDEMIOLOGY

The female to male ratio is 8:1 during the reproductive years. The first symptoms usually occur between the second and fourth decades of life. The disease seems to be less severe in the elderly. In SLE with onset at an older age, the female to male ratio is equal. The frequency of SLE is increased in African Americans, Native Americans, and Asians.

- The female to male ratio in SLE is 8:1 during the reproductive years.

- The frequency of SLE is increased in African Americans, Native Americans, and Asians.

- The first symptoms of SLE present between the second and fourth decades of life.

ETIOLOGY

In human disease, viral-like particles in glomeruli of patients with SLE have been reported; however, attempts to isolate viruses have been unsuccessful. Therefore, a direct causal relationship between viral infection and SLE has not been established.

- In SLE, there are increased viral antibody titers to a wide range of antigens without specificity for a particular viral agent.

GENETICS

Among relatives of patients with SLE, 25% have antinuclear antibodies, circulating immune complexes, antilymphocyte antibodies, or a false-positive result on the VDRL test without clinical disease. Concordance for SLE among monozygotic twins is much greater than among dizygotic twins. Multiple genetic and environmental factors are important in the development of SLE.

- In SLE, the frequency of HLA-B8, HLA-DR2, and HLA-DR3 is increased.

- Multiple genetic and environmental factors are important in the development of SLE.

PATHOGENESIS

There is a change in the activity of the cellular immune system with an absolute decrease in T-suppressor cells. There is

[a] Portions previously published in Ginsburg WW. Drug-induced systemic lupus erythematosus. Semin Respir Med. 1980;2:51–8. Used with permission.

an increase in the activity of the humoral immune system with B-cell hyperactivity resulting in polyclonal activation and antibody production.

Circulating immune complexes (antibodies to native DNA [anti–native DNA]) contribute to glomerulonephritis and skin disease. Immune complexes bind complement, which initiates the inflammatory process. Organ-specific autoantibodies also contribute to the pathophysiology of the disease and include antibodies that are 1) antierythrocyte, 2) antiplatelet, 3) antileukocyte, 4) antineuronal, and 5) antithyroid.

- Circulating immune complexes (anti–native DNA) contribute to glomerulonephritis and skin manifestations in SLE.

- Organ-specific autoantibodies also contribute to the pathophysiology of the disease and include antibodies that are 1) antierythrocyte, 2) antiplatelet, 3) antileukocyte, 4) antineuronal, and 5) antithyroid.

- Late complications of SLE are related to vascular damage, sometimes in the relative absence of active immunologic disease. Damage to the intima during active disease ultimately may result in various thrombotic, ischemic, and hypertensive manifestations.

CLINICAL MANIFESTATIONS

General

Fever in SLE usually is caused by the disease, but infection must be ruled out. Shaking chills and leukocytosis strongly suggest infection.

Articular

The arthritis of SLE is characteristically inflammatory but nondeforming and nonerosive. Avascular necrosis of bone occurs, and not only in patients taking steroids. The femoral head, navicular bone, and tibial plateau are most commonly affected.

- The arthritis of SLE is inflammatory but nondeforming and nonerosive.

Dermatologic

An erythematous malar rash (butterfly rash) often exacerbated by sunlight occurs during flares of SLE. Discoid lupus involves the face, scalp, and extremities. There is follicular plugging with atrophy leading to scarring. Subacute cutaneous LE is a subset of SLE that primarily has skin involvement with psoriasiform or annular erythematous lesions. Patients may be negative for antinuclear antibodies but frequently are positive for antibodies to the extractable nuclear antigen Sjögren syndrome A (SS-A) (Ro).

Cardiopulmonary

Cardiac involvement in SLE is manifested by pericarditis, myocarditis, valvular involvement, accelerated coronary atherosclerosis, and coronary vasculitis. An association between SLE and premature coronary artery disease has also been established. Therefore, in a young woman with chest pain, coronary artery disease must be strongly considered. Besides known cardiovascular risk factors such as hypertension and hyperlipidemia, SLE itself is an independent risk factor, possibly through immune-mediated chronic vascular inflammation common to the pathogenesis of SLE and atherosclerosis.

Pulmonary involvement in SLE is manifested by any of the following: pleurisy, pleural effusions, pneumonitis, pulmonary hypertension, hemorrhage, and diaphragmatic dysfunction.

Neuropsychiatric

Central nervous system lupus is a variable and unpredictable phenomenon. Manifestations such as impaired cognitive function, seizures, long tract signs, cranial neuropathies, psychosis, and migraine-like attacks occur with little apparent relationship to each other or to other systemic manifestations. Patients may have increased cerebrospinal fluid protein immunoglobulin (Ig) G, pleocytosis, and antineuronal antibodies.

Results of electroencephalography may be abnormal. Magnetic resonance imaging can show areas of increased signal in the periventricular white matter, similar to those found in multiple sclerosis. Magnetic resonance imaging findings are often nonspecific, as sometimes occurs in patients who have SLE without central nervous system manifestations. On pathologic examinations of autopsy specimens, findings are usually microinfarcts, nerve cell loss, rarely vasculitis, or no detectable abnormalities.

Psychosis caused by steroid therapy is probably rarer than previously thought. When there is doubt about the cause of psychosis in patients with SLE, the steroid dose should be increased and the patient observed. Patients rarely can have isolated central nervous system involvement and normal results of cerebrospinal fluid examination and no other organ involvement.

Particularly with neuropsychiatric symptoms or respiratory symptoms, secondary causes must be considered, especially infection, hypertension, anemia, and hypoxia. Fever should be considered due to infection until proved otherwise.

- Central nervous system lupus is a variable and unpredictable phenomenon.
- Particularly with neuropsychiatric symptoms or respiratory symptoms, secondary causes must be considered, especially infection, hypertension, anemia, and hypoxia.
- Fever should be considered due to infection until proved otherwise.

PREGNANCY AND SLE

Women with SLE who become pregnant have a high prevalence of spontaneous abortion. Because abortion may lead to a flare of the disease, therapeutic abortion ordinarily is not recommended after the first trimester. Flares of disease should be treated with steroids, particularly during the postpartum period.

In infants of mothers with SLE, thrombocytopenia and leukopenia can develop from passive transfer of antibodies. They also can have transient cutaneous lesions and complete heart block. Mothers usually have anti–SS-A (Ro), which crosses the placenta and is transiently present in the infant. Mothers usually are HLA-B8/DR3–positive, but there is no HLA association in the child.

RENAL INVOLVEMENT

The types of renal disease in SLE are 1) mesangial, 2) focal glomerulonephritis, 3) membranous glomerulonephritis, 4) diffuse proliferative glomerulonephritis, 5) interstitial nephritis with defects in the renal tubular handling of K+, and 6) renal vein thrombosis with nephrotic syndrome.

Treatment of renal disease depends in part on the results of renal biopsy. Patients with high activity indices on biopsy such as active inflammation, proliferation, necrosis, and crescent formation are considered for aggressive therapy. Patients with high chronicity indices such as tubular atrophy, scarring, and glomerulosclerosis are less likely to respond to aggressive therapy. Patients with mesangial changes alone do not require aggressive therapy. Active diffuse proliferative glomerulonephritis is treated with high-dose steroids and cyclophosphamide. Recently, mycophenolate mofetil has shown efficacy equivalent to cyclophosphamide with fewer adverse effects and can be considered an alternative to induction and maintenance therapy in lupus nephritis.

In patients with chronic proteinuria even without evidence of active renal disease, angiotensin-I converting enzyme inhibitors should be used. They have been shown to lower proteinuria and have renoprotective effects.

- Renal biopsies are helpful for directing therapy in renal disease associated with SLE.
- Patients with mesangial changes alone do not require aggressive therapy.

- Active diffuse proliferative glomerulonephritis is treated with high-dose steroids and immunosuppressive agents.
- Patients with chronic proteinuria should be treated with angiotensin-I converting enzyme inhibitors.

LABORATORY FINDINGS

Anemia of chronic disease and hemolytic anemia (Coombs positive) may occur. Leukopenia usually does not predispose to infection. Anti-lymphocyte antibodies cause lymphopenia in SLE. Idiopathic thrombocytopenic purpura with the presence of platelet antibodies can be the initial manifestation of SLE. Polyclonal gammopathy due to hyperactivity of the humoral immune system is common. The erythrocyte sedimentation rate usually correlates with disease activity.

Hypocomplementemia (CH50, C3, C4) usually correlates with active disease. Hypocomplementemia with increased anti–native DNA antibodies usually implies renal disease. A total complement value too low to measure with normal C3 and C4 values suggests a hereditary complement deficiency. Familial C2 deficiency is the most common complement deficiency in SLE, but C1r, C1s, C1q, C4, C5, C7, and C8 deficiencies also have been reported.

Patients with SLE may have false-positive results of the VDRL test as a result of antibody to phospholipid, which cross-reacts with the phospholipid antibody used in the VDRL test. Patients with SLE also can have false-positive results of the fluorescent treponemal antibody test, but they usually have the "beaded" pattern of fluorescence. LE cells are present in approximately 70% of patients with SLE and are caused by antibody to deoxyribonucleoprotein. This test is not specific and is no longer performed in many centers.

Anti–native DNA levels fluctuate with disease activity, whereas levels of other autoantibodies (ribonucleoprotein [RNP], Smith [Sm], antinuclear antibody) show no consistent relationship to levels of anti–native DNA or disease activity.

Although all patients with SLE should have positive results of antinuclear antibody tests, a positive result is by no means specific for SLE. Antinuclear antibody patterns are outlined in Table 26.1. Other autoantibodies and disease associations are outlined in Table 26.2.

Table 26.1 ANTINUCLEAR ANTIBODY PATTERNS

FLUORESCENT PATTERN	ANTIGEN	DISEASE ASSOCIATION
Rim, peripheral, shaggy	nDNA	SLE
Homogeneous	DNP	SLE, others
Speckled	ENA	MCTD, SLE, others
Nucleolar	RNA	Scleroderma

Abbreviations: DNP, deoxyribonucleoprotein; ENA, extractable nuclear antigen; MCTD, mixed connective tissue disease; nDNA, native DNA; SLE, systemic lupus erythematosus.

Table 26.2 AUTOANTIBODIES IN RHEUMATIC DISEASES

ANTIBODY	DISEASE ASSOCIATION
Anti–nDNA	SLE, 50%-60%
Anti-Sm (Smith)	SLE, 30%
Anti-RNP (ribonucleoprotein)	MCTD, 100% high titer SLE, 30% Scleroderma, low frequency, low titer
Anti–SS-A (Sjögren syndrome A)	Sjögren, 70% SLE, 35% Scleroderma + MCTD, low frequency, low titer
Anti–SS-B (Sjögren syndrome B)	Sjögren, 60% SLE, 15%
Antihistone	Drug-induced SLE, 95% SLE, 60% RA, 20%
Anti–Scl-70 (antitopoisomerase I)	Scleroderma, 25%
Anticentromere	CREST, 70%-90% Scleroderma, 10%-15%
Anti-PM1 (polymyositis)	PM, 50%
Anti-Jo1 (antisynthetase)	PM/interstitial lung disease, 30%

Abbreviations: CREST, syndrome of *c*alcinosis cutis, *R*aynaud phenomenon, *e*sophageal dysmotility, *s*clerodactyly, *t*elangiectasia; MCTD, mixed connective tissue disease; nDNA, native DNA; RA, rheumatoid arthritis; SLE, systemic lupus erythematosus.

- Hemolytic anemia (Coombs positive) can occur in SLE.

- Idiopathic thrombocytopenic purpura can be the initial manifestation of SLE.

- Hypocomplementemia (CH50, C3, C4) usually correlates with active disease.

- Hypocomplementemia with increased anti–native DNA antibodies usually implies renal disease (or skin disease).

- Anti–native DNA levels fluctuate with disease activity, but other associated antibodies do not.

- A positive result of an antinuclear antibody test is not specific for lupus.

TREATMENT

Treatment should match the activity of SLE in the individual patient. Serial monitoring of organ function and appropriate laboratory evaluation (anti–native DNA, C3, erythrocyte sedimentation rate) allow rapid recognition and treatment of flares and appropriate tapering of steroid dose during periods of disease quiescence. Table 26.3 provides guidelines for treatment, and Table 26.4 outlines the complications of treatment. Belimumab, a monoclonal antibody that inhibits the

Table 26.3 TREATMENT OF MANIFESTATIONS OF SYSTEMIC LUPUS ERYTHEMATOSUS

MANIFESTATION	TREATMENT
Arthritis, fever, mild systemic symptoms	ASA, NSAID
Photosensitivity, rash	Avoidance of sun, use of sunscreens
Rash, arthritis	Hydroxychloroquine (Plaquenil)
Significant thrombocytopenia, hemolytic anemia	Steroids
Renal disease, CNS disease, pericarditis, other significant organ involvement	Steroids
Rapidly deteriorating renal function	Cyclophosphamide, mycophenolate mofetil

Abbreviations: ASA, acetylsalicylic acid; CNS, central nervous system; NSAID, nonsteroidal anti-inflammatory drug.

B-lymphocyte stimulator, was recently approved for cutaneous and articular manifestations nonresponsive to conventional therapy.

OUTCOME

The 10-year survival rate is 90% in newly diagnosed SLE. Prognosis is worse in blacks and Hispanics than in whites. Prognosis is worse in patients with creatinine values more than 3.0 mg/dL. The major causes of death are 1) active disease, 2) infection, and 3) cardiovascular disease.

- The 10-year survival rate is 90% in newly diagnosed SLE.

- Among patients with SLE, the prognosis is worse in African Americans and Hispanics.

Table 26.4 COMPLICATIONS OF TREATMENT FOR SYSTEMIC LUPUS ERYTHEMATOSUS

TREATMENT	COMPLICATION
Ibuprofen	Aseptic meningitis (headache, fever, stiff neck, CSF pleocytosis)
NSAID	Decreased renal blood flow
ASA	Salicylate hepatitis (common), benign
Cyclophosphamide	Hemorrhagic cystitis, alopecia, opportunistic lymphomas, infection, increased incidence of lymphomas (CNS)
Hydroxychloroquine (Plaquenil)	Retinal toxicity

Abbreviations: ASA, acetylsalicylic acid; CNS, central nervous system; CSF, cerebrospinal fluid; NSAID, nonsteroidal anti-inflammatory drug.

DRUG-INDUCED LUPUS

Many drugs have been implicated in drug-induced lupus. The most common drugs are listed in Box 26.2. The clinical syndrome of drug-induced lupus must be differentiated from only a positive antinuclear antibody result without clinical symptoms. Only hydralazine and procainamide have been *strongly* implicated in drug-induced lupus. A drug-induced lupus syndrome develops in 5% to 10% of persons taking hydralazine and in 15% to 25% of those taking procainamide. Virtually all patients taking procainamide for 2 years have a positive result of the antinuclear antibody test.

- Only hydralazine and procainamide are *strongly* implicated in drug-induced lupus.
- Virtually all patients taking procainamide for 2 years have a positive result of the antinuclear antibody test.

CLINICAL FEATURES

The clinical manifestations of drug-induced lupus include arthralgias and polyarthritis, which occur in approximately 80% of cases. Malaise is common, and fever has been reported in up to 40% of cases. Approximately 30% of patients have pleural-pulmonary manifestations as their presenting symptoms. Pericarditis has been reported in approximately 20% of cases. Diffuse interstitial pneumonitis has been noted. Asymptomatic pleural effusions may be found on routine chest radiography. In contrast to SLE, the incidence of renal and central nervous system involvement is low in drug-induced lupus.

- In drug-induced lupus, arthralgias and polyarthritis occur in about 80% of cases.
- Malaise is common in drug-induced lupus, and fever occurs in up to 40% of cases.
- About 30% of patients have pleural-pulmonary manifestations on presentation.
- Pericarditis is reported in about 20% of cases.
- The incidence of renal and central nervous system involvement is low.

SLE is predominantly a disease of premenopausal females, whereas drug-induced disease has an almost equal sex distribution and occurs in an older population. This disparity in age reflects the use of hydralazine and procainamide in primarily an older population.

LABORATORY ABNORMALITIES

Virtually all patients with SLE and drug-induced lupus have antinuclear antibodies. Anti–native DNA is found in only a small percentage of cases of drug-induced lupus but in approximately 60% of cases of SLE. Serum total hemolytic complement, C3, and C4 values are usually normal in drug-induced disease, in contrast to SLE. Antibodies such as anti-Sm, SS-A, SS-B, and RNP are also unusual in drug-induced lupus. The frequency of antihistone antibodies in drug-induced lupus is high (>95% of cases), but these also occur in approximately 60% of cases of SLE.

METABOLISM

Drugs involved in drug-induced lupus have different chemical structures, but 3 of them—isoniazid, procainamide, and hydralazine—contain a primary amine that is acetylated by the hepatic *N*-acetyltransferase system. Persons taking 1 of these drugs and who are slow acetylators have a much higher incidence of serologic abnormalities and clinical disease than rapid acetylators.

- Slow acetylators have a much higher incidence of serologic abnormalities and clinical disease.

TREATMENT

When possible, patients with drug-induced lupus should stop using the offending drug. Symptoms usually subside within several weeks, although the duration for complete resolution varies depending on the drug. Serologic abnormalities can remain for years after resolution of clinical symptoms. Treatment depends on the clinical manifestations and could include nonsteroidal anti-inflammatory drugs or possibly low-dose prednisone, if needed.

- Patients with drug-induced lupus should stop using the offending drug.

MIXED CONNECTIVE TISSUE DISEASE

This is a distinct disease with variable features of SLE, polymyositis, systemic sclerosis, and rheumatoid arthritis. The incidence of renal disease is low. It is serologically characterized by a positive antinuclear antibody and by a high titer of anti-RNP. Anti–native DNA usually is not present. Raynaud phenomenon is common.

- Patients with mixed connective tissue disease have a high titer of anti-RNP.

UNDIFFERENTIATED CONNECTIVE TISSUE DISEASE

In this category, patients have symptoms that do not fulfill the diagnostic criteria for a definite or specific connective tissue disease. Common symptoms include Raynaud phenomenon, arthralgias, fatigue, and variable joint or soft tissue swelling. The antinuclear antibody may be positive, but other autoantibodies are not present. Patients need to be observed to determine whether progression to a distinct connective tissue disease occurs.

ANTIPHOSPHOLIPID ANTIBODY SYNDROME

Antiphospholipid antibody syndrome is diagnosed on the basis of clinical criteria and laboratory criteria. The clinical criteria include a history of venous or arterial thrombosis, fetal loss after 10 weeks' gestation, or recurrent fetal loss before 10 weeks' gestation. The laboratory criteria are 1) the presence of medium to high levels of IgG or IgM antiphospholipid antibodies or the lupus anticoagulant on 2 occasions at least 12 weeks apart, 2) medium to high levels of IgG or IgM anticardiolipin in serum or plasma (ie, >40 IgG phospholipid units/mL or >40 IgM phospholipid units or >99th percentile) on 2 or more occasions at least 12 weeks apart, or 3) anti-β_2-glycoprotein I on 2 occasions at least 12 weeks apart. At least 1 clinical criterion and 1 laboratory criterion must be present for a patient to be classified as having antiphospholipid antibody syndrome.

The hallmark of the antiphospholipid antibody syndrome is prolongation of the activated partial thromboplastin time. The failure of normal plasma to correct this distinguishes the lupus anticoagulant and antiphospholipid antibody from clotting factor deficiencies (Box 26.3).

- Antiphospholipid antibodies are of either the IgG or the IgM class.

- An activated partial thromboplastin time that is prolonged and not corrected by adding normal plasma is the laboratory hallmark of the lupus anticoagulant.

Box 26.3 **COAGULATION TEST RESULTS CHARACTERIZING THE LUPUS ANTICOAGULANT**

Screening tests
 Prothrombin time normal
 aPTT prolonged
 Plasma clot time prolonged
Test identifying the lupus anticoagulant
 Prolonged aPTT not corrected by adding normal plasma

Abbreviation: aPTT, activated partial thromboplastin time.

Many, but not all, patients with the lupus anticoagulant also have increased IgG or IgM antiphospholipid antibody levels.

The lupus anticoagulant and antiphospholipid antibodies are associated with SLE, but they also have been reported in various other autoimmune, malignant, infectious, and drug-induced diseases. The antibodies are also found in persons with no apparent disease but in whom recurrent thrombosis develops; these patients have primary antiphospholipid antibody syndrome, which represents approximately 50% of cases in which the antibodies are present.

- Lupus anticoagulant and antiphospholipid antibodies also have been reported in various autoimmune, malignant, infectious, and drug-induced diseases.

- The primary antiphospholipid antibody syndrome represents 50% of cases in which the antibodies are present.

CLINICAL FEATURES

Thrombotic events described have included stroke, transient ischemic attacks, myocardial infarctions, brachial artery thrombosis, deep venous thrombophlebitis, retinal vein thrombosis, hepatic vein thrombosis resulting in Budd-Chiari syndrome, and pulmonary hypertension. Other manifestations include recurrent fetal loss, thrombocytopenia, positive results of Coombs test, migraines, chorea, epilepsy, chronic leg ulcers, livedo reticularis, and progressive dementia resulting from cerebrovascular accidents. Acquired valvular heart disease, especially aortic and mitral insufficiency, has also been described.

Although many patients with lupus and other diseases can have a lupus anticoagulant or antiphospholipid antibodies, thrombosis will not necessarily develop. In general, patients with the highest levels of antiphospholipid antibodies are more prone to thrombosis than those with lower levels. Also, the IgG antiphospholipid antibody is more strongly associated with recurrent thrombosis than is the IgM antiphospholipid antibody. In patients with a lupus anticoagulant or increased antiphospholipid antibodies without a history of thrombosis, no treatment is required other than aspirin. In patients with either antiphospholipid antibodies or the lupus anticoagulant, even if they have not had a thrombotic event, the use of estrogen-containing oral contraceptive pills should be avoided because they may put the patient at higher risk for thrombosis.

- There is an association between the presence of the lupus anticoagulant and antiphospholipid antibodies and recurrent venous or arterial thrombosis.

- Other manifestations include recurrent fetal loss, thrombocytopenia, positive Coombs test, migraines, chorea, epilepsy, chronic leg ulcers, livedo reticularis, and progressive dementia from cerebrovascular accidents.

- Patients with the highest levels of antiphospholipid antibodies are more prone to thrombosis.

- IgG antiphospholipid antibody is more strongly associated with recurrent thrombosis.

TREATMENT

For most patients who have recurrent thrombosis and high-titer anticardiolipin antibody, warfarin is prescribed in doses sufficient to yield international normalized ratio values close to 3 and will need to be taken for life. Low-dose aspirin and subcutaneous heparin have been used in pregnant women to prevent fetal loss. Corticosteroids have not been clearly shown to be efficacious for preventing thrombosis.

RAYNAUD PHENOMENON

This is biphasic or triphasic color changes (pallor, cyanosis, erythema) accompanied by pain and numbness in the hands or feet. Cold is a common precipitating agent. Associated factors are listed in Box 26.4.

Box 26.4 CAUSES OF SECONDARY RAYNAUD PHENOMENON

Chemotherapeutic agents
  Bleomycin
  Vinblastine
Toxins
  Vinyl chloride
Vibration-induced injuries
  Jackhammer use
Vascular occlusive disorders
  Thoracic outlet obstruction
  Atherosclerosis
  Vasculitis
Connective tissue diseases
  Scleroderma, 90%-100%
  Mixed connective tissue disease, 90%-100%
  Systemic lupus erythematosus, 15%
  Rheumatoid arthritis, <10%
  Polymyositis
Miscellaneous
  Cryoglobulinemia
  Cold agglutinins
  Increased blood viscosity

- Cold is a common precipitating agent for Raynaud phenomenon.

Raynaud phenomenon is related to an abnormality of the microvasculature associated with intimal fibrosis. In male patients with Raynaud phenomenon, a rare occurrence, a connective tissue disease may develop. Although Raynaud phenomenon is common in females, it usually is not associated with a connective tissue disease unless the patient has positive results for antinuclear antibody, which suggest that a connective tissue disease may develop in the future.

Skin capillary microscopy reveals tortuous, dilated capillary loops in systemic sclerosis, mixed connective tissue disease, and polymyositis. They also may be present in patients with Raynaud phenomenon who will go on to have systemic sclerosis, polymyositis, or mixed connective tissue disease.

Treatment involves smoking cessation, wearing gloves, biofeedback, 2% nitrol paste, and antihypertensive agents (prazosin or the calcium channel blockers amlodipine besylate or nifedipine). A stellate ganglion block, digital nerve block, or surgical digital sympathectomy is used if ischemia is severe. β-Adrenergic blockers and serotonin agonists such as sumatriptan can increase spasm and should be avoided.

SYSTEMIC SCLEROSIS (SCLERODERMA)

Systemic sclerosis (scleroderma) can be subdivided into several categories: 1) diffuse systemic sclerosis (diffuse scleroderma); 2) limited cutaneous scleroderma, which includes the CREST (calcinosis cutis, Raynaud phenomenon, esophageal dysmotility, sclerodactyly, telangiectasias) syndrome; 3) localized scleroderma, which includes morphea and linear scleroderma; and 4) overlap and undifferentiated connective tissue diseases, which include some component of scleroderma in conjunction with a manifestation of another connective tissue disease. For the diagnosis of systemic sclerosis, 1 major criterion or 2 or more minor criteria need to be present. The major criterion is symmetric induration of the skin of the fingers and the skin proximal to metacarpophalangeal or metatarsophalangeal joints. The minor criteria are sclerodactyly, digital pitting scars or loss of substance from the finger pad, and bibasilar pulmonary fibrosis. The pathologic hallmark of the disease is an obliterative noninflammatory vasculopathy and the accumulation of collagen in the skin and other organs that leads to fibrosis.

- Systemic sclerosis is characterized by symmetric induration of the skin of the fingers and the skin proximal to metacarpophalangeal or metatarsophalangeal joints, sclerodactyly, fingertip pitting or scarring, and bibasilar pulmonary fibrosis.

CLINICAL MANIFESTATIONS

Skin

Patients with rapidly progressive acral and trunk skin thickening are at risk for early visceral abnormalities.

Raynaud Phenomenon

Raynaud phenomenon occurs in almost all patients with scleroderma. It usually occurs more than 2 years before skin changes. If Raynaud phenomenon is not present but skin findings are suggestive of scleroderma, another disease such as eosinophilic fasciitis should be considered.

- Almost all patients with scleroderma have Raynaud phenomenon.

Articular

Nondeforming symmetric polyarthritis similar to rheumatoid arthritis may precede cutaneous manifestations by 12 months. Patients can have both articular erosions and nonarticular bony resorptive changes of ribs, mandible, radius, ulna, and distal phalangeal tufts, which are unique to systemic sclerosis. Up to 60% of patients have "leathery" crepitation of the tendons of the wrist.

Pulmonary

A considerable decrease in diffusing capacity can be present with a normal chest radiograph. Diffuse interstitial fibrosis occurs in approximately 70% of patients and is the most common pulmonary abnormality. Patients who have active alveolitis demonstrated by 1) bronchopulmonary lavage, 2) high-resolution computed tomography showing ground-glass appearance without honeycombing, or 3) lung biopsy are most likely to respond to prednisone and cyclophosphamide therapy with improvement of pulmonary function. Pleuritis (with effusion) is very rare. Pulmonary hypertension is more common in patients with CREST variant. Patients with pulmonary hypertension can have an isolated decrease in the diffusing capacity of the lung for carbon monoxide (Dlco). Although echocardiography is helpful for making a diagnosis, right heart catheterization should always be performed to confirm the diagnosis and to obtain accurate measurements of pulmonary artery and capillary wedge pressures.

- Patients with pulmonary hypertension can have an isolated decrease in Dlco.

- Diffuse interstitial fibrosis occurs in approximately 70% of patients and is the most common pulmonary abnormality.

- Pulmonary hypertension is more common in patients with CREST variant.

Cardiac

Cardiac abnormalities occur in up to 70% of patients. Conduction defects and supraventricular arrhythmias are most common. Pulmonary hypertension with cor pulmonale is the most serious problem.

- Cardiac abnormalities occur in up to 70% of patients.

- Pulmonary hypertension with cor pulmonale is a serious potential problem.

Gastrointestinal

Esophageal dysfunction is the most frequent gastrointestinal abnormality. It occurs in 90% of patients and often is asymptomatic. Lower esophageal sphincter incompetence with acid reflux may produce esophageal strictures or ulcers. Medications to reduce acid production are important. Reduced esophageal motility may respond to therapy with metoclopramide, cisapride, or erythromycin. Small bowel hypomotility may be associated with pseudo-obstruction, bowel dilatation, bacterial overgrowth, and malabsorption. Treatment with tetracycline may be helpful, but promotility agents are less effective. Colonic dysmotility also occurs, and wide-mouthed diverticuli may be found.

- Esophageal dysmotility occurs in more than 90% of patients with scleroderma.

Renal

Renal involvement may result in fulminant hypertension, renal failure, and death if not treated aggressively. Proteinuria, newly diagnosed mild hypertension, microangiopathic hemolytic anemia, vascular changes on renal biopsy, and rapid progression of skin thickening may precede overt clinical findings of renal crisis. Renal involvement with hyperreninemia necessitates the use of angiotensin-converting enzyme inhibitors. Aggressive early antihypertensive therapy can extend life expectancy.

- Renal involvement in scleroderma may be life-threatening.

LABORATORY FINDINGS

Antinuclear antibodies are found in 95% or more of patients. Antitopoisomerase I antibody (anti-Scl-70) is found in approximately 25% of patients with scleroderma and is usually associated with more severe disease. Anticentromere antibody occurs in 10% to 20%.

TREATMENT

No remissive or curative therapy is available. Aggressive nutritional support, including hyperalimentation, may be required for extensive gastrointestinal disease.

- No remissive or curative therapy is available for systemic sclerosis.

CREST SYNDROME

This is characterized by *c*alcinosis cutis, *R*aynaud phenomenon, *e*sophageal dysmotility, *s*clerodactyly, and *t*elangiectasias. Skin involvement progresses slowly and is limited to

Table 26.5 CLINICAL FINDINGS IN LIMITED AND DIFFUSE SCLERODERMA

| CLINICAL FINDING | CUTANEOUS DISEASE | |
	Limited	*Diffuse*
Raynaud phenomenon	Precedes other symptoms by years	Onset associated with other symptoms within 1 y
Nailfold capillaries	Dilated	Dilated with dropout
Skin changes	Distal to elbow	Proximal to elbow with involvement of trunk
Telangiectasia, digital ulcers, calcinosis	Frequent	Rare early, but frequent later in the course
Joint & tendon involvement	Uncommon	Frequent (tendon rubs)
Visceral disease	Pulmonary hypertension	Renal, intestinal, & cardiac disease; pulmonary interstitial fibrosis
Autoantibodies	Anticentromere (70%-90%)	Antitopoisomerase 1 (anti-Scl-70) (25%)
10-year survival	>70%	<70%

the extremities. Development of internal organ involvement occurs but is delayed. Lung involvement occurs in 70% of patients. Diffusing capacity may be low, and pulmonary hypertension can develop. The latter is more common in CREST than in diffuse scleroderma. Bosentan and sildenafil were recently approved for pulmonary hypertension in scleroderma and CREST syndrome. Anticentromere antibody is found in 70% to 90% of patients and anti-Scl-70 antibody in 10%. The incidence of primary biliary cirrhosis is increased.

- In CREST syndrome, 70% of patients have lung involvement.
- The diffusing capacity may be low, and pulmonary hypertension can develop.
- Anticentromere antibody is present in 70%-90% of patients.
- There is an increased incidence of primary biliary cirrhosis.

The clinical manifestations of limited and systemic scleroderma are listed in Table 26.5.

SCLERODERMA-LIKE SYNDROMES

DISORDERS ASSOCIATED WITH OCCUPATION OR ENVIRONMENT

This group includes polyvinyl chloride disease, organic solvents, jackhammer disease, silicosis, and toxic oil syndrome.

EOSINOPHILIC FASCIITIS

Clinical features of this disorder include tight bound-down skin of the extremities, characteristically sparing the hands and feet. Peau d'orange skin changes can develop. Onset after vigorous exercise is common. Raynaud phenomenon does not occur, and there is no visceral involvement. Flexion contractures and carpal tunnel syndrome can develop.

Laboratory findings are peripheral eosinophilia, increased sedimentation rate, and hypergammaglobulinemia. The diagnosis is based on the findings of inflammation and thickening of the fascia on deep fascial biopsy. Treatment is with prednisone (40 mg daily). The response is usually good. Associated conditions are aplastic anemia and thrombocytopenia (both antibody-mediated) and leukemia and myeloproliferative diseases.

- Eosinophilic fasciitis is characterized by tight bound-down skin of the extremities, usually sparing the hands and feet.
- Raynaud phenomenon does not occur.
- There is no visceral involvement.
- Laboratory findings include peripheral eosinophilia.
- Treatment with prednisone provides good response.

METABOLIC CAUSES

This group includes porphyria, amyloidosis, carcinoid, and diabetes mellitus (flexion contractures of the tendons in the hands, cheiropathy, can develop).

OTHER CAUSES

As a manifestation of graft-versus-host disease, skin induration develops in up to 30% of patients who receive a bone marrow transplant. Drug-induced disorders are caused by carbidopa, bleomycin, and bromocriptine. Eosinophilic myalgia syndrome is associated with ingestion of contaminated L-tryptophan. Eosinophilia, myositis, skin induration, fasciitis, and peripheral neuropathy develop. Skin changes are similar to those of eosinophilic fasciitis. There is a poor response to steroids. Scleredema frequently occurs after streptococcal upper respiratory tract infection in children. It is usually self-limiting. Swelling of the head and neck is common. In adults, diabetes mellitus is often an associated condition. Scleromyxedema is associated with IgG mono-clonal protein. Cocaine use and appetite suppressants also cause scleroderma-like illness. Nephrogenic systemic fibrosis, a recently described cutaneous fibrosing disorder, is caused by exposure to gadolinium-containing contrast agents during magnetic resonance imaging, especially in patients with renal insufficiency.

THE INFLAMMATORY MYOPATHIES

Inflammatory myopathies can be classified into several categories, including polymyositis, dermatomyositis, myositis associated with malignancy, childhood-type, and overlap connective tissue disease. Polymyositis is an inflammatory myopathy characterized by proximal muscle weakness. Patients with dermatomyositis have an associated rash that includes a heliotrope hue of the eyelids, a rash on the metacarpophalangeal and proximal interphalangeal joints (Gottron papules), and photosensitivity dermatitis of the face. Most patients have an increased creatine kinase level, a characteristic electromyogram, and a characteristic muscle biopsy.

Electromyography is characteristic but not diagnostic of inflammatory myopathies. It shows decreased amplitude and increased spike frequency, it is polyphasic, and conduction speed is normal. Fibrillation potentials are not specific for inflammatory myopathies, but when present they indicate active disease. Loss of fibrillation potentials usually means the inflammatory myopathy is under control, but if the electromyographic result is still myopathic, it suggests an associated steroid myopathy caused by treatment. The muscle biopsy, which is mandatory in all patients with inflammatory myopathy, shows degeneration, necrosis, and regeneration of myofibrils with lymphocytic and monocytic infiltrate in a perivascular or interstitial distribution.

In patients older than 40 years, perhaps 10% to 20% of those with dermatomyositis and polymyositis have an associated malignancy. The antibody anti-Jo1 is associated with polymyositis and dermatomyositis in approximately 25% of cases. This antibody is associated with inflammatory arthritis, progressive interstitial lung disease, Raynaud phenomenon, and increased mortality primarily due to respiratory failure. "Mechanic's hands," characterized by fissuring or cracking of the distal skin pads in the fingers, can also occur. The autoantibody anti-Mi-2 is associated with dermatomyositis in 2% to 20% of patients.

- Polymyositis is an inflammatory myopathy characterized by proximal muscle weakness.

- Dermatomyositis is an inflammatory myopathy associated with a rash that includes heliotrope hue of the eyelids.

- Electromyography is characteristic but not diagnostic of polymyositis.

- Perhaps 10%-20% of patients >40 years with dermatomyositis and polymyositis have associated malignancy.

- Anti-Jo1 is associated with polymyositis, dermatomyositis, pulmonary disease, and increased mortality.

Treatment of polymyositis includes prednisone (60 mg daily), usually for 1 to 2 months, until the muscle enzyme values normalize. The dosage is slowly reduced thereafter, and the clinical course and creatine kinase values are monitored. In severe or steroid-resistant cases, either azathioprine (1–2 mg/kg daily), methotrexate, or intravenous immunoglobulin can be used.

Aspiration pneumonia can occur as a result of pharyngeal weakness. If so, a liquid diet, feeding tube, or feeding gastrostomy is needed until there is clinical improvement.

INCLUSION BODY MYOSITIS

This usually occurs in the elderly. The onset of weakness is more insidious, occurring over many years. The creatine kinase value often is only minimally to several times increased, and distal and proximal weakness occur. The electromyogram, besides showing a myopathic picture, also has an associated neuropathic picture. The diagnosis of inclusion body myositis is made from biopsy. Histopathologic findings are indistinguishable from those of polymyositis except for the presence of eosinophilic inclusions and rimmed vacuoles with basophilic enhancement. Inclusion body myositis responds poorly to prednisone and immunosuppressive therapy, and the course is one of slow, progressive weakness.

- Inclusion body myositis usually occurs in the elderly.

- Diagnosis is made from biopsy.

- It responds poorly to prednisone.

DRUG-INDUCED MYOPATHIES

Drugs may cause an inflammatory myopathy. The myopathy associated with colchicine mimics polymyositis, and patients have muscle weakness and an increased creatine kinase level. This often occurs in the setting of a patient with gout and renal insufficiency receiving long-term therapy with colchicine. Lipid-lowering drugs such as the statins; other drugs including zidovudine, D-penicillamine, and hydroxychloroquine; and addictive drugs such as heroin or cocaine have all been associated with myopathy. Corticosteroids cause a steroid myopathy with proximal muscle weakness and a normal creatine kinase value.

INFECTIOUS ARTHRITIS

An infectious cause should be ruled out immediately in a patient with acute monarticular arthritis. Approximately 5% to 10% of patients with septic arthritis present with multiple joint involvement.

- Infectious causes should be ruled out in patients with acute monarticular arthritis.

BACTERIAL ARTHRITIS

Nongonococcal bacterial arthritis is caused by hematogenous spread of bacteria, direct inoculation (which is usually traumatic), or extension of soft tissue infection with osteomyelitis into the joint space. Large joints are more commonly affected. Patients who are elderly or immunosuppressed are predisposed to septic arthropathy. The possibility of septic arthritis should be considered in patients with a preexisting polyarthritis who have a single joint flare that is out of proportion to the rest of their joint symptoms. In any patient with a septic joint, the possibility of infectious endocarditis or a disk space infection should be considered.

Septic arthritis is a medical emergency. Joint aspiration is required. Typically, patients with nongonococcal septic arthritis have a leukocyte value of more than 50,000/mcL and a low glucose concentration in the synovial fluid. Blood cultures should be performed when septic arthritis is considered. Radiographs of an involved joint may show an associated osteomyelitis or previous local trauma, but radiographic findings of infection usually lag considerably behind clinical symptoms.

Staphylococcus aureus is the most common pathogen in adults with nongonococcal bacterial arthritis. In sickle cell anemia, *Salmonella* is the organism commonly causing septic arthritis. *Pseudomonas* should be considered in the context of cat or dog bites, and an anaerobic infection should be considered in cases of human bites. Intravenous drug users may have bacteremia with unusual organisms, such as *Pseudomonas* or *Serratia*, and this may present with septic arthritis in unusual locations, such as the sternoclavicular or sacroiliac joints. Gram-negative bacilli, such as *Escherichia coli* and *Klebsiella*, may cause septic arthritis in older patients with gastrointestinal or genitourinary infections or instrumentation.

Broad-spectrum antibiotics should be used until culture results are available. Daily aspiration and lavage of the affected joint should be performed. Synovial fluid leukocytes and volume should decrease, or orthopedic arthroscopic or even open drainage should be considered. Such drainage usually is indicated in joints such as the hip, which are not readily accessible. The duration of treatment depends on the virulence of the organisms, but antibiotics usually are given intravenously for at least 2 weeks.

- Nongonococcal bacterial arthritis is caused by hematogenous spread of bacteria, direct inoculation (which is usually traumatic), or extension of soft tissue infection or osteomyelitis.

- Synovial fluid Gram stain and culture are essential.

- The portal of entry may predict the organism causing septic arthritis.

- Antibiotic therapy should be initiated even before culture results are available.

- If repeated aspiration and antibiotics do not lead to clinical improvement and a decrease in synovial fluid volume and leukocytosis, then arthroscopic or open drainage and débridement may be necessary.

GONOCOCCAL ARTHRITIS

Disseminated gonococcal infection develops in approximately 0.2% of patients with gonorrhea. The male to female ratio is 3:1. This is the most common form of septic arthritis in younger, sexually active persons who may be asymptomatic carriers of gonococci. When gonococcal infection is suspected, specimens from the pharynx, joints, rectum, blood, and genitourinary tract should be cultured. Females present with gonococcal arthritis commonly during pregnancy or within 1 week after onset of menses, possibly related to the pH of vaginal secretions. The most common form of gonococcal arthritis is the disseminated gonococcal arthritis syndrome with fever, dermatitis, and an inflammatory tenosynovitis. Approximately 50% of patients with this syndrome present with an inflammatory arthritis, commonly of the knee, wrist, or ankle. Tenosynovitis is more common than large joint effusions. Rash, sometimes with pustules or hemorrhagic vesicles, is common. The second form of gonococcal arthritis commonly begins as a migratory polyarthralgia, which subsequently localizes to 1 or more joints.

Synovial fluid cultures are positive in only 30% of patients with known disseminated gonococcal infection. Culture of the skin lesion is positive for gonococcus in 40% to 60% of patients with disseminated gonococcal infection. Rare patients who have recurrent disseminated gonococcal infection may have an associated terminal complement component deficiency (C5-C9).

Most patients with disseminated gonococcal arthritis are treated as outpatients. Current treatment recommendations suggest a later third-generation cephalosporin, such as ceftriaxone, 1.0 g daily. Treatment involves a minimal 7-day course. Treatment should include an antichlamydial antibiotic.

- Gonococcal arthritis develops in 0.2% of patients with gonorrhea.

- In the disseminated gonococcal arthritis syndrome, fever, dermatitis, and tenosynovitis are common.

- In the nonbacteremic form of gonococcal arthritis, migratory polyarthralgias are followed by inflammation localizing to 1 or more joints.

- Synovial fluid cultures are positive in 30% of patients with known disseminated gonococcal infection.

- Joint fluid leukocyte counts may be lower than in other types of septic arthritis.

- Joint effusions may be related to a reactive or postinfectious arthritis.

- Treatment recommendations are the use of a later third-generation cephalosporin (eg, ceftriaxone).

- Treatment should include an antichlamydial antibiotic.

MYCOBACTERIAL AND FUNGAL JOINT INFECTIONS

These types of organisms usually cause chronic bone and joint infections. A synovial biopsy and culture may be required to document these infections. Tuberculous arthritis is often otherwise asymptomatic and usually is caused by direct extension from adjacent bony infection. Atypical mycobacterial infection may cause an inflammatory arthritis and tenosynovitis frequently involving the hand and wrist. Sporotrichosis and blastomycosis are the fungi most likely to have skeletal manifestations. The classic presentation in sporotrichosis is a gardener with a rose-thorn penetration in whom a monarthritis develops.

- Tuberculous arthritis is often otherwise asymptomatic and is caused by direct extension from adjacent bony infection.
- Atypical mycobacterial infection may cause an inflammatory arthritis and tenosynovitis most commonly affecting the hand and wrist.
- Sporotrichosis and blastomycosis are the fungi most likely to have skeletal manifestations.

SPINAL SEPTIC ARTHRITIS

This condition should be suspected in patients with acute or chronic, unrelenting back pain associated with fever and marked local tenderness. The thoracolumbar region is most commonly affected. An antecedent infection or procedure predisposing to bacteremia may help suggest this diagnosis. Imaging studies usually have evidence for infection crossing the disk space. In tuberculous spinal septic arthritis (Pott disease), the site of involvement is most commonly T10-L2, and there is usually an associated paraspinal abscess.

Intravertebral disk infection is often a difficult diagnosis to establish because pain patterns may be unusual and localizing signs may be absent. Bone scanning may be helpful, but magnetic resonance imaging may be very helpful, particularly because of the ability to show extension of infection into surrounding tissues.

INFECTED JOINT PROSTHESES

Infection in joint prostheses occurs in 1% to 5% of all joint replacements. Fever may not be present, and laboratory findings are often unhelpful, although the erythrocyte sedimentation rate may be increased. There may or may not be evidence of loosening of the cement holding the new joint in place, and radiographs may reveal lytic changes around the prosthesis. A negative bone scan is reassuring. Aspiration of fluid from the prosthetic joint is necessary to confirm infection. Prosthetic joint infection usually is caused by gram-positive organisms, particularly *Staphylococcus aureus* and *Staphylococcus epidermidis*, in the first 6 months after the replacement operation and by gram-negative and fungal organisms after 6 months. Patients with prosthetic joints do not require antibiotic prophylaxis before invasive dental, gastrointestinal, or genitourinary procedures according to the recent guidelines, unless obvious immunosuppression is present.

- Prosthetic joint infection usually is caused by a gram-positive organism within the first 6 months after joint replacement.
- Prosthetic joint infections usually are caused by gram-negative or fungal organisms beyond the initial 6 months after joint replacement.

RHEUMATIC FEVER AND POSTSTREPTOCOCCAL REACTIVE ARTHRITIS

Arthritis affects two-thirds of all patients with rheumatic fever. One-third of patients with acute rheumatic fever have no obvious antecedent pharyngitis. In adults, arthritis may be the only clinical feature of acute rheumatic fever. The arthritis may be migratory, with each joint remaining inflamed for approximately 1 week. The arthritis of rheumatic fever is nonerosive; however, repeated attacks may result in a Jaccoud deformity, in which the metacarpophalangeal joints are in ulnar deviation as a result of tendon laxity rather than bony damage.

Patients with joint symptoms without carditis may be treated with high-dose salicylates (3–6 g daily). Corticosteroids may be required if patients do not respond to salicylates. Joint symptoms may rebound when anti-inflammatory therapy is discontinued.

- The arthritis in rheumatic fever may be migratory and usually involves the large joints, particularly the knees, ankles, elbows, and wrists.
- Repeated attacks of rheumatic fever may result in Jaccoud deformity.
- The mainstay treatment for the arthritis of rheumatic fever is high-dose salicylates (3–6 g daily).

VIRAL ARTHRITIS

Viruses associated with arthralgia and arthritis include human immunodeficiency virus (HIV), hepatitis B, rubella, parvovirus, and, less commonly, mumps, adenovirus, herpesvirus, and enterovirus. Most viral-related arthritides have joint symptoms with a semiacute onset, but fortunately they are usually of brief duration. The arthritis is nondestructive.

Although parvovirus infection is usually mild in children, associated arthralgias and arthritis are common in adults, usually without an associated rash, and may mimic rheumatoid arthritis. The diagnosis of parvovirus infection is made by demonstrating the presence of anti-B19 IgM antibodies. Treatment is usually conservative and includes anti-inflammatory medications, but in more chronic infections more aggressive treatment such as low-dose corticosteroids may be warranted. Parvovirus infection also has been associated with cytopenias.

Hepatitis B virus infection has been associated with an immune complex-mediated arthritis, which can be dramatic. The arthritis is usually limited to the pre-icteric prodrome. Polyarteritis nodosa has been associated with hepatitis B. Hepatitis B and, more commonly, hepatitis C are associated with mixed cryoglobulinemia. Hepatitis C virus infections can mimic autoimmune diseases, including rheumatoid arthritis, Sjögren syndrome, and SLE, both clinically and serologically. Numerous autoantibodies may be detected in hepatitis C virus infection, including a positive rheumatoid factor, antinuclear antibody, anti–SS-A and –SS-B, and antiphospholipid antibodies. Rubella virus infection is frequently associated with joint complaints in young adults. In a few patients, the symptoms have persisted for months to years. Joint symptoms may occur just before or after the appearance of the characteristic rash.

- Parvovirus infection in adults may cause a symmetric polyarthritis mimicking rheumatoid arthritis.

- Parvovirus infection can be documented by demonstrating the presence of anti-B19 IgM antibodies.

- Hepatitis B virus infection has been associated with an arthritis limited to the pre-icteric prodrome.

- Hepatitis B and C viremia have been associated with cryoglobulinemia and vasculitis.

- Rubella virus infection frequently is associated with joint complaints in young adults.

RHEUMATOLOGIC MANIFESTATIONS OF HIV INFECTION

Musculoskeletal complaints can be among the first manifestations of HIV infection (Box 26.5). Articular manifestations can be extremely debilitating. Epidemiologic studies have not concluded whether HIV infection predisposes to

---

Box 26.5 **RHEUMATOLOGIC MANIFESTATIONS OF HUMAN IMMUNODEFICIENCY VIRUS (HIV)**

Arthralgia
Painful articular syndrome
HIV arthropathy
Reactive arthritis
Psoriatic arthritis
Undifferentiated spondyloarthropathy
Myositis
Vasculitis
Raynaud phenomenon
Sjögren-like syndrome (diffuse infiltrative lymphocytosis syndrome)
Septic arthritis
Fibromyalgia
Serologic abnormalities

---

arthritis or whether other viral or new mechanisms associated with HIV infection have a role in the pathogenesis of arthritis.

REACTIVE ARTHRITIS AND UNDIFFERENTIATED SPONDYLOARTHROPATHY

Signs and symptoms of reactive arthritis, psoriatic arthritis, or a nonspecific enthesopathy may occur before or simultaneously with the onset of HIV infection. These HIV-associated spondyloarthropathies have a predisposition for patients who are HLA-B27–positive and frequently are associated with severe enthesopathy and dactylitis. Progressive axial involvement is less common in HIV-associated arthritides. Most HIV-infected patients with reactive arthritis have skin and mucocutaneous manifestations, including urethritis, keratoderma blennorrhagicum, circinate balanitis, or painless oral ulcers, but conjunctivitis is unusual. In approximately one-third of patients, the onset of HIV-associated reactive arthritis has been linked to a documented infection with specific enteric organisms known to precipitate reactive arthritis.

- Enthesopathy and dactylitis may be severe in HIV-infected patients.

- Mucocutaneous features are common, but conjunctivitis is unusual.

LUPUS-LIKE ILLNESSES IN HIV INFECTION

Some of the features of SLE are similar to those of HIV infection. Fever, lymphadenopathy, mucous membrane lesions, rashes, arthritis, and hematologic abnormalities are common to both lupus and HIV infection. HIV infection also may be associated with polyclonal B-cell activation resulting in autoantibody production, including antinuclear and antiphospholipid antibodies. HIV infection should be considered in the differential diagnosis of SLE in any patient who is at risk for HIV. Antinuclear antibodies in high titer have not been found in HIV infection, and antibodies to double-stranded DNA are absent.

- Although some features of HIV infection may resemble those of SLE, antinuclear antibodies are present in low titer only, and antibodies to double-stranded DNA are absent.

HIV-ASSOCIATED VASCULITIS

Primary angiitis of the central nervous system, angiocentric lymphoproliferative vasculopathies, and polyarteritis nodosa have been reported. Any person with known HIV infection who presents with new mononeuritis should be evaluated for vasculitis.

The diffuse, infiltrative lymphocytosis syndrome is manifested by xerostomia, xerophthalmia, and salivary gland swelling mimicking Sjögren syndrome. The glands are infiltrated with CD8 lymphocytes. In contrast to Sjögren syndrome, HIV-positive patients usually do not have antibodies to SS-A or SS-B and are usually rheumatoid factor-negative.

There is an inflammatory articular syndrome associated with HIV infection that is distinct from any resemblance to spondyloarthropathy. Usually this is an oligoarthritis affecting joints of the lower extremities and is short-lived.

There is an acquired immunodeficiency syndrome–associated myopathy that may be viral. There is also a myopathy due to zidovudine therapy. Fibromyalgia also has been reported in up to 25% of HIV-infected patients.

OTHER TYPES OF INFECTIOUS ARTHRITIS

Whipple disease is a rare cause of arthropathy and usually is associated with constitutional symptoms, fever, neurologic symptoms, malabsorption, lymphadenopathy, and hyperpigmentation. There may be a slow, progressive dementia. The arthritic symptoms may precede the gastrointestinal manifestations. The infectious agent is *Tropheryma whipplei*. Polymerase chain reaction on small bowel or synovial biopsy or synovial fluid may be necessary to establish the diagnosis. Treatment is usually with doxycycline or trimethoprim-sulfamethoxazole, often required for a year.

SUMMARY

- A positive result of antinuclear antibody test alone is not specific for SLE.

- Mixed connective tissue disease is defined by overlap symptoms and a strongly positive titer of anti-RNP.

- A history of thrombosis and the presence of antiphospholipid antibodies define the antiphospholipid antibody syndrome.

- Scleroderma is defined by indurated skin of the fingers and the skin proximal to the metacarpophalangeal joints.

- Polymyositis is characterized by proximal muscle weakness, increased creatine kinase value, and myopathic findings on electromyography.

- Hepatitis C infection can cause arthritis, vasculitis, cryoglobulinemia, and a positive rheumatoid factor.

- Parvovirus in adults can mimic rheumatoid arthritis. It is diagnosed by demonstrating the presence of anti-B19 IgM antibodies.

- HIV infection is associated with a wide variety of rheumatologic conditions, including spondyloarthropathies, vasculitis, and Sjögren and lupus-like syndromes. It should be considered in patients at risk for the disease.

PART VI

ENDOCRINOLOGY

27.

DISORDERS OF THE THYROID GLAND

Marius N. Stan, MD

GOALS

- Review tests to assess thyroid function.
- Summarize the evaluation, causes, and management of hyperthyroidism and hypothyroidism.
- Recognize thyroid-related medical emergencies and review their management.
- Explain the evaluation of thyroid nodules.
- Describe thyroid malignancies.

LABORATORY ASSESSMENT OF THYROID FUNCTION

SERUM THYROTROPIN

Current assays measure thyrotropin (ie, thyroid-stimulating hormone) concentrations as low as 0.01 mIU/L, allowing differentiation between low-normal values and suppressed values. Thyrotropin levels are increased in primary hypothyroidism, during recovery from nonthyroid illness, and with thyroid hormone resistance. Thyrotropin levels are low in hyperthyroidism, in nonthyroid illness, and with use of drugs such as somatostatin, dopamine, and glucocorticoids. Measurement of the thyrotropin level is the best single test of thyroid function. However, thyrotropin levels are unreliable in cases of pituitary disease since values can be inappropriately normal in relation to thyroid hormone concentrations. Thus, thyrotropin levels may be normal or increased with thyrotropin-producing tumors and normal or decreased in central hypothyroidism.

THYROXINE

Free Thyroxine

Although free thyroxine (T_4) is frequently measured, there is substantial variability in the accuracy of the various assays available for clinical use. Serum free T_4 is decreased in hypothyroidism and nonthyroid illness and increased in hyperthyroidism, nonthyroid illness, and thyroid hormone resistance.

Total Thyroxine

Total T_4 concentration is a measurement of T_4 after displacement from the thyroid hormone–binding proteins such as thyroxine-binding globulin (TBG). Therefore, conditions that affect TBG concentration will also affect total T_4 measurements. Androgens, anabolic steroids, glucocorticoids, chronic liver disease, niacin, and familial TBG deficiency decrease total TBG. Estrogens, pregnancy, acute hepatitis, and familial TBG excess increase TBG and, therefore, total T_4 concentrations.

TOTAL TRIIODOTHYRONINE

Similar to total T_4, serum total triiodothyronine (T_3) concentration is decreased in hypothyroidism, nonthyroid illness, and caloric deprivation and by drugs such as propranolol, amiodarone, and glucocorticoids. Serum T_3 levels are increased in thyrotoxicosis and thyroid hormone resistance. Serum T_3 concentrations should be measured to establish or exclude the diagnosis of T_3 thyrotoxicosis in a patient who has a decreased thyrotropin level and a normal T_4 level. In subclinical hyperthyroidism, the thyrotropin level is suppressed, but T_3 and T_4 levels are normal; in subclinical hypothyroidism, the thyrotropin level is elevated, but T_3 and T_4 levels are normal (Table 27.1).

THYROID HORMONE–BINDING PROTEINS

Measurement of thyroid hormone–binding proteins can be helpful when there is a discrepancy between the total thyroid hormone concentrations and the other thyroid test results. The concentration of these proteins can be altered by medications (eg, increased by estrogens and decreased by androgens). In addition, the concentration of available protein for binding can be affected by changes in thyroid function (increased in hypothyroidism and decreased in hyperthyroidism) and by substances that interfere with the binding of thyroid hormones to the proteins (eg, carbamazepine and certain nonsteroidal anti-inflammatory drugs [NSAIDs]).

Table 27.1 **INTERPRETATION OF THYROID FUNCTION TEST RESULTS**

SERUM CONCENTRATION

Thyrotropin	Free T_4	T_3	DIAGNOSIS
Normal	Normal	Normal	Normal
High	Low	Normal or low	Primary hypothyroidism
High	Normal	Normal	Subclinical hypothyroidism
Low	High or normal	High	Hyperthyroidism
Low	Normal	Normal	Subclinical hyperthyroidism

Abbreviations: T_3, triiodothyronine; T_4, thyroxine.

THYROID SCANNING

Thyroid scanning displays the distribution of functioning thyroid tissue. It differentiates between hyperthyroidism caused by Graves disease and toxic thyroid nodules, ectopic thyroid tissue, and metastatic disease in the follow-up of patients with differentiated thyroid cancer.

RADIOACTIVE IODINE UPTAKE

Results of the radioactive iodine uptake (RAIU) test represent the percentage of radioactive iodine retained for a specific time after it is administered (usually 24 hours). RAIU is indicated during the evaluation of hyperthyroidism to distinguish between low- and high-uptake states and to aid in dose calculations when radioactive iodine is used to treat Graves disease.

SERUM THYROGLOBULIN

Thyroglobulin is used as a tumor marker in patients who have differentiated thyroid carcinoma. It is also useful in the differential diagnosis of hyperthyroidism to distinguish between an endogenous hormone source (increased thyroglobulin) and an exogenous hormone source (suppressed thyroglobulin).

THYROTROPIN RECEPTOR ANTIBODIES

Thyrotropin receptor antibodies (TRAbs) are a mixture of stimulating, inhibitory, and neutral antibodies. Some laboratories measure the stimulating fraction of TRAbs, called thyroid-stimulating immunoglobulins. They are markers of autoimmunity and are useful to diagnose Graves disease in patients who cannot undergo RAIU testing (eg, pregnant women). In women with active Graves disease or a history of it, an elevated TRAb level in the last trimester of pregnancy predicts an increased risk of neonatal hyperthyroidism.

THYROGLOBULIN AND THYROPEROXIDASE ANTIBODIES

Thyroglobulin and thyroperoxidase antibodies are used as markers of autoimmune thyroid disease. However, their absence does not exclude autoimmune thyroid disease. Conversely, they can also be found in healthy persons. High titers occur in more than 90% of patients with Hashimoto thyroiditis. When thyroglobulin antibodies are present, the measurement of thyroglobulin is unreliable for follow-up of thyroid malignancies.

THYROID ULTRASONOGRAPHY

Ultrasonography is used for the anatomical assessment of thyroid nodules and goiter and for the follow-up of patients after thyroid cancer treatment.

HYPERTHYROIDISM

ETIOLOGY

The etiology of primary thyroid disorders that cause hyperthyroidism can be divided into those characterized by increased production and release of T_4 (high RAIU) and those characterized by unregulated release of T_4 because of gland destruction (low RAIU) (Box 27.1).

The most common thyroid-related cause of hyperthyroidism in the United States is Graves disease. Other common causes are toxic nodular goiter and thyroiditis (lymphocytic or subacute). Exogenous hyperthyroidism is a common cause of nonthyroid hyperthyroidism, particularly in patients receiving combination T_4 and T_3 treatment.

- Primary causes of hyperthyroidism are related to increased production and release of T_4 (high-RAIU causes) or unregulated release of T_4 because of gland destruction (low-RAIU causes).

- Graves disease is the most common thyroid-related cause of hyperthyroidism in the United States.

- Toxic nodular goiter and thyroiditis are common causes of hyperthyroidism.

Box 27.1 **ETIOLOGY OF HYPERTHYROIDISM ACCORDING TO RADIOACTIVE IODINE UPTAKE (RAIU)**

Normal or elevated RAIU over the neck
  Graves disease
  Toxic nodule or toxic multinodular goiter
  Thyrotropin-producing pituitary adenoma
  Thyroid hormone resistance
  Trophoblastic disease
Low or nearly absent RAIU over the neck
  Painless lymphocytic thyroiditis
  Subacute painful thyroiditis
  Amiodarone-induced thyroiditis
  Iatrogenic thyrotoxicosis
  Struma ovarii

Box 27.2 **SYMPTOMS AND SIGNS OF HYPERTHYROIDISM**

Symptoms
  Heat intolerance
  Palpitations
  Nervousness
  Irritability
  Insomnia
Signs
  Tachycardia
  Increased sweating
  Diarrhea
  Weight loss
  Muscle weakness (proximal)

- Exogenous hyperthyroidism commonly causes nonthyroid hyperthyroidism in patients taking thyroid hormone replacement.

CLINICAL FEATURES

Most clinical features reflect the effects of excess thyroid hormone. Typical symptoms and signs are listed in Box 27.2. Most patients with hyperthyroidism have a small, firm goiter.

Graves ophthalmopathy is specific for Graves disease. Ocular manifestations include findings due to sympathetic overactivity from hyperthyroidism of any cause (retraction of the upper lid, stare, and lid lag) or findings unique to Graves ophthalmopathy (lid edema, conjunctival injection, chemosis, proptosis, and extraocular muscle weakness). Patients with Graves ophthalmopathy may complain of a gritty sensation in the eyes, excessive lacrimation, photophobia, and diplopia.

Elderly patients with hyperthyroidism may present with atypical findings. Findings in patients with apathetic thyrotoxicosis, for example, include apathy, weight loss, supraventricular tachyarrhythmia, and congestive heart failure. Gynecomastia may develop in younger men.

- Clinical features reflect the hypermetabolic state due to excess thyroid hormone.

- Sympathetic overreactivity due to thyroid hormone excess causes upper eyelid retraction, stare, and lid lag.

- In elderly patients, findings of apathy, weight loss, supraventricular tachyarrhythmia, and heart failure may be from apathetic thyrotoxicosis.

DIAGNOSIS

The diagnosis of hyperthyroidism is biochemical:

- Overt hyperthyroidism—suppressed thyrotropin and elevated levels of T_4 or T_3 (or both).

- Subclinical hyperthyroidism—suppressed thyrotropin with normal levels of T_4 and T_3.

- Pituitary thyrotropin-secreting tumor—inappropriately *normal* or *high* thyrotropin level with elevated levels of T_4 or T_3 (or both).

A low serum thyrotropin level alone is not diagnostic of hyperthyroidism because a low level can also be encountered in nonthyroid illness, glucocorticoid therapy, dopamine therapy, and secondary hypothyroidism.

- Biochemical parameters establish the diagnosis and lead to the cause of hyperthyroidism.

SPECIFIC CAUSES

Graves Disease

Graves disease is characterized by hyperthyroidism with diffuse RAIU and the presence of TRAbs and thyroid-stimulating immunoglobulins, which have a stimulatory effect on the receptor causing the hyperthyroidism. The disease is more common in young women and causes the thyroid to be mildly enlarged and firm.

Graves ophthalmopathy and pretibial dermopathy are usually associated with Graves disease. TRAbs are the pathophysiologic link between them. Treating hyperthyroidism is an important first step in the management of these conditions. The conditions associated with Graves (ophthalmopathy and dermopathy) respond to treatment of hyperthyroidism when initiated early in the disease process.

- Graves disease is defined as hyperthyroidism with *diffuse* RAIU and TRAbs.

- Young women are more commonly affected than men.

- Associated conditions include a mildly enlarged and firm thyroid, Graves ophthalmopathy, and pretibial dermopathy.

Painless Lymphocytic Thyroiditis (Postpartum Thyroiditis or Silent Thyroiditis)

Painless lymphocytic thyroiditis is usually a self-limiting disease that occurs most commonly in the postpartum period and tends to recur with subsequent pregnancies. However, it can also occur unrelated to pregnancy and in males.

The classic presentation is a sequential triphasic pattern: hyperthyroid phase (suppressed thyrotropin, low RAIU, and increased levels of free T_4) is followed by a hypothyroid phase, which is followed by a recovery phase with normal thyroid function. This triphasic pattern may not be seen.

Treatment is symptomatic. β-Blockers may be needed during the hyperthyroid phase, and temporary thyroid hormone replacement may be necessary during the hypothyroid phase. In some cases, the hypothyroidism may be permanent.

There is no indication for antithyroid medications or radioactive iodine therapy because the hyperthyroidism results from the release of preformed thyroid hormone, not increased production.

- Painless lymphocytic thyroiditis is a self-limited illness that occurs most often in the postpartum period but which may occur unrelated to pregnancy or in males.
- The classic triphasic presentation includes a hyperthyroid phase followed by a hypothyroid phase followed by the recovery of thyroid function.

Subacute Painful Thyroiditis (de Quervain Thyroiditis)

Subacute thyroiditis is characterized by a painful, tender goiter. Patients often complain of fever, malaise, myalgia, and a history of upper respiratory tract infection. Transient hyperthyroidism (low RAIU) is often present at diagnosis and may be followed by transient hypothyroidism. The erythrocyte sedimentation rate is invariably increased.

Treatment is symptomatic. β-Blockers and thyroid hormone replacement are used as discussed for painless thyroiditis. NSAIDs and corticosteroids are useful for pain. The response to corticosteroid therapy is dramatic, typically with relief of symptoms within 24 hours.

- Transient hyperthyroidism (at diagnosis) followed by transient hypothyroidism may occur.
- Erythrocyte sedimentation rate is always elevated.
- Symptomatic treatment is provided with β-blockers and thyroid hormone replacement; NSAIDs and corticosteroids are used to manage pain.

Multinodular Goiter

Toxic multinodular goiter occurs in patients with a long-standing nodular goiter, in which autonomous functioning nodules develop. The hyperthyroidism is usually mild, yet cardiovascular manifestations tend to dominate. The goiter is large, nodular, and asymmetric. The thyroid may be difficult to palpate in some patients because of substernal extension or a short neck. Patients are at risk for symptom exacerbation from iodine-induced hyperthyroidism due to exposure to iodinated contrast media.

- Toxic multinodular goiter results from the development of autonomous functioning nodules in a long-standing nodular goiter.
- Palpating the thyroid gland may be difficult because of a substernal extension or a short neck.

Toxic Thyroid Adenoma

Toxic thyroid nodules are follicular adenomas with autonomously increased thyroid hormone production. The nodule is solitary, usually larger than 3 cm, and found in middle-aged women. It is easy to palpate and has a firm consistency. A radioisotope scan demonstrates intense uptake in the nodule, with suppressed uptake in the rest of the gland.

- This condition is characterized by a large, solitary nodule and most commonly occurs in middle-aged women.
- The nodule demonstrates intense radioisotope uptake, with suppressed uptake in the rest of the gland.

Exogenous Hyperthyroidism

Exogenous hyperthyroidism can result from the use of T_4 or T_3 (or both). It should be suspected if thyrotoxic patients have low RAIU and no palpable goiter. Low serum levels of thyroglobulin help to differentiate this disorder from painless lymphocytic thyroiditis.

- Thyrotoxic patients with low RAIU and a nonpalpable goiter should be suspected of having exogenous hyperthyroidism.
- Low thyroglobulin levels differentiate this from painless lymphocytic thyroiditis.

THERAPY

Thionamides

Methimazole and propylthiouracil can be used to treat hyperthyroidism due to increased production of thyroid hormone. They act by blocking thyroid hormone synthesis. Thionamides are used in Graves disease to control hyperthyroidism, with the hope that the disease will undergo spontaneous remission during therapy. Treatment is given for 12 to 18 months and then discontinued. The effect of thionamides is temporary, and hyperthyroidism often recurs after discontinuation. In more than 50% of patients, the disease relapses within the first 3 to 6 months after treatment is stopped.

Potentially serious adverse effects include agranulocytosis and hepatitis. Agranulocytosis can develop abruptly (within a few hours). It typically manifests initially with a severe sore throat. Hepatitis is more common with propylthiouracil; therefore, methimazole is the drug of choice.

- Methimazole and propylthiouracil block thyroid hormone synthesis.
- These drugs are used to treat the hyperthyroidism of Graves disease; spontaneous remission may result.
- Hyperthyroidism often recurs after use of the medication is stopped; in 50% of patients, the disease relapses within the first 3–6 months.

Radioactive Iodine

Radioactive iodine therapy effectively ablates the thyroid gland and is the most commonly used therapy in the United States for high-RAIU hyperthyroidism. The goal of therapy is to render the patient hypothyroid. The maximal effect is apparent within 2 to 3 months. Treatment of toxic multinodular goiter requires higher doses of radioactive iodine and often more than 1 course of treatment. Radioactive iodine therapy has not been associated with long-term risks, but pregnancy and breast-feeding are contraindications. Radioactive iodine can worsen the course of active Graves ophthalmopathy, but that worsening can be avoided with the prophylactic use of glucocorticoids.

- Hypothyroidism is the goal of therapy.

- Pregnancy and breast-feeding are contraindications to the use of radioactive iodine, but overall no long-term risks have been associated with the use of radioactive iodine.

- Active Graves ophthalmopathy may be worsened by radioactive iodine, but that worsening can be avoided with the prophylactic use of glucocorticoids.

Surgery

Near-total or total thyroidectomy is usually unnecessary for treatment of Graves disease or toxic multinodular goiter. If nodules appear suspicious with fine-needle aspiration (FNA), surgery should be strongly considered. Thyroid lobectomy is used for toxic thyroid adenoma. In addition, surgery is usually considered when *rapid* restoration of a euthyroid state is desired, when the patient is pregnant, or when the patient has a large, compressive goiter. Damage to the recurrent laryngeal nerves or parathyroid glands is uncommon (<1%-2%) with experienced surgeons. To prevent thyroid storm and excessive bleeding from the overactive friable gland, the patient should be treated preoperatively with stable iodine solution in combination with antithyroid drug therapy and β-blockers. This approach should render the patient euthyroid or nearly euthyroid at surgery.

- When nodules appear suspicious on FNA, surgery is recommended.

- Toxic thyroid adenoma is treated with thyroid lobectomy.

- Surgical treatment is recommended when rapid restoration of a euthyroid state is desired, when the patient is pregnant, or when the patient has a large, compressive goiter.

- Thyroid storm and excessive bleeding (the gland is friable) can be prevented with preoperative use of antithyroid drugs, β-blockers, and stable iodine solution.

Supportive Therapy

Symptomatic patients should be given β-blockers to control adrenergic manifestations of hyperthyroidism while waiting for definitive therapy to take effect.

THYROID STORM

Thyroid storm is a state of life-threatening hyperthyroidism with severe multisystem manifestations. It develops in patients who have acute illness superimposed on uncontrolled thyrotoxicosis and in patients who have a sudden increase in thyroid hormone levels from postoperative manipulation or radiation-induced thyroiditis. Thyroid storm is characterized by delirium, fever, tachycardia, hypotension, vomiting, diarrhea, and, eventually, coma. Treatment should be initiated immediately in the intensive care unit. Antithyroid therapy with propylthiouracil is preferred. Iodine solution is added to inhibit the release of preformed thyroid hormone and decrease peripheral conversion of T_4 to T_3. β-Blocker therapy, supportive therapy directed at systemic disturbances, and therapy directed at the precipitating event should be delivered in parallel.

- Thyroid storm is a medical emergency with multisystem manifestations.

- Delirium, fever, tachycardia, hypotension, diarrhea, vomiting, and coma characterize thyroid storm.

- Propylthiouracil is the preferred treatment, with the addition of iodine solution to inhibit the release of preformed thyroid hormone and decrease peripheral conversion of T_4 to T_3.

- β-Blocker therapy and supportive therapy should be directed at end-organ toxicities.

HYPOTHYROIDISM

Hypothyroidism can be primary (intrinsic thyroid disease) or secondary (hypothalamic-pituitary disease). Primary hypothyroidism accounts for more than 99% of all cases.

- Nearly all cases of hypothyroidism result from intrinsic thyroid disease.

ETIOLOGY

The most common cause in the United States is Hashimoto thyroiditis, an autoimmune thyroid disease. It tends to cluster in families and is more common in women. Other causes of hypothyroidism include hypothyroidism after radioactive iodine treatment of hyperthyroidism, thyroidectomy, radiotherapy for neck malignancies, and transient hypothyroidism during the course of subacute or painless thyroiditis.

- Causes of hypothyroidism include radioactive iodine treatment, thyroidectomy, radiotherapy for neck cancers, and subacute or painless thyroiditis, which causes transient hypothyroidism.

CLINICAL FEATURES

The clinical manifestation of hypothyroidism depends on the degree and duration of the deficiency. When symptoms are present, they are nonspecific. Many patients are asymptomatic at presentation, with hypothyroidism having been diagnosed through routine screening. The most common signs and symptoms are listed in Box 27.3.

Macrocytic anemia (due to pernicious anemia or autoimmune disease) or microcytic anemia (iron deficiency due to menorrhagia) may be present. Patients with dramatic increases in thyrotropin may experience galactorrhea (thyrotropin stimulates prolactin secretion). Rarely, patients may have psychosis, deafness, or cerebellar ataxia (or any combination of these). If patients have respiratory depression, central hypoventilation and apnea may be observed. Hyponatremia due to syndrome of inappropriate secretion of antidiuretic hormone may be present. Associated laboratory findings include hyperlipidemia and increased levels of aspartate aminotransferase, lactate dehydrogenase, or creatine kinase. The possibility of associated endocrinopathies as part of a polyglandular autoimmune syndrome (Addison disease, type 1 diabetes mellitus, hypoparathyroidism, or pernicious anemia) should be considered when hypothyroidism is identified. It may also be associated with vitiligo and other autoimmune or connective tissue diseases.

- Symptoms of hypothyroidism, when present, are generally nonspecific.

- Hypothyroidism may be associated with a polyglandular autoimmune syndrome, other autoimmune diseases, or connective tissue diseases.

DIAGNOSIS

Low T_4 and increased thyrotropin levels are diagnostic of overt primary hypothyroidism if nonthyroid illness has been excluded. Subclinical hypothyroidism is identified when the thyrotropin level is elevated, but the T_4 level is normal. The decision to treat depends on the degree of thyrotropin elevation. Hashimoto thyroiditis is usually associated with a firm goiter and a high titer of antimicrosomal (thyroid peroxidase) antibodies. A low T_4 and inappropriately normal or low thyrotropin indicate secondary hypothyroidism. Magnetic resonance imaging of the head and pituitary function tests should be performed.

- Increased thyrotropin with low T_4 is diagnostic of primary hypothyroidism in the absence of nonthyroid illness as a potential cause.

- Subclinical hypothyroidism is present when thyrotropin is elevated but T_4 is normal; therapy depends on the degree of thyrotropin elevation.

- Secondary hypothyroidism is present when T_4 is low but thyrotropin is low or normal. Magnetic resonance imaging of the head and pituitary function tests should be done.

THERAPY

Thyroid hormone replacement therapy is initiated with synthetic T_4 (levothyroxine). The goals of therapy are to normalize thyrotropin in primary hypothyroidism and to normalize T_4 in secondary hypothyroidism. Failure to normalize thyrotropin concentrations may indicate poor adherence to drug therapy, decreased absorption due to concomitant use of interfering medications (eg, sucralfate, calcium supplements, ferrous sulfate), or gastrointestinal tract disease. Other possibilities include progressive thyroid disease, increased thyroid-binding proteins (as with pregnancy or estrogen use), and increased hormone clearance (eg, with phenytoin or carbamazepine). It is important to assess thyrotropin annually or as indicated by the patient's symptoms.

- In primary hypothyroidism, the goal of therapy is to normalize thyrotropin.

- In secondary hypothyroidism, the goal of therapy is to normalize T_4.

- When thyrotropin cannot be normalized, possible causes include poor adherence to drug therapy, decreased drug absorption, gastrointestinal tract disease, progressive thyroid disease, use of other drugs leading to increased hormone clearance, and states of increased thyroid-binding protein availability.

MISCELLANEOUS CIRCUMSTANCES

T_4 Replacement Therapy in Pregnancy

Most women with primary hypothyroidism require an increase in the dose of levothyroxine during pregnancy (average increase, 25%-30%). Women receiving T_4 replacement therapy should be counseled about the importance of ensuring adequate replacement *before* conception because of the multiple potential complications for both mother and fetus, including first-trimester spontaneous abortion, preterm delivery, and perinatal morbidity and mortality. Thyrotropin levels should be assessed periodically during pregnancy, and the T_4 dose should be adjusted as necessary to maintain a normal thyrotropin.

- The levothyroxine dose usually needs to be increased during pregnancy.

- Adequate T_4 replacement therapy before conception is important, and patients require counseling.

T₄ Replacement Therapy in Patients With Cardiac Disease and in Elderly Patients

Replacement therapy for elderly patients and patients who have coronary artery disease should start at a low dose (25–50 mcg daily) and increase gradually until thyrotropin is normal. Hypothyroidism does not contraindicate cardiac intervention, although there is an increased risk of hyponatremia and other perioperative complications.

- For elderly patients and patients with cardiac disease, initiate *low*-dose thyroid hormone replacement therapy, and gradually increase the dose until thyrotropin is normal.
- Cardiac interventions are *not* contraindicated in patients with hypothyroidism, but patients should be assessed for hyponatremia and other perioperative complications.

Subclinical Hypothyroidism

Subclinical hypothyroidism is a relatively common disorder, affecting 5% to 15% of elderly patients. The risk of progression to overt hypothyroidism increases with age, the presence of thyroid antibodies, and thyrotropin levels greater than 10 mIU/L. A trial of replacement therapy is indicated for symptomatic patients and for patients at risk of progressive disease.

- Risk of progression to overt hypothyroidism increases with age, the presence of thyroid antibodies, and elevated thyrotropin levels.
- Symptomatic patients and patients at risk of progressive disease should receive a trial of replacement therapy.

Myxedema Coma

Myxedema coma is severe, life-threatening hypothyroidism. It occurs in patients who have severe, untreated hypothyroidism with a superimposed acute illness (eg, infection, surgery, or myocardial infarction), exposure to cold, or the use of sedatives or opiates. The onset is insidious, with progressive stupor culminating in coma. Seizures, hypothermia, hypotension, hypoventilation, hyponatremia, and hypoglycemia may be present. The mortality rate is high (20%-50%). Treatment should be initiated promptly with intravenous T₄ and supportive measures.

- Patients with myxedema coma become progressively stuporous and eventually lapse into a coma.
- Seizures, hypothermia, hypotension, hypoventilation, hyponatremia, and hypoglycemia are possible findings.
- Mortality is high, and treatment with intravenous T₄ and supportive therapy must be initiated promptly.

THYROID NODULES

Thyroid nodules are extremely common and increase in frequency with age. They may be noticed by the patient, detected during a routine medical examination, or detected during neck imaging performed for other reasons. When nodules are identified, the primary concern is whether they are benign or malignant. At least 95% of palpable thyroid nodules are benign. The likelihood of malignancy increases with solitary nodules, older age, male sex, and a history of radiotherapy to the head and neck (especially during childhood).

- Factors increasing the likelihood of malignancy include solitary nodule, older age, male sex, and a history of head and neck radiotherapy.

Evaluation should begin with thyrotropin measurement to determine whether the nodule functions autonomously. Malignancy is substantially less likely if the thyrotropin level is suppressed, in which case ultrasonography of the thyroid and RAIU should be performed. A nonautonomous nodule should be sampled by ultrasound-guided FNA if the nodule is palpable or larger than 1 cm. Thyroid nodule FNA has high sensitivity and specificity for excluding malignancy if performed and interpreted by experienced personnel. If the aspirate is benign, annual follow-up with palpation, thyroid ultrasonography, and thyrotropin measurement is adequate. A change in nodule size requires consideration of another biopsy. A nondiagnostic aspirate requires additional aspiration. If the aspirate is interpreted as suspicious or compatible with malignancy, surgical intervention is required. Compressive symptoms (dysphonia, dysphagia, and dyspnea) should prompt surgical intervention even if the nodule is benign.

- A thyroid nodule is likely benign if the thyrotropin level is suppressed.
- RAUI and thyroid ultrasonography should be performed when the nodule is autonomous.
- Nonautonomous nodules should be sampled by FNA if they are palpable or >1 cm.
- Surgical intervention should be undertaken if FNA findings are suspicious or compatible with malignancy, or if the patient has compressive symptoms even if the nodule is benign.

THYROID CANCER

DIFFERENTIATED THYROID MALIGNANCIES

Papillary Thyroid Carcinoma

Papillary thyroid carcinoma is the most common type of thyroid cancer (80%-90% of cases). It has a bimodal incidence distribution, with increased incidence in early adulthood and again in late adulthood. Dissemination is typically lymphatic. Lung and bone metastases may occur. Usually found as a thyroid nodule, papillary thyroid carcinoma may also manifest as cervical adenopathy or as an incidental finding in an excised thyroid gland.

Follicular Carcinoma

Follicular carcinoma is the diagnosis in 10% to 15% of thyroid cancer cases. It typically spreads hematogenously. The usual manifestation is a thyroid mass or metastases to the lungs, bones, or brain. Rarely, it causes thyrotoxicosis if the tumor burden is large.

- Papillary thyroid cancer has a bimodal incidence distribution: early and late adulthood.
- Follicular carcinoma usually manifests as a thyroid mass or metastases to the lung, bones, or brain.

OTHER THYROID CANCERS

Anaplastic Carcinoma

Anaplastic carcinoma typically manifests as a rapidly enlarging thyroid mass that causes pain and compressive local neck symptoms. It is highly undifferentiated and the prognosis is extremely poor, carrying a median survival of less than 3 months after diagnosis.

Medullary Thyroid Carcinoma

Medullary thyroid carcinoma is a neuroendocrine tumor that produces calcitonin. It is part of a familial syndrome in 25% of cases (multiple endocrine neoplasia type 2); it typically manifests as either a solitary nodule or a dominant nodule in a multinodular goiter; and it is frequently metastatic at diagnosis, with 50% of patients having lymph node involvement. Tumor production of hormonal substances can lead to diarrhea and facial flushing or Cushing syndrome. Because there are *RET* proto-oncogene mutations in the familial form, patients with medullary thyroid carcinoma should be offered genetic testing. Median survival is less than that for differentiated thyroid malignancies, but significantly better than for anaplastic carcinoma.

- Anaplastic carcinoma usually manifests as a rapidly enlarging, painful thyroid mass that causes compressive symptoms.
- Medullary thyroid carcinoma is a neuroendocrine tumor that produces calcitonin and may produce other hormones.
- Medullary thyroid carcinoma produces hormones that may cause Cushing syndrome or carcinoid-like symptoms.

MANAGEMENT OF THYROID MALIGNANCY

Surgical excision is the therapy of choice for differentiated thyroid cancer and medullary thyroid carcinoma. Excision of anaplastic carcinoma may be undertaken to palliate tracheal compression. Papillary cancer carries the best prognosis of all thyroid malignancies. Factors associated with a poorer prognosis include age greater than 45 years at diagnosis, incomplete

resection, extensive local invasion, large size of primary tumor, and presence of distant metastases. Cervical lymph node involvement does not affect prognosis.

- Differentiated thyroid cancers and medullary thyroid cancer should be treated surgically.
- Papillary thyroid cancer carries the best prognosis of all thyroid malignancies.
- Poor prognostic indicators include age greater than 45 years, incomplete resection, extensive local invasion, large size of primary tumor, and distant metastases.

Patients at high risk for recurrence often undergo radioactive iodine therapy to ablate the thyroid remnant. Suppressive therapy is then initiated, with the target thyrotropin level less than 0.1 mIU/L. Patients at low risk for recurrence do not require thyroid remnant ablation and are treated with thyroid hormone replacement to maintain thyrotropin at the low end of the reference range (0.1–0.5 mIU/L). Patients should be reevaluated 3 to 6 months later and annually thereafter. Most differentiated thyroid malignancies synthesize and secrete thyroglobulin, which can be used as a marker of recurrent or persistent disease. Whole-body iodine scanning and neck ultrasonography are also used widely to follow patients after treatment of thyroid cancer. Recurrences are treated with excision or radioactive iodine, depending on location.

- Postoperatively, patients at low risk for recurrence begin thyroid hormone replacement to maintain thyrotropin at 0.1–0.5 mIU/L; these patients do not require remnant ablation.
- Thyroglobulin can be used as a marker of recurrent or persistent disease in patients with differentiated malignancies.

MISCELLANEOUS THYROID DISORDERS

SICK EUTHYROID SYNDROME

Patients with systemic illness frequently have abnormal thyroid function test results without identifiable intrinsic thyroid disease. The abnormalities resolve with recovery from the acute illness. Specific therapy is not required. The main challenge is to distinguish between nonthyroid illness and intrinsic thyroid or pituitary disease, since thyrotropin may be normal or low initially but increase during recovery. In the absence of specific features suggestive of thyroid disease (eg, goiter, extrathyroidal manifestations of Graves disease, hypopituitarism, and arrhythmias), thyroid testing should be avoided in the inpatient setting.

- Sick euthyroid syndrome occurs when patients with systemic illness have abnormal thyroid function test results and no identifiable thyroid disease.

- Avoid thyroid testing in the inpatient setting unless patients have clinical features suggestive of intrinsic thyroid disease.

AMIODARONE AND THE THYROID

With its high iodine content, amiodarone causes thyroid dysfunction in about 15% of patients; amiodarone-associated thyroid dysfunction is more likely in patients with thyroid abnormalities. The most common abnormality in iodine-replete geographic areas is hypothyroidism. Hyperthyroidism may be caused by an increase in thyroid hormone production (type 1) or a destructive thyroiditis (type 2). Medical therapy is less effective than for other causes of hyperthyroidism; in some cases, thyroidectomy is needed. Periodic monitoring of thyroid function is essential for patients treated with amiodarone, particularly elderly patients.

- Amiodarone may lead to thyroid dysfunction due to its high iodine content.
- Hyperthyroidism due to amiodarone may occur because of increased thyroid hormone production (type 1) or destructive thyroiditis (type 2).
- Thyroidectomy may be needed to treat hyperthyroidism since medical therapy is often less effective for amiodarone-induced hyperthyroidism.

SUMMARY

- Primary causes of hyperthyroidism are related to increased production and release of T_4 (high-RAIU causes) or unregulated release of T_4 because of gland destruction (low-RAIU causes).
- Graves disease is the most common thyroid-related cause of hyperthyroidism in the United States.
- Biochemical parameters establish the diagnosis and lead to the cause of hyperthyroidism.
- Thyroid storm is a medical emergency with multisystem manifestations: delirium, fever, tachycardia, hypotension, diarrhea, vomiting, and coma.
- Causes of hypothyroidism include radioactive iodine treatment, thyroidectomy, radiotherapy for neck cancers, and subacute or painless thyroiditis, which causes transient hypothyroidism.
- In primary hypothyroidism, the goal of therapy is to normalize thyrotropin; in secondary hypothyroidism, the goal of therapy is to normalize T_4.
- A thyroid nodule is likely benign if the thyrotropin level is suppressed.
- Papillary thyroid cancer carries the best prognosis of all thyroid malignancies.

28.

LIPID DISORDERS AND DIABETES MELLITUS

Maria L. Collazo-Clavell, MD

GOALS

- Review the various lipid disorders.

- Recognize other cardiovascular disease risk factors that affect lipid management.

- Enumerate management strategies for lipid disorders.

- Understand the goals of lipid-lowering treatment based on patient characteristics.

- Review type 1 and type 2 diabetes mellitus.

- Recognize clinical manifestations of diabetes mellitus.

- Enumerate management strategies for diabetes mellitus.

- Understand acute and chronic complications of diabetes mellitus and management strategies.

LIPID DISORDERS

ETIOLOGY

Disorders of lipoprotein metabolism predispose to premature coronary heart disease (CHD) and vascular disease. *Primary hyperlipidemia* is an increase in lipoprotein concentration. It may be caused by genetic defects (eg, absence of the low-density lipoprotein [LDL] receptor) or acquired defects (eg, interactions of aging, weight gain, poor diet, sedentary lifestyle, and genetic predisposition). Features of primary hyperlipidemias are outlined in Table 28.1. *Secondary hyperlipidemia* may be caused by a coexisting disorder (eg, poorly controlled diabetes mellitus, hypothyroidism, nephrotic syndrome) or the use of drugs (eg, corticosteroids, antirejection agents) (Box 28.1).

- Hyperlipidemia can be secondary to drugs or diseases.

- Hyperlipidemia may be genetic or acquired (or both).

CLINICAL FEATURES

Hyperlipidemia is usually diagnosed on screening. Patients usually do not have physical findings directly attributable to hyperlipidemia; however, some patients have eyelid xanthelasmata and arcus corneae. Extreme increases in LDL cholesterol (LDL-C) may cause tendon xanthomas. Increased intermediate-density lipoprotein (IDL) may result in palmar tuboeruptive xanthomas. Hyperchylomicronemia can cause eruptive xanthomas on the buttocks.

Increased LDL-C, IDL, and Lp(a) lipoprotein and decreased high-density lipoprotein cholesterol (HDL-C) all confer increased risk of atherosclerotic vascular disease. Increased HDL-C is associated with decreased atherogenic risk. Hypertriglyceridemia may be atherogenic by inducing alterations in other lipoproteins. Triglycerides have an unidentified direct atherogenic action. Pancreatitis may develop with very high triglyceride concentrations (generally >1,000 mg/dL).

- Patients with hyperlipidemia are often asymptomatic.

- Hyperlipidemia may lead to pathognomonic physical findings, depending on which fraction is elevated and the degree and duration of elevation.

- Classic physical findings are tendon xanthomas, eruptive xanthomas involving the buttocks, and palmar eruptive xanthomas; such changes are uncommon and are attributable to specific lipid fractions.

- Clinical sequelae of hyperlipidemia include ischemic vascular disease and pancreatitis for severe hypertriglyceridemia.

DIAGNOSIS

The Third Adult Treatment Panel of the National Cholesterol Education Program recommends that adults older than 20 years be evaluated for hypercholesterolemia. LDL-C concentrations can be reliably estimated if plasma triglyceride concentrations are less than 400 mg/dL. Nonmodifiable risk factors for CHD include the following:

1. Age older than 45 (men) or 55 (women)

Table 28.1 FEATURES OF PRIMARY HYPERLIPIDEMIAS

FEATURE	FAMILIAL HYPERCHOLESTEROLEMIA	FAMILIAL COMBINED HYPERLIPIDEMIA	FAMILIAL DYSBETALIPOPROTEINEMIA	FAMILIAL HYPERTRIGLYCERIDEMIA	SEVERE HYPERTRIGLYCERIDEMIA Early Onset	SEVERE HYPERTRIGLYCERIDEMIA Adult Onset
Pathophysiology	Defective LDL receptor or defective apo B-100; impaired catabolism of LDL	Overproduction of hepatic VLDL–apo B-100 but not of VLDL-Tg	Defective or absent apo E; excess of CM remnants & VLDL in fasting state	Overproduction of hepatic VLDL–Tg but not of apo B-100	Lipoprotein lipase deficiency Apo C-II deficiency; defect in CM & VLDL catabolism	Overproduction of hepatic VLDL–Tg Delayed catabolism of CMs & VLDL
Mode of inheritance	Autosomal codominant	Autosomal dominant	Autosomal recessive	Autosomal dominant	Autosomal recessive	Autosomal recessive
Estimated population frequency	1:500	1:50	1:5,000	1:50	<1:10,000	Rare
Risk of CHD	+++	++	+	+ In families in which HDL-C is deficient	−	+
Physical findings	Arcus senilis Tendinous xanthomas	Arcus senilis	Arcus senilis Tuberoeruptive & palmar xanthomas	None	Lipemia retinalis Eruptive xanthomas	Milky plasma Lipemia retinalis Eruptive xanthomas Pancreatitis
Associated findings		Obesity Glucose intolerance Hyperuricemia HDL-C deficiency	Obesity Glucose intolerance Hyperuricemia	Obesity Glucose intolerance Hyperuricemia HDL-C deficiency	HDL-C deficiency Recurrent abdominal pain Pancreatitis Hepatosplenomegaly	Obesity Glucose intolerance Hyperuricemia HDL-C deficiency Pancreatitis
Treatment	Diet Niacin & resin Statin & resin Probucol & resin	Diet Drugs singly or in combination with niacin, statin, gemfibrozil, resin	Diet Niacin Gemfibrozil Statin	Diet Niacin Gemfibrozil Abstain from alcohol, estrogen	Diet Fish oil	Diet Control diabetes when present Avoid alcohol, estrogen Gemfibrozil Fish oil

Abbreviations: apo, apolipoprotein; CHD, coronary heart disease; CM, chylomicron; HDL-C, high-density lipoprotein cholesterol; LDL, low-density lipoprotein; Tg, triglyceride; VLDL, very low-density lipoprotein; +++, very high; ++, high; +, moderate; −, no increased risk.

Box 28.1 CAUSES OF SECONDARY HYPERLIPIDEMIA

Increased LDL-C
    Hypothyroidism
    Dysglobulinemia
    Nephrotic syndrome
    Obstructive liver disease
    Progestins
    Anabolic steroids, glucocorticoid therapy
    Anorexia nervosa
    Acute intermittent porphyria
Increased triglycerides
    Obesity
    Diabetes mellitus
    Hypothyroidism
    Sedentary lifestyle
    Alcohol
    Renal insufficiency
    Estrogens
    β-Blockers
    Thiazides, steroids
    Dysglobulinemia
    Systemic lupus erythematosus
Decreased HDL-C
    Hypertriglyceridemia
    Obesity
    Diabetes mellitus
    Cigarette smoking
    Sedentary lifestyle
    β-Blockers
    Progestins
    Anabolic steroids

Abbreviations: HDL-C, high-density lipoprotein cholesterol; LDL-C, low-density lipoprotein cholesterol.

2. Family history of premature CHD (parent or sibling with myocardial infarction or sudden death before age 55)

Modifiable risk factors for CHD include the following:

1. Smoking

2. Hypertension

3. Diabetes mellitus

4. HDL-C <35 mg/dL (HDL-C >60 mg/dL is protective)

Lp(a) lipoprotein is an independent risk factor for vascular disease and should be measured in patients with a strong family history of premature ischemic heart disease without conventional risk factors and in patients with established CHD with disease progression despite control of conventional risk factors.

- The decision to measure Lp(a) lipoprotein should be based on individual patient risk factors.

THERAPY

Therapy is guided with use of the National Cholesterol Education Program guidelines (Table 28.2). Specific therapy and LDL-C goals depend on the need to treat concurrent ischemic heart disease or a CHD risk equivalent such as type 2 diabetes mellitus (both considered secondary prevention) or risk factors for ischemic heart disease (primary prevention). Patients with a CHD risk equivalent have a risk greater than 20% for a cardiovascular event in 10 years.

- CHD risk equivalents include type 2 diabetes mellitus, symptomatic carotid artery disease, peripheral artery disease, abdominal aortic aneurysm, and chronic kidney disease.

- High-risk patients have 2 or more risk factors.

- Very high-risk patients have type 2 diabetes mellitus or poorly controlled risk factors.

Treatment includes therapeutic lifestyle changes, correction of secondary causes (eg, treatment of hypothyroidism or diabetes mellitus), and use of lipid-lowering agents to achieve lipid goals when clinically indicated.

THERAPEUTIC LIFESTYLE CHANGES

Therapeutic lifestyle changes are first-line therapies to reduce the risk associated with lipid disorders. These therapies include smoking cessation, healthy dietary changes, regular exercise, and weight management. Smoking cessation lowers the risk for CHD events in both primary and secondary prevention and is associated with an increase in HDL-C. The American Heart Association step I diet recommends limiting dietary fat intake (≤30% of total calories, with <10% of calories from saturated fat and avoidance of trans fats). Alcohol restriction can decrease triglyceride concentrations. At least 150 minutes of moderate-intensity aerobic activity weekly is recommended.

Weight measurement, body mass index (BMI) calculation (weight in kilograms divided by height in meters squared), and waist circumference measurement are recommended. A 10% weight loss is associated with many health benefits for patients with BMI greater than 25 kg/m² and waist circumference greater than 35 inches (88 cm) (women) or greater than 40 inches (100 cm) (men). Weight loss enhances the cholesterol-lowering effect of an appropriate diet, decreases triglycerides, increases HDL-C, decreases blood pressure, and improves glucose tolerance.

- Limiting dietary fat intake, exercising regularly, and achieving and maintaining a healthy weight are cornerstones of lipid management.

DRUG THERAPY

Drug therapy for hyperlipidemia usually needs to be continued indefinitely and thus should be initiated only after vigorous

Table 28.2 OVERVIEW OF THERAPY FOR HYPERLIPIDEMIA[a]

CLINICAL RISK ASSESSMENT	INITIATE THERAPEUTIC LIFESTYLE CHANGES	CONSIDER DRUG THERAPY	GOAL OF THERAPY
No CHD; <2 risk factors[b]	≥160 mg/dL	≥190 mg/dL (160–189 mg/dL: drug optional)	<160 mg/dL
No CHD; ≥2 risk factors (10-y risk ≤20%)	≥130 mg/dL	10-y risk 10%-20%: ≥130 mg/dL 10-y risk <10%: ≥160 mg/dL	<130 mg/dL
CHD or CHD risk equivalents (10-y risk >20%)	≥100 mg/dL	≥130 mg/dL (100–129 mg/dL: drug optional)[c]	<100 mg/dL
Very high risk	≥100 mg/dL	≥130 mg/dL	<70 mg/dL

Abbreviations: CHD, coronary heart disease; LDL, low-density lipoprotein.

[a] Values reported as milligrams per deciliter are LDL cholesterol levels.

[b] Almost all people with <2 risk factors have a 10-year risk <10%; thus, 10-year risk assessment for people with <2 risk factors is not necessary.

[c] Some authorities recommend use of LDL-lowering drugs in this category if an LDL cholesterol <100 mg/dL cannot be achieved by therapeutic lifestyle changes. Others prefer use of drugs that primarily modify triglycerides and high-density lipoprotein (eg, nicotinic acid or fibrate). Clinical judgment also may call for deferring drug therapy in this subcategory.

Adapted from ATP III guidelines at-a-glance quick desk reference. National Cholesterol Education Program. Bethesda (MD): National Institutes of Health Publication No. 01–3305; c2001.

efforts at dietary and lifestyle modification. Appropriate lifestyle modifications must be continued. The teratogenic potential of most of these drugs should be considered when prescribing for women of childbearing age. Patients should be monitored for potential side effects and for the efficacy of the medication in reaching the predetermined goals. Lipid concentrations should be checked approximately 3 months after therapy is started. Modification of lipid-lowering therapy may be warranted if goals are not met. Combination therapy may need to be considered for some patients, especially for secondary prevention, including CHD risk equivalents. Combination therapy should be reserved for secondary prevention in established cardiovascular disease because of the risk of myositis and hepatitis.

TREATMENT OF INCREASED LDL-C

A statin is usually the drug of choice for elevated LDL-C. In estrogen-deficient women, estrogen replacement therapy is effective in decreasing LDL-C and increasing HDL-C, and it is appropriate for women until menopause; however, estrogen replacement therapy may increase the risk of cardiovascular events, at least among women at high risk. There is insufficient evidence on whether ezetimibe or a resin reduces cardiovascular event risk. Niacin reduces LDL-C levels, but side effects (flushing and worsening glucose tolerance) make it difficult to tolerate. Flushing can be reduced by taking the drug 30 to 60 minutes after low-dose aspirin.

TREATMENT OF HYPERTRIGLYCERIDEMIA

Extreme hypertriglyceridemia (>1,000 mg/dL) may cause pancreatitis and thus requires treatment, including cessation of oral estrogen or alcohol use, improved control of diabetes, and restriction of caloric intake, especially sources of simple carbohydrates. Fibrates are the drugs of choice. Glucose intolerance or diabetes mellitus is common in patients with hypertriglyceridemia, and insulin treatment may be helpful. Omega-3 fatty acids (docosahexaenoic acid [DHA] and eicosapentaenoic acid [EPA]) effectively reduce triglycerides. Prescription formulations are nearly 100% omega-3 fatty acid, allowing for more effective dosing compared with over-the-counter formulations.

TREATMENT OF LOW HDL-C

In the absence of heart disease, lifestyle modification is the intervention of choice. The use of drugs that can lower HDL-C (eg, androgens) should be discontinued when possible. Niacin, statins, and, to a lesser extent, fibrates increase HDL-C.

TREATMENT OF INCREASED LP(A) LIPOPROTEIN

Niacin may produce some modest decrease, but there is no proven treatment for increased Lp(a) lipoprotein. Consider lowering LDL-C to less than 100 mg/dL in these patients.

- Drug therapy should be reserved for patients with insufficient lipid lowering after therapeutic lifestyle changes. Tailor the drug choice to the elevated lipid fraction and reserve combination therapy for patients with clear indications.

DIABETES MELLITUS

ETIOLOGY AND CLASSIFICATION

Diabetes mellitus is characterized by increased levels of fasting and postprandial serum glucose and is the most common metabolic disorder, affecting approximately 10% of the US population. Type 1 diabetes mellitus (T1D) is characterized by loss of function of insulin-producing beta cells of the islets of Langerhans because of autoimmune destruction. Ten percent to 20% of diabetic patients have T1D. T1D often manifests at a young age but can develop at any age. Approximately one-third of patients with T1D present with acute hyperglycemic symptoms or diabetic ketoacidosis.

A complex interaction between genes and the environment leads to the development of T1D. Antibodies to islet cells or some constituent of the islets are frequently present and may help to differentiate T1D from type 2 diabetes mellitus (T2D). A "honeymoon" period may occur soon after disease onset, with restoration of euglycemia. The duration of this phase is highly variable, and all patients eventually require insulin.

- T1D is characterized by immune destruction of the islets, leading to insulin deficiency.

- Specific antibodies are frequently present in the early stages of the disease.

- All patients will require insulin at some point.

T2D is characterized by abnormalities of insulin action and insulin secretion in target tissues (eg, muscle and adipose tissue). The ability of glucose itself to stimulate glucose uptake and suppress glucose release is also defective. Suppression of glucagon secretion after eating is also impaired, contributing to postprandial hyperglycemia. T2D is more common among certain ethnic groups, and compared with T1D, the pathogenesis of T2D has a significant genetic contribution. Environmental factors contributing to obesity, and obesity itself, have a definite role in the development of the disease.

- T2D is characterized by defective insulin action and secretion.

- Obesity and environmental factors contributing to obesity are important in T2D development.

- T2D can occur at any age; certain ethnic groups are at higher risk.

Secondary causes of diabetes include pancreatic disease, endocrinopathies, drugs or chemicals, and infections. Certain genetic syndromes are sometimes associated with diabetes (eg, Down syndrome, Klinefelter syndrome, Turner syndrome).

Gestational diabetes mellitus is glucose intolerance that develops or is first recognized in pregnancy. Therapy may involve insulin or only dietary modification. Gestational diabetes mellitus may or may not persist after pregnancy.

CLINICAL FEATURES

The onset of T1D is usually rapid, with weight loss, polyuria, and polydipsia due to abrupt, severe insulin deficiency. Manifestation is often precipitated by infection or other severe physical stress. Severe dehydration and ketoacidosis may be present.

T2D usually has a more insidious onset and is often diagnosed during routine laboratory testing by the presence of glycosuria or hyperglycemia. Patients may report blurry vision, myopia, recurrent skin infections, or candidal vaginitis (females) or balanitis (males). Patients occasionally present with chronic diabetic complications (eg, neuropathy, nephropathy, retinopathy, or vascular disease) but without symptoms of glucose intolerance. Polyuria, polydipsia, and polyphagia may develop only at times of increased insulin resistance (eg, pregnancy, infection, or corticosteroid use). Patients occasionally present with hyperosmolar nonketotic coma.

- T1D has a rapid onset due to abrupt, severe insulin deficiency, with polyuria, polydipsia, and weight loss despite polyphagia, severe dehydration, and ketoacidosis.

- T2D has an insidious onset, and patients may present with complications. Under certain conditions, polyuria, polydipsia, and polyphagia may develop.

DIAGNOSIS

The normal fasting plasma glucose concentration is less than 100 mg/dL. Impaired fasting glucose, or prediabetes, is defined by fasting glucose values from 100 to 125 mg/dL. A glucose tolerance test is not required for the diagnosis.

- The diagnosis of diabetes mellitus is confirmed with the following:

  a. Fasting plasma glucose values ≥126 mg/dL documented on ≥2 occasions

  b. Casual plasma glucose ≥200 mg/dL in the presence of classic symptoms of hyperglycemia

  c. Plasma glucose ≥200 mg/dL 2 hours after a 75-g oral glucose load

  d. Hemoglobin A_{1c} values ≥6.5% documented on 2 occasions (values of 5.7%-6.4% are consistent with impaired glycemia)

The diagnosis of gestational diabetes mellitus requires an oral glucose tolerance test (see the "Diabetes and Pregnancy" section).

THERAPY FOR T1D

Insulin replacement is necessary for T1D treatment; oral agents have no role in its management. Therapy is aimed at preventing acute and chronic complications of diabetes while allowing the patient to maintain a healthy and active lifestyle, with optimal glycemic control and minimal hypoglycemia. Intensive insulin therapy requires considerable commitment from the patient to self-monitor plasma glucose concentrations and adjust the insulin dosage accordingly. Intensive therapy with tight glycemic control prevents or markedly decreases the risks of chronic microvascular complications of diabetes and reduces mortality.

An amylin analogue (pramlintide) can be used to manage both T1D and T2D. Amylin is a peptide that is cosecreted with insulin by beta cells. It has several mechanisms for lowering glucose levels, including delaying gastric emptying, regulating postprandial glucagon secretion, and decreasing appetite. It is injected before meals of at least 250 kcal and always as an adjunct to insulin therapy. It shows modest efficacy at improving glycemic control (lowering hemoglobin A_{1c} <1%), with nausea being the most common side effect. Pramlintide therapy is weight neutral and does not increase the risk of hypoglycemia. However, insulin doses should be decreased by 50% when pramlintide therapy is initiated.

- An amylin analogue can be used as an adjunct to insulin therapy, allowing insulin doses to be decreased by 50%.

- Pramlintide therapy is weight neutral and does not cause hypoglycemia.

NUTRITION

Intake should allow for maintenance of a healthy weight, with 10% to 20% of the total calories from protein, less than 30% of calories from fat (saturated fat <10%), and the remainder from complex carbohydrates. Insulin doses for meals depend on carbohydrate content of the meal. Patients are advised to maintain a consistent intake of carbohydrates or adjust the insulin dose according to carbohydrate intake at each meal ("carbohydrate counting").

EXERCISE

The glycemic response to exercise depends on glucose level, duration and type of exercise, physical fitness, and relationship of exercise to meals and insulin injections. Glucose levels should be monitored before and after exercise. If strenuous exercise is initiated while the patient is hyperglycemic, the serum glucose concentration may increase further. Patients should always carry appropriate identification and have access to glucose or sugar.

INSULIN THERAPY

Intensive insulin therapy mimics insulin secretion by the healthy pancreas. Short-acting insulin (regular, lispro, aspart, or glulisine) is injected at mealtimes, and a once- or twice-daily long-acting insulin (glargine or detemir insulin) replaces basal insulin secretion.

An insulin pump provides programmable continuous subcutaneous insulin infusion and is used to provide meal-stimulated insulin secretion. It allows the patient to adjust the infusion rate of basal insulin (during exercise or at night).

The insulin dosage required for a typical patient with T1D (within 20% of ideal body weight and without intercurrent illness) is approximately 0.5 to 1.0 U/kg daily. Insulin requirements may increase markedly during illness.

Glycemic goals are individualized according to the presence of other disease (ischemic heart disease or cerebrovascular disease), diabetic complications, and the ability to perceive hypoglycemia. For women with T1D who are considering pregnancy, tight glucose control starting weeks to months before pregnancy is critical to decrease the risk of birth defects. Tight glycemic control during pregnancy prevents macrosomia.

- For T1D patients, intensive insulin therapy simulates normal insulin secretion with a combination of short- and long-acting insulin.

- An insulin pump allows the patient to adjust basal insulin levels as needed.

- Glucose and insulin management of T1D patients who are considering childbearing or who are pregnant is essential to prevent birth defects and other complications.

GLYCEMIC GOALS OF OPTIMAL THERAPY

The blood glucose target fasting level is 70 to 130 mg/dL, and the target bedtime level is 100 to 140 mg/dL. Hemoglobin A_{1c} should be less than 7.0%. Higher target levels are required for patients at risk of hypoglycemia because of their inability to recognize hypoglycemic symptoms.

MONITORING

Glucose concentration should be self-monitored 4 times daily—before meals and at bedtime. If the patient has unexplained morning hypoglycemia or hyperglycemia, blood glucose should be measured between 2 AM and 4 AM. Hemoglobin A_{1c} should be measured every 3 months.

THERAPY FOR T2D

Most patients with T2D are obese, have a sedentary lifestyle, and often have multiple cardiovascular risk factors such as hypertension and dyslipidemia. Therapy should include risk factor modification, including exercise, weight loss and improved nutrition, and achievement of appropriate glycemic control with a near-normal hemoglobin A_{1c} in the absence of hypoglycemia.

An initial goal of losing 5% to 10% of initial body weight is recommended for patients with BMI values greater than 25. Exercise improves insulin action, facilitates weight loss, reduces cardiovascular risks (increases HDL-C and decreases very low-density lipoprotein [VLDL]-triglycerides), and increases a sense of well-being. Exercise recommendations should be modified appropriately for patients with preexisting coronary or peripheral vascular disease.

- The treatment goals for T2D include appropriate lifestyle modification, cardiovascular risk factor modification, and optimal glycemic control.

- Calorie restriction is appropriate to promote weight reduction of 5% to 10% of initial body weight.

- A prudent exercise program facilitates weight reduction and improves insulin action, cardiovascular fitness, and sense of well-being.

DRUG THERAPY FOR T2D

Metformin is the first-line agent for managing T2D. It improves insulin-mediated glucose use in the liver. It is effective as monotherapy and in combination therapy with other glucose-lowering drugs. The main side effect is diarrhea. Metformin provides multiple benefits, including less weight gain compared with other oral agents and lower risk of CHD events and mortality. The risk of lactic acidosis had been a concern, but there is no reliable evidence that metformin increases this risk. Metformin may lead to vitamin B$_{12}$ deficiency due to decreased absorption. The drug should generally be held when patients are hospitalized. Metformin is contraindicated in the presence of the following:

- Renal impairment (creatinine ≥1.5 mg/dL for men and ≥1.4 mg/dL for women).
- Cardiac or respiratory disease likely to cause central hypoxia or reduced peripheral perfusion.
- History of lactic acidosis.
- Severe infection that could lead to reduced tissue perfusion.
- Liver disease.
- Alcohol abuse with binge drinking.
- Use of intravenous radiographic contrast agents.

Sulfonylureas are insulin secretagogues. Their efficacy depends on the presence of endogenous insulin secretion. Primary failure occurs in the absence of endogenous insulin secretion. Secondary failure occurs with progression of disease, when sulfonylureas become ineffective. The risk of hypoglycemia from sulfonylureas increases with a longer-acting sulfonylurea (glyburide) and in the presence of renal failure.

Repaglinide and *nateglinide* have extremely short half-lives and act in a fashion similar to sulfonylureas. These agents are taken before each meal, and the dose is skipped if the patient misses a meal.

Thiazolidinediones (TZDs) improve hepatic and peripheral insulin action and do not cause hypoglycemia. Pioglitazone causes marked fluid retention, increasing the risk of heart failure, and should not be prescribed for patients who have congestive heart failure. Pioglitazone has not been associated with other cardiovascular risks. Significant weight gain and osteoporosis have been reported with TZD use.

α-Glucosidase inhibitors (acarbose, miglitol) inhibit upper intestinal glucosidases, limiting the conversion of complex carbohydrates to monosaccharides. Modest efficacy (lowering hemoglobin A$_{1c}$ <1%) and significant gastrointestinal tract side effects (flatulence in 70% of users) limit clinical use. Glucose is necessary to treat hypoglycemia in patients taking an α-glucosidase inhibitor.

Glucagon-Like Peptide-1 (GLP1) *analogues* (exenatide, liraglutide) augment insulin secretion and glucagon suppression in response to glucose. They also slow gastric emptying, reduce appetite, and lead to moderate weight loss. They are approved for use with metformin and sulfonylureas. Nausea and vomiting occur in a substantial proportion of users early in therapy but often subside. Used in combination with sulfonylurea, these agents can lead to hypoglycemia. Although all the newer agents seem to be effective in improving hemoglobin A$_{1c}$, the effect on clinical outcomes (vascular disease and microvascular complications) is unknown. Generally, until more data are available, these agents should be reserved for patients whose therapy with more traditional drugs has failed.

Dipeptidyl-peptidase-4 (DPP4) *inhibitors* (sitagliptin, saxagliptin) potentiate the effect of GLP1 by inhibiting degradation by DPP4. Glucose lowering occurs by enhancing GLP1-mediated insulin secretion. DPP4 inhibitors do not have a strong effect on gastric emptying or food intake and are considered weight neutral. They are associated with a lower risk of hypoglycemia and are approved for use as monotherapy and combination therapy with sulfonylureas, metformin, and TZDs.

- Metformin is the preferred therapy for the patient with T2D.
- Sulfonylureas stimulate insulin secretion, so their efficacy depends on the presence of endogenous insulin secretion. Hypoglycemia is the most important side effect.
- TZDs are associated with fluid retention, weight gain, and osteoporosis.
- Repaglinide and nateglinide are short acting and increase insulin secretion; doses are taken before meals and skipped when fasting.
- GLP1 analogues are associated with weight loss and lower risk of hypoglycemia except when used in combination with sulfonylureas.
- DPP4 inhibitors promote GLP1-mediated insulin secretion and are associated with lower risk of hypoglycemia. They are weight neutral.

Insulin is often reserved for patients with T2D when diet and oral agents (monotherapy and combination therapy) provide inadequate glycemic control, for sick patients when oral agents may be contraindicated, or for patients who require rapid glycemic control. Insulin is preferred for patients who are pregnant, under perioperative care, or severely ill. Patients with T2D often have some degree of meal-stimulated endogenous insulin secretion, which allows treatment with simpler insulin regimens than for T1D. Once-daily injections of intermediate-acting insulin in combination with an oral agent or twice-daily injections of intermediate-acting insulin are commonly used to manage T2D. Insulin therapy is associated with some degree of weight gain in most patients. Insulin can also be given in combination with metformin. Patients who have a more severe insulin deficiency may use an intensive insulin program, as in T1D. Intensive insulin therapy with basal and bolus doses gives more flexibility with meal schedules, while the split-mix regimen requires scheduled meals.

- Simple insulin regimens are useful for patients with T2D who have had treatment failure with oral agents.

- Prescribe an intensive insulin program or a split-mix program for patients with severe insulin deficiency.

An *amylin analogue* (pramlintide) is also approved for T2D patients receiving insulin therapy (see "Therapy for T1D" section).

HYPOGLYCEMIA IN DIABETES

Hypoglycemia may result from unplanned exercise, inappropriate dosing of insulin, or inadequate carbohydrate intake. Patients with long-standing T1D are prone to hypoglycemia unawareness due to repeated neuroglycopenia. Prevention of hypoglycemia has been shown to reverse or ameliorate hypoglycemia unawareness in some patients. Hypoglycemia can occur at night (*nocturnal hypoglycemia*) and may not be apparent if glucose is checked at bedtime and at breakfast. Patients may report symptoms such as nightmares, morning headache, or night sweats. Periodic monitoring of blood glucose between 1 AM and 3 AM, especially if the patient is taking intermediate insulin in the evenings, is essential. Preventive strategies include increasing the bedtime snack or modifying the insulin regimen.

In patients with long-standing T1D, inability to secrete glucagon leads to defective counter-regulation and patients become dependent on the autonomic nervous system to respond to hypoglycemia. The use of β-blockers in these situations can abolish warning palpitations with hypoglycemia.

Lower doses of insulin may be needed in patients with renal impairment. Alcohol may interfere with gluconeogenesis and the perception of hypoglycemic symptoms. Hypoglycemia may also be a manifestation of cortisol deficiency (eg, Addison disease or autoimmune hypophysitis).

- Patients with T1D are especially prone to hypoglycemia.

- Episodes of severe hypoglycemia may occur during the night—check the blood glucose level between 1 AM and 3 AM.

- Hypoglycemia may be precipitated by unplanned exercise, decreased carbohydrate intake, renal insufficiency, and cortisol deficiency.

- Insulin and sulfonylureas are associated with the highest risk of hypoglycemia.

- Metformin, TZDs, GLP1 analogues, and DPP4 inhibitors are associated with less hypoglycemia.

- Hypoglycemia with use of α-glucosidase inhibitors must be treated with glucose.

ACUTE COMPLICATIONS OF DIABETES MELLITUS

DIABETIC KETOACIDOSIS

Diabetic ketoacidosis may be the initial presentation in patients with T1D. When diabetic ketoacidosis occurs in patients with T2D, the patients usually also have infection, myocardial infarction, or other major stresses. Diabetic ketoacidosis is characterized by polyuria, polydipsia, dehydration, anorexia, nausea and vomiting, abdominal pain, tachypnea, mental obtundation, and coma. Physical findings include evidence of dehydration, decreased mentation, deep and rapid Kussmaul respiration, and a characteristic breath odor (fruity odor of acetone). Diabetic ketoacidosis can be precipitated by a failure to take insulin or to increase the insulin dose and consume extra fluids during acute illness, infection, or other illness such as myocardial infarction, pancreatitis, stroke, or trauma.

The diagnosis is based on the demonstration of moderate or severe hyperglycemia, ketonemia, and metabolic acidosis. Associated biochemical abnormalities include hyponatremia, azotemia, and hyperamylasemia. Large body losses of electrolytes occur, but often serum levels of potassium, phosphate, and magnesium are normal. Concentrations of these ions often decrease precipitously as the acidosis is corrected.

- Diabetic ketoacidosis occurs with severe insulin deficiency and is often precipitated by intercurrent illness.

- It may be the initial manifestation of T1D.

- Diagnosis requires the presence of pronounced hyperglycemia, ketonemia, and metabolic acidosis.

- Serum levels of potassium and other electrolytes may be normal despite large body losses; significant shifts can occur with correction of acidosis.

- Precipitating factors should be identified and corrected.

Treatment

Treatment of diabetic ketoacidosis requires administration of fluids and insulin to correct metabolic acidosis and electrolyte depletion. Electrolyte levels should be carefully monitored and corrected and precipitating factors ameliorated. The average fluid deficit in adults is 5 to 8 L. The risk of cerebral edema is decreased through careful rehydration and correction of ketoacidosis to avoiding a rapid decrease in osmolality.

Insulin infusion doses should be modified according to the degree of glycemia and continued until the acidosis resolves. This approach suppresses lipolysis and ketogenesis and stimulates glucose uptake.

The potassium deficit is typically 300 to 500 mEq, reflecting low total body stores. Serum potassium levels decrease with correction of the acidosis. Potassium should be added to the intravenous fluids as soon as renal perfusion and urine flow are assured. Phosphate repletion is indicated by phosphate levels less than 1 mg/dL. The serum level of phosphate must be monitored carefully owing to the risk of hypocalcemia, seizures, and death.

The mortality rate is 5% to 15% among patients with coma associated with diabetic ketoacidosis. For most patients, death is due to an associated precipitating illness such as myocardial infarction, stroke, or sepsis. After successful therapy, the goal is to avoid recurrence by educating the patient.

- Diabetic ketoacidosis is accompanied by significant fluid and electrolyte deficits that must be corrected while avoiding serious complications of too rapid or excessive replacement.

HYPERGLYCEMIC HYPEROSMOLAR NONKETOTIC COMA

Hyperglycemic hyperosmolar nonketotic coma is characterized by hyperglycemia and hyperosmolar dehydration *without* ketoacidosis. This typically occurs in poorly treated T2D when insulin levels are sufficient to inhibit excess lipolysis and ketogenesis but not to suppress hepatic glucose production or to stimulate glucose use. High concentrations of urinary glucose provoke an osmotic diuresis, with marked dehydration and decreased renal function. It is commonly precipitated by acute illness such as myocardial infarction, pancreatitis, infection, or surgery.

Diagnosis

Hyperglycemic hyperosmolar nonketotic coma should be suspected in any patient with diabetes who presents with an altered level of consciousness and severe dehydration. Laboratory abnormalities include hyperglycemia (blood glucose often >600 mg/dL), absence of ketones, and plasma hyperosmolarity (>320 mOsm/L). Always correct the underlying disorder.

- Hyperglycemic hyperosmolar nonketotic coma is characterized by hyperglycemia and dehydration without ketoacidosis.

- The disorder should be suspected in any patient with diabetes who has altered sensorium and severe dehydration.

- Laboratory evaluation demonstrates marked hyperglycemia (>600 mg/dL), no significant ketosis, and plasma hyperosmolarity (>320 mOsm/L).

- Always search for and correct the precipitating disorder.

Therapy

The objectives for treatment are to restore volume and osmolarity and to control the hyperglycemia. Total fluid loss is often larger in hyperglycemic hyperosmolar nonketotic coma than in diabetic ketoacidosis. Fluid resuscitation and insulin infusion are necessary and must be done with caution. Renal failure can complicate electrolyte replacement. Repeated neurologic evaluation is essential because focal deficits or seizures may become apparent during therapy. Complications include vascular events such as myocardial infarction or stroke, cerebral edema, and hypokalemia. The mortality rate can be up to 50%.

- Treatment of hyperglycemic hyperosmolar nonketotic coma includes fluid and electrolyte replacement and management of hyperglycemia.

- Hyperglycemic hyperosmolar nonketotic coma has a significant mortality rate.

CHRONIC COMPLICATIONS OF DIABETES MELLITUS

MICROVASCULAR DISEASE IN DIABETES

The microcirculation is damaged by chronic hyperglycemia and other metabolic abnormalities associated with diabetes. Clinical manifestations include retinopathy, nephropathy, and neuropathy. Diabetic retinopathy occurs in most patients with T1D within 10 years of diagnosis. Diabetic retinopathy is present in 15% to 20% of patients at the time of diagnosis of T2D and reaches 50% by 15 years. Background diabetic retinopathy is characterized by microaneurysms, hard exudates, hemorrhages, and macular edema. Retinal ischemia leads to proliferative retinopathy, stimulating the growth of new vessels that are fragile and prone to hemorrhage; loss of vision may result. It is treated with panretinal laser photocoagulation. Patients should undergo a dilated ophthalmic examination annually. Treatment of hypertension, hyperglycemia, glaucoma, and dyslipidemia is also important.

- Diabetic patients are at significant risk of neuropathy, including peripheral and autonomic neuropathy, and nephropathy, which often leads to chronic renal impairment and renal failure.

- Diabetes leads to microvascular disease and can cause retinopathy, neuropathy, and nephropathy.

INFECTIONS AND DIABETES

Skin infections can be a presenting feature of poorly controlled T2D. They include carbuncles (*Staphylococcus aureus*), malignant external otitis (*Pseudomonas*), and, in diabetic ketoacidosis, mucormycosis (*Mucor* species). Candidiasis and furunculosis also occur more frequently with poorly controlled diabetes.

- Specific infections are common in diabetic patients.

ATHEROSCLEROTIC VASCULAR DISEASE IN DIABETES

Ischemic cardiovascular disease appears earlier and is more extensive in diabetic patients than in the general population. CHD accounts for about 70% of deaths among persons with diabetes, and patients may present with sudden cardiac death.

Persons with T2D have the same risk of myocardial infarct as patients with prior myocardial infarction. Treatment of dyslipidemia is therefore considered secondary prevention in this population. Patients with ischemic heart disease may present with atypical symptoms; angina may manifest as epigastric distress, heartburn, and neck or jaw pain. Myocardial infarction may be silent (in 15% of patients), and patients may present with sudden onset of left ventricular failure. Patients with diabetes have a higher risk of cerebrovascular and peripheral arterial diseases, but the role of screening for vascular disease in asymptomatic patients with diabetes is uncertain.

- Diabetic patients have a significant risk of cardiovascular disease, and diabetes is considered a coronary heart disease risk equivalent.

HYPERLIPIDEMIA IN DIABETES

In poorly controlled T2D, the concentrations of triglyceride-rich lipoproteins are increased owing to overproduction of VLDL and decreased lipoprotein lipase activity. HDL-C levels are low, and control of glucose and triglyceride levels leads to levels that are improved but usually not normalized. Compositional changes in LDL (small, dense LDL) that increase the atherogenicity of these particles are more likely to occur in patients with T2D. Aggressive management of hyperlipidemia and low HDL-C is warranted in diabetic patients because they have a high risk of cardiovascular disease.

DIABETES AND PREGNANCY

Both fasting and postprandial glucose concentrations decrease in normal pregnancy, and insulin secretion increases owing to increased levels of circulating hormones (eg, human placental lactogen, estrogen, progesterone, and cortisol), which increase insulin resistance.

Pregnancy is a diabetogenic state and may worsen glucose control in women with diabetes. Inadequate glycemic control early in pregnancy increases the risk of congenital malformations; poor control in late pregnancy increases the risk of macrosomia, neonatal hypoglycemia, hypocalcemia, polycythemia, hyperbilirubinemia, and respiratory distress. Pregnancy may exacerbate diabetic retinopathy, and nephropathy may lead to pregnancy-induced hypertension and toxemia.

Gestational diabetes complicates 2% to 3% of all pregnancies. All pregnant women older than 25 years should be evaluated at 24 to 28 weeks with a 50-g oral glucose tolerance test. A glucose level higher than 140 mg/dL 1 hour after ingestion of the glucose drink should trigger formal testing with a 100-g glucose drink. Gestational diabetes is diagnosed if the fasting glucose is greater than 105 mg/dL and if the glucose is greater than 190 mg/dL at 1 hour, greater than 165 mg/dL at 2 hours, and greater than 145 mg/dL at 3 hours. Earlier evaluations are often needed for high-risk patients.

- Early detection and optimal management of diabetes during pregnancy can prevent congenital malformations and decrease neonatal morbidity and mortality.

- Gestational diabetes complicates 2%-3% of all pregnancies.

- All pregnant women older than 25 years should be evaluated at 24–28 weeks.

TREATMENT

Home monitoring for blood glucose and urine ketones is important in gestational diabetics. Postprandial glucose concentrations are closely associated with macrosomia and neonatal complications, so they are often used to guide therapy. The fasting blood glucose concentration should be between 60 and 90 mg/dL and the postprandial level should be 70 to 140 mg/dL (1 hour after a meal).

Women with gestational diabetes who become euglycemic in the postpartum state should institute lifestyle changes to prevent onset of T2D, and they should be periodically evaluated. They are at high risk of T2D (diabetes develops in >50% within the 15 years after diagnosis of gestational diabetes) and should be encouraged to exercise, consume an appropriate diet, and lose weight if appropriate.

- Periodic follow-up of patients with gestational diabetes is necessary because of the high incidence of T2D.

HYPOGLYCEMIA IN NONDIABETIC PATIENTS

ETIOLOGY

Hypoglycemic disorders may be classified as *insulin mediated* and *noninsulin mediated*. Causes of insulin-mediated hypoglycemia include insulinoma, sulfonylurea or exogenous insulin use, and autoimmune hypoglycemia mediated by insulin antibodies, which prevent insulin degradation. Noninsulin-mediated hypoglycemia may be related to drugs, alcohol use, or cortisol insufficiency. Renal failure, liver failure, and sepsis are common causes of noninsulin-mediated hypoglycemia in hospitalized patients. Insulinlike growth factor (IGF)-producing tumors, such as mesenchymal or epithelial tumors, may cause hypoglycemia.

- Insulin-mediated causes of hypoglycemia include insulinoma, exogenous insulin use, sulfonylurea use, and autoimmune hypoglycemia.

- Noninsulin-mediated causes of hypoglycemia include alcohol use, cortisol deficiency, renal failure, liver failure, sepsis, and tumors secreting IGF-2.

CLINICAL FEATURES

Hypoglycemia may result in hyperadrenergic symptoms (palpitations, sweating, tremor, and nervousness) and neuroglycopenic symptoms (confusion, inappropriate affect, blurred vision, diplopia, seizures, and loss of consciousness). Symptoms are relieved promptly after oral carbohydrate intake. Patients with fasting hypoglycemia often learn to reduce symptoms by increasing the frequency of their meals; as a result, they may gain weight.

- Hypoglycemia may cause symptoms related to activation of the sympathoadrenal system and neuroglycopenia.

DIAGNOSIS

For all patients with suspected hypoglycemia, it is essential to investigate the Whipple triad: low plasma glucose, symptoms of hypoglycemia, and prompt resolution of symptoms after normalization of plasma glucose level.

- Capillary blood glucose monitors should not be used to confirm hypoglycemia owing to inaccuracy.

- Plasma insulin levels should be measured to determine the mechanism of hypoglycemia; insulin is not appropriately suppressed in insulin-mediated causes of hypoglycemia.

- C-peptide levels distinguish between exogenous and endogenous insulin; if the patient is injecting insulin, C-peptide levels are undetectable.

- C-peptide levels in endogenous hyperinsulinemic hypoglycemia caused by insulinoma are indistinguishable from those in sulfonylurea use. Consequently, plasma sulfonylurea levels should be measured in all cases of insulin-mediated hypoglycemia (while the patient is hypoglycemic).

INSULINOMA

Diagnostic criteria for insulinoma are plasma insulin level at least 6 mU/mL and C peptide level at least 200 pmol/L when plasma glucose is less than 50 mg/dL and plasma sulfonylurea is undetectable. Ultrasonography and spiral computed tomography of the pancreas are performed to identify and localize the insulinoma; localization is successful in approximately 60% of cases. Arteriography and selective arterial catheterization with calcium stimulation of insulin release identify the region of the pancreas that is the source of insulin. The key to successful removal is surgical exploration of the pancreas by an experienced surgeon combined with intraoperative ultrasonography. Almost all insulinomas can be identified and excised in this manner. Patients with insulinoma who decline surgical excision or who have persistent or recurrent malignant insulinoma may be treated with diazoxide, which inhibits insulin secretion, but side effects (edema and malaise) limit its tolerability.

- Preoperative abdominal ultrasonography and spiral computed tomography of the pancreas localize approximately 60% of insulinomas.

- Intraoperative ultrasonography of the pancreas is a useful localization tool.

POSTPRANDIAL HYPOGLYCEMIA

Postprandial symptoms are not always caused by postprandial hypoglycemia. *Postprandial hypoglycemia* is defined as symptomatic hypoglycemia occurring 1 to 5 hours after a meal. Patients with noninsulinoma pancreatogenous hypoglycemia syndrome can have postprandial hypoglycemia. The oral glucose tolerance test is not reliable for diagnosing reactive hypoglycemia. Insulinoma usually causes fasting hypoglycemia.

THERAPY

Treatment is directed at correcting both the hypoglycemia and the underlying cause. For patients with serious hypoglycemia who cannot eat or drink, 1 mg of glucagon can be administered to stimulate endogenous glucose production. Alternatively, intravenous dextrose can be given, although this may be associated with superficial phlebitis and pain.

- Injected glucagon may be used to treat hypoglycemia if the oral route is not available.

SUMMARY

- Hyperlipidemia can be secondary to drugs or diseases; it can be genetic or acquired (or both).

- Patients with hyperlipidemia are often asymptomatic.

- The decision to measure Lp(a) lipoprotein should be based on individual patient risk factors.

- Limiting dietary fat intake, exercising regularly, and achieving and maintaining a healthy weight are cornerstones of lipid management.

- Drug therapy should be reserved for patients with insufficient lipid lowering after therapeutic lifestyle changes. Tailor the drug choice to the elevated lipid fraction and reserve combination therapy for patients with clear indications.

- T1D has a rapid onset due to abrupt, severe insulin deficiency, with polyuria, polydipsia, and weight loss despite polyphagia, severe dehydration, and ketoacidosis.

- T2D has an insidious onset, and patients may present with complications. Under certain conditions, polyuria, polydipsia, and polyphagia may develop.

- For T1D patients, intensive insulin therapy simulates normal insulin secretion with a combination of short- and long-acting insulin.

- The treatment goals for T2D include appropriate lifestyle modification, cardiovascular risk factor modification, and optimal glycemic control.

- Metformin is the preferred therapy for the patient with T2D.

- Diabetic ketoacidosis occurs with severe insulin deficiency and is often precipitated by intercurrent illness. It may be the initial manifestation of T1D.

- Diabetes leads to microvascular disease and can cause retinopathy, neuropathy, and nephropathy.

SUGGESTED READING

American Diabetes Association. Diagnosis and classification of diabetes mellitus. Diabetes Care. 2010 Jan;33 Suppl 1:S62–9. Erratum in: Diabetes Care. 2010 Apr;33(4):e57.

Bell DS. Metformin-induced vitamin B12 deficiency presenting as a peripheral neuropathy. South Med J. 2010 Mar;103(3):265–7.

Chiasson JL, Josse RG, Hunt JA, Palmason C, Rodger NW, Ross SA, et al. The efficacy of acarbose in the treatment of patients with non-insulin-dependent diabetes mellitus: a multicenter controlled clinical trial. Ann Intern Med. 1994 Dec 15;121 (12):928–35.

Hollander PA, Levy P, Fineman MS, Maggs DG, Shen LZ, Strobel SA, et al. Pramlintide as an adjunct to insulin therapy improves long-term glycemic and weight control in patients with type 2 diabetes: a 1-year randomized controlled trial. Diabetes Care. 2003 Mar;26(3):784–90.

Ratner RE, Dickey R, Fineman M, Maggs DG, Shen L, Strobel SA, et al. Amylin replacement with pramlintide as an adjunct to insulin therapy improves long-term glycaemic and weight control in Type 1 diabetes mellitus: a 1-year, randomized controlled trial. Diabet Med. 2004 Nov;21(11):1204–12.

Raz I, Hanefeld M, Xu L, Caria C, Williams-Herman D, Khatami H; Sitagliptin Study 023 Group. Efficacy and safety of the dipeptidyl peptidase-4 inhibitor sitagliptin as monotherapy in patients with type 2 diabetes mellitus. Diabetologia. 2006 Nov;49(11):2564–71. Epub 2006 Sep 26.

Richter B, Bandeira-Echtler E, Bergerhoff K, Lerch C. Emerging role of dipeptidyl peptidase-4 inhibitors in the management of type 2 diabetes. Vasc Health Risk Manag. 2008;4(4):753–68.

29.

OBESITY

Maria L. Collazo-Clavell, MD

GOALS

- Identify overweight and obese patients, and identify their health risks.

- Review the management of overweight and obesity.

- Identify complications of bariatric surgery and understand management strategies.

- Recognize when nutritional supplementation is appropriate (for micronutrients and macronutrients) and the role of different routes of administration.

INTRODUCTION

Body mass index (BMI) (calculated as weight in kilograms divided by height in meters squared) is used to assess the health risk of body weight. Waist circumference (WC), another variable used to predict health risk, is a surrogate for visceral fat. WC is most useful for persons who have a BMI between 25 and 35. Persons who have an increased BMI in combination with an increased WC, which indicates excess visceral fat, have a greater health risk than if the BMI alone is increased. BMI values greater than 35 are associated with high health risk anyway, so in that BMI range, WC is less meaningful (Table 29.1).

The prevalence of overweight and obesity continues to increase in the United States and the westernized world. Many factors contribute to overweight and obesity, particularly excess caloric intake and low physical activity. Additional risk factors include smoking cessation, sleep deprivation, contributory social networks, lower socioeconomic status, medications, and, less commonly, health conditions.

HEALTH RISK ASSESSMENT

Overweight and obesity are associated with increased morbidity and mortality (Box 29.1). Some of the increased mortality may be negated by cardiovascular fitness. Screening for weight-related medical complications is indicated (measurement of blood pressure, fasting blood glucose or hemoglobin

A_{1c}, lipid profile, and thyrotropin and evaluation for obstructive sleep apnea).

OBESITY MANAGEMENT

Implementation of healthy lifestyle changes is the key factor to managing overweight and obesity. Dietary changes with caloric restriction (by 250–500 kcal daily) is needed to achieve weight loss. Macronutrient composition has minimal impact on weight loss at 12 months. Regular physical activity promotes weight loss by creating an additional caloric deficit but is insufficient alone. However, regular physical activity is a key determinant to maintaining weight loss.

Achieving an initial weight loss goal of 5% to 10% of initial body weight is associated with multiple benefits, including prevention of type 2 diabetes mellitus. Predictors of weight loss success include having a higher initial body weight, engaging in more minutes of physical activity weekly, recording caloric intake, and participating in group behavioral therapy. Considerable weight loss occurs with aggressive dietary restriction (very low-calorie diets of <800 kcal daily) and bariatric surgery. With very low-calorie diets, the prevalence of weight regain is high.

- Caloric restriction of 250–500 kcal daily is the main determinant of successful weight loss.

- Macronutrient composition without calorie restriction has no significant impact.

- Initial weight loss of 5%-10% of initial body weight is recommended.

- Predictors of success include having a higher initial weight, engaging in more minutes of physical activity weekly, recording caloric intake, and participating in group behavioral therapy.

MEDICATIONS FOR WEIGHT LOSS

Use of medication improves the likelihood of losing 5% to 10% of initial body weight. The 2 medications available for obesity

Table 29.1 BODY MASS INDEX, WAIST CIRCUMFERENCE, AND HEALTH RISK

BMI	BMI CLASSIFICATION	WC	HEALTH RISK BMI Alone	BMI + WC
<18.5	Underweight			
18.5–24.9	Normal			
25.0–29.9	Overweight		Increased	
		Women: >88		High
		Men: >102		High
30.0–34.9	Class I obesity		High	
		Women: >88		Very high
		Men: >102		Very high
35.0–39.9	Class II obesity		Very high	
>40.0	Class III obesity		Extremely high	

Abbreviations: BMI, body mass index (calculated as weight in kilograms divided by height in meters squared); WC, waist circumference in centimeters.

Adapted from National Institutes of Health, National Heart, Lung, and Blood Institute, North American Association for the Study of Obesity. The practical guide: identification, evaluation, and treatment of overweight and obesity in adults. Bethesda (MD): National Institutes of Health; c2000. NIH Publication No. 00-4084.

are phentermine and orlistat. Medications are generally reserved for patients who are obese (BMI ≥30.0) or overweight (BMI 25.0–29.9) and have weight-related medical complications.

Phentermine is a sympathomimetic agent that suppresses appetite. Few long-term studies (>12 weeks) have been performed, and there are insufficient data detailing efficacy and safety. It has *not* been implicated in the development of cardiac valve abnormalities and pulmonary hypertension. Patients previously treated with fenfluramine or dexfenfluramine should be evaluated for cardiac valve abnormalities. Sibutramine was removed from the market after it was reported to increase the risk of nonfatal heart attacks and stroke in a high-risk population.

Orlistat is a lipase inhibitor that limits dietary fat absorption. Administered with a low-fat diet (fat <30% of calories),

it is associated with greater weight loss than placebo. The main side effects involve the gastrointestinal tract; diarrhea and flatulence often limit compliance. A daily multivitamin is recommended to prevent vitamin deficiencies. Concurrent use with medications influenced by fat absorption (eg, cyclosporine, amiodarone, warfarin) can limit the efficacy of those drugs.

- Medications for weight loss are reserved for patients who meet criteria for obesity or overweight and have weight-related medical problems.

- There are insufficient long-term data on the efficacy and safety of phentermine.

- Patients with a history of fenfluramine or dexfenfluramine use should be evaluated for cardiac valve abnormalities.

- Orlistat limits dietary fat absorption and should be used along with a low-fat diet. Patients should take a daily multivitamin.

- Orlistat can limit the efficacy of medications influenced by fat absorption.

Box 29.1 **HEALTH RISKS ASSOCIATED WITH OBESITY**

Type 2 diabetes mellitus
Hypertriglyceridemia
Hypertension
Obstructive sleep apnea
Coronary artery disease
Congestive heart failure
Atrial fibrillation
Thromboembolic disease
Degenerative joint disease
Gastroesophageal reflux disease
Nonalcoholic steatohepatitis
Cancer
Death

BARIATRIC SURGERY

- The indications for bariatric surgery include the following:

  a. BMI >40 *or*

  b. BMI >35 *and* weight-related medical comorbidities, documented efforts at medically supervised weight management, absence of psychologic contraindications, and life expectancy >5 years

Mechanisms for weight loss after bariatric surgery vary. They include the following:

1. Dietary restriction—vertical banded gastroplasty, laparoscopic adjustable gastric banding

2. A combination of restriction and maldigestion—Roux-en-Y gastric bypass (RYGB)

3. Malabsorption—biliopancreatic diversion with a duodenal switch (BPD-DS)

The most commonly performed operation is the RYGB, and data have demonstrated its beneficial effects, including prevention and resolution of type 2 diabetes mellitus. Resolution rates have been reported for other medical problems, including obstructive sleep apnea, gastroesophageal reflux disease, hypertriglyceridemia, and hypertension. Restrictive operations are generally associated with less weight loss and lower resolution rates for most obesity-related complications, and BPD-DS is associated with the greatest reported weight loss and the greatest effect on the complications of excess weight.

- Several bariatric procedures are being used with very low overall perioperative mortality.

- Weight loss after surgery leads to reduction and possible resolution of obesity-related health problems.

EARLY COMPLICATIONS OF BARIATRIC SURGERY

Perioperative mortality is reported as less than 1%. The most common cause of death is pulmonary embolism. Anastomotic leak with subsequent peritonitis is the second most common cause of death for RYGB and BPD-DS. A high index of awareness is critical when assessing an ill patient presenting with dyspnea or abdominal pain within weeks after a bariatric operation. Sinus tachycardia is the most common physical finding in patients with an anastomotic leak. Risk factors associated with higher perioperative morbidity and mortality are male sex, age older than 60 years, BMI greater than 60, smoking, untreated obstructive sleep apnea, inactivity, and surgeon inexperience.

Anastomotic complications are also common after RYGB. Anastomotic ulcerations and stricture of the gastrojejunal anastomosis are the most common. Risk factors include use of nonsteroidal anti-inflammatory drugs, prior *Helicobacter pylori* infection, and smoking. Presenting symptoms include epigastric pain with or without nausea and vomiting. Esophagogastroduodenoscopy is the diagnostic study of choice; balloon dilation of a stricture can be performed. Anastomotic ulcers are effectively treated with proton pump inhibitors with or without sucralfate.

- The most common causes of death after bariatric surgery are pulmonary embolism and anastomotic leaks.

- If a patient presents with epigastric pain, nausea, and vomiting after bariatric surgery, anastomotic ulceration or stricture should be suspected.

NUTRITION AFTER BARIATRIC SURGERY

Nutritional deficiencies are recognized complications of bariatric surgery; therefore, empirical vitamin supplementation is recommended for all patients after surgery and should include vitamin B_{12}, a multivitamin, and calcium with vitamin D.

After any bariatric procedure, acute thiamine deficiency can occur in a patient who is vomiting and cannot maintain adequate oral intake over several days. In addition to gastrointestinal tract symptoms, neurologic complaints are common. Wernicke-Korsakoff encephalopathy may occur, so thiamine must be supplemented before intravenous infusion of dextrose-containing fluids.

- Bariatric surgery patients should receive vitamin B_{12}, a multivitamin, and calcium with vitamin D.

- Acute thiamine deficiency should be suspected in the patient who, within weeks after bariatric surgery, presents with severe nausea and vomiting of several days' duration.

Anemia is the most common manifestation of deficiencies of iron, vitamin B_{12}, or folate and normalizes with appropriate supplementation. Iron deficiency anemia is the most common vitamin deficiency reported, especially among menstruating women. Folate and vitamin B_{12} deficiencies are less common owing to empirical supplementation, but a high index of awareness is needed owing to variable adherence to vitamin supplementation regimens. Neurologic complications resulting from vitamin B_{12} deficiency may not resolve. Care must be taken to assess folate status before supplementation. Measuring the ferritin level is a reliable screening test for iron deficiency. Low vitamin B_{12} levels should be confirmed with a methylmalonic acid level.

- Iron deficiency anemia is the most common nutritional deficiency after bariatric surgery, particularly among menstruating women. Measuring the ferritin level is the recommended screening test.

- Vitamin B_{12} deficiency is less common owing to empirical supplementation, but it should be suspected in patients who have a history of bariatric surgery and present with macrocytic anemia. Folate status should be checked before vitamin B_{12} supplementation begins.

Inadequate diet, inadequate supplementation, and, often, persistent gastrointestinal tract symptoms such as diarrhea can lead to chronic nutritional deficiencies. Vitamin D deficiency is common among obese patients seeking bariatric surgery and may worsen during rapid weight loss after surgery. Hypocalcemia is a late finding and is often absent with mild or moderate deficiencies. The most common early findings may be increased parameters of bone turnover (bone alkaline phosphatase) and secondary hyperparathyroidism with an elevated parathyroid hormone level. Secondary hyperparathyroidism is also influenced by decreased dietary calcium. Calcium deficiency can be detected early only by identifying hypocalciuria in a 24-hour urine collection. Long-term vitamin D deficiency can lead to metabolic bone disease with low bone mineral density or mineralization defects (or both) resulting in osteomalacia.

Other fat-soluble vitamin deficiencies (ie, vitamin A or E deficiency) are less common but may occur. Vitamin A deficiency is associated with night blindness. Protein malnutrition is a worrisome complication of BPD-DS, which must be reversed in 1% to 2% of patients.

- Vitamin D and calcium deficiencies are common in the obese population and can worsen after bariatric surgery.

- Malabsorptive operations (BPD-DS) carry the highest risk of fat-soluble vitamin and protein malnutrition.

LATE COMPLICATIONS OF BARIATRIC SURGERY

Cholelithiasis develops in one-third of patients; 40% become symptomatic. Prophylactic cholecystectomy was commonly performed at bariatric surgery when it was an open abdominal operation (before the laparoscopic approach became common). Administration of ursodeoxycholic acid for 6 months after surgery decreases the prevalence of gallstone development and is gaining popularity. Therefore, prophylactic cholecystectomy is no longer indicated.

Bacterial overgrowth is common after RYGB and BPD-DS. Abdominal pain and bloating associated with diarrhea are common symptoms. Esophagogastroduodenoscopy with small bowel aspirates for culture or breath tests are usually diagnostic. When bacterial overgrowth is suspected or confirmed, antibiotic therapy should be instituted; various regimens are available. Resolution of symptoms occurs within 1 week. Bacterial overgrowth can recur, worsening the malabsorption of nutrients and increasing the risk of vitamin deficiencies.

Other complications include renal stone disease (primarily calcium oxalate stones). Fat malabsorption and dietary calcium allow increased absorption of intestinal oxalate, increasing the risk of calcium oxalate stone formation. Insulin-mediated hypoglycemia may occur in patients who have postprandial symptoms that suggest hypoglycemia. Symptoms may be difficult to differentiate from those of classic dumping. Further evaluation requires documentation of hypoglycemia (blood glucose <55 mg/dL), endogenous hyperinsulinemia (insulin >3 μIU/mL; C-peptide >0.2 ng/mL), and a negative sulfonylurea screen while the patient is symptomatic.

- Cholelithiasis is common after bariatric surgery. Prophylactic administration of ursodeoxycholic acid for 6 months after surgery decreases the risk of gallstone formation.

- Bacterial overgrowth should be suspected in patients presenting with abdominal pain and diarrhea.

- Reported complications of RYGB and BPD-DS include renal stone disease with predominantly calcium oxalate stones and rarely insulin-mediated hypoglycemia.

NUTRITION

Ideal weight is reflected by BMI values from 18.5 to 24.9. Persons with BMI values less than 18.5 are considered underweight, and the risk of morbidity and mortality increases with BMI values less than 15.

An optimal diet should provide the caloric requirements to maintain a weight within an ideal BMI range and minimize the risk of illness. High intakes of fruits and vegetables have been consistently shown to provide multiple health benefits, particularly in lowering the risk of cardiovascular disease (Box 29.2).

MICRONUTRIENT SUPPLEMENTATION

Multivitamin supplementation has not been shown to provide health benefits to the population at large, and it is recommended only for persons not meeting their nutritional needs orally owing to illness or self-imposed dietary restriction.

The benefits of empirical vitamin supplementation have been reported for folic acid in women of childbearing age (to prevent neural tube defects) and for vitamin D to prevent metabolic bone disease.

Empirical supplementation of antioxidant vitamins (beta carotene and vitamin E) to prevent cardiovascular disease is no longer advised owing to a lack of benefit and the potential risk of lung cancer in smokers and patients who have a history of asbestos exposure. Folic acid supplementation to decrease homocysteine levels is no longer advised owing to a lack of benefit in preventing cardiovascular disease.

ω-3 Fatty acid (docosahexaenoic acid [DHA] and eicosapentaenoic acid [EPA]) supplementation lowers cardiovascular mortality. Eating at least 1 serving of a fatty fish (rich in ω-3 fatty acids) weekly or supplementing with DHA and EPA is beneficial, with studies suggesting that antiarrhythmic properties contribute to a lower risk of cardiovascular death. Higher doses lower triglyceride levels.

Box 29.2 **DIETARY GUIDELINES TO DECREASE THE RISK OF CARDIOVASCULAR DISEASE**

Dietary protein <20% of total calories
    Prefer lean meats
Dietary fat <35% of total calories
    Avoid *trans* fats
    Restrict saturated fats to 10% of total calories
    Restrict dietary cholesterol to <300 mg daily
    Prefer polyunsaturated fats
Dietary carbohydrates <55% of total calories
    Prefer fruits, vegetables, and whole grains
    Restrict refined carbohydrates, processed grains, and starches

- Multivitamin supplementation is advised for persons who do not meet their nutritional needs orally or who have a self-imposed dietary restriction.

- Benefits of vitamin D and folic acid supplementation have been reported.

- Empirical supplementation with antioxidant vitamins and folic acid does not provide cardiovascular health benefits.

- ω-3 Fatty acids lower cardiovascular mortality and, at higher doses, triglycerides.

MICRONUTRIENT DEFICIENCIES

In the general population, nutritional deficiencies of calcium, vitamin D, vitamin B_{12}, and iron are common. Current dietary intake of dairy products and other food sources of calcium is low. Recommended calcium intake varies by age, and calcium supplementation is effective. Various calcium preparations are available. Calcium carbonate requires gastric acid for optimal absorption, so dosing is advised with meals; efficacy may be lower with medications that decrease gastric acid secretion. Calcium citrate is generally better absorbed and preferred if a patient has a gastrointestinal tract illness.

Vitamin D deficiency is associated with decreased sun exposure. Vitamin D status is reflected by 25-hydroxyvitamin D levels (reference range, 25–80 ng/mL). Mild to moderate deficiencies (10–25 ng/mL) are common, are often asymptomatic, and can be associated with secondary hyperparathyroidism. Severe deficiency (<10 ng/mL) increases the risk of bone mineralization defects and osteomalacia. Patients often report deep bone pain and proximal muscle weakness.

- Dietary intake of calcium often does not meet the recommended intake.

- The 25-hydroxyvitamin D level is the best reflection of vitamin D status.

The cause of vitamin B_{12} deficiency can be 1) autoimmune (eg, pernicious anemia), 2) gastrointestinal tract disease impairing vitamin B_{12} absorption (eg, surgery or inflammatory bowel disease), or 3) medications (eg, metformin). A low vitamin B_{12} level (<100 ng/L) is consistent with a deficiency. Low normal values should be evaluated by methylmalonic acid measurement; a deficiency is indicated by an elevated level of methylmalonic acid. Macrocytic anemia is the most common presenting abnormality. Neurologic symptoms can occur and may not fully resolve if identification and supplementation is delayed. Anti-parietal cell antibodies are present in pernicious anemia. Any gastrointestinal tract surgery or illness affecting the gastric antrum or ileum can lead to vitamin B_{12} deficiency. Parenteral supplementation is advised, particularly if the patient is symptomatic or the underlying cause is abnormal gastrointestinal tract absorption. Monitoring of vitamin B_{12} levels is advised with oral supplementation. Folate levels should be checked before supplementing vitamin B_{12}.

Iron deficiency is also common, and it is the most common abnormality in patients with celiac sprue. Persons with self-imposed dietary restrictions (including vegetarians and vegans), patients who have gastrointestinal tract illness or have had surgery affecting the duodenum, where iron is absorbed, and women with heavy menses are also at risk. Unless more aggressive treatment with packed cell transfusion is needed or the patient is intolerant of oral iron, oral supplementation is sufficient.

- Vitamin B_{12} deficiency must be suspected in any condition (medical or surgical) that impairs absorption of intrinsic factor or vitamin B_{12}.

- Iron deficiency anemia is the most common nutritional abnormality in patients with celiac sprue.

NUTRITIONAL SUPPORT

During illness, patients often do not meet their nutritional needs orally. A weight loss of more than 5% of initial body weight suggests inadequate nutrition, and the need for nutritional support should be assessed.

If adequate oral intake can be resumed within 7 to 14 days, previously healthy patients generally do not benefit from nutritional support. Intravenous fluid hydration is adequate for most patients in an uncomplicated hospital setting. The potential need for nutritional support should be considered for critically ill patients and for patients with a BMI less than 18.5, a loss of 5% of initial body weight in 1 month, a loss of 10% of initial body weight in 6 months, more than 14 days of not meeting nutritional needs, or multiple organ failure.

- Nutritional support should be considered for critically ill patients and for patients who have a BMI <18.5, a weight loss >5%-10% of initial body weight, or an inability to meet their nutritional needs for 14 days.

Enteral feedings (delivered into the stomach with a nasogastric tube or as postpyloric feedings) are preferred unless contraindicated. Patients who benefit include perioperative patients with chronic liver disease, critically ill patients, and malnourished geriatric patients. Enteral feedings also reduce the risk of sepsis.

Gastric feedings are preferred but should be avoided in settings that may promote intolerance or potential complications, including any conditions that impair gastric emptying or increase the risk of aspiration. Most medications can be provided by this route.

Patients with contraindications or intolerance to gastric feedings or concerns with potential complications from gastric feeding should receive postpyloric feedings. Fewer medications can be safely administered by this route.

- In the absence of contraindications, enteral nutritional support is preferred. Gastric feedings should be avoided in patients with suspected delayed gastric emptying or at increased risk of aspiration. Postpyloric feedings should then be considered.

Parenteral nutrition is advised for patients who do not meet their nutritional needs for 7 to 14 days and have contraindications or intolerance to enteral feedings. Parenteral nutrition is associated with risks, and patients must be monitored appropriately.

Hyperglycemia is the most common complication, and glucose monitoring is advised. Hypertriglyceridemia is a recognized complication; limiting calories provided as fat is advised for patients with triglyceride levels greater than 300 mg/dL. An increased risk of bloodstream infection (bacterial and fungal organisms) is associated with parenteral nutrition. Patients receiving parenteral nutrition have up to a 5-fold greater risk of fungal infection. Common risk factors include poor hygiene in managing venous access and formula, severity of illness, and duration of catheter insertion.

- Parenteral nutrition is advised for patients who do not meet their nutritional needs for 7–14 days and have contraindications or intolerance to enteral feedings. Hyperglycemia, hypertriglyceridemia, and bloodstream infection are recognized complications of parenteral nutrition.

Ideally, nutritional needs are calculated with an accurate body weight, which is often difficult to measure if the patient is critically ill. Protein needs are higher in critically ill patients, but caution must taken if patients have comorbidities contraindicating a high-protein load (eg, renal insufficiency, liver disease).

- Calculation of nutritional needs is based on weight and clinical situation. Current weight is used for patients with a BMI ≤29.9; 75% of calculated calories are provided for patients with a BMI ≥30.
- Common recommendations for nutritional support based on patient need:

  a. Critically ill patient: 20 kcal/kg with 1.5–2.0 g/kg protein

  b. Clinically stable patient: 25–35 kcal/kg with 1.0 g/kg protein

  c. Weight gain: >35 kcal/kg 1.0 g/kg protein

Refeeding syndrome is a recognized complication of aggressive nutritional support. It is most frequently observed in the significantly underweight patient (BMI <15) who is receiving parenteral nutrition. Abnormalities due to hyperinsulinemia occur in response to feedings and include hypokalemia, hypophosphatemia, hypomagnesemia, volume overload, and edema, with hypophosphatemia being very common. Severe hypophosphatemia is associated with heart failure, arrhythmias, impaired diaphragmatic contractility, liver function test abnormalities, delirium, and seizures. The patient at risk of refeeding syndrome must be recognized so that the necessary precautions can be taken. Prevention includes gradual caloric progression, monitoring of clinical status, and correction of electrolyte abnormalities identified before the initiation of nutrition.

- It is important to recognize the patient at risk of refeeding syndrome so that precautions can be taken to avoid potentially fatal complications.

SUMMARY

- Caloric restriction of 250–500 kcal daily is the main determinant of successful weight loss.

- Medications for weight loss are reserved for patients who meet criteria for obesity or overweight and have weight-related medical problems.

- The most common causes of death after bariatric surgery are pulmonary embolism and anastomotic leaks.

- Cholelithiasis is common after bariatric surgery. Prophylactic administration of ursodeoxycholic acid for 6 months after surgery decreases the risk of gallstone formation.

- Nutritional support should be considered for critically ill patients and for patients who have a BMI <18.5, a weight loss >5%-10% of initial body weight, or an inability to meet their nutritional needs for 14 days.

- In the absence of contraindications, enteral nutritional support is preferred.

- Parenteral nutrition is advised for patients who do not meet their nutritional needs for 7–14 days and have contraindications or intolerance to enteral feedings. Hyperglycemia, hypertriglyceridemia, and bloodstream infection are recognized complications of parenteral nutrition.

SUGGESTED READING

Aasheim ET. Wernicke encephalopathy after bariatric surgery: a systematic review. Ann Surg. 2008 Nov;248(5):714–20.

Ascherio A, Rimm EB, Giovannucci EL, Spiegelman D, Stampfer M, Willett WC. Dietary fat and risk of coronary heart disease in men: cohort follow up study in the United States. BMJ. 1996 Jul 13;313(7049):84–90.

Barba CA, Butensky MS, Lorenzo M, Newman R. Endoscopic dilation of gastroesophageal anastomosis stricture after gastric bypass. Surg Endosc. 2003 Mar;17(3):416–20. Epub 2002 Dec 4.

Buchwald H, Avidor Y, Braunwald E, Jensen MD, Pories W, Fahrbach K, et al. Bariatric surgery: a systematic review and meta-analysis. JAMA. 2004 Oct 13;292(14):1724–37. Erratum in: JAMA. 2005 Apr 13;293(14):1728.

Dickey RA, Bartuska DG, Bray GW, Callaway CW, Davidson ET, Feld S, et al; AACE/ACE Obesity Task Force. AACE/ACE position statement on the prevention, diagnosis, and treatment of obesity (1998 revision). Endocr Pract 1998 Sept/Oct;4(5):297–350.

Di Stefano M, Miceli E, Missanelli A, Mazzocchi S, Corazza GR. Absorbable vs. non-absorbable antibiotics in the treatment of small intestine bacterial overgrowth in patients with blind-loop syndrome. Aliment Pharmacol Ther. 2005 Apr 15;21(8):985–92.

Flum DR, Salem L, Elrod JA, Dellinger EP, Cheadle A, Chan L. Early mortality among Medicare beneficiaries undergoing bariatric surgical procedures. JAMA. 2005 Oct 19;294(15):1903–8.

Hamilton EC, Sims TL, Hamilton TT, Mullican MA, Jones DB, Provost DA. Clinical predictors of leak after laparoscopic Roux-en-Y gastric bypass for morbid obesity. Surg Endosc. 2003 May;17(5):679–84. Epub 2003 Mar 7.

Huang HY, Caballero B, Chang S, Alberg AJ, Semba RD, Schneyer CR, et al. The efficacy and safety of multivitamin and mineral supplement use to prevent cancer and chronic disease in adults: a systematic review for a National Institutes of Health state-of-the-science conference. Ann Intern Med. 2006 Sep 5;145(5):372–85. Epub 2006 Jul 31.

Janssen I, Katzmarzyk PT, Ross R. Body mass index, waist circumference, and health risk: evidence in support of current National Institutes of Health guidelines. Arch Intern Med. 2002 Oct 14;162(18):2074–9.

Jeejeebhoy KN. Permissive underfeeding of the critically ill patient. Nutr Clin Pract. 2004 Oct;19(5):477–80.

Koretz RL, Lipman TO, Klein S; American Gastroenterological Association. AGA technical review on parenteral nutrition. Gastroenterology. 2001 Oct;121(4):970–1001.

Kraft MD, Btaiche IF, Sacks GS. Review of the refeeding syndrome. Nutr Clin Pract. 2005 Dec;20(6):625–33.

Law MR, Morris JK. By how much does fruit and vegetable consumption reduce the risk of ischaemic heart disease? Eur J Clin Nutr. 1998 Aug;52(8):549–56.

Love AL, Billett HH. Obesity, bariatric surgery, and iron deficiency: true, true, true and related. Am J Hematol. 2008 May;83(5):403–9.

Maggard MA, Shugarman LR, Suttorp M, Maglione M, Sugerman HJ, Livingston EH, et al. Meta-analysis: surgical treatment of obesity. Ann Intern Med. 2005 Apr 5;142(7):547–59.

Marik PE, Zaloga GP. Early enteral nutrition in acutely ill patients: a systematic review. Crit Care Med. 2001 Dec;29(12):2264–70. Erratum in: Crit Care Med. 2002 Mar;30(3):725.

Mechanick JI, Kushner RF, Sugerman HJ, Gonzalez-Campoy JM, Collazo-Clavell ML, Spitz AF, et al; American Association of Clinical Endocrinologists; Obesity Society; American Society for Metabolic & Bariatric Surgery. American Association of Clinical Endocrinologists, The Obesity Society, and American Society for Metabolic & Bariatric Surgery medical guidelines for clinical practice for the perioperative nutritional, metabolic, and nonsurgical support of the bariatric surgery patient. Obesity (Silver Spring). 2009 Apr;17 Suppl 1:S1–70, v. Erratum in: Obesity (Silver Spring). 2010 Mar;18(3):649.

Mozaffarian D, Rimm EB. Fish intake, contaminants, and human health: evaluating the risks and the benefits. JAMA. 2006 Oct 18;296(15):1885–99. Erratum in: JAMA. 2007 Feb 14;297(6):590.

National Institutes of Health, National Heart, Lung, and Blood Institute, North American Association for the Study of Obesity. The practical guide: identification, evaluation, and treatment of overweight and obesity in adults. Bethesda (MD): National Institutes of Health; c2000. NIH Publication No. 00–4084.

Rasmussen JJ, Fuller W, Ali MR. Marginal ulceration after laparoscopic gastric bypass: an analysis of predisposing factors in 260 patients. Surg Endosc. 2007 Jul;21(7):1090–4. Epub 2007 May 19.

Report at a glance: report brief. Dietary reference intakes for calcium and vitamin D [Internet]. Washington, DC: Institute of Medicine of the National Academies. c2010 – [cited 2012 Jul 17]. Available from: http://www.iom.edu/Reports/2010/Dietary-Reference-Intakes-for-Calcium-and-Vitamin-D/Report-Brief.aspx.

Roldan CA, Gill EA, Shively BK. Prevalence and diagnostic value of precordial murmurs for valvular regurgitation in obese patients treated with dexfenfluramine. Am J Cardiol. 2000 Sep 1;86(5):535–9.

Sapala JA, Wood MH, Schuhknecht MP, Sapala MA. Fatal pulmonary embolism after bariatric operations for morbid obesity: a 24-year retrospective analysis. Obes Surg. 2003 Dec;13(6):819–25.

Schneider BE, Villegas L, Blackburn GL, Mun EC, Critchlow JF, Jones DB. Laparoscopic gastric bypass surgery: outcomes. J Laparoendosc Adv Surg Tech A. 2003 Aug;13(4):247–55.

Service GJ, Thompson GB, Service FJ, Andrews JC, Collazo-Clavell ML, Lloyd RV. Hyperinsulinemic hypoglycemia with nesidioblastosis after gastric-bypass surgery. N Engl J Med. 2005 Jul 21;353(3):249–54.

Sinha MK, Collazo-Clavell ML, Rule A, Milliner DS, Nelson W, Sarr MG, et al. Hyperoxaluric nephrolithiasis is a complication of Roux-en-Y gastric bypass surgery. Kidney Int. 2007 Jul;72(1):100–7. Epub 2007 Mar 21.

Snow V, Barry P, Fitterman N, Qaseem A, Weiss K; Clinical Efficacy Assessment Subcommittee of the American College of Physicians. Pharmacologic and surgical management of obesity in primary care: a clinical practice guideline from the American College of Physicians. Ann Intern Med. 2005 Apr 5;142(7):525–31.

Sugerman HJ, Brewer WH, Shiffman ML, Brolin RE, Fobi MA, Linner JH, et al. A multicenter, placebo-controlled, randomized, double-blind, prospective trial of prophylactic ursodiol for the prevention of gallstone formation following gastric-bypass-induced rapid weight loss. Am J Surg. 1995 Jan;169(1):91–6.

Tribble DL. AHA Science Advisory. Antioxidant consumption and risk of coronary heart disease: emphasis on vitamin C, vitamin E, and beta-carotene: a statement for healthcare professionals from the American Heart Association. Circulation. 1999 Feb 2;99(4):591–5.

Yang J, Lee HR, Low K, Chatterjee S, Pimentel M. Rifaximin versus other antibiotics in the primary treatment and retreatment of bacterial overgrowth in IBS. Dig Dis Sci. 2008 Jan;53(1):169–74. Epub 2007 May 23.

30.

PITUITARY DISORDERS

Charles F. Abboud, MB, ChB, Bryan McIver, MB, ChB, PhD, and Pankaj Shah, MD

GOALS

- Summarize hypothalamic and pituitary disorders.
- Review water metabolism.
- Describe pituitary-related emergencies.

HYPOPITUITARISM

ETIOLOGY

Hypopituitarism usually results from a deficiency of anterior pituitary hormones or, rarely, from tissue resistance to these hormones. Deficiency may be from primary pituitary disease, pituitary stalk disorders, or hypothalamic disease or from an extrasellar disorder impinging on, or infiltrating, the hypothalamic-pituitary unit.

Primary pituitary disease results from the loss of anterior pituitary cells and may be congenital or acquired. Common causes are pituitary tumors and their surgical or radiotherapeutic ablation. Infrequent causes include pituitary infarction (eg, postpartum pituitary necrosis, also known as Sheehan syndrome), pituitary apoplexy, lymphocytic hypophysitis, infiltrative diseases (eg, hemochromatosis), and metastatic disease (eg, from breast or lung).

Hypothalamic hypopituitarism results from hypothalamic or pituitary stalk disease associated with the loss of hypophysiotropic regulatory hormones of the anterior pituitary cells. Primary hypothalamic diseases are relatively rare and include disorders that are genetic (Kallmann syndrome), traumatic (accidental, surgical, or radiotherapeutic), inflammatory or infiltrative (eg, tuberculosis, sarcoidosis, and histiocytosis X), vascular (eg, bleeding disorders and vasculitis), or neoplastic, including primary neoplasms (eg, glioma, ependymoma, hamartoma, and gangliocytoma) or metastatic neoplasms.

Functional hypothalamic disorders are common and include the following:

1. Functional suppression of gonadotropin-releasing hormone (GnRH) related to disorders of weight, exercise, psychiatric disorder, systemic disease, or endocrinopathy (eg, hyperprolactinemia, thyroid [or adrenal] disorders, and uncompensated diabetes mellitus)

2. Functional lack of growth hormone (GH) as occurs in emotional deprivation syndrome

3. Functional lack of corticotropin (ACTH) as occurs after withdrawal of prolonged supraphysiologic glucocorticoid therapy

4. Functional lack of thyrotropin (TSH) as occurs for a few weeks after correction of a hyperthyroid state. A structural hypothalamic disorder is not evident in a functional hypothalamic disorder, and normal endocrine function is ultimately restored after the cause is managed or removed.

Extrasellar disorders impinge on and impair the function of the hypothalamic-pituitary unit. Examples include craniopharyngioma (most common), optic glioma, meningioma, nasopharyngeal carcinoma, sphenoid sinus mucocele, and carotid artery aneurysms.

- Hypopituitarism can result from primary pituitary disorders, hypothalamic–pituitary stalk disorders, or extrasellar disorders.

- Most common causes of primary hypopituitarism: pituitary tumors and their surgical or radiotherapeutic ablation.

- Most common causes of hypothalamic hypopituitarism: reversible functional disorders, accidental or surgical or radiotherapeutic trauma, and infiltrative disorders.

- Most common cause of hypopituitarism due to extrasellar disorder: craniopharyngioma.

CLINICAL FEATURES

Patients with hypopituitarism can present with features of deficiency of 1 or more of the anterior pituitary hormones. The clinical picture depends on the age at onset, hormones affected, extent and duration of deficiency, and acuteness of the process. The most common presentation is that of a chronic process of insidious onset.

Chronic Illness

Gonadotropin Deficiency

The features of gonadotropin deficiency are those of the loss of the steroidogenic and gametogenic functions of the gonads. Female patients may have infertility, oligomenorrhea or amenorrhea, loss of libido, vaginal dryness and dyspareunia, involution of the uterus and genitalia, and atrophy or loss of secondary sex characteristics. Male patients may have loss of libido, potency impairment, infertility, atrophy or loss of secondary sex characteristics, atrophy of the testes and prostate, and, occasionally, gynecomastia. In both sexes, fine wrinkling of the skin may be seen radially around the mouth or eyes and osteoporosis may occur.

ACTH Deficiency

The features of ACTH deficiency result primarily from a lack of cortisol and loss of the pigmentary functions of ACTH and related peptides. Such features may include ill health, anorexia, weight loss, gastrointestinal tract disturbances, rheumatologic aches and pains, hypoglycemia, hyponatremia, susceptibility to adrenocortical crises, pallor, and inability to tan or maintain a tan. The features of mineralocorticoid deficiency are typically absent because aldosterone secretion depends on the renin-angiotensin system, not on ACTH. Therefore, hyperkalemia and hypovolemia with orthostatism are typically absent. Partial ACTH deficiency may cause symptoms only during periods of acute medical or surgical illness.

TSH Deficiency

TSH deficiency results in a lack of thyroid hormones (triiodothyronine [T_3] and thyroxine [T_4]) and the characteristic features of slowing of emotional, mental, and physical functions. The thyroid gland is atrophic.

Prolactin Deficiency

Postpartum women who have prolactin deficiency cannot lactate.

GH Deficiency

The features of GH deficiency in adults include ill health and asthenia, fatigue, muscle weakness, osteopenia, obesity, psychosocial difficulties, and increased cardiovascular risk.

- Gonadotropin deficiency: failure of production of sex steroids and gametes; main features are hypogonadism and infertility.

- ACTH deficiency: cortisol deficiency and loss of pigmentary effects of ACTH and related peptides. Lack of cortisol is manifested as chronic ill health, hypoglycemia, hyponatremia, and susceptibility to adrenocortical crises. Aldosterone secretion is basically normal; hyperkalemia and hypovolemia are characteristically absent.

- TSH deficiency: hypothyroidism and absence of goiter.

- Prolactin deficiency: failure of lactation in postpartum women.

- GH deficiency: ill-defined syndrome of asthenia, weakness, and ill health.

Acute Illness

Adrenocortical crisis may be precipitated by the following:

1. Withdrawal of prolonged glucocorticoid therapy without proper glucocorticoid coverage during recovery of the hypothalamic-pituitary-adrenal axis

2. Pituitary surgery without optimal glucocorticoid stress coverage

3. Acute medical or surgical illness in a patient who has a lack of cortisol that is unrecognized or poorly managed

4. Pituitary apoplexy

5. Thyroid hormone replacement therapy in a patient who has an associated and unrecognized deficiency of ACTH

Other acute manifestations are fasting hypoglycemia syndrome (decreased hepatic neoglucogenesis due to lack of cortisol and GH), hyponatremic syndrome (renal water conservation due to decreased glomerular filtration rate [GFR] and unchecked secretion of antidiuretic hormone [ADH]—ie, syndrome of inappropriate secretion of ADH [SIADH]), and increased sensitivity to central nervous system (CNS) depressants (decreased metabolism and clearance due to lack of ACTH and TSH).

- Acute manifestations of hypopituitarism: adrenocortical crisis, fasting hypoglycemia syndrome, hyponatremic syndrome, and increased sensitivity to CNS depressants.

DIAGNOSIS

Diagnosis requires documenting the presence of hypopituitarism *and* identifying the cause. In the appropriate clinical setting, provocative tests are used to accurately diagnose deficiencies of nontropic hormones, which act directly on target cells (eg, prolactin, oxytocin, GH). For deficiencies of tropic hormones, which act on other endocrine glands (eg, TSH, ACTH, luteinizing hormone [LH], follicle-stimulating hormone [FSH], GH), target gland function is evaluated. GH has both tropic and nontropic functions. If target gland failure is present, tropic hormone levels must be determined to distinguish between primary target gland failure and failure due to hypothalamic-pituitary disease. Increased pituitary tropic hormone levels indicate target gland failure; normal or low tropic hormone levels indicate hypopituitarism.

- In diagnosing hypopituitarism: hypopituitarism must be documented and its cause delineated.

- Use a provocative test in the appropriate clinical setting to evaluate nontropic hormone deficiency.

- Evaluate target gland function for suspected tropic hormone deficiency; test the tropic hormone level if target gland failure is present to distinguish between primary target gland failure and hypothalamic-pituitary disease.

Gonadotropin Axis

Male patients have a low serum testosterone level, inappropriately low serum LH and FSH levels, and a low sperm count. Female patients have a low serum estradiol level and inappropriately low serum LH and FSH levels. Provocative tests for LH and FSH with GnRH or clomiphene are rarely needed in clinical practice.

- Male patients: low sperm count, low serum testosterone level, and inappropriately low serum LH and FSH levels.

- Female patients: low serum estradiol and inappropriately low serum LH and FSH levels.

ACTH Axis

A morning plasma cortisol of less than 3 μg/dL, repeated on 2 occasions, confirms adrenocortical failure. A level of more than 18 μg/dL indicates a normal axis. Values of 3 to 18 μg/dL require a provocative test to assess adrenal function.

In chronic ACTH deficiency, the adrenal cortices are atrophic and do not secrete cortisol in response to the short-acting exogenous ACTH stimulation test (ie, the cosyntropin test). Primary adrenocortical failure is confirmed by an increased serum level of ACTH or by a lack of adrenocortical responsiveness to prolonged exogenous ACTH stimulation if cosyntropin testing is not available. In adrenocortical failure due to hypothalamic-pituitary disease, the levels of serum ACTH are inappropriately low.

- The cosyntropin test (ie, the short ACTH stimulation test) usually shows absence of cortisol secretory response.

- In adrenocortical failure due to hypothalamic-pituitary disease, serum levels of ACTH are inappropriately low.

TSH Axis

Low serum free thyroxine (FT_4) (or FT_4 index) and an inappropriately "normal" or low serum level of TSH support the diagnosis of central hypothyroidism. In hypothyroid patients, a high serum level of TSH or the presence of goiter points to primary hypothyroidism, and an inappropriately low serum level of TSH confirms the diagnosis of TSH deficiency.

- TSH deficiency: low serum level of FT_4 or FT_4 index and an inappropriately "normal" or low serum TSH.

Growth Hormone

GH deficiency is likely present in the patient with demonstrable structural disease of the pituitary gland; deficiencies of gonadotropins, ACTH, and TSH; and a low age-specific serum level of insulinlike growth factor 1 (IGF-1). In the absence of other pituitary hormone deficiency, a provocative test is indicated. The preferred test uses arginine plus GH-releasing hormone (GHRH). The insulin hypoglycemia test is not safe and is contraindicated in patients who have seizures or cerebrovascular or cardiovascular disease.

GH deficiency is indicated by low serum levels of IGF-1 with documented structural pituitary disease and loss of other pituitary hormones. In the absence of other indicators, GH deficiency is confirmed by a low serum GH response to stimulation. The insulin-hypoglycemia test can be hazardous and should not be done.

Prolactin

Provocative tests for prolactin are not needed in clinical practice.

- A low serum level of prolactin is diagnostic.

Radiologic Evaluation

Radiologic evaluation includes imaging of the hypothalamic-pituitary region by computed tomography (CT) or magnetic resonance imaging (MRI) and, in the presence of suprasellar disease, neuro-ophthalmologic evaluation to assess visual fields, visual acuity, and optic discs. MRI is preferred.

- Anatomical evaluation: imaging with CT or MRI (preferred) and neuro-ophthalmologic evaluation.

In determining the cause of hypopituitarism, suspected functional causes must be removed or corrected. Normalization of pituitary function after correction of a functional cause lends support to "functional" hypopituitarism. If the functional causes are excluded, or if hypopituitarism persists despite removal or correction of a functional cause, evaluation for structural hypothalamic-pituitary disease is mandatory. This evaluation is based on the clinical setting and appropriate endocrine and anatomical studies.

- Suspected functional causes must be removed or corrected.

- If hypopituitarism persists after removal or correction of possible functional causes, evaluate for structural hypothalamic-pituitary disease on the basis of the clinical setting and appropriate laboratory and radiologic studies.

THERAPY

Therapy includes correction of the cause and, when applicable, administration of the hormones of the target glands or, in selected cases, pituitary hormones.

- Treat the cause and, if needed, administer pituitary hormones or target gland hormones.

ACTH Deficiency

For ACTH deficiency, glucocorticoid replacement is critical. Instruct patients in dose modification during acute illness. In patients with a deficiency of both ACTH and TSH, initiate glucocorticoid therapy *before* thyroid hormone therapy to avoid a thyroid hormone–induced increased need for cortisol and precipitation of an acute adrenocortical crisis. Adequacy of therapy is judged by clinical criteria, resolution of symptoms, and the absence of signs and symptoms of supraphysiologic replacement. Serum ACTH levels cannot be used to assess adequacy of therapy.

- Instruct patients about dose modification during acute illness.

- In patients with a deficiency of both ACTH and TSH, initiate glucocorticoid therapy *before* thyroid hormone therapy.

TSH Deficiency

For TSH deficiency, the drug of choice is T_4. Assess the adequacy of therapy by the feeling of well-being and the serum level of FT_4. Serum TSH level should not be used to monitor the adequacy of the T_4 dosage since it is low in untreated persons.

- T_4 is the drug of choice.

Gonadotropin Deficiency

Gonadotropin deficiency is treated with sex steroids. In female patients, estrogen therapy is used. Progestagens must be used for patients with an intact uterus.

In male patients, testosterone is used to try to restore full androgenicity. Assess status of the prostate in middle-aged and elderly men before therapy and follow annually. For restoration of fertility, FSH and LH (or GnRH therapy in patients with hypothalamic disorders) may be indicated. Evaluate the patient's psychosexual needs and lifestyle to assess the effect of therapy.

- In hypogonadal female patients, use estrogen therapy. Use supplemental progestagens for patients with an intact uterus.

- In hypogonadal male patients, use testosterone.

- For restoration of fertility, consider the use of exogenous gonadotropins (or, if feasible, GnRH therapy in patients with hypothalamic disease).

GH Deficiency

For GH deficiency, short-term GH therapy enhances a sense of well-being, normalizes body composition, increases muscle strength and exercise capacity, increases bone mineral density, and improves cardiac function. GH therapy may be considered for patients with hypothalamic-pituitary disease and a poor GH response to a standard stimulus. The goal of therapy is to restore serum IGF-1 to normal levels and to avoid side effects. The long-term effects of such therapy are unknown; thus, a benefit-risk profile cannot be determined.

PITUITARY TUMORS

Pituitary tumors can be described according to size as microadenomas (≤ 10 mm) or macroadenomas (>10 mm), by extent as sellar or sellar/extrasellar, and by type as functioning or nonfunctioning. *Functioning pituitary tumors* include prolactinomas (40%-50%), GH tumors (10%-15%), ACTH tumors (10%-15%), and TSH tumors (<5%). *Nonfunctioning tumors* (30%-40%) include the gonadotropinomas and null-cell adenomas. Pituitary tumors are usually sporadic; rarely, they may be part of syndromes such as multiple endocrine neoplasia type 1 (MEN-1), McCune-Albright syndrome, or Carney complex.

- Tumor size: microadenoma (≤ 10 mm) or macroadenoma (>10 mm).

- Tumor extent: sellar or sellar/extrasellar.

- Tumor type: functioning or nonfunctioning.

- Tumor may be isolated or part of a syndrome such as MEN-1.

CLINICAL FEATURES

The usual manifestation of a pituitary tumor is that of a chronic, slowly evolving disorder. Mass effects include headaches and evidence of tumor extension beyond the confines of the sella as follows:

1. *Superior tumor extension* may cause the following:

    a. Chiasma syndrome (impaired visual acuity and visual field defects)

    b. Hypothalamic syndrome (vegetative disturbance in thirst, appetite, satiety, sleep, and temperature regulation and the endocrine disorder of diabetes insipidus or SIADH)

    c. Obstructive hydrocephalus

    d. Frontal lobe dysfunction

2. *Lateral tumor extension* may cause impairment of cranial nerves III, IV, V, and VI, with diplopia, facial pain, and temporal lobe dysfunction.

3. *Inferior tumor extension* may cause nasopharyngeal mass or cerebrospinal fluid (CSF) rhinorrhea.

Endocrine effects include the following:

1. *Hypersecretory states*, in which hyperpituitarism leads to gigantism or acromegaly (GH excess), hyperprolactinemic syndrome (prolactin excess), Cushing disease and Nelson-Salassa syndrome (ACTH excess), and thyrotoxicosis (TSH excess). Generally, LH or FSH excess is clinically silent.

2. *Hypopituitarism* can be caused by tumor growth that destroys the pituitary gland.

3. *Endocrine associations* of pituitary tumors include MEN-1, that is, parathyroid tumor or hyperplasia (primary hyperparathyroidism), endocrine pancreas tumor or hyperplasia (various endocrine pancreatic syndromes), other endocrine gland tumors (thyroid, adrenal), and lipomas.

Rarely, pituitary tumors manifest acutely with pituitary apoplexy (acute hemorrhage into the pituitary gland), which may be the first clinical expression of the underlying tumor.

- Mass effects include headaches and extrasellar effects due to tumor extension beyond the sella.
- Endocrine effects result from hypersecretory states or hypopituitarism.
- Endocrine associations of pituitary tumors include MEN-1.
- Pituitary apoplexy may complicate the course or be the initial manifestation of the tumor.

DIAGNOSIS

The presence of a pituitary tumor is suggested by the clinical features and confirmed by pituitary imaging. MRI is the preferred imaging technique. Neuro-ophthalmologic evaluation is important, particularly if suprasellar extension is present. Endocrine evaluation includes evaluation for hormonal excess or deficiency and for the presence of MEN-1. A pituitary tumor is diagnosed if a sellar mass is associated with an excess of anterior pituitary hormone (except for mild hyperprolactinemia, which can occur with nonpituitary masses and the "stalk effect"). Otherwise, the diagnosis is confirmed at surgical exploration.

- The presence of a pituitary tumor is suggested by clinical assessment and radiologic imaging findings.
- Neuro-ophthalmologic evaluation is important, particularly with suprasellar extension.
- Endocrine evaluation should assess for hormonal excess or deficiency and the presence of MEN-1.

TREATMENT

Pituitary tumors generally are treated with surgical excision or radiotherapy. Drug therapy is available for prolactin-, GH-, or TSH-producing tumors. Medical therapy is the primary therapy for prolactinomas and is an adjunct to ablative therapy. Conservative noninterventional therapy is an option for small tumors with no effect on quality or quantity of life.

- Treatment options for pituitary tumors include surgical excision, radiotherapy, or drug therapy.
- Drug therapy is the primary therapy for prolactinomas and is a useful adjunctive therapy in the treatment of GH or TSH tumors.
- Noninterventional therapy is an option for a small, nonfunctioning tumor or for a microprolactinoma not associated with clinical features that impinge on quality of life.

Transsphenoidal surgery is the operation of choice for most tumors; the transcranial approach is used for large suprasellar tumor extension. Surgical morbidity and mortality and the available neurosurgical expertise should be considered. Morbidity (eg, bleeding, infection, transient diabetes insipidus, and CSF rhinorrhea) is less than 1% for microadenomas and less than 4% for macroadenomas, and mortality is less than 1% with an experienced surgeon. Persistence or recurrence of the tumor is less than 20% to 30% for microadenomas and 50% to 70% for macroadenomas.

- Transsphenoidal surgery is the operation of choice.
- Morbidity and mortality are low with an experienced surgeon.
- Persistence or recurrence of the tumor is moderately high.

Radiotherapy results in a long latent period (a few months to years) and postradiation hypopituitarism (in 10 years, >50% of patients, or a smaller percentage with a highly focused modality). CNS damage and development of CNS tumors are rare.

- A majority of patients have postradiation hypopituitarism.
- CNS damage and CNS tumors due to radiotherapy are rare.

Dopamine agonists are used for the management of prolactinomas or GH-producing tumors. Somatostatin analogues are used for the management of GH- or TSH-producing tumors. Pegvisomant, a GH-receptor blocker, is used in the management of GH-producing tumors refractory to other management options.

- Drug therapy may be first-line (dopamine agonists for prolactinomas) or adjunctive.

Follow-up is essential to monitor for persistence or recurrence of the tumor, development of hypopituitarism in patients treated surgically or with radiotherapy, and the possible occurrence of MEN-1 in familial cases.

PROLACTINOMA AND THE HYPERPROLACTINEMIC SYNDROME

Pituitary tumors associated with hyperprolactinemia may be prolactinomas, mixed tumors (eg, GH- and prolactin-producing tumors), or nonfunctioning tumors with suprasellar extension and the stalk effect. In stalk-effect hyperprolactinemia, impingement of the mass on the pituitary stalk interferes with the access of hypothalamic dopamine to the anterior pituitary and results in disinhibition of prolactin secretion by normal lactotrophs.

- Pituitary tumors associated with hyperprolactinemia: prolactinomas, mixed tumors, or any tumor or mass lesion with suprasellar extension and the stalk effect.

CLINICAL FEATURES

Mass effects include hypopituitarism and expressions of extrasellar extension of the pituitary tumor. Persons with hyperprolactinemia may be asymptomatic but are usually symptomatic. Hyperprolactinemia suppresses GnRH secretion and causes a lactogenic effect on the breasts.

In women, hyperprolactinemia is usually expressed as galactorrhea, ovulatory and menstrual dysfunction (short luteal phase or anovulation leading to infertility), oligomenorrhea or amenorrhea and hypogonadism, and decreased libido. In some women, hyperprolactinemia may be associated with hirsutism and acne.

In men, hyperprolactinemia results in hypogonadism, infertility due to oligospermia, and, rarely, galactorrhea or gynecomastia. The recognition of hyperprolactinemia frequently is delayed in men because decreased libido and impaired potency may be dismissed by the patient and physician and attributed to psychiatric factors. In men with a pituitary tumor, marked hyperprolactinemia and a macroprolactinoma are common at presentation.

- Endocrine effects include the effects of hyperprolactinemia, associated pituitary dysfunction, and associated MEN-1.

- Hyperprolactinemia exerts its clinical effects dominantly on GnRH secretion and the breasts.

- Women may have ovulatory or menstrual dysfunction, galactorrhea, and hirsutism.

- Men may have decreased libido and impotence.

- In men, recognition of hyperprolactinemia is frequently delayed, and a macroprolactinoma is common at diagnosis.

DIAGNOSIS

Prolactinoma must be distinguished from other causes of hyperprolactinemia and from other pituitary area masses. Hyperprolactinemia can be physiologic or pathologic in origin:

1. *Physiologic hyperprolactinemia* may occur in pregnancy and the postpartum state and in conditions of stress, such as surgery or acute illness.

2. *Pathologic hyperprolactinemia* may be eutopic (pituitary) or ectopic (extrapituitary). Eutopic hyperprolactinemia may occur in primary pituitary disease or in hypothalamic or stalk disease resulting in loss of dopaminergic influence and disinhibition of prolactin secretion by normal lactotrophs. Primary pituitary causes include prolactinoma, "mixed tumors," nonfunctioning pituitary tumors with suprasellar extension and stalk effect hyperprolactinemia, hypophysitis, and primary empty sella.

- Hyperprolactinemia may be physiologic or pathologic.

- Physiologic hyperprolactinemia may occur in pregnancy, the postpartum state, and conditions of stress.

- Pathologic hyperprolactinemia may be eutopic (pituitary) or ectopic (extrapituitary) in origin.

- Pituitary causes: most common is prolactinoma.

Hypothalamic or stalk disorders can be functional or organic. *Functional hypothalamic disorders* lead to hyperprolactinemia because of interference with the synthesis, secretion, or action of dopamine or other hypothalamic regulators of prolactin secretion. These disorders may be caused by the following:

1. Drugs (eg, neuroleptics, antidepressants, narcotics, and estrogens)

2. Primary hypothyroidism (15%-30%)

3. Chest wall irritative lesions (eg, herpes zoster, dermatitis, and thoracotomy)

4. Renal failure

5. Cirrhosis or hepatic encephalopathy

Organic hypothalamic disorders include traumatic disorders (eg, surgery or radiotherapy), inflammatory disorders (eg, sarcoidosis or histiocytosis X), or neoplastic disorders (eg, craniopharyngioma, optic glioma, meningioma, or metastases such as those from the breast or lungs). Ectopic hyperprolactinemia (very rare) has been reported with hypernephroma, gonadoblastoma, and ovarian teratomas.

- Hypothalamic causes of hyperprolactinemia are functional or organic.

- Functional disorders may be caused by drugs, primary hypothyroidism, chest wall lesions, and chronic renal or hepatic failure.

- Organic causes include hypothalamic disorders due to trauma, inflammation, and infiltrative processes.

Female patients with hyperprolactinemia must have pregnancy excluded. The morning basal fasting serum level of prolactin should be measured.

The diagnosis of a prolactinoma is established with serum levels of prolactin greater than 10 times the upper end of the reference range. However, prolactinomas, particularly microprolactinomas, may be associated with lower prolactin levels.

If the prolactin level is less than 10 times the upper end of the reference range, rule out functional causes. If a functional cause is present, remove it or treat it if possible. If hyperprolactinemia does not resolve in about 3 months, evaluate for hypothalamic-pituitary disease. If a functional cause is not present, rule out organic hypothalamic-pituitary disease by imaging the hypothalamic-pituitary region, preferably by MRI, and by evaluating other pituitary functions and the visual fields, if appropriate.

If a cause is not found, the hyperprolactinemia is considered to be of indeterminate origin. Follow-up evaluation is critical because some patients may harbor microadenomas or other hypothalamic-pituitary space-occupying lesions that are below the limit of radiologic detection, and follow-up examinations may show evidence of a mass. The serum level of prolactin should be checked every 6 to 12 months and imaging should be repeated in 1 to 2 years or earlier if new symptoms develop.

Macroprolactinemia may account for up to 10% of patients presenting with hyperprolactinemia. Rarely, glycosylated prolactin circulating in aggregates (macroprolactin) accounts for most of the circulating prolactin. These aggregates are not cleared well by the kidneys. This appears to be a benign condition requiring no specific therapy. However, it can be misdiagnosed and treated inappropriately.

TREATMENT

Microprolactinoma or Idiopathic Hyperprolactinemia

Treatment is indicated for management of infertility, hypogonadism, or significant galactorrhea. Treatment options for infertility include dopamine agonist therapy and transsphenoidal surgery for microprolactinoma. If fertility is not an issue, estrogen therapy is indicated to prevent hypoestrogenic manifestations, including bone loss. Otherwise, observe and check the serum level of prolactin annually and reimage every 2 to 3 years.

Macroprolactinoma

Therapy is indicated for all patients because of the threat of a mass lesion and the effects of hyperprolactinemia. Drug therapy with a dopamine agonist is the preferred treatment. Surgical excision or radiotherapy is reserved for the drug-intolerant or drug-resistant cases (10%-20% for bromocriptine; 3%-7% for cabergoline).

Dopamine Agonists

Dopamine agonists are the mainstay of prolactinoma therapy. They suppress prolactin secretion and proliferation of prolactin-producing cells, restore gonadal function (70%-80%), and decrease tumor size (>50%). Patients with Parkinson disease who receive cabergoline should be monitored clinically and by echocardiography biannually because of the possible development of cardiac valvular disease. Therapy with dopamine agonists is temporizing, and discontinuation usually leads to recurrence of tumor growth and endocrine dysfunction. However, in some patients who have the outcomes of normoprolactinemia and significantly smaller tumor, use of the drug can be withdrawn after 1 to 2 years. In these patients, the tumor may have a long remission but need careful monitoring.

Dopamine agonist therapy should be stopped at the earliest sign of pregnancy. In pregnancy, the risk of microprolactinoma growth is less than 5%, and the risk of macroprolactinoma growth, 20% to 40%. Observe patients closely; if tumor growth is suspected, confirm with imaging (do not use gadolinium during pregnancy). If significant tumor growth complicates pregnancy, consider surgical excision or reinstitution of dopamine agonist therapy.

- Dopamine agonists suppress hyperprolactinemia, restore gonadal function (70%-80%), and decrease tumor size (>50%).

- Bromocriptine and cabergoline are safe and effective drugs. Cabergoline appears to be more effective, is more convenient to use, and is associated with lesser degrees of drug intolerance or resistance.

- Discontinuation of the use of the dopamine agonist usually leads to resumption of tumor growth and endocrine dysfunction.

- Use of dopamine agonists should be stopped at the earliest sign of pregnancy.

- During pregnancy, the risk of microprolactinoma growth is <5%, and the risk of macroprolactinoma growth, 20%-40%.

- If significant tumor growth complicates pregnancy, consider surgical excision or reinstitution of drug therapy.

Surgical Treatment of Prolactinomas

For microadenomas, the surgical cure rates are 60% to 80%; for macroadenomas, 0% to 30%.

GH TUMORS: ACROMEGALY AND GIGANTISM

ETIOLOGY

Acromegaly is nearly always caused by a benign GH-producing pituitary tumor. These tumors usually secrete only GH; infrequently, they may simultaneously secrete prolactin, α-glycoprotein, ACTH, or TSH. Rarely, acromegaly may be caused by ectopic GH-producing tumors or hypothalamic or extrahypothalamic GHRH-producing tumors.

GH-producing pituitary tumors are usually sporadic; rarely, they are familial and may occur in association with MEN-1, McCune Albright syndrome, or Carney complex.

CLINICAL FEATURES

The clinical presentations are related to excess levels of GH and IGF-1, the pituitary tumor, and the associations of acromegaly. Excess levels of GH and IGF-1 lead to gigantism in a child and to the characteristic acromegalic features in an adult. These include the following:

1. Bone and soft-tissue overgrowth, with coarsening of the facial features; frontal bossing; prognathism; widened spaces between teeth; macroglossia; increased hat, glove, ring, or shoe size; acroparesthesias; and nerve entrapment syndromes

2. Hyperhidrosis, heat intolerance, skin tags, and increased skin oiliness

3. Carbohydrate intolerance (20%) and, rarely, frank diabetes mellitus, hypercalciuria, and hyperphosphatemia

4. Fibromas or acanthosis nigricans

5. Sleep apnea, obstructive and central

6. Cardiovascular effects, including hypertension, left ventricular hypertrophy, diastolic dysfunction, cardiomyopathy, arrhythmias, and coronary artery disease

7. Propensity to early and severe degenerative joint disease

Pituitary mass–related manifestations include hypopituitarism, stalk-effect hyperprolactinemia, and anatomical effects related to extrasellar extension of a macroadenoma.

Compared with survival among age-matched controls, survival among patients with untreated or poorly treated acromegaly is reduced by an average of 10 years (excess mortality primarily results from cardiovascular, cerebrovascular and respiratory deaths). Patients with acromegaly have a 2- to 3-fold increased risk of cancer and a 3- to 8-fold increased risk of colon cancer and premalignant colon polyps.

- Clinical presentation of GH-producing tumors: related to excess levels of GH and IGF-1, the pituitary tumor, and associations of acromegaly.

- Acromegaly is associated with increased risk of premalignant colon polyps, colon cancer, and other malignancies: screen with colonoscopy at diagnosis and every 2 or 3 years.

Endocrine Diagnosis

Serum IGF-1 provides the best screening test for the diagnosis of acromegaly. Age- and sex-matched serum IGF-1 levels are almost universally increased. (IGF-1 levels are normally increased in pregnancy and in adolescence.) The diagnosis is confirmed by the demonstration of abnormal GH suppressibility within 1 to 2 hours after a 75-g glucose load (failure of GH suppression to <1 ng/mL or a paradoxical increase in GH secretion). A random serum level of GH is not helpful because of the pulsatile nature of GH secretion.

Radiologic Diagnosis

When the diagnosis is documented biochemically, imaging of the sella is indicated. MRI is the imaging study of choice. If a pituitary tumor is not delineated (a rare event), serum GHRH levels are measured to exclude a GHRH-producing tumor and a search is made for evidence of an ectopic GH-producing tumor.

- Serum IGF-1: The best screening test. Age- and sex-matched serum IGF-1 is increased in all patients with active acromegaly.

- Glucose tolerance–GH suppressibility test: failure of GH to suppress to <1 ng/mL is diagnostic of acromegaly.

- When acromegaly is documented biochemically, proceed with imaging the sella. If no tumor is visible, measure the serum level of GHRH and look for evidence of an ectopic GH-producing tumor.

THERAPY

Because of the increased morbidity and mortality associated with untreated acromegaly, active management is indicated for all patients. Optimal therapy is directed at normalization of GH and IGF-1 levels, preservation or normalization of pituitary functions, control of comorbidities, and normalization of mortality rates. No single line of treatment can accomplish all these goals in all patients. Often one has to use several forms of therapy for patients with acromegaly.

Pituitary Tumor

Surgical Therapy

Transsphenoidal adenomectomy is the treatment of choice, and the cure rate depends on the size of the tumor (70%-80% with microadenomas; <50% with macroadenomas). For persistent disease, consideration is given to radiotherapy or pharmacotherapy (or both).

Radiotherapy

External beam conventional or stereotactic radiotherapy is usually used if surgical therapy fails. However, this therapy has also been used as primary ablative therapy in some patients. Radiotherapy has a cure rate of 50% to 70% after 10 years. Hypopituitarism occurs in most patients after 10 years; other morbidity is rare. The major disadvantage of radiotherapy is its long latent period (months to years) before it controls disease activity.

Medical Therapy

Medical treatment is used only infrequently as a primary mode of therapy. It is usually used if surgical therapy fails. If surgical therapy is unsuccessful, medical treatment can be used alone, as an interim therapy when postoperative radiotherapy is given, or while awaiting the results of radiotherapy. Three lines of medical therapy are available: somatostatin analogues, dopamine agonists, and pegvisomant. It is important to remember that the effects of pharmacotherapy are temporizing: they are effective only as the drug is being taken. Cessation of drug therapy leads to recrudescence of disease activity.

- Therapy of choice: surgical excision. For persistent disease: radiotherapy or pharmacologic therapy.

- Radiotherapy may be used as alternative ablative therapy.

- Drug therapy: somatostatin analogues, dopamine agonists, and GH-receptor blocker, alone or in combination, are temporizing. These are mainly used while awaiting the full effects of primary or adjunctive radiotherapy or when surgical therapy has been unsuccessful or declined.

Comorbidities

Therapy is directed at the management of associated comorbities such as hypopituitarism, hypertension, secondary diabetes, obstructive sleep apnea, or degenerative joint disease.

Ectopic GH or GHRH Tumor

Surgical resection is the therapy of choice for ectopic GH or GHRH tumors. For persistent disease, consider pharmacotherapy (see above).

ACTH-PRODUCING TUMORS

ACTH-producing tumors are discussed in Chapter 31 ("Gonadal and Adrenal Disorders").

GONADOTROPIN-PRODUCING TUMORS

Gonadotropin-producing tumors constitute the largest fraction of nonfunctioning pituitary tumors. Although more than 80% of them can synthesize the gonadotropins or their subunits, increased serum levels of FSH, LH, or their subunits are found in less than 35% of affected patients. Clinically, the tumors are macroadenomas at presentation; patients may present at any age, but they are usually middle-aged or elderly male patients. Extrasellar effects dominate the clinical picture, and some degree of hypopituitarism is usually present. The tumor mass may be associated with stalk-effect hyperprolactinemia. CT or MRI reveals the sellar mass with extrasellar extension. Currently, no effective medical therapy is available. Treatment is usually surgical, with or without postoperative radiotherapy. Endocrine replacement therapy is given for management of hypopituitarism.

THYROTROPIN-PRODUCING TUMORS

The characteristic clinical presentations of patients who have primary TSH tumors are diffuse goiter and hyperthyroidism. Other presentations include extrasellar mass effects and hypopituitarism. Laboratory evaluation reveals that, in a thyrotoxic patient, the sensitive TSH value is normal or high, α-glycoprotein subunit levels are high, and TSH responsiveness to thyrotropin-releasing hormone is absent. CT or MRI shows a sellar mass with or without extrasellar extension. The main differential diagnosis is Graves disease. Among patients with TSH-producing tumors, in contrast to Graves disease, one finds equal incidence between the sexes, absence of ophthalmopathy and dermopathy, and normal or high sensitive TSH values in the presence of hyperthyroidism. Treatment options include ablation (surgically or with irradiation), pharmacologic therapy with octreotide, and ancillary measures for the management of thyrotoxicosis.

PITUITARY INCIDENTALOMAS

Pituitary incidentalomas are a relatively common entity. Autopsy studies suggest that 10% to 20% of persons harbor small pituitary tumors. CT or MRI of the head performed for nonendocrine reasons shows mass lesions in the sella larger than 3 mm in 4% to 20% of persons. Potential threats to health from these incidentalomas include functioning pituitary tumors and incidentalomas with actual or potential mass effects. Masses larger than 10 mm are more likely to be associated with mass effects (hypopituitarism, stalk-effect hyperprolactinemia, or chiasma syndrome) and are more likely to enlarge during observation.

The diagnostic approach includes assessing for functioning pituitary tumors and mass effects. Assessing for functioning pituitary tumors may include 1-mg overnight dexamethasone suppression test or 24-hour urinary free cortisol test and measurement of prolactin, IGF-1, FT_4 and TSH, and FSH, LH, and their subunits. In the asymptomatic patient, only a serum prolactin level is measured. The other pituitary hormones are assessed only when suspicion is supported by clinical findings.

Active intervention is dictated by finding a functioning pituitary tumor that can cause morbidity or mortality (ie, all functioning pituitary tumors except a small microprolactinoma in a postmenopausal female patient) or identifying an incidentaloma larger than 1 cm in diameter with extrasellar extension. Otherwise, observe and repeat the imaging study in 6 to 12 months and then later at less frequent intervals. An increase in the size of the nonfunctioning incidentaloma under observation requires surgical intervention.

MISCELLANEOUS PITUITARY DISORDERS

CRANIOPHARYNGIOMA

Craniopharyngioma is a slow-growing encapsulated squamous cell tumor originating from remnants of the Rathke pouch. It is the most common tumor in the pituitary region in childhood but can occur at any age. Two-thirds of the tumors are suprasellar, and one-third originate in or extend into the sella. Most are cystic, and some are solid or mixed. These tumors have a propensity to calcify. The clinical presentation includes obstructive hydrocephalus, hypothalamic syndrome (diabetes insipidus and hyperprolactinemia), chiasmal defects, hypopituitarism, or calcification in or around the sella, as seen incidentally on radiography. Radiography shows calcification in intrasellar or suprasellar regions (75% of children; 25% of adults). CT or MRI reveals a solid or cystic mass, calcification (on CT), and low attenuation values (cholesterol content).

Surgical excision is possible for only small craniopharyngiomas. Larger craniopharyngiomas are decompressed. A ventriculoperitoneal shunt is used for obstructive hydrocephalus. Other treatments include postoperative radiotherapy and management of endocrine dysfunction.

PITUITARY APOPLEXY

Pituitary apoplexy refers to hemorrhagic infarction of the pituitary gland, with or without underlying disease. The usual clinical setting is that of a pituitary tumor, irradiated pituitary tumor, pregnancy, anticoagulation therapy, increased intracranial pressure, vascular disease (eg, diabetes mellitus), or vasculitis (eg, temporal arteritis). Persons are asymptomatic if the bleeding is small or gradual. In the acute condition, hemorrhage is sudden or large, with features such as severe headache, ophthalmoplegia, visual defects, meningismus, depressed sensorium, and acute adrenocortical crisis. Death may occur. Diagnosis is made on the basis of the characteristic clinical, radiologic, and surgical findings. Therapy includes neurosurgical decompression and hormonal support. Late sequelae may include hypopituitarism, secondary empty sella syndrome, or regression of hypersecretory syndrome in an infarcted functioning pituitary tumor.

LYMPHOCYTIC HYPOPHYSITIS

Lymphocytic hypophysitis is presumed to be of autoimmune origin. It usually occurs in association with other autoimmune endocrinopathies and affects adults, predominantly women, especially during pregnancy and the postpartum period. The clinical presentation may include hypopituitarism or the presence of a sellar mass associated with hyperprolactinemia. The major differential diagnoses are prolactinoma and Sheehan syndrome. The diagnosis depends on the associations and the results of surgical exploration. No specific therapy is available. Hormonal replacement is given as needed.

ADH DEFICIENCY: DIABETES INSIPIDUS

ETIOLOGY

Renal water output is dependent on the presence of ADH and a responsive distal nephron. Therefore, diabetes insipidus (DI) may result from 1 of 2 pathophysiologic defects:

1. Decreased production of ADH in response to normal osmotic stimulation
2. Decreased responsiveness of the distal nephron to ADH (nephrogenic or vasopressin-resistant DI).

Decreased Production of ADH

ADH production decreases in response to normal osmotic stimulation most commonly from organic disorders of the anterior hypothalamus, median eminence, or upper stalk (hypothalamic, neurogenic, central, or ADH-sensitive DI). Infrequently, it results from functional suppression of ADH production by the ingestion of excessive volumes of fluid (primary polydipsia or dipsogenic DI).

Hypothalamic or Central DI

Hypothalamic or central DI may result from genetic or acquired disorders of the anterior hypothalamus, median eminence, or upper pituitary stalk. Genetic disorders are rare. Causes of acquired disorders include traumatic (closed head trauma or neurosurgery); inflammatory or granulomatous (sarcoidosis, tuberculosis, or histiocytosis X); primary neoplasms such as craniopharyngioma, germinoma, and optic glioma; or metastatic neoplasms primarily from the breast or lung. Idiopathic hypothalamic DI is probably the most common cause of the syndrome and may be an autoimmune disorder.

Dipsogenic DI

Dipsogenic DI may be idiopathic or associated with psychosis or, rarely, organic disorders of the anterior hypothalamus such as sarcoidosis or neoplasms.

Nephrogenic DI

Nephrogenic DI, or decreased responsiveness of the distal nephron to ADH, may also be caused by genetic or acquired disorders, the most common being chronic renal disease, electrolyte abnormalities (hypercalcemia or hypokalemia), and ADH-antagonist drugs such as lithium and demeclocycline.

- DI may result from decreased production of ADH or from renal unresponsiveness to ADH.

- Hypothalamic DI: genetic or acquired loss of ADH-secreting neurons. The most common cause is idiopathic DI. Other causes include traumatic, idiopathic, and neoplastic primary or metastatic neoplasms.

- Dipsogenic DI: inappropriate excessive fluid intake and functional suppression of ADH secretion due to idiopathic, psychogenic, or organic causes.

- Nephrogenic DI: genetic or acquired renal unresponsiveness to ADH. Common causes: chronic renal disease, hypercalcemia, hypokalemia, and use of ADH-antagonists.

The clinical manifestations include those of DI and the etiologic disorder. Polyuria and polydipsia, often with preference for ice-cold water, are characteristic. Nocturia is usually present and enuresis may be the presenting complaint in children. An abrupt onset of symptoms usually points to central DI. Absence of nocturia, variable intensity or intermittency of symptoms, and a 24-hour urine output greater than 18 L suggest primary polydipsia. It is important to remember that because patients with hypothalamic or nephrogenic DI rely on their thirst mechanism to regulate water balance, no other ill effects may be apparent unless the patient becomes unconscious for any reason, is unable to obtain fluids, or has an impaired thirst mechanism. In such circumstances, extreme hyperosmolar dehydration and hypertonic encephalopathy may develop.

- DI is characterized by polyuria (2.5–20 L daily) and polydipsia, often with preference for ice-cold water.

- Abrupt onset of symptoms usually suggests central DI, and absence of nocturia suggests primary polydipsia.

- When thirst sensation is impaired or access to water is restricted, a hyperosmolar state may ensue and may be complicated by hypertonic encephalopathy and circulatory collapse.

ENDOCRINE DIAGNOSIS

The diagnosis depends on the use of random plasma osmolality (or serum level of sodium) and urine osmolality levels under conditions of unrestricted fluid intake and on the use of provocative tests. The induction of plasma hyperosmolality (either by water deprivation or by administration of hypertonic saline) is used to assess the patient's ability to produce ADH and to respond to it. The patient's response can be assessed 1) indirectly by measurements of urine volume and osmolality before and after the administration of exogenous ADH or 2) directly by measurements of plasma levels of ADH in addition to plasma and urine osmolalities.

Although the diagnosis of severe DI of any cause can be straightforward, the diagnostic process is often difficult because the extent of the disorder may be only partial and because prolonged periods of polyuria, regardless of the primary cause, may decrease the maximal urine-concentrating ability (renal medullary washout), in effect adding a nephrogenic DI component to the basic disease process.

In a patient with polyuria and dilute urine, a random plasma osmolality >295 mOsm/kg points to neurogenic or nephrogenic DI. These can be differentiated by the response to exogenous ADH. A random plasma osmolality <280 mOsm/kg, in an untreated patient, points to primary polydipsia.

- Obtain random plasma and urine osmolality values: a random plasma osmolality >295 mOsm/kg points to neurogenic or nephrogenic DI. These can be differentiated by the response to exogenous ADH. A random plasma osmolality <280 mOsm/kg, in an untreated patient, points to primary polydipsia.

ETIOLOGIC DIAGNOSIS

Look for clinical evidence of hypothalamic-pituitary or systemic disorders, examine the visual fields, assess anterior pituitary functions, and perform MRI. The most common causes of central DI are idiopathic DI, trauma (accidental or neurosurgical), metastases from breast or lung cancers, and hypothalamic area tumors. Systemic diseases with hypothalamic or stalk involvement must be considered.

THERAPY

Therapy, whenever possible, is directed at the cause. For mild central DI, free access to water is the treatment. Desmopressin is used for moderate to severe central DI. For partial central DI, use ADH agonists such as chlorpropamide (250–500 mg daily). For nephrogenic DI, thiazides are the only treatment available.

ADH EXCESS: SIADH

ETIOLOGY

ADH excess, in the absence of a hyperosmolar stimulus, may be appropriate when it occurs in response to hypovolemia or hypotension and inappropriate when it occurs in the absence of a hypovolemic or hypotensive stimulus. SIADH can result from exogenous or endogenous disorders.

Exogenous ADH excess may result from the inappropriate administration of ADH (or its analogues such as desmopressin) or oxytocin. *Endogenous ADH excess* may originate from a eutopic hypothalamic or an ectopic extrahypothalamic source. *Eutopic ADH excess* may be a consequence of the following:

1. CNS or hypothalamic disorders of various causes (eg, traumatic, inflammatory, degenerative, vascular, or neoplastic disorders)

2. Use of agonist drugs that enhance ADH secretion or action (chlorpropamide, carbamazepine, vincristine, vinblastine, cyclophosphamide, phenothiazines, monoamine oxidase inhibitors, tricyclic antidepressants, and clofibrate)

3. Neurogenic influences such as pain or nausea

Ectopic extrahypothalamic ADH excess may result from the following:

1. Malignancies (cancers of the bronchus, pancreas, ureter, prostate, or bladder; lymphoma; leukemia; thymoma; or mesothelioma)

2. Benign pulmonary disorders (pneumonia, lung abscess, empyema or pneumothorax, tuberculosis, cystic fibrosis, and the use of positive-pressure ventilation)

Continued water intake and ADH hypersecretion in the absence of a hyperosmolar stimulus leads to the following:

1. Increased renal water retention, hyponatremia, and hypo-osmolality of body fluids with inappropriately concentrated urine

2. Expansion of body fluid compartments, including extracellular fluid volume

3. Homeostatic adjustments that promote "renal escape" and natriuresis, including increased GFR, increased atrial natriuretic hormones, and suppression of the renin-angiotensin-aldosterone axis. Natriuresis exacerbates plasma hypo-osmolality, thus explaining the absence of edema despite an expanded extracellular fluid volume.

- Physiologic or appropriate ADH hypersecretion occurs in response to plasma hyperosmolality, hypovolemia, or hypotension.

- Pathophysiologic or inappropriate ADH excess occurs in the absence of physiologic stimuli and can have either an exogenous or an endogenous cause. Endogenous ADH excess can be from a eutopic hypothalamic source or an ectopic extrahypothalamic source.

- SIADH is characterized by hypervolemia, hyponatremia, and hypo-osmolality of body fluids, inappropriately concentrated urine, natriuresis, absence of edema, and low serum creatinine and uric acid levels (a result of increased GFR).

CLINICAL FEATURES

The clinical features are a composite of the effects of the underlying disorder and those of the hyponatremic syndrome that depend on the degree and rapidity of its development. Patients with SIADH may be asymptomatic if the hyponatremia is mild or has developed gradually over weeks and months. When patients are symptomatic, the most frequent symptoms are lethargy, fatigue, ill health, anorexia, nausea and vomiting, and irritability or confusion. Severe or rapidly developing hyponatremia can lead to a behavioral change, a change in the level of consciousness, or seizures.

- Clinical features depend on the degree and rapidity of the development of hyponatremia and range from asymptomatic to neurologically impaired.

DIAGNOSIS

1. Confirm true hyponatremia. Exclude pseudohyponatremia associated with hyperlipidemia or hyperlipoproteinemia (clinical and biochemical features and normal plasma osmolality indicate pseudohyponatremia).

2. Exclude hyperosmolar states and loss of intracellular water to the hyperosmolar extracellular fluid, as in hyperglycemia and the use of mannitol (plasma glucose, history of mannitol use, and increased plasma osmolality).

3. In the absence of advanced renal failure, the differential diagnosis is SIADH and appropriate ADH excess associated with decreased cardiac output (volume and pressure stimuli). Establish the appropriateness or inappropriateness of ADH hypersecretion. If the findings point to SIADH, identify the cause. If an exogenous source is not apparent, search for a eutopic or ectopic source of ADH hypersecretion.

4. The main diagnostic challenge is to differentiate SIADH from subclinical hypovolemia. Consider urinary sodium concentration, serum creatinine or uric acid levels, and plasma renin activity and aldosterone level. In contrast to findings in SIADH, subclinical hypovolemia is associated with a urinary sodium concentration less than 20 mEq/L, increased serum creatinine and uric acid levels, and an increased plasma renin activity and plasma aldosterone level.

- Confirm true hyponatremia and exclude hyperosmolar states, advanced renal failure, and states of appropriate ADH excess.

- The main diagnostic challenge is to differentiate SIADH from subclinical hypovolemia; consider urinary sodium, serum creatinine and uric acid, and plasma renin activity and aldosterone.

THERAPY

Therapy for SIADH includes identifying and managing the underlying disorder, restricting water intake to 800 to 1,000 mL daily, and monitoring the patient's weight and serum sodium level. Combined therapy with furosemide and salt tablets often can increase the plasma sodium concentration in SIADH. Treatment with demeclocycline, a direct cell toxin and ADH antagonist (900–1,200 mg daily), may be useful. This drug can be nephrotoxic, particularly in patients with chronic liver disease. Specific ADH antagonists, the vaptans, have become recently available (tolvaptan for oral use and conivaptan for intravenous use); these will have an increasing role in the management of SIADH in the future.

When acute neurologic sequelae are present, give hypertonic saline intravenously (200–300 mL of 5% saline over 3–4 hours). Achieve a gradual increase in serum sodium (do not exceed 0.5 mEq/h or 12 mEq in 24 hours). Continue giving hypertonic saline until the neurologic symptoms cease and a "safe" serum sodium level of 120 mEq/L is reached. Rapid correction of hyponatremia can lead to central pontine myelinolysis, which often is fatal.

- Identify and treat the underlying disorder and manage the hyponatremia.

- Therapy for hyponatremia: water restriction and, if needed, an ADH antagonist (ie, demeclocycline).

- For acute neurologic sequelae: hypertonic saline to increase serum sodium by 0.5 mEq/h to control symptoms and achieve a "safe" serum sodium level of 120 mEq/L.

- Rapid correction of hyponatremia can lead to potentially fatal central pontine myelinolysis.

SUMMARY

- Hypopituitarism can result from primary pituitary disorders, hypothalamic–pituitary stalk disorders, or extrasellar disorders.

- Acute manifestations of hypopituitarism: adrenocortical crisis, fasting hypoglycemia syndrome, hyponatremic syndrome, and increased sensitivity to CNS depressants.

- Use a provocative test in the appropriate clinical setting to evaluate nontropic hormone deficiency.

- Evaluate target gland function for suspected tropic hormone deficiency; test the tropic hormone level if target gland failure is present to distinguish between primary target gland failure and hypothalamic-pituitary disease.

- Treatment options for pituitary tumors include surgical excision, radiotherapy, or drug therapy.

- SIADH is characterized by hypervolemia, hyponatremia, and hypo-osmolality of body fluids, inappropriately concentrated urine, natriuresis, absence of edema, and low serum creatinine and uric acid levels (a result of increased GFR).

GONADAL AND ADRENAL DISORDERS

Charles F. Abboud, MB, ChB, Bryan McIver, MB, ChB, PhD, and Pankaj Shah, MD

GOALS

- Summarize adrenal disorders.
- Identify adrenal emergencies.
- Describe gonadal disorders.

DISORDERS OF THE ADRENAL GLANDS

ADRENOCORTICAL FAILURE

Etiology

Adrenocortical failure most commonly is due to a decrease in production of 1 or more adrenal hormones. It may involve the zona fasciculata and zona reticularis (cortisol and sex-steroid deficiency) or the zona glomerulosa (aldosterone deficiency) or all 3. Decreased production of adrenocortical hormones may be a consequence of adrenocortical disease (primary failure) or tropic hormone loss (secondary failure).

Primary Adrenocortical Failure (Addison Disease)

Primary adrenocortical failure is associated usually with deficiencies of all 3 hormones. It may be due to organ-specific autoimmune adrenalitis; granulomatous adrenalitis such as tuberculosis or histoplasmosis; bilateral adrenal hemorrhage with anticoagulant use, trauma, or sepsis (particularly meningococcemia); AIDS; metastatic malignancies; congenital adrenal enzyme deficiency; or use of steroidogenesis-blocking drugs such as aminoglutethimide. In the United States, the most common causes are autoimmune adrenalitis and bilateral adrenal hemorrhage. Adrenal failure associated with infections may be due to the combined effects of adrenalitis and the use of drugs that inhibit steroidogenesis (eg, ketoconazole) or those that accelerate cortisol clearance (eg, rifampin and phenytoin).

Secondary Adrenocortical Failure

Secondary adrenocortical failure is due to lack of corticotropin (ACTH). Therefore, it affects cortisol and sex-steroid production but leaves aldosterone secretion intact.

Lack of ACTH may occur as an isolated deficiency or, more commonly, in association with other features of hypopituitarism. It may occur in association with pituitary tumors, hypothalamic or extrasellar disease, surgery or radiotherapy to the hypothalamic-pituitary region, or head injury. Functional central ACTH deficiency, the most common cause of ACTH deficiency, is a consequence of suppression of the axis by the prolonged use of glucocorticoids in pharmacologic doses for nonendocrine purposes. The deficiency becomes clinically manifest after withdrawal of the glucocorticoid therapy.

Hypoaldosteronism can occur independently of cortisol deficiency. It may result from a primary disorder of the zona glomerulosa, or it may be secondary to angiotensin II deficiency, which may be a consequence of renin deficiency or angiotensin-converting enzyme deficiency.

- Adrenocortical failure most commonly is due to a decrease in production of 1 or more adrenal hormones.

- Primary adrenocortical failure is associated with cortisol, sex steroids, and aldosterone deficiencies. It has many organic and functional causes; in the United States, the most common causes are autoimmune adrenalitis and bilateral adrenal hemorrhage; worldwide, tuberculosis-associated adrenalitis is common.

- Secondary adrenal failure is due to ACTH deficiency. It affects production of cortisol and sex steroids, whereas aldosterone secretion is basically intact; it is most commonly due to functional suppression of the axis by prolonged glucocorticoid therapy.

Clinical Features

The clinical features of adrenocortical failure depend on the extent of the hormone deficiency, whether the failure is partial or complete, whether 1 or all hormones are involved, the rapidity of development of the deficiency, and, when present, changes in the levels of circulating ACTH.

The usual manifestation of adrenocortical failure is that of a chronic, slowly evolving disorder.

1. *Cortisol deficiency*: decreased vitality, energy, and stamina; muscle weakness; anorexia, weight loss, nausea, vomiting, or diarrhea (may mimic abdominal malignancy); mood changes; hyponatremia, fasting hypoglycemia, transient hypercalcemia, anemia, lymphocytosis, and eosinophilia

2. *Aldosterone deficiency*: hypovolemia, orthostatic hypotension, hyperkalemia, hyperchloremic acidosis, and azotemia

3. *Androgen deficiency*: not significant in males; associated with decreased libido and thinning of sexual hair in females

4. *ACTH-related symptoms*: ACTH excess in Addison disease is associated with hyperpigmentation; pallor and the inability to tan result from ACTH deficiency in hypothalamic-pituitary disease

Acute Adrenocortical Failure or Adrenal Crisis

Adrenal crisis is suggested in the presence of dehydration, hypotension, or shock out of proportion to the severity of the current illness; nausea and vomiting with a history of anorexia and weight loss; abdominal pain (may mimic acute abdomen); unexplained fever; and hyponatremia, hyperkalemia, azotemia, hypercalcemia, eosinophilia, and hypoglycemia. It often is precipitated by an illness in a patient who has unrecognized adrenocortical failure and who recently had glucocorticoid therapy withdrawn or has sustained bilateral hemorrhage of the adrenals.

- Addison disease usually manifests as a chronic, slowly evolving syndrome; manifestations are a composite of the effects of a lack of cortisol, sex steroids, and aldosterone and an excess of ACTH.

- Adrenal crisis is precipitated by an illness in a patient who has unrecognized adrenocortical failure and who recently had glucocorticoid therapy withdrawn or has sustained bilateral hemorrhage of the adrenals.

Diagnosis

Endocrine Diagnosis

The symptoms and signs of adrenocortical failure are variable and nonspecific, and diagnosis requires a high degree of clinical awareness. Plasma cortisol levels (reference range, 7–27 µg/dL) may be helpful in diagnosis. A value less than 3 µg/dL indicates adrenocortical failure, and a value greater than 18 µg/dL excludes the diagnosis.

The diagnosis is confirmed most reliably and effectively by the cosyntropin test, which assesses the cortisol response to a synthetic, rapidly acting ACTH (250 µg). The normal response to cosyntropin is an absolute value of plasma cortisol greater than 18 µg/dL. An impaired response to cosyntropin establishes the diagnosis of adrenocortical failure but does not specify the type. Defining whether the failure is primary or

secondary rests on the measurement of serum ACTH: a high ACTH level indicates Addison disease, and a low or "inappropriately normal" level indicates secondary failure.

A normal response to cosyntropin rules out Addison disease but does not exclude ACTH deficiency that is partial or of recent onset. If the diagnosis is still suspected, a metyrapone test or an insulin-hypoglycemia test is performed: a normal response to the provocative test excludes adrenocortical failure; an impaired response in a patient who has a normal response to cosyntropin indicates secondary failure. A low-dose cosyntropin test (1 µg) has been advocated as a reliable alternative for the diagnosis of recent or partial ACTH deficiency, but its value for this purpose is debatable.

- A plasma cortisol value <3 µg/dL indicates adrenocortical failure, whereas a value >18 µg/dL excludes the diagnosis.

- Cosyntropin test: a subnormal cortisol response establishes the diagnosis of adrenocortical failure but cannot differentiate Addison disease from failure due to hypothalamic-pituitary disease. This differentiation is based on serum ACTH measurements or, if not available, on the long ACTH stimulation test.

- Normal cortisol response to cosyntropin excludes Addison disease but does not rule out secondary adrenocortical failure that is partial or of recent onset. A metyrapone test or an insulin-hypoglycemia test is performed.

Etiologic Diagnosis

In Addison disease, an etiologic diagnosis depends on clinical assessment and a search for other autoimmune disorders, infections, and neoplasms. Autoimmune adrenalitis is diagnosed by measuring antibodies against the steroidogenic enzyme 21-hydroxylase (*CYP21A2*). Computed tomographic (CT) imaging of the adrenal glands is helpful in the diagnosis of inflammatory disorders, adrenal hemorrhage, or malignancy. In secondary failure, pituitary function is assessed and magnetic resonance imaging (MRI) or CT imaging of the head is performed to look for a space-occupying lesion in the hypothalamic-pituitary region.

Therapy

Primary adrenocortical failure requires glucocorticoid and mineralocorticoid replacement therapy, whereas secondary failure requires only glucocorticoid replacement. Patient education is critical and must cover several topics: the need for disciplined daily lifelong therapy, the manner of dosage adjustments during acute illness, the use of injectable glucocorticoids when oral replacement therapy is not possible, and the use of an identification bracelet or necklace.

Primary Adrenocortical Failure

Glucocorticoid therapy consists of hydrocortisone (10–20 mg in the morning and 5–10 mg in the afternoon) or prednisone (5 mg in the morning and 0–2.5 mg in the afternoon). The adequacy of therapy is assessed by the patient's sense of well-being, the decrease in pigmentation, and the absence of manifestations of excessive glucocorticoid replacement; ACTH levels are not always reliable for monitoring the adequacy of therapy.

Mineralocorticoid therapy consists of fludrocortisone (0.05–0.2 mg orally) and liberal salt intake. The adequacy of replacement is monitored by measurement of the supine and standing blood pressure, presence of edema, serum potassium level, and, if needed, plasma renin activity.

- Primary adrenocortical failure requires glucocorticoid and mineralocorticoid therapy.

- Secondary failure requires only glucocorticoid therapy.

- Patient education is a critical component of effective management.

- Therapy for primary adrenocortical failure: hydrocortisone (10–20 mg in the morning and 5–10 mg in the afternoon) or the equivalent; fludrocortisone (0.05–0.2 mg orally); and liberal salt intake.

Acute Illness

In mild to moderate acute illness, the glucocorticoid dosage is doubled or tripled and given at that increased dosage for the duration of the illness. In the presence of severe illness or vomiting, patients should seek medical attention promptly and be treated with parenteral dexamethasone (4 mg intramuscularly) or other parenteral glucocorticoid. For minor procedures performed under local anesthesia and for most radiologic procedures, no special preparation is required. For moderately stressful procedures such as endoscopy, hydrocortisone (100 mg intravenously) or another glucocorticoid in an equivalent dose should be given 1 hour before the procedure. For major surgery, 100 mg of hydrocortisone is given intravenously before the induction of anesthesia and repeated every 6 to 8 hours for the first 24 hours, after which the dose is tapered at a rate that depends on the patient's recovery (usually a decrease in dosage by 50% daily to maintenance levels). Because this stress-dosage of hydrocortisone has adequate mineralocorticoid effect, the use of a specific mineralocorticoid during the acute illness is not necessary.

- Glucocorticoid replacement needs to be modified in acute medical or surgical illness and when oral therapy is not possible.

Adrenal Crisis

An adrenal crisis requires prompt management, with treatment beginning immediately—as soon as the diagnosis is suspected—rather than waiting for test results. Establish intravenous access and collect blood samples for measuring electrolyte, glucose, plasma cortisol, and serum ACTH levels. Infuse saline and dextrose (to restore blood and extracellular fluid volume) and hydrocortisone (100 mg every 6 hours). Specific mineralocorticoid therapy usually is not necessary. After the patient's condition has stabilized, continue infusions, but at a lower rate. Search for and treat possible infections and other precipitating causes. After the acute illness is over, switch the glucocorticoid therapy to dexamethasone (it will not interfere with plasma cortisol measurements) and perform the cosyntropin stimulation test to initiate the adrenocortical diagnostic process. Taper the dosage of glucocorticoids to a maintenance dosage and begin mineralocorticoid replacement, if needed, after the saline infusion is stopped.

- Prompt management is critical.

- Collect blood samples for measuring electrolytes, glucose, plasma cortisol, and serum ACTH, but do not wait for the results; begin treatment as soon as the diagnosis is suspected.

- Parenteral glucocorticoids are critical. Ensure adequate fluid, electrolyte, and volume replacement. Search for and treat any underlying precipitating disorder such as infection.

- After the patient's condition has stabilized, continue infusions at a lower rate and perform the cosyntropin test.

- With recovery, taper the glucocorticoid dosage to a maintenance dosage; if patients have primary adrenocortical failure, add mineralocorticoid replacement.

CUSHING SYNDROME

Etiology

Cushing syndrome may have an exogenous or endogenous origin. *Exogenous Cushing syndrome* is more common and is usually caused by long-term use of supraphysiologic doses of cortisol or, more commonly, its analogues (eg, prednisone) in the management of inflammatory, allergic, or neoplastic disorders. It rarely is caused by the surreptitious use of these agents.

Endogenous Cushing syndrome is caused by cortisol overproduction by the adrenal cortex. Cortisol overproduction may result from the following:

1. Primary adrenal, autonomous, and ACTH-independent disorders, such as an adrenal adenoma (a small differentiated tumor <3 cm in diameter) that produces a "pure glucocorticoid excess" syndrome; an undifferentiated adrenal carcinoma (usually >6 cm in diameter) that is inefficient in steroidogenesis and produces (in addition to cortisol) large quantities of adrenal androgens; or, rarely, macronodular or micronodular adrenal hyperplasia.

2. Excessive secretion of ACTH causes *ACTH-dependent Cushing syndrome*, which may be caused by a pituitary corticotroph cell adenoma or, rarely, hyperplasia (the condition is then called *Cushing disease*). The adenoma usually is small; more than 50% of these tumors are not detected on MRI. The most common causes of endogenous Cushing syndrome are Cushing disease (75%), ectopic-ACTH tumors (15%), and adrenal tumors (10%).

- Exogenous glucocorticoid therapy is the most common cause of Cushing syndrome.

- Endogenous Cushing syndrome is best classified into ACTH-independent and ACTH-dependent disorders.

- ACTH-independent disorders: adrenal tumors (10%) and, rarely, nodular hyperplasias.

- ACTH-dependent disorders: Cushing disease (75%), ectopic-ACTH tumors (15%), adrenal tumors (10%), and, rarely, ectopic corticotropin-releasing hormone tumors.

Clinical Features

Features of cortisol excess are the dominant features of the syndrome and are those of chronic indolent cortisol excess: weight gain and central obesity, thin skin with easy bruisability and wide violaceous striae, plethora, muscle weakness, osteoporosis, cessation of linear growth in growing children or adolescents, lanugo hair, hypertension, insulin resistance and secondary diabetes, hypercalciuria and renal stones, and propensity to fungal infections.

Features of adrenal androgen excess may be modest and lead to acne, hirsutism, and menstrual irregularities, as in the usual cases of Cushing disease and ACTH-producing bronchial carcinoids, or they may be more severe and lead to virilization, as in adrenal carcinoma. These features may be absent in patients with glucocorticoid-producing adrenal adenoma.

ACTH produced in significant quantities, as in the usual malignant causes of ectopic-ACTH tumors, may lead to hyperpigmentation.

Anatomical effects of the underlying tumor include extrasellar effects with pituitary macroadenomas, bronchopulmonary effects of lung cancer, and abdominal pain caused by adrenocortical carcinoma or metastatic effects of malignant causal tumors.

- Features of cortisol excess dominate the clinical picture; variably, one may see the features of adrenal androgen excess, ACTH excess, and the mass effects of the underlying tumor. Occasionally, attention may be drawn to the syndrome by the finding of a pituitary or adrenal incidentaloma.

- Features of cortisol excess are usually chronic and slowly evolving, giving rise to the typical cushingoid features.

- The clinical features of malignant ectopic ACTH tumors may be dominated by weight loss, weakness, edema, hyperkalemia, hypertension, and secondary diabetes.

Diagnosis

The diagnostic approach to a patient with suspected Cushing syndrome has 2 central components: confirming the diagnosis of Cushing syndrome and identifying its cause. The following issues make establishing the diagnosis complex:

1. Many non-Cushing disorders can increase cortisol production and impair hypothalamic-pituitary-adrenal homeostatic mechanisms. These include acute illness of any type, stress, nutritional disorders, alcoholism, and depression.

2. Many drugs can alter diagnostic tests for cortisol overproduction, such as oral contraceptives, which can increase cortisol-binding globulin, and drugs that alter dexamethasone metabolism.

3. No single test is completely reliable to confirm or exclude the diagnosis. Clinicians usually rely on repeated measurements of several tests, which are sometimes repeated over an extended period.

4. Some patients with the syndrome have only cyclic expression of the disease, with periods of activity extending over several weeks to months, interspersed with periods of disease inactivity. Laboratory results during periods of disease inactivity may be erroneously "normal." Only repeated testing over several months may point to the underlying disease.

Identification of Cushing Syndrome

The best screening tests for Cushing syndrome are the 1-mg overnight dexamethasone suppression test, a 24-hour urine collection for free cortisol, and late-night salivary cortisol testing. The demonstration of abnormal dexamethasone suppressibility or significantly increased late-night salivary cortisol and urinary free cortisol results indicate a diagnosis of Cushing syndrome.

The 1-mg dexamethasone suppression test is a reliable screening test. The normal response is a plasma cortisol value less than 5 μg/dL. Patients with Cushing syndrome usually have values greater than 10 μg/dL. False-positive test results occur in 13% of patients with simple obesity and in 25% of patients who are chronically ill. Sensitivity of this test has been improved by reducing the plasma cortisol cut-off value, and a value less than 2 μg/dL is believed to exclude Cushing syndrome.

Urinary free cortisol is increased in more than 97% of patients with Cushing syndrome. It can be increased in states of high urinary output. Importantly, it can be modestly increased in simple obesity, but a value greater than 300 μg per 24 hours usually indicates Cushing syndrome.

- Screening tests: 1-mg dexamethasone test, urinary free cortisol (most reliable), or late-night salivary cortisol.

- Definitive test: urinary free cortisol >300 μg/24 h or failure of normal suppression in the 2-day low-dose dexamethasone (2 mg daily) suppression/corticotropin-releasing hormone test.

- Exclude acute illness, alcoholism, and depression.

Etiologic Diagnosis

Serum ACTH level is the test that differentiates between ACTH-dependent and ACTH-independent causes. Plasma ACTH levels are suppressed (<5 pg/mL) in patients with adrenal tumors; "normal" (20–80 pg/mL) or modestly increased (<200 pg/mL) in patients with Cushing disease or ectopic ACTH caused by bronchial carcinoids; and very high (>200 pg/mL) in most patients with the usual ectopic ACTH tumor.

- The most important tests to delineate the cause: serum ACTH and radiologic evaluation.
- Cushing syndrome caused by adrenal tumor: low or undetectable ACTH level and an adrenal mass found on abdominal CT.
- Cushing syndrome caused by ectopic ACTH tumor: evident ectopic tumor, rapid clinical course, very high ACTH levels (>200 pg/mL), and nonsuppressibility.
- Cushing disease: ACTH values are normal or moderately increased (<200 pg/mL), and CT or MRI of the sella may show a pituitary tumor. About 50% of patients have normal sellar radiographic features.

Therapy

For Cushing disease, the treatment of choice is transsphenoidal surgical adenomectomy or subtotal hypophysectomy. For postoperative persistent disease, the therapeutic options include pituitary radiotherapy and the interim use of steroidogenesis blockers, such as ketoconazole, or bilateral adrenalectomy and postoperative pituitary radiotherapy. The treatment for adrenal adenoma is unilateral adrenalectomy. For adrenal carcinoma, the treatment is unilateral adrenalectomy; mitotane and steroidogenesis blockers are indicated for persistent or recurrent disease. Tumor excision is indicated for ectopic ACTH tumor; if the tumor is incurable, steroidogenesis blockers are used short-term. Bilateral adrenalectomy is recommended for tumors with a more indolent course.

In all cases of Cushing syndrome, surgical excision of the causative tumor is followed by cortisol deficiency caused by the suppressed hypothalamic-pituitary adrenal axis. It may take up to 1 or 2 years for the axis to recover; during this period, the patient needs glucocorticoid replacement therapy.

- After removal of a causative tumor of Cushing syndrome, a period of suppression of the normal axis follows and may last up to 1–2 years. During this period, treat with glucocorticoids, as in adrenocortical failure.
- Patients who undergo bilateral adrenalectomy require lifelong glucocorticoid and mineralocorticoid replacement.

PRIMARY ALDOSTERONISM

Etiology

Primary aldosteronism results from an autonomous renin-angiotensin–independent disorder of the zona glomerulosa. It may be caused by idiopathic bilateral hyperplasia (65%), an aldosterone-producing adenoma (30%), unilateral adrenal hyperplasia (<5%), adrenocortical carcinoma (<3%), and, very rarely, the familial disorder glucocorticoid-remediable aldosteronism.

Clinical Features

The prevalence of primary aldosteronism in the hypertensive population is about 10% (5%-13%). Most patients present with hypertension that is mild to severe (malignant hypertension is extremely rare) and hypokalemia (>30% have normokalemia). Hypokalemia is typically unprovoked, but it may be provoked significantly and rapidly with diuretic therapy. Most patients are asymptomatic, but a few report the effects of hypokalemic alkalosis (fatigue and muscle weakness, paresthesias, orthostatic hypotension, nephrogenic diabetes insipidus, and glucose intolerance). Edema typically is absent.

- Presentation: usually asymptomatic hypertension and unprovoked or easily provoked hypokalemia. However, >30% of patients are normokalemic.
- Absence of edema because of "escape" from the salt-retaining effects; no escape occurs from the potassium and hydrogen ion-losing state.

Diagnosis

The diagnosis of primary aldosteronism rests on documenting autonomous aldosterone hypersecretion and on defining the underlying cause.

Endocrine Diagnosis

Hypokalemia is a classic finding in primary aldosteronism; however, it may be absent (>30%) and is nonspecific. In a patient with hypokalemia, a urinary potassium level greater than 30 mEq/24 h suggests renal potassium wasting and increases the likelihood that the patient has aldosteronism.

The characteristic endocrine abnormalities in primary aldosteronism are increased production of aldosterone that is autonomous of regulation by the renin-angiotensin system and suppressed plasma renin activity. The best screening procedure is to obtain plasma measurements of aldosterone (PA) (in nanograms per deciliter) and renin activity (PRA) (in nanograms per milliliter per hour) and to calculate the PA:PRA ratio. It is important to remember that hypokalemia should be corrected before measurements of aldosterone levels, because hypokalemia may reduce the aldosterone production in primary aldosteronism. The test can be done with the patient receiving antihypertensive drugs except spironolactone and eplerenone, which are aldosterone-receptor blockers. An increased PA and a suppressed PRA, with a PA:PRA ratio greater than 20, and a plasma aldosterone concentration greater than 15 μg/dL, suggest primary aldosteronism. An increased PA and an increased PRA with a PA:PRA ratio less than 10 indicate secondary aldosteronism. A low PA and a low PRA suggest that another mineralocorticoid is the cause of hypertension and hypokalemia.

The diagnosis of primary aldosteronism is confirmed by demonstrating the unsuppressible autonomous secretion of aldosterone despite salt loading (oral salt loading, saline infusion, or fludrocortisone suppression test).

- Unprovoked or easily provoked hypokalemia is characteristic of primary aldosteronism.

- Exclude extrarenal potassium loss by checking urinary potassium; a value >30 mEq/24 h in a patient with hypokalemia suggests a renal potassium-losing state, which includes mineralocorticoid excess.

- The best screening test for primary aldosteronism is the PA:PRA ratio.

- PA:PRA ratio >20: primary aldosteronism.

- PA:PRA ratio <10: secondary aldosteronism.

- Confirm the diagnosis by demonstrating autonomous aldosterone production (salt loading fails to suppress aldosterone production).

Etiologic Diagnosis

The major challenge is to differentiate between a unilateral adrenal disorder (an aldosterone-producing adenoma or unilateral adrenal hyperplasia) and bilateral adrenal hyperplasia. This differentiation has important therapeutic implications. Unilateral adrenal disease is treated surgically by unilateral adrenalectomy. However, bilateral hyperplasia is treated medically by the use of an aldosterone antagonist (see below). This differentiation relies on CT of the adrenals and selective venous sampling.

CT of the adrenals is used most frequently. An adrenal mass usually indicates an aldosterone-producing adenoma. However, CT may be misleading because adenomas are small and many may be missed, an adrenal mass seen on CT may not be an aldosteronoma but an adrenal incidentaloma, and the mass may be a hyperplastic nodule in macronodular bilateral adrenal hyperplasia.

Selective venous sampling is the most accurate localizing procedure. A unilateral gradient suggests unilateral disease, and the absence of a gradient suggests bilateral hyperplasia. However, this procedure is technically difficult and requires radiologic expertise.

- Primary aldosteronism is due to unilateral adenoma or hyperplasia or to bilateral adrenal hyperplasia.

- The most reliable localizing test is selective venous sampling; a unilateral gradient suggests an adenoma. The test is difficult to perform and requires expertise.

- CT may demonstrate an adrenal mass but has several pitfalls.

Differential Diagnosis

The main considerations in the differential diagnosis are hypertensive variants of secondary aldosteronism and other causes of mineralocorticoid-induced hypertension.

Secondary aldosteronism associated with hypertension results from increased renin production as a consequence of renal artery stenosis, malignant hypertension, or a renin-producing tumor. Plasma renin activity, angiotensin II, and aldosterone production are increased, and patients present with renin-dependent hyperaldosteronism with hypertension and hypokalemia.

- Secondary aldosteronism: hypertension, hypokalemia, increased aldosterone, increased plasma renin activity.

- Other types of mineralocorticoid-induced hypertension: hypertension with hypokalemia, low aldosterone, and suppressed plasma renin activity.

Therapy

Therapy has 3 objectives: control or reverse hypertension, correct hypokalemia, and prevent the noxious effects of excess aldosterone on the cardiovascular system.

Unilateral adrenalectomy is the treatment of choice for aldosteronoma or unilateral hyperplasia unless the patient is at high surgical risk. Surgery corrects the hypokalemia in all patients and normalizes the blood pressure or significantly improves the hypertension in most (70%). Patients with persistent postoperative hypertension should be treated with standard antihypertensive drug therapy.

Medical treatment is indicated for bilateral adrenal hyperplasia and for aldosteronoma if the patient is at high surgical risk. (Surgical treatment of hyperplasia requires bilateral adrenalectomy to normalize the serum potassium level, but it rarely restores blood pressure to normal levels.) Spironolactone, an aldosterone antagonist, is given in a dosage of 25 to 100 mg every 8 to 12 hours. It restores normokalemia and normalizes blood pressure in most patients. Adverse effects include gastrointestinal tract upset, menstrual irregularity, and, in men, gynecomastia and impaired libido and potency. Women of childbearing age who take spironolactone should use oral contraceptives because the drug may cause feminization of the male fetus through its androgen-blocking effects. Eplerenone, a highly selective mineralocorticoid receptor antagonist with fewer side effects, has been used as an alternative to spironolactone; it has not been approved by the US Food and Drug Administration for the management of primary aldosteronism.

- Surgery: unilateral adrenalectomy for patients with aldosteronoma or unilateral adrenal hyperplasia unless the patient declines surgery or is at high surgical risk.

- Medical therapy: for patients with hyperplasia and for those with aldosteronoma who are at high surgical risk or who decline surgery.

- Medical treatment: spironolactone, an aldosterone antagonist, is most commonly used. Eplerenone has been used as an alternative.

PHEOCHROMOCYTOMA AND PARAGANGLIOMA

Etiology

Catecholamine-producing chromaffin tumors usually arise in the adrenal medulla (pheochromocytomas); they arise infrequently along the sympathetic chain in the abdomen, thorax, or neck (paragangliomas), and they arise rarely in sympathetic tissue in the walls of the urinary bladder. They are important because, although rare and occurring in less than 1% of all hypertensive patients, they usually occur with a distinctive recognizable clinical syndrome, they are curable, and, if untreated, they can be lethal; 10% of these tumors are malignant, and 10% are familial. More than 90% of pheochromocytomas are sporadic, adrenal in location, unilateral, and benign. Familial pheochromocytomas are more likely to be intra-adrenal, bilateral, and malignant. Extra-adrenal tumors are usually located in the abdomen. Less than 1% of paragangliomas are located in the chest or neck.

Clinical Features

Pheochromocytomas can be asymptomatic (10%-50%), especially with adrenal incidentalomas or genetic syndromes. More commonly, they are suspected because of the presence of hypertension (particularly if it is labile, paroxysmal, or refractory to treatment) or paroxysmal symptoms of headaches, palpitations, sweating, anxiety with a feeling of impending doom, and pallor. In most patients, the paroxysmal symptoms are stereotyped and vary only in severity or frequency.

- Pheochromocytomas can be asymptomatic and discovered incidentally on abdominal imaging. More commonly, they are suspected because of hypertension or paroxysmal symptoms.

- Common symptoms: headache, palpitations, and sweating. Symptoms may be paroxysmal. In most patients, the paroxysmal symptoms are stereotyped and vary only in severity or frequency.

- Other presentations: heat intolerance, sweating, weight loss, unexplained abdominal or chest pain, paradoxical response to some antihypertensive agents, orthostatic hypotension, and unexplained shock.

- Family history of pheochromocytoma, multiple endocrine neoplasia type 2A or 2B, or other neuroectodermal syndromes.

Diagnosis

Endocrine Diagnosis

The biochemical diagnosis of pheochromocytoma is based on measured levels of 24-hour urinary fractionated catecholamines and total metanephrines, and fractionated plasma metanephrines. In pheochromocytoma, these values are typically elevated more than 2-fold. A 24-hour urine collection for metanephrines and catecholamines has 90% sensitivity and 98% specificity. (In all urine collections, creatinine is measured to ensure the adequacy of the collection.) Plasma metanephrine levels have 97% to 99% sensitivity but only 85% to 89% specificity; they provide the best test for patients who have high pretest probability of disease, such as those with

genetic syndromes. Normal values of plasma metanephrines exclude the diagnosis of pheochromocytoma; increased values, unless markedly elevated, need further confirmation with more specific urinary catecholamines and metanephrines. If patients have paroxysmal symptoms, the diagnostic yield can be significantly increased by initiating collection during or shortly after a paroxysm.

- Document catecholamine hypersecretion. Check urinary catecholamines and metanephrines. Normal values in a hypertensive patient exclude the diagnosis. In patients with paroxysmal symptoms, the diagnostic yield is increased significantly by initiating collection during or shortly after a paroxysm.

- Plasma metanephrines provide the best test for patients who have high pretest probability of disease, such as those with genetic syndromes. Normal values of plasma metanephrines exclude the diagnosis of pheochromocytoma; increased values, unless markedly elevated, need further confirmation with more specific urinary catecholamines and metanephrines.

- Increased values in hypertensive patients establish the diagnosis only with the exclusion of interfering drugs (especially tricyclic antidepressants) and disorders associated with hypertension and catecholamine excess (eg, severe stress, intercurrent illness, acute myocardial ischemia, abrupt withdrawal of clonidine, hypoglycemia, and obstructive sleep apnea).

Radiologic Localization

Radiologic evaluation should be initiated only after catecholamine excess has been confirmed biochemically. CT and MRI of the abdomen (and, if findings are negative, the pelvis, thorax, and neck) are the mainstay of radiologic localization. They have a sensitivity and specificity greater than 90%. CT has better spatial resolution. MRI is better at characterizing the mass, with pheochromocytomas showing high-signal intensity on T2-weighted images. MRI is considered the radiologic procedure of choice.

- Radiologic localization of the pheochromocytoma is attempted only after biochemical confirmation.

- CT or MRI of the abdomen (if findings are negative, image the pelvis and thorax) are the mainstay of radiologic localization.

- MRI is the radiologic procedure of choice; pheochromocytomas appear as high-intensity signal masses on T2-weighted images.

Therapy

Surgical excision of the tumor is curative. Medical treatment is used in preoperative preparation to diminish perioperative morbidity and mortality and on a long-term basis if surgical excision is not successful. α-Adrenergic blockade is the cornerstone of medical therapy and should be instituted as soon as the diagnosis is made. Phenoxybenzamine is the drug of choice to control the hypertension and to restore the plasma volume (a high-salt diet is also important). Its major side effect is postural hypotension. Alternate drugs include prazosin, terazosin, labetalol, nifedipine, and angiotensin-converting enzyme inhibitors. β-Adrenergic blockers may be necessary to control tachyarrhythmias, but these drugs should be used only after adequate α-blockade to prevent exacerbation of the hypertension. For hypertensive emergencies, phentolamine, an α-blocker, is the drug of choice and can be given in 5- to 10-mg doses every 5 to 15 minutes as needed. Alternatively, nitroprusside or labetalol can be used. For an inoperable pheochromocytoma, add metyrosine, a competitive inhibitor of tyrosine hydroxylase, to the treatment.

Postoperatively, in the surgically cured patient, the urinary catecholamine and metabolite levels normalize in 2 weeks. Long-term follow-up is important to assess for persistence, recurrence, or development of other manifestations of the genetic syndromes mentioned above.

- Surgical excision of the tumor is curative.

- Medical treatment is used in preoperative preparation to diminish perioperative morbidity and mortality and on a long-term basis if surgical excision is not successful.

- α-Adrenergic blockade is the cornerstone of medical therapy. It should be instituted as soon as the diagnosis is made.

- β-Blockade may be necessary to control tachyarrhythmias; use only after adequate α-blockade.

- For hypertensive emergencies, use phentolamine (an α-blocker).

ADRENAL INCIDENTALOMA

Etiology

Small (1–6 cm) adrenal masses are found in up to 9% of unselected autopsies and in more than 2% of all abdominal imaging studies. Most are nonfunctioning adenomas; a few are functioning adenomas or carcinomas of the adrenal cortex or medulla. Metastatic disease to the adrenal glands is common. Identification of the nature of the mass is important: nonfunctioning adenomas are harmless, a functioning adenoma or a carcinoma requires surgery, and a metastasis requires oncologic care.

Diagnosis

The diagnosis of a functioning adrenal tumor rests on clinical evaluation, the use of screening tests, and, when appropriate, confirmatory tests. For all patients, hormonal evaluation should screen for pheochromocytoma (24-hour urinary fractionated catecholamines and metanephrines) and Cushing syndrome (in this context, a 1-mg overnight dexamethasone

suppression test is considered superior to measuring the 24-hour urinary free cortisol level).

With the exception of an adrenal myelolipoma, which is benign and has characteristic fat-density images, imaging studies with CT or MR may not differentiate between benign and malignant neoplasms. However, certain imaging characteristics make a benign disorder very likely: size less than 4 cm, density less than 10 Hounsfield units on CT, homogeneous density, lack of vascularity, and a well-defined border. Bright T2 images on MRI suggest pheochromocytoma or adrenal cancer.

The only place for needle aspiration in the diagnosis of an adrenal mass is if adrenal metastases are a possibility. Pheochromocytoma must be excluded before aspiration.

Therapy

Therapy is based on observation and follow-up. Every patient with an adrenal mass that is not resected should have another CT scan within 3 to 6 months to assess for growth of the mass. If the mass size is stable after 3 to 6 months, additional scans are performed 12 and 24 months after the diagnosis. Every mass lesion that demonstrably increases in size during the observation period should be surgically excised after appropriate biochemical studies are performed.

- Exclude pheochromocytoma and a subclinical cortisol-producing tumor before proceeding with any proposed surgery for an adrenal mass.

- Surgical excision is indicated for a functioning adrenal mass, a large solid or solid-cystic mass (>6 cm), and cystic masses with blood contents on CT-guided needle aspiration.

- Otherwise, observation is indicated with subsequent scans done 3–6, 12, and 24 months after the diagnosis. A demonstrable increase in size of the mass at any time dictates surgical removal after appropriate screening endocrine tests.

DISORDERS OF THE TESTIS

MALE HYPOGONADISM IN THE ADULT

Male hypogonadism refers to the clinical presentations resulting from testosterone deficiency. Such deficiency usually is associated with defects in spermatogenesis and infertility. However, spermatogenic failure may exist independently of any testosterone deficiency.

Etiology

Testosterone deficiency may result from decreased testosterone production by the testes or target tissue resistance to testosterone action. Decreased testosterone production may be the consequence of primary testicular failure (*hypergonadotropic hypogonadism*) or luteinizing hormone (LH) deficiency resulting from a central hypothalamic-pituitary disorder (*hypogonadotropic hypogonadism*).

Among the causes of *primary hypergonadotropic testicular failure* are genetic disorders such as Klinefelter syndrome; traumatic disorders such as those resulting from physical, radiotherapeutic, or chemotherapeutic agents; inflammatory disorders such as those due to mumps or autoimmune endocrinopathy; and degenerative disorders such as myotonia dystrophica.

Central hypogonadotropism may be a consequence of functional hypothalamic hypogonadotropism, as in constitutional delay in puberty, or the use of neuroleptic or antidepressant drugs, nutritional disorders, systemic illness, stress, or other endocrinopathies such as hyperprolactinemia, hyperestrogenic states, and thyroid or adrenal disorders.

Androgen resistance may be genetic or acquired. Acquired androgen resistance may occur with the use of androgen-receptor blockers such as spironolactone or flutamide.

- Testosterone deficiency may result from decreased testosterone production or target tissue resistance.

- Decreased testosterone production may result from primary testicular failure (hypergonadotropic failure) or central hypothalamic-pituitary disorder (hypogonadotropic failure).

- Primary testicular failure is a consequence of organic diseases of the testes.

- Central hypogonadotropism may result from functional or organic hypothalamic disorders or from organic diseases of the anterior pituitary gland.

- Target tissue resistance to testosterone action may be genetic or acquired.

Clinical Features

The clinical manifestations of hypogonadism in men include decreased libido and potency, decreased ejaculate volume, infertility, decreased energy and stamina, decreased sexual hair growth, and gynecomastia. Hot flushes may occur if the testosterone deficiency has a rapid onset. In men with chronic or severe testosterone deficiency, physical findings may include the classic hypogonadal facies (with pallor and fine wrinkling around the mouth and eyes), altered feminine-like fat distribution, testicular atrophy, decrease in prostate size, osteoporosis, and gynecomastia.

The testes must be examined for size (using an orchidometer), consistency, and evidence of structural disease such as trauma, infiltrative lesions, infections, or masses. Men with estrogen-secreting Leydig cell tumors may present with hypogonadism. For men with long-standing hypogonadism, bone densitometry is recommended.

- Characteristic manifestations of hypogonadism in men include decreased libido and potency, decreased ejaculate volume, gynecomastia, and secondary osteoporosis.

- In severe cases, men may have the characteristic facies, loss of secondary sex characteristics, and testicular and prostate atrophy.

- The testes must be examined carefully.

- Bone densitometry is recommended for men with long-standing hypogonadism.

Diagnosis

The diagnosis is suspected on the basis of the clinical picture and is confirmed by the finding of low serum levels of testosterone. Low serum levels of total testosterone may reflect hypogonadism or abnormalities of sex hormone–binding globulin. Most commonly, abnormal testosterone binding is related to obesity (decreased binding) or aging (increased binding). Low serum levels of free testosterone define hypogonadism. When convenient and possible, a semen analysis is performed. In almost all cases, a normal semen analysis indicates a normal hypothalamic-pituitary-gonadal axis.

The etiologic diagnosis is suspected on the basis of the clinical picture and is confirmed by measurements of the serum levels of LH and follicle-stimulating hormone (FSH). In primary testicular failure, the serum levels of FSH and LH are increased (hypergonadotropic hypogonadism). Additional tests are not indicated except for determining karyotype (to confirm Klinefelter syndrome or its variants or mosaics) or evaluation for other endocrinopathies (in patients with autoimmune testicular failure). In central hypothalamic-pituitary hypogonadism, serum levels of LH and FSH are low or "inappropriately normal" in relation to the low level of serum testosterone (hypogonadotropic hypogonadism). Otherwise, hypogonadotropism dictates a complete clinical evaluation, determination of serum prolactin level and other pituitary function tests, and an MRI of the head to exclude mass lesions or other organic forms of hypothalamic-pituitary disease.

- Suspicion depends on clinical evaluation and the characteristic finding of low serum levels of testosterone.

- A normal semen analysis excludes hypogonadism.

- Low serum levels of testosterone may reflect hypogonadism or sex hormone–binding globulin abnormalities. Check serum level of free testosterone. Low free testosterone defines hypogonadism.

- Serum levels of LH and FSH: determine whether the hypogonadism is primary testicular (hypergonadotropic) or secondary to hypothalamic-pituitary (hypogonadotropic) disease.

- The cause of hypogonadotropism is usually obvious from the clinical setting.

- Hypogonadotropic hypogonadism should prompt assessment of the other pituitary functions, MRI of the head, and consideration of functional hypogonadotropism.

Therapy

In adults, androgen therapy is aimed at restoring and maintaining androgenic functions. In hypogonadal pubertal males, it is designed to initiate and induce full pubertal development. Androgen replacement may be given in the form of parenteral long-acting 17-hydroxyl esters of testosterone (enanthate or cypionate esters). They are effective and safe. The usual dosage for an adult male is 200 mg intramuscularly every 15 days. Alternately, testosterone may be administered transdermally either in the form of a patch (2.5–7.5 mg) or gel (2.5–7.5 mg) applied daily. This therapy is associated with stable physiologic serum testosterone concentrations. Buccal testosterone given twice daily is also available but experience with it is limited. Oral preparations available in the United States are all 17α-alkylated derivatives of testosterone. They are less effective and more costly, and they can be associated with the potentially serious side effects of hepatotoxicity, induction of peliosis hepatis, and hepatic tumors. Assessment of the adequacy of therapy is best done clinically and by measurement of serum testosterone 2 to 3 months after the institution of therapy. If the patient has primary hypogonadism, normalization of serum LH is also used as an indicator of adequacy of therapy.

Absolute contraindications to androgen therapy include androgen-dependent tumors of the prostate and male breast. Relative contraindications include mental retardation, psychopathy, and obstructive prostatism. Side effects include acne, mild weight gain, edema, increased erythropoiesis, and induction or worsening of obstructive sleep apnea. Androgens may worsen obstructive uropathy due to benign prostatic hypertrophy. It is important to remember that prostate cancer is at least partially an androgen-dependent tumor. A digital rectal examination, a serum prostate-specific antigen level measurement, and a complete blood cell count should be done before the initiation of therapy, 3 months after the initiation of therapy, and yearly thereafter.

- In adults, the aims of androgen therapy are to restore and maintain androgenic function. In hypogonadal pubertal males, the objectives are to initiate and induce full pubertal development.

- Androgen replacement therapy includes intramuscular testosterone enanthate or cypionate or use of a transdermal testosterone patch or gel.

- Oral preparations are all 17α-alkylated derivatives of testosterone. These agents have potentially serious side effects.

- Absolute contraindications for testosterone therapy are androgen-dependent tumors of the prostate and male breast.

- Testosterone therapy may induce erythropoiesis and aggravate sleep apnea and obstructive prostatism.

GYNECOMASTIA

Etiology

Gynecomastia refers to a benign enlargement of the male breast caused by an increase in glandular and stromal tissues. It is the most common disorder of the male breast, accounting for more than 85% of male breast masses. The basic pathophysiologic mechanism is an increase in the estrogen to androgen ratio, which may result from androgen deficiency, exposure to exogenous estrogen, or an endogenous increase in estrogen production. Gynecomastia may have a benign or sinister cause. It is always important to attempt to identify a specific cause. In young pubertal males, the most likely cause is physiologic gynecomastia. In adults, the most common causes are drugs and alcohol-related liver disease. In about 10% of cases, the cause of gynecomastia is indeterminate or idiopathic.

Diagnosis

If gynecomastia is bilateral, exclude pseudogynecomastia (fatty enlargement). If it is unilateral, exclude cancer of the breast. Signs that should arouse suspicion of malignancy include an eccentric location in relation to the areola, unusual firmness, fixation, ulceration, bloody discharge from the nipple, and the presence of axillary lymphadenopathy. Mammography and excisional biopsy may be necessary for definitive diagnosis. A complete medical history, physical examination, and appropriate laboratory studies should rule out physiologic, pharmacologic, alcohol-related, and refeeding types of gynecomastia. Endocrine tests may include measurement of the serum levels of testosterone, estradiol, LH and FSH, β-human chorionic gonadotropin, sensitive thyrotropin, dehydroepiandrosterone sulfate (DHEAS), and prolactin.

- If gynecomastia is bilateral, rule out pseudogynecomastia. If unilateral, rule out tumors.

- Signs that arouse suspicion of malignancy: eccentric location in relation to the areola, unusual firmness, fixation, ulceration, bloody discharge from the nipple, and axillary lymphadenopathy.

- A complete medical history, physical examination, and appropriate laboratory studies should rule out physiologic, pharmacologic, alcohol-related, and refeeding types of gynecomastia.

- Endocrine tests may include measurement of the serum levels of testosterone, estradiol, LH and FSH, β-human chorionic gonadotropin, sensitive thyrotropin, DHEAS, and prolactin.

DISORDERS OF THE OVARY

AMENORRHEA

Primary amenorrhea is present when menarche has not occurred by age 16 in a young female patient with normal secondary sex characteristics or by age 14 in the absence of secondary sex characteristics. *Secondary amenorrhea* is present when a woman with previously established menstrual function experiences the absence of menstruation for more than 3 of her previous cycle intervals or for 6 months.

Etiology

The requirements for normal regular menstrual function are the following:

1. Normal cyclic secretion of hypothalamic gonadotropin-releasing hormone (GnRH) and the pituitary gonadotropins LH and FSH

2. Normal ovarian follicular apparatus that responds to cyclic gonadotropin stimulation by ovulation and production of estrogen and progesterone in a cyclic fashion

3. Normal endometrium capable of responding to estradiol (follicular proliferative endometrium) and progesterone (luteal secretory endometrium) and then to their declining concentrations by the initiation of menstrual shedding

Amenorrhea can be physiologic or pathologic. The most common causes of amenorrhea are physiologic (pregnancy, lactation, and prepubertal and perimenopausal states). Pathologic amenorrhea may result from the following:

1. A functional or organic hypothalamic disorder leading to loss of cyclic GnRH production

2. An organic pituitary disorder resulting in loss of the gonadotrope population

3. An organic ovarian disorder resulting in loss of the follicular apparatus, or in anovulation, and loss of the normal sequential estradiol and progesterone secretion

4. Organic uterine disorders and loss of the endometrium or genital tract disorders preventing egress of the shed endometrium

- Amenorrhea can result from impaired function of any component of the hypothalamic-pituitary-gonadal axis or from an anatomical abnormality of the genital tract.

- The most common causes of amenorrhea are physiologic: pregnancy, postpartum lactation, and prepubertal and perimenopausal states.

- The common causes of primary amenorrhea are gonadal dysgenesis, constitutional delay in puberty, and müllerian agenesis.

- The most common causes of secondary amenorrhea are ovarian disorders, hypothalamic dysfunction, and pituitary disease.

Primary Amenorrhea

Outflow tract abnormalities are uncommon causes of primary amenorrhea. Developmental anomalies include imperforate hymen, isolated absence of the uterus, and vaginal aplasia or atresia. Ovarian disorders, including developmental and acquired disorders, account for most of the causes of primary amenorrhea. Hypothalamic-pituitary disease can cause gonadotropin deficiency and amenorrhea by the following:

1. Destruction of pituitary gonadotrophs or the hypothalamic GnRH cell population by organic diseases of various origins

2. Functional suppression of these cells, commonly by a nutritional or psychiatric disorder, prolonged heavy exercise, systemic illness, and other endocrinopathies such as uncontrolled diabetes mellitus, hyperprolactinemic states, and thyroid and adrenal disorders

- Outflow tract disorders are uncommon causes and include developmental abnormalities.

- Ovarian disorders are the most common cause of primary amenorrhea; they may be genetic or acquired.

- Hypothalamic-pituitary disease may be organic and caused by destructive processes affecting the endocrine hypothalamus or the anterior pituitary, or it may be functional and caused by functional suppression of GnRH secretion by nutritional or psychiatric disorders, systemic disease, and other endocrinopathies.

Secondary Amenorrhea

Ovarian disorders are common causes of secondary amenorrhea. The most common disorder is polycystic ovary syndrome (PCOS). Ovarian destructive processes are an uncommon cause of secondary amenorrhea and premature menopause. These processes include autoimmune oophoritis, abdominal radiotherapy, chemotherapy with agents such as cyclophosphamide and vincristine, and ovarian tumors that cause secondary amenorrhea by hormonal abnormalities (hypersecretion of estrogen, androgen, or human chorionic gonadotropin) or, if bilateral, by destruction of the ovarian tissue.

Hypothalamic-pituitary disorders are the most common pathologic causes of secondary amenorrhea and may be either functional or organic. *Functional hypogonadotropism* results from hypothalamic dysfunction caused by a defect in the cyclic center, inhibition of the mid-cycle surge of GnRH and LH, and the failure of ovulation. Mild disorders of GnRH release may be triggered by situational stresses or mild weight loss. Moderate or severe disorders of GnRH release may occur with severe weight loss, severe emotional stresses, competitive athletics, systemic disease, thyroid disorders, uncontrolled diabetes mellitus, or a hyperandrogenic state caused by an adrenal or ovarian disorder. In *organic hypothalamic-pituitary disorder*, hypogonadotropism can be the only manifestation or it can occur in association with other pituitary function abnormalities. Hypogonadotropism can occur as a result of pituitary disorders, hypothalamic disorders, or disorders of extrasellar structures impinging on the hypothalamic-pituitary unit. Hyperprolactinemia is a common cause of secondary amenorrhea, accounting for 25% to 40% of all cases. Postpartum pituitary necrosis (Sheehan syndrome), previously a common cause, has declined in incidence with improvements in obstetric care.

- Acquired outflow tract abnormalities are uncommon causes of secondary amenorrhea.

- Ovarian disorders are common causes of secondary amenorrhea. The most common disorder is PCOS. Ovarian destructive processes are an uncommon cause of secondary amenorrhea and premature menopause.

- Hypothalamic-pituitary disorders are the most common pathologic causes of secondary amenorrhea. They may be functional or organic.

Clinical Features

In addition to amenorrhea, findings of a hypoestrogenic state may be present: decreased vaginal secretions and dyspareunia, hot flushes, osteopenia, and lack of development or loss of the secondary sex characteristics. Other findings are related to the etiologic disorder, such as hyperandrogenic features, expressible or spontaneous galactorrhea, shortness of stature or Turner stigmata, thyroid dysfunction and goiter, or other manifestations of hypopituitarism.

Diagnosis

The diagnostic approach to secondary amenorrhea is summarized as follows:

- Rule out physiologic amenorrhea (pregnancy test), genital tract outflow disorders (clinical evaluation, hysteroscopy), and hyperandrogenic state (clinical evaluation, serum levels of testosterone and DHEAS).

- Measure serum levels of estradiol, LH, and FSH to distinguish ovarian disease from hypothalamic-pituitary disease.

- Low serum levels of estradiol and increased levels of FSH and LH suggest primary ovarian failure. Obtain a karyotype if the patient is younger than 30 years.

- Low serum levels of estradiol and inappropriately low levels of FSH and LH suggest a hypothalamic-pituitary disorder. Rule out a functional disorder and organic hypothalamic-pituitary disease.

- If organic disease is not identified, consider amenorrhea to be of indeterminate cause and pursue long-term follow-up.

Therapy

Management is directed at the underlying disorder and restoration of a eugonadal state. It is important to identify and treat the cause. If the cause cannot be treated successfully, estrogen replacement and, if feasible, restoration of ovulation and fertility potential are indicated.

- Identify and treat the cause.

- If the cause cannot be treated successfully, provide estrogen replacement therapy and, if feasible, restore ovulation and reproductive potential.

Estrogen Replacement

The goals of estrogen therapy include control of vasomotor instability, prevention of genitourinary atrophy, preservation of secondary sex characteristics, prevention of osteoporosis, reduction of the risk of coronary artery disease, and restoration of a sense of well-being.

Absolute contraindications to estrogen therapy include known or suspected estrogen-dependent neoplasm (breast or uterus), cholestatic hepatic dysfunction, active thromboembolic disorder, history of thromboembolic disorder associated with previous estrogen use, neuro-ophthalmologic vascular disease, and undiagnosed vaginal bleeding.

Estrogen therapy must be individualized and administered only after a thorough discussion with the patient about the benefits and risks of the therapy. Therapy is initiated as soon as possible after the diagnosis of estrogen deficiency and is continued indefinitely or until the cause has been reversed.

Estrogen preparations include oral estradiol (0.5–2 mg daily); conjugated estrogens (0.625–1.25 mg daily); or transdermal estradiol patch (0.025–0.1 mg estradiol daily). Use progestational agents for a woman with an intact uterus (medroxyprogesterone acetate, 10 mg daily, or oral progesterone, 200 mg daily) for days 1 to 12 of each month. Oral and transdermal hormonal combinations are also available.

Complications of estrogen replacement include an increased risk (4- to 8-fold) of endometrial cancer (usually stage I, with no excess mortality), which is dose- and duration-dependent. This risk is prevented by progestin supplementation. Other possible adverse effects include a slightly increased risk of breast cancer (breast examination and mammography before treatment and annually thereafter are essential) and increased risk of surgical gallbladder disease.

- The goal of estrogen therapy is to restore the estrogenic state.

- Exclude the absolute contraindications.

- Individualize the therapy.

- Initiate therapy as soon as the diagnosis of hypoestrogenism is made.

- Continue therapy indefinitely unless the cause is reversed or a significant side effect or contraindication develops.

- Use progestin supplementation in the woman who still has her uterus.

- Complications of estrogen replacement therapy include an increased risk of endometrial cancer, a possibly slightly increased risk of breast cancer, and an increased risk of surgical gallbladder disease.

Ovulation Induction

Hypogonadal women who desire fertility can be given clomiphene citrate, exogenous gonadotropin, or GnRH therapy. The drug of choice for hyperprolactinemic infertility is the dopamine-agonist bromocriptine.

POLYCYSTIC OVARY SYNDROME

PCOS is the most common cause of nonvirilizing hyperandrogenicity. It is characterized by oligo-ovulation or anovulation, clinical or biochemical evidence of hyperandrogenism, and polycystic changes in the ovaries:

1. In each ovary, ≥12 follicles measuring 2–9 mm in diameter

2. Increased ovarian volume (>10 mL)

3. Increased stromal volume

The pathogenesis is poorly understood. Gonadotropin dynamics are abnormal, with loss of the LH surge and increased LH levels. Hyperandrogenicity is mild to moderate and LH-dependent.

In many patients, there is associated obesity and insulin resistance and consequent hyperinsulinism, which further contribute to the androgen excess. Insulin resistance may be present without obesity. The degree of insulin resistance varies. Many women have a mild form; severe insulin resistance is usually appreciated clinically by the presence of acanthosis nigricans.

The onset of the disorder is at puberty, and its progression is slow and of mild degree. Hirsutism (70% of patients), menstrual abnormality (88%), infertility and anovulation (75%), and obesity (50%) are usually present. The serum level of testosterone is normal or modestly increased (70% of patients) and is nearly always less than 200 ng/dL. DHEAS levels are normal or mildly increased in 25% of patients. Changes seen on pelvic ultrasonography are characteristic (70%); hyperprolactinemia may be present in 25% to 30% of patients. It is important to note that anovulation exposes the endometrium to unopposed estrogen, which increases the risk of endometrial hyperplasia and cancer.

The diagnosis of PCOS is one of exclusion of other causes of hyperandrogenism, such as late-onset congenital adrenal hyperplasia, Cushing syndrome, and androgen-secreting tumors of the ovaries or adrenals.

- PCOS is the most common cause of hyperandrogenicity.

- Hyperandrogenicity in PCOS is mild to moderate and LH-dependent.

- Features: onset at puberty, slow progression, hirsutism (70% of patients), menstrual abnormality (88%), infertility and anovulation (75%), and obesity (50%).

- Serum level of testosterone: normal or modestly increased (70%); it almost always is <200 ng/dL.

- Serum level of DHEAS: normal or mildly increased.

- Modest degree of hyperprolactinemia occurs in 25%-30% of patients.

- The diagnosis of PCOS is one of exclusion of other causes of hyperandrogenism.

SUMMARY

- Primary adrenocortical failure is associated with cortisol, sex steroids, and aldosterone deficiencies. It has many organic and functional causes; in the United States, the most common causes are autoimmune adrenalitis and bilateral adrenal hemorrhage; worldwide, tuberculosis-associated adrenalitis is common.

- Secondary adrenal failure is due to ACTH deficiency. It affects production of cortisol and sex steroids, whereas aldosterone secretion is basically intact; it is most commonly due to functional suppression of the axis by prolonged glucocorticoid therapy.

- Adrenal crisis is precipitated by an illness in a patient who has unrecognized adrenocortical failure and who recently had glucocorticoid therapy withdrawn or has sustained bilateral hemorrhage of the adrenals.

- Testosterone deficiency may result from decreased testosterone production or target tissue resistance.

- Decreased testosterone production may result from primary testicular failure (hypergonadotropic failure) or central hypothalamic-pituitary disorder (hypogonadotropic failure).

- Amenorrhea can result from impaired function of any component of the hypothalamic-pituitary-gonadal axis or from an anatomical abnormality of the genital tract.

- The most common causes of amenorrhea are physiologic: pregnancy, postpartum lactation, and prepubertal and perimenopausal states.

32.

DISORDERS OF CALCIUM AND BONE METABOLISM

Marius N. Stan, MD

GOALS

- Review the causes, evaluation, and management of hypercalcemia.

- Summarize the causes, evaluation, and management of hypoparathyroidism.

- Describe osteoporosis and osteomalacia.

- Define Paget disease of bone.

HYPERCALCEMIA

The causes of hypercalcemia are categorized as either parathyroid hormone (PTH) dependent or PTH independent.

PTH-DEPENDENT HYPERCALCEMIA

Primary Hyperparathyroidism

Etiology

Primary hyperparathyroidism is the most common cause of hypercalcemia in ambulatory patients. A single parathyroid adenoma is the cause in 85% of patients, and multiglandular disease is the cause in the remainder. Parathyroid carcinoma is a rare cause of hypercalcemia. Primary hyperparathyroidism may be sporadic or familial. Familial hyperparathyroidism is usually multiglandular and most commonly a manifestation of multiple endocrine neoplasia (MEN) type 1 (MEN-1) or type 2 (MEN-2) syndromes.

- Parathyroid carcinoma is a rare cause of hypercalcemia.

- Familial hyperparathyroidism is most often due to MEN-1 or MEN-2 and is usually multiglandular.

Clinical Features

Most patients with hyperparathyroidism are asymptomatic and are identified with routine laboratory testing. Symptoms of hypercalcemia include polyuria, polydipsia, constipation, fatigue, and abdominal pain. Hypercalciuria can cause nephrolithiasis and nephrocalcinosis. Skeletal manifestations include osteopenia or osteoporosis and, in severe disease, bone pain, fractures, and osteitis fibrosa cystica (bone pain and characteristic areas of periosteal bone resorption).

- Nephrolithiasis and nephrocalcinosis may result from hypercalciuria.

- Osteopenia and osteoporosis, bone pain, fractures, and osteitis fibrosa cystica are potential skeletal manifestations.

Diagnosis

Elevated serum calcium and PTH levels are hallmarks of primary hyperparathyroidism. The serum PTH level is usually increased but may be inappropriately normal for the degree of hypercalcemia. Serum phosphate concentrations are normal or low. Urinary calcium excretion is high-normal or elevated; this test is also useful to assess risk for nephrolithiasis and exclude disorders characterized by low urinary calcium excretion (eg, familial hypocalciuric hypercalcemia and thiazide use). Characteristic skeletal radiographic changes include subperiosteal bone resorption, a salt-and-pepper appearance of the skull, and osteitis fibrosa cystica. Renal stones or nephrocalcinosis may be visible on abdominal radiographs.

- The hallmark laboratory findings are elevated serum calcium and PTH levels.

- Serum phosphate is usually normal or low.

- Urinary calcium is high-normal or elevated; this test can also help assess risk for renal stones and exclude disorders characterized by low urinary calcium excretion.

Therapy

Surgical parathyroidectomy is the treatment of choice. Conservative therapy may be indicated for mild uncomplicated disease, especially in the elderly. Indications for surgical intervention are listed in Box 32.1. Imaging studies are helpful for guiding the surgeon, but they do not help in diagnosis.

Preoperative imaging (parathyroid sestamibi scanning or ultrasonography) often identifies a solitary parathyroid adenoma, allowing minimally invasive surgery. Transient, mild hypocalcemia is common in the early postoperative period. However, in patients with severe preexisting parathyroid-induced bone disease, correction of hyperparathyroidism may lead to marked and prolonged hypocalcemia due to hungry bone syndrome.

- Surgical parathyroidectomy is the treatment of choice, but conservative therapy is reasonable for mild, uncomplicated disease, particularly in the elderly.

- Imaging studies help guide the surgeon; they are not used in diagnosis.

Familial Hypocalciuric Hypercalcemia

Familial hypocalciuric hypercalcemia (FHH) is an autosomal dominant disorder resulting from an altered set point of the calcium-sensing receptor in the parathyroid glands and renal tubules. It manifests as mild, asymptomatic hypercalcemia in a patient with a normal or slightly increased level of PTH, low urinary calcium, and often a family history positive for hypercalcemia. The diagnosis is strongly supported by a ratio of urinary calcium to creatinine clearance that is less than 0.01, distinguishing it from primary hyperparathyroidism. Genetic testing is clinically available. Parathyroid surgery is not indicated because complications associated with hyperparathyroidism do not develop.

- A ratio of urinary calcium to creatinine clearance <0.01 supports a diagnosis of FHH.

Thiazide-Induced Hypercalcemia

Mild hypercalcemia may occur in patients taking thiazide diuretics. The hypercalcemia is multifactorial (dehydration, decreased renal calcium clearance, and possibly increased PTH secretion). PTH levels are inappropriately normal or mildly increased. The hypercalcemia usually resolves within a few weeks of discontinuation of the drug unless it is coexistent with primary hyperparathyroidism.

- Thiazide diuretics may cause mild hypercalcemia, which is generally multifactorial.

- PTH is inappropriately normal or mildly increased.

Lithium

Lithium raises the threshold for serum calcium's inhibition of PTH secretion. PTH levels are inappropriately normal or mildly increased. The hypercalcemia resolves after discontinuation of lithium therapy.

- Discontinuation of lithium leads to normalization of the serum calcium.

PTH-INDEPENDENT HYPERCALCEMIA

Hypercalcemia of Malignancy

Hypercalcemia of malignancy often develops acutely and may be severe and life-threatening. It is the most common cause of hypercalcemia in hospitalized patients. It results from the destructive effects of skeletal metastases through local cytokines or the paraneoplastic effect of a malignancy through PTH-related peptide. Serum PTH is suppressed in all cases of hypercalcemia due to malignancy.

- Serum PTH is always suppressed in hypercalcemia of malignancy.

Vitamin D Intoxication

Hypercalcemia, hypercalciuria, renal insufficiency, and soft tissue calcification can result from prolonged intake of high levels of vitamin D. Because vitamin D is stored in fat, this condition may persist for months after the vitamin D supplementation has been discontinued.

- The manifestations of vitamin D intoxication may persist for months after supplementation is discontinued, because vitamin D is stored in fat.

Sarcoidosis, Granulomatous Disorders, and Lymphoma

The hypercalcemia and hypercalciuria in sarcoidosis, granulomatous disorders, and lymphoma are due to increased 1α-hydroxylase enzyme activity within the cells of the granuloma or lymphoma, which can autonomously generate 1,25-dihydroxyvitamin D (the active form of vitamin D). The serum 25-hydroxyvitamin D level is normal, whereas the 1,25-dihydroxyvitamin D level is increased. The PTH level is low and the serum phosphorus level may be normal or elevated. The hypercalcemia is responsive to treatment of the underlying disease and glucocorticoid therapy.

- The autonomous production of 1,25-dihydroxyvitamin D and the 1α-hydroxylase activity in granulomas or lymphoma lead to hypercalcemia and hypercalciuria.

- The serum 25-hydroxyvitamin D level is normal, 1,25-dihydroxyvitamin D is elevated, PTH is low, and phosphorus is normal or elevated.

Miscellaneous Causes

Hyperthyroidism enhances bone turnover and may lead to net bone loss. Hypercalcemia and, more often, hypercalciuria may be present. The hypercalcemia resolves with the treatment of thyrotoxicosis.

- Treatment of thyrotoxicosis leads to resolution of hypercalcemia.

Addison disease can cause symptomatic hypercalcemia related to dehydration and increased albumin concentration. The hypercalcemia is reversible with glucocorticoid therapy.

- Dehydration and hyperalbuminemia may cause symptomatic hypercalcemia in patients with Addison disease.

MANAGEMENT OF HYPERCALCEMIA

When feasible, treatment of the primary cause is the best intervention. Glucocorticoids are the drugs of choice for the hypercalcemia of granulomatous disorders. Humoral hypercalcemia of malignancy may respond to complete resection of the tumor. In severe hypercalcemia or hypercalcemia in which the primary cause is not immediately treatable, calcium concentrations should be decreased. Aggressive rehydration with volume expansion promotes calciuresis. Loop diuretics promote renal calcium excretion (*after* volume expansion). A single-dose, intravenous infusion of pamidronate inhibits bone resorption and mobilization of calcium from bone and has a marked, prolonged effect on calcium concentrations. Dialysis is reserved for patients with renal failure.

- Treatment of the underlying cause, rehydration with volume expansion to promote calciuriesis, and administration of pamidronate are cornerstones of therapy for patients with hypercalcemia.

HYPOPARATHYROIDISM

ETIOLOGY

Hypoparathyroidism may be due to decreased PTH production or to resistance of the target tissue to the actions of PTH. The parathyroid glands may be damaged during thyroidectomy, or they may be excised completely for the treatment of primary hyperparathyroidism due to parathyroid hyperplasia. Postoperative hypoparathyroidism may be transient or permanent. It appears within hours after the operation and, if transient, can take days to weeks for full recovery. Other causes of decreased PTH secretion are an autoimmune or infiltrative process involving the parathyroid glands (hemochromatosis or Wilson disease), congenital defect (DiGeorge syndrome), or hypomagnesemia (due to diuretic use, malabsorption, or malnutrition), which impairs the secretion and action of PTH.

- Surgical damage or excision can cause transient or permanent postoperative hypoparathyroidism.

- Autoimmune or infiltrative processes, congenital defect, or hypomagnesemia may lead to decreased PTH secretion.

Pseudohypoparathyroidism is characterized by end-organ (kidney and bone) resistance to the actions of PTH as a result of a receptor or postreceptor defect. In one type, patients have a characteristic appearance: short stature, round face, short metacarpals and metatarsals, and mild mental retardation (Albright hereditary osteodystrophy). A defect in the Gs subunit of the receptor is commonly identified. Patients have hypocalcemia, hyperphosphatemia, and elevated PTH. *Pseudopseudohypoparathyroidism* is a variant in which patients have the same characteristic phenotype as patients with Albright hereditary osteodystrophy but do not have the biochemical abnormalities.

- Receptor or postreceptor defects leading to end-organ resistance to PTH result in pseudohypoparathyroidism.

CLINICAL FEATURES

Hypoparathyroidism leads to decreased mobilization of calcium from bone, decreased renal calcium reabsorption, decreased renal phosphate excretion, and decreased renal production of 1,25-dihydroxyvitamin D with subsequent hypocalcemia and hyperphosphatemia. In hypoparathyroidism, the PTH level is low or inappropriately normal in the presence of hypocalcemia. In contrast, the PTH level is increased in pseudohypoparathyroidism.

- Hypocalcemia, hyperphosphatemia, and low PTH level are the common findings in hypoparathyroidism.

Hypocalcemia often is manifested by tingling in the fingers, perioral numbness, muscle cramping, or a positive Chvostek sign (facial nerve hyperirritability) or Trousseau sign (characteristic hand posture after blood pressure cuff inflation due to nerve hyperirritability and muscle spasm). Symptoms of hypocalcemia reflect its degree and rate of development. Laryngeal stridor and convulsions can occur when hypoparathyroidism is severe. Basal ganglia calcification, cataract formation, and benign intracranial hypertension can result from chronic hypoparathyroidism. QT-interval prolongation may be present. Mucocutaneous candidiasis may develop as a manifestation of polyglandular autoimmune syndrome type I (hypoparathyroidism, adrenal insufficiency, and mucocutaneous candidiasis).

- Symptoms of hypocalcemia include a positive Chvostek sign or Trousseau sign.

- Severe hypoparathyroidism may lead to laryngeal stridor and convulsions.

- Polyglandular autoimmune syndrome type I is a cause of hypoparathyroidism.

DIFFERENTIAL DIAGNOSIS

The differential diagnosis of hypocalcemia includes hypoparathyroidism, decreased vitamin D production, vitamin D resistance, and disorders associated with decreased mobilization of calcium from bone or increased calcium deposition in tissues. Vitamin D deficiency may be caused by malnutrition, malabsorption, and liver or kidney disease. In acute or chronic renal failure, the pathogenesis of hypocalcemia is thought to be multifactorial, resulting from hyperphosphatemia and decreased 1,25-dihydroxyvitamin D production. In vitamin D deficiency, hypocalcemia triggers secondary hyperparathyroidism with renal phosphate wasting. Increased tissue deposition occurs in osteoblastic metastases (eg, prostate cancer) and in the hungry bone syndrome occurring after parathyroidectomy for hyperparathyroidism with severe bone disease. Hypocalcemia and soft tissue calcification may also occur in acute pancreatitis. Increased calcium elimination is associated with the use of loop diuretics.

- The differential diagnosis of hypocalcemia includes hypoparathyroidism, disorders leading to vitamin D deficiency or resistance, and disorders associated with decreased mobilization of calcium from bone or increased calcium deposition in tissues.

DIAGNOSTIC APPROACH

Correct assessment of calcium requires a mathematical correction of the total calcium value based on serum albumin level or the measurement of ionized calcium. This assessment should be followed by measurement of the serum PTH level. In a hypocalcemic patient, a low PTH level is diagnostic of hypoparathyroidism. A high PTH level suggests vitamin D deficiency or pseudohypoparathyroidism. Serum concentrations of creatinine and magnesium help identify renal failure and magnesium deficiency states.

- Mathematical correction of the total calcium value based on serum albumin level or the measurement of ionized calcium provides an accurate assessment of the serum calcium level.

- Renal insufficiency and hypomagnesemia should be excluded.

THERAPY

For acute, severe hypocalcemia, urgent treatment with intravenous calcium is indicated to prevent tetany, laryngeal stridor, or convulsions. Extravasation of calcium can cause severe tissue necrosis, so central (*not* peripheral) administration is urged. Intravenous calcium should be infused slowly, over 5 to 10 minutes. Continuous electrocardiographic monitoring is essential. For long-term treatment of hypocalcemia, oral calcium supplements (2.0–3.0 g daily) and vitamin D are given. In hypoparathyroidism and renal insufficiency, the PTH-mediated conversion of 25-hydroxyvitamin D to 1,25-dihydroxyvitamin D does not occur. Therefore, the preferred form of vitamin D therapy is calcitriol (the active form of vitamin D). Thiazide diuretics are used to decrease the risk of marked hypercalciuria, and oral phosphate binders may be given to control hyperphosphatemia. It is critical to monitor therapy closely since patients are at risk of hypercalciuria, nephrolithiasis, and nephrocalcinosis. Therapeutic doses are adjusted to keep the serum level of calcium just below the lower limits of normal and the urinary level of calcium at less than 300 mg in 24 hours.

- Acute, severe hypocalcemia requires urgent therapy with intravenous calcium.

- Calcitriol is necessary to treat hypoparathyroidism and renal insufficiency.

- Thiazide diuretics and oral phosphate binders are needed.

OSTEOPOROSIS

Osteoporosis is the most common skeletal disorder encountered in clinical practice. It is characterized by decreased bone mass, leading to bone fragility and increased risk of fracture. Bone density can be quantified with dual energy x-ray absorptiometry (DEXA). *Osteopenia* is defined as bone mass that is between 1.0 and 2.5 standard deviations below the mean peak bone mass of a sex-matched control population and is designated by a T score of −1.0 to −2.5. *Osteoporosis* is defined as bone mass of at least 2.5 standard deviations below the peak bone mass of a sex-matched control population and is designated by a T score of −2.5 or less.

- Osteoporosis is characterized by decreased bone mass, leading to bone fragility and increased fracture risk.

ETIOLOGY

Osteoporosis may be primary or secondary. Primary osteoporosis (postmenopausal osteoporosis and senile osteoporosis, which occurs in older men and women) is the most common. Secondary osteoporosis may result from endocrine, nutritional, intestinal, neoplastic, or genetic disorders or from certain drugs and immobilization (Box 32.2).

Box 32.2 **CAUSES OF SECONDARY OSTEOPOROSIS**

Endocrine: hypogonadism, hyperparathyroidism, hyperthyroidism, hypercortisolism

Nutritional and intestinal: calcium deficiency, protein malnutrition, alcoholism, malabsorption, current smoking

Neoplastic disorders: multiple myeloma, leukemia, lymphoma, systemic mastocytosis

Genetic disorders: osteogenesis imperfecta

Culprit drugs: corticosteroids, heparin, anticonvulsants, gonadotropin-releasing hormone analogues (suppress sex steroid production), aromatase inhibitors

Fractures can occur with minor trauma. Osteoporotic fractures heal normally. Vertebral fractures lead to loss of height and spinal deformity. Serum levels of calcium, phosphate, and alkaline phosphatase are normal.

- Serum levels of calcium, phosphate, and alkaline phosphatase are normal in osteoporosis.

DIAGNOSIS

The diagnosis of osteoporosis is based on the finding of low bone mass by DEXA (T score ≤−2.5) or the presence of insufficiency fractures. Other causes of low bone mass, such as osteomalacia, multiple myeloma, and metastatic disease, must be excluded. Osteomalacia may coexist with osteoporosis. Myeloma or metastatic disease should be excluded as a cause of pathologic fracture.

Secondary causes of osteoporosis should be excluded. Evaluation should include serum levels of calcium, 25-hydroxyvitamin D, testosterone (free, bioavailable, and total) for males, and thyrotropin. There should be a low threshold for ruling out Cushing syndrome and multiple myeloma. DEXA should be used as a screening study for patients at risk of osteoporosis (eg, women ≥65 years of age or younger women or men with risk factors for osteoporosis or osteoporotic fracture). Routine screening in other populations (eg, men >70 years of age) is currently debated.

- Other causes of low bone mass (eg, osteomalacia, multiple myeloma, and metastases) must be excluded.
- Causes of secondary osteoporosis should be considered, and levels of calcium, 25-hydroxyvitamin D, testosterone (in males), and thyrotropin should be measured.

PREVENTION AND TREATMENT OF OSTEOPOROSIS

Bone loss can be prevented through adequate lifestyle activities, including regular weight-bearing exercise, tobacco avoidance, and avoidance of excessive alcohol use. All adults should consume an adequate amount of vitamin D (400–800 international units) and calcium (1,000–1,200 mg) daily. Estrogen replacement in women at or after menopause is effective but must be balanced against its known risks.

- Weight-bearing exercise, tobacco avoidance, nonexcessive alcohol intake, and intake of adequate amounts of calcium and vitamin D are all essential components of therapy.

Therapy requires adequate calcium and vitamin D supplementation, similar to preventive approaches. Bisphosphonates are considered first-line therapies for osteoporosis. Alendronate, risedronate, and ibandronate are oral bisphosphonates with potent antiresorptive effects that prevent bone loss. They reduce fracture risk and are effective in preventing steroid-induced bone loss. Side effects include dyspeptic

symptoms and esophagitis, particularly if the medication is taken incorrectly. Ibandronate and zoledronic acid are intravenous bisphosphonates approved for treatment of osteoporosis when oral forms are not tolerated or cannot be administered. Osteonecrosis of the jaw is a rare complication of bisphosphonate therapy; the risk is significantly higher among patients given intravenous bisphosphonates while being treated for a malignancy. Bisphosphonates should not be given to patients who have creatinine clearances of less than 30 to 35 mL/min because of the risk of renal osteodystrophy.

- Treatment requires adequate calcium and vitamin D supplementation.
- Bisphosphonates are first-line therapy for osteoporosis; they reduce fracture risk and prevent steroid-induced bone loss.

Estrogen replacement is effective for preventing and treating osteoporosis in postmenopausal women. However, the use of estrogen for osteoporosis treatment should be balanced against the risks of breast cancer, venous thrombosis, and cardiovascular disease. Raloxifene is a selective estrogen receptor modulator (SERM) effective in the prevention of both osteoporosis and breast cancer. It is less effective than bisphosphonates and estrogens with regards to bone benefits, and it increases the risk of thrombotic events. Recombinant PTH (teriparatide) is a potent enhancer of bone formation by increasing bone turnover. Patients who have increased bone turnover (eg, Paget disease) or an increased risk of osteosarcoma (eg, prior radiotherapy to bone) are not candidates for this therapy. It is administered as a daily subcutaneous injection for a maximum of 2 years. Nasal calcitonin is a weak antiresorptive agent with some analgesic properties.

- Raloxifene can be used to prevent osteoporosis and breast cancer, but it is less effective than both bisphosphonates and estrogen in terms of bone benefits.
- Recombinant PTH enhances bone formation but should not be used in patients with conditions of increased bone turnover or increased risk for osteosarcoma.

OSTEOMALACIA

DEFINITION AND ETIOLOGY

Osteomalacia is characterized by inadequate mineralization of newly formed bone. Normal bone mineralization requires adequate calcium and phosphate concentrations, functional osteoblasts, and optimal conditions for the mineralization of mature osteoid. Osteomalacia ensues when these conditions are not met. Vitamin D deficiency is the most common cause of osteomalacia. It results from inadequate oral intake, malabsorption (celiac disease), limited sun exposure, or decreased liver production of 25-hydroxyvitamin D (due to liver disease or drug side effect). Renal disease and inherited disorders affecting activation or action of vitamin D can also cause osteomalacia. Phosphate deficiency may result from malnutrition or increased renal losses. This is seen in inherited conditions such as hypophosphatemic rickets. An acquired tubular phosphate leak can occur with some mesenchymal tumors (oncogenic osteomalacia) or with multiple myeloma (generalized tubular defect in renal Fanconi syndrome).

- Vitamin D deficiency is the most common cause of osteomalacia.

CLINICAL FEATURES

Typical symptoms of osteomalacia include diffuse bone pain and tenderness along with muscle weakness. Calcium and phosphorus levels are low or low-normal, and the serum alkaline phosphatase level is usually increased. With vitamin D deficiency, secondary hyperparathyroidism also occurs. Radiographs can display pseudofractures in later stages of osteomalacia. These are narrow lines of radiolucency perpendicular to the cortical bone surface; they are typically bilateral and symmetrical. They are found most commonly in the pubic rami and the medial aspect of the femur near the femoral head.

- Calcium and phosphorus levels are low or low-normal, and the serum alkaline phosphatase level is increased.
- Secondary hyperparathyroidism occurs with vitamin D deficiency.

THERAPY

Effective therapy requires treating the underlying disorder and providing adequate calcium and phosphate to the areas of inadequate mineralization. This usually is achieved with calcium, vitamin D, and, when indicated, phosphate supplementation. Vitamin D dosing regimens vary, but a common approach is 50,000 IU weekly for 8 weeks followed by 800 IU daily for maintenance. Osteomalacia is considered adequately treated when urinary calcium excretion and bone density start to increase. The goal of therapy is to achieve bone healing while normalizing the serum concentrations of calcium, phosphate, vitamin D, and alkaline phosphatase. Alkaline phosphatase can remain elevated for several months after correction of vitamin D deficiency. During therapy, serum and urinary calcium levels should be closely monitored to avoid hypercalcemia, hypercalciuria, and nephrocalcinosis.

- When urinary calcium excretion and bone density start to increase, osteomalacia is considered adequately treated.
- The goal of therapy is bone healing and normalization of calcium, phosphate, vitamin D, and alkaline phosphatase levels.

PAGET DISEASE

Paget disease affects 3% of the population older than 45 years and is characterized by increased bone resorption with disorganized bone remodeling. Its pathogenesis is not fully understood.

CLINICAL FEATURES

Most patients present with increased serum levels of alkaline phosphatase or a radiographic abnormality. Serum alkaline phosphatase is the most useful marker of disease activity and response to therapy. The main clinical features are bone pain and deformity. Disorganized bone remodeling results in decreased tensile strength, skeletal pain, and bone deformities. Pain may also be related to fracture, degenerative changes in adjoining joints, or, rarely, the development of osteosarcoma. Commonly affected sites include the sacrum, spine, femur, tibia, skull, and pelvis. Other complications include nerve entrapment, hydrocephalus due to the development of platybasia, and high-output cardiac failure due to increased vascularity of affected bones.

- Alkaline phosphatase is a useful marker of disease activity and response to therapy.
- The most commonly affected sites are the sacrum, spine, femur, tibia, skull, and pelvis.

DIAGNOSIS

Paget disease should be suspected if the serum alkaline phosphatase level is increased and the serum calcium, phosphate, and 25-hydroxyvitamin D levels are normal. A bone scan is the most sensitive test for identifying bone lesions of Paget disease. Plain radiographs are best for further definition of the affected bones (expansion, sclerosis, deformity) and surrounding joints.

- Consider Paget disease if the alkaline phosphatase level is elevated while calcium, phosphate, and 25-hydroxyvitamin D levels are normal.
- A bone scan is the most sensitive test to identify lesions of Paget disease.

THERAPY

Many patients require only monitoring of alkaline phosphatase levels. The decision to initiate therapy relates to the presence of symptoms, the location of the bone lesions, and the disease activity. Indications for therapy are bone pain, disease involving bones where complications could occur (skull, spine, weight-bearing bone, or near joints) or a significant increase in the serum alkaline phosphatase level. Medical therapy consists of oral or intravenous bisphosphonates. Alkaline phosphatase levels are used to monitor therapy. Orthopedic surgery may be needed to treat deformity, fracture, or degenerative joint disease. Neurosurgical intervention may be required for nerve entrapment syndromes.

- Monitoring alkaline phosphatase levels is sufficient for most patients.
- Bisphosphonates are the mainstay of therapy; monitor therapy with alkaline phosphatase levels.

SUMMARY

- Primary hyperparathyroidism: elevated serum calcium and PTH levels, normal or low serum phosphate, and high-normal or elevated urinary calcium.

- Serum PTH is always suppressed in hypercalcemia of malignancy.

- Treatment of the underlying cause, rehydration with volume expansion to promote calciuriesis, and administration of pamidronate are cornerstones of therapy for patients with hypercalcemia.

- Hypocalcemia, hyperphosphatemia, and low PTH level are the common findings in hypoparathyroidism.

- The differential diagnosis of hypocalcemia includes hypoparathyroidism, disorders leading to vitamin D deficiency or resistance, and disorders associated with decreased mobilization of calcium from bone or increased calcium deposition in tissues.

- Osteoporosis: serum levels of calcium, phosphate, and alkaline phosphatase are normal.

- Osteomalacia: calcium and phosphorus levels are low or low-normal, and the serum alkaline phosphatase level is increased.

- Consider Paget disease if the alkaline phosphatase level is elevated while calcium, phosphate, and 25-hydroxyvitamin D levels are normal.

PART VII

ONCOLOGY

33.

ONCOLOGY

Timothy J. Moynihan, MD, and Michelle A. Neben Wittich, MD

GOALS

- Understand the natural history, diagnosis, and treatment of solid tumors involving the breast, cervix, colon, lung, ovary, prostate, and testicle.

- Understand the diagnosis and treatment of malignancies of unknown primary origin.

- Recognize the paraneoplastic syndromes.

- Identify oncologic complications and emergencies.

- Review the risks, treatment options, and follow up for the most common head and neck cancers.

BREAST CANCER

MAGNITUDE OF THE PROBLEM

In the United States, approximately 200,000 new cases of breast cancer are diagnosed annually. Breast cancer will develop in approximately 1 in 8 women who achieve a normal life expectancy and is the second most common cause of cancer death among women in the United States (lung cancer is the most common). The incidence has decreased steadily during the past 3 years.

- Breast cancer will develop in 1 in 8 American women.

- The incidence of breast cancer has decreased for the past 3 years.

- Breast cancer is the second most common cause of cancer death in American women.

RISK FACTORS

The risk factors for breast cancer are outlined in Table 33.1. Breast cancer-associated genes (*BRCA1* and *BRCA2*) occur in fewer than 5% to 10% of cases of breast cancer, but those women who carry these genes have a 50% to 80% chance for breast cancer developing in their lifetime. Less than 25% of women with breast cancer have known high-risk factors.

- Less than 25% of women with breast cancer have known high-risk factors.

SCREENING

The use of screening mammography in the age group 50 years or older has been associated with decreased breast cancer mortality (20%-30%). The use of screening mammography in women aged 40 to 50 years is controversial. There is general consensus that women 50 years or older should be screened with annual clinical examinations and mammography. For women at high risk for breast cancer, screening should begin at an appropriate earlier age, generally 5 to 10 years before the earliest diagnosis of breast cancer in affected first-degree relatives. Currently, mammography misses about 10% of breast cancers detectable on physical examination. Thus, any palpable breast mass should be evaluated with ultrasonography. If ultrasonography shows a simple cyst, it can be either closely observed or aspirated. For a palpable lesion that shows a solid component on ultrasonography, biopsy should be done, even in the presence of a normal mammogram. Current recommendations for screening magnetic resonance imaging (MRI) are confined to women at very high risk of breast cancer based on family history or prior exposure to radiation therapy (eg, upper mantle radiation for Hodgkin disease) and possibly for women with very dense breast tissue on mammography, because high breast density is an independent risk factor for breast cancer.

For women with newly diagnosed breast cancer, one-time MRI is also highly controversial. MRI in this setting has been shown to find additional lesions in both the ipsilateral and the contralateral breasts. Many of these lesions are benign but require biopsy, surgical resection, or close follow-up. There are no data that show MRI improves outcomes or decreases future risks. MRI in women with newly diagnosed breast cancer has been associated with a higher rate of mastectomy.

- Screening for breast cancer can reduce mortality.

- Women 50 years old should be screened with annual clinical breast examinations and mammography.

- Screening women aged 40–50 years is controversial.

Table 33.1 **RISK FACTORS FOR BREAST CANCER**

HIGH RISK: RELATIVE RISK >4.0	MODERATE RISK: RELATIVE RISK 2–4	LOW RISK: RELATIVE RISK 1–2
Older age	Any first-degree relative with breast cancer	Menarche before age 12 y
Personal history of breast cancer	Personal history of ovarian or endometrial cancer	Menopause after age 55 y
Family history of premenopausal bilateral breast cancer or familial cancer syndrome	Age at first full-term pregnancy >30 y	White race
Known *BRCA* mutation	Nulliparous	Moderate alcohol intake
Breast biopsy showing proliferative disease with atypia	Obesity in postmenopausal women	Long-duration (≥15 y) estrogen replacement therapy
Dense breast tissue on mammography	Upper socioeconomic class Prior history of radiation therapy (eg, Hodgkin disease or lymphoma)	

- Ten percent of breast cancers found on physical examination are missed by mammography.

- Ultrasonography is recommended for a suspicious palpable lump, even if mammography is negative.

- Biopsy should be done for lumps with a solid component on ultrasonography.

- MRI is recommended for women at very high risk for breast cancer and women with dense breast tissue on mammography, but it is controversial in women with newly diagnosed breast cancer.

PATHOLOGY

Breast cancer can be invasive or noninvasive (in situ). Ninety-five percent of breast cancers are classified as ductal (70%) or lobular (25%), corresponding to the ducts and lobules of the normal breast (Figure 33.1). Invasive (sometimes called infiltrating) breast cancer has the potential for systemic spread, as opposed to carcinoma in situ, which does not have metastatic potential because by definition it has not invaded through the basement membrane. Infiltrating ductal carcinoma is the most common histologic type (70% of breast cancers) of invasive breast cancer. Invasive lobular carcinoma makes up 25% of breast cancers, is more frequently multifocal and bilateral, and is less likely to be seen on mammography.

Ductal carcinoma in situ is noninvasive, does not have the potential for systemic spread, and is primarily treated with local therapy only, including resection with or without breast irradiation. However, if left untreated, ductal carcinoma in situ can progress to invasive disease. Lobular carcinoma in situ is not believed to be a precursor for invasive disease, but it is a marker for increased risk for future development of invasive carcinoma in the ipsilateral or contralateral breast. Use of the selective estrogen-receptor modulator tamoxifen after resection of estrogen-receptor–positive or progesterone-receptor–positive ductal carcinoma in situ is frequently considered. This drug does decrease the risk of a subsequent breast event (defined as either recurrent carcinoma in situ or development of an invasive breast cancer in the ipsilateral or contralateral breast) in the subsequent 10 years from 13% to 8%; however, there is no evidence of increased survival with use of tamoxifen and it is associated with a substantial potential for adverse effects.

- Infiltrating ductal carcinoma is the most common histologic type of breast cancer.

- Lobular disease is more frequently multifocal and bilateral.

- Ductal carcinoma in situ is noninvasive and does not have the potential for systemic spread.

- Use of tamoxifen after resection of estrogen-receptor–positive or progesterone-receptor–positive ductal carcinoma in situ is worth considering.

STAGING

The staging system of the American Joint Committee on Cancer is shown in Box 33.1.

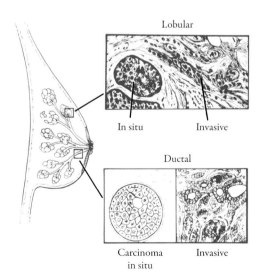

Figure 33.1 Breast Carcinomas: Ductal and Lobular, In Situ and Invasive.

Primary tumor (T)

TIS	Carcinoma in situ
T1	T = ≤2 cm
T2	T = 2.1–5 cm
T3	T = >5 cm
T4	T of any size with direct extension to chest wall or skin

Regional nodes (N)

N0	No involved nodes
N1	Movable ipsilateral axillary nodes
N2	Matted or fixed nodes, or in clinically apparent ipsilateral internal mammary nodes in the absence of clinically evident axillary lymph node metastasis
N3	Metastasis in ipsilateral infraclavicular lymph nodes

Distant metastasis (M)

M0	None detected
M1	Distant metastasis present (includes ipsilateral supraclavicular nodes)

Stage grouping

Stage I	T1 N0	
Stage IIA	T0 N1	
	T1 N1	
	T2 N0	= Operable disease
Stage IIB	T2 N1	
	T3 N0	
Stage IIIA	T0 N2	
	T1 N2	
	T2 N2	= Locally advanced disease
	T3 N1,N2	
Stage IIIB	T4, Any N	
Stage IIIC	Any T N3	= Advanced disease
Stage IV	Any T Any N M1	= Advanced or metastatic

Data from Singletary SE, Allred C, Ashley P, Bassett LW, Berry D, Bland KI, et al. Revision of the American Joint Committee on Cancer staging system for breast cancer. J Clin Oncol. 2002 Sep 1;20(17):3628–36.

NATURAL HISTORY AND PROGNOSTIC FACTORS

Nodal Status

The number of involved axillary lymph nodes is the most important predictor of outcome (Figure 33.2).

Tumor Size

After nodal status, tumor size is the most important prognostic factor (Table 33.2).

Hormone Receptor Status

In general, patients with estrogen-receptor–positive tumors have a better prognosis, especially in the first 5 to 10 years after initial diagnosis. However, the difference in recurrence rates at 5 years is only 8% to 10% when compared with receptor-negative disease. After 5 years, the recurrence rate

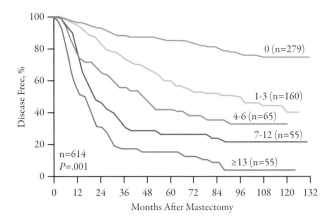

Figure 33.2 Relation of Disease-Free Survival to Numbers of Nodal Metastases. Data are for more than 600 women with breast cancer treated with radical mastectomy alone in the early 1970s. (From Fisher ER, Sass R, Fisher B. Pathologic findings from the National Surgical Adjuvant Project for Breast Cancers [protocol no. 4]. X. Discriminants for tenth year treatment failure. Cancer. 1984 Feb 1;53[3 Suppl]:712–23. Used with permission.)

for estrogen-receptor–positive disease is higher than that for estrogen-receptor–negative disease. Extent of hormone positivity may be very important in treatment outcome; patients with more than 90% of tumor cells staining positive for estrogen receptor respond very well to hormonal therapies and may be able to avoid adjuvant chemotherapy, whereas those whose tumors are weakly positive or negative for estrogen receptor may benefit from adjuvant chemotherapy.

HER2/neu

HER2/neu is a transmembrane protein that is overexpressed in approximately 20% to 30% of breast cancers. Without the use of anti-HER2/neu–directed therapy, tumors that are HER2/neu-positive are associated with a higher risk of recurrence and an overall worse prognosis. Women with HER2/neu-positive disease are usually recommended to receive adjuvant chemotherapy, even in the presence of otherwise good risk features (such as small tumor size and negative nodes). In addition, the

Table 33.2 LONG-TERM RESULTS[a] IN PATIENTS WITH NODE-NEGATIVE BREAST CANCER TREATED SURGICALLY

TUMOR SIZE, CM	NO. OF PATIENTS	% FREE OF RECURRENCE	% DEAD OF DISEASE
<1	171	88	10
1.1–2.0	303	74	24
2.1–3.0	188	72	24
3.1–5.0	105	61	36

[a] Median duration of follow-up was 18 years.

Data from Rosen PP, Groshen S, Kinne DW. Survival and prognostic factors in node-negative breast cancer: results of long-term follow-up studies. J Natl Cancer Inst Monogr. 1992;(11):159–62.

use of therapies directed against the HER2/neu pathway such as trastuzumab (Herceptin) greatly improve the prognosis. HER2/neu tumors also seem to have a significantly increased risk of recurrence within the central nervous system.

Triple-Negative Breast Cancer

A recently described subset of breast cancer is known as "triple negative," meaning that the cancer cells show no evidence of overexpression of estrogen receptors, progesterone receptors, or HER2/neu. Triple-negative tumors tend to have a better response to chemotherapy than other subtypes, yet they are associated with a poorer overall prognosis. Patients with triple-negative disease who show no evidence of recurrence after 5 years are at lower risk of late, distant recurrence.

Grade

Most breast cancers are high-grade. Patients with low-grade tumors have fewer recurrences and longer survivals.

- The number of involved axillary nodes is the most important predictor of outcome.

- After nodal status, tumor size is the most important prognostic factor.

- Patients with receptor-positive tumors have a better prognosis.

- Overexpression of HER2/neu confers a poorer prognosis if not treated with anti-HER2/neu therapies and alters recommendations for adjuvant therapy.

- All breast cancers should be tested for status of estrogen receptors, progesterone receptors, and HER2/neu.

- Patients with low-grade tumors have a better prognosis.

TREATMENT

Primary or Local-Regional Treatment

Primary local treatment for invasive breast cancer is either lumpectomy (also known as wide local excision or breast conservation) followed by radiation or mastectomy. Several randomized controlled clinical trials have shown therapeutic equivalence for breast conservation compared with mastectomy in terms of overall survival, whereas mastectomy has a slightly lower local recurrence rate. The outcome for women with invasive breast cancer depends more on the presence of distant microscopic metastatic disease rather than on the treatment of local disease. The most important predictor for the presence of micrometastatic disease is involvement of axillary lymph nodes. All women with invasive breast cancer should have axillary lymph node dissection or a newer procedure called a sentinel lymph node biopsy. If the sentinel lymph node shows histologic signs of cancer, then a complete axillary lymph node dissection should be considered based on features that predict for involvement of additional lymph nodes. If

the sentinel lymph node does not have metastatic tumor cells, then the probability of other lymph nodes being affected is less than 5%. When compared with axillary lymph node dissection, sentinel lymph node biopsy decreases late complications such as lymphedema.

- Breast conservation plus radiation is equivalent to mastectomy in terms of overall survival.

- Compared with axillary lymph node dissection, sentinel lymph node biopsy is associated with less risk of lymphedema.

Adjuvant Treatment

After primary treatment of the breast, additional systemic treatment (adjuvant) has been shown to decrease the risk of systemic recurrence and improve overall survival. The number of involved axillary lymph nodes is the single most important predictor of outcome. Women with metastatically involved axillary lymph nodes should generally be offered adjuvant treatment: chemotherapy or hormonal therapy or both. Women with negative lymph nodes have a 25% or less chance of microscopic metastatic disease. Adjuvant systemic treatment should generally be offered to women in the intermediate- and high-risk groups. Chemotherapy has been shown to decrease the risk of recurrence and improve overall survival in both node-negative and node-positive cancer, but it is associated with more toxicity than hormonal therapy. Women with node-negative tumors of more than 1 centimeter and with node-positive cancers that overexpress HER2/neu should also be offered adjuvant trastuzumab (Herceptin) therapy.

Long-term follow-up of women with breast cancer (especially hormone-receptor–positive disease) is essential because there are as many recurrences 5 to 15 years after diagnosis as there are in the first 5 years after diagnosis, and metastatic disease can first become apparent 30 or more years later.

- Women with node-positive disease are at high risk of systemic disease and should be offered adjuvant treatment.

- Women with node-negative disease have a 25% or less chance of systemic disease.

- Adjuvant therapy decisions should be individualized on the basis of each person's risk of recurrence.

Treatment of Advanced Disease

We currently lack curative therapy for recurrent metastatic breast cancer. The median duration of survival with recurrent disease is 2.5 years, but the spectrum of survival is very wide. Survival is generally longer with bone-only or soft tissue recurrence than with visceral recurrence. Because treatment is not curative, the initial systemic treatment for patients with estrogen-receptor–positive advanced disease is usually hormonal. Chemotherapy is used once disease has progressed in patients with hormone-receptor–positive disease while receiving hormonal therapy or in patients with estrogen-receptor–negative breast cancer.

- There is no curative therapy for recurrent metastatic breast cancer.

- The average survival with recurrent breast cancer is 2.5 years.

Chemotherapy

Several drugs are active against breast cancer. Notably, there is a very small, but real, increased risk for secondary leukemias in women receiving adjuvant chemotherapy, especially anthracycline-based chemotherapy, and this may be increased in women who also receive growth factors to accelerate leukocyte recovery.

Hormonal Treatment

Tamoxifen is a hormonal agent that is commonly used to treat breast cancer. On some tissues tamoxifen acts like an antiestrogen (breast tissue), but on other tissue it acts like an estrogen (bones, lipids, uterus). Its benefits include 1) antitumor effects on breast cancer cells, 2) decreased risk (by 40%) of contralateral breast cancer, 3) improved bone density, and 4) favorable effects on lipid profiles. Tamoxifen also has adverse effects, including 1) hot flashes, 2) thromboembolism (1%-2%), 3) increased risk of endometrial cancer, and 4) increased risk of cataracts. Women who are currently taking CYP2D6 inhibitors (such as paroxetine, cimetidine, citalopram) should ideally have these medications changed to eliminate drug interactions.

A newer class of hormonal agents, known as the aromatase inhibitors, is being used for treatment of breast cancer in postmenopausal women. These drugs show a slight superiority to tamoxifen in reducing the risk for recurrence of breast cancer, and they are not associated with an increased risk for thrombotic or endometrial events. The aromatase inhibitors do increase the risks for osteoporosis, arthralgias, and vaginal dryness and are more expensive than tamoxifen. These drugs are useful only in women in a postmenopausal state, and premenopausal women who undergo chemotherapy-induced amenorrhea should not routinely receive these drugs because they have the ability to cause resumption of menstrual cycles and increase native estrogen production.

- Tamoxifen has both antiestrogen and estrogen-like activity.

- Beneficial effects of tamoxifen are antitumor effects, increased bone density, improved lipid profile, and decreased risk of contralateral breast cancer.

- Adverse effects of tamoxifen are hot flashes, venous thromboembolism, and increased risk of endometrial cancer.

- Aromatase inhibitors are useful only for postmenopausal women.

- Aromatase inhibitors increase the risk of osteoporosis, severe arthralgias, and vaginal dryness, but they do not increase the risk of thromboembolism risk or endometrial cancer.

- Premenopausal women with hormonally sensitive disease may also benefit from oophorectomy (either chemical or surgical).

Other Agents

Herceptin

About 25% of breast cancers overexpress HER2/neu. A monoclonal antibody directed against HER2/neu (trastuzumab, Herceptin) has been shown to have activity against these cancers. In the adjuvant setting, use of trastuzumab therapy for 1 year has shown a roughly 50% decrease in the risk for breast cancer recurrence in women with HER2/neu-positive breast cancer.

Lapatinib

Lapatinib (Tykerb) is an oral agent that also interferes with the HER2/neu signaling pathway. As opposed to trastuzumab, which acts on the membrane-bound, extracellular domain of the HER2/neu pathway, lapatinib acts intracellularly and is effective in women with trastuzumab-refractory HER2/neu-positive breast cancer.

Zoledronic Acid (Zometa) and Pamidronate (Aredia).

The use of the bisphosphonates can reduce the need for palliative radiation, bone fixation, and pain medicine in women with lytic bone metastases. Some, but not all, recent data suggest that zoledronic acid may also lead to a decrease in the recurrence rate of breast cancer.

FOLLOW-UP AFTER CURATIVE THERAPY

After definitive therapy for breast cancer, patients are at risk for recurrence of their disease or development of a new primary lesion. Current recommendations for follow-up include annual mammography and history, review of systems, and physical examination every 6 months.

Routine follow-up blood tests, including tumor marker tests, liver function tests, or complete blood counts, and imaging studies such as chest radiography and bone scanning, have not been shown to be helpful in improving survival or outcomes and are not recommended. Testing should be done based on history and physical examination findings. MRI examination in patients with a prior history of breast cancer and physical examination and mammography have been shown to detect abnormalities in up to 25% of patients, and 1% of patients actually have a cancer or carcinoma in situ. There is no evidence that MRI leads to improved outcomes, and the associated very high false-positive rate does not justify routine MRI surveillance in breast cancer survivors.

Patients who have had treatment for breast cancer should be followed for late adverse effects of therapy. These include altered sexual function, osteoporosis, myelodysplastic syndrome, and late cardiac toxicity. Exercise and maintenance of ideal body weight, while not definitively proven to decrease cancer recurrence, should be recommended.

PATTERNS OF RECURRENCE

Breast cancer tends to recur in bones, liver, lungs, or brain or locally in the chest wall or residual breast. Recurrences can occur decades after initial diagnosis, and this possibility must always be kept in mind in any patient with a history of breast cancer. Hormone receptor–negative disease and HER2/neu-positive disease are more aggressive, and these both tend to recur earlier than hormone receptor–positive disease. Recent data suggest that women with HER2/neu-positive tumors who have treatment with trastuzumab (Herceptin) have a higher chance of recurrence in the central nervous system. Hormone receptor–positive disease is more indolent; only about 20% of recurrences happen within the first 5 years after initial diagnosis, and metastatic recurrences can occur decades later.

CERVICAL CANCER

BACKGROUND

In recent decades, the incidence of cervical cancer has decreased by 30% and mortality associated with cervical cancer has decreased by 40%. These changes have been attributed to widespread use of cytologic (Papanicolaou) smear screening. In US women each year, there are 12,200 new cases of cervical cancer and 4,100 associated deaths. In addition, more than 50,000 cases of carcinoma in situ of the cervix are diagnosed annually. Risk factors for cervical cancer include first intercourse at an early age, a greater number of sexual partners, smoking, history of sexually transmitted disease, especially herpesvirus or human papillomavirus, and lower socioeconomic class. It is now understood that human papillomavirus is an etiologic agent for cervical carcinogenesis.

If a Papanicolaou smear shows dysplasia or malignant cells, colposcopy with directed biopsy should be done. The Papanicolaou smear has limited sensitivity; false-negative rates of 20% frequently are quoted. The American Cancer Society recommends that asymptomatic, low-risk women 20 years of age or older and those younger than 20 years who are sexually active have a Papanicolaou smear annually for 2 consecutive years and, if the results are negative, at least 1 every 3 years.

TREATMENT

Treatment for carcinoma in situ of the cervix is usually total hysterectomy. If childbearing is desired, a more conservative approach, such as a therapeutic conization, is another option. Early invasive carcinoma of the cervix is usually treated with total hysterectomy. For patients with higher-stage disease, a combination of chemotherapy (cisplatin-based) and radiation therapy is recommended.

PREVENTION

The majority of cases of cervical cancer are associated with human papillomavirus. A recently approved vaccine (Gardasil) can provide protection against the 4 most common strains of the virus and has shown efficacy in decreasing the risk of cervical cancer. The American Cancer Society recommends this vaccine for all females before onset of sexual activity. In 2011, the US Food and Drug Administration approved use of this vaccine for males to help prevent spread of human papillomavirus and to prevent the relatively rare penile cancer. Other methods for prevention include decreasing high-risk behavior, such as limiting sexual partners and use of condoms.

COLORECTAL CANCER

BACKGROUND

Colorectal cancer is diagnosed in approximately 148,000 Americans and causes 57,000 deaths each year. Colorectal cancer is the second most common cause of cancer death in North America and Europe. The incidence of colorectal cancer has declined during the past few years, following its peak in the late 1990s. It is associated with high-fat, low-fiber diets. Decreased levels of physical activity and obesity are also associated with an increased risk of colorectal cancer. Population screening with fecal occult blood testing remains problematic. Although one study showed a reduction in mortality from colorectal cancer with fecal occult blood screening, any participants who had positive results went on to have colonoscopy. Another study showed that fecal occult blood tests failed to detect 70% of colorectal cancers and 80% of large (≥2 cm) polyps. Although specific screening recommendations vary, some form of screening should be initiated by age 50 years regardless of risk. For high-risk patients, such as those with a family history of colorectal cancer or a prior colorectal cancer, structural studies of the entire large bowel, such as colonoscopy (every 5–10 years) or (less preferable) rectosigmoidoscopy plus barium enema, should be performed at appropriate intervals (such as every 1–3 years).

- Colorectal cancer is associated with high-fat, low-fiber diets, decreased physical activity, and obesity.

- Although specific screening recommendations vary, some form of screening process should be initiated by age 50 years regardless of risk.

- For high-risk patients, the entire large bowel should be studied at appropriate intervals.

RISK FACTORS

Approximately 10% of colorectal cancer is related to either defined or as yet undefined familial syndromes. High-risk groups include persons with 1) familial polyposis syndromes (familial adenomatous polyposis—for which a gene recently was identified on chromosome 5—and Gardner syndrome—gut polyps plus desmoid tumors, lipomas, sebaceous cysts, and other abnormalities), accounting for 1% of colorectal cancer; 2) familial cancer syndromes without polyps (hereditary nonpolyposis colorectal cancer or Lynch syndrome, which are marked by colon cancer with or without endometrial, breast, and other cancers), accounting for 3% to 4% of colorectal cancer; and 3) inflammatory bowel disease (incidence, 12% after 25 years).

- High-risk factors for colorectal cancer are familial polyposis syndromes, including familial adenomatous polyposis and Gardner syndrome, both inherited as an autosomal dominant trait; select familial cancer syndromes without polyps; and inflammatory bowel disease.

TREATMENT

Surgery

Surgical resection is the preferred method of curative treatment for carcinomas of the colon or rectum for all but the very earliest cancers. Surgical exploration and resection allow for pathologic determination of tumor depth of penetration through the bowel wall and assessment of regional lymph nodes. Prognosis is directly related to the stage of disease (Table 33.3). Five-year survival rates for locoregional disease have improved in recent decades as a result of many factors, including improvements in preoperative staging, surgical technique, adequate lymph node retrieval, and the use of neoadjuvant (preoperative) and adjuvant (postoperative) therapy.

- Surgical resection is the preferred treatment for colorectal cancer.

- Prognosis is directly related to the stage of disease.

- Five-year survival rates are improving.

Adjuvant Therapy

For colon cancers, adjuvant chemotherapy with a multidrug regimen that includes oxaliplatin, 5-fluorouracil (5-FU), and leucovorin, given for 6 months, is recommended for node-positive (stage III) disease. Controversy exists about standard recommendations for deeply invasive but lymph-node negative (stage II) colon carcinomas. For rectal cancers, a combination of chemotherapy (5-FU–based) and pelvic irradiation, preferably administered preoperatively (neoadjuvant), is standard for stage II and III disease followed by adjuvant chemotherapy after surgery.

- For stage III colon cancers, adjuvant chemotherapy is indicated.

- For rectal cancer, a preoperative combination of chemotherapy and radiotherapy is the standard recommendation.

Metastatic Disease

Certain patients with metastatic colorectal cancer may be candidates for an attempt at curative resection of their metastatic disease. Of carefully selected patients with minimal metastatic disease, limited to the liver or lung, 30% to 40% survive beyond 5 years, many without further evidence of disease recurrence, after resection of metastatic lesions and systemic chemotherapy.

Palliative chemotherapy is the only option for the vast majority of patients with advanced metastatic colorectal cancer. The median duration of survival for patients given medical therapy is about 24 months.

- Surgical resection of metastatic disease can result in long-term disease-free survival in a select subset of patients.

- Palliative conventional chemotherapy is the only option for advanced colorectal carcinoma.

Carcinoembryonic Antigen

Until recently, routine monitoring of carcinoembryonic antigen (CEA) after curative resection of colon cancer was not recommended. Current American Society of Clinical Oncology guidelines do recommend that the CEA level be checked preoperatively if it would assist in staging and surgical planning. After curative treatment for colon cancer, the guidelines recommend that the CEA level be checked every

Table 33.3 **STAGING OF COLORECTAL CANCER AND SURVIVAL**

DUKES STAGE	AJCC STAGE	DEPTH OF PENETRATION	NODAL STATUS	5-YEAR SURVIVAL, %
A	I	Submucosa or muscularis	Negative	90
B	II	Through muscularis or to other organs	Negative	60–80
C	III	Any	Positive	30–60

Abbreviation: AJCC, American Joint Committee on Cancer.

3 months for at least 3 years in patients with stage II and III disease, as long as the patient's general medical condition is such that the patient would be a candidate for surgical intervention or chemotherapy. Monitoring of CEA may be useful for determining the response of metastatic disease to therapy.

LUNG CANCER

MAGNITUDE OF THE PROBLEM

Approximately 172,000 new cases of lung cancer are diagnosed in the United States annually, and approximately 157,000 deaths from lung cancer occur. Thus, only approximately 15% of patients with lung cancer survive the disease. Lung cancer is the leading cause of cancer mortality in both men and women.

RISK FACTORS

About 95% of lung cancers in men and about 80% of lung cancers in women result from cigarette smoking. Men who smoke 1 to 2 packs per day have up to a 25-fold increased risk for lung cancer compared with men who have never smoked. The risk for lung cancer in an ex-smoker declines with time. Passive smoking is associated with an increased risk of lung cancer. Certain occupations (eg, smelter and iron workers), chemicals (eg, arsenic and methylethyl ether), and exposure to radioactive agents and asbestos are associated with increased risks for lung cancer.

- 95% of lung cancers in men and 80% in women result from cigarette smoking.
- Men who smoke 1 to 2 packs a day have a 25-fold increased risk for lung cancer compared with men who have never smoked.
- Passive smoking is associated with an increased risk for lung cancer.

SCREENING

Several large, randomized trials have tested the utility of chest radiography and sputum cytology in screening for lung cancer. None of these studies have shown that either sputum cytology or regular chest radiography improves survival from lung cancer. Thus, such screening is not currently recommended. The National Lung Screening Trial has shown a survival advantage to screening high-risk smokers with low-dose computed tomography. This study, however, found a very large number of false-positive results for every case of lung cancer, which in turn resulted in additional tests with concern for overdiagnosis bias. Computed tomography screening for lung cancer remains controversial, and additional trial data are necessary to define the role for screening computed tomography.

HISTOLOGIC TYPES AND CHARACTERISTICS

Lung cancer is divided into small cell and non–small cell types. Small cell lung cancer occurs almost exclusively in smokers. The primary tumors are often small but are associated with bulky mediastinal adenopathy. They may be associated with paraneoplastic syndromes, including the syndrome of inappropriate secretion of antidiuretic hormone, and various neurologic abnormalities. Non–small cell lung cancers can be divided into squamous, adenocarcinoma, and large cell types. Squamous cell carcinomas may be associated with hypercalcemia due to the secretion of a parathyroid hormone-like peptide. Squamous carcinomas tend to occur centrally, whereas large cell and adenocarcinoma types tend to be more peripheral. Adenocarcinoma is the most frequent histologic subtype in nonsmokers. Bronchoalveolar carcinoma is a low-grade non–small cell carcinoma that frequently presents as a patchy infiltrate. It may be multifocal.

STAGING

The classic Tumor-Node-Metastasis (TNM) system is simplified in Table 33.4.

NATURAL HISTORY

The natural history of surgically treated lung cancer, by stage, is shown in Figure 33.3.

TREATMENT

Non–Small Cell Lung Cancer

Resection is the treatment of choice for clinical stages I, II, and selected IIIA non–small cell lung cancer. The use of adjuvant chemotherapy has been shown to improve survival by 10% to 12% compared with operation alone. The use of adjuvant

Table 33.4 **STAGING OF LUNG CANCER**

NON–SMALL CELL TYPE	
Stage I	Primary tumor >2 cm from carina; node negative
Stage II	Primary tumor >2 cm from carina; hilar nodes positive
Stage IIIA	Tumor <2 cm from carina, or invading a resectable structure, or ipsilateral mediastinal nodes positive
Stage IIIB	Tumor invading an unresectable structure, supraclavicular or contralateral mediastinal nodes positive or cytologically positive pleural effusion
Stage IV	Metastatic disease
SMALL CELL TYPE	
Limited	Limited to 1 hemithorax less supraclavicular lymph nodes. Can be encompassed within a tolerable radiation port
Extensive	All other disease (metastatic disease)

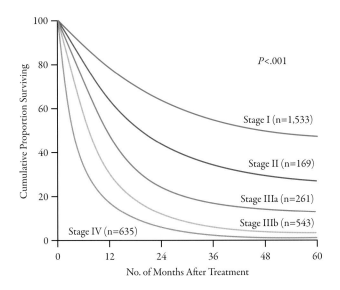

Figure 33.3 Survival Curves for Patients With Lung Cancer by Stage. (From Mountain CF. A new international staging system for lung cancer. Chest. 1986 Apr;89[4 Suppl]:225S–33S. Used with permission.)

radiation does not improve survival in resected stage II and III disease, but it is able to decrease the likelihood of local recurrence. In patients with locally advanced unresectable non–small cell lung cancer, the use of concurrent chemotherapy and radiation improves long-term survival compared with radiation alone. Although patients with metastatic disease are not cured, studies have shown that the use of chemotherapy improves overall survival by several weeks and quality of life compared with best supportive care. These studies, however, are hampered by lack of uniform definitions of what constitutes best supportive care.

- Operation is the treatment of choice for stages I and II and selected IIIA non–small cell lung cancer.

- There is some improvement in survival with adjuvant chemotherapy.

- Chemotherapy is not curative for metastatic non–small cell lung cancer.

- Chemotherapy improves overall survival by several weeks and may improve quality of life for patients with metastatic non–small cell lung cancer.

Small Cell Lung Cancer

Treatment of limited-stage small cell lung cancer consists of both chemotherapy and chest radiation. Surgical resection has not been shown to improve survival. For patients who have a complete response to chemotherapy and chest radiation therapy, prophylactic cranial irradiation is used to decrease the frequency of recurrence in the central nervous system, although there is controversy about whether this treatment improves overall survival. Prophylactic cranial irradiation is associated with risk for delayed leukoencephalopathy, but this risk can be reduced by the administration of radiation in

small-dose fractions without concomitant chemotherapy. For limited-stage small cell disease, the median duration of survival is approximately 18 months; 30% to 40% of patients survive 2 years, and 10% to 20% survive 5 years.

- For small cell lung cancer, treatment of limited-stage disease consists of both chemotherapy and chest radiation.

- Prophylactic cranial irradiation decreases the frequency of recurrence in the central nervous system.

- Median survival is 18 months with limited-stage disease.

Chemotherapy is used for extensive-stage (stage IV) small cell lung cancer. Combination chemotherapy is favored over single-agent therapy. Active drugs include etoposide, cisplatin, cyclophosphamide, doxorubicin, and vincristine. High-dose chemotherapy with or without autologous bone marrow transplant or marrow colony-stimulating factors has not yet been proved superior to standard chemotherapy. The median duration of survival is approximately 9 months; about 10% of patients survive 2 years, and 1% or fewer survive 5 years.

- For extensive-stage small cell lung cancer, treatment is chemotherapy.

- High-dose chemotherapy has not yet been proved superior to standard chemotherapy.

- Median survival for patients with extensive-stage small cell lung cancer is 9 months.

OVARIAN CANCER

Ovarian cancer is diagnosed in 25,400 American women annually. It is the leading cause of death due to gynecologic cancer, resulting in 14,300 deaths annually. There are no early warning signs; most patients present with vague gastrointestinal complaints such as bloating, nausea, constipation, voiding problems, and pain. Most patients (75%) present with advanced disease (ie, stages III and IV, disease spread beyond the pelvis). The term *ovarian cancer* refers to tumors derived from the ovarian surface epithelium, not germ cell tumors.

- Ovarian cancer is the leading cause of death due to gynecologic cancer.

- There are no early warning signs.

- Most patients (75%) present with advanced disease.

STAGING

Stage I is confined to the ovary, stage II is confined to the pelvis, stage III includes spread to the upper abdomen, and stage IV includes spread to distant sites.

CANCER ANTIGEN 125

Cancer antigen 125 (CA 125) is expressed by approximately 85% of epithelial ovarian tumors and released into the circulation. However, it is detectable in only 50% of patients with stage I disease. The highest serum levels of CA 125 are found in patients with ovarian cancer, but the serum CA 125 level also may be increased in other malignancies and in pregnancy, endometriosis, and menstruation. Measurement of CA 125 for monitoring the course of ovarian cancer is currently controversial. There is no clear role for CA 125 for screening purposes.

- CA 125 is expressed by about 85% of epithelial ovarian tumors.
- The CA 125 level also may be increased in other malignancies and in pregnancy, endometriosis, and menstruation.

SCREENING

Pelvic ultrasonography and serum CA 125 testing are inadequate for screening for ovarian cancer in the general female population. Screening for ovarian cancer is difficult for several reasons. The incidence of the disease is low, and there are no recognized pre-invasive lesions. Moreover, pelvic ultrasonography and CA 125 testing lack sufficient sensitivity and specificity. The cause of epithelial ovarian cancer is unknown. A small subset of patients (<5%) has an inherited predisposition to this disease. Generally, this predisposition occurs in families with both breast and ovarian cancer.

- Population screening for ovarian cancer is not recommended.
- Pelvic ultrasonography and CA 125 testing lack sufficient sensitivity and specificity to be routinely recommended for screening.

TREATMENT

The initial management of patients with epithelial ovarian cancer includes a thorough surgical staging and debulking procedure. Outcome in this disease depends on the amount of tumor tissue remaining after initial operation. Patients with only microscopic residual disease fare better than those with less than optimally debulked tumors. Subsequently, patients receive chemotherapy.

- Management of ovarian cancer includes thorough surgical staging and debulking followed by chemotherapy, both systemic and intraperitoneal.
- The outcome depends on the amount of tumor tissue remaining after initial operation.

OUTCOME

Outcome depends on the stage of disease. At 5 years, 90% of patients with stage I disease are alive and 80% of those with stage II disease are alive. Unfortunately, survival with advanced disease is poor: 15% to 20% of patients with stage III disease are alive at 5 years and only 5% of patients with stage IV disease are alive.

PROSTATE CANCER

BACKGROUND

There are approximately 186,000 new cases of prostate cancer annually in the United States. It is the most common cancer in US men and is the second leading cause of death from cancer in US men (29,000 deaths annually). Risk factors for prostate cancer include older age, race (African American), family history (first-degree relative), and possibly dietary fat. The American Cancer Society recommends a digital rectal examination in men 40 years or older and determination of the prostate-specific antigen (PSA) value in men 50 years or older. Use of PSA for prostate cancer screening is controversial and has not been shown to reduce mortality. Screening in older men should be discontinued when they have a life expectancy of less than 10 years due to age or other comorbidities.

- Prostate cancer is the most common cancer and the second leading cause of death from cancer in US men.
- Risk factors for prostate cancer include older age, race (African American), family history, and a high-fat diet.
- Screening should be stopped when advanced age or comorbid conditions suggest a life expectancy of <10 years.

PROSTATE-SPECIFIC ANTIGEN

PSA is produced by normal and neoplastic prostatic ductal epithelium. Its concentration is proportional to the total prostatic mass. The inability to differentiate benign prostatic hyperplasia from carcinoma on the basis of the PSA level renders it inadequate as the sole screening method for prostate cancer. PSA is useful for monitoring response to therapy in cases of known prostate cancer, particularly after radical prostatectomy, when PSA should be undetectable.

- The concentration of PSA is proportional to the total prostatic mass.
- The PSA test is inadequate as the sole screening test for prostate cancer.
- PSA is useful for monitoring response to therapy.

Prognostic factors for prostate cancer include stage of disease, grade of tumor, and pretreatment PSA level. Table 33.5 simplifies the staging of prostate cancer, including the TNM classification. The Gleason scoring system is used for pathologic grading of tumors. The surgical specimen is graded by the most predominant pattern of differentiation added to the secondary architectural pattern (eg, 3+5=8). Gleason grades 2 through 6 are associated with a better prognosis. Retrospective results indicate that the pretreatment PSA value is a strong predictor of disease outcome after operation or radiotherapy.

Table 33.5 STAGING OF PROSTATE CANCER

WHITMORE	TNM[a]	CRITERIA
A1	T1A	Incidental focus of tumor in ≤5% of resected tissue
A2	T1B	Incidental tumor in >5% of resected tissue
B0	T1C	Tumor identified by needle biopsy (performed on basis of increased PSA value)
B1	T2A	Tumor ≤1/2 of 1 lobe
B2	T2B	Tumor >1/2 of 1 lobe but not both lobes
	T2C	Tumor involvement of both lobes
C	T3 or T4	Extracapsular local disease or local invasion
D1	N1	Pelvic node involvement
D2	M1	Distant disease

Abbreviation: PSA, prostate-specific antigen.

[a] *Tumor-Node-Metastasis system.*

- Prognostic factors for the outcome of prostate cancer include tumor stage, grade, and pretreatment PSA value.

- Gleason grades 2 through 6 have a better prognosis.

MANAGEMENT

Management of Specific Stages

Considerable controversy surrounds the primary treatment of prostate cancer in nearly all stages of the disease. Because this is a disease of older men, comorbid conditions, age, and performance status need to be considered when selecting a therapy because more men will die *with* prostate cancer than *of* prostate cancer. In general, patients with T1A prostate tumors are observed without treatment. For organ-confined prostate cancer (T1B, T1C, and T2 tumors), both radiation therapy and radical prostatectomy are equally viable options. For stage C (T3 or T4) disease (locally advanced), radiotherapy is generally used. For stage D1 disease (positive pelvic nodes), the management is controversial. Divergent approaches include androgen deprivation alone, x-ray therapy with or without androgen deprivation, close observation with androgen deprivation at progression, or, infrequently, prostatectomy with androgen deprivation.

Prostatectomy

Prostatectomy is reserved for patients with localized disease. The 15-year disease-specific survival rate after prostatectomy is 85% to 90% for stage A2 or B disease. Nerve-sparing prostatectomy is able to spare potency in 68% to 86% of patients. Risk for impotency increases with increasing age, size of tumor, extent of spread, and preoperative sexual function. Total urinary incontinence is rare (<2% of patients), although many men have some degree of incontinence after prostatectomy.

- Prostatectomy is used for localized disease.

- The 15-year survival rate is 85%-90% for stage A2 or B disease.

- Nerve sparing operations preserve sexual function in a majority of men.

Radiation Therapy

External beam radiotherapy is considered the equivalent of prostatectomy for overall survival. It is preferred for stage C disease at most centers. Impotence can occur, but less often than with prostatectomy. Chronic radiation proctitis is not uncommon.

Patients with organ-confined prostate cancer may also be candidates for brachytherapy. In this procedure, hundreds of radioactive seeds are placed in the prostate gland through a transrectal approach. This treatment works as well as external beam radiation therapy in appropriately selected patients, is less likely to cause radiation proctitis or impotence, but is less likely to adequately treat patients with extraprostatic spread of disease. Brachytherapy also requires fewer treatments and thus is often attractive to patients who live a long distance from the radiation center.

- External beam radiotherapy is considered the equivalent of prostatectomy for overall survival.

- Impotence is less frequent with radiotherapy than prostatectomy.

Androgen Deprivation

For advanced (D2) disease, bone is the most frequent site of metastatic disease. Although hormonal therapy is effective and produces a response in most patients, it is noncurative. The average duration of response to initial hormonal therapy is 18 months. The average duration of survival is 2 to 3 years after diagnosis of symptomatic metastatic disease, but many patients live for years with metastatic prostate cancer.

- Bone is the most frequent site of metastatic disease from the prostate.

- Hormonal therapy is effective and produces PSA response, but it is noncurative and is associated with considerable adverse effects.

- The average duration of survival with advanced prostatic cancer is 2–3 years.

The 2 sources of androgens in men are the testes (testosterone, 95%) and adrenal glands (5%). Androgen deprivation can be accomplished surgically with orchiectomy or medically. Potential agents include luteinizing hormone-releasing hormone agonists such as leuprolide, buserelin, and goserelin. They decrease androgen levels through continuous binding of the luteinizing hormone-releasing hormone receptor and subsequent decrease of luteinizing hormone and thus testosterone. They are administered as a depot injection once monthly. Androgen deprivation therapy, although typically well tolerated, is associated with considerable adverse effects, including decreased libido, impotence, gynecomastia, osteoporosis, and an increased risk of myocardial infarction.

- Androgen deprivation is accomplished with orchiectomy or medically.
- Luteinizing hormone-releasing hormone agonists decrease androgen levels.

Chemotherapy

Prostate cancer had previously been considered refractory to most chemotherapy regimens. Newer combinations using docetaxel (Taxotere) and prednisone have shown not only considerable responses but also improved survival in men with metastatic, hormone-refractory prostate cancer.

Bisphosphonates

The use of bisphosphonates in men with prostate cancer metastatic to bone remains controversial and does not improve overall survival. Bisphosphonates, however, can be a useful adjunct for treatment of painful metastases.

- Chemotherapy and bisphosphonates can be used for palliative effects in men with prostate cancer.

FOLLOW-UP RECOMMENDATIONS

After curative therapy for prostate cancer (ie, prostatectomy or radiation), the PSA level can be used as a marker for recurrence. PSA should be undetectable after successful primary surgical therapy, but some level will persist after radiation treatment. After definitive local therapy, the median time between increased PSA level (biochemical recurrence) and development of symptoms from metastatic prostate cancer in patients receiving no ongoing therapy is 8 years, and median time to death from recurrent prostate cancer is 13 years. Thus, how closely any individual patient is monitored depends on overall health, comorbid conditions, and overall life expectancy.

- After curative treatment of prostate cancer, the median time from biochemical recurrence of prostate cancer to first symptom from metastatic disease is 8 years and the median time to death from prostate cancer is 13 years.

TESTICULAR CANCER

BACKGROUND

This cancer is diagnosed in 7,600 men annually. It is the most common carcinoma in males 15 to 35 years old. It is highly curable, even when metastatic. At high risk are males with cryptorchid testes (40-fold relative risk) and Klinefelter syndrome (also increased risk of breast cancer). The 2 broad

categories of testicular cancer are seminomas (40%) and nonseminomas. Types of nonseminomas include embryonal carcinoma, mature and immature teratoma, choriocarcinoma, yolk sac tumor, and endodermal sinus tumor. There is often an admixture of several cell types within nonseminomas. Any nonseminomatous component plus seminoma is treated as a nonseminoma.

- Testicular cancer is the most common carcinoma in males 15–35 years old.
- Testicular cancer is highly curable, even when metastatic.
- High-risk factors for testicular cancer are cryptorchid testes and Klinefelter syndrome.
- The 2 broad categories of testicular cancer are seminomas (40%) and nonseminomas.

Evaluation includes determination of β-human chorionic gonadotropin and α-fetoprotein values and computed tomography of the abdomen (retroperitoneal nodes) and chest (mediastinal nodes or pulmonary nodules).

STAGING

Stage I disease is confined to the testis, stage II includes infradiaphragmatic nodal metastases, and stage III is spread beyond retroperitoneal nodes. About 85% of nonseminomas are associated with an increased β-human chorionic gonadotropin or α-fetoprotein value. Approximately 10% of seminomas are associated with an increased β-human chorionic gonadotropin level. The α-fetoprotein value is never increased in pure seminoma; if it is increased, the tumor is nonseminoma and should be treated as such.

- 85% of nonseminomas are associated with an increased β-human chorionic gonadotropin or α-fetoprotein value.
- 10% of seminomas are associated with an increased β-human chorionic gonadotropin value.
- The α-fetoprotein value is never increased in pure seminoma.

MANAGEMENT

Radical inguinal orchiectomy is the definitive procedure for both pathologic diagnosis and local control. Scrotal orchiectomy or biopsy is associated with a high incidence of local recurrence or spread to inguinal nodes.

- Radical inguinal orchiectomy is the definitive initial procedure for testicular cancer.

HEAD AND NECK MALIGNANCY

DIAGNOSIS

The most common head and neck cancer is squamous cell carcinoma. Head and neck squamous cell carcinoma can occur in the nasopharynx, oropharynx, larynx or hypopharynx, oral cavity, and sinuses. Uncommon cancers of the head and neck include salivary gland cancers, esthesioneuroblastoma, melanoma, lymphoma, sarcoma, and paraganglioma. Symptoms at presentation are related to the head and neck and can include throat pain, ear pain, hoarseness, trouble swallowing, and enlarged lymph nodes.

RISK FACTORS

Traditional risk factors for the development of head and neck squamous cell carcinoma include tobacco abuse, alcohol use, and chewing betel nuts. Nasopharyngeal cancer is often associated with Epstein-Barr virus. Recently, human papillomavirus has been implicated in oropharynx and oral cavity squamous cell carcinoma in nonsmokers. Human papillomavirus–related tumors have a better prognosis than smoking- and alcohol-related tumors.

SCREENING

There are no published guidelines on screening for head and neck malignancy. Patients at increased risk should have a thorough head and neck examination, including palpation for masses in the mouth and tongue. Palpation for enlarged cervical lymph nodes should also be done.

TREATMENT AND FOLLOW-UP

Treatment of head and neck cancers includes surgical resection and organ preservation with chemotherapy and radiation. Recurrence can be local or distant and generally occurs within 5 years. However, follow-up by the patient's oncologist or otorhinolaryngologist should be lifelong. Patients with one head and neck cancer have a 25% chance for development of a second head and neck cancer due to a field cancerization effect. Late adverse effects from treatment include skin fibrosis, decreased neck range of motion, lymphedema, xerostomia, dental problems, and swallowing difficulties.

- The most common head and neck cancer is squamous cell carcinoma.

- Human papillomavirus has been implicated in oropharynx and oral cavity squamous cell carcinoma in nonsmokers.

- Recurrence can be local or distant and generally occurs within 5 years.

CARCINOMA OF UNKNOWN PRIMARY ORIGIN

BACKGROUND

Patients presenting with metastatic carcinoma with an unknown primary lesion make up 5% to 10% of general oncologic practice. The first principle of management is to establish the diagnosis with a sufficient histologic specimen. In general,

open biopsy is preferable to fine-needle aspiration, because a larger specimen allows optimal histologic and immunohistochemical analysis. All patients should have a careful history and complete physical examination, including pelvic and rectal examinations. Most patients, approximately 60%, have an adenocarcinoma. In 35% of patients, poorly differentiated carcinoma is diagnosed. Once a pathologic diagnosis is established, additional evaluation should be tailored according to the patient's risk factors (eg, smoking, breast cancer risk), symptoms and signs, sites of metastasis, and the histologic diagnosis. Special consideration should be given to rule out possible curable malignancies such as germ cell tumors or lymphoma or treatable malignancies such as breast, ovarian, or prostate cancer. Women presenting with axillary adenocarcinomas, with no clear breast primary lesion, should receive treatment for breast cancer. Women with peritoneal carcinomatosis generally have exploratory laparotomy with surgical cytoreduction, as for ovarian carcinoma. Men presenting with bone metastases, particularly osteoblastic metastases, should have a PSA test and their tumor material stained for PSA expression.

TREATMENT

If a potentially treatable neoplasm is ruled out, most patients with metastatic cancer of an unknown primary lesion have a very poor prognosis, with expected survival of 4 to 6 months. Some may benefit from palliative treatment (radiation or chemotherapy); many are managed best with supportive care and hospice care.

PARANEOPLASTIC SYNDROMES

BACKGROUND

These conditions are the effects of a cancer occurring at a distance from the tumor; they are called remote effects. They do not necessarily indicate metastatic disease. Common paraneoplastic syndromes and associated tumor types are listed in Table 33.6.

CARCINOID SYNDROME

This is caused by peptide mediators secreted by carcinoid tumors that most frequently arise in the small intestine and that may have metastasized to the liver. It is less frequent with primary carcinoid tumors arising from other sites such as lung, thymus, or ovary. The most common symptoms are episodic flushing and diarrhea; bronchospasm may occur. Flushing and diarrhea may occur spontaneously or be precipitated by emotional factors or ingestion of food or alcohol. Carcinoid heart disease (right-sided valvular disease) is a potential late complication.

LAMBERT-EATON SYNDROME

This consists of muscle weakness (proximal) and gait disturbance. Strength is increased with exercise. It is associated with small cell lung cancer.

Table 33.6 CLASSIFICATION OF PARANEOPLASTIC SYNDROMES

SYNDROME	MEDIATOR	TUMOR TYPE
Endocrine		
Cushing syndrome[a]	ACTH	Small cell lung cancer
SIADH[a]	ADH	Lung, especially small cell
Hypercalcemia[a]	PTH-like peptide	Lung, especially squamous; breast; myeloma
Carcinoid syndrome	? Serotonin	Gut neuroendocrine tumors
	? Subtance P	
Hypoglycemia	Insulin	Gut neuroendocrine tumors; other
	Insulin-like growth factors	
Neuromuscular		
Cerebellar degeneration	Anti-Purkinje cell antibodies	Lung, especially small cell; ovarian; breast
Dementia	?	Lung
Peripheral neuropathy[a]	Autoantibodies	Lung, gastrointestinal, breast
Lambert-Eaton	Antibodies to cholinergic receptor	Small cell lung cancer
Dermatomyositis	?	Lung, breast
Skin		
Dermatomyositis	?	Lung, breast
Acanthosis nigricans	? TGF-α	Intra-abdominal cancer, usually gastric
Hematologic		
Venous thrombosis[a]	Activators of clotting cascade & platelets	Various adenocarcinomas, especially pancreatic & gastric
Nonbacterial thrombotic endocarditis	Activators of clotting cascade & platelets	Various adenocarcinomas, especially pancreatic & gastric

Abbreviations: ACTH, adrenocorticotropic hormone; ADH, antidiuretic hormone; PTH, parathyroid hormone; SIADH, syndrome of inappropriate secretion of antidiuretic hormone; TGF-α, transforming growth factor-α

[a] Most common types.

DERMATOMYOSITIS

The female to male ratio is 2:1. Findings include muscle weakness (proximal), inflammatory myopathy, and increased creatine kinase values. Skin changes are variable and include heliotrope rash, periorbital edema, and Gottron papules. An underlying malignancy (lung, breast, gastrointestinal) is common in patients older than 50 years.

ONCOLOGIC COMPLICATIONS AND EMERGENCIES

HYPERCALCEMIA

The most common causes of hypercalcemia are malignancies and primary hyperparathyroidism. Patients with primary hyperparathyroidism have increased serum parathyroid hormone (PTH) values, but PTH is usually suppressed in cancer-associated hypercalcemia. Cancer-related hypercalcemia is often mediated by the tumor secreting a PTH-related protein (PTHrP), which can be measured with current assays. Local osteolytic effects by tumors within bone can cause hypercalcemia in metastatic breast cancer and multiple myeloma, but only rarely in prostate cancer metastases. Tumors can also cause hypercalcemia by secreting other bone-resorbing substances or by enhancing conversion of 25-hydroxyvitamin D to 1,25-dihydroxyvitamin D, a mechanism closely associated with lymphomas.

Effects on bone and kidney contribute to hypercalcemia. Accelerated bone resorption is due to activation of osteoclasts by various mediators, primarily the PTHrP. The same factors that induce osteoclast-mediated bone resorption also stimulate renal tubular resorption of calcium. The hypercalcemic state interferes with renal resorption of sodium and water, leading to polyuria and eventual depletion of extracellular fluid volume. This reduces the glomerular filtration rate, further increasing the serum calcium level. Immobilization tips the balance toward bone resorption, worsening the hypercalcemia.

- PTH is usually suppressed in cancer-associated hypercalcemia.

- Malignancy-associated hypercalcemia is often mediated by PTHrP secreted by a tumor.

- Bone and kidney pathophysiologic effects lead to an increased calcium level.

Symptoms and signs of hypercalcemia include gastrointestinal (anorexia, nausea, vomiting, constipation), renal (polyuria, polydipsia, dehydration), central nervous system (cognitive difficulties, apathy, somnolence, or even coma), and cardiovascular (hypertension, shortened QT interval, arrhythmia, enhanced sensitivity to digitalis).

Cancers associated with hypercalcemia include squamous cell carcinomas of the lung and head and neck, breast cancer, renal cell carcinoma, multiple myeloma, and lymphoma. Breast cancer and myeloma patients are the most likely to have bony involvement with their disease.

The magnitude of the hypercalcemia and the degree of symptoms are key considerations for the treatment of hypercalcemia. Generally, patients with a serum calcium value more than 14 mg/dL, mental status changes, or an inability to maintain adequate hydration should be hospitalized for immediate treatment. However, there is no absolute value of serum calcium at which all patients become symptomatic, and relatively high levels may be well tolerated if the rate of increase has been gradual. The serum calcium value should be adjusted if the serum albumin value is abnormal. The conversion formula is 0.8 mg/dL of serum total calcium for every 1 g of serum albumin more or less than 4 g/dL. If the serum albumin value is increased (as with dehydration), the total calcium value should be adjusted downward; if the serum albumin value is reduced (as in chronic illness), the total calcium value should be adjusted upward.

Patients with clinically symptomatic hypercalcemia are almost always intravascularly volume-depleted. Initial therapy therefore includes vigorous hydration with intravenously administered normal saline (up to 500 mL/h if heart function is normal). Loop diuretics are not used until after intravascular volume expansion has been completed. Furosemide facilitates urinary excretion of calcium by inhibiting calcium resorption in the thick ascending loop of Henle. Thiazide diuretics should be avoided because they can worsen hypercalcemia.

Intravenous bisphosphonates (pamidronate or zoledronic acid) are helpful in the treatment of hypercalcemia of malignancy. Oral agents should be avoided because gastrointestinal absorption is poor. Bisphosphonates bind to hydroxyapatite and inhibit osteoclasts. In addition to fluids, bisphosphonates have become the mainstay of treatment for hypercalcemia. They must be used cautiously and infused over longer periods in the setting of renal failure.

Calcitonin is given subcutaneously or intramuscularly; it is not effective at reducing calcium in its intranasal form. It has a rapid onset of action, often lowering calcium within 12 to 24 hours; thus, it is useful in immediate life-threatening situations. However, calcitonin is a relatively weak agent with short-lived effect, and it should not be used as a single agent due to rebound hypercalcemia. Salmon-derived calcitonin is associated with a risk of hypersensitivity reaction, and epinephrine should be given for any allergic sequelae beyond flushing. However, anaphylaxis is so rare that a test dose is no longer recommended.

Glucocorticoids are useful in hypercalcemia associated with calcitriol production by hematologic malignancies and can have a direct antitumor effect on neoplastic lymphoid tissue. Calcium-free hemodialysis may be the fastest and least hazardous method of correcting hypercalcemia in patients with diminished kidney function. Dialysis also allows calcium-lowering in the setting of congestive heart failure or other conditions that prevent high-volume fluid infusion.

- In patients with hypercalcemia, volume expansion must precede administration of furosemide.
- Furosemide inhibits calcium resorption in the thick ascending loop of Henle.
- Bisphosphonates bind to hydroxyapatite and inhibit osteoclasts.

- Calcitonin is a relatively weak agent with a rapid, short-lived effect.
- Dialysis should be considered in hypercalcemia associated with renal failure, especially if the creatinine value is more than 3.0 mg/dL.

TUMOR LYSIS SYNDROME

This syndrome occurs as a result of the overwhelming release of tumor cell contents into the bloodstream such that concentrations of certain substances become life-threatening. It most commonly occurs in cancers with large tumor burdens and high proliferation rates that are exquisitely sensitive to chemotherapy. Tumor lysis syndrome can rarely occur spontaneously before antitumor therapy begins. Examples include high-grade lymphomas, leukemia, and, much less commonly, solid tumors (small cell lung cancer, anaplastic thyroid cancer, and germ cell tumors). The syndrome is characterized by an increased uric acid value, which leads to renal complications; acidosis; an increased potassium value, which can cause lethal cardiac arrhythmias; an increased phosphate value, which leads to acute renal failure; and a decreased calcium value, which causes muscle cramps, cardiac arrhythmias, and tetany. The syndrome can be prevented with adequate hydration, alkalinization, and administration of allopurinol before chemotherapy. Allopurinol does not lower uric acid levels that are already increased, and severe hyperuricemia can be treated with rasburicase.

- Tumor lysis syndrome is a result of the overwhelming release of tumor cell contents into the bloodstream.
- It is most common in cancers with large tumor burdens and high proliferation rates that are exquisitely sensitive to chemotherapy.
- It is characterized by increased uric acid, potassium, and phosphate values, acidosis, and decreased calcium value.

FEBRILE NEUTROPENIA

This condition is defined as a temperature of 38.3°C or more on 1 occasion or 2 episodes of 38°C at least 1 hour apart and an absolute neutrophil count of 500×10^9/L or less (or $<1{,}000 \times 10^9$/L with a predicted decline to <500 within 48 hours). The risk of neutropenia is dependent on the type and dose of chemotherapy administered. Although a source of infection is identified in a minority of patients, at least 2 sets of peripheral blood samples for culture should be drawn in each patient with neutropenic fever, preferably before antibiotics are given. In addition, at least 1 culture should be drawn through each lumen of a multiple-port vascular catheter to determine whether the infection is device-related.

Although management of febrile neutropenia generally involves hospitalization and institution of parenteral broad-spectrum antibiotics, recent extensive clinical experience and multiple randomized clinical trials have shown the safety and efficacy of outpatient therapy for select patients.

Table 33.7 MEDICAL AND SOCIAL CONTRAINDICATIONS TO OUTPATIENT TREATMENT OF FEBRILE NEUTROPENIA

Medical contraindications
  Anticipated duration of neutropenia of >7 d (typically patients with leukemia or lymphoma)
  Absolute neutrophil count <100/10^9 per L
  Comorbid medical conditions
    Hypertension (systolic blood pressure <90 mm Hg)
    Hypoxia or tachypnea (respiratory rate >30 breaths/min)
    Altered mental status
    Renal insufficiency (creatinine >2.5 mg/dL)
    Hyponatremia (sodium <124 mg/dL)
    Bleeding
    Dehydration
    Poor oral intake
Social contraindications
  History of noncompliance or being unreliable with prior medical therapy follow-up
  Geographically remote (>30 miles from 24-h emergency medical care)
  Unable to care for self & lack of reliable caregiver
  No telephone
  No transportation

All patients need to be evaluated by a physician for both medical and social contraindications to outpatient treatment (Table 33.7). Patients who have no contraindication to outpatient treatment should receive oral amoxicillin/clavulanate (Augmentin) 875 mg twice daily and oral ciprofloxacin 500 mg every 8 hours. All patients should be reevaluated within 24 hours either by telephone contact or in person.

For inpatient management of febrile neutropenia, monotherapy is acceptable only with a sufficiently broad-spectrum agent such as the fourth-generation cephalosporins (eg, cefepime), a carbapenem, or piperacillin-tazobactam, all of which offer anti-pseudomonal activity. Vancomycin can be added for skin and soft tissue infections, pneumonia, or suspicion of an infected device, but it should not be used as monotherapy.

Multiple randomized, placebo-controlled clinical trials have shown that the use of colony-stimulating factors at the time of febrile neutropenia is not indicated, although these factors can be used prophylactically more than 24 hours after chemotherapy has been completed.

- Not all patients with febrile neutropenia need to be admitted to the hospital.

- Growth factors should not be used once neutropenia has developed.

- Growth factors may prevent the development of febrile neutropenia, but they must be used more than 24 hours after the chemotherapy.

SPINAL CORD COMPRESSION

Acute spinal cord compression is a neurologic emergency. It results most commonly from epidural extension of vertebral body metastases. The most common tumors include lung,

Table 33.8 REFLEXES AND THEIR CORRESPONDING ROOTS AND MUSCLES

REFLEX	ROOT(S)	MUSCLE
Biceps	C5–6	Biceps
Triceps	C7–8	Triceps
Knee jerk	L2–4	Quadriceps
Ankle jerk	S1	Gastrocnemius

breast, prostate, myeloma, and kidney. Occasionally, compression can occur from neighboring nodal involvement and tumor infiltration through intervertebral foramina (eg, lymphoma, sarcomas, lung cancer). The locations are cervical in 10% of cases, thoracic in 70%, and lumbar in 20%. Multiple noncontiguous levels are involved in 10% to 40%. The most important prognostic factor in preserving neurologic function is early diagnosis, before neurologic deficits have developed.

More than 90% of patients present with pain. Cervical pain may radiate down the arm. Thoracic pain radiates around the rib cage or abdominal wall; it may be described as a compressing band bilaterally around the chest or abdomen. Lumbar pain may radiate into the groin or down the leg. Pain may be aggravated by coughing, sneezing, or straight-leg raising. Focal neurologic signs depend on the level affected. Paresthesias (tingling, numbness), weakness, and altered reflexes also can be present (Table 33.8). Tenderness over the spine may help localize the level, but absence does not exclude the possibility of cord involvement. Autonomic changes of urinary or fecal retention or incontinence are very concerning and may predict development of motor function loss in the near future.

Imaging studies include bone scanning or plain radiography, which show vertebral metastases in approximately 85% of patients with epidural compression. MRI of the entire spine is generally recommended. Computed tomographic myelography can be used in patients who cannot undergo MRI.

Treatment usually includes an initial bolus of 10 to 100 mg of dexamethasone intravenously, depending on the severity of block. Thereafter, dexamethasone is given (4 mg 4 times daily), although some physicians favor higher doses for a few days followed by a rapid taper. Radiation therapy is applied to the involved area(s). Surgical resection and stabilization may lead to an increased chance at neurologic recovery in select patients who present with weakness or paralysis or in patients who present with no prior cancer diagnosis (Table 33.9). Patients with extensive organ involvement, progressive malignancies,

Table 33.9 OUTCOME OF PATIENTS WITH SPINAL CORD COMPRESSION, BY NEUROLOGIC STATUS

STATUS AT PRESENTATION	% AMBULATORY AFTER RADIATION
Ambulatory	>80
Paraparetic	<50
Paraplegic	<10

or poor performance status are unlikely to be able to tolerate an extensive operative procedure and should be treated more conservatively.

- Early diagnosis of spinal cord compression, before development of neurologic deficit, improves outcome.
- Surgical therapy is indicated for select patients with neurologic deficit and spinal cord compression.

CANCER PAIN

More than 70% of patients with cancer have substantial pain during the course of their disease. Multiple studies have shown that patients with cancer-related pain are not given adequate analgesic therapy. Barriers to optimal management of cancer pain include inadequate pain assessment by health care professionals, physician reluctance and inadequate knowledge of how to prescribe opioids, and patient reluctance to take opioids. Physician reluctance to prescribe opioids stems from concern about addiction, lack of familiarity with the agents, problems with management of adverse effects of opioids, and legal or regulatory concerns. Psychological addiction to opioids in cancer patients is very rare, occurring in less than 1% of patients.

Evaluation

Evaluation should include 1) a history regarding onset, quality, severity, and location of pain; exacerbating and relieving factors; and associated symptoms and 2) physical examination, which should include a complete neurologic examination. Diagnostic studies are determined by the results of the history and physical examination. Administration of analgesia should not be delayed while awaiting diagnostic studies or other tests.

Treatment

Three-Tiered Approach

Step 1: For mild pain, administer acetaminophen or a nonsteroidal anti-inflammatory drug around the clock. Studies of nonsteroidal anti-inflammatory drugs for cancer pain have shown that these agents are 1.5 to 2 times more effective than placebo.

Step 2: When step 1 fails to provide adequate analgesia, or for moderate pain, add codeine or oxycodone.

Step 3: For severe pain or inadequate pain relief with steps 1 and 2, agents include a strong opioid such as morphine, hydromorphone, oxycodone, methadone, and fentanyl.

General Principles

For most cancer pain, opioids are the main treatment approach. Mild to moderate pain (4–7 on a scale of 1–10) can often be effectively treated with oral medications. Severe pain (>7/10) should be treated with intravenous medications because they allow for much more rapid titration of dose and more prompt pain relief. If an intravenous access is not available, subcutaneous administration usually works well as long as the patient is reasonably well hydrated. Intramuscular administration is strongly discouraged because it is painful and absorption of drug is very erratic. Treatment should always begin with immediate-release oral or parenteral administration until the opioid requirements and effective dose for the individual patient are determined. Once the opioid dose required to relieve the pain is known, then a long-acting form should be added.

The dose of opioid used to treat acute pain is highly dependent on whether the patient is already using opioids because many cancer patients are opioid-tolerant. Patients who are opioid-naïve should be treated with 5 to 15 mg of oral, immediate-release morphine, which is equianalgesic to 2 to 5 mg given intravenously. Other opioids are equally effective when compared with morphine. Equianalgesic tablets are readily available and should be used to calculate an equivalent dose. For patients already taking opioids, the total amount of opioids taken in the preceding 24 hours should be calculated. An immediate-release form of opioid equivalent to 10% to 20% of the 24-hour total dose should be administered as initial dose to try to relieve pain. Doses will then need to be adjusted to achieve adequate analgesia. Before adjusting the dose, one must wait until the time to peak effect has passed. For immediate-release oral agents, this is typically 1 hour, for intravenous agents, 6 to 10 minutes, and for subcutaneous agents, 20 to 30 minutes. Shortly after the time to peak effect, the patient should be reevaluated. If pain has decreased substantially, the same dose may be repeated on an as-needed basis, and the duration of the effect would be expected to be 3 to 4 hours for most immediate-release forms. If the pain has decreased only a small amount, then the same dose should be repeated and the patient reassessed after time to peak effect. If the pain has not changed at all, the next dose should be increased by 50% to 100% and the patient again reevaluated shortly after the time to peak effect has passed. Using such an algorithm has been shown to allow for rapid control of pain with minimal risk of adverse events (Figures 33.4 and 33.5).

There is no standard opioid dosage. The dose must be increased until analgesia is achieved or adverse effects occur. Because for most patients with cancer-associated pain the source of the pain is unlikely to be soon eliminated, scheduled, around-the-clock dosing is necessary. Once the effective dose is determined, then sustained-release or continuous-infusion intravenous opioid should be given. When the algorithms are followed, the last short-acting dose given that resulted in substantial diminishment of pain should be used to calculate the long-acting dose. This is considered the effective 4-hour dose because the duration of analgesia (not to be confused with time to peak effect) would be expected to be 3 to 4 hours for both immediate-release oral and intravenous administration. The effective 4-hour dose should be used to calculate the 24-hour equivalent. This can then be given as either a continuous infusion intravenously or as a sustained-release oral form. An immediate-release form of an opioid should continue to be made available to the patient for unexpected exacerbations of pain. This "breakthrough" dose is calculated by using 10% to 20% of the total daily dose of opioid being given. Appropriate equianalgesic conversions should be made when changing the

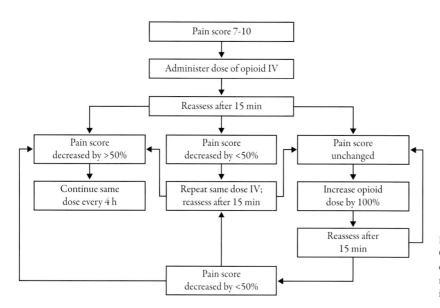

Figure 33.4 Algorithm for Treatment of Severe Cancer Pain With Intravenous Opioid. Dose of opioid should be determined from patient's status regarding pain and prior use of opioids. IV indicates intravenously.

route or drug. Patients who require 4 or more breakthrough doses in a 24-hour period should have their long-acting opioid dose adjusted. Each time the 24-hour dose is adjusted, the breakthrough dose should likewise be adjusted by using 10% to 20% of the 24-hour total.

Adverse effects of opioids include sedation, nausea, constipation, respiratory depression, and myoclonus. Tolerance to opioid-induced sedation and nausea usually develops within a few days. For opioid-induced constipation, docusate sodium and senna should be used. Methylnaltrexone (Relistor) is a new medication for the treatment of opioid-induced constipation. It is administered as a subcutaneous injection and is effective for producing laxation in a substantial proportion of patients, but it is not a medication used for prevention of constipation. Respiratory depression typically follows sedation; if a patient is excessively somnolent and has a very low respiratory rate, doses should be held. No opioid is more or less likely to result in a particular adverse-effect profile. However, one opioid may produce an adverse effect in a patient whereas another will not. Thus, sequential trials of different opioids

may be needed to determine the one best suited for any individual patient. The fentanyl patch (a transdermal formulation) delivers drug continuously over 72 hours. It is especially useful for patients with poor tolerance of orally administered opioids or those unable to take medications orally. Because subcutaneous fat is required for absorption of the drug, this may not be a good choice in patients with severe cachexia. Likewise, patients who are severely dehydrated will not have adequate skin perfusion to absorb the drug. Hydromorphone, fentanyl, and methadone are the opioids preferred for use in patients with renal insufficiency.

- Pain is common in patients with cancer and is often undertreated.

- The appropriate opioid dose for any one patient is that which relieves pain without excessive adverse effects.

- Acute pain exacerbations should be treated with immediate release or parenteral opioids until the effective dose is determined.

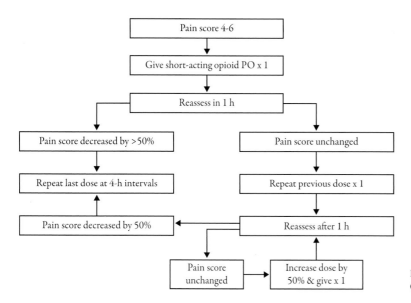

Figure 33.5 Algorithm for Treatment of Mild to Moderate Cancer Pain With Oral Opioids. PO indicates orally.

- Once the effective opioid dose is known, scheduled, long-acting opioids should be given along with as-needed immediate-release opioids for breakthrough pain.

- Early referral to palliative care or hospice can improve quality of life.

OTHER SYMPTOMS

Patients with cancer face numerous other symptoms and challenges as they progress through the course of their illness. Dyspnea, nausea, fatigue, weight loss, depression, difficulty concentrating or thinking, and sexual dysfunction are all common. Careful attention to symptoms and anticipation of expected symptoms can help alleviate many of these. Early referral to palliative care or hospice specialists can greatly enhance a patient's quality of life. Delineation of a patient's goals for care and development of advanced directives can allow the patient to remain in control and avoid unnecessary, painful, and, at times, harmful procedures.

SUMMARY

- MRI is recommended for women at very high risk for breast cancer and women with dense breast tissue on mammography, but it is controversial in women with newly diagnosed breast cancer.

- High-risk factors for colorectal cancer are familial polyposis syndromes, including familial adenomatous polyposis and Gardner syndrome, both inherited as an autosomal dominant trait; select familial cancer syndromes without polyps; and inflammatory bowel disease.

- For small cell lung cancer, treatment of limited-stage disease consists of both chemotherapy and chest radiation.

- CA 125 is expressed by about 85% of epithelial ovarian tumors.

- Risk factors for prostate cancer include older age, race (African American), family history, and a high-fat diet.

- Testicular cancer is the most common carcinoma in males 15–35 years old.

ACKNOWLEDGMENTS

The authors gratefully acknowledge Charles L. Loprinzi, MD, Steven R. Alberts, MD, Roxana S. Dronca, MD, Svetomir N. Markovic, MD, PhD, Brian A. Costello, MD, Mark Lewis, MD, and Heidi D. (Gunderson) Finnes, PharmD for their thoughtful comments and edits to the current edition.

PART VIII

HEMATOLOGY

34.

BENIGN HEMATOLOGY

Alexandra P. Wolanskyj, MD

GOALS

- Describe the approach to evaluation of microcytic, macrocytic, and normocytic anemias.

- Differentiate causes of hemolytic anemia.

- Review various types of transfusion reactions.

ANEMIAS

EVALUATION OF ANEMIA

Anemia is a reduction in the mass of healthy circulating red blood cells (RBCs). Anemia occurs as a result of 1 of 3 mechanisms: 1) inadequate production of RBCs by the bone marrow (ie, marrow failure, intrinsic RBC synthetic defects, or lack of essential RBC components such as vitamins); 2) blood loss; and 3) premature destruction of RBCs (ie, hemolysis). After a complete history and physical examination, evaluation of anemia includes a complete blood cell count, so that anemia can be classified as microcytic, macrocytic, or normocytic on the basis of mean corpuscular volume (MCV).

MICROCYTIC ANEMIAS

Microcytic anemia indicates the presence of small RBCs (MCV <80 fL). The most common forms of anemia are microcytic (Tables 34.1 and 34.2).

The causes of hypochromic microcytic anemias can be remembered with the mnemonic *TAILS* (*t*halassemia, *a*nemia of chronic disease, *i*ron deficiency, *l*ead poisoning, and *s*idero-blastic anemia). Other, less common causes of microcytosis include vitamin C deficiency, vitamin B_6 deficiency, copper deficiency, sirolimus or mycophenolate, primary myelofibrosis, renal cell carcinoma, and Hodgkin lymphoma.

A complete blood cell count and iron parameters aid in making a diagnosis (Table 34.2). Blood loss should be considered in all patients with anemia, especially those with microcytic anemia. Investigating the gastrointestinal tract is essential in the work-up of microcytic anemia, since it is the most common site of occult blood loss.

- Use *TAILS* (*t*halassemia, *a*nemia of chronic disease, *i*ron deficiency, *l*ead poisoning, and *s*ideroblastic anemia) to remember causes of microcytic anemia.

Iron Deficiency

Iron deficiency is the most common cause of anemia in the world and is especially common among menstruating women and the elderly (Figure 34.1).

Mechanisms of iron deficiency include the following:

1. Blood loss, including gastrointestinal tract disorders (eg, ulcers, malignancy, telangiectasia, arteriovenous malformations, hiatal hernia, and long-distance runner's anemia); respiratory disorders (eg, malignancy and pulmonary hemosiderosis); menstruation; phlebotomy (eg, blood donation, diagnostic phlebotomy, treatment of polycythemia vera or hemochromatosis, and self-inflicted or factitious injury); trauma; and surgery

2. Increased requirements in relation to intake (as in pregnancy)

3. Decreased absorption, including partial gastrectomy and malabsorption syndromes (eg, celiac disease)

Patients with early iron deficiency may have a normal MCV. Patients with iron deficiency may also have a normal MCV if they have a condition that causes macrocytosis (eg, iron deficiency in combination with folate deficiency).

The serum ferritin test is the most useful initial test for iron deficiency. A ferritin level less than 15 ng/mL almost always indicates iron deficiency. Ferritin testing is useful in pregnant women, in whom transferrin saturation is often elevated. Ferritin is an acute phase reactant, and the level is increased in inflammatory states. Thus, patients with these conditions may have iron deficiency even if the ferritin level is normal or increased. Notably, an elevated soluble transferrin receptor (sTfR) measurement, which is not an acute-phase reactant, also signifies iron deficiency.

Table 34.1 TYPICAL FEATURES OF UNCOMPLICATED MICROCYTIC ANEMIAS (DECREASED MCV)

	TYPE OF ANEMIA	
VARIABLE	*Thalassemia*	*Iron Deficiency*
RBC count, $\times 10^{12}$/L	≥5.0	<5.0
RBC distribution width, %	<16	≥16

Abbreviations: MCV, mean corpuscular volume; RBC, red blood cell.

- The serum ferritin test is the most useful initial test for iron deficiency.

- When iron deficiency anemia is discovered, identify the underlying cause.

Oral iron replacement therapy is the treatment of choice for iron deficiency. Gastric acid is required for optimal iron absorption; thus, antacids may interfere with absorption. Reticulocytosis is seen in 4 to 7 days after initiating oral iron replacement therapy, improvement in anemia in 3 to 4 weeks, and correction of anemia in 6 weeks—if the cause of anemia is solely iron deficiency. Continue iron replacement therapy for another 6 months to replenish bone marrow reserves.

Indications for intravenous iron therapy include renal dialysis (with recombinant erythropoietin) and inability to tolerate or absorb iron taken orally.

- Oral iron replacement therapy is the treatment of choice for iron deficiency.

Thalassemias

The thalassemias are common single-gene disorders. β-Thalassemia results when β-globin chains are decreased or absent in relation to α-globin. In α-thalassemia, the converse is true: excess β-globin chains precipitate as tetramers called *hemoglobin H*. Genetic counseling is indicated after the diagnosis of α- or β-thalassemia has been established.

β-Thalassemia

Point mutations result in β-thalassemia of varying severity. Clinically, β-thalassemia is categorized as follows:

1. *β-Thalassemia trait*—microcytosis and either normal hemoglobin or mild anemia

2. *β-Thalassemia intermedia*—microcytosis and moderate anemia without long-term transfusion dependence

3. *β-Thalassemia major* (also known as Cooley anemia)—profound anemia and lifelong transfusion dependence

In β-thalassemia, the hemoglobin A_2 level is elevated (Figure 34.2). However, if the patient has iron deficiency, the hemoglobin A_2 level may be normal, since iron deficiency decreases the hemoglobin A_2 level.

α-Thalassemia

Normally, a person has 4 α-globin genes, but only 2 β-chain loci. α-Thalassemia is classifed as follows:

1. *α-Thalassemia minor* (*α-thalassemia trait*)—absence of 1 or 2 of the 4 α-globin genes (patients are asymptomatic, usually with a low-normal MCV and normal hemoglobin)

2. *Hemoglobin H disease*—absence of 3 α-globin genes (patients have chronic hemolytic anemia of moderate severity, and they may benefit from splenectomy if hemolysis becomes problematic)

3. Absence of all 4 α-globin genes is not compatible with life and results in stillbirth

Vitamin C Deficiency

Patients with vitamin C deficiency (scurvy) present with microcytic anemia, purpura, gingival disease, and peripheral edema.

SIDEROBLASTIC ANEMIAS

The sideroblastic anemias are characterized by microcytic, normocytic, or macrocytic anemia and ring sideroblasts in the bone marrow (Figure 34.3), which are abnormal erythroid

Table 34.2 COMPARISON OF THE MOST COMMON HYPOCHROMIC MICROCYTIC ANEMIAS

DISEASE STATE	MCV	RED BLOOD CELL COUNT	TIBC	TRANSFERRIN SATURATION	SERUM FERRITIN	MARROW IRON
Iron deficiency anemia	Decreased	Decreased	Increased	Low	Low	Absent
Anemia of chronic disease	Normal or decreased	Decreased	Normal	Normal or increased	Normal or increased	Normal or increased
Thalassemia minor	Decreased	Usually increased	Normal	Normal	Normal or increased	Normal

Abbreviations: MCV, mean corpuscular volume; TIBC, total iron-binding capacity.

Adapted from Savage RA. Cost-effective laboratory diagnosis of microcytic anemias of complex origin. ASCP check sample H84-10(H-153). Used with permission.

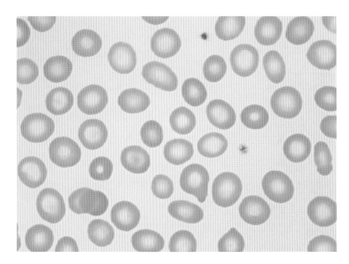

Figure 34.1 Hypochromic Microcytic Anemia. The erythrocytes are small with increased central pallor and assorted aberrations in size (anisocytosis) and shape (poikilocytosis). This pattern is characteristic of iron deficiency rather than thalessemia; in thalassemia, red blood cells are small but more uniform. If a mature lymphocyte is available for reference, the diameter of a normal erythrocyte (7 μm) should be similar to the diameter of the nucleus of the lymphocyte (peripheral blood smear; Wright-Giemsa). (Courtesy of Curtis A. Hanson, MD, Mayo Clinic, Rochester, Minnesota. Used with permission.)

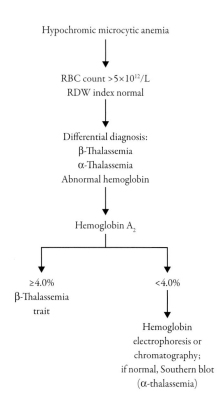

Figure 34.2 Algorithm for Approach to Diagnosis of Hypochromic Microcytic Anemia With an Increased Total Red Blood Cell (RBC) Count and a Normal RBC Distribution Width (RDW) Index. (Adapted from Savage RA. Cost-effective laboratory diagnosis of microcytic anemias of complex origin. ASCP check sample H84-10[H-153]. Used with permission.)

precursors ineffective at heme synthesis and often seen in myelodysplastic syndromes. Reactive causes include alcohol, zinc toxicity, and drugs such as isoniazid and pyrazinamide. Several forms of congenital sideroblastic anemia may respond to vitamin B_6 (pyridoxine) therapy.

MACROCYTIC ANEMIAS

Macrocytic anemia indicates the presence of large RBCs (MCV >100 fL). The differential diagnosis of macrocytic anemias includes vitamin B_{12} deficiency, folate deficiency, drugs, liver disease, alcohol abuse, hypothyroidism, heavy tobacco use, myelodysplasia or other primary bone marrow disorders, cold agglutinin disease (artifactual clumping of cells in an automated counter), and reticulocytosis (reticulocytes are larger than mature RBCs). A laboratory approach to macrocytic anemias is outlined in Figure 34.4. An MCV greater than 115 fL almost always indicates a deficiency of either vitamin B_{12} or folate or an artifact due to RBC agglutination. Common drug-related causes of macrocytosis are chemotherapy drugs that inhibit purine or pyrimidine synthesis (eg, azathioprine and 5-fluorouracil), deoxyribonucleotide synthesis (hydroxyurea and cytarabine), and dihydrofolate reductase (methotrexate).

- An MCV >115 fL almost always indicates a deficiency of either vitamin B_{12} or folate or an artifact due to RBC agglutination.
- Multiple drugs cause macrocytosis.

Vitamin B_{12} Deficiency

Vitamin B_{12} (cobalamin) is present in animal products and in small quantities in some plant-derived foods. Hydrochloric

acid is necessary to free cobalamin from food; thus, patients with achlorhydria cannot absorb vitamin B_{12}. Free cobalamin is immediately bound by R-binders, which protect cobalamin from the acidic gastric environment. As the complex passes into the duodenum, pancreatic proteases facilitate release of the R-binders. The free cobalamin combines with

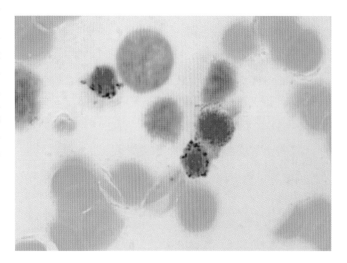

Figure 34.3 Ring Sideroblasts. Seen on iron staining of a bone marrow aspirate, ring sideroblasts can be reactive, congenital, or part of a myelodysplastic syndrome or other clonal myeloid disorder (bone marrow aspirate; iron stain with potassium ferrocyanide and nuclear fast red counterstain). (Courtesy of Curtis A. Hanson, MD, Mayo Clinic, Rochester, Minnesota. Used with permission.)

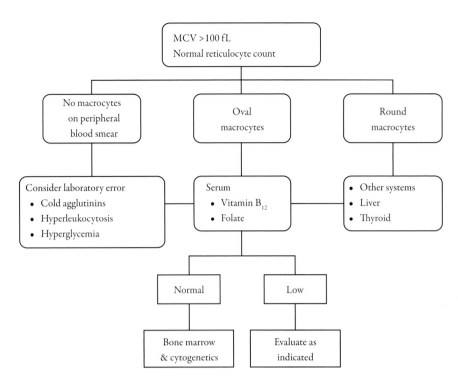

```
        ┌─────────────────────────┐
        │   MCV >100 fL           │
        │ Normal reticulocyte count│
        └─────────────────────────┘
```

Figure 34.4 Laboratory Approach to Macrocytic Anemias. MCV indicates mean corpuscular volume. (Adapted from Colon-Otero G, Menke D, Hook CC. A practical approach to the differential diagnosis and evaluation of the adult patient with macrocytic anemia. Med Clin North Am. 1992 May;76[3]:581–97. Used with permission.)

intrinsic factor and is absorbed in the ileum. Thus, sufficient ileal mucosal surface and a normally functioning pancreas are required for adequate absorption of vitamin B$_{12}$.

Causes of vitamin B$_{12}$ deficiency include pernicious anemia (defective production of intrinsic factor, usually due to auto-immune production of anti–intrinsic factor or anti–parietal cell antibodies), atrophic gastritis, total or partial gastrectomy, ileal resection or Crohn disease involving the ileum, bacterial overgrowth syndromes, infection with *Diphyllobothrium latum*, and pancreatic insufficiency (most commonly from chronic pancreatitis or cystic fibrosis). Nitrous oxide inactivates vitamin B$_{12}$, and abuse of this anesthetic (eg, by dentists or dental office workers) can lead to rapid development of severe vitamin B$_{12}$ deficiency. Vitamin B$_{12}$ deficiency due to inadequate dietary intake is very rare.

The symptoms and signs of vitamin B$_{12}$ deficiency include a beefy and atrophic tongue, diarrhea, and neurologic signs (eg, paresthesias, gait disturbance, mental status changes ["B$_{12}$ madness"], vibratory/position sense impairment [dorsal column "dropout"], the absence of ankle reflexes, and extensor plantar responses).

The MCV is increased, and hypersegmented neutrophils are usually present (Figure 34.5). As in folate deficiency, serum homocysteine levels are increased; however, unlike in folate deficiency, serum and urinary levels of methylmalonic acid are also increased. A serum vitamin B$_{12}$ level less than 200 pg/mL strongly suggests vitamin B$_{12}$ deficiency. Vitamin B$_{12}$ levels of 200 to 400 pg/mL (borderline or low-normal range) can also indicate deficiency; if clinical suspicion is high, methylmalonic acid levels can help establish the diagnosis. When present, an abnormal intrinsic factor antibody confirms pernicious anemia as the cause of vitamin B$_{12}$ deficiency. Serum gastrin levels are typically high. The Schilling test is frequently described in textbooks but rarely performed in clinical practice.

Vitamin B$_{12}$ deficiency, including pernicious anemia, is treated with oral or intramuscular vitamin B$_{12}$. Lifelong maintenance treatment is required. Vitamin B$_{12}$ levels may be spuriously low in patients who are pregnant or using oral contraceptives and are falsely elevated in patients who have myeloproliferative disorders, because of alterations in levels of vitamin B$_{12}$-binding proteins.

- Homocysteine levels are elevated in both folate deficiency and vitamin B$_{12}$ deficiency.

- Methylmalonic acid levels are increased only in vitamin B$_{12}$ deficiency.

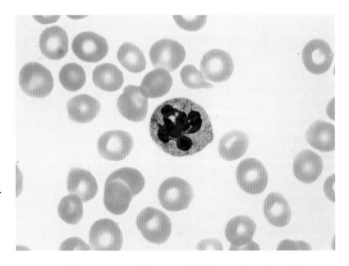

Figure 34.5 Hypersegmented Neutrophil. Polymorphonuclear leukocytes with 5 or more nuclear lobes are characteristic of vitamin B$_{12}$ or folate deficiency and are not typically seen in other causes of macrocytic anemia (peripheral blood smear; Wright-Giemsa).

Folate Deficiency

In contrast to anemia caused by vitamin B_{12} deficiency, macrocytic anemia caused by folate deficiency develops quickly (ie, within months) in patients with inadequate dietary intake of folic acid. Folate is present in green leafy vegetables and some fruits. It is absorbed in the duodenum and proximal jejunum. Notably, folate deficiency has decreased in the United States with folic acid fortification of grain products. Mechanisms of folate deficiency include increased requirements (eg, pregnancy, hemolytic anemia), poor folate intake (eg, alcoholics, persons following extremely restrictive diets), poor absorption, and interference with the recycling of folate from liver stores to tissue (eg, alcohol).

Anemia due to folate deficiency is indistinguishable from anemia due to vitamin B_{12} deficiency. The possibility of coexistent vitamin B_{12} or iron deficiency should be considered if response to replacement folate therapy is not optimal. Folate helps convert homocysteine to methionine; thus, folate deficiency leads to an increased homocysteine level. In contrast to vitamin B_{12} deficiency, in folate deficiency the level of methylmalonic acid is normal. RBC folate levels are more accurate than serum folate levels in detecting true folate deficiency, since serum folate levels fluctuate quickly with dietary changes. A single day of healthy meals in the hospital may normalize a patient's serum folate level and lead to a false-negative result.

- If anemia due to folate deficiency does not respond optimally to folate replacement, consider coexistent vitamin B_{12} or iron deficiency.

- Unlike vitamin B_{12} deficiency, folate deficiency develops quickly with inadequate dietary intake.

NORMOCYTIC ANEMIAS

Normocytic anemia is defined as anemia with an MCV of 80 to 100 fL. Diagnosing the cause of a normochromic normocytic anemia can be challenging. The differential diagnosis includes mixed nutritional deficiency (eg, concomitant folate and iron deficiency), erythropoietic failure (aplastic anemia and RBC aplasia), marrow replacement (malignancy and fibrosis), kidney disease with lack of erythropoietin production, hemolysis, acute hemorrhage, some myelodysplastic syndromes, chemotherapy, anemia of acute disease, and anemia of chronic disease (eg, infections, neoplasia, rheumatoid arthritis, and other inflammatory rheumatologic conditions).

Anemia of Chronic Disease

Anemia of chronic disease (ACD) is usually moderate (ie, hemoglobin 9–11 g/dL), MCV is normal or modestly decreased, and the reticulocyte count is low. ACD is sometimes called anemia of chronic inflammation, since it results from the inhibitory effects of inflammatory cytokines on the bone marrow. A peptide produced by the liver, hepcidin, is elevated in ACD. Hepcidin sequesters iron and decreases iron absorption. As a consequence, serum iron levels are low in ACD, but unlike in iron deficiency, total iron-binding capacity is normal or low and ferritin is usually normal or elevated (Table 34.2).

In evaluating patients with suspected ACD, it is important to exclude hemolysis and gastrointestinal tract blood loss early in the evaluation. No single blood test confirms ACD, but diagnosis is probable if 1) inflammatory markers are present; 2) results of iron studies are typical (ie, normal total iron-binding capacity, normal or increased serum ferritin, and normal or increased transferrin saturation); 3) another cause for the normocytic anemia is not apparent; and 4) the clinical setting is appropriate. The sTfR concentration is normal in ACD in contrast to iron deficiency anemia, in which sTfR is usually elevated. Patients with ACD do not benefit from iron therapy.

APLASTIC ANEMIA

Aplastic anemia is a rare disorder characterized by pancytopenia, bone marrow hypocellularity, and absence of another disorder that would explain the hypocellularity (eg, myelodysplastic syndrome, T-cell clonal disorders, or other congenital bone marrow failure syndromes). Acquired aplastic anemia is often idiopathic. Common causes include drugs (eg, chloramphenicol, sulfonamides, gold, and benzene), toxins, radiation, infections (eg, hepatitis A, Epstein-Barr virus [EBV], cytomegalovirus, human immunodeficiency virus [HIV], and human parvovirus B19), and autoimmune marrow suppression. The criteria for severe aplastic anemia include less than 25% of expected marrow cellularity and 2 of the following: 1) neutrophil count less than $0.5 \times 10^9/L$, 2) platelet count less than $20 \times 10^9/L$, and 3) a corrected reticulocyte count less than 1%.

- Aplastic anemia is characterized by pancytopenia, hypocellular bone marrow, and absence of another cause of marrow hypoplasia.

- Common causes of aplastic anemia include autoimmune marrow suppression, idiopathic causes, drug reaction, toxins, radiation, and viral infections.

Allogeneic hematopoietic stem cell transplant is the therapy of choice for patients with an identical twin and patients younger than 20 years, or high-risk patients between the ages of 20 and 40 who have an HLA match. For patients older than 40, the treatment of choice is antithymocyte globulin in combination with corticosteroids and cyclosporine, although it is usually not curative. Without treatment, 80% of patients who have severe aplastic anemia die within 2 years of diagnosis.

- Full recovery in aplastic anemia is uncommon without treatment.

SICKLE CELL DISORDERS

CLASSIFICATION AND PATHOPHYSIOLOGY

The sickle cell disorders include sickle cell anemia (homozygous hemoglobin S), sickle cell trait (heterozygous

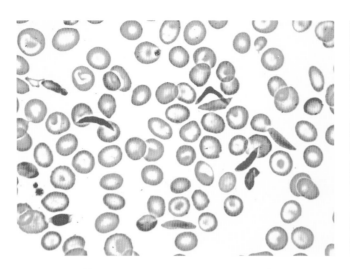

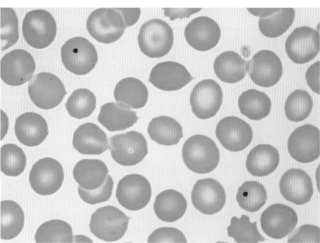

Figure 34.6 Sickle Cell Anemia. Several irreversibly sickled cells are seen. Abundant target cells indicate hyposplenism from autoinfarction of the spleen. Liver disease due to transfusional hemosiderosis was also a contributing factor to these target cells (peripheral blood smear; Wright-Giemsa).

Figure 34.7 Howell-Jolly Bodies. These small, round blue inclusions are seen with Wright-Giemsa or a comparable stain. These are characteristic of hyposplenism due to splenectomy or to a functionally defective spleen. Howell-Jolly bodies should not be confused with Heinz bodies, which require a special preparation (Heinz body preparation) to observe and are not seen on a conventional peripheral smear (peripheral blood smear; Wright-Giemsa).

hemoglobin S), and compound states (hemoglobin S with thalassemia or other hemoglobinopathies).

Sickle cell anemia occurs in persons of sub-Saharan African descent and, less commonly, in persons of Middle Eastern or South Asian origin. Approximately 1 of every 8 African Americans carries 1 copy of the sickle cell gene, with sickle cell disease occurring in 1 of 500. Hemoglobin S substitutes valine for glutamic acid at the sixth position of the β chain. Deoxygenated hemoglobin S distorts the cell into a sickle shape and injures the cell membrane (Figure 34.6). Vasoocclusion is a function of decreased RBC deformability, increased viscosity, and increased RBC adherence to altered endothelium.

Sickling is inhibited by hemoglobin F, and symptoms are not apparent until after 6 months of age owing to high levels of fetal hemoglobin in early life. The first episode of vasoocclusive disease typically develops between the ages of 12 months and 6 years and results from obstruction of the microcirculation by intravascular sickling.

Acute complications of sickle cell anemia include vasoocclusive episodes, acute chest syndrome, dactylitis, splenic sequestration, stroke, aplastic crisis, infection, acute cholecystitis, priapism, and renal papillary necrosis. Acute chest syndrome, accounting for up to 25% of deaths, is the leading cause of death in sickle cell anemia; clinical features include fever, chest pain, tachypnea, leukocytosis, and pulmonary infiltrates. When infection is present, causative organisms include pneumococci, *Mycoplasma*, *Haemophilus*, *Salmonella*, and *Escherichia coli*. Aplastic crises usually follow a febrile illness and are often associated with human parvovirus B19 infection in adults. In sickle cell patients, osteomyelitis is caused by *Salmonella*, *Staphylococcus*, and pneumococci.

Chronic complications include hemolytic anemia, growth retardation, pulmonary hypertension, folate deficiency, retinopathy, chronic renal insufficiency, accelerated cardiovascular disease, transfusional hemochromatosis, nonhealing skin ulcers, osteopenia, avascular necrosis, and growth retardation.

Although disease manifestations do not increase during pregnancy, maternal mortality is 5% to 8% and fetal mortality 20%.

Laboratory findings include severe anemia (hemoglobin, 5.5–9.5 g/dL), sickled cells, ovalocytes, target cells, basophilic stippling, polychromatophilia, reticulocytosis (3%-12%), and hyposplenia with Howell-Jolly bodies (Figure 34.7). A persistent increase in the white blood cell count to 12×10^9/L to 15×10^9/L (in the absence of infection) with eosinophilia is characteristic. Evidence of chronic hemolysis may be present. Liver test results are often increased. Routine diagnostic tests include the sickle solubility test, electrophoresis, and chromatography.

- Acute complications of sickle cell anemia include vasoocclusive episodes, acute chest syndrome, dactylitis, splenic sequestration, aplastic crisis, infection, priapism, renal papillary necrosis, and cerebrovascular accidents.

- Chronic complications include hemolytic anemia, pulmonary hypertension, folate deficiency, retinopathy, chronic renal insufficiency, accelerated cardiovascular disease, transfusional hemosiderosis, nonhealing skin ulcers, osteopenia, and growth retardation.

- Acute chest syndrome is the leading cause of death in sickle cell anemia.

- Maternal and fetal mortality are increased.

TREATMENT

Many sickle cell crises can be prevented by avoiding infection, fever, dehydration, acidosis, hypoxemia, cold, and high altitude. Most patients with sickle cell disease undergo autosplenectomy through recurrent infarction by age 5. Immunizations for encapsulated organisms, penicillin prophylaxis, and folate supplementation are indicated. For painful crises, the cornerstone of treatment includes gentle hydration and pain control. Analgesics, including opioids, are essential and should not be withheld because of concern about drug-seeking behavior. Acetaminophen is used for fever because aspirin contributes to acid load. A temperature greater than 40.6°C implies infection rather than just infarction. Blood transfusion and exchange transfusions are the most effective means of treatment for severe complications. Exchange transfusion is indicated for stroke, stroke prevention in patients at high risk, acute chest syndrome, priapism, and progressive retinopathy. For life-threatening complications, exchange transfusion is recommended with a goal for the hemoglobin S fraction of less than 30%. Posttransfusion increases in hemoglobin to more than 10 to 11 g/dL should be avoided except preoperatively. Iron chelation is recommended if the transfusion requirement is high and the ferritin level is elevated.

Treatment with hydroxyurea decreases the frequency of painful vasoocclusive crises (by about 50%), the frequency of acute chest syndrome, and the number of transfusions and hospitalizations. It is indicated for patients who have had severe complications such as acute chest syndrome and for patients who have frequent, painful crises.

Hematopoietic stem cell transplant with marrow or umbilical cord blood from HLA-identical siblings may be curative. The present indications for transplant include stroke and recurrent acute chest syndrome.

- Hydroxyurea decreases the frequency of painful vasoocclusive crises by 50% and decreases the frequency of acute chest syndrome.

- Death in sickle cell disease is associated with acute pain, acute chest syndrome, stroke, and infection.

- Achieving a hemoglobin S level of <30% with exchange transfusion is recommended for life-threatening complications, including acute chest syndrome and stroke.

- A posttransfusion increase in hemoglobin to >10 g/dL should be avoided except before elective surgery.

SICKLE CELL TRAIT AND COMPOUND STATES

Sickle cell trait (heterozygous hemoglobin S) is not associated with anemia, RBC abnormalities, increased risk of infections, or increased mortality. Associations with sickle cell trait include hematuria due to renal papillary necrosis, splenic infarction at high altitude (>3,030 m), hyposthenuria, pyelonephritis in pregnancy, and pulmonary embolism. Compound states such as sickle cell–hemoglobin C disease and hemoglobin S/β-thalassemia are generally milder than sickle cell disease, depending on the hemoglobin concentrations.

HEMOLYTIC ANEMIAS

There are many causes of hemolysis. If hemolytic anemia is suspected, the first step is to confirm the presence of hemolysis. Hemolytic anemias are characterized as follows:

1. Increased RBC destruction

    a. Elevated indirect bilirubin level (>8 mg/dL suggests concomitant liver disease)

    b. Elevated lactate dehydrogenase (LDH) level

    c. Decreased haptoglobin level (haptoglobin is a scavenger of free hemoglobin and may be transiently decreased after transfusion or hemodialysis)

2. Increased RBC production

    a. Elevated reticulocyte count

    b. Marrow erythroid hyperplasia

Peripheral smear findings such as the following can assist in making a diagnosis:

1. *Spherocytes* (Figure 34.8) are associated with hereditary spherocytosis, alcohol, and autoimmune hemolytic anemia.

2. *Basophilic stippling* occurs in lead poisoning, β-thalassemia, and arsenic poisoning.

3. *Hypochromia* occurs in thalassemia, sideroblastic anemia, and lead poisoning.

4. *Target cells* are present in thalassemia and liver disease and after splenectomy (Figure 34.9).

5. *Agglutination* is present in cold agglutinin disease (Figure 34.10).

6. *Stomatocytes* are associated with acute alcoholism; they also occur as an artifact.

7. *Spur cells* (*acanthocytes*) (Figure 34.11) are present in chronic severe liver disease, abetalipoproteinemia, and malabsorption.

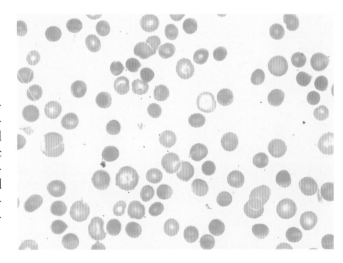

Figure 34.8 Spherocytes. Spherocytes are the smooth, small, and spheroidal darkly stained cells with minimal or no central pallor. They are most commonly seen in hereditary spherocytosis or autoimmune hemolytic anemia (peripheral blood smear; Wright-Giemsa). (Courtesy of Curtis A. Hanson, MD, Mayo Clinic, Rochester, Minnesota. Used with permission.)

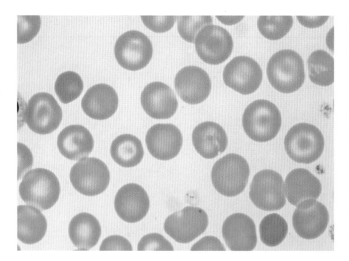

Figure 34.9 Target Cells. Target cells are the red blood cells with a broad diameter and dark center with a pale surrounding halo. They are most commonly seen in hemoglobin C disease, thalassemia, or liver disease or after splenectomy (peripheral blood smear; Wright-Giemsa). (Courtesy of Curtis A. Hanson, MD, Mayo Clinic, Rochester, Minnesota. Used with permission.)

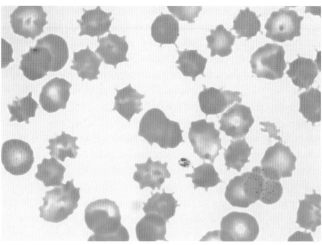

Figure 34.11 Spur Cells (Acanthocytes). Note the thin, thorny, or finger-like projections. Spur cells are characteristic of advanced liver disease and must be distinguished from burr cells (echinocytes) (see Figure 34.12) (peripheral blood smear; Wright-Giemsa). (Courtesy of Curtis A. Hanson, MD, Mayo Clinic, Rochester, Minnesota. Used with permission.)

8. *Burr cells* (*echinocytes*) occur in uremia (Figure 34.12) and disappear with hemodialysis.

9. *Heinz bodies* are present in glucose-6-phosphate dehydrogenase (G6PD) deficiency; they are seen with supravital stain.

10. *Howell-Jolly bodies* indicate hyposplenism (Figure 34.7).

11. *Polychromasia* indicates reticulocytosis (Figure 34.13).

12. *Intraerythrocytic parasitic inclusions* occur in malaria and babesiosis (Figure 34.14).

Hemolytic anemias may result from factors that are intrinsic or extrinsic to the RBC and may be direct Coombs-negative or Coombs-positive (Figure 34.15). A positive direct

Coombs test (also called the direct antiglobulin test [DAT]) indicates the presence of complement component C3 or IgG (or both) on the surface of RBCs. Notably, an aplastic crisis may occur in chronic hemolytic anemia and usually results from the development of folate deficiency or infection with parvovirus.

- Hemolytic anemias may be hereditary or acquired, from factors intrinsic or extrinsic to the RBC, and Coombs-positive or Coombs-negative.

- Evidence of increased RBC destruction includes elevated LDH, indirect hyperbilirubinemia, and a low haptoglobin level.

- Reticulocytosis is the normal marrow response to hemolysis.

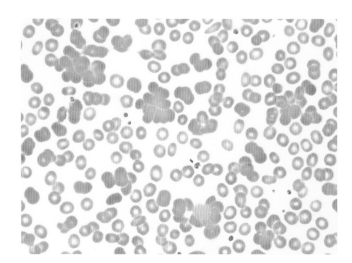

Figure 34.10 Agglutination. The random clumping of red blood cells most commonly indicates cold agglutinin disease or laboratory artifact. It is important to distinguish agglutination from rouleaux (see Figure 34.16) (peripheral blood smear; Wright-Giemsa).

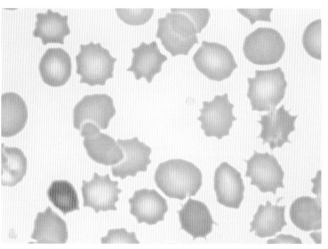

Figure 34.12 Burr Cells (Echinocytes). Burr cell projections are much smaller and more uniform in size than spur cell projections. Burr cells are characteristic of uremia, and the membrane abnormality is reversible with hemodialysis (peripheral blood smear; Wright-Giemsa).

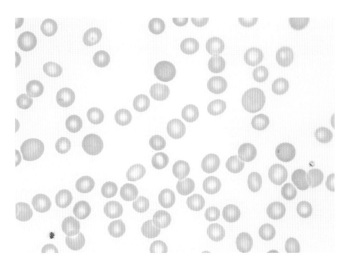

Figure 34.13 Polychromasia. The larger cells are reticulocytes. These are often seen in high numbers during recovery from blood loss or hemolysis (peripheral blood smear; Wright-Giemsa).

INTRAVASCULAR HEMOLYSIS COMPARED WITH EXTRAVASCULAR HEMOLYSIS

In intravascular hemolysis, RBCs are destroyed while circulating within blood vessels. Their destruction releases free hemoglobin into the bloodstream, leading to hemoglobinemia, hemoglobinuria, and hemosiderinuria, all of which occur exclusively with intravascular hemolysis. Hemosiderinuria indicates that desquamated renal tubular cells absorbed free hemoglobin days to weeks earlier. Causes of intravascular hemolysis include transfusion reactions from ABO blood group antibodies, microangiopathic hemolytic anemia, paroxysmal nocturnal hemoglobinuria, paroxysmal cold hemoglobinuria, cold agglutinin syndrome, immune-complex drug-induced hemolytic anemia, infections (including falciparum malaria and clostridial sepsis), and G6PD deficiency. All other forms of hemolysis are primarily extravascular, in which the RBCs are lysed in the macrophages of the spleen and liver.

- Hemoglobinuria and hemosiderinuria are signs of intravascular hemolysis.
- Most hemolysis is extravascular.

AUTOIMMUNE HEMOLYTIC ANEMIA

Mechanisms of Drug-Induced Hemolytic Anemia

There are 3 distinct mechanisms of drug-induced hemolytic anemia:

1. *Autoantibody mechanism*—Methyldopa may form autoantibodies that can induce hemolysis. Direct Coombs test results are positive in 3 to 6 months. Discontinuing the use of methyldopa usually leads to a rapid reversal in hemolysis.

2. *Drug adsorption mechanism*—The use of high doses of penicillins or cephalosporins for more than 7 days may lead to immunohemolytic anemia due to antibodies formed against the drug–RBC membrane antigen complex. In 3% of patients, the direct Coombs test is positive.

3. *Immune complex mechanism*—Exposure to quinidine may cause an antidrug antibody to form and create an immune complex, which is adsorbed on the RBCs and may activate complement. The direct Coombs test is positive because of the complement on the RBC surface.

- Autoantibody mechanism: methyldopa.
- Drug adsorption mechanism: penicillin.
- Immune-complex mechanism: quinine and quinidine.
- Typical clinical scenario: A patient has evidence of hemolysis (increased reticulocyte count, LDH, and indirect bilirubin), positive Coombs test with or without splenomegaly, and jaundice with a history of exposure to a common offending drug.

Cold Agglutinin Syndrome (Primary Cold Agglutinin Disease)

Cold agglutinin syndrome is characterized by chronic hemolytic anemia, agglutination, and a positive direct Coombs test (anti–complement component C3). IgM autoantibodies are reactive at temperatures below 37°C. The cause is most commonly idiopathic but can also be secondary to infection (most commonly *Mycoplasma pneumoniae* and EBV) or malignancy (B-cell lymphoma, chronic lymphocytic leukemia, multiple myeloma, and Waldenström macroglobulinemia).

Clinical signs and symptoms relate to small-vessel occlusion, including acrocyanosis of the finger, toes, ears, and tip of the nose. All digits may be affected equally in contrast to

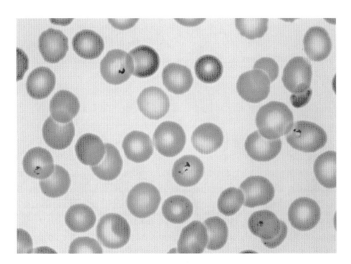

Figure 34.14 Intraerythrocytic Ring-Shaped Parasites of Babesiosis. Malaria is the other common disease with an intraerythrocytic parasite (peripheral blood smear; Wright-Giemsa).

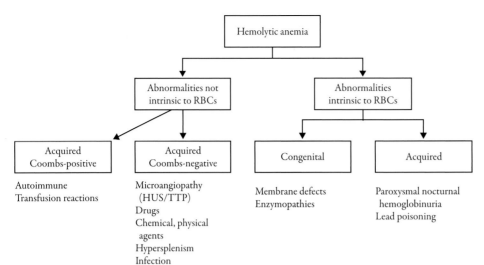

Figure 34.15 Differential Diagnosis of Hemolytic Anemia. HUS indicates hemolytic uremic syndrome; RBC, red blood cell; TTP, thrombotic thrombocytopenic purpura.

Raynaud phenomenon, in which 1 or 2 fingers turn from white to blue to red.

The peripheral blood smear shows RBC agglutination that disappears if prepared at 37°C (Figure 34.10). Agglutinated RBCs clump together, spuriously elevating the MCV. Therapy includes avoidance of the cold. In severe cases rituximab and cytotoxic agents are used. Agglutination should not be confused with rouleaux, in which RBCs stack in a linear pattern (Figure 34.16).

- Cold agglutinins are often associated with *Mycoplasma pneumoniae*, EBV (infectious mononucleosis), and malignancy.

- Differentiate from Raynaud phenomenon with Coombs-positive hemolytic anemia.

- Typical clinical scenario: The patient has hemolytic anemia and acrocyanosis of the ears, tip of the nose, toes, and

fingers. The diagnosis of cold agglutinin syndrome is made by finding RBC agglutination on a peripheral blood smear only if prepared at temperatures <37°C.

Autoimmune Hemolytic Anemia: Warm Agglutinins

Warm agglutinins are IgG antibodies that bind to RBCs at physiologic temperatures rather than primarily in the cold. The direct Coombs test is positive for both IgG and complement component C3. Associated causes include autoimmune disorders (systemic lupus erythematosus), lymphoproliferative disorders (chronic lymphocytic leukemia), drugs, and transfusion. The first general principle in the treatment of warm agglutinin autoimmune hemolytic anemia is to treat the underlying disease (if one can be identified) and to discontinue the use of drugs that have been implicated in hemolysis.

Paroxysmal Cold Hemoglobinuria (Complement-Mediated Lysis)

Paroxysmal cold hemoglobinuria is the least common cause of autoimmune hemolytic anemia. A positive Donath-Landsteiner test is diagnostic; it detects an IgG antibody that binds to RBCs at low temperatures, causing hemolysis. Paroxysmal cold hemoglobinuria is often idiopathic and can be associated with syphilis (congenital and late), mononucleosis, mycoplasma, and childhood exanthems. The overall prognosis is good, and the condition usually resolves after the infection clears.

COOMBS-NEGATIVE HEMOLYTIC ANEMIA

The differential diagnosis of Coombs-negative hemolytic anemia is broad and includes hereditary RBC disorders such as enzymopathies (eg, G6PD deficiency and pyruvate kinase deficiency), hemoglobinopathies, and membrane disorders; paroxysmal nocturnal hemoglobinuria; Wilson disease; and microangiopathic conditions, including thrombotic thrombocytopenic purpura (TTP). Rarely, warm autoimmune hemolytic anemia is Coombs-negative owing to low antibody titers.

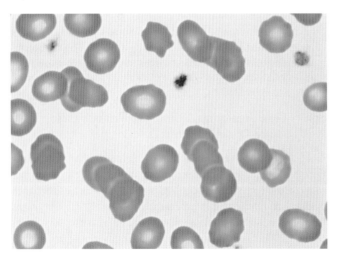

Figure 34.16 Rouleaux. Stacking of red blood cells in a linear pattern distinguishes rouleaux from agglutination (see Figure 34.10). Rouleaux are most commonly associated with hypergammaglobulinemia, especially in human immunodeficiency virus infection or monoclonal plasma cell disorders (peripheral blood smear; Wright-Giemsa). (Courtesy of Curtis A. Hanson, MD, Mayo Clinic, Rochester, Minnesota. Used with permission.)

G6PD DEFICIENCY

G6PD deficiency is the most common RBC enzyme deficiency. It causes decreased levels of glutathione (an antioxidant), making RBCs more sensitive to oxidative damage by infections, toxins (eg, naphthalene in mothballs), or drugs. Except for G6PD and phosphoglycerate kinase deficiences, which are sex-linked, all other RBC enzymopathies are autosomal recessive. Rarely, a female who is heterozygous for abnormal G6PD may be clinically affected because of unfavorable lyonization. G6PD deficiency confers some protection against falciparum malaria and extends to both males and heterozygous females.

Anemia or RBC defects do not occur in the steady state with the most common G6PD variants. Risk of hemolysis increases with concurrent kidney or liver disease, viral or bacterial infection, diabetic ketoacidosis, ingestion of fava beans (seen only in G6PD Mediterranean), and drugs. Even mild infections can cause hemolytic anemia; this occurs more often than drug-induced hemolysis. Drugs that commonly cause hemolytic anemia in G6PD deficiency include antimalarial agents (eg, primaquine and chloroquine), dapsone, sulfonamides, nitrofurantoin, high-dose aspirin, probenecid, and nitrites.

Abnormal laboratory findings include intravascular hemolysis, methemoglobinemia, and methemalbuminemia (specific for intravascular hemolysis due to enzymopathy). Supravital staining for Heinz bodies is a good screening test, but their absence does not rule out the diagnosis. The G6PD assay is the definitive test but should not be done during acute hemolysis in patients of African ancestry. Therapy includes treating the underlying infection and withdrawing use of the offending drug.

- G6PD deficiency is the most common RBC enzyme deficiency and is inherited on the X chromosome.

- G6PD deficiency provides some protection against falciparum malaria.

- Anemia or RBC defects do not occur in the steady state with the most common G6PD variants.

- Hemolysis is induced by infection more commonly than by drugs.

- A good screening test: Heinz bodies seen on supravital staining of peripheral blood.

- Treat underlying infections and withdraw the use of offending drugs.

HEREDITARY SPHEROCYTOSIS

Hereditary spherocytosis is typically an autosomal dominant disorder, but it can be autosomal recessive or sporadic. It is caused by an underlying defect in the RBC cytoskeleton because of a partial gene deficiency (eg, in ankyrin or spectrin). The osmotic fragility test is almost always abnormal and is the most reliable diagnostic test. Features include jaundice, splenomegaly, negative direct Coombs test, spherocytes, and increased osmotic fragility. Pigment gallstones are present in

most patients by age 50. Treatment is splenectomy after the first decade of life for moderate or severe hemolysis, which invariably reduces hemolysis. Asymptomatic adults may be observed if the hemoglobin concentration is greater than 11 g/dL and the reticulocyte count is less than 6%.

- Hereditary spherocytosis: mostly autosomal dominant but may be autosomal recessive or sporadic.

- Splenomegaly is invariably present; pigment gallstones are common.

- Features include negative direct Coombs test and increased osmotic fragility.

- Treatment: splenectomy after the first decade of life for patients with moderate or severe hemolysis.

- Asymptomatic adults with hemoglobin >11 g/dL and a reticulocyte count <6% may be observed.

PAROXYSMAL NOCTURNAL HEMOGLOBINURIA

Paroxysmal nocturnal hemoglobinuria (PNH) is an acquired, chronic, clonal, hematologic stem cell disorder. Blood cells are unusually sensitive to activated complement and are lysed, primarily at night when plasma is more acidotic from sleep-related physiology (eg, relative hypoxia). The disorder is characterized by abnormal hematopoietic stem cells, reticulocytopenia, leukopenia, or thrombocytopenia due to lysis by complement-mediated mechanisms.

A mutation in the *PIGA* gene causes cells in PNH to have a decrease or absence of glycosylphosphatidylinositol (GPI)-linked proteins, including CD14, CD55, and CD59. Clinically, PNH is characterized by chronic intravascular hemolytic anemia, episodic abdominal pain, and venous thrombosis of the portal system, brain, and extremities. Budd-Chiari syndrome (hepatic vein thrombosis) is the main cause of death. In up to 10% of patients, myelodysplasia or acute myeloid leukemia develops. PNH and aplastic anemia can coexist.

The most useful assay for diagnosis of PNH is flow cytometry to establish the absence of the GPI-linked antigens. Up to 60% of patients respond to prednisone; eculizumab is a monoclonal antibody that can be used for long-term therapy for hemolysis in PNH.

- PNH is associated with venous thrombosis, especially Budd-Chiari syndrome, and is the main cause of death.

- Acute myelogenous leukemia or myelodysplasia occurs in 5%-10% of patients.

- Diagnosis: flow cytometry studies for GPI-linked proteins.

THROMBOTIC MICROANGIOPATHIES: DIFFERENTIAL DIAGNOSIS

In microangiopathic hemolytic anemia, RBCs are fragmented and deformed by fibrin deposits in the peripheral

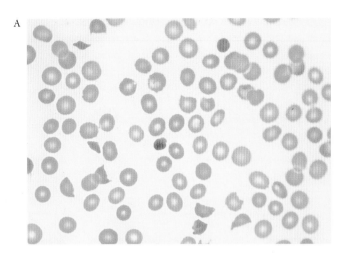

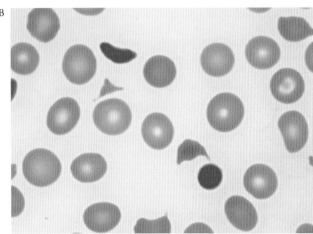

Figure 34.17 Schistocytes. A and B, Fragmented red blood cells are shaped like helmets, triangles, or kites. These are characteristic of any microangiopathic hemolytic process (peripheral blood smear; Wright-Giemsa). (Courtesy of Curtis A. Hanson, MD, Mayo Clinic, Rochester, Minnesota. Used with permission.)

blood (Figure 34.17). Direct Coombs testing is negative. The associated disorders, characterized by widespread microvascular thrombosis leading to end-organ injury, include TTP, hemolytic uremic syndrome (HUS), malignant hypertension, pulmonary hypertension, acute glomerulonephritis, renal allograft rejection, obstetric catastrophes, HELLP syndrome (*h*emolysis, *e*levated *l*iver function tests, and *low* *p*latelet count), disseminated intravascular coagulopathy, collagen vascular diseases, vascular malformations including Kasabach-Merritt syndrome (giant hemangiomas that trap platelets), viral infections (HIV), bacterial infections (*E coli* O157:H7), drug-induced disorders (eg, mitomycin C, quinine, ticlopidine, tacrolimus, cisplatin, and cyclosporine), acute radiation nephropathy, bone marrow transplant, and solid organ transplant.

Thrombotic Thrombocytopenic Purpura

The features of TTP include the pentad of microangiopathic hemolytic anemia, thrombocytopenia, neurologic signs, fever, and kidney abnormalities. Most patients do not manifest all 5 features before the diagnosis is made. The primary criteria

are thrombocytopenia and microangiopathy, and these are sufficient to establish the diagnosis. The anemia is normochromic normocytic, with microangiopathic hemolytic features (Figure 34.17). Direct Coombs test results are negative. Results of coagulation studies are normal or only mildly abnormal, in contrast to results in disseminated intravascular coagulopathy. The cause of TTP is unknown in more than 90% of the patients. TTP is associated with pregnancy and the use of oral contraceptives, HIV infection, cancer, bone marrow transplant, certain chemotherapy drugs (especially mitomycin C and bleomycin), and other drugs (eg, crack cocaine, ticlopidine, and cyclosporine).

Clinically, thrombocytopenia is associated with bleeding in 96% of patients. Neurologic signs often wax and wane and include headache, coma, mental changes, paresis, seizure and coma, aphasia, syncope, visual symptoms, dysarthria, vertigo, agitation, confusion, and delirium. Kidney abnormalities include abnormal urinary sediment and elevated creatinine level. Patients with TTP are deficient in the von Willebrand factor–cleaving protease ADAMTS13. Even when ADAMTS13 assays are available, results can take days to return; thus, the assay is not useful for initial treatment decisions.

Without treatment, more than 90% of patients die of multiorgan failure, but with treatment, 70% to 80% survive the disease and have few or no sequelae. The treatment of choice is plasma exchange. Relapses are also managed with plasma exchange. The management of refractory TTP includes intravenous vincristine, rituximab, splenectomy, or intravenous high-dose γ-globulin. Platelet transfusion should be used only when required for an invasive procedure since it can exacerbate the disease.

- TTP: the pentad of microangiopathic hemolytic anemia, fever, thrombocytopenia, neurologic signs, and renal abnormalities.

- The treatment of choice is plasma exchange.

Hemolytic Uremic Syndrome

HUS is characterized by microangiopathic hemolytic anemia, thrombocytopenia, and acute kidney injury. Fever and neurologic signs are usually not present. It is associated with infections (*E coli* O157:H7, *Shigella dysenteriae*), pregnancy, bone marrow transplant, chemotherapy, and immunosuppressive medications such as cyclosporine. HUS is usually not associated with a decrease in ADAMTS13 activity. Management of HUS is supportive. In adults, treatment with plasma exchange is indicated, but response is variable.

- HUS: hemolytic anemia, thrombocytopenia, and acute kidney injury.

TRANSFUSION REACTIONS

The primary cause of major transfusion reactions and transfusion-related deaths is medical error, which includes

Table 34.3 RISKS OF COMPLICATIONS FROM TRANSFUSIONS IN THE UNITED STATES

COMPLICATION	RISK PER UNIT
Minor allergic reaction	3/100
Circulatory overload	Variable
Febrile, nonhemolytic	3/100
Delayed hemolytic transfusion reaction	1/4,000
TRALI	1/10,000
Acute hemolytic transfusion reaction	$1/2.5 \times 10^4$ to $1/1.0 \times 10^6$
HIV infection	$1/2.1 \times 10^6$
Hepatitis B virus infection	$1/2.0 \times 10^5$
Hepatitis C virus infection	$1/1.9 \times 10^5$
HTLV type I or II infection	$1/2.0 \times 10^5$
West Nile virus infection	Unknown
Bacterial infections	$1/2,000$ to $1/5.0 \times 10^5$
IgA-related anaphylaxis	$1/1.0 \times 10^5$
Graft-vs-host disease	Rare
Immunosuppression	Unknown
Posttransfusion purpura	Rare
Prion infection	Unknown

Abbreviations: HIV, human immunodeficiency virus; HTLV, human T-cell leukemia virus; TRALI, transfusion-related acute lung injury.

bypassed safeguards, similar patient names, and verbal or faxed communications. The major transfusion reactions include acute hemolytic transfusion reactions, transfusions associated with anti-IgA antibodies, transfusion-related acute lung injury (TRALI), adult respiratory distress syndrome, delayed hemolytic transfusion reactions, febrile transfusion reactions, urticarial (allergic) transfusion reactions, and circulatory overload (Table 34.3).

ACUTE HEMOLYTIC TRANSFUSION REACTIONS

Acute hemolytic transfusion reactions are the most life-threatening tranfusion reactions and occur within minutes to hours. The recipient's RBC antibodies (usually IgM) react against the donor's RBCs and cause complement-mediated hemolysis. The most common cause is human error, especially when blood is released emergently. Mortality rate is about 20%; of the fatal transfusion reactions, 85% involve ABO incompatibility. ABO compatibility is illustrated in Table 34.4. Other, nonclerical causes include antibodies not detected before transfusion, such as Kell, Duffy (Fy[a]), and Kidd (Jk[a]). Clinically, patients experience pain at the intravenous site, a sense of impending doom, back pain, abdominal pain, fever, chills, chest pain, hypotension, nausea, flushing, and dyspnea. Direct Coombs testing is positive in most cases.

Complications include oliguria, acute kidney injury, and disseminated intravascular coagulation. Treatment includes immediate termination of the transfusion, vigorous administration of fluids, and furosemide to increase renal cortical blood flow.

- The most common cause of acute hemolytic transfusion reaction is human error.

- Most mortality is related to ABO incompatibility.

ALLERGIC TRANSFUSION REACTIONS

Allergic transfusion reactions are a complication in 3% of transfusions and are caused by a recipient's antibody against foreign-donor serum proteins. Transfusion reactions can also be associated with anti-IgA antibodies. These include anaphylactic reactions, which occur most commonly in patients with IgA deficiency who may have circulating complement-binding anti-IgA antibodies that react with donor IgA. Clinical features are similar to those of an acute hemolytic transfusion reaction. Treatment includes stopping the transfusion and giving antihistamines and conventional antianaphylactic drugs. Transfusion protocols for patients include use of washed RBCs and IgA-deficient plasma.

Table 34.4 BLOOD PRODUCT COMPATIBILITY IN THE ABO SYSTEM[a]

RECIPIENT ABO GROUP	ACCEPTABLE DONOR ABO GROUPS		
	Packed Red Blood Cells	*Platelets & Fresh Frozen Plasma*	*Whole Blood (Rarely Used)*
O	O	AB, A, B, or O	O
A	A or O	A or AB	A
B	B or O	B or AB	B
AB	AB, A, B, or O	AB	AB

[a] Natural alloimmunization against A and B antigens occurs in people lacking these antigens. Upon transfusion of ABO-incompatible blood, preformed antibodies serve as hemagglutinins, resulting in life-threatening acute hemolysis and complement activation. Hemagglutinins are found primarily in plasma; platelets are considered similar to plasma products with respect to ABO compatibility.

- Allergic transfusion reactions are often associated with anti-IgA antibodies.

TRANSFUSION-RELATED ACUTE LUNG INJURY

Transfusion-associated acute respiratory distress syndrome or TRALI results from an interaction between the recipient's leukocytes and donor antileukocyte antibodies. TRALI often is unrecognized and ranks third among causes of transfusion-related deaths. It is characterized by acute respiratory distress during transfusion or within 6 hours after completion of transfusion, hypotension, bilateral pulmonary infiltrates, normal or low pulmonary capillary wedge pressure, no evidence of circulatory overload, and fever. With appropriate supportive care, recovery is rapid, occurring in 24 to 48 hours.

- Treatment of TRALI is primarily supportive care.

DELAYED HEMOLYTIC TRANSFUSION REACTIONS

Delayed hemolytic transfusion reactions (occurring in 1 in 4,000 transfusions) occur because of the inability to detect clinically significant recipient antibodies before transfusion. They usually occur 5 to 10 days after transfusion and are less dangerous than an acute hemolytic reaction. The recipient's plasma contains antibody before transfusion because of a previous transfusion or previous pregnancy. There is evidence of hemolysis and direct Coombs testing is positive. One-third of the patients are asymptomatic, and the reactions are detected by the recurrence of laboratory-detected anemia without clear cause; other patients present with symptoms of anemia, chills, jaundice, and fever. Management consists of monitoring hemoglobin concentration and renal output and avoiding the use of units with the offending antigen in the future.

- Delayed hemolytic transfusion reactions usually occur 5–10 days after transfusion and are less dangerous than acute hemolytic reactions.

FEBRILE TRANSFUSION REACTIONS

Febrile transfusion reactions are characterized by chills, fever, flushing, headache, tachycardia, myalgias, and arthralgias. They usually begin about 1 hour after the transfusion starts and last for 8 to 10 hours. They occur in 1% of all transfusions. Causes include cytokines from leukocytes and platelets against donor antigens and antiserum protein antibodies. Treatment consists of stopping the transfusion to evaluate the patient; initially, a febrile reaction cannot be distinguished from a hemolytic transfusion reaction. Preventive methods include leukoreduction.

- Febrile transfusion reactions usually begin about 1 hour after the start of a transfusion.

CIRCULATORY OVERLOAD

Circulatory overload may cause tightness in the chest, dry cough, and acute edema. It occurs in patients who already have an increased intravascular volume or decreased cardiac reserve, with symptoms generally developing within several hours after transfusion. Management includes slowing the transfusion to 100 mL per hour, placing the patient in the sitting position, and giving diuretics.

- Symptoms of circulatory overload develop within hours of transfusion and affect patients with increased intravascular volume or decreased cardiac reserve.

POSTTRANSFUSION PURPURA

Posttransfusion purpura is a rare syndrome in which the recipient makes antiplatelet antibodies, which cause an abrupt onset of severe thrombocytopenia 5 to 10 days after blood transfusion. Most cases involve patients who lack human platelet antigen 1a and who have an antibody from a previous pregnancy or transfusion.

- Posttransfusion purpura usually occurs in patients who have an antibody from a previous pregnancy or transfusion.

INFECTION

Pathogen transmission may occur with transfusions. These risks and other risks of transfusion are summarized in Table 34.3.

PORPHYRIA

The porphyrias are enzyme disorders that are autosomal dominant with low disease penetrance, except for congenital erythropoietic porphyria (which is autosomal recessive) and porphyria cutanea tarda (which may be acquired and is associated with hepatitis C and hemochromatosis). Most persons remain biochemically and clinically normal throughout most of their lives. Clinical expression is linked to environmental and acquired factors.

Disease manifestations depend on the type of excess porphyrin intermediate. When there is an excess of the earlier precursor molecules (δ-aminolevulinic acid and porphobilinogen), the clinical manifestations are neuropsychiatric, including autonomic dysfunction (abdominal pain, vomiting, constipation, tachycardia, and hypertension), psychiatric symptoms, fever, leukocytosis, and paresthesias. If the excess is in the distal intermediates (uroporphyrins, coproporphyrins, and protoporphyrins), the manifestations are cutaneous (photosensitivity, blister formation, facial hypertrichosis, and hyperpigmentation). If there is excess of both early and late porphyrins, there are both neuropsychiatric and cutaneous manifestations.

Porphobilinogen production and excretion are increased during marked symptoms caused by the 3 neuropathic porphyrias, which include acute intermittent porphyria, hereditary

Table 34.5 COMPARISON OF PORPHYRIAS

PORPHYRIA CUTANEA TARDA	ACUTE INTERMITTENT PORPHYRIA	PORPHYRIA VARIEGATA
Features		
Most common type of porphyria Iron overload Skin lesions on light-exposed areas Hypertrichosis (usually mild) Increased uroporphyrins in urine No neuropathic features	Increased urinary δ-aminolevulinic acid & porpho-bilinogen during acute symptomatic episodes; often normal levels between episodes Neurologic symptoms: abdominal pain of 3–5 days' duration without anatomical cause, focal neuro-logic problems such as polyneuropathy & motor paresis, psychiatric problems with hallucinations, confusion, psychosis, seizures Decreased porphobilinogen deaminase activity Normal protoporphyrin & coproporphyrin in stool	Clinically: photosensitivity, abdom-inal pain, neurologic problems (similar to acute intermittent porphyria) Increased protoporphyrin & coproporphyrin in stool
Associations		
Alcoholic liver disease, chronic hepatitis C, hemochromatosis Estrogens: females, males treated for prostatic carcinoma Hexachlorobenzene	Drugs can precipitate crises (eg, sulfonamides, barbi-turates, alcohol) Menstrual cycle can exacerbate symptoms Infection or surgery can precipitate crisis Inadequate nutrition can precipitate crisis	Common in South Africa (due to founder effect), Holland
Treatment		
Phlebotomy to remove iron Chloroquine Low-dose antimalarials	Avoid prolonged fasting & crash diets Large amounts of carbohydrate (400 g daily) Intravenous hematin Luteinizing hormone–releasing hormone agonists for suppression of hormonal fluctuation	Same as for acute intermittent porphyria

coproporphyria, and porphyria variegata. In hereditary coproporphyria and porphyria variegata, there is an accumu-lation of coproporphyrinogen/coproporphyrin or protopor-phyrinogen/protoporphyrin and a concomitant increase in δ-aminolevulinic acid and porphobilinogen. In the acute por-phyrias, determine the 24-hour urinary porphobilinogen level during an attack. Patients with acute intermittent porphyria lack skin lesions. It is important to check fecal porphyrins in protoporphyria, porphyria variegata, and coproporphyria. An elevated coproporphyrin level alone, therefore, does not sup-port a diagnosis of porphyria. The porphyrias are compared in Table 34.5.

- In suspected acute porphyria, determine the 24-hour urinary porphobilinogen level during the acute episode.

- Mild coproporphyrin elevation is nonspecific and not diagnostic of porphyria.

- Porphyria cutanea tarda is associated with chronic hepatitis C and with hemochromatosis.

SUMMARY

- Iron deficiency anemia should prompt a search for the underlying cause.

- Hemolytic anemias may be hereditary or acquired, from factors intrinsic or extrinsic to the RBC, and Coombs-positive or Coombs-negative.

- The most common cause of acute hemolytic transfusion reaction is human error.

35.

HEMATOLOGY: HEMOSTASIS[a]

Rajiv K. Pruthi, MBBS

GOALS

- Understand the approach to laboratory evaluation of a bleeding patient.

- Understand how to recognize, diagnose, and treat congenital and acquired bleeding disorders.

- Understand how to differentiate between various causes of thrombocytopenia, and know how to manage the conditions.

OVERVIEW OF COAGULATION SYSTEM

The 2 essential functions of the coagulation system (maintaining hemostasis and preventing and limiting thrombosis) are served by the procoagulant and anticoagulant components. Vascular injury results in activation of the phases of hemostasis, including vasospasm, platelet plug formation (platelet activation, adhesion, and aggregation), and fibrin clot formation (by activation of coagulation factors in the procoagulant system). The anticoagulant system controls excessive clot formation, while the fibrinolytic system breaks down and remodels blood clots.

EVALUATION FOR A BLEEDING DISORDER

The best screening tool to evaluate for a bleeding disorder is a thorough clinical evaluation (personal and family hemostatic history and physical examination). Inquiry into the presence and age at onset of spontaneous bleeding (epistaxis, easy bruising, joint bleeding, etc), unusual or unexpected posttraumatic or surgical bleeding (including dental extractions), and family history may suggest the presence of a bleeding disorder. A thorough clinical evaluation should also include review of

medications and coexisting medical problems to identify clinical risk factors for thrombosis.

- The best screening tool to evaluate for a bleeding disorder is a thorough personal and family hemostatic history and physical examination.

LABORATORY TESTING TO EVALUATE A BLEEDING PATIENT

Tests include a complete blood cell count (CBC), prothrombin time (PT), activated partial thromboplastin time (aPTT), and fibrinogen. Additional testing that may not be generally available includes assays for von Willebrand disease (vWD), coagulation factor assays, factor XIII (FXIII) assays, and platelet function tests.

PT (International Normalized Ratio)

The PT assesses the extrinsic and final common pathways of the procoagulant cascade (Figure 35.1). Prolonged PT results from deficiencies or inhibitors of clotting factors. The PT is mainly useful as a monitoring test for warfarin anticoagulation and as an initial screening test for patients who have bleeding symptoms. The international normalized ratio reduces interlaboratory variation of the PT and is calculated and reported by the laboratory. There is no role for routine PT testing in the preoperative patient.

- The PT assesses the extrinsic and final common pathways.

- The main utility of the international normalized ratio is for monitoring warfarin anticoagulation.

Activated Partial Thromboplastin Time

The aPTT assesses the intrinsic and final common pathways (Figure 35.1); deficiencies or inhibitors of clotting factors within the intrinsic and final common pathways result in prolongation of the aPTT. The aPTT is commonly used to monitor unfractionated heparin (UFH) therapy and direct thrombin inhibitor (DTI) therapy (eg, argatroban and lepirudin) and as

---

[a] Portions previously published in Pruthi RK. A practical approach to genetic testing for von Willebrand disease. Mayo Clin Proc. 2006 May;81(5):679–91; and Kamal AH, Tefferi A, Pruthi RK. How to interpret and pursue an abnormal prothrombin time, activated partial thromboplastin time, and bleeding time in adults. Mayo Clin Proc. 2007 Jul;82(7):864–73. Used with permission of Mayo Foundation for Medical Education and Research.

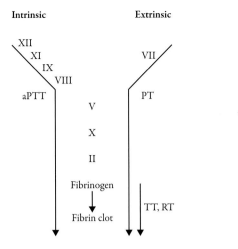

Figure 35.1 Coagulation Cascade. aPTT indicates activated partial thromboplastin time; PT, prothrombin time; RT, reptilase time; TT, thrombin time.

an initial screening test for the presence of lupus anticoagulant or for patients who have bleeding symptoms.

- The aPTT assesses the intrinsic pathway.
- The aPTT is commonly used to monitor UFH and DTI therapy.

Bleeding Time

Use of the bleeding time (BT) test has been discontinued in many hospitals. A review of multiple studies led to the following conclusions:

1. In the absence of the clinical history of a bleeding disorder, BT is not a useful predictor of risk of hemorrhage with surgical procedures.

2. Normal BT does not exclude the possibility of excessive hemorrhage with invasive procedures.

3. BT cannot reliably identify patients exposed to aspirin or nonsteroidal anti-inflammatory drugs.

Approach to a Prolonged PT or aPTT

Step 1: Exclude artifactual causes (elevated hematocrit; nonfasting, lipemic sample; or heparin contamination of the specimen).

Step 2: Perform a mixing study in a 1:1 ratio with normal pooled plasma.

Step 3a: Correction of the clotting time (ie, the aPTT normalizes) implies a coagulation factor deficiency; follow-up factor assays are then performed.

Step 3b: Inhibition of the aPTT (ie, aPTT may shorten but does not normalize) implies the presence of an inhibitor, including the following:

1. Medications (eg, heparins and DTIs)

2. Specific factor inhibitors (eg, factor VIII [FVIII] or factor V inhibitors)

3. Nonspecific inhibitors (eg, lupus anticoagulants)

Appropriate follow-up testing typically leads to the diagnosis of the underlying cause of the prolongation of the PT and aPTT.

Bleeding Disorders Not Detected With PT and aPTT

Disorders that are not detected with the PT and aPTT include the following:

1. Qualitative platelet defects (requires specialized platelet function testing)

2. vWD (requires assays for von Willebrand factor [vWF])

3. FXIII deficiency (requires specialized FXIII screening or functional assays)

4. Deficiency of antiplasmin and plasminogen activator inhibitor 1 (requires specific assays)

OVERVIEW OF BLEEDING DISORDERS

Bleeding disorders consist of the following:

1. Clotting factor deficiencies or inhibitors

2. Vascular bleeding disorders

3. Platelet disorders (quantitative and qualitative)

Each of these is broadly classified into congenital disorders and acquired disorders.

CONGENITAL PLASMATIC BLEEDING DISORDERS (FACTOR DEFICIENCIES)

Of the congenital plasmatic bleeding disorders, vWD is the most common. Others include hemophilia A, hemophilia B, and hemophilia C. Other factor deficiency states are rare (Table 35.1). All clotting factors are produced by the liver except vWF, which is produced by vascular endothelial cells and megakaryocytes.

von Willebrand Disease

Definition
vWD refers to a deficiency or dysfunction of vWF.

Classification
vWD is classified according to whether the defect is quantitative (types I and III) or qualitative (types IIA, IIB, IIM, and IIN).

Table 35.1 CONGENITAL BLEEDING DISORDERS

CONGENITAL DISORDER	DEFICIENT FACTOR	PT	aPTT	PREVALENCE	MODE OF INHERITANCE
Hemophilia A	Factor VIII	NL	Prol	1:5,000[a]	X-linked recessive
Hemophilia B	Factor IX	NL	Prol	1:30,000[a]	X-linked recessive
Hemophilia C	Factor XI	NL	Prol	Up to 4%[b]	Autosomal recessive
von Willebrand disease	von Willebrand factor	NL	NL or Prol	Up to 1%	Autosomal dominant or recessive
Factor VII deficiency		Prol	NL	1:500,000	Autosomal recessive
Rare coagulation factor deficiencies					
Factor V		Prol	Prol	1:1 million	Autosomal recessive
Factor II		Prol	NL or Prol	Rare	Autosomal recessive
Factor X		Prol	NL or Prol	1:500,000	Autosomal recessive
Factor XIII		NL	NL	Rare	Autosomal recessive
Combined factors VIII & V		Prol	Prol	Rare	Autosomal recessive

Abbreviations: aPTT, activated partial thromboplastin time; NL, normal; Prol, prolonged; PT, prothrombin time.

[a] Live male births.

[b] Among Ashkenazi Jews.

Biochemistry

Endothelial cells and platelets store vWF. After secretion, the ultra-large-molecular-weight multimers of vWF, the most hemostatically active, are cleaved into multimers of smaller size by a protease, ADAMTS13 (ADAM metallopeptidase with thrombospondin type 1 motif, 13).

Function of vWF

vWF mediates platelet adhesion and aggregation. It acts as a carrier protein for FVIII, protecting it from proteolytic inactivation.

Clinical Features

Patients who have mild vWD may be asymptomatic and bleed only when challenged with trauma or minor surgery (eg, dental extraction) or major surgery.

Patients who have severe vWD may have spontaneous bleeding. Spontaneous bleeding is typically mucocutaneous (bruising, epistaxis, hematuria, gastrointestinal tract hemorrhage); in type III vWD, bleeding occurs in joints and soft tissue. Bleeding may be exacerbated by the use of aspirin or nonsteroidal analgesics.

Laboratory Testing

Laboratory testing (Table 35.2) includes testing for vWF antigen (vWF:Ag), vWF activity, and FVIII activity. If initial results are abnormal, vWF multimer analyses are performed to subtype vWD:

1. Type I vWD—mild to moderate reduction in vWF:Ag level and activity

2. Type II vWD—disproportionate reduction in activity of the vWF called the *ristocetin cofactor* (RCoF) compared with vWF:Ag

3. Type III vWD—absent vWF

Variables Affecting vWF Levels

Healthy people with blood group O have vWF levels that are 25% to 30% lower than in people with blood groups A, B, or AB and thus may receive a misdiagnosis of vWD. Therefore, ABO typing should be part of the initial testing.

Acquired defects of vWF (ie, *acquired von Willebrand syndrome*) may be seen in patients with aortic stenosis, myeloproliferative disorders, and monoclonal protein disorders. The syndrome mimics congenital type II vWD.

Table 35.2 STEPWISE APPROACH TO ASSESSMENT FOR VON WILLEBRAND DISEASE

1. Bleeding history

2. Complete blood cell count

3. vWD profile testing
   vWF:Ag
   RCoF
   VIII:c

4. ABO blood group

5. Optional tests if initial data suggest vWD
   vWF multimers
   vWF:CBA
   vWF:VIIIB
   RIPA

6. Genetic tests if indicated

Abbreviations: Ag, antigen; CBA, collagen-binding assay; VIIIB, factor VIII binding assay; VIII:c, factor VIII coagulant activity; RCoF, ristocetin cofactor; RIPA, ristocetin-induced platelet aggregation: vWD, von Willebrand disease; vWF, von Willebrand factor.

Short-term physical exertion, inflammation, malignancy, hyperthyroidism, estrogens, and pregnancy increase vWF levels to normal and may mask a diagnosis of vWD. Hypothyroidism is associated with reduced vWF levels.

Type IIB vWD is associated with thrombocytopenia. Type IIN vWD results from mutations in the FVIII binding domain of vWF. This subtype may be mistaken for mild hemophilia A.

- Type I vWD: mild to moderate reduction in vWF:Ag level and activity.
- Type II vWD: disproportionate reduction in activity of RCoF compared with vWF:Ag.
- Type III vWD: vWF is absent.
- ABO typing should be part of the initial testing.

Inheritance of vWD

Type I vWD is inherited as an autosomal dominant trait with variable penetrance. Types IIA, IIB, and IIM vWD are inherited as autosomal dominant traits. Type III vWD and type IIN (Normandy) vWD are inherited as autosomal recessive traits.

Management

Upon establishment of a diagnosis of vWD, a desmopressin acetate (DDAVP) treatment trial should be performed for patients with types I, IIA, or IIM vWD. Intravenous (IV) infusion of 0.3 mcg/kg body weight releases vWF from its storage sites; measure levels 60 minutes after infusion.

- Side effects include facial flushing, headache, mild decrease in blood pressure, mild tachycardia, and hyponatremia. Doses repeated at intervals shorter than 24 hours may result in a decrease or loss of response (tachyphylaxis) and syndrome of inappropriate antidiuresis.

Desmopressin is generally not helpful for patients with type IIB vWD since the release of endogenous vWF worsens thrombocytopenia. Patients with type III vWD do not respond to desmopressin and should not undergo a desmopressin trial.

For patients who do respond, desmopressin is a reasonable alternative for prevention or treatment of minor bleeding, for minor procedures such as dental extraction, and for the management of menorrhagia in women with vWD. An intranasal formulation of desmopressin is also available. For patients who do not respond to desmopressin and for those in whom it is contraindicated, administration of purified plasma-derived vWF concentrates is the therapy of choice.

The goals for managing vWD include preventing and treating hemorrhage. General measures include the following:

1. Provide patient education
2. Recommend a medical condition identification tag

3. Generate treatment guidelines for managing bleeding
4. Refer to a comprehensive hemophilia treatment center for periodic follow-up

Specific measures include the following:

1. Administer desmopressin
2. Administer adjunctive ε-aminocaproic acid or vWF concentrates preoperatively to prevent bleeding or to manage bleeding
3. Administer vWF concentrates

- A desmopressin treatment trial should be performed for patients with types I, IIA, or IIM vWD.
- Desmopressin is generally not helpful for patients with type IIB vWD and should not be used in patients with type III vWD.
- For patients who do not respond to desmopressin and for those in whom it is contraindicated, administration of purified plasma-derived vWF concentrates is the therapy of choice.

Hemophilia A and Hemophilia B

Hemophilia A and hemophilia B are clinically indistinguishable X-linked recessive bleeding disorders. Hemophilia A is due to a deficiency in blood coagulation FVIII, and hemophilia B is due to a deficiency in factor IX (FIX).

Classification

Hemophilia is classified according to levels of FVIII and FIX:

1. Severe (<1%)
2. Moderate (1%-5%)
3. Mild (>5%-40%)

Clinical Features

Patients who have mild hemophilia seldom experience spontaneous hemorrhage but will bleed after trauma or surgery; rarely, they may not receive a diagnosis of hemophilia until adulthood.

Patients who have moderate hemophilia infrequently experience spontaneous bleeding but typically bleed after minor trauma and surgery.

Patients who have severe hemophilia frequently experience spontaneous bleeding, including hemarthrosis, soft tissue hematomas, and intracranial hemorrhage in addition to minor hemorrhage such as epistaxis and ecchymoses. Regular prophylactic administration of vWF concentrates to patients with severe disease has reduced the frequency and associated chronic complications related to bleeding.

Management

At the initial diagnosis of mild or moderate hemophilia A, as with vWD, a desmopressin trial is performed; FVIII levels are checked before and 1 hour after infusion. For patients who have hemophilia A and respond to desmopressin, administer desmopressin for minor hemorrhage or for prophylaxis and treatment of minor surgical hemorrhage. Use recombinant or plasma-derived FVIII concentrates as therapy for *major* hemorrhages and as prophylaxis for major surgery.

Desmopressin is not used for hemophilia B; instead, recombinant or plasma-derived FIX concentrates are used.

Inheritance

Hemophilia A and hemophilia B are X-linked recessive bleeding disorders.

Complications of Treatment

Transfusion-transmitted viral infections (eg, viral hepatitis, human immunodeficiency virus [HIV] infection) occur, although with contemporary clotting factor manufacturing processes and the introduction of recombinant factors, these are rare.

Recurrent hemarthrosis (in severe hemophilia and in patients who have FVIII or FIX inhibitors) leads to premature degenerative joint disease.

Development of FVIII and FIX inhibitors is the most serious complication. Standard FVIII and FIX concentrates are ineffective, and bypassing agents (eg, recombinant factor VIIa or activated prothrombin complex concentrates) are required for management of surgical bleeding and hemorrhage.

Factor VII Deficiency

Factor VII (FVII) deficiency is typically a mild bleeding disorder that is usually detected with a preoperative prolonged PT. FVII levels as low as 10% of normal may be undetected for many years. Bleeding symptoms are similar to those of hemophilia. Recombinant factor VIIa is the treatment of choice for preventing and treating hemorrhage; however, fresh frozen plasma is also an option.

Factor XI Deficiency (Hemophilia C)

Factor XI (FXI) deficiency is a rare autosomal recessive disorder that is prevalent in Ashkenazi Jews. It is a mild bleeding disorder; patients usually present after surgery or trauma or after starting therapy with antiplatelet agents or anticoagulants.

Bleeding symptoms do not correlate well with FXI levels (ie, patients with mild deficiencies may have significant bleeding symptoms, whereas patients with more severe deficiencies may remain asymptomatic until after surgery or initiation of an anticoagulant or antiplatelet agent).

Fresh frozen plasma is the treatment of choice for prevention and treatment of hemorrhage. FXI concentrates are in clinical trials.

FXIII Deficiency

Severe FXIII deficiency has an autosomal recessive inheritance pattern and is characterized by significant bleeding but normal screening test results (PT, aPTT). Other characteristics include umbilical cord bleeding, delayed wound healing, delayed hemorrhage, and recurrent pregnancy loss. Cryoprecipitate and FXIII concentrates are the treatment of choice for prevention and treatment of hemorrhage.

- With significant bleeding and normal screening tests, think of severe FXIII deficiency.

- Cryoprecipitate and FXIII concentrates are the treatment of choice for prevention and treatment of hemorrhage.

Factor Deficiencies That Prolong the aPTT But Do Not Result in Hemorrhage

Deficiencies of factor XII, high-molecular-weight kininogen, and prekallikrein can result in a marked prolongation of the aPTT, yet even severe deficiencies are not risk factors for hemorrhage. Their roles in hemostasis are being defined.

ACQUIRED BLEEDING DISORDERS

Acquired bleeding disorders can result from decreased production of coagulation factors by the liver (as in liver disease), increased consumption of coagulation factors (as in disseminated intravascular coagulation [DIC] and fibrinolysis), or the development of inhibitors against coagulation factors (Table 35.3).

Liver Disease

Since most coagulation factors (except vWF) are produced in the liver, hepatocellular damage and liver failure lead to decreased production of clotting factors and a bleeding tendency. Supportive management includes replenishment of the deficient coagulation factors with fresh frozen plasma (cryoprecipitate is a more concentrated form for fibrinogen and FXIII) until the liver recovers or is replaced by a transplanted liver.

Disseminated Intravascular Coagulation

DIC is a dynamic process with various causes that result in microvascular thrombosis and consumption of clotting factors (Box 35.1).

Clinical Features

DIC should be suspected in a patient presenting with underlying conditions known to predispose to DIC (Box 35.1). Most patients present with new onset of bleeding; occasionally, patients present with thrombosis or both bleeding and thrombosis.

Table 35.3 CAUSES OF ACQUIRED COAGULATION FACTOR DEFICIENCIES

CAUSE OF DEFICIENCY	DEFICIENT FACTOR
Warfarin	Vitamin K–dependent factors
Decreased nutritional intake or malabsorption	Vitamin K–dependent factors
Liver failure	Multiple factors
Amyloid	Factor X
Myeloproliferative disease	Factor V
Acquired von Willebrand syndrome	von Willebrand factor & factor VIII
Disseminated intravascular coagulation	Multiple factors

Bleeding manifestations include bleeding from surgical wounds and venipuncture sites, ecchymoses, petechiae, hematomas, vaginal bleeding, or hemorrhage from the gastrointestinal tract or genitourinary system.

Thrombotic manifestations occur less frequently than bleeding and include necrotic skin lesions, venous thromboembolism (deep vein thrombosis and pulmonary embolism), and acute arterial occlusions (stroke and myocardial infarction).

Pathophysiology

An understanding of the pathophysiology of DIC helps with understanding laboratory testing and management. The

---

Box 35.1 CAUSES OF DIC

Acute & subacute DIC
   Malignancies (hematologic & solid organ)
   Infection or sepsis (bacterial)
   Obstetric complications (placental abruption, amniotic fluid embolism)
   Massive trauma
   Burns
   Advanced liver disease
   Snake bite
   Hemolytic transfusion reaction
Chronic DIC
   Solid tumors
   Obstetric complications (retained dead fetus)
   Advanced liver disease
Localized causes of systemic DIC
   Aortic aneurysm
   Giant hemangiomas

Abbreviation: DIC, disseminated intravascular coagulation.

---

underlying disease (Box 35.1) stimulates the procoagulant system, generating thrombin and resulting in consumption of coagulation factors and platelets. The fibrinolytic system also is activated, converting plasminogen to plasmin. Plasmin prevents stabilization of fibrin clots (resulting in circulating fibrin monomers) and degrades existing fibrin clots and fibrinogen-releasing cleavage products called D-dimers. The circulating fibrin monomers are soluble and thus form weak clots.

Laboratory Testing

Laboratory findings in suspected DIC vary, and there is no single diagnostic laboratory test. Clinical findings need to be interpreted along with laboratory data. Typical laboratory findings in DIC include thrombocytopenia, prolonged PT and aPTT, low fibrinogen due to consumption, and increased D-dimers and soluble fibrin monomer complexes.

Management

Principles of management include identifying and treating underlying disease while managing the coagulopathy.

Blood Component Replacement Therapy

Observation may be reasonable for patients who have low-grade compensated DIC with mild coagulopathy and no bleeding.

For patients who have symptomatic hemorrhage or abnormal laboratory results and for those at risk for bleeding, therapy includes transfusion of blood components:

1. If fibrinogen is low (<100 mg/dL), give cryoprecipitate.

2. If PT and aPTT are markedly prolonged (suggesting significant coagulation factor deficiency states), give fresh frozen plasma.

3. If the platelet count is low (<30×10^9/L or <50×10^9/L for bleeding patients), give platelet concentrates.

The target platelet count is greater than 20×10^9/L to 30×10^9/L, especially if the patient is bleeding or undergoing procedures. Monitor transfusion therapy with a CBC, PT, aPTT, and fibrinogen level 60 minutes after a transfusion and every 6 to 8 hours thereafter.

Ancillary Therapies for DIC

Although *UFH* inhibits thrombin and interrupts the cycle of consumptive coagulopathy, it is also associated with hemorrhage, including intracranial hemorrhage. Thus, in acute DIC, heparin usually has a limited role, if any (except with acute DIC associated with promyelocytic leukemia), but it may have a role in chronic DIC as seen with solid tumors, the retained dead fetus syndrome, aortic aneurysm, and giant hemangiomas. *Recombinant activated protein C* improves mortality among patients with severe sepsis.

Antithrombin concentrate has not been shown to improve mortality among patients with DIC. *Fibrinolysis inhibitors*, such as ε-aminocaproic acid or tranexamic acid, are generally contraindicated in DIC.

Acquired von Willebrand Syndrome

Acquired von Willebrand syndrome is an acquired quantitative or qualitative abnormality of vWF that is associated with monoclonal protein disorders, myeloproliferative disease, hypothyroidism, and other malignancies. Occasionally no underlying disease is found. Management consists of infusion of vWF concentrates to prevent and treat hemorrhage; desmopressin is seldom effective.

Acquired (Autoimmune) Hemophilia

In acquired (autoimmune) hemophilia, the development of FVIII inhibitors in previously healthy people results in a potentially life-threatening bleeding disorder. Management consists of maintaining hemostasis with special factor concentrates (activated prothrombin complex concentrates or recombinant FVIIa) and immunosuppression (glucocorticoids, cytotoxic chemotherapy, and anti-CD20 antibody [rituximab]).

Platelets are produced in the bone marrow and, after circulating for about 7 to 10 days, are destroyed in the reticuloendothelial system. Thrombocytopenia is most commonly acquired and poses a risk of bleeding. It commonly occurs as a result of decreased production or accelerated destruction. When thrombocytopenia occurs for the first time, the diagnosis of pseudothrombocytopenia should be excluded with examination of a peripheral blood smear. Rarely, thrombocytopenia is congenital.

Pseudothrombocytopenia

Pseudothrombocytopenia is due to EDTA-induced platelet clumping; platelets range from 50×10^9/L to 100×10^9/L. Repeat the CBC in a citrate tube to prevent clumping. A peripheral blood smear (Figure 35.2) is useful to detect clumping.

After exclusion of pseudothrombocytopenia, other causes are broadly classified as accelerated platelet destruction, decreased platelet production, or splenic sequestration (careful physical examination for splenomegaly will help exclude this possibility) (Box 35.2). Potentially serious causes for thrombocytopenia should be excluded, including heparin-induced thrombocytopenia (HIT), thrombotic thrombocytopenic purpura, and the HELLP syndrome (*h*emolysis, *e*levated *l*iver enzymes, and *l*ow *p*latelet count) occurring in pregnancy.

Abnormally large platelets (Figure 35.3) are seen in immune thrombocytopenia, clonal myeloid disorders (eg,

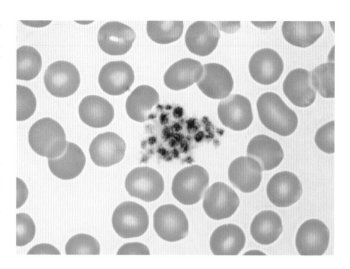

Figure 35.2 Platelet Clumping (Agglutination). Agglutination is a cause of artifactual thrombocytopenia. Drawing the blood in a citrate tube rather than an EDTA-anticoagulated tube usually eliminates this in vitro phenomenon (Wright-Giemsa). (Courtesy of Curtis A. Hanson, MD, Mayo Clinic. Used with permission.)

essential thrombocythemia), and congenital disorders of platelet synthesis and function (eg, conditions associated with mutations of the *MYH9* gene [eg, May-Hegglin anomaly] and Bernard-Soulier syndrome).

Thrombocytopenia Due to Increased Platelet Destruction

Autoimmune Thrombocytopenic Purpura

Autoimmune thrombocytopenic purpura, formerly called idiopathic thrombocytopenic purpura, is an autoimmune disease characterized by thrombocytopenia, usually with a normal white blood cell count and hemoglobin concentration (Table 35.4).

The diagnosis of autoimmune thrombocytopenic purpura is a diagnosis of exclusion:

1. Examine a peripheral blood smear to exclude microangiopathy.

2. In mild to moderate thrombocytopenia, exclude congenital thrombocytopenia. (Type IIB vWD is typically associated with thrombocytopenia, but these patients usually have a lifelong personal and family history of bleeding and bruising.)

3. Evaluate for heavy alcohol use and drugs associated with thrombocytopenia.

4. Test for HIV in patients with risk factors.

Clinical Manifestations

In adults, autoimmune thrombocytopenic purpura has an insidious onset, often with incidental diagnosis on routine CBC. Patients present with petechiae and purpura, mucous membrane hemorrhage, and cerebromeningeal bleeding. Up

Pseudothrombocytopenia
Dilutional
    Massive transfusion
    Pregnancy
Increased destruction
    Immune
        Autoimmune
        Idiopathic
        Secondary (drug-induced, connective tissue diseases)
    Nonimmune
        Consumptive (DIC)
        Sepsis
Decreased production
    Bone marrow failure syndromes
        Primary: anaplastic anemia
        Secondary: metastatic disease, hematologic malignancies
    Nutritional
        Vitamin B_{12} & folate deficiency
    Infections
        Viral (HIV infection, CMV infection, viral hepatitis)

Abbreviations: CMV, cytomegalovirus; DIC, disseminated intravascular coagulation; HIV, human immunodeficiency virus.

to 60% of adults progress to a chronic state of autoimmune thrombocytopenic purpura. Only 10% of patients have splenomegaly. If splenomegaly is present, one should think of other causes.

Laboratory Findings
In most patients, the platelet count is less than 50×10^9/L, and in 30% it is less than 10×10^9/L (spontaneous bleeding may occur at this level). The mean platelet volume is increased.

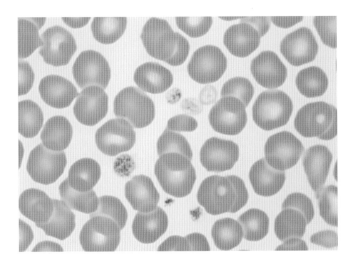

Figure 35.3 Giant Platelets. Giant platelets may be associated with congenital platelet synthesis disorders, acquired clonal myeloid disorders, or immune thrombocytopenia (Wright-Giemsa). (Courtesy of Curtis A. Hanson, MD, Mayo Clinic. Used with permission.)

Antibodies to specific platelet-membrane glycoproteins, usually the glycoprotein IIb/IIIa complex, and platelet-associated IgG can be detected in most patients but are not necessary for diagnosis or treatment.

In patients older than 60, a bone marrow examination is appropriate to rule out another disorder causing thrombocytopenia (such as a myelodysplastic syndrome, which is more common in older patients). Bone marrow examination in autoimmune thrombocytopenic purpura shows a normal to increased number of megakaryocytes.

Treatment
The American Society of Hematology guidelines for treatment are as follows:

1. Patients with platelet counts of 50×10^9/L or higher do not routinely require treatment.

2. Patients with platelet counts less than 50×10^9/L but greater than 30×10^9/L should be treated if there is mucous membrane bleeding or risk factors for bleeding, including hypertension, peptic ulcer disease, and a vigorous lifestyle.

3. Patients with platelet counts less than 30×10^9/L should be treated.

   a. Prednisone is the mainstay of initial treatment; initially, 70% of patients respond, with a 40% chance of long-term remission (prednisone 1 mg/kg daily for up to 1 month).

   b. If bleeding is severe, treat with IV immunoglobulin (1 g/kg daily for 2 days) and platelets; high-dose IV corticosteroids can also be considered (eg, methylprednisolone, 1 g daily for 2–3 consecutive days; initial response rate is 80%).

Splenectomy, the treatment of choice for steroid-refractory autoimmune thrombocytopenic purpura, removes the predominant site of antibody production and platelet destruction; the likelihood of remission is 75%, with about 60% of patients remaining in long-term remission. Pneumococcal, meningococcal, and *Haemophilus influenzae* vaccines should be administered 2 weeks before splenectomy. Absence of Howell-Jolly bodies on a postsplenectomy peripheral blood smear suggests an accessory spleen, and accessory splenectomy can result in remission. Pulsed dexamethasone (40 mg daily for 4 sequential days every 28 days for 12 months) is an option for the treatment of resistant autoimmune thrombocytopenic purpura or disease relapse. Other agents used in refractory cases include azathioprine, cyclophosphamide, colchicine, cyclosporine, rituximab, vincristine, vinblastine, anti-Rh_O(D) immune globulin, danazol, and immunoadsorption apheresis on staphylococcal protein A columns.

Novel agents approved for use in patients with corticosteroid-refractory autoimmune thrombocytopenic purpura include oral (eltrombopag) and parenteral (romiplostim) thrombopoietin receptor agonists.

Table 35.4 AUTOIMMUNE THROMBOCYTOPENIC PURPURA

CHARACTERISTIC	ACUTE	CHRONIC
Presentation	Abrupt onset of petechiae, purpura, mucosal bleeding	Insidious petechiae, menorrhagia
Usual age	Children (2–6 y)	Adults (20–40 y)
Female to male ratio	1:1	3:1
Antecedent infection	Common (85%) Typically an upper respiratory tract infection	Uncommon
Platelet count, ×10⁹/L	<20	30–80
Duration	2–6 wk	Months to years
Spontaneous remission	80% within 6 mo	Uncommon, fluctuates

Adapted from Thienelt CD, Calverley DC. Thrombocytopenia caused by immunologic platelet destruction. In: Greer JP, Foerster J, Rodgers GM, Paraskevas F, Glader B, Arber DA, Means RT Jr, editors. 12th ed. Vol 2. Wintrobe's clinical hematology. Philadelphia (PA): Wolters Kluwer Health/Lippincott Williams & Wilkins; c2009. p. 1292–1313. Used with permission.

- Spontaneous bleeding may occur with platelet counts <10×10⁹/L.

- Autoimmune thrombocytopenic purpura is a diagnosis of exclusion.

- Examine the peripheral blood smear (exclude microangiopathy).

- Consider discontinuing use of any drug that may cause the disease.

- A bone marrow examination is appropriate to establish the diagnosis of autoimmune thrombocytopenic purpura in patients older than 60 years.

- In autoimmune thrombocytopenic purpura with severe bleeding, IV immunoglobulin is the treatment of choice, with platelet transfusions and high-dose corticosteroids.

- Corticosteroids are the initial treatment, followed by splenectomy in relapsed or refractory cases.

Drug-Induced Thrombocytopenia

Drug-induced thrombocytopenia is caused by direct marrow toxicity or by haptens bound to a carrier protein. Common drugs include heparin, quinidine, quinine, valproic acid, gold, trimethoprim-sulfamethoxazole, amphotericin B, carbamazepine, chlorothiazide, chlorpropamide, procainamide, rifampin, and vancomycin. Glycoprotein IIb/IIIa antagonists have also been implicated. HIT is one of the most lethal drug-induced thrombocytopenias.

Drug-induced thrombocytopenia subsides in 4 to 14 days after use of the drug is discontinued—except for gold-induced

thrombocytopenia, which may take much longer. In contrast, viral-induced thrombocytopenia resolves in 2 weeks to 3 months.

Heparin-Induced Thrombocytopenia

Type I

Type I HIT is a benign, nonimmune-mediated thrombocytopenia that occurs in association with UFH, typically in the first 4 days of heparin therapy.

Type II

Type II HIT is a more serious, immune-mediated thrombocytopenia.

Incidence

The incidence of HIT is 1% to 7.8% with UFH (the incidence is lower with low-molecular-weight heparin [LMWH]). It can develop at any dose of heparin, including low-dose prophylaxis for venous thrombosis postoperatively.

Clinical Presentation

HIT is more common with UFH than with LMWH. The onset of thrombocytopenia varies:

1. Typical: 4 to 14 days after initiating heparin administration

2. Rapid: less than 4 days in patients with recent (within the preceeding 3 months) heparin exposure

3. Delayed: 2 to 3 weeks after discontinuation of heparin administration

The platelet count decreases 50% from baseline (ie, from before heparin administration). Thrombosis may or may not occur and may be venous (more common) or arterial.

Pathophysiology

IgG antibodies to platelet factor 4–heparin complexes result in platelet activation, generation of thrombin, and a high risk of thrombosis.

Rare Presentations and Complications

1. Warfarin-induced venous gangrene with limb damage

2. Acute platelet activation syndromes (fevers, chills, or transient amnesia) 5–30 minutes after an IV bolus of heparin

3. Painful, necrotic skin lesions at the site of the injection of heparin

Laboratory Testing

1. Functional assays (serotonin release assay)

2. Antigen assays (heparin-dependent antibody against platelet factor 4)

Anticoagulant Management
Administer a DTI: lepirudin, bivalirudin, or argatroban (Box 35.3). Argatroban is the treatment of choice for patients with renal insufficiency because of hepatic elimination; in contrast, for patients with hepatic failure, lepirudin (renally excreted) is preferred.

- Heparin is the drug that most commonly causes thrombocytopenia.
- HIT type II requires discontinuation of the use of *all* heparin, including LMWH.
- Given the high risk of thrombosis, initiation of a DTI should be strongly considered.

Chemotherapy-Associated Thrombocytopenia

The threshold for platelet transfusion is 10×10^9/L unless other risk factors for bleeding (eg, fever, mucosal lesion) are present. Interleukin 11 (oprelvekin) is modestly effective but is associated with fluid retention and atrial dysrhythmias. Pharmacologic agents stimulating the thrombopoietin receptor are likely to be approved soon.

Thrombocytopenia Due to Decreased Platelet Production

Thrombocytopenia caused by decreased platelet production typically occurs as the result of disorders affecting the bone marrow. These can be broadly classified as follows:

1. Primary marrow or metastatic malignancy (eg, solid tumor, leukemia, lymphoma) or infections (eg, HIV infection, cytomegalovirus infection, sepsis, viral hepatitis)

---

2. Inflammatory or autoimmune states (eg, connective tissue diseases such as systemic lupus erythematosus and rheumatoid arthritis)

3. Nutritional deficiencies (eg, vitamin B_{12} or folate deficiencies)

4. Bone marrow failure states such as myelodysplastic syndrome or aplastic anemia

Management consists of identifying and treating the underlying disease.

Congenital Platelet Disorders

Congenital abnormalities of the platelet receptor glycoproteins lead to platelet dysfunction and thrombocytopenia. Lifelong mucocutaneous bleeding and postoperative bleeding are typical. Platelet transfusions are used for prevention and treatment of hemorrhage. A risk of frequent transfusions is platelet alloimmunization. Diagnosis is based on platelet function testing as follows:

1. Bernard-Soulier syndrome
   a. Due to abnormalities in the glycoprotein Ib/IX complex receptor
   b. Characterized by large platelets
   c. Platelet aggregation is decreased with ristocetin but normal with adenosine diphosphate, epinephrine, collagen, and arachidonate

2. Glanzmann thrombasthenia
   a. Due to abnormalities in the glycoprotein IIb/IIIa complex
   b. Platelet aggregation is normal with ristocetin but decreased with adenosine diphosphate, epinephrine, collagen, and arachidonate

3. Wiskott-Aldrich syndrome
   a. Associated with small platelets

Thrombocytopenia in Pregnancy

Mild thrombocytopenia (platelets $>70\times10^9$/L) occurs in 6% to 8% of pregnant women at term and in 25% of women with preeclampsia. The most common causes of thrombocytopenia in pregnancy are physiologic gestational thrombocytopenia and nonphysiologic benign gestational thrombocytopenia, which account for 75% of cases. No treatment is required. Platelet counts generally recover within 72 hours after delivery without adverse maternal or fetal outcomes. The diagnosis is one of exclusion.

Other common causes include preeclampsia (including the HELLP syndrome), idiopathic autoimmune thrombocytopenia (or autoimmune thrombocytopenic purpura), DIC, acute fatty liver of pregnancy, HIV infection, antiphospholipid antibodies, drugs (quinine and quinidine, cocaine, and heparin), nutritional deficiency, and thrombotic thrombocytopenic purpura.

The primary treatment of the HELLP syndrome is stabilization of the patient's condition and delivery of the fetus.

- Platelet aggregation is decreased with ristocetin in Bernard-Soulier syndrome but normal with adenosine diphosphate, epinephrine, collagen, and arachidonate. The opposite is true in Glanzmann thrombasthenia: platelet aggregation is normal with ristocetin but decreased with adenosine diphosphate, epinephrine, collagen, and arachidonate.

- Most thrombocytopenia in pregnancy is physiologic and does not require treatment.

- Treat HELLP syndrome by stabilizing the patient and facilitating delivery of the fetus if possible.

SUMMARY

- Tests for evaluating a bleeding patient include a CBC, PT, aPTT, and fibrinogen.

- The most common congenital plasmatic bleeding disorder is vWD.

- Acquired bleeding disorders result from a decrease in the production of coagulation factors by the liver, an increase in the consumption of coagulation factors, or the inhibition of coagulation factors.

- Most thrombocytopenia is acquired and results from decreased production or increased destruction of platelets.

36.

HEMATOLOGY: THROMBOSIS

Rajiv K. Pruthi, MBBS

GOALS

- Understand the diagnostic testing and risks associated with thrombophilic conditions.
- Review the evaluation and treatment of patients with venous thromboembolism (VTE).

THROMBOPHILIA: THE HYPERCOAGULABLE STATES

Thrombophilia refers to the tendency for thromboembolism (ie, having risk factors for thromboembolism), which may be inherited or acquired (Box 36.1). The presence of increasing numbers of risk factors further increases the risk of venous thrombosis. Lupus anticoagulant and hyperhomocysteinemia are associated with arterial thrombosis.

Thrombophilic defects can be broadly classified into abnormalities of the procoagulant system and abnormalities of the anticoagulant system.

DEFECTS IN THE PROCOAGULANT SYSTEM

Inherited Risk Factors

Factor V Leiden

The most common inherited defect is activated protein C (APC) resistance due to the factor V Leiden mutation (R506Q). This causes activated factor V to be resistant to inactivation by APC.

1. Heterozygous mutation

    a. Prevalence of 5%-7% in the healthy white population and 20%-50% among persons with VTE.

    b. Heterozygotes have a 2- to 4-fold increased risk of VTE.

    c. Risk of VTE is increased 30-fold for heterozygous carriers taking estrogen-containing oral contraceptives compared with oral contraceptive users without factor V Leiden.

2. Homozygotes have an 80-fold increased risk of VTE

Laboratory testing consists of performing the APC resistance assay and, if the results are abnormal, follow-up DNA-based testing for factor V Leiden to determine whether the person is heterozygous or homozygous.

- The most common inherited defect of the procoagulant system is APC resistance due to the factor V Leiden mutation.
- Heterozygotes have an approximately 2- to 4-fold increased risk of VTE, and the risk is increased 30 times when they take estrogen-containing oral contraceptives.

Prothrombin G20210A

The next most common defect is the prothrombin G20210A mutation, which results in an elevated plasma prothrombin level. The heterozygous mutation has a prevalence of approximately 3% in the healthy white population and 6% to 18% among persons with VTE. Heterozygotes have an approximately 2-fold increased risk of VTE. These defects are common among white people and rare among people of Asian or African ancestry. Laboratory testing consists of DNA-based testing for the presence or absence of the mutation.

Other Risk Factors

Additional abnormalities of procoagulant proteins that confer an increased risk of VTE include increased levels of factors VIII, IX, and XI. Currently, there is no established cutoff for this increased risk and there is no known genetic basis for these abnormalities.

DEFECTS IN THE ANTICOAGULANT SYSTEM

Congenital deficiencies of the anticoagulants antithrombin, protein C, and protein S confer an increased risk of VTE. In the majority of patients, VTE develops by 50 years of age. Rare congenital abnormalities of fibrinogen (dysfibrinogenemias) pose a risk of thrombosis rather than hemorrhage.

VTE (deep vein thrombosis [DVT] and pulmonary embolism) affects 1:1,000 people in the western hemisphere and is a major cause of morbidity. The annual mortality rate is 50,000, which is higher than that for breast cancer.

Risk Factors for VTE

Acquired Risk Factors

Antiphospholipid antibodies (eg, lupus anticoagulant, anticardiolipin antibodies, anti–β_2-glycoprotein I antibodies) pose a significant risk of both venous thrombosis and arterial thrombosis. Antiphospholipid antibody syndrome is characterized by clinical and laboratory criteria that include the following:

1. Vascular thrombosis (venous or arterial) or recurrent miscarriage, or both

2. Presence and persistence (on subsequent testing after 12 weeks) of lupus anticoagulant or medium to high titers of anticardiolipin or anti–β_2-glycoprotein I antibody

If testing of asymptomatic patients shows the presence of antiphospholipid antibodies, prophylactic anticoagulant therapy is not recommended. Patients with vascular thrombosis should be treated with long-term anticoagulation, and women with recurrent fetal loss benefit from heparin (unfractionated heparin [UFH] or low-molecular-weight heparin [LMWH]) in combination with aspirin during pregnancy.

- Asymptomatic patients with antiphospholipid antibodies do not need anticoagulant therapy.

- Patients with antiphospholipid antibodies and vascular thrombosis should be treated with long-term anticoagulation.

Other acquired risk factors for VTE include immobilization (hospitalization, paralysis, etc), orthopedic or general surgery, and estrogen-containing drugs, which pose a significant risk of VTE. When any of these risk factors is combined with an underlying inherited risk factor (eg, factor V Leiden), the chances of symptomatic VTE increase significantly.

Mixed Inherited and Acquired Risk Factors

In selected situations (eg, hyperhomocysteinemia), genetic determinants (eg, MTHFR C677T mutation) pose a risk that may be compounded by acquired determinants (eg, dietary deficiencies of folate and vitamins B_6 and B_{12}), resulting in an increased risk of VTE. Patients with inherited risk factors have a baseline increased risk; symptomatic VTE develops when the inherited risk factors are present in combination with acquired risk factors, such as pregnancy, estrogen use, or surgery.

Prevention of VTE

All hospitalized medical, surgical, and trauma patients should be assessed for the risk of VTE and given appropriate prophylaxis. The risk of VTE must be balanced against the risk of hemorrhage and the presence of contraindications to anticoagulation (Table 36.1). Although the benefits of mechanical and pharmacologic prophylaxis have been demonstrated, only 30% of patients at risk receive prophylaxis. The risk of VTE in surgical patients varies with the site of surgery, surgical technique, duration, type of anesthesia, complications (infection, shock, etc), and degree of immobilization. High-risk surgical procedures include open abdominal or urologic surgery, neurosurgery, gynecologic surgery, and orthopedic surgery of the lower extremities (joint replacement and hip fracture repair). In addition, patient-related risk factors include intensive care unit admission, age, cardiac dysfunction, acute myocardial infarction, congestive heart failure, cancer and its treatment, paralysis, prolonged immobility, prior VTE, obesity, varicose veins, central venous catheters, inflammatory bowel disease, lobar pneumonia, nephrotic syndrome, pregnancy, and estrogen use.

Suggested Strategies for Prophylaxis

1. Education and early ambulation—Educate all patients about the signs and symptoms of VTE and the role of prophylaxis. Encourage patients to ambulate as early and as often as feasible.

2. Low-risk patients—Focus on education and early ambulation.

3. Moderate-risk or high-risk patients—Same as for low-risk patients, with the additions of elastic graded compression stockings (below-knee), intermittent

Table 36.1 **RISK FACTORS AND INCIDENCE OF VTE**

			INCIDENCE, %			
LEVEL OF RISK	SURGERY	ADDITIONAL RISK FACTORS	*CVT*	*Proximal DVT*	*Clinical PE*	*Fatal PE*
Low	Minor	None	2	0.4	0.2	0.002
Moderate	Minor	Yes	10–20	2–4	1–2	0.1–0.4
	Major	None				
High	Major	Yes	20–40	4–8	2–4	0.4–1.0
Very high	Major (hip or knee arthroplasty, hip fracture, major trauma, spinal cord injury)	Prior VTE, active malignancy	40–80	10–20	4–10	0.2–0.5

Abbreviations: CVT, calf vein thrombosis; DVT, deep vein thrombosis; PE, pulmonary embolism; VTE, venous thromboembolism.

pneumatic compression if immobilized, and pharmacologic prophylaxis (UFH and LMWH are equivalent).

4. Very high-risk patients—Same as for moderate- or high-risk patients but with the following differences: UFH is not recommended; LMWH, fondaparinux, and adjusted-dose warfarin are used to keep the international normalized ratio (INR) between 2.0 and 3.0; and extended out-of-hospital prophylaxis may be needed.

5. Patients with a previous history of VTE or thrombophilia—Same as the strategies for very high-risk patients.

Evaluation of the Patient for VTE

Upon radiologic testing, more than 75% of ambulatory patients who present with symptoms worrisome for DVT are found not to have the disease. Thus, a sensitive and specific strategy to reduce excess radiologic imaging studies without compromising patient safety is required. A history of the presence or absence of acquired risk factors for VTE should be obtained. Considerations in the clinical evaluation include patient and family history of VTE, pregnancy, recurrent miscarriage, estrogen use, recent trauma, surgery, hospitalization, malignancy, and travel. A physical examination should include evaluation for venous stasis and for detection of an underlying malignancy. The most critical initial component of the examination is to determine the presence or absence of venous limb gangrene (phlegmasia cerulea dolens), in which severe obstruction of extremity venous drainage leads to congestion and eventual obstruction of arterial inflow. If venous limb gangrene is present, thrombolytic therapy, fasciotomy, or thrombectomy may be indicated.

Although important, clinical findings alone are poor predictors of the presence or severity of VTE, and objective diagnostic testing may eventually be required. Initial steps, however, consist of estimating the clinical pretest probability of VTE and using the D-dimer assay with further diagnostic testing as indicated.

Step 1: Determine the Clinical Pretest Probability

The Wells model (Table 36.2) categorizes the pretest probability of DVT as high (≥3 points), moderate (1 or 2 points), or low (<1 point). A similar model has been applied to pulmonary embolism (Table 36.3), which stratifies patients according to whether pulmonary embolism is less likely (≤4) or likely (>4). For patients in the low-risk category, further imaging studies are probably not needed, and determining the level of D-dimer, a breakdown product from cross-linked stabilized fibrin clots, is recommended.

Step 2: Determine the D-Dimer Level

In ambulatory outpatients, a negative D-dimer test has a high negative predictive value for DVT, thus avoiding unnecessary additional diagnostic tests. It is most useful for ambulatory outpatients, and it should not be used to exclude VTE in hospitalized patients, patients with malignancy or recent trauma, surgery, or hemorrhage. In these patients, proceeding with imaging studies is appropriate.

Table 36.2 **WELLS MODEL FOR PREDICTING CLINICAL PRETEST PROBABILITY OF DEEP VEIN THROMBOSIS**

CLINICAL VARIABLE	POINTS
Active cancer	1
Paralysis or recent limb casting	1
Recent immobility for >3 d	1
Local vein tenderness	1
Limb swelling	1
Lateral calf swelling >3 cm	1
Pitting edema	1
Collateral superficial vein	1
Alternative diagnoses likely	−2

Table 36.3 WELLS MODEL FOR PREDICTING CLINICAL PRETEST PROBABILITY OF PULMONARY EMBOLISM

CLINICAL VARIABLE	POINTS
Clinical signs & symptoms of DVT	3
Alternative diagnoses less likely	3
Heart rate >100 beats per minute	1.5
Immobilization or surgery in previous 4 wk	1.5
Previous DVT or PE	1.5
Hemoptysis	1
Malignancy	1
Collateral superficial vein	1

Abbreviations: DVT, deep vein thrombosis; PE, pulmonary embolism.

For patients with objectively confirmed VTE, initial laboratory testing should include a complete blood cell count, blood smear, serum chemistry studies, baseline prothrombin time and activated partial thromboplastin time (before initiation of anticoagulants), and urinalysis. Further investigations (eg, radiologic studies) should be reserved for further investigation of initial history and examination findings and patient risk factors (eg, smoking). Testing should also include age-appropriate cancer screening.

Thrombophilia Testing

It is reasonable to perform thrombophilia testing with the recognition that selected assays are affected by acute thrombotic events, heparin, and warfarin. Testing should be considered if results will affect long-term management of anticoagulation (Box 36.1). Thrombophilia testing can be performed before initiation of anticoagulation or after completion of anticoagulation appropriate for a thrombotic event if certain caveats are recognized and appropriate follow-up testing is performed.

- Effects of acute thrombosis: Rarely, protein C, protein S, or antithrombin levels may be falsely decreased owing to acute thrombosis. Follow-up testing to confirm abnormal results is important.

- Effects of anticoagulants (heparin and wafarin): Anticoagulants can produce false-positive results for lupus anticoagulants. Warfarin typically reduces protein C and protein S levels, and heparin can falsely decrease antithrombin levels.

DNA-based testing (eg, factor V Leiden and prothrombin G20210A mutation) is not affected by acute thrombosis, heparin anticoagulation, or warfarin. However, the optimal time for thrombophilia testing is 4 to 6 weeks after completion of anticoagulation.

Thrombophilia does not alter acute management of VTE except in 2 circumstances. If the baseline activated partial thromboplastin time is prolonged in association with lupus anticoagulants, monitoring of UFH complex, use of the heparin assay (anti-Xa levels), or use of LMWH (which requires no monitoring) should be considered. With congenital deficiency of protein C or protein S, the risk of warfarin skin necrosis increases, especially if heparin therapy (with UFH or LMWH) is prematurely discontinued (see "Treatment of VTE" section). For thrombophilic conditions that impart a high risk of recurrence, a longer duration of anticoagulation is needed.

Diagnostic Approach for DVT

1. Low clinical pretest probability and negative D-dimer results—DVT is effectively ruled out and no further testing is needed unless new or progressive symptoms occur. With this approach, VTE subsequently develops in less than 1% of patients.

2. Moderate or high clinical pretest probability—Patients in this category should have diagnostic imaging studies performed (eg, duplex ultrasonography with compression). If the imaging study results are negative, checking the D-dimer level is reasonable. If the level is elevated, further imaging studies are indicated.

Diagnostic Approach for Pulmonary Embolism

Pulmonary embolism should be considered in patients with dyspnea, pleuritic chest pain, and tachypnea. Assess hemodynamic stability. Alternative therapies such as thrombolytic therapy or surgical thrombectomy may be indicated. If pulmonary embolism is less likely (Wells score ≤4), the D-dimer level should be determined; if it is within the reference range, alternative diagnoses should be considered, and if it is elevated, imaging studies (eg, computed tomographic pulmonary angiography) should be performed. If pulmonary embolism is likely (Wells score >4), proceed directly to imaging studies.

Treatment of VTE

Initial Management of VTE

For established VTE, the aims of initial therapy include preventing extension or embolization of the thrombus and reducing postphlebitic syndrome, and the aim of long-term therapy is secondary prevention or reducing the risk of recurrence. Patients who are hemodynamically unstable should be hospitalized. For most hemodynamically stable patients, however, outpatient anticoagulation is reasonable. After excluding contraindications to anticoagulation, initiate therapeutic doses of LMWH subcutaneously, and simultaneously initiate oral warfarin therapy. LMWH does not need monitoring, but the INR is used to assess the warfarin effect. Continue therapy with both agents for at least 5 days or until the INR is in the therapeutic range (ie, 2–3) for at least 48 hours before discontinuing the LMWH doses. Use of knee-high compression stockings has been shown to reduce the incidence of postphlebitic syndrome.

Long-term Management of VTE

Warfarin therapy is continued for an appropriate duration. INR is monitored every 4 to 6 weeks. Long-term outcomes have been shown to be superior when VTE is managed in anticoagulation clinics and with home INR devices.

Calf Vein Thrombosis

Asymptomatic calf vein thrombosis can be observed if the patient is willing and able to return for follow-up compression ultrasonography to document stability or progression of the clot. For symptomatic or progressive calf vein thrombosis, anticoagulation should be initiated.

Proximal DVT

LMWH and warfarin should be administered as described above.

Pulmonary Embolism

Patients with pulmonary embolism should be hospitalized for at least 24 hours to assess clinical stability. Selected asymptomatic, clinically stable patients may be treated as outpatients with LMWH and warfarin as described above.

Duration of Warfarin Anticoagulation

Treat with warfarin for at least 3 months for DVT and pulmonary embolism. For DVT occurring without risk factors (idiopathic), an additional 3 months of warfarin for secondary prevention is recommended. For recurrent DVT, consider secondary prevention with warfarin for a total of 12 months of treatment. For hemodynamically significant or idiopathic pulmonary embolism, long-term treatment with warfarin is reasonable. Long-term treatment with warfarin is also reasonable for VTE in patients who have underlying thrombophilia (eg, from lupus anticoagulant or deficiency of protein C, protein S, or antithrombin) or for patients who are compound heterozygous for factor V Leiden and prothrombin G20210A mutation. Continuing warfarin anticoagulation should be balanced with the risk of hemorrhage.

SUMMARY

- Estimating pretest probability is important in determining a diagnostic approach for VTE.

- Treat DVT and pulmonary embolism for a minimum of 3 months.

- Unprovoked or recurrent VTE requires longer treatment; weigh risks and benefits of anticoagulation.

37.

MALIGNANT HEMATOLOGY

Carrie A. Thompson, MD

GOALS

- Describe common presentations, diagnostic features, and treatment of lymphoproliferative disorders.

- Identify key features of various plasma cell disorders.

- Describe the recognition, diagnosis, and treatment of acute leukemias.

- Review the approach to chronic myeloid neoplasms, including myeloproliferative disorders and myelodysplastic syndromes.

INTRODUCTION

The hematologic neoplasms include the following:

1. Lymphoproliferative disorders—for example, chronic lymphocytic leukemia (CLL), large granular lymphocyte (LGL) leukemia, hairy cell leukemia (HCL), Hodgkin lymphoma, non-Hodgkin lymphoma (NHL)

2. Plasma cell disorders—multiple myeloma, light chain amyloidosis, Waldenström macroglobulinemia, plasmacytoma

3. Chronic myeloid neoplasms—chronic myeloid leukemia (CML), myeloproliferative neoplasms, myelodysplastic syndromes (MDSs)

4. Acute leukemia—acute myeloid leukemia (AML), acute lymphocytic leukemia (ALL)

LYMPHOPROLIFERATIVE DISORDERS

CHRONIC LYMPHOCYTIC LEUKEMIA

CLL is a clonal disorder of mature lymphocytes (Figure 37.1) that is primarily seen in older patients (median age, 65–70 years). Median survival is about 10 years.

The diagnosis of CLL requires a B-lymphocyte count of more than 5,000/μL; a smaller B-cell clone is also considered CLL if accompanied by lymphadenopathy, splenomegaly, marrow infiltration, or cytopenias attributable to CLL. A small B-cell clone may be detected incidentally by flow cytometry in about 5% of patients older than 60 without accompanying cytopenias, adenopathy, or splenomegaly; these patients have monoclonal B-cell lymphocytosis (MBL) and should be observed.

The peripheral blood smear in CLL classically shows *smudge cells*, which are lymphocytes that break apart during slide processing (Figure 37.1). Interphase fluorescence in situ hybridization (FISH) testing identifies the characteristic CLL immunophenotype: clonal light-chain expression, CD5+ (also expressed in mantle cell lymphoma), CD19+, CD23+, and CD20+. The 2 widely used staging classifications are outlined in Tables 37.1 and 37.2.

Favorable prognosis factors include early stage, mutation of the variable region of immunoglobulin heavy chain (IGVH), and isolated deletion of chromosome 13. Poor risk factors include advanced clinical stage, deletion of chromosome 17p13 or 11q22, unmutated *IGVH*, and expression of CD38 and ZAP-70.

- CLL diagnosis requires a B-lymphocyte count >5,000/μL; smaller clones can be CLL if associated with clinical disease.

- FISH testing is useful in CLL. Isolated chromosome 13q deletion imparts a favorable prognosis (median survival, 11 years); a chromosome 17p deletion predicts the most unfavorable outcome (median survival, 2 years).

Recurrent infections are a common complication, in part because of hypogammaglobulinemia. Prophylactic γ-globulin may reduce infection rates and should be considered for patients with recurrent serious infections. About 5% of patients have autoimmune hematologic complications, including hemolytic anemia, thrombocytopenia, and pure red cell aplasia. Patients with CLL also are at increased risk for second malignancies, including evolution to more aggressive B-cell malignancy (ie, *Richter transformation*, which occurs in

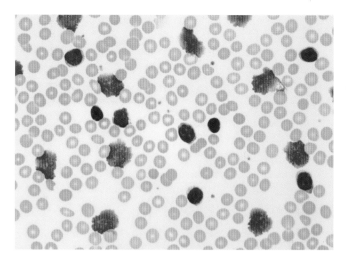

Figure 37.1 Chronic Lymphocytic Leukemia. There are a large number of small and mature lymphocytes with nuclei approximately the same size as red blood cells. Smudge cells are also characteristic of this disorder (peripheral blood smear; Wright-Giemsa). (Courtesy of Curtis A. Hanson, MD, Mayo Clinic, Rochester, Minnesota. Used with permission.)

about 5% of cases), skin cancer, and solid organ malignancies. In CLL patients with fever, infection and transformation to diffuse large B-cell lymphoma (DLBCL) should be excluded before attributing fever to progressive CLL.

- Autoimmune complications occur in about 5% of patients.

- In CLL, fever should prompt concern for infection or Richter transformation.

For patients with early-stage CLL and good-risk prognostic factors, the standard practice is observation. Treatment indications include disease-related cytopenias, progressive adenopathy or splenomegaly, constitutional symptoms, or rapid lymphocyte doubling time. Chemotherapy in combination

Table 37.1 STAGING OF CHRONIC LYMPHOCYTIC LEUKEMIA: RAI CLASSIFICATION

STAGE	CHARACTERISTICS	MEDIAN SURVIVAL TIME, MO
0	Peripheral lymphocytosis ($>15\times10^9$/L), bone marrow lymphocytosis (>40%)	>150
I	Lymphocytosis, lymphadenopathy	101
II	Lymphocytosis, splenomegaly	71
III	Lymphocytosis, anemia (hemoglobin <11 g/dL), excluding AIHA	19
IV	Lymphocytosis, thrombocytopenia	19

Abbreviation: AIHA, autoimmune hemolytic anemia.

Data from Rai KR, Sawitsky A, Cronkite EP, Chanana AD, Levy RN, Pasternack BS. Clinical staging of chronic lymphocytic leukemia. Blood. 1975 Aug;46(2):219–34.

Table 37.2 STAGING OF CHRONIC LYMPHOCYTIC LEUKEMIA: INTERNATIONAL WORKSHOP ON CHRONIC LYMPHOCYTIC LEUKEMIA CLASSIFICATION

CLINICAL STAGE	FEATURES
A	No anemia or thrombocytopenia & <3 areas of lymphoid enlargement (spleen, liver, & lymph nodes in cervical, axillary, & inguinal regions)
B	No anemia or thrombocytopenia but with ≥3 involved areas of lymphoid enlargement
C	Anemia (hemoglobin <10 g/dL) or thrombocytopenia (or both)

Adapted from International Workshop on CLL. Chronic lymphocytic leukaemia: proposals for a revised prognostic staging system. Br J Haematol. 1981 Jul;48(3):365–7. Used with permission.

with immunotherapy (ie, *chemoimmunotherapy*), including a purine analogue (fludarabine or pentostatin) in combination with rituximab (an anti-CD20 monoclonal antibody), is the initial treatment of choice for most patients. Patients with chromosome 17p deletion do not respond well and alternative therapies should be used. The major adverse effects of chemoimmunotherapy are myelosuppression and immunosuppression, which predisposes to infection. Allogeneic bone marrow transplant is used in selected patients with high-risk or relapsed disease.

- Observe asymptomatic patients who have early- to intermediate-stage CLL.

- Treat patients who have symptoms, cytopenias, progressive adenopathy or splenomegaly, or rapid lymphocyte doubling time (<6 months).

- The optimal initial treatment of CLL is chemoimmunotherapy with a purine analogue (such as fludarabine) plus rituximab.

HAIRY CELL LEUKEMIA

HCL is a rare mature B-cell neoplasm characterized by an insidious onset of cytopenias and the presence of cells with "hairy" cytoplasmic projections. The male to female ratio is 4:1 (Figure 37.2).

The symptoms are related to cytopenias, infections, and splenomegaly. The bone marrow often yields a "dry tap" (ie, no liquid marrow is obtained); core biopsy specimens are hypercellular, with diffuse infiltration by neoplastic cells and fibrosis. With treatment, most patients live for more than 10 years. HCL causes immunosuppression and an increased risk of infection. Atypical mycobacterial infections are a classic association.

- Cytopenias and splenomegaly are common in patients with HCL.

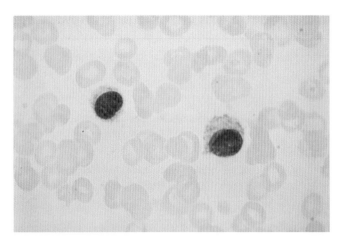

Figure 37.2 Hairy Cell Leukemia. These mature lymphocytes have eccentrically placed nuclei, pale cytoplasm, and characteristic projections (bone marrow aspirate smear; Wright-Giemsa).

- Peripheral blood smear shows atypical mononuclear cells with irregular projections.

- The bone marrow biopsy yields a "dry tap."

- Infection is a major cause of death among patients with HCL, and atypical mycobacterial infections are classically associated.

LARGE GRANULAR LYMPHOCYTE SYNDROME

LGLs are cytotoxic T cells or natural killer cells (Figure 37.3). Clonal expansion of LGLs is called LGL leukemia or LGL syndrome. T-cell LGL leukemia is associated with neutropenia, splenomegaly, anemia, and a normal to mildly elevated lymphocyte count. It occurs most commonly in older patients (median age, 60 years). The diagnosis is suggested by flow cytometry and can be confirmed by T-cell receptor gene rearrangement studies.

Up to one-third of T-cell LGL leukemia patients have rheumatoid arthritis (RA), and there is overlap

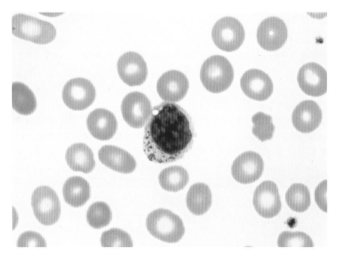

Figure 37.3 Large Granular Lymphocyte. The pale blue cytoplasm contains azurophilic granules (peripheral blood smear; Wright-Giemsa)

with Felty syndrome (ie, triad of neutropenia, RA, and splenomegaly).

T-cell LGL leukemia is a chronic disorder that requires treatment only if symptoms are present. Immunosuppressive therapy with methotrexate, cyclophosphamide, or cyclosporine is often effective.

- T-cell LGL leukemia is a chronic, indolent disorder of clonal T cells.

- T-cell LGL leukemia is associated with RA and Felty syndrome (ie, RA, neutropenia, and splenomegaly).

- Immunosuppressive therapy is often effective.

HODGKIN LYMPHOMA

Treatment of Hodgkin lymphoma is a major success of modern cancer therapy. With treatment, more than 80% of patients with Hodgkin lymphoma are now cured.

The age at presentation has a bimodal distribution, with the first peak at a median age of 25 years and the second peak after age 60. Patients with Hodgkin lymphoma usually present with locally limited disease. The typical finding at presentation is lymphadenopathy; less common presentations include pruritus, cytopenias, abnormal liver function test results, and pain in involved lymph nodes after alcohol consumption.

The most important unfavorable prognostic factors are low levels of hemoglobin (<10.5 g/dL) and serum albumin (<4 g/dL), male sex, age older than 45 years, stage IV disease (Table 37.3), high white blood cell (WBC) count ($>15\times10^9/L$), and lymphocytopenia (lymphocyte count $<0.6\times10^9/L$).

The diagnosis of Hodgkin lymphoma is based on the presence of Reed-Sternberg cells, which typically have 2 or more nuclei with prominent nucleoli that give the cells the appearance of owl eyes (Figure 37.4).

Disease stage is the principal factor in selecting treatment (Table 37.3 and Box 37.1). The disease is routinely staged with use of computed tomography of the chest, abdomen, and pelvis and positron emission tomography. Currently, the treatment of choice for localized disease (stages IA and IIA) is a short course of combination chemotherapy with ABVD (doxorubicin [Adriamycin], bleomycin, vinblastine, and dacarbazine) and low doses of radiotherapy. Most patients with localized disease are cured. The treatment of choice for advanced disease is combination chemotherapy; cure rates are up to 65%. Autologous stem cell transplant is considered for relapses after chemotherapy (Box 37.1).

Late complications of Hodgkin lymphoma therapy are substantial. They include infertility, amenorrhea, hypothyroidism, avascular necrosis, cardiomyopathy, coronary artery disease, pericarditis, pulmonary fibrosis, and secondary malignancies. Potential secondary malignancies include AML, MDS, non-Hodgkin lymphoma, and solid tumors (eg, breast, lung, and thyroid cancer, if those areas are included in the irradiated field).

Table 37.3 COTSWOLDS STAGING CLASSIFICATION OF HODGKIN LYMPHOMA

CLASSIFICATION	DESCRIPTION
Stage I	Involvement of a single lymph node region or lymphoid structure
Stage II	Involvement of ≥2 lymph node regions on the same side of the diaphragm (the mediastinum is considered a single site, whereas hilar lymph nodes are considered bilaterally)
Stage III	Involvement of lymph node regions or structures on both sides of the diaphragm
Stage III-1	With or without involvement of splenic, hilar, celiac, or portal nodes
Stage III-2	With involvement of para-aortic, iliac, & mesenteric nodes
Stage IV	Involvement of 1 or more extranodal sites in addition to a site for which the designation "E" has been used

Designations Applicable to Any Disease Stage

A	No symptoms
B	Fever (temperature >38°C), drenching night sweats, unexplained loss of >10% of body weight within the preceding 6 mo
X	Bulky disease (a widening of the mediastinum by more than one-third or the presence of a nodal mass with a maximal dimension >10 cm)
E	Involvement of a single extranodal site that is contiguous or proximal to the known nodal site
CS	Clinical stage
PS	Pathologic stage (as determined by laparotomy)

Adapted from Lister TA, Crowther D. Staging for Hodgkin's disease. Semin Oncol. 1990 Dec;17(6):696–703. Used with permission.

- Diagnosis of Hodgkin lymphoma requires the presence of Reed-Sternberg cells in a biopsy specimen.
- Disease stage is the principal factor in selecting treatment for Hodgkin lymphoma.
- Autologous stem cell transplant is indicated after a first relapse.
- Late complications of treatment are common and may include AML, solid tumors, hypothyroidism, and cardiac disease.

NON-HODGKIN LYMPHOMAS

NHL is a diverse group of lymphoproliferative disorders (Box 37.2). The Ann Arbor Staging System, which is very similar to the staging system for Hodgkin lymphoma in Table 37.3, has traditionally been used for NHL.

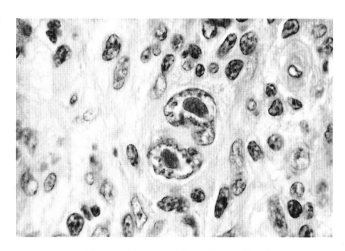

Figure 37.4 Hodgkin Lymphoma. Reed-Sternberg cell is a large binuclear cell (bone marrow biopsy section; hematoxylin-eosin). (Courtesy of Curtis A. Hanson, MD, Mayo Clinic, Rochester, Minnesota. Used with permission.)

Low-Grade (Indolent) Lymphomas

Low-grade (indolent) lymphomas may remain in a chronic phase for many years or transform into aggressive lymphomas. Patients with follicular lymphoma, the most common type of indolent lymphoma, often have a t(14;18) translocation resulting in amplification of the antiapoptotic *BCL2* gene.

Low-grade NHLs are not curable unless they are stage I disease, which can sometimes be cured with radiotherapy. At diagnosis, most patients have stage III or IV disease, which is not curable; however, median survival is 8 years. Observation is an option for asymptomatic patients with no evidence of bulky disease. Treatment is indicated for patients with symptoms, bulky disease, or progressive disease. Many therapeutic regimens exist, including CVP (*c*yclophosphamide, *v*incristine, and *p*rednisone) with rituximab; rituximab alone; R-CHOP (*r*ituximab, *c*yclophosphamide, *h*ydroxydaunomycin [Adriamycin], vincristine [*O*ncovin], and *p*rednisone); bendamustine with rituximab; and fludarabine.

Gastric mucosa–associated lymphoid tissue (MALT) lymphomas are associated with *Helicobacter pylori* infections. Up to 70% of patients respond to a regimen of antibiotics in

Box 37.1 STAGING PROCEDURES FOR LYMPHOMA

History & examination: identification of *B* symptoms (see designations in Table 37.3) & sites of palpable adenopathy

Imaging procedures: plain chest radiography; computed tomography of thorax, abdomen, & pelvis

Hematologic procedures: CBC with differential, determination of erythrocyte sedimentation rate, & bilateral bone marrow aspiration & biopsy (not always necessary in Hodgkin lymphoma)

Biochemical procedures: liver function tests; measurement of serum albumin, lactate dehydrogenase, & calcium

Special procedures: PET scan

Abbreviations: CBC, complete blood cell count; PET, positron emission tomographic.

WHO CLASSIFICATION OF THE MATURE B-CELL, T-CELL, AND NK-CELL NEOPLASMS (2008)

Mature B-Cell Neoplasms

Chronic lymphocytic leukemia/small lymphocytic lymphoma
B-cell prolymphocytic leukemia
Splenic marginal zone lymphoma
Hairy cell leukemia
Splenic lymphoma/leukemia, unclassifiable[a]
    Splenic diffuse red pulp small B-cell lymphoma[a]
    Hairy cell leukemia-variant[a]
Lymphoplasmacytic lymphoma
Waldenström macroglobulinemia
Heavy chain diseases
    Alpha heavy chain disease
    Gamma heavy chain disease
    Mu heavy chain disease
Plasma cell myeloma
Solitary plasmacytoma of bone
Extraosseous plasmacytoma
Extranodal marginal zone lymphoma of mucosa-associated lymphoid tissue (MALT lymphoma)
Nodal marginal zone lymphoma
Pediatric nodal marginal zone lymphoma[a]
Follicular lymphoma
Pediatric follicular lymphoma[a]
Primary cutaneous follicle center lymphoma
Mantle cell lymphoma
DLBCL, NOS
    T-cell/histiocyte-rich large B-cell lymphoma
    Primary DLBCL of the central nervous system
    Primary cutaneous DLBCL, leg type
    EBV-positive DLBCL of the elderly[a]
DLBCL associated with chronic inflammation
Lymphomatoid granulomatosis
Primary mediastinal (thymic) large B-cell lymphoma
Intravascular large B-cell lymphoma
ALK-positive large B-cell lymphoma
Plasmablastic lymphoma
Large B-cell lymphoma arising in HHV8-associated multicentric Castleman disease
Primary effusion lymphoma
Burkitt lymphoma
B-cell lymphoma, unclassifiable, with features intermediate between diffuse large B-cell lymphoma & Burkitt lymphoma
B-cell lymphoma, unclassifiable, with features intermediate between diffuse large B-cell lymphoma & classical Hodgkin lymphoma

Mature T-Cell & NK-Cell Neoplams

T-cell prolymphocytic leukemia
T-cell large granular lymphocytic leukemia
Chronic lymphoproliferative disorder of NK cells[a]
Aggressive NK cell leukemia
Systemic EBV-positive T-cell lymphoproliferative disease of childhood
Hydroa vacciniforme–like lymphoma

Adult T-cell leukemia/lymphoma
Extranodal NK/T-cell lymphoma, nasal type
Enteropathy-associated T-cell lymphoma
Hepatosplenic T-cell lymphoma
Subcutaneous panniculitis-like T-cell lymphoma
Mycosis fungoides
Sézary syndrome
Primary cutaneous CD30[+] T-cell lymphoproliferative disorders
    Lymphomatoid papulosis
    Primary cutaneous anaplastic large cell lymphoma
Primary cutaneous γ-δ T-cell lymphoma
Primary cutaneous CD8[+] aggressive epidermotropic cytotoxic T-cell lymphoma[a]
Primary cutaneous CD4[+] small/medium T-cell lymphoma[a]
Peripheral T-cell lymphoma, NOS
Angioimmunoblastic T-cell lymphoma
Anaplastic large cell lymphoma, ALK-positive
Anaplastic large cell lymphoma, ALK-negative

Hodgkin Lymphoma

Nodular lymphocyte-predominant Hodgkin lymphoma
Classical Hodgkin lymphoma
    Nodular sclerosis classical Hodgkin lymphoma
    Lymphocyte-rich classical Hodgkin lymphoma
    Mixed cellularity classical Hodgkin lymphoma
    Lymphocyte-depleted classical Hodgkin lymphoma

PTLDs

Early lesions
Plasmacytic hyperplasia
Infectious mononucleosis–like PTLD
Polymorphic PTLD
Monomorphic PTLD (B- & NK/T-cell types)[b]
Classical Hodgkin lymphoma type PTLD[b]

Abbreviations: ALK, anaplastic lymphoma kinase; DLBCL, diffuse large B-cell lymphoma; EBV, Epstein-Barr virus; HHV8, human herpesvirus 8; NK, natural killer; NOS, not otherwise specified; PTLD, posttransplant lymphoproliferative disorder; WHO, World Health Organization.

[a] Provisional entities for which the WHO Working Group felt there was insufficient evidence to recognize as distinct diseases at this time.

[b] These lesions are classified according to the leukemia or lymphoma to which they correspond.

Adapted from Jaffe ES, Harris NL, Stein H, Isaacson PG. Classification of lymphoid neoplasms: the microscope as a tool for disease discovery. Blood. 2008 Dec 1;112(12):4384–99. Used with permission.

combination with a proton pump inhibitor. If this is unsuccessful, chemotherapy and irradiation are typically administered.

Aggressive Lymphomas

In contrast to low-grade lymphomas, aggressive lymphomas are potentially curable, but the duration of survival is short if the patient does not have remission. Patients typically present with symptomatic disease, including *B* symptoms (as in Table

37.3: fevers, drenching night sweats, and weight loss). For patients with aggressive lymphoma that relapses after complete remission, autologous stem cell transplant is the standard therapy.

The standard therapy for DLBCL is R-CHOP (>50% are cured). The International Prognostic Factor Index uses age, lactate dehydrogenase level, performance status scores, disease stage, and extranodal involvement to predict survival of patients who have DLBCL. Five-year survival ranges from 26% to 73%, depending on risk factors.

Mantle cell lymphoma is characterized by a CD5+ and CD20+ immunophenotype and a t(11;14) translocation, with overexpression of the cyclin D1 oncogene. Unlike other aggressive lymphomas, mantle cell lymphoma is not curable; thus, stem cell transplant is usually incorporated early.

Very aggressive lymphomas, such as Burkitt lymphoma and lymphoblastic lymphoma, are treated with regimens similar to those used for ALL. These subtypes carry a high risk of central nervous system involvement and tumor lysis syndrome.

Patients with human immunodeficiency virus (HIV)-related lymphoproliferative disorders with a CD4 cell count less than 200/mL have a poor response to standard treatment. Primary central nervous system lymphoma occurs with or without HIV infection, carries a poor prognosis, and is generally treated with high-dose methotrexate.

- The most common low-grade NHL is follicular lymphoma. Low-grade lymphomas respond to treatment but are incurable.

- DLBCL is the most common aggressive lymphoma. Aggressive lymphomas are curable but cause death if they do not respond to treatment.

- Gastric MALT lymphomas may respond to antibiotic and proton-pump inhibitor therapy directed at *H pylori*.

- Patients with HIV-related lymphoproliferative disorders and a CD4 cell count <200/mL have a poor response to treatment.

- Lymphoblastic lymphoma and Burkitt lymphoma carry a higher risk of central nervous system involvement and tumor lysis syndrome.

PLASMA CELL DISORDERS (MONOCLONAL GAMMOPATHIES)

The plasma cell disorders (monoclonal gammopathies) are characterized by clonal proliferation of plasma cells, usually associated with the presence of monoclonal immunoglobulins (M proteins) in the serum or urine (or both). The differential diagnosis of monoclonal gammopathies includes monoclonal gammopathy of undetermined significance (MGUS) and multiple myeloma, Waldenström macroglobulinemia, and immunoglobulin light chain (AL) amyloidosis.

MONOCLONAL GAMMOPATHIES OF UNDETERMINED SIGNIFICANCE

In MGUS, the most common form of dysproteinemia involves the serum M-protein level (typically <3 g/dL). The bone marrow has less than 10% plasma cells. The serum creatinine, calcium, and hemoglobin levels are normal, and the urine has either no M protein or only a small amount. Osteolytic bone lesions are absent, and patients are usually asymptomatic.

MGUS is common. In population-based studies, an M protein was found in the serum of 3.2% of adults older than 50 years, 5.3% of those older than 70, and 7.5% of those 85 or older. MGUS progresses to a malignant monoclonal gammopathy at an annual rate of about 1%. On free light-chain analysis, an abnormal κ:λ ratio is a risk factor for progression. Patients with MGUS should be observed.

- In MGUS, the serum M protein is typically <3 g/dL; bone marrow has <10% plasma cells; and serum hemoglobin, creatinine, and calcium levels are normal.

- Patients are observed without therapy.

- Typical clinical scenario: A patient without symptoms has a serum M-protein spike <3 g/dL and bone marrow plasma cells <10%. Blood counts, serum creatinine level, and bone radiographs are normal.

MULTIPLE MYELOMA

The median age at onset of multiple myeloma is 65 years. It is more common in men and in African Americans. By definition, patients must have 10% or more clonal plasma cells in the bone marrow (Figure 37.5), an M protein in the serum or urine, and signs of end-organ damage that are felt to be related to the plasma cell proliferative disorder (mnemonic, *CRAB*): hypercalcemia, renal failure, anemia, or osteolytic bone lesions. The presence of more than 10% clonal plasma cells in the bone marrow without end-organ damage or symptoms is called "smoldering" multiple myeloma.

Clinical features of multiple myeloma include fatigue, bone pain, anemia, renal insufficiency, hypercalcemia, and spinal cord compression. Anemia is normochromic and normocytic and a peripheral blood smear may show rouleaux. Radiographs may show lytic lesions, osteoporosis, and fractures. Bone scans are rarely helpful because lytic lesions do not usually show up. Renal failure may be caused by hypercalcemia, dehydration, or light chain nephropathy (myeloma kidney). Light chain nephropathy may respond to plasmapheresis.

The median survival has been 3 to 4 years, although this is improving with newer treatments. The International Staging System for myeloma is useful for prognostication, with median survival ranging from 29 to 62 months (Table 37.4). Patients should be observed if they have smoldering myeloma.

The standard treatment is evolving. For transplant-eligible patients, current therapy involves "induction" of a response with dexamethasone in combination with lenalidomide, thalidomide, or bortezomib before stem cell collection. Autologous

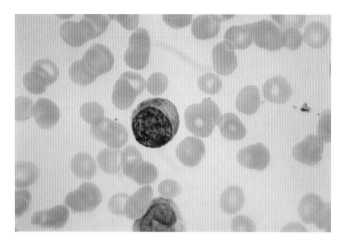

Figure 37.5 Plasma Cell. Note the eccentrically placed round nucleus; the copious, dark blue cytoplasm has a characteristic pale-staining area adjacent to the nucleus (bone marrow aspirate smear; Wright-Giemsa).

stem cell transplant improves survival. For patients who are older than 70 years or who have poor performance status, melphalan is used in combination with prednisone, often with thalidomide or bortezomib. Palliative radiotherapy is effective in managing bone pain. Bisphosphonate therapy delays the onset of skeletal-related events and reduces bone pain. The most worrisome side effect of bisphosphonate therapy is osteonecrosis of the jaw.

- Multiple myeloma: differentiated from MGUS and smoldering myeloma by the presence of end-organ damage (mnemonic, *CRAB*: hyper*c*alcemia, *r*enal failure, *a*nemia, osteolytic *b*one lesions).

- Lytic bone lesions do not show up on bone scans; skeletal surveys (plain radiographs) are a better test.

- Bisphosphonates can prevent skeletal complications. Osteonecrosis of the jaw is associated with bisphosphonate therapy.

- Typical clinical scenario: A patient presents with bone pain, anemia, renal insufficiency, and hypercalcemia. Bone survey shows lytic bone lesions, and serum and urine protein electrophoresis studies demonstrate M protein. Bone marrow biopsy contains >10% plasma cells.

WALDENSTRÖM MACROGLOBULINEMIA

Waldenström macroglobulinemia is characterized by an IgM paraprotein, clonal lymphoplasmacytic cells in the bone marrow, and anemia, hyperviscosity, lymphadenopathy, or hepatosplenomegaly. Bence Jones proteinuria may be present, and hyperviscosity syndrome occurs in 15%.

Hyperviscosity syndrome is characterized by fatigue, dizziness, blurred vision, bleeding, sausage-shaped retinal veins, and papilledema. The initial treatment of hyperviscosity is plasmapheresis followed by chemotherapy. Active drugs include rituximab, alkylating agents, and purine nucleoside analogues such as fludarabine.

- Waldenström macroglobulinemia: IgM paraprotein, ≥10% infiltration of the bone marrow by lymphoplasmacytic cells, and anemia, hyperviscosity, lymphadenopathy, or hepatosplenomegaly.

- Hyperviscosity syndrome is treated initially with plasmapheresis.

- Typical clinical scenario: A 65-year-old patient has fatigue, epistaxis, and visual and neurologic symptoms. Serum protein electrophoresis demonstrates an IgM M protein, and bone biopsy shows a lymphoplasmacytic infiltration.

AMYLOIDOSIS

The amyloidoses comprise a group of diseases that are characterized by extracellular deposition of insoluble fibrillar proteins that stain with Congo red. The amyloidoses are classified as follows:

1. Primary—AL amyloidosis; 90% of amyloidosis in the United States is the AL type

2. Secondary—AA amyloidosis, which is caused by chronic infections such as osteomyelitis or by autoimmune disease

3. Familial—associated with mutations in transthyretin or other proteins

4. Senile—amyloidosis associated with aging

5. Localized—skin, bladder, or other organs

6. Dialysis-associated—deposits of β_2-microglobulin

The amyloid fibrils in AL amyloidosis are fragments of immunoglobulin light chains. The bone marrow usually has less than 20% plasma cells (unless there is associated multiple myeloma), and there are no lytic bone lesions. Initial biopsies should include fat aspiration of the abdominal wall (80% positive) and bone marrow biopsy (50% positive).

Table 37.4 INTERNATIONAL STAGING SYSTEM FOR MULTIPLE MYELOMA

STAGE	SERUM β_2-MICROGLOBULIN, mg/L	SERUM ALBUMIN, g/dL	MEDIAN SURVIVAL, mo
I	<3.5	≥3.5	62
II	3.5–5.5	<3.5	44
III	>5.5	...	29

Adapted from Greipp PR, San Miguel J, Durie BG, Crowley JJ, Barlogie B, Blade J, et al. International staging system for multiple myeloma. J Clin Oncol. 2005 May 20;23(15):3412–20. Epub 2005 Apr 4. Erratum in: J Clin Oncol. 2005 Sep 1;23(25):6281. Harousseau, Jean-Luc [corrected to Avet-Loiseau, Herve]. Used with permission.

Patients with AL amyloidosis may present with fatigue, weight loss, hepatomegaly, macroglossia, renal insufficiency, proteinuria, nephrotic syndrome, congestive heart failure, orthostatic hypotension, carpal tunnel syndrome, or peripheral neuropathy. When patients have cardiac involvement, electrocardiography may show low voltage or Q waves. The echocardiogram is abnormal in 60%, with concentrically thickened ventricles or a thickened intraventricular septum and sometimes a "speckled" appearance. Peripheral neuropathy is often associated with autonomic failure, as manifested by diarrhea, pseudo-obstruction of the bowel, or orthostatic syncope.

For AL amyloidosis, treatment with melphalan and dexamethasone is modestly effective. Autologous stem cell transplant provides benefit in carefully selected patients. The median survival for all patients with AL amyloidosis is 13 months. With overt congestive heart failure, the median survival is less than 6 months.

Treatment of AA amyloidosis involves correcting the underlying disease. Liver transplant may be valuable in familial cases in which an amyloidogenic protein is made by the liver.

- The amyloidoses are characterized by deposition of insoluble fibrils in tissues, leading to organ dysfunction.

- AL amyloidosis is the most common form.

- Associated clinical features: fatigue, nephrotic syndrome, congestive heart failure, sensorimotor neuropathy, and macroglossia.

- Typical clinical scenario: A 64-year-old man has weakness, weight loss, congestive heart failure, carpal tunnel syndrome, peripheral neuropathy, and orthostatic hypotension. An M protein is detected on serum electrophoresis.

ACUTE LEUKEMIAS

Acute leukemia is defined by the presence of at least 20% undifferentiated blast cells in the bone marrow. If the cells exhibit myeloid differentiation, the diagnosis is AML; if the cells have lymphoid markers, the diagnosis is ALL.

ACUTE MYELOID LEUKEMIA

The cause of AML is unknown in most cases, but there are many associations: previous myeloproliferative neoplasm or MDSs; exposure to radiation or benzene; prior chemotherapy; and congenital disorders such as Down syndrome, Fanconi syndrome, and ataxia-telangiectasia.

The median age of patients with AML (Figure 37.6) is about 65 years. Patients may present with nonspecific symptoms, such as fatigue and headache, or with complications of cytopenias. By definition, patients have 20% or more undifferentiated blasts in the bone marrow. Good prognostic signs include being younger than 40 years; having chromosomal

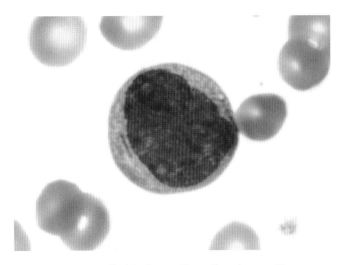

Figure 37.6 Acute Myeloid Leukemia. Blast cells are large and have an open, granular nuclear chromatin, often with 1 or more nucleoli. The presence of an Auer rod means that the blast is myeloid rather than lymphoid (bone marrow aspirate smear; Wright-Giemsa).

abnormalities of t(8;21), t(15;17), or inv(16); and achieving complete remission with 1 cycle of induction chemotherapy. Poor prognostic signs include age older than 40 years (especially >60 years); an antecedent hematologic disorder; previous chemotherapy or radiotherapy; high-risk chromosomal abnormalities (chromosome 5, 7, or 11q23, or a complex karyotype); and poor general physical condition.

For patients who present with extreme leukocytosis (WBC count $>80\times10^9$/L) and acute leukemia, the initial complication of most concern is cerebral hemorrhage due to leukostasis. Emergency treatment includes hydration, allopurinol, hydroxyurea, and leukapheresis, followed by treatment of the specific type of leukemia. Patients with acute promyelocytic leukemia (AML-M3) (Figure 37.7) typically have t(15;17) and often present with disseminated intravascular coagulation (DIC).

Treatment for AML is divided into 1) induction therapy (cytarabine and an anthracycline agent) and 2) consolidation therapy (high-dose cytarabine). Relapse occurs eventually in most patients with AML, usually within 3 years. In patients with relapsed AML, reinduction of remission is followed by hematopoietic stem cell transplant, if feasible. The 5-year survival for younger patients with a good cytogenetic profile is 60%, but for patients who have poor cytogenetics or who are older (especially older than 70), the 5-year survival is less than 10%.

All-*trans*-retinoic acid (ATRA) is the treatment of choice in AML-M3 with t(15;17). Induction chemotherapy is with ATRA and an anthracycline-based program, followed by consolidation therapy. Maintenance therapy includes ATRA for 1 to 2 years.

- AML: median age of patients is about 65 years.

- Good prognosis: being younger than 40 years; having chromosomal abnormalities t(8;21), t(15;17), or inv(16); and achieving complete remission with 1 cycle of induction chemotherapy.

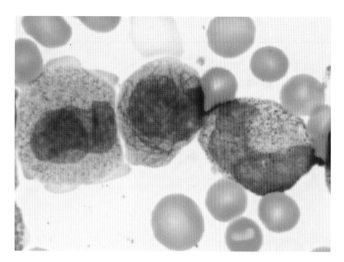

Figure 37.7 Leukemic Cells in Acute Promyelocytic Leukemia (AML-M3). There are abundant cytoplasmic granules and Auer rods (bone marrow aspirate smear; Wright-Giemsa). (Courtesy of Curtis A. Hanson, MD, Mayo Clinic, Rochester, Minnesota. Used with permission.)

- A peripheral blood smear shows numerous immature WBC precursors (blasts).

- Typical clinical scenario for AML-M3: A patient who has circulating blasts presents with DIC. Cytogenetics show t(15;17).

ACUTE LYMPHOCYTIC LEUKEMIA

ALL is most common in children; their complete remission rates are greater than 90%. In adults, however, ALL is less common and outcomes are much poorer. Remission rates in adults are up to 75%, but relapse occurs in most patients.

Bone pain, lymphadenopathy, splenomegaly, and hepatomegaly are more common in ALL than in AML. Poor prognostic factors include advanced age (especially older than 60), WBC count greater than 30×10^9/L, null cell phenotype, specific chromosomal abnormalities, and failure to achieve remission within the first 4 weeks of chemotherapy.

Most adults with ALL have chromosomal abnormalities; t(9;22), t(4;11), t(8;14), and t(1;19) carry the poorest prognoses. Patients with normal chromosomes have the best prognosis. All patients receive intrathecal therapy because of the risk of relapse in the central nervous system. Allogeneic transplant in the first remission is recommended for patients with t(9;22) and t(4;11) because their prognosis with chemotherapy alone is poor. For patients with relapsed disease, allogeneic transplant is the only potentially curative therapy.

CHRONIC MYELOID DISORDERS

Chronic myeloid disorders include MDSs, CML, and myeloproliferative neoplasms. Patients with these disorders have less than 20% bone marrow blasts, which distinguishes them from AML. Chronic myeloid disorders often evolve into AML.

MYELODYSPLASTIC SYNDROMES

MDSs are heterogeneous and share 3 common features: peripheral blood cytopenia, abnormal "dysplastic" bone marrow morphology, and a tendency to evolve to AML. Important prognostic factors include the proportion of bone marrow blasts, the karyotype, and the number of blood lineages affected by cytopenias.

Transformation to acute leukemia occurs in about 25% to 30% of patients; patients with MDS who have more than 10% marrow blasts or a poor-risk karyotype have the highest risk. Infection is the most common cause of death, followed by complications of AML progression and hemorrhage.

Clonal karyotypic abnormalities have been reported in 40% to 50% of patients who have de novo disease and in 70% to 80% of patients who have MDS as a consequence of prior chemotherapy or radiotherapy. Patients with del(5q) MDS have a favorable prognosis and respond well to lenalidomide treatment. The standard of care for most patients is supportive. Those who are eligible should be considered for allogeneic bone marrow transplant.

- Patients with MDS present with cytopenias.

- The most common cause of death in MDS is infection. About 25% of patients progress to AML.

- Lenalidomide therapy is most effective in patients with del(5q) MDS.

CHRONIC MYELOID LEUKEMIA

CML constitutes 20% of all leukemias. The Philadelphia chromosome, t(9;22), is the hallmark of this disease. The molecular equivalent of the Philadelphia chromosome is the abnormal *BCR-ABL* fusion (Figure 37.8).

Symptoms include malaise, dyspnea, anorexia, fever, night sweats, weight loss, abdominal fullness, easy bruising, gout, and priapism. Splenomegaly is present in 85% of patients.

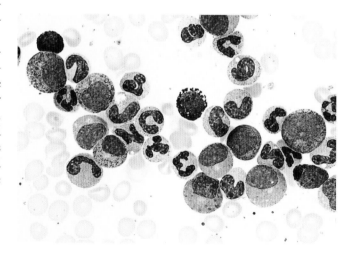

Figure 37.8 Chronic Myeloid Leukemia. Normal-appearing myeloid cells show all stages of maturation, with a decreased number of erythropoietic cells and 1 basophil precursor in the center (bone marrow aspirate smear; Wright-Giemsa). (Courtesy of Curtis A. Hanson, MD, Mayo Clinic, Rochester, Minnesota. Used with permission.)

Characteristic laboratory findings include leukocytosis. WBC counts of 100×10^9/L are common, but leukapheresis is not usually required since the leukocytes are mature and do not cause leukostasis. Granulocytes in all stages of maturation are present on peripheral blood smear, with basophilia and eosinophilia and a characteristic *myelocyte bulge* (ie, increased numbers of myelocytes in relation to other stages of granulocyte differentiation). The bone marrow is hypercellular.

- CML: clonal neoplasm due to acquired *BCR-ABL* fusion.

- Philadelphia chromosome, t(9;22), results in *BCR-ABL* fusion.

- Typical complete blood cell count finding: increased WBC count, with granulocytes in all stages of maturation and basophilia.

Patients who are resistant to tyrosine kinase inhibitors may be eligible for allogeneic stem cell transplant or interferon and cytarabine. Untreated, the chronic phase eventually progresses to an accelerated phase and then a blast crisis, which is characterized by blast counts greater than 20%. Blast crisis is treated like AML.

- Imatinib, a potent BCR-ABL inhibitor, is the treatment of choice in CML.

PHILADELPHIA CHROMOSOME–NEGATIVE MYELOPROLIFERATIVE NEOPLASMS

The classic myeloproliferative neoplasms include polycythemia vera, primary myelofibrosis, and essential thrombocythemia. Their characteristic features are listed in Table 37.5. These disorders are interrelated: polycythemia vera progresses to postpolycythemic myelofibrosis in 10% of patients, and essential thrombocythemia progresses to postthrombocythemic myelofibrosis in 5%. AML is a complication of polycythemia vera (10% of patients), essential thrombocythemia (<5%), and primary myelofibrosis (10%-20%) and is usually refractory to therapy. Each of these disorders carries a risk of thrombosis and hemorrhage.

Activating mutations involving JAK2 tyrosine kinase are present in almost all patients with polycythemia vera and in about half of those with primary myelofibrosis or essential thrombocythemia.

- Myeloproliferative neoplasms include polycythemia vera, primary myelofibrosis, and essential thrombocythemia.

- *JAK2* mutations are universal in polycythemia vera and are common in other myeloproliferative neoplasms.

- Polycythemia vera and essential thrombocythemia may progress to myelofibrosis. All myeloproliferative neoplasms can progress to AML.

Primary Myelofibrosis, Postpolycythemic Myelofibrosis, and Postthrombocythemic Myelofibrosis

Splenomegaly occurs in virtually all patients and is a hallmark of primary myelofibrosis. Other features are a leukoerythroblastic peripheral blood smear, including nucleated red blood cells and dacrocytes (teardrop cells), and hypercellular marrow with increased fibrosis (Figure 37.9).

Foci of extramedullary hematopoiesis can occur in any area of the body but are most common in the spleen, liver, lung and pleural space, skin, eye, and central nervous system. The median survival is 3 to 5 years.

- The median survival of patients with myelofibrosis is 3–5 years.

- Primary myelofibrosis: hallmark is splenomegaly, often massive.

- Leukoerythroblastic peripheral blood smear includes teardrop cells.

Asymptomatic patients should be observed. Medical therapy for anemia includes transfusion with packed red blood cells, androgens, or erythropoietin. Some patients respond to thalidomide or lenalidomide.

Symptoms related to the spleen, such as early satiety, infarcts, and pressure, can be treated with splenectomy, hydroxyurea, or splenic irradiation. DIC is common and increases the risk of a complication at splenectomy. Hydroxyurea is indicated for symptomatic hepatosplenomegaly, leukocytosis, and

Table 37.5 **CHARACTERISTIC FEATURES OF CHRONIC MYELOPROLIFERATIVE NEOPLASMS**

CHARACTERISTIC	POLYCYTHEMIA VERA	PRIMARY MYELOFIBROSIS	ESSENTIAL THROMBOCYTHEMIA	CHRONIC MYELOID LEUKEMIA
Increased red cell mass	Yes	No	No	No
Myelofibrosis	Later	Yes	Rare	Later
Leukocytosis	Variable	Variable	Variable	Yes
Thrombocytosis	Variable	Variable	Yes	Variable
BCR-ABL oncogene	No	No	No	Yes
JAK2 V617F mutation	>95%	50%	50%	Never

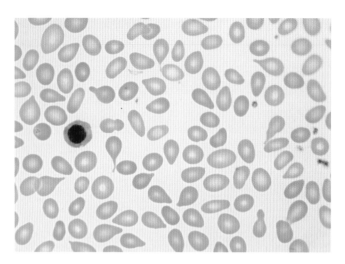

Figure 37.9 Leukoerythroblastic Blood Smear. The teardrop-shaped erythrocytes (dacrocytes) and nucleated red blood cell are characteristic of marrow fibrosis, whether due to primary myelofibrosis or a reactive cause (peripheral blood smear; Wright-Giemsa).

thrombocytosis. Bone marrow transplant may be helpful in some young patients.

Essential Thrombocythemia

Essential thrombocythemia (also called *essential thrombocytosis*) is a clonal hematologic disorder in which patients present with thrombocytosis and sometimes leukocytosis. Patients may be asymptomatic, or they may have thrombosis or hemorrhage. Patients have a relatively long life expectancy (>10 years). Young females have a higher risk of miscarriage than age-matched controls. The risk of acute leukemic transformation is less than 5% at 15 years.

Diagnostic features of essential thrombocythemia include a sustained platelet count greater than 450×10^9/L, megakaryocytic hyperplasia in the bone marrow, and absence of the Philadelphia chromosome. It may be challenging to distinguish essential thrombocythemia from reactive thrombocytosis or iron deficiency.

Treatment depends on the clinical situation. All patients who can tolerate aspirin should receive low-dose aspirin. Platelet apheresis should be used only for emergent management of acute bleeding or thrombosis and is not indicated from the platelet count alone. Cytoreductive therapy (hydroxyurea is the treatment of choice; anagrelide is an alternative) is recommended for patients with acute thrombosis or a previous history of thrombosis and for patients older than 60 years. Patients who are asymptomatic and young may be observed. In patients with very high platelet counts (>$1,000\times10^9$/L), acquired von Willebrand disease can develop. For these patients, the bleeding risk is greater than the thrombotic risk.

- Essential thrombocythemia: elevated platelet count with secondary causes excluded; half of the patients have JAK2 V617F.

- Cytoreductive therapy is indicated for patients older than 60 years or for patients who have had prior thrombosis.

- Relatively benign prognosis: <5% leukemic transformation rate at 15 years.

Polycythemia Vera

Polycythemia vera is a myeloproliferative disorder that results from activating mutations involving JAK2 tyrosine kinase. Clinical features include postbathing pruritus, fatigue, erythromelalgia (acral dysesthesias and erythema), headache, dizziness, and weight loss. More than 50% of patients have leukocytosis and thrombocytosis in addition to erythrocytosis. Polycythemia vera should be considered in the evaluation of an idiopathic thrombosis, especially in an atypical site such as an abdominal vessel or a dural sinus in the brain.

Bone marrow findings in polycythemia vera typically include trilineage hyperplasia. Most bone marrow specimens lack iron stores because the erythrocyte proliferation outstrips the iron supply. The leukocyte alkaline phosphatase score is not often measured anymore, but it is increased in polycythemia vera and primary myelofibrosis and low in CML. Erythropoietin levels are low or low normal. The mainstay of therapy for all patients with polycythemia vera is phlebotomy, with the goal of maintaining the hematocrit at less than 45%. Low-dose aspirin therapy is indicated for all patients who do not have a contraindication.

For patients who are older than 60 or who have had prior thrombosis, cytoreductive therapy is indicated. Hydroxyurea is often the first choice. Interferon alfa is the treatment of choice for younger patients and women of childbearing age. Radiophosphorus may be useful in older patients, but it increases the risk of AML.

- Polycythemia vera: low erythropoietin and universal finding of *JAK2* mutation.

- Pruritus, unusual thrombosis, and erythromelalgia.

- For polycythemia vera, phlebotomy is the cornerstone of treatment.

- For patients older than 60 years or with a history of thrombosis, add hydroxyurea.

SUMMARY

- With treatment, more than 80% of patients with Hodgkin lymphoma are now cured.

- NHL is a diverse group that includes low-grade lymphomas (which are usually not curable by the time they are diagnosed) and aggressive lymphomas (which are potentially curable).

- Multiple myeloma is distinguished from MGUS and smoldering myeloma by the presence of end-organ damage; treatment is evolving.

- The median age of patients with AML is about 65 years; the prognosis may be good if patients are younger than 40.

PART IX

NEPHROLOGY

38.

ACID–BASE AND ELECTROLYTE DISORDERS

Qi Qian, MD

GOALS

- Define fluid, electrolyte, and acid–base disorders.
- Cite treatments for fluid, electrolyte, and acid–base disorders.
- Apply these concepts to clinical scenarios.

DISORDERS OF SODIUM BALANCE AND VOLUME REGULATION

Volume expansion can be general (as in patients with congestive heart failure, cirrhosis, and nephrotic syndrome) or regional (as in patients with regional capillary leak, venous insufficiency, and lymphatic obstruction). Volume depletion is associated primarily with gastrointestinal tract (GI) fluid loss, excessive sweating, and renal sodium loss related to diuretic use or, rarely, renal salt wasting.

DIAGNOSIS

The cause of a volume disorder can be determined by physical examination. Elevated systemic blood pressure with or without edema signifies total body sodium excess. In congestive heart failure and cirrhosis, the kidneys are stimulated to retain sodium because the systemic blood pressure is low from low arterial effective volume (arterial underfill) due to pump failure and circulation derangements. Sodium retention leads to a net positive sodium balance and edema. Regional volume expansion is typically obvious on physical examination, showing normal vital signs and confined areas of fluid retention. Volume depletion is manifested by hypotension and tachycardia.

THERAPY

Management of volume disorders is 2-fold:

1. Volume repletion for hypovolemia and volume removal for hypervolemia with diuretics or dialysis (or both) when appropriate

2. Correction of the underlying causes

For patients with volume depletion, infusion of isotonic fluids and oral sodium restores volume status. In patients with congestive heart failure, measures that optimize cardiac function may improve renal perfusion and, therefore, facilitate diuresis. In cirrhosis, interventions that reduce portal hypertension and the need for liver transplant improve hemodynamics. In nephrotic syndrome, correcting proteinuria restores sodium homeostasis and volume balance. Diuresis, in general, is unnecessary in patients with regional fluid retention (except for regional edema involving the airway).

- Sodium balance reflects the body's volume status. Total body sodium excess equates with volume expansion (hypervolemia), and total body sodium deficiency equates with volume depletion (hypovolemia).

DISORDERS OF WATER BALANCE

HYPONATREMIA (WATER EXCESS)

Hyponatremia can be categorized as hypovolemic, euvolemic, or hypervolemic. Hypovolemia is a potent stimulator for arginine vasopressin (AVP)-mediated renal water retention, which leads to hyponatremia. Euvolemic hyponatremia includes 1) psychogenic polydipsia and beer potomania, in which water or hypotonic beer ingestion exceeds the capacity of renal water excretion; 2) syndrome of inappropriate secretion of antidiuretic hormone (SIADH), in which AVP-mediated water retention is independent of serum osmolality and volume status; and, rarely, 3) hypothyroidism and adrenal insufficiency. Hypervolemic hyponatremia mainly occurs in patients with congestive heart failure or cirrhosis. Arterial underfill in both conditions signals volume depletion, and activates AVP-mediated water retention, resulting in hyponatremia. In patients with moderate to advanced renal failure, dilutional hyponatremia may develop because of the diminished capacity of renal water excretion.

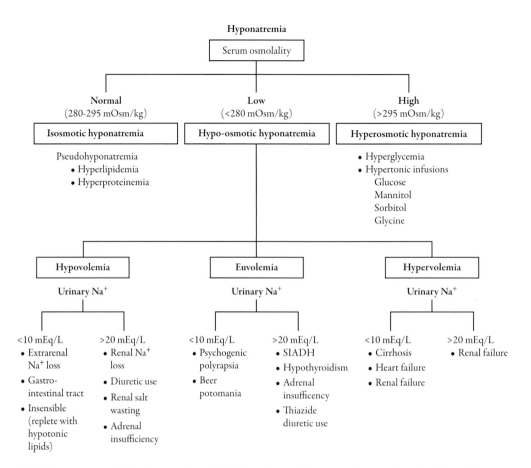

Figure 38.1 Diagnosis of Hyponatremia. Na⁺ indicates sodium; SIADH, syndrome of inappropriate secretion of antidiuretic hormone.

Diagnosis

The initial step in evaluating patients with hyponatremia is to determine the serum osmolality. As shown in Figure 38.1, depending on the serum osmolality, the differential diagnosis is narrowed to 3 categories.

If hypo-osmolality is confirmed, the diagnosis can be further narrowed to hypovolemic, euvolemic, or hypervolemic hyponatremia on the basis of the patient's volume status, determined by physical examination. Urine osmolality and urinary sodium concentration can then further help with delineating the underlying cause of hyponatremia.

In patients with euvolemic hyponatremia, if the urine is not maximally diluted (>150 mOsm/kg) and the urinary sodium concentration is greater than 20 mEq/L (on a regular Western diet), thyroid disease and adrenal insufficiency must be ruled out before considering the diagnosis of SIADH.

Patients with thiazide diuretic–induced hyponatremia may present with euvolemic hyponatremia that is indistinguishable from SIADH. Clinical history is critical in establishing causation. Postoperative pain can be associated with transient SIADH. Drugs associated with euvolemic hyponatremia include selective serotonin reuptake inhibitors, carbamazepine, chlorpromazine, vasopressin analogues, and, rarely, theophylline and amiodarone. Ecstasy intoxication can cause hyponatremia.

Therapy

For isosmotic and hyperosmotic hyponatremia, management should be directed toward correcting the underlying cause.

For hypovolemic hyponatremia, restoring intravascular volume eliminates the stimulatory signal for AVP. For patients with normal renal clearance, renal water unloading normalizes serum sodium concentration and osmolality.

For hypervolemic hyponatremia, symptomatic treatment directed toward reducing both total body water and sodium (aquaresis more than natriuresis) is necessary. Loop diuretics with or without vasopressin V2 receptor antagonists (vaptans) are usually effective. Correcting the underlying cardiac and hepatic abnormalities, if possible, will ultimately correct the water dysregulation.

For euvolemic hyponatremia, SIADH, treatment options include free water restriction, vasopressin V2 receptor blocker, and, when symptomatic, high-concentration (3%) saline. Specific attention should be paid to the rate of serum sodium correction. If hyponatremia developed over more than 2 days, correction should be gradual (<10 mEq daily). Rapid correction could lead to central pontine myelinolysis, a devastating neurologic complication of the "locked-in" state. Underlying causes of SIADH should always be sought and, when possible, corrected.

- Hyponatremia can be categorized as hypovolemic, euvolemic, or hypervolemic.

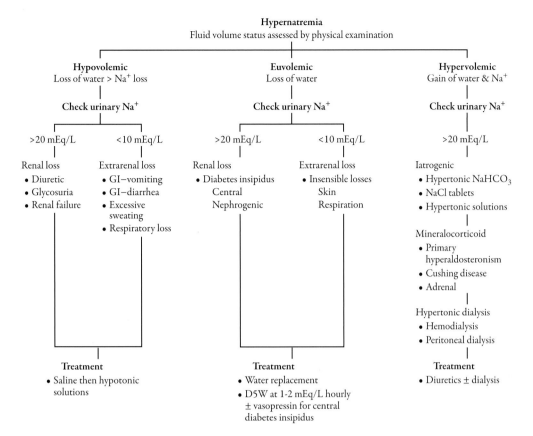

Figure 38.2 Diagnosis and Management of Hypernatremia. D5W indicates 5% dextrose in water; GI, gastrointestinal tract; Na⁺, sodium; NaCl, sodium chloride; NaHCO₃, sodium bicarbonate.

HYPERNATREMIA (WATER DEFICIENCY)

Hypernatremia (Figure 38.2) occurs in the following settings:

1. Decreased oral water intake (insufficient water provision or impairment of central nervous system thirst response

2. Increased renal water loss (diabetes insipidus [DI] or diuretic or aquaretic medications), GI water loss (osmotic diarrhea), or insensible water loss (sweat and respiration)

3. Hypertonic sodium–containing fluid administration (intravenous administration of concentrated sodium bicarbonate solution)

There is almost always a degree of overlap in excessive water loss and insufficient water intake. Hypernatremia occurs mostly in the elderly and infants and increases mortality among hospitalized patients.

Diagnosis

Unlike hyponatremia, for which confirmation of hypo-osmolality is necessary, hypernatremia is always associated with hyperosmolality; hence, there is no need to measure serum osmolality.

Urine osmolality and volume help differentiate renal from extrarenal water loss. Renal water wasting is typically associated with dilute urine and high urine volume (>3 L daily), whereas extrarenal water loss is associated with a maximally concentrated urine (>900 mOsm/kg) and urine output is usually low normal (<1.0–1.5 L daily).

Renal water wasting can be confirmed by determining random urine sodium and potassium concentrations. Renal water wasting is signified if the sum of the urinary sodium and urinary potassium concentrations is less than the serum sodium concentration. Investigations for osmotic diuresis and diabetes insipidus are indicated.

- Hypernatremia occurs in the setting of 1) decreased oral water intake; 2) increased renal water loss, GI water loss, or insensible water loss; or 3) hypertonic sodium–containing fluid administration.

OSMOTIC DIURESIS

Patients with osmotic diuresis may present with polyuria and hypernatremia. The osmolality of their urine is typically nearly isotonic to the plasma osmolality. Osmotic diuresis can be confirmed by calculating the total daily solute excretion. Normal solute excretion for an adult is approximately 700 to 1,000 mOsm daily (or about 10 mOsm/kg daily). If solute excretion in a 24-hour urine sample is greater than normal, the presence of osmotic diuresis is confirmed.

DIABETES INSIPIDUS

DI can be classified into 2 major types: central DI and nephrogenic DI. *Central DI* is due to insufficiency or absence of endogenous AVP. *Nephrogenic DI* is due to a partial or complete unresponsiveness of the renal tubular cells to AVP. Nephrogenic DI can be caused by genetic disorders, but more commonly it is caused by various acquired conditions. Lithium, demeclocycline, and amphotericin B are well-known drugs that can cause renal concentration defect and nephrogenic DI.

In addition, a rare type of gestational DI exists. It occurs in approximately 1 of every 300,000 pregnancies and is caused by placental production of vasopressinase, which degrades endogenous AVP and results in DI.

Diagnosis

DI is diagnosed with a water deprivation study, during which the combination of high serum sodium concentration (>145 mEq/L) and low urine osmolality (<150 mOsm/kg) constitutes a positive result and is diagnostic for DI.

If patients present with both hypernatremia (>145 mEq/L) and dilute urine (<150 mOsm/kg) without receiving any aquaretic medications, those findings are sufficient to establish a diagnosis of DI. A water deprivation study is not necessary.

After a diagnosis of DI is made, intranasal or intravenous desmopressin may be administered to differentiate central DI from nephrogenic DI. Desmopressin should be administered only when the serum sodium concentration is greater than 145 mEq/L. Central DI is diagnosed if the urine osmolality increases in response to desmopressin. Nephrogenic DI is diagnosed if there is no change in urine osmolality with desmopressin.

DI-associated polyuria should be differentiated from psychogenic polydipsia. The serum sodium concentration helps with the differentiation. In patients with psychogenic polydipsia, polyuria is driven by excessive water intake; thus, serum sodium concentration is typically in the lower end of the reference range (<140 mEq/L). Patients with DI, however, typically have serum sodium concentrations that are in the upper end of the reference range (>140 mEq/L) or elevated.

Therapy

The same principles for correcting hyponatremia apply to correcting hypernatremia. When hypernatremia develops over the course of more than 2 days, correction of sodium concentration should be gradual (≤10–12 mEq daily).

In gestational DI, placenta vasopressinase is inefficient in degrading exogenous desmopressin. Thus, desmopressin is efficacious in treating severe and symptomatic cases. It is important to recognize that gestational DI is a transient condition; placental vasopressinase typically dissipates within days post partum. Accordingly, treatment should be transient.

- Central DI is due to insufficiency or absence of endogenous AVP.

- Nephrogenic DI is due to a partial or complete unresponsiveness of the renal tubular cells to AVP.

DISORDERS OF POTASSIUM BALANCE

HYPOKALEMIA

Hypokalemia can be associated with pseudohypokalemia, transcellular shift, inadequate intake or GI loss, and renal loss. Hypokalemia (excluding pseudohypokalemia) can cause cellular hyperpolarization. Manifestations of hypokalemia include electrocardiographic (ECG) changes (blunted T wave and appearance of U wave), muscle weakness, ileus, polyuria (functional nephrogenic DI), and, in severe cases, rhabdomyolysis and asystole.

Diagnosis

Pseudohypokalemia due to active cellular potassium uptake in the test tube (leukocytosis or leukemia) should be ruled out when appropriate. If the plasma is immediately separated from the blood sample, this error can be avoided.

Hypokalemia caused by transcellular shift is typically transient. Pertinent clinical history provides key diagnostic clues, especially for rare hereditary types of hypokalemic paralysis.

As shown in Figure 38.3, quantifying urinary potassium is a key step in delineating the underlying (GI or renal) causes of hypokalemia.

Therapy

Potassium repletion can be achieved with oral or intravenous supplementation. Intravenous potassium infusion is indicated for patients who have severe symptomatic hypokalemia or who lack GI access. Intravenous potassium should be given in a saline-based solution rather than a dextrose-containing solution because sugar stimulates insulin secretion, shifting potassium intracellularly and exacerbating hypokalemia. A central line is preferred for the infusion since potassium can be corrosive to peripheral vessels. The rate of potassium infusion should not exceed 10 mEq hourly.

- Hypokalemia can be associated with pseudohypokalemia, transcellular shift, inadequate intake or GI loss, and renal loss.

- Manifestations of hypokalemia include ECG changes, muscle weakness, ileus, polyuria, rhabdomyolysis, and asystole.

HYPERKALEMIA

Hyperkalemia (Figure 38.4) can be associated with pseudohyperkalemia, excessive potassium intake, transcellular shift, and impaired secretion of renal potassium. Hyperkalemia (excluding pseudohyperkalemia) can cause cellular depolarization. Clinical manifestations include ECG changes (peaked T wave, shortened QT interval, and prolonged PR interval

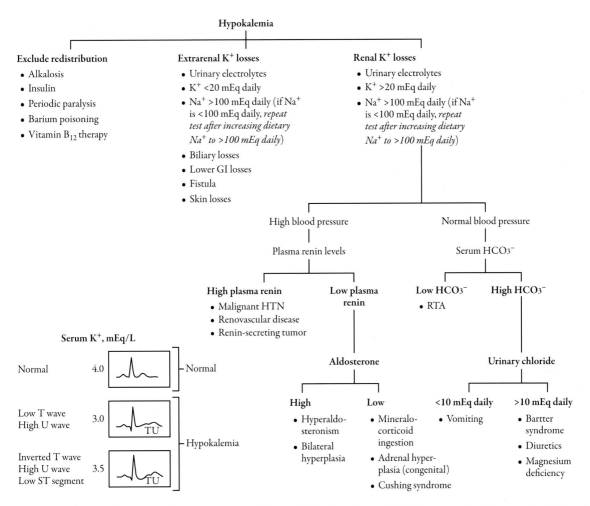

Figure 38.3 Diagnosis of Hypokalemia. GI indicates gastrointestinal tract; HCO$_3^-$, bicarbonate; HTN, hypertension; K$^+$, potassium; Na$^+$, sodium; RTA, renal tubular acidosis.

with widened QRS), and muscle weakness or frank paralysis. These manifestations may occur when the serum potassium concentration exceeds 6.5 to 7.0 mEq/L. Severe hyperkalemia can cause lethal cardiac arrhythmia (sine wave or complete absence of electrical activity—cardiac standstill), although a clear correlation between the ECG changes and serum potassium concentration has not been established.

Diagnosis

- Rule out pseudohyperkalemia due to cell lysis during or after blood sampling from using a small needle and inadequate technique. Use of a needle of appropriate size and optimal technique can mitigate the problem.

- Impaired excretion of renal potassium occurs primarily in patients with kidney failure and is a major cause of persistent hyperkalemia.

- Hyperkalemia caused by increased intake of potassium is seen typically in patients with some degree of kidney dysfunction.

- Cellular breakdown (rhabdomyolysis and tumor lysis syndrome) can acutely release cellular potassium into

the circulation. Hyperosmolality (hyperglycemia or administration of osmotically active solutions) can shift intracellular potassium out to the extracellular compartments through solvent drag.

- Hyperkalemia due to impaired potassium excretion from the collecting duct cells is common in patients with urinary outlet obstruction (eg, benign prostatic hypertrophy).

- Other conditions that can cause hyperkalemia include hyporeninemic hypoaldosteronism and medications such as potassium-sparing diuretics, nonsteroidal anti-inflammatory drugs, calcineurin inhibitors, angiotensin-converting enzyme inhibitors, angiotensin receptor blockers, and heparin.

Therapy

Therapy is dictated by the severity and underlying causes of hyperkalemia. For patients with ECG changes, urgent intravenous administration of calcium is indicated to stabilize the myocardium. Simultaneously, intravenous insulin, dextrose solution (5% or 10%), and inhaled β-agonist should be administered to promote an intracellular potassium shift.

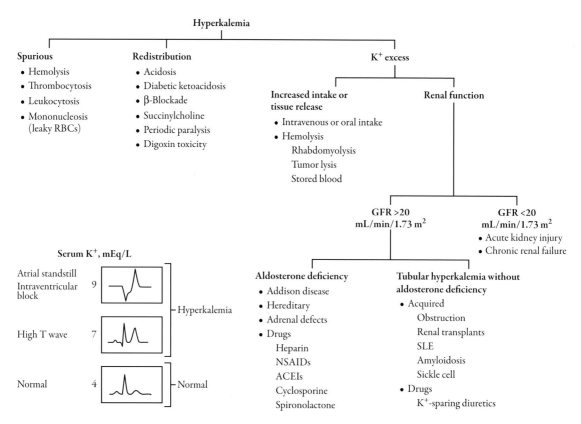

Figure 38.4 Diagnosis of Hyperkalemia. ACEI indicates angiotensin-converting enzyme inhibitor; GFR, glomerular filtration rate; K+, potassium; NSAID, nonsteroidal anti-inflammatory drug; RBC, red blood cell; SLE, systemic lupus erythematosus.

Box 38.1 **EXAMPLE OF ACID–BASE DETERMINATION**

Patient: A 37-year-old woman with a history of Sjögren syndrome and hypothyroidism was admitted for shortness of breath. Evaluation showed significant electrolyte and acid–base imbalance. Physical examination findings were unremarkable except for mild tachypnea. Laboratory test results were the following: sodium 134 mEq/L, potassium 2.6 mEq/L, chloride 115 mEq/L, bicarbonate (HCO_3) 10 mEq/L, and creatinine 0.6 mg/dL. Arterial blood gas results were pH 7.25 and Pco_2 25 mm Hg.

Question: What is the patient's acid–base status?

Answer: With the Henderson-Hasselbalch equation, first look at the blood pH. The patient's blood pH is decreased, indicating acidemia. Next identify which of the 2 variables (Pco_2 or HCO_3) decreases like the blood pH. Her serum HCO_3 is decreased, like the blood pH (low HCO_3 and low blood pH), indicating metabolic acidosis. Then look at whether the patient has an appropriate degree of compensation, which indicates a singular metabolic acidosis without any other primary abnormality. If the compensation is much more or much less than expected, there is likely a second, primary respiratory abnormality. For example, if the Pco_2 is lower than the expected compensation, there is a primary respiratory alkalosis in addition to a primary metabolic acidosis; a Pco_2 higher than expected indicates the existence of an additional primary respiratory acidosis.

One of 2 methods is used to determine the expected respiratory compensation (Pco_2):

1. Winter formula: Expected $Pco_2 = (1.5 \times HCO_3) + 8 \pm 2$. For this patient, expected $Pco_2 = 23 \pm 2$ mm Hg. This formula is used when the patient's serum HCO_3 is in the acidemic range (<20 mEq/L).

2. Rule of +15: Expected $Pco_2 = HCO_3 + 15$. The value (25 for this patient) should equal the last 2 digits of the pH if the patient has a single acidosis with adequate respiratory compensation. The rule of +15 is relatively simple and applicable when the HCO_3 ranges between 10 and 40 mEq/L.

On the basis of the calculation, this patient has a pure non–anion gap acidosis with appropriate compensation.

When appropriate, non–potassium-sparing diuretics and potassium-exchange resin (sodium polystyrene) may be used to promote renal and GI potassium excretion. For asymptomatic patients with mild to moderate hyperkalemia (<6 mEq/L), dietary potassium restriction, non–potassium-sparing diuretics, and potassium-exchange resin may suffice. For patients with advanced renal failure or hyperkalemia that is refractory to conservative measures, dialysis is necessary.

While the above measures mitigate hyperkalemia, steps should be taken to correct the underlying causes. Correcting a urinary tract obstruction can lead to kaliuresis. Medication-induced hyperkalemia should be corrected by adjusting the medication regimen.

- Hyperkalemia can be associated with pseudohyperkalemia, excessive potassium intake, transcellular shift, and impaired secretion of renal potassium.
- Therapy is dictated by the severity and underlying causes of hyperkalemia.

ACID–BASE DISORDERS

DETERMINATION OF ACID–BASE STATUS

Examination of acid–base status should begin with the Henderson-Hasselbalch equation:

$$pH = pK_a + \log \frac{[A^-]}{[HA]},$$

where pK_a is the negative logarithm of the acid dissociation constant and A^- is the concentration of the ionized form of the acid HA. Blood pH is derived from the ratio of 2 variables, serum bicarbonate (HCO_3) (base) and Pco_2 (acid). Under conditions in which 1 of these variables increases or decreases, the other variable predictably and compensatorily also increases or decreases and minimizes the change in the ratio, hence minimizing blood pH alterations. An example of acid–base determination with the Winter formula and the rule of +15 is shown in Box 38.1.

NON–ANION GAP ACIDOSIS

Metabolic acidoses, defined as a primary decrease in serum HCO_3 and a compensatory reduction in Pco_2, are classified as normal anion gap (non–anion gap) and increased anion gap acidoses. Non–anion gap acidosis may be caused by renal tubular acidosis (RTA) (renal hydrogen ion retention or HCO_3 wasting or both), diarrhea (GI HCO_3 wasting), early-stage chronic kidney failure (low serum HCO_3 associated with serum creatinine elevation), ureterosigmoid fistula (enteric chloric-HCO_3 exchange), and certain medications, such as carbonic anhydrase inhibitors (eg, acetazolamide).

Renal Tubular Acidoses

There are 3 main types of RTA (Table 38.1):

1. Type 1—distal tubular acidosis due to defects in hydrogen ion excretion in the collecting duct
2. Type 2—proximal tubular acidosis due to defects in proximal tubular HCO_3 reclamation
3. Type 4—hyporeninemic hypoaldosteronism

- Non–anion gap acidosis may be caused by RTA, diarrhea, early-stage chronic kidney failure, ureterosigmoid fistula, and certain medications (eg, carbonic anhydrase inhibitors).

Table 38.1 **FEATURES OF RENAL TUBULAR ACIDOSES**

FEATURE	TYPE 1: DISTAL	TYPE 2: PROXIMAL	TYPE 4: HYPORENINEMIC HYPOALDOSTERONISM
Defect	H^+ excretion in distal tubule	HCO_3 reabsorption in proximal tubule	Low renin, low aldosterone
Etiology & clinical setting	Acquired: connective tissue diseases, interstitial renal diseases Drug: Amphotericin B Hereditary: rare	Acquired: dysproteinemia (MM), interstitial renal diseases (less frequently), lead or mercury toxicity Drug: ifosfamide Hereditary: glycogen storage disease, hereditary fructose intolerance, mitochondrial diseases, cystinosis, Wilson disease	DM, mild to moderate CKD
Serum potassium	Low	Low	High
Urine pH	Always high (>5.3)	Low (when $HCO_3 <$ Tm)	Variable
Urinary loss of glucose, amino acids, & phosphate (Fanconi syndrome)	No	Yes	No
Nephrocalcinosis or nephrolithiasis	Yes	No	No
Acidemia	Severe without treatment	Self-limited	Mild
Alkali treatment	Small requirement	Large requirement; treat the cause	Small requirement
FE-HCO_3	<5%	Can be high with alkali treatment	Variable

Abbreviations: CKD, chronic kidney disease; DM, diabetes mellitus; FE, fractional excretion; H^+, hydrogen ion; HCO_3, bicarbonate; MM, multiple myeloma; Tm, tubular transport maximum.

Table 38.2 METABOLIC ALKALOSIS

CAUSES	PATHOPHYSIOLOGY	DIAGNOSTIC FEATURES IN ADDITION TO METABOLIC ALKALOSIS	THERAPY
Vomiting & gastric secretions	Net acid loss Enhanced renal proximal tubular HCO_3 absorption	↓ or normal BP Low urinary chloride (<20 mEq/L)	Normal saline
Hyperaldosteronism: primary hyperaldosteronism; secondary hyperaldosteronism (renal artery stenosis, volume depletion, & use of diuretics)	↑ Renal H^+ excretion ↑ Proximal renal tubular HCO_3 absorption	↑ BP in primary hyperaldosteronism (high urinary chloride [>20 mEq/L]) & renal artery stenosis ↓ BP in volume depletion & diuretic use Hypokalemia	Correction of the causes
Severe hypokalemia	↑ Renal H^+ excretion ↑ Renal HCO_3 absorption ↑ Ammonium genesis	Normal BP Hypokalemia Polyuria	Potassium repletion
Exogenous alkali intake ($CaHCO_3$ & $NaHCO_3$)	Analogous to milk alkaline syndrome	Hypercalcemia Usually in patients with CKD	Discontinue alkaline intake
Posthypercapnic state	Net loss of carbonic acid	Mechanical ventilation in patients with severe COPD	↓ Ventilation
Liddle syndrome	Autosomal dominant inheritance Epithelial sodium channel mutation Defective retrieval of sodium channels from apical surface of renal epithelial cells	↑ BP Hypokalemia	Potassium repletion
Glucocorticoid-remediable aldosteronism	Autosomal dominant inheritance Aldosterone synthesis is stimulated by corticotropin	↑ BP ↑ Aldosterone Hypokalemia ↓ Serum renin activity	Glucocorticoids
Apparent glucocorticoid excess	Defects in 11β-hydroxysteroid dehydrogenase Genetic defect (autosomal recessive inheritance), acquired (excessive licorice intake), or Cushing syndrome	↑ BP Hypokalemia ↓ Serum renin activity ↓ Aldosterone level ↑ Urinary cortisol to cortisone ratio	Mineralocorticoid receptor blockade Symptomatic treatment
Bartter syndrome	Autosomal recessive inheritance with 5 types of genetic defects	Neonatal or childhood onset ↓ BP Hypokalemia Hypercalciuria High urinary chloride (>20 mEq/L)	Sodium and potassium repletion
Gitelman syndrome	Autosomal recessive inheritance Mutations in distal sodium-chloride cotransporters	Adolescence or adulthood onset ↓ or normal BP Hypokalemia Hypocalciuria High urinary chloride (>20 mEq/L)	Sodium and potassium repletion

Abbreviations: ↓, decreased; ↑, increased; BP, blood pressure; $CaHCO_3$, calcium bicarbonate; CKD, chronic kidney disease; COPD, chronic obstructive pulmonary disease; H^+, hydrogen ion; HCO_3, bicarbonate; $NaHCO_3$, sodium bicarbonate.

ANION GAP ACIDOSIS

Anion gap metabolic acidoses can be grouped according to underexcretion and overgeneration of nonvolatile acids. Underexcretion occurs mainly in patients with renal failure in which nonvolatile acids from regular metabolism cannot be excreted. Overgeneration is related to excessive generation of nonvolatile acid, as in lactic acidosis, ketoacidosis, and ingestion of toxic acids from toxic alcohol or drugs (eg, salicylate).

In recent years, several new anion gap–generating acids have been added to the list as causes of anion gap metabolic acidosis. Accordingly, the new mnemonic for the major causes of anion gap metabolic acidosis is GOLDMARK: *g*lycerose (ethylene and propylene), *o*xoproline, *L*-lactate, *D*-lactate, *m*ethanol, *a*spirin, *r*enal failure, and *k*etoacidosis.

L-lactic acidoses can be subdivided into type A and type B lactic acidoses. Type A lactic acidosis develops with tissue hypoxia, as in shock, severe anemia, and hypoxia from pulmonary diseases. Type B lactic acidosis refers to conditions of mitochondrial oxidative impairment, including MELAS syndrome, cyanide intoxication, and use of certain medications (metformin, linezolid, and reverse transcriptase inhibitors).

D-lactic acidosis mainly occurs in patients with short gut syndrome and overgrowth of gut bacteria. The bacteria generate D-lactate, which causes anion gap acidosis. Notably, most clinical laboratories test for only L-lactate. Therefore, when D-lactic acidosis is suspected, measurement of D-lactate must be requested specifically.

Diagnosis and Therapy

In most cases, clinical scenarios will reveal the cause of acidosis. In addition to its use for acid–base disturbances, the osmolal gap should be calculated when toxic alcohol ingestion is suspected. The toxic alcohols (especially methanol and ethylene glycol) are osmotically active molecules. Before their conversion to toxic acids, the alcohols generate an osmolal gap (measured serum osmolality is greater than the calculated serum osmolality by more than 10 mOsm/kg). When the osmolal gap is elevated, treatment should be instituted immediately to block the toxic alcohols (parent compounds) from being metabolized. Inhibitors of alcohol dehydrogenase (eg, 4-methylpyrazole) effectively block alcohol metallization. In severe cases, hemodialysis is necessary.

Salicylate intoxication in adults typically causes anion gap acidosis and respiratory alkalosis. Anion gap acidosis is caused by salicylic acid, its metabolites, and lactate; respiratory alkalosis is caused by stimulation of the central nervous system respiratory center.

- Anion gap metabolic acidoses can be grouped according to underexcretion and overgeneration of nonvolatile acids.

- A mnemonic for the major causes of anion gap metabolic acidosis is GOLDMARK: *g*lycerose (ethylene and propylene), *o*xoproline, *L*-lactate, *D*-lactate, *m*ethanol, *a*spirin, *r*enal failure, and *k*etoacidosis.

METABOLIC ALKALOSIS

Metabolic alkalosis can result from a net loss of acid or a net gain of bicarbonate (generation phase). Alkalosis is then perpetuated by hypovolemia, hypokalemia, or excessive mineralocorticoid stimulation. These conditions prevent the kidney from unloading the accumulated bicarbonate (maintenance phase). Clinical manifestations include weakness, muscle cramps, hyperreflexia, alveolar hypoventilation, and arrhythmias. The major causes, pathophysiology, diagnostic features, and therapy are summarized in Table 38.2.

Diagnosis and Therapy

Metabolic alkalosis associated with hypovolemia is characterized by a low urine chloride concentration (<20 mEq/L) and

---

Box 38.2 RESPIRATORY ACID–BASE ALTERATIONS

Causes of respiratory acidosis
  CNS respiratory depression
    Injury: trauma, infarct, hemorrhage, tumor
    Drugs: opiates, sedatives, anesthetics
    Hypoventilation of obesity (eg, pickwickian syndrome)
    Cerebral hypoxia
  Nerve or muscle
    Guillain-Barré syndrome, myasthenia gravis, various myopathies
    Diaphragmatic factors: paralysis or splinting, muscle relaxants
    Toxins (eg, organophosphates, snake venom)
  Chest wall airway lung
    Airway: upper and lower airway obstruction
    Chest wall trauma: flail chest, contusion, hemothorax, pneumothorax
    Lung: pulmonary edema, ARDS, aspiration
  Carbon dioxide excess
    Hypercatabolic states: malignant hyperthermia
    Addition of CO_2 to inspired gas
    Insufflation of CO_2 into body cavity (eg, for laparoscopic surgery)
Causes of respiratory alkalosis
  CNS respiratory stimulation
    Pain, hyperventilation syndrome, anxiety, psychosis, infection, trauma, cerebrovascular accident
  Hypoxia
    High altitude, severe anemia, right-to-left shunts
  Drugs
    Progesterone, methylxanthines, salicylates, catecholamines, nicotine
  Endocrine conditions
    Progesterone (pregnancy)
  Pulmonary conditions
    Pneumonia, edema, embolism, asthma
  Miscellaneous
    Sepsis, hepatic failure, recovery phase of metabolic acidosis

Abbreviations: ARDS, acute respiratory distress syndrome; CNS, central nervous system; CO_2, carbon dioxide.

---

is responsive to volume expansion with isotonic saline infusion or oral salt tablets. Metabolic alkalosis associated with primary mineralocorticoid excess is usually hypervolemic, exhibits a high urine chloride concentration (>20 mEq/L), and is resistant to saline or salt but responsive to acetazolamide diuresis and mineralocorticoid antagonizers. These treatments should be given only after serum potassium is repleted, since both alkalosis and treatment with acetazolamide are associated with kaliuresis.

- Metabolic alkalosis can result from a net loss of acid or a net gain of bicarbonate (generation phase).

RESPIRATORY ACID–BASE ALTERATIONS

Alterations of P_{CO_2} mark respiratory acid–base dysregulation. P_{CO_2}, determined by tidal volume and respiratory rate, is regulated by the ventilatory system. The key components of the ventilatory system include the respiratory center in the central nervous system, the chest wall (ribs, nerves, and muscles), and lung parenchyma. Central nervous system respiratory drive can be affected by medications, hormones (progesterone during pregnancy), and toxins (in patients with hepatic failure, uremia, or sepsis); chest wall function can be affected by neuromuscular diseases, paralysis, and trauma (flail chest); and lung parenchyma can be affected by infection, edema as in acute respiratory distress syndrome, and chronic obstructive pulmonary disease.

Causes of respiratory acid–base alterations and expected metabolic compensations for acute and chronic respiratory acid–base alterations are summarized in Box 38.2.

Diagnosis and Therapy

Respiratory acidosis is characterized by a decrease in blood pH, an increase in Pco_2, and a compensatory increase in serum HCO_3. Respiratory alkalosis features an increase in blood pH, a decrease in Pco_2, and a compensatory decrease in serum HCO_3. Therapy for respiratory acid–base alterations is directed to the specific causes.

- Respiratory acidosis is characterized by a decrease in blood pH, an increase in Pco_2, and a compensatory increase in serum HCO_3.

- Respiratory alkalosis features an increase in blood pH, a decrease in Pco_2, and a compensatory decrease in serum HCO_3.

SUMMARY

- In this chapter, fluid, electrolyte, and acid–base disorders were defined. Additionally, treatments for fluid, electrolyte, and acid–base disorders were explored.

ACUTE KIDNEY INJURY, GLOMERULAR DISEASE, AND TUBULOINTERSTITIAL DISEASE

Suzanne M. Norby, MD, Kianoush B. Kashani, MD, and Fernando C. Fervenza, MD, PhD

GOALS

- Discuss the differential diagnosis, etiology, and pathophysiology of acute kidney injury (AKI).

- Recognize features of nephritic syndrome and nephrotic syndrome.

- Cite the various types of glomerular and tubulointerstital diseases along with their diagnosis and management.

ACUTE KIDNEY INJURY

AKI is a term that has replaced *acute renal failure* in contemporary medical literature. AKI denotes a rapid deterioration of kidney function (glomerular filtration rate [GFR]) within hours to weeks, resulting in the accumulation of nitrogenous metabolites and fluid, electrolyte, and acid-base imbalances.

DEFINITION AND DIAGNOSIS

The definition of *AKI* was refined by the Acute Kidney Injury Network (AKIN) to a 3-stage definition (Table 39.1) and includes 1) an absolute or relative increase in serum creatinine (SCr) from baseline and 2) decreased urine output (Figure 39.1). Use of SCr as a marker of AKI, however, has disadvantages, including the following:

1. Baseline level of SCr is often unknown.

2. Creatinine is eliminated by the kidneys through both glomerular filtration and tubular secretion. As GFR decreases, tubular secretion of creatinine increases.

3. Changes in SCr unrelated to GFR can occur when tubular excretion of SCr is affected by other factors.

- AKI denotes a rapid deterioration of kidney function (GFR) within hours to weeks, resulting in the

accumulation of nitrogenous metabolites and fluid, electrolyte, and acid-base imbalances.

Increased SCr without changes in GFR, resulting in *underestimation* of actual GFR, can occur when tubular secretion of creatinine is blocked by drugs (eg, trimethoprim, cimetidine, amiloride, probenecid, spironolactone, and triamterene). Drugs and substances such as cefoxitin, glucose, ketone bodies, proline, and flucytosine may interfere with older SCr assays and increase the measured SCr value. In addition, rhabdomyolysis, vigorous exercise, and ingestion of cooked meat increase production of creatinine without changing GFR.

Decreased SCr without changes in GFR, resulting in *overestimation* of actual GFR, can also be caused by substances that interfere with older SCr assays (eg, bilirubin, α-methyldopa, and methimazole) and occur in persons with low creatinine production, such as those with low muscle mass (small women, amputees, elderly patients, and patients with end-stage liver disease), muscle wasting disorders, malnutrition, and dietary protein restriction.

Changes in serum urea nitrogen (SUN) level are less reliable for diagnosing AKI than changes in SCr. In acute illness, alterations in protein metabolism, dietary habits, and volume status affect SUN. *Increased* SUN without changes in GFR can occur with tissue trauma, use of diuretics or glucocorticoids, high-protein meals, and gastrointestinal tract bleeding. *Decreased* SUN without changes in GFR can occur in patients with advanced liver disease and in persons consuming low-protein diets.

The traditional classification subdivides AKI into prerenal, intrinsic renal, and postrenal categories. Although 1 main cause of AKI can be found in some patients, multiple factors contribute to the development of AKI in many patients. The key diagnostic tests are urinalysis with microscopy and renal ultrasonography.

- Certain drugs and endogenous compounds may affect the reliability of SCr and SUN levels.

- The key diagnostic tests for evaluating AKI are urinalysis with microscopy and renal ultrasonography.

Table 39.1 CLASSIFICATION AND STAGING SYSTEM FOR ACUTE KIDNEY INJURY

STAGE	SERUM CREATININE CONCENTRATION	URINE OUTPUT
1	Increase of ≥0.3 mg/dL *or* Increase to ≥ 150%-200% from baseline	<0.5 mL/kg per hour for >6 h
2	Increase to >200%-300% from baseline	<0.5 mL/kg per hour for >12 h
3	Increase to >300% from baseline *or* Concentration ≥4.0 mg/dL, with a recent increase of ≥0.5 mg/dL *or* Need for renal replacement therapy	<0.3 mL/kg per hour for 24 h *or* anuria for 12 h

Adapted from Mehta RL, Kellum JA, Shah SV, Molitoris BA, Ronco C, Warnock DG, et al; Acute Kidney Injury Network. Acute Kidney Injury Network: report of an initiative to improve outcomes in acute kidney injury. Crit Care. 2007;11(2):R31. This article is online at: http://ccforum.com/content/11/2/R31. ©2007 Mehta et al. This is an open access article distributed under the terms of the Creative Commons Attribution License (http://creativecommons.org/licenses/by/2.0), which permits unrestricted use, distribution, and reproduction in any medium, provided the original work is properly cited.

PRERENAL AKI

Prerenal AKI is defined as decreased GFR due to decreased renal perfusion *without* ischemic injury to tubules, resulting from volume depletion, low cardiac output, drugs, or peripheral vasodilation (eg, sepsis). It is characterized by 1) increased reabsorption of sodium and water leading to concentrated urine, 2) increased reabsorption of urea resulting in elevation of SUN out of proportion to creatinine (>20:1), and 3) reversibility within 3 to 4 days if the underlying cause is treated.

One cause of prerenal AKI is intravascular volume depletion from external loss of fluids and electrolytes (vomiting, diarrhea, and dehydration), loss of plasma volume (burns), internal fluid losses (third spacing, as occurs in severe pancreatitis), and hemorrhage. Physical findings of volume depletion include orthostatic hypotension, dry mucous membranes, and decreased skin turgor. Management involves administration of oral liquids or intravenous fluids, such as normal saline, albumin, or blood, depending on the clinical situation.

A second cause of prerenal AKI is volume overload or decreased cardiac output (or both) as occurs in congestive heart failure (cardiorenal syndrome). Physical findings include elevated jugular venous pressure, bibasilar crackles in the lungs, peripheral edema, and a third heart sound gallop. Management includes optimization of hemodynamics, often with diuretics.

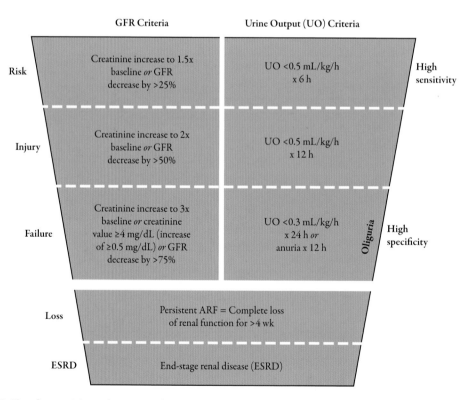

Figure 39.1 The RIFLE Classification Scheme for Acute Kidney Injury. ARF indicates acute renal failure; GFR, glomerular filtration rate; RIFLE, *r*isk, *i*njury, *f*ailure, *l*oss, and *E*SRD. (Adapted from Bellomo R, Ronco C, Kellum JA, Mehta RL, Palevsky P; Acute Dialysis Quality Initiative workgroup. Acute renal failure: definition, outcome measures, animal models, fluid therapy and information technology needs: the Second International Consensus Conference of the Acute Dialysis Quality Initiative [ADQI] Group. Crit Care. 2004 Aug;8[4]:R204–12. Epub 2004 May 24. Critical Care 2004;8:R204–R212. This article is online at: http://ccforum.com/content/8/4/R204. ©2004 Bellomo et al. This is an Open Access article: verbatim copying and redistribution of this article are permitted in all media for any purpose, provided this notice is preserved along with the article's original URL.)

A third cause of prerenal AKI is renal artery occlusion. It is characterized by a sudden occlusion (thrombosis, stenosis, emboli, vasculitis of the main renal arteries, or several intrarenal arteries) of the arteries supplying blood to the kidneys and the resultant rapid decline in renal function. If not promptly addressed, renal artery occlusion causes ischemic acute tubular necrosis (ATN).

Vasoactive drugs can cause intrarenal hemodynamic changes that decrease renal blood flow, leading to prerenal AKI. Nonsteroidal anti-inflammatory drugs (NSAIDs) inhibit cyclooxygenase and decrease vasodilatory prostaglandin production. Patients who take NSAIDs and have underlying renal insufficiency, volume depletion, advanced liver disease, or congestive heart failure are at risk of AKI. Angiotensin-converting enzyme inhibitors (ACEIs) and angiotensin receptor blockers (ARBs) increase the risk of AKI when renal blood flow is decreased. These medications interfere with the action of angiotensin II, which serves to maintain GFR when renal blood flow is decreased. If AKI develops while a patient is taking an ACEI or ARB, use of these medications should be withheld until renal function improves. Also, the calcineurin inhibitors cyclosporine and tacrolimus cause renal vasoconstriction.

Hepatorenal syndrome (HRS), another cause of prerenal AKI, occurs in patients with end-stage liver disease. HRS is a functional renal failure induced by intrarenal vasoconstriction in the setting of circulatory dysfunction with splanchnic vasodilation and relatively insufficient cardiac output leading to effective hypovolemia. Precipitating events may be worsening liver function, bleeding, infection (such as spontaneous bacterial peritonitis), and large-volume paracentesis without albumin replacement. Diagnostic criteria include the following:

1. Cirrhosis with ascites

2. SCr >1.5 mg/dL

3. No improvement in SCr after 2 days of diuretic withdrawal and volume expansion with albumin

4. No recent administration of nephrotoxic drugs

5. Normal findings on renal ultrasonography

6. Absence of shock

7. Absence of renal parenchymal disease (defined as proteinuria >500 mg/daily and microhematuria >50 red blood cells [RBCs] per high-power field)

Type 1 HRS occurs with rapid decline in renal function. Type 2 HRS manifests with a more gradual decline in renal function and often refractory ascites. Administration of albumin and vasoconstrictors (such as vasopressin analogues) or midodrine plus octreotide may improve the historically poor short-term prognosis. Transjugular intrahepatic portosystemic shunt may also improve HRS. Liver transplant is the preferred therapy for appropriate candidates.

- *Prerenal AKI* is defined as decreased GFR due to decreased renal perfusion *without* ischemic injury to tubules,

resulting from volume depletion, low cardiac output, drugs, or peripheral vasodilation (eg, sepsis).

- Causes of prerenal AKI include volume overload, renal artery occlusion, vasoactive drugs, and HRS.

INTRINSIC RENAL AKI

Glomerular Disease and Vasculitis

Glomerular disease occurring in combination with AKI, called rapidly progressive glomerulonephritis (GN), and vasculitis are discussed later in this chapter in the "Glomerular Disease" section.

Acute Tubular Necrosis (ATN)

The natural history of ATN depends on its etiology and can be caused by ischemia (decrease in oxygen delivery), inflammation or nephrotoxic injury. Many toxins, both endogenous and exogenous, can cause tubular damage. Since hospital-acquired AKI is usually multifactorial, the timeline of development and recovery of ATN is based on the clinical picture. If prerenal ischemia lasts long enough, tubular damage begins. Extension of the injury after reperfusion is usually from the infiltration of inflammatory cells. The typical course of ischemic ATN begins with a rapid decrease in urine output, accompanied by an increase in the SCr level (Figure 39.2). During the maintenance phase, oliguria is usually followed by polyuria before tubules regain their concentrating capacity. The longer the duration of the oliguric phase before recovery, the smaller the chance of complete recovery of kidney function. In the recovery phase, the SCr level begins to decrease and urine output normalizes.

Contrast-induced nephropathy (CIN) is typically defined as an increase in SCr of 0.5 mg/dL or 25% within 3 days after administration of a contrast agent if there is no other cause. In

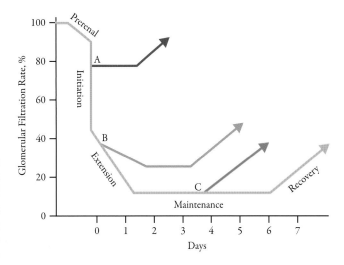

Figure 39.2 Time Course of Acute Tubular Necrosis. A, B, and C indicate therapy to prevent (A) or limit (B) the extension phase and therapy for established acute tubular necrosis (C). (Adapted from Molitoris BA. Transitioning to therapy in ischemic acute renal failure. J Am Soc Nephrol. 2003 Jan;14[1]:265–7. Used with permission.)

most patients, urine output decreases and SCr increases 24 to 48 hours after administration of the dye and returns to normal within 7 to 10 days. Risk factors for CIN are diabetes mellitus, chronic kidney disease (CKD) (especially with estimated GFR <30 mL/min), congestive heart failure, acute myocardial infarction within 24 hours, peripheral vascular disease, dehydration, concomitant use of other nephrotoxins, or advanced age. In high-risk patients, the following steps are thought to reduce the incidence or decrease the severity of CIN: using low-osmolar contrast agents, limiting the dose of contrast agent, spacing repeated dye loads, and withholding the use of medications that alter renal blood flow or intrarenal hemodynamics (ACEIs, ARBs, and NSAIDs). Intravenous hydration with normal saline is the accepted therapy for preventing CIN. Administration of *N*-acetylcysteine and intravenous hydration with fluid containing sodium bicarbonate have also been advocated as preventive measures, but results of studies that have assessed these agents have been inconsistent.

Tubular cells can be directly damaged by many medications and agents, including aminoglycosides, amphotericin B, vancomycin, calcineurin inhibitors, cisplatin, methotrexate, ifosfamide, pentamidine, contrast agents, foscarnet, and cidofovir. Toxicity is usually dose dependent. Amphotericin B lowers GFR through vasoconstriction and is also associated with distal tubular dysfunction (nephrogenic diabetes insipidus and type 4 renal tubular acidosis). Toxicity occurs after a cumulative amphotericin B dose of 2 to 3 g. Avoiding volume depletion and using the liposomal form of amphotericin B decreases the chance of nephrotoxicity. Aminoglycoside renal toxicity occurs after 5 to 7 days of treatment and correlates with a cumulative dose. Patients are often nonoliguric and have potassium and magnesium wasting. Once-daily dosing regimens decrease the incidence of aminoglycoside nephrotoxicity.

Pigment nephropathy can occur with rhabdomyolysis or intravascular hemolysis when abnormal amounts of free hemoglobin or myoglobin in the serum are filtered by the kidney. These pigments are directly toxic to renal tubular cells and can also form casts inside the tubular lumens. Urine dipstick testing is positive for blood in the urine, but RBCs are not apparent with urine microscopy. During rhabdomyolysis or hemolysis, the patient should be aggressively hydrated to achieve a high rate of urine flow (200–300 mL/h). Urine alkalinization has been advocated but is controversial.

Myeloma cast nephropathy is discussed later in this chapter in the "Glomerular Disease" section.

- The natural history of ATN depends on its cause (ischemia from a decrease in oxygen delivery, inflammation, or nephrotoxic injury).

Atheroembolic Disease

Atheroembolic disease usually occurs after vascular manipulations during arterial catheterization or vascular operations in patients who have severe atherosclerosis. The timeline for development of atheroembolic disease after the procedure is variable, ranging from hours to weeks. About 20% of patients

with atheroembolic disease do not report a history of vascular procedures. Unstable atheromatous plaques release a shower of cholesterol crystals into the arterial bloodstream, where they embolize in small vessels, causing blockage and distal necrosis. Livedo reticularis may be seen on the back, flank, abdomen, or extremities. On ophthalmoscopic examination, the atheroemboli manifest as Hollenhorst plaques. Other clinical manifestations are bowel ischemia and necrosis in addition to AKI. Although the diagnosis is mostly clinical, the definitive diagnosis of atheroembolic disease is by kidney or skin biopsy and observation of cholesterol crystals in small arterioles with distal necrosis. A high erythrocyte sedimentation rate or C-reactive protein level and decreased complement levels are suggestive of atheroembolic disease. The prognosis for kidney recovery after atheroembolic disease is poor and recovery is usually incomplete. The treatment is supportive, including cholesterol-lowering agents and renal replacement therapy (RRT) as needed. Anticoagulation is contraindicated since it can destabilize the atheromatous plaques and, therefore, cause additional cholesterol emboli.

- Atheroembolic disease usually occurs after vascular manipulations during arterial catheterization or vascular operations in patients who have severe atherosclerosis.

Acute Interstitial Nephritis

Acute interstitial nephritis (AIN) is an inflammatory process characterized by a mononuclear cell infiltrate within the renal interstitium. Relatively common, AIN accounts for approximately 10% to 15% of cases of AKI. AIN is idiopathic in 10% to 20% of cases, but it is most frequently associated with the following (Box 39.1):

1. Drugs, particularly antibiotics and NSAIDs
2. Infections
3. Autoimmune systemic diseases
4. Malignancies

Diagnosis of AIN may require renal biopsy. Clinically, AIN has a sudden onset (usually after the patient has had several days of exposure if the cause is related to a medication). Systemic manifestations of a hypersensitivity reaction in patients with drug-induced AIN include fever, maculopapular rash, and arthralgias (25% of patients). Flank pain caused by distention of the renal capsule occurs in about 50% of patients. Abnormal renal function, occurring in about 60% of patients, varies from a mild increase in SCr level to severe AKI that requires dialysis. Tubular damage can impair the urinary concentration mechanism and result in polyuria. Peripheral eosinophilia is common (about 50% of patients). Urinary abnormalities include the following:

1. Pyuria (in nearly 100% of patients)
2. Microscopic hematuria

COMMON CAUSES OF ACUTE INTERSTITIAL NEPHRITIS

Drugs

    Antibiotics—penicillin, methicillin (anti–tubular basement membrane antibodies), ampicillin, rifampin, sulfa drugs, ciprofloxacin, pentamidine

    NSAIDs—interstitial nephritis with nephrotic syndrome & renal insufficiency may have a latent period; not dose-dependent; recurs; possibly T-cell–mediated; allergic signs & symptoms are absent

    Diuretics—thiazides, furosemide, bumetanide (sulfa derivatives)

    Cimetidine

    Proton pump inhibitors

    Allopurinol, phenytoin, phenindione

    Cyclosporine

Infections

    Bacteria—*Legionella, Brucella, Streptococcus, Staphylococcus, Pneumococcus*

    Virus—Epstein-Barr, CMV, *Hantavirus*, HIV, hepatitis B, *Polyomavirus*

    Fungus—*Candida, Histoplasma*

    Parasites—*Plasmodium, Toxoplasma, Schistosoma, Leishmania*

Systemic diseases

    Systemic lupus erythematosus

    Sjögren syndrome

    Sarcoidosis

    Lymphoma, leukemic infiltration

    Renal transplant rejection

Idiopathic

Abbreviations: CMV, cytomegalovirus; HIV, human immunodeficiency virus; NSAID, nonsteroidal anti-inflammatory drug.

3. Eosinophiluria (>1% eosinophils)—suggestive of AIN but also seen in other unrelated renal diseases

4. Proteinuria that is usually mild (<1 g/1.73 m² per 24 hours)

Therapy for AIN is primarily supportive. Identification and elimination of inciting factors is important. Treatment with corticosteroids (prednisone 60 mg every other day) for 2 to 4 weeks may hasten recovery of renal function and may benefit patients who do not regain renal function within 1 week after discontinuing use of the offending agent. Corticosteroids are not indicated in infection-related AIN. Although AIN has traditionally been considered to be a reversible process, recent studies have shown that impaired renal function can persist long-term in up to 40% of patients.

- Therapy for AIN is primarily supportive. Identification and elimination of inciting factors is important.

Acute Phosphate Nephropathy

Acute phosphate nephropathy occurs in patients who receive oral sodium phosphate–based laxatives, commonly when preparing for colonoscopy. The main risk factors are older age, hypertension, preexisting CKD, volume depletion, and the use of ACEIs or ARBs. Calcium phosphate precipitation is promoted by high serum phosphate concentrations that are induced rapidly by ingestion of oral sodium phosphate–based laxatives. AKI is caused by AIN due to precipitation of calcium phosphate in the renal tubules and interstitium.

The treatment is hydration, and in the majority of cases removal of phosphorus is recommended. Seizures and tetany may result from severe hypocalcemia, and calcium must be replaced cautiously since it may increase the chance of calcium phosphate crystal precipitation. Initially, the episode of acute phosphate nephropathy may be unrecognized clinically, and it may not be diagnosed until weeks to months later. Renal biopsy shows acute and chronic tubulointerstitial nephritis with tubular and interstitial deposits of calcium phosphate. In the majority of patients, CKD develops after an episode of acute phosphate nephropathy; the chance of recovery is poor.

- Acute phosphate nephropathy occurs in patients who receive oral sodium phosphate–based laxatives.

Acute Uric Acid Nephropathy

Acute uric acid nephropathy is associated with the tumor lysis syndrome that develops after chemotherapy, myeloproliferative disorders, heat stroke, status epilepticus, and Lesch-Nyhan syndrome. AKI is caused by uric acid crystal formation in the renal tubular lumens, causing intrarenal tubular obstruction. This condition is generally completely reversible. The serum uric acid level is often greater than 15 mg/dL, the 24-hour urinary uric acid is greater than 1,000 mg, and the ratio of spot urinary uric acid concentration to the spot urinary creatinine concentration is often greater than 1.0. Prevention includes alkaline diuresis, allopurinol, and, sometimes, hemodialysis.

Crystal Deposition Due to Medications or Toxins

Medications that cause crystal deposition include acyclovir, indinavir, sulfonamide, methotrexate (doses >50 mg/kg), and triamterene. AKI is caused by renal tubular obstruction due to crystal formation in the renal tubular lumens and by interstitial inflammation due to deposition in the interstitium. Crystal deposition is mainly a pH-dependent process, and treatment includes adequate hydration, urine alkalinization, and discontinued use of the offending medication. Excessive oxalate production occurs following ethylene glycol ingestion. Precipitation of calcium oxalate crystals contributes to AKI, which is also mediated by direct tubular toxicity of glycolate, another ethylene glycol metabolite. Treatment consists of urine alkalinization, administration of the alcohol dehydrogenase inhibitor fomepizole, and hemodialysis.

- Crystal deposition due to medications or toxins causes AKI by renal tubular obstruction due to crystal formation in the renal tubular lumens and by interstitial inflammation due to deposition in the interstitium.

Hypercalcemia

Hypercalcemia induces nephrogenic diabetes insipidus. If patients do not drink enough water, they can present with AKI due to hypovolemia. In addition, hypercalcemia can cause interstitial nephritis by precipitating in the renal tubules and interstitium. Treatment is directed at lowering the serum calcium level and addressing the underlying cause of hypercalcemia.

- Causes of intrinsic renal disease include glomerular disease, ATN, atheroembolic disease, AIN, acute phosphate nephropathy, acute uric acid nephropathy, and hypercalcemia.

POSTRENAL AKI

Postrenal AKI is defined as obstruction to urine flow at any level of the urinary tract. This obstruction can result from any of the following:

1. Bladder outlet obstruction (eg, prostate cancer or benign prostatic hypertrophy in men and genitourinary cancer in women)

2. Neurogenic bladder

3. Ureteral obstruction (eg, urolithiasis, tumor, necrosed renal papillae, and blood clots)

4. Extrinsic compression of the genitourinary tract (eg, malignancies and retroperitoneal fibrosis)

5. Inadvertent surgical ligation of a ureter

6. Intratubular precipitation of crystals (eg, uric acid crystals in tumor lysis syndrome and drugs, such as acyclovir, indinavir, methotrexate, sulfonamide, and triamterene)

Postrenal AKI is often accompanied by pain, hypertension, and normal anion gap acidosis. Postrenal causes should be excluded in all patients with anuria. For this purpose, ultrasonography is recommended because it is noninvasive, it is widely available, and it is the best method to evaluate for hydronephrosis. With ultrasonography, though, early obstruction may be missed. Postrenal AKI is usually reversible with prompt relief of the obstruction. Additionally, partial or unilateral obstruction may occur without an increase in SCr.

- Postrenal AKI is defined as obstruction to urine flow at any level of the urinary tract.

DIAGNOSTIC APPROACH TO AKI

Medical history and physical examination are the first steps in differentiating the causes of AKI. Laboratory studies, including urinalysis, can help distinguish between prerenal, intrinsic, and postrenal causes.

The medical history should include past medical history, family history, and identification of risk factors such as diabetes mellitus, hypertension, allergies, and medications. Urinary symptoms such as polyuria, oliguria, anuria, hematuria, and dysuria provide diagnostic clues and should be investigated. Hemoptysis can suggest a pulmonary renal syndrome. Other clinical manifestations of AKI are metabolic acidosis (with increased respiratory rate due to respiratory compensation), hypervolemia, hypertension, and hyperkalemia.

The physical examination should assess fluid balance to distinguish between prerenal causes and intrinsic or postrenal causes. A maculopapular rash may indicate allergic interstitial nephritis, and palpable purpura suggests vasculitis involving skin and kidneys. Livedo reticularis suggests atheroemboli. A palpable bladder or flank tenderness suggests postrenal AKI.

Laboratory Studies

Findings on urinalysis and urine chemistries can help to distinguish between causes of AKI (Table 39.2). In prerenal AKI, urine osmolality is increased and the urinary sediment is usually benign, with only hyaline casts. Urinary sodium and fractional excretion of sodium (FENa) are low because sodium is avidly retained by the kidney in states of low renal perfusion.

In ATN, urine is usually isosmotic with the serum and urinary sediment may contain renal tubular epithelial cells, granular casts, and epithelial cell casts. Damaged tubules have a decreased ability to reabsorb sodium, causing FENa to increase. FENa is useful in differentiating between prerenal AKI and intrinsic renal AKI due to ATN in oliguric patients.

In AIN, leukocytes are usually present along with leukocyte casts and, often, urinary eosinophils. Inflammation of the renal tubules can occur along with inflammation of the interstitium; therefore, renal tubular epithelial cells and epithelial

Table 39.2 **COMPARISON OF TEST RESULTS IN PRERENAL FAILURE AND ACUTE TUBULAR NECROSIS**

LABORATORY TEST OR URINARY INDEX	PRERENAL FAILURE	ACUTE TUBULAR NECROSIS
Urine osmolality, mOsm/kg	>500	<400
Urine specific gravity	>1.018	Approximately 1.010
Urinary sodium level, mEq/L	<20	>40
Fractional excretion of sodium, %[a]	<1	>2
Fractional excretion of urea, %	<35	>35
Urinary sediment	Normal; occasional hyaline or fine granular casts	Renal tubular epithelial cells; granular and muddy brown casts

[a] Fractional Excretion of Sodium $= \dfrac{[\text{Urinary Sodium}] \times [\text{Plasma Creatinine}]}{[\text{Plasma Sodium}] \times [\text{Urinary Creatinine}]} \times 100$

Adapted from Schrier RW, Wang W, Poole B, Mitra A. Acute renal failure: definitions, diagnosis, pathogenesis, and therapy. J Clin Invest. 2004 Jul;114(1):5–14. Erratum in: J Clin Invest. 2004 Aug;114(4):598. Used with permission.

Table 39.3 USE OF ULTRASONOGRAPHY IN ACUTE KIDNEY INJURY

ULTRASONOGRAPHIC FINDING	DIAGNOSIS
Shrunken kidneys	Chronic kidney disease
Normal-sized kidneys	
Echogenic	Acute glomerulonephritis
	Acute tubular necrosis
Normal	Prerenal
	Acute renal artery occlusion
Enlarged kidneys	Malignancy
	Renal vein thrombosis
	Diabetic nephropathy
	Human immunodeficiency virus
Hydronephrosis	Obstructive nephropathy

Adapted from Lameire N, Van Biesen W, Vanholder R. Epidemiology, clinical evaluation, and prevention of acute renal failure. In: Feehally J, Floege J, Johnson RJ, editors. Comprehensive clinical nephrology. 3rd ed. Philadelphia (PA): Mosby Elsevier; c2007. p. 771–85. Used with permission.

cell casts are sometimes seen with AIN. Dysmorphic RBCs and RBC casts indicate GN. With severe glomerular inflammation, leukocytes and leukocyte casts may also be seen. RBCs that are not dysmorphic can be a clue to obstruction related to genitourinary cancer or urolithiasis.

Notably, diuretic use causes an increase in FENa, even in prerenal azotemia, since loop and thiazide diuretics act by increasing the urinary excretion of sodium. The fractional excretion of urea is not altered by diuretics; as a result, an FENa of less than 35% indicates a prerenal state.

Imaging

Ultrasonography can be helpful in differentiating between the causes of AKI (Table 39.3). In postrenal AKI, ultrasonography is the test of choice to determine whether hydronephrosis is present, although it may not detect early obstruction. To improve the ability to detect the presence of obstruction and also to determine its cause, noncontrast computed tomography may be used in combination with ultrasonography.

MANAGEMENT OF AKI

The therapeutic approach to patients with AKI is mostly supportive. Determining and managing the risk factors are essential steps to decrease the extent of the injury. Management should include the following:

1. Avoid intravascular volume depletion.

2. Optimize cardiac function. While use of diuretics to maintain urine output does not expedite renal recovery, diuretics help with volume management in some patients with AKI. Low-dose dopamine is not considered beneficial.

3. Relieve urinary obstruction, which may be followed by polyuria. Therapy is aimed at preventing a new prerenal

component to the AKI by closely monitoring fluid intake, urine output, and renal function. Replacing two-thirds of the postobstructive diuresis volume is indicated if SCr increases after relief of the obstruction.

4. Avoid the use of nephrotoxic medications and intravenous contrast media.

5. Identify medications that affect renal blood flow (ACEIs, ARBs, cyclosporine, tacrolimus, cyclooxygenase 2 inhibitors, and NSAIDs) and withhold their use or carefully monitor changes in renal function while they are being used.

6. Adjust dosages of medications eliminated by the kidneys as renal function changes. Monitor drug levels when indicated.

7. Maintain nutritional requirements. Patients who are seriously ill are usually catabolic. Adjust the patient's diet to limit potassium, sodium, phosphorus, and fluid intake. If serum phosphorus levels increase despite dietary phosphorus restriction, phosphate binders should be administered with meals.

• The therapeutic approach to patients with AKI is mostly supportive.

Renal Replacement Therapy

The goals for RRT in AKI are the following:

1. Maintain fluid, electrolyte, acid-base, and solute balance

2. Prevent further insult and promote healing

3. Permit the use of other support measures, such as intravenous medications and parenteral nutrition

RRT should be considered for patients who have fluid overload unresponsive to diuretics, severe electrolyte disorders (typically hyperkalemia with electrocardiographic changes), severe acid-base disorders, and uremic symptoms (metabolic encephalopathy or other evidence of nervous system toxicity, pericarditis and bleeding believed to be due to uremic platelet dysfunction).

The choice of RRT must be customized to the needs of the patient:

1. Conventional intermittent hemodialysis with high- or low-flux membranes—This treatment is used for severe metabolic abnormalities (eg, hyperkalemia with electrocardiographic changes and severe acidosis) that require rapid, immediate correction for a short period. Hemodynamically stable patients who can tolerate rapid fluid and electrolyte shifts can undergo conventional intermittent dialysis.

2. Continuous RRT—Continuous RRT is used for severely ill and catabolic patients who require intravenous fluids and nutrition, continuous or frequent intravenous

administration of medications, and intravenous fluid resuscitation. Daily intermittent hemodialysis or continuous dialysis therapy is best to avoid large fluid gains and to maintain solute homeostasis. Hemodynamically unstable patients who require RRT are best treated with a form of continuous dialysis (continuous venovenous hemodialysis [CVVHD], continuous venovenous hemofiltration [CVVH], or continuous venovenous hemodiafiltration [CVVHDF]). These methods with continuous gentle fluid and solute removal improve hemodynamic stability by decreasing osmolar and solute concentration changes and limiting fluid shifts.

3. Peritoneal dialysis

• In RRT, the goals are to maintain fluid, electrolyte, acid-base, and solute balance; prevent further insult and promote healing; and permit the use of other supportive measures, such as intravenous medications and parenteral nutrition.

GLOMERULAR DISEASE

CLINICAL MANIFESTATIONS OF GLOMERULAR DISEASE

Clinical manifestations of glomerular injury vary. They include the occurrence of asymptomatic hematuria or proteinuria with urinary protein excretion greater than 300 mg/1.73 m² per 24 hours and less than 3.5 g/1.73 m² per 24 hours (nonnephrotic proteinuria). Proteinuria can be transient or hemodynamic. Fixed nonnephrotic proteinuria is usually due to glomerular disease, although tubulointerstitial diseases can be associated with proteinuria (usually <1.5 g/1.73 m² per 24 hours). In these patients, a urine dipstick test detects albumin and will be negative when proteinuria is due to immunoglobulin light chains.

Hematuria also occurs (defined as ≥3 RBCs per high-power field in a centrifuged urinary sediment sample). Glomerular hematuria is characterized by the presence of dysmorphic RBCs or RBC casts (or both). Macroscopic hematuria due to glomerular disease is painless. Urine is often brown, rather than bright red, as a result of methemoglobin formation in acidic urine.

Renal biopsy is usually indicated in the presence of any of the following:

1. Active urinary sediment (dysmorphic RBCs, RBC casts, or white blood cell casts)

2. Proteinuria (usually >1 g/1.73 m² per 24 hours)

3. Reduced GFR

4. AKI lasting more than 3 to 4 weeks

5. Atypical course of diabetic nephropathy

6. A suspicion of systemic diseases associated with renal manifestations (eg, systemic lupus erythematosus [SLE],

paraproteinemias and amyloidosis, systemic vasculitis, Alport syndrome, or Fabry disease)

Renal biopsy is rarely indicated in patients with small, shrunken kidneys because of increased risk of bleeding and the low probability of providing a diagnosis.

• Renal biopsy is indicated in the presence of active urinary sediment, proteinuria, reduced GFR, AKI lasting >3–4 weeks, atypical course of diabetic nephropathy, or a suspicion of systemic diseases associated with renal manifestations.

NEPHROTIC SYNDROME

Nephrotic syndrome is defined as the presence of urinary protein greater than 3.5 g/1.73 m² per 24 hours, hypoalbuminemia (<3.0 g/dL), peripheral edema, hypercholesterolemia, and lipiduria. Edema can be prominent. Urinalysis shows waxy casts, free fat, oval fat bodies, and lipiduria ("Maltese crosses").

Complications of nephrotic syndrome include the following:

1. Hypogammaglobulinemia, which increases the risk of infection, especially cellulitis and spontaneous peritonitis

2. Vitamin D deficiency due to loss of vitamin D–binding protein

3. Iron deficiency anemia due to hypotransferrinemia

4. Thrombotic complications because of increased levels of prothrombotic factors and decreased antithrombin III and antiplasmin

5. Renal vein thrombosis

General management of nephrotic syndrome includes using diuretics to manage edema, controlling blood pressure, limiting dietary protein and sodium, and treating hyperlipidemia.

• Nephrotic syndrome is defined as the presence of urinary protein >3.5 g/1.73 m² per 24 hours, hypoalbuminemia (<3.0 g/dL), peripheral edema, hypercholesterolemia, and lipiduria.

NEPHRITIC SYNDROME

Nephritic syndrome is defined as the presence of urinary protein <3.5 g/1.73 m² per 24 hours, hypoalbuminemia (<3.0 g/dL), peripheral edema, hypercholesterolemia, and lipiduria. It is characterized by oliguria, edema, hypertension, proteinuria (usually <3.5 g/1.73 m² per 24 hours), and an active urinary sediment. General management includes sodium restriction and use of loop diuretics to reduce the risk of fluid overload and to help control hypertension.

• Nephritic syndrome is characterized by oliguria, edema, hypertension, proteinuria (usually <3.5 g/1.73 m² per 24 hours), and an active urinary sediment.

Postinfectious GN

Classically, poststreptococcal GN develops after pharyngitis (1–3 weeks) or skin infection (2–4 weeks) due to specific ("nephritogenic") strains of group A β-hemolytic streptococci. Cultures are usually negative. Titers for antistreptolysin O (ASO) and antideoxyribonuclease B (anti-DNAse B) may provide evidence of recent streptococcal infection. Postinfectious GN can occur after other infections, such as staphylococcal, meningococcal, and pneumococcal infections; bacterial endocarditis; and infections of ventriculoatrial shunts.

A typical manifestation is the abrupt onset of nephritic syndrome with active urinary sediment and proteinuria that is usually less than 3 g/1.73 m^2 per 24 hours. Treatment is supportive with appropriate antibiotic therapy for persistent infections and for persons who are contacts (to prevent new cases). In adults, microscopic hematuria, proteinuria, hypertension, and renal dysfunction may persist for years.

IgA Nephropathy

IgA nephropathy (IgAN) is a mesangial proliferative GN characterized by diffuse deposition of IgA in the mesangium of glomeruli. It is the most common glomerulopathy worldwide, with an incidence approaching 1:100 in some countries (eg, Japan).

Patients are typically young adults in the second and third decades of life who present with episodic macroscopic hematuria, often accompanying an upper respiratory tract infection ("synpharyngitic hematuria"). The majority of patients are asymptomatic, and the disease may be identified when microscopic hematuria, with or without proteinuria, is found on routine urinalysis. Proteinuria is common, but nephrotic syndrome occurs in less than 10% of all patients. Patients with nephrotic syndrome may have minimal change nephropathy (MCN) superimposed on IgAN or another glomerulopathy.

Patients who are normotensive and have proteinuria less than 500 mg/1.73 m^2 per 24 hours and normal renal function at presentation usually have a good long-term prognosis. However, in 20% to 40% of patients, the disease progresses to end-stage renal disease (ESRD) within 10 to 25 years. Progression to ESRD in patients at high risk has been shown to be slowed by angiotensin II blockade (with ACEIs or ARBs or both) and administration of high doses of corticosteroids. The use of fish oil to prevent progression of IgAN is controversial. Persistent proteinuria of more than 1 g/1.73 m^2 per 24 hours, uncontrolled hypertension, impaired renal function at diagnosis, and glomerular or interstitial fibrosis identified in renal biopsy specimens are the most important predictors of a poor outcome. Patients with IgAN and concomitant MCN typically respond to corticosteroid therapy. For patients with rapidly progressive renal failure due to crescentic IgAN, a regimen of corticosteroids and cyclophosphamide, with the addition of plasma exchange or pulse methylprednisolone, has been tried with variable results.

- IgAN is a mesangial proliferative GN characterized by diffuse deposition of IgA in the mesangium of glomeruli.

- IgAN is the most common glomerulopathy worldwide.

Henoch-Schönlein Purpura

Henoch-Schönlein purpura is a systemic form of IgAN. Patients usually present with microscopic or gross hematuria (or both), RBC casts, purpura, and abdominal pain. Generally, the prognosis is good for children and variable for adults. In patients with normal renal function, treatment is supportive only. Patients with progressive renal failure should be considered for treatment with high-dose corticosteroids with or without cytotoxic medication.

Membranoproliferative GN

Clinical presentations of all forms of membranoproliferative GN (MPGN) are variable and include nephrotic and nephritic features. Approximately one-third of patients present with a combination of asymptomatic hematuria and proteinuria. Another third present with nephrotic syndrome and preserved renal function. Some patients (10%-20%) present with nephritic syndrome. Hypertension is common (50%-80% of patients). The prognosis is worse with hypertension, poor renal function, and proteinuria greater than 3 g/1.73 m^2 per 24 hours. There are 2 main types of MPGN: type I and type II.

In adults with MPGN type I, secondary forms associated with the following conditions tend to predominate: monoclonal gammopathies, cryoglobulinemia in patients with hepatitis C virus infection, hepatitis B virus infection, subacute bacterial endocarditis, infections of shunts used to manage hydrocephalus, malaria, SLE, sickle cell disease, α_1-antitrypsin deficiency, and recently described abnormalities in the alternative pathway of complement activation (C3 glomerulopathy). Levels of C3, C4, and total hemolytic complement (CH50) may be low in cases of MPGN type I secondary to activation of the classical complement pathway, whereas cases due to activation of the alternative pathway of complement activation will have low C3 but normal C4. Management includes treatment of the underlying cause. Corticosteroids, with or without cyclophosphamide, may be used in "idiopathic" MPGN type I with nephrotic syndrome or rapidly progressive GN.

The pathogenesis of MPGN type II involves abnormalities of factors comprising the alternate pathway of complement activation, or antibodies to those factors, resulting in persistent breakdown of C3. Low levels of C3 and normal levels of C4 are present. MPGN type II is associated with monoclonal gammopathies, partial lipodystrophy, and macular degeneration. Management of MPGN type II involves plasma exchange. Pulse intravenous corticosteroids followed by tapered administration of prednisone may be considered in patients who present with a rapidly progressive course.

- MPGN occurs as a complication of other systemic infectious and inflammatory diseases.

Rapidly Progressive GN—Crescentic GN

Rapidly progressive GN is defined as an acute, rapidly progressive (days to weeks or months) deterioration of renal function associated with an active urinary sediment and a focal necrotizing crescentic GN seen on light microscopic examination of renal biopsy specimens. Oliguria is common. The immunofluorescence pattern seen on renal biopsy specimens shows 3 patterns:

1. Type I—linear IgG deposition (Goodpasture disease or anti–glomerular basement membrane [GBM] antibody–mediated)

2. Type II—granular immune complexes (SLE)

3. Type III—pauci-immune, with negative or weak immunofluorescence (antineutrophil cytoplasmic autoantibody [ANCA] vasculitis)

Pulmonary-renal syndrome is frequent and can be due to Goodpasture disease, ANCA vasculitis (microscopic polyangiitis, granulomatosis with polyangiitis [Wegener granulomatosis]), Churg-Strauss syndrome, SLE, cryoglobulinemia, pulmonary edema, or other conditions.

- Rapidly progressive GN is an acute, rapidly progressive (days to weeks or months) deterioration of renal function associated with an active urinary sediment and a focal necrotizing crescentic GN seen on light microscopic examination of renal biopsy specimens.

ANCA Vasculitides

The ANCA vasculitides are characterized by inflammation and necrosis of small blood vessels of the kidney and other organs in association with autoantibodies against antigens present in lysosomal granules in the cytoplasm of neutrophils: myeloperoxidase (MPO) and proteinase 3. Patients with ANCA vasculitis, which is the most common cause of rapidly progressive GN in patients older than 60, have a wide range of signs and symptoms (Box 39.2).

Microscopic polyangiitis is a necrotizing vasculitis of small vessels (ie, capillaries, venules, and arterioles) with few or no immune deposits (pauci-immune) on immunofluorescence. Necrotizing GN with crescents is common, and pulmonary capillaritis often occurs. A necrotizing arteritis involving small and medium-sized arteries can be present. Fifty percent of patients are MPO-ANCA–positive, 40% are PR3-ANCA–positive, and a few are ANCA-negative.

Granulomatosis with polyangiitis is a granulomatous inflammation involving the respiratory tract and necrotizing vasculitis affecting small and medium-sized vessels (ie, capillaries, venules, arterioles, and arteries). Necrotizing GN is common. Seventy-five percent of patients are PR3-ANCA–positive and 20% are MPO-ANCA–positive.

Churg-Strauss syndrome is characterized by peripheral blood eosinophilia, asthma or other form of atopy, an eosinophil-rich granulomatous inflammation involving the respiratory tract, and a necrotizing vasculitis affecting small and medium-sized vessels. Sixty percent of patients are MPO-ANCA–positive.

Treatment of ANCA vasculitis includes a combination of high-dose corticosteroids and cyclophosphamide until remission is achieved (3–6 months). Rituximab (anti-CD20 monoclonal antibody) may be equivalent to cyclophosphamide for induction therapy, although long-term outcomes for patients initially treated with rituximab are not yet available. Patients with pulmonary hemorrhage or severe renal failure (SCr >5.5 mg/dL or receiving dialysis) or both should also receive plasma exchange. Patients with granulomatosis with polyangiitis who are nasal carriers of *Staphylococcus aureus* benefit from long-term treatment with trimethoprim-sulfamethoxazole.

A drug-induced ANCA vasculitis syndrome has been reported with the use of propylthiouracil, methimazole, carbimazole, hydralazine, minocycline, and penicillamine. While uncommon, drug-induced ANCA vasculitis should be considered in patients with ANCA vasculitis. Clinical presentation is similar to the presentation in cases that are not drug related (Box 39.2). Most patients have MPO-ANCA, frequently in very high titers, and antibodies to elastase or to lactoferrin.

- Granulomatosis with polyangiitis (Wegener granulomatosis) is a granulomatous inflammation involving the respiratory tract and necrotizing vasculitis affecting small and medium-sized vessels (ie, capillaries, venules, arterioles, and arteries).

- Churg-Strauss syndrome is characterized by peripheral blood eosinophilia, asthma or other form of atopy, an eosinophil-rich granulomatous inflammation involving the respiratory tract, and a necrotizing vasculitis affecting small and medium-sized vessels.

Polyarteritis Nodosa

Polyarteritis nodosa (PAN) is a rare disease characterized by necrotizing inflammation of medium-sized or small arteries without GN or vasculitis in arterioles, capillaries, or venules. It affects males and females equally, with onset most frequently between the ages of 40 and 60 years. PAN is ANCA-negative. In some patients, it is associated with hepatitis B virus

---

Box 39.2 **SIGNS AND SYMPTOMS OF ANCA VASCULITIS**

Cutaneous purpura, nodules, & ulcerations
Peripheral neuropathy (mononeuritis multiplex)
Abdmoninal pain & blood in stools
Hematuria, proteinuria, & renal failure
Hemoptysis & pulmonary infiltrates or nodules
Necrotizing (hemorrhagic) sinusitis
Myalgias & arthralgias
Muscle & pancreatic enzymes in blood

Abbreviation: ANCA, antineutrophil cytoplasmic autoantibody.

infection. Diagnosis is made by finding aneurysms on angiography or nerve biopsy. Treatment of patients who do not have evidence of hepatitis B virus infection includes high-dose corticosteroids and cyclophosphamide. Patients with hepatitis B–associated PAN should be treated with a short course of corticosteroids in combination with antiviral therapy and plasma exchange.

Anti-GBM Antibody–Mediated GN (Goodpasture Disease)

Goodpasture disease is a pulmonary-renal syndrome caused by circulating anti-GBM antibodies and linear staining seen along the GBM and alveolar basement membrane on immunofluorescence staining of a renal biopsy specimen. The antibody is directed against the α3 chain of type IV collagen. Approximately 25% to 30% of patients with anti-GBM antibodies are also ANCA-positive. Pulmonary hemorrhage may be absent or not clinically apparent.

Treatment is with high-dose corticosteroids (oral prednisone or pulse intravenous methylprednisolone) in combination with oral cyclophosphamide (2–3 mg/kg daily up to 200 mg daily; the dose should be decreased by 25% for patients older than 55 or with SCr >5 mg/dL) and plasma exchange. Patients who have 100% circumferential crescents and are receiving dialysis do not recover renal function and should not be treated with the immunosuppressive regimen outlined above, except in the presence of pulmonary hemorrhage. The prognosis for patients depends on the percentage of circumferential crescents of the renal biopsy specimen, the presence of oliguria, and the need for dialysis. Anti-GBM disease rarely recurs.

- Goodpasture disease is a pulmonary-renal syndrome caused by circulating anti-GBM antibodies and linear staining seen along the GBM and alveolar basement membrane on immunofluorescence staining of a renal biopsy specimen.

GLOMERULAR DISEASE USUALLY MANIFESTING AS NEPHROTIC SYNDROME

Minimal Change Nephropathy

MCN is defined by the absence of structural glomerular abnormalities, except for the widespread fusion of epithelial cell foot processes seen on electron microscopy, in a patient with nephrotic syndrome. It is the most common cause of nephrotic syndrome in children. The presence of nephrotic syndrome in a child with normal urinalysis results indicates MCN until proved otherwise. Among patients with nephrotic syndrome, MCN is the cause in 70% to 90% of children younger than 10 years (although rarely before the first year of life), 50% of adolescents and young adults, and less than 20% of adults with primary nephrotic syndrome.

The typical presentation is abrupt onset of nephrotic syndrome. Hematuria is unusual. In adults, hypertension and renal insufficiency may be present. The pathogenesis of MCN is unknown and may be a consequence of T-lymphocyte abnormalities, with T cells producing a lymphokine that is toxic to glomerular epithelial cells. In some patients, MCN may have a secondary cause, such as viral infections, drugs, tumors, or allergies.

Treatment includes high-dose corticosteroid therapy continued for 4 to 8 weeks after remission is achieved. In adolescents and adults, response to therapy is high (>80%), but the response is slow and some patients may require up to 16 weeks of treatment to achieve remission. Of the patients who have a response to corticosteroid therapy, 25% have a long-term remission, whereas others have at least 1 relapse. Other immunosuppressive agents are used in patients with frequent relapses or corticosteroid dependence or resistance. The overall prognosis is excellent, with patients maintaining long-term renal function. If there is no response to therapy or if progressive renal failure develops, an alternative diagnosis (such as focal segmental glomerulosclerosis [FSGS]) must be considered.

- MCN is defined by the absence of structural glomerular abnormalities, except for the widespread fusion of epithelial cell foot processes seen on electron microscopy, in a patient with nephrotic syndrome.
- MCN is the most common cause of nephrotic syndrome in children.

Focal Segmental Glomerulosclerosis

FSGS accounts for about 25% of cases of adult nephrotic syndrome. It is the most common form of idiopathic nephrotic syndrome in African Americans. FSGS is associated with variations in the apolipoprotein AI gene. Secondary causes of FSGS include drugs (heroin abuse, pamidronate, anabolic steroids, and interferon), infection (eg, human immunodeficiency virus [HIV] and parvovirus), sickle cell disease, obesity, vesicoureteral reflux, unilateral renal agenesis, remnant kidneys, healed lesions of other inflammatory disorders in glomeruli, and aging.

Patients with FSGS present with either asymptomatic proteinuria or full-blown nephrotic syndrome. Treatment includes prolonged (>4 months) high-dose corticosteroid therapy. The remission rate for nephrotic syndrome is up to 40% to 60%, with preservation of long-term renal function. For patients who do not respond to corticosteroids, alternative therapy includes the use of cytotoxic drugs (either alone or in combination with corticosteroids) or a low-dose calcineurin inhibitor (cyclosporine or tacrolimus). For patients with secondary forms of FSGS, treatment should target the primary cause, if possible. In all patients, treatment with an ACEI or an ARB, alone or in combination, may substantially reduce proteinuria and prolong renal survival. For patients who have protein excretion of less than 3 g/1.73 m² per 24 hours, treatment with an ACEI or angiotensin II receptor antagonist (or both) may be sufficient to reduce proteinuria and improve renal survival. The prognosis is better for patients with a smaller degree of proteinuria and for those who respond to corticosteroids.

- FSGS is the most common form of idiopathic nephrotic syndrome in African Americans.

Membranous Nephropathy

Membranous nephropathy (MN) occurs in persons of all ages and races. It is the most common cause of nephrotic syndrome in white adults; it is most often diagnosed in middle age, with the incidence peaking during the fourth and fifth decades of life. The male to female ratio is 2:1. Patients present with the following:

1. High-grade proteinuria (>2.0 g/1.73 m² per 24 hours in >80% of patients and >10 g/1.73 m² per 24 hours in as many as 30%)

2. Initially, preserved renal function in the majority of patients

3. Absence of hypertension in >80% of patients at diagnosis

4. Microscopic hematuria in approximately 30% of patients

5. Thrombotic complications

Secondary causes include autoimmune diseases (SLE), infections (eg, hepatitis B, hepatitis C, and syphilis), drugs (eg, NSAIDs, penicillamine, and gold), and malignancies (solid tumors such as colon, breast, and lung cancer). The association with malignancy increases with the patient's age, reaching up to 20% among patients older than 60.

Initial therapy should be directed to the control of edema, treatment of hypertension, treatment of hyperlipidemia, dietary protein restriction, and reduction of proteinuria through inhibition of the renin-angiotensin system with the use of ACEIs and ARBs. The probability of renal survival is more than 80% at 5 years and 60% at 15 years. Without additional treatment, nearly 25% of patients have spontaneous complete remission and 50% have partial remission. Immunosuppressive therapies should be considered for patients who remain nephrotic after a 6-month trial of maximal angiotensin II blockade and should include combined use of corticosteroids and cytotoxic agents, cyclosporine, or tacrolimus. Overall, the prognosis is worse for nephrotic patients.

- MN is the most common cause of nephrotic syndrome in white adults.

OTHER GLOMERULAR DISORDERS

Diabetic Nephropathy

Diabetic nephropathy (DN) is the most common cause of ESRD in the United States. It occurs in both type 1 diabetes mellitus (30%-40% of patients) and type 2 diabetes mellitus (20%-30% of patients). In type 1 diabetes mellitus, the peak onset of nephropathy is between 10 and 15 years after the initial presentation with diabetes. DN is unlikely to develop in patients who do not have proteinuria after 25 years of diabetes. The main risk factors for DN developing are a positive family history of DN, hypertension, and poor glycemic control. The risk is greater in some ethnic groups (eg, Pima Indians and African Americans).

The initial manifestation of DN is the onset of microalbuminuria (defined as urinary albumin excretion of 20–200 μg/min or 30–300 mg/1.73 m² per 24 hours). Microalbuminuria can evolve into overt proteinuria (>300 mg/1.73 m² per 24 hours) and subsequent full-blown nephrotic syndrome. After overt proteinuria develops, the progression toward ESRD is relentless, although rates of decline vary among patients (over a period of 5–15 years). The degree of proteinuria correlates approximately with the renal prognosis. In patients with type 1 diabetes mellitus, there is a strong correlation (95%) between the development of nephropathy and other signs of diabetic microvascular compromise, such as diabetic retinopathy and DN. This correlation is weaker for patients with type 2 diabetes mellitus; nephropathy develops in up to one-third of these patients without evidence of diabetic retinopathy.

Other renal manifestations of diabetes include the following:

1. Hypertension in approximately 75% of patients with proteinuria

2. Papillary necrosis

3. Frequent urinary tract infections, which may be complicated by the development of acute pyelonephritis and perinephric abscess

4. Functional obstruction due to neurogenic bladder

5. Renal artery stenosis, related to the accelerated rate of atherosclerosis in diabetic patients

6. Type 4 renal tubular acidosis

The pathogenesis of DN involves increased glycosylation of proteins, with accumulation of advanced glycosylation end products that cross-link with collagen, in combination with glomerular hyperfiltration and hypertension. In patients with long-term diabetes, especially if retinopathy is present and other causes of proteinuria are excluded, renal biopsy may not be necessary. Renal biopsy is indicated for patients if the disease has an atypical course or if progressive loss of renal function occurs rapidly.

Progression of DN can be slowed by tight glycemic control (glycated hemoglobin <7.0%) and the use of ACEIs or ARBs (target systolic blood pressure <125–130 mm Hg). Use of ACEIs or ARBs should be started in patients who have diabetes and microalbuminuria even if they are normotensive. Patients with ESRD due to DN are candidates for a solitary kidney or combined kidney-pancreas transplant, which afford better long-term survival and quality of life than the alternatives of hemodialysis and peritoneal dialysis.

- DN is the most common cause of ESRD in the United States.

- Progression of DN can be slowed by tight glycemic control (glycated hemoglobin <7.0%) and the use of ACEIs or ARBs (target systolic blood pressure <125–130 mm Hg).

Lupus Nephritis

Approximately 25% of patients with SLE have substantial renal involvement. Renal involvement usually occurs early in the course of the disease and is rarely the sole manifestation of SLE. For patients with severe lupus nephritis (LN) (classified by renal biopsy showing focal or diffuse proliferative LN), the use of a high-dose corticosteroid (either orally or "pulse" intravenous methylprednisolone) in combination with intravenous cyclophosphamide was the most effective form of therapy until recent studies demonstrated that mycophenolate mofetil in combination with oral prednisone resulted in fewer side effects and was as effective as cyclophosphamide in combination with prednisone. A subtype of membranous LN is characterized by proteinuria, weakly positive or negative antinuclear antibody, and no erythrocyte casts. Initial therapy is supportive, using ACEIs or ARBs to reduce proteinuria. Immunosuppressive treatment should be considered for patients who remain nephrotic for more than 6 months.

Cryoglobulinemic GN Associated With Hepatitis Infection

Type II or mixed essential cryoglobulins (Table 39.4) are commonly found in patients with hepatitis C virus infection. Cryoglobulins contain hepatitis C virus RNA and anti–hepatitis C virus IgG, which precipitate in the glomeruli, bind complement, activate a cytokine cascade, and trigger an inflammatory response. Patients may present with proteinuria, microscopic hematuria, nephrotic syndrome, or renal impairment. Hypertension is common and may be severe, particularly with acute nephritic syndrome. Cryoglobulinemic GN is usually associated with low levels of C3 and C4. Cryocrits correlate poorly with disease activity, and 30% to 40% of patients do not have detectable cryoglobulins. Combination treatment with interferon alfa and ribavirin is effective in clearing the virus from the circulation and results in improvement of proteinuria and renal function. Relapses after discontinuation of the antiviral therapy are common. Treatment with prednisone, cytotoxic agents, and plasmapheresis is indicated for patients with acute nephritis. The renal prognosis is usually good, with few patients progressing to ESRD.

HIV-Associated Nephropathy

HIV-associated nephropathy (HIV-AN) is characterized by progressive renal insufficiency in patients with nephrotic-range proteinuria (frequently massive) but often little edema. Ultrasonography shows large echogenic kidneys. Renal biopsy specimens show a collapsing form of FSGS. HIV-AN is more common and clinically more severe in African Americans than in whites. Treatment includes the use of highly active antiretroviral therapy (HAART), treatment of underlying infections, and ACEIs to reduce proteinuria.

Other types of renal disease can be encountered in HIV-infected patients. These include IgAN, MPGN, MCN, MN, postinfectious GN, thrombotic microangiopathy, and a lupus-like and immune complex–mediated GN. Intratubular obstruction results from crystal precipitation after the administration of sulfadiazine or intravenous acyclovir. Renal calculi or nephropathy (or both) can occur after administration of indinavir.

- Treatment of HIV-AN includes the use of HAART, treatment of underlying infections, and use of ACEIs to reduce proteinuria.

Thrombotic Microangiopathies

Thrombotic microangiopathies are characterized by microangiopathic hemolytic anemia and thrombocytopenia; renal thrombotic microangiopathies have various causes. It is debated whether hemolytic uremic syndrome (HUS) and thrombotic thrombocytopenic purpura (TTP) are distinct disorders, although they share a spectrum of common findings and are often considered together as HUS-TTP. Features include anemia with schistocytes on peripheral blood smear, high reticulocyte count, elevated levels of indirect bilirubin and lactate dehydrogenase, decreased haptoglobin level, and presence of urinary hemoglobin without RBCs on microscopy.

Hemolytic Uremic Syndrome

The sporadic or diarrhea-associated form (D+HUS) is strongly linked to ingestion of meat or other foods contaminated with *Escherichia coli* O157:H7, which produces a Shiga-like toxin that binds to a glycolipid receptor on renal endothelial cells and triggers endothelial damage. The treatment is supportive, and antibiotics should not be used.

The non–diarrhea-associated form (D−HUS) occurs in association with the use of various medications (oral contraceptives, cyclosporine, tacrolimus, mitomycin C, bleomycin, ticlopidine, or quinine), antiphospholipid antibody syndrome, underlying malignancy, or radiotherapy.

Table 39.4 **CRYOGLOBULINS AND ASSOCIATED DISEASES**

CRYOGLOBULIN TYPE	IMMUNOGLOBULIN CLASS	ASSOCIATED DISEASES
I. Monoclonal immunoglobulins	M>G>A>BJP	Myeloma, Waldenström macroglobulinemia
II. Mixed cryoglobulins with monoclonal immunoglobulins	M/G>>G/G	Sjögren syndrome, Waldenström macroglobulinemia, lymphoma, essential cryoglobulinemia
III. Mixed polyclonal immunoglobulins	M/G	Infection, SLE, vasculitis, neoplasia, essential cryoglobulinemia

Abbreviations: BJP, Bence Jones protein; SLE, systemic lupus erythematosus.

Atypical HUS results from various inherited and acquired abnormalities of the proteins involved in the alternate pathway of complement activation. Episodes of atypical HUS may recur. The treatment is plasma exchange.

Thrombotic Thrombocytopenic Purpura

Typically, fluctuating neurologic signs and symptoms along with purpura are more commonly associated with TTP. TTP may result from autoantibody to the von Willebrand factor–cleaving protease ADAMTS13 (acute form) or from deficiency of ADAMTS13 (chronic form). TTP can occur in association with drugs (eg, cocaine, quinidine, and ticlopidine), malignancies, SLE, antiphospholipid antibody syndrome, scleroderma renal crisis, and HIV infection. In general, treatment is plasma exchange, although scleroderma renal crisis is treated with ACEIs.

- Thrombotic microangiopathies are characterized by microangiopathic hemolytic anemia and thrombocytopenia; renal thrombotic microangiopathies have various causes.

- Thrombotic microangiopathies include HUS and TTP.

DISEASES WITH GBM ABNORMALITIES

ALPORT SYNDROME

Alport syndrome is characterized by a progressive nephritis manifested by persistent or intermittent hematuria. It is frequently associated with sensorineural hearing loss and ocular abnormalities. Patients have proteinuria that increases with age. In virtually all male patients, the syndrome progresses to ESRD, often by age 16 to 35. It is usually mild in heterozygous females, although ESRD develops in some women, usually after age 50. The rate of progression to ESRD is fairly constant among affected males within individual families, but it varies markedly from family to family.

The diagnostic abnormality occurring only in patients with Alport syndrome is the absence of $\alpha3(IV)$, $\alpha4(IV)$, and $\alpha5(IV)$ chains from the GBM and distal tubular basement membrane in immunohistochemical studies of type IV collagen. More than 50% of patients have a mutation in the gene (*COL4A5*) that codes for the $\alpha5$ chain of type IV collagen, $\alpha5(IV)$. It is X-linked in at least 80% of the patients. Additionally, autosomal recessive and autosomal dominant patterns of inheritance have been described.

No specific treatment is available. Tight control of blood pressure and moderate dietary protein restriction are recommended to retard the progression of renal disease, but the benefits of these are unproven. Peritoneal dialysis, hemodialysis, and renal transplant are used successfully for long-term RRT. If the defect is in the $\alpha5(IV)$ chain, these patients do not express the $\alpha3(IV)$ chain. Thus, among patients with Alport syndrome who receive a kidney transplant, there is a 5% to 10% risk of Goodpasture disease developing because of the presence of the $\alpha3(IV)$ chain (the location of the "Goodpasture antigen") in the transplanted kidney.

- The diagnostic abnormality occurring only in patients with Alport syndrome is the absence of $\alpha3(IV)$, $\alpha4(IV)$, and $\alpha5(IV)$ chains from the GBM and distal tubular basement membrane in immunohistochemical studies of type IV collagen.

THIN BASEMENT MEMBRANE NEPHROPATHY

Thin basement membrane nephropathy (TBMN), sometimes referred to as benign familial hematuria, is a relatively common condition characterized by isolated glomerular hematuria associated with the renal biopsy finding of an excessively thin GBM. Patients with TBMN can be considered carriers of the autosomal recessive Alport syndrome since mutations (homozygous or compound heterozygous) in both alleles of *COL4A3* or *COL4A4* cause autosomal recessive Alport syndrome. TBMN is transmitted in a dominant fashion.

The clinical presentation includes persistent or intermittent hematuria first detected in childhood or during a routine urinalysis. Sometimes TBMN is not manifested until adulthood. Macroscopic hematuria is not uncommon and may occur in association with an upper respiratory tract infection. Blood pressure is typically normal. When TBMN is first detected in young adults, 60% have proteinuria less than $500 \text{ mg}/1.73 \text{ m}^2$ per 24 hours. In contrast to patients with Alport syndrome, patients with TBMN do not have hearing loss, ocular abnormalities, or a strong family history of ESRD. The diagnosis of TBMN requires a renal biopsy and electron microscopy with measurement of GBM thickness. For the majority of patients who have isolated hematuria and a negative family history of ESRD, the condition is benign, requires no specific treatment, and carries an excellent long-term prognosis. In some patients, progressive proteinuria and renal failure may develop and can eventually result in ESRD. TBMN has been reported to occur in association with other glomerular diseases.

- TBMN, sometimes referred to as benign familial hematuria, is a relatively common condition characterized by isolated glomerular hematuria associated with the renal biopsy finding of an excessively thin GBM.

PARAPROTEINEMIA-ASSOCIATED RENAL DISEASES

MULTIPLE MYELOMA

Multiple myeloma has renal manifestations that may manifest as AKI or as chronic progressive disease occurring at any time during the course of the disease. Other renal manifestations include pseudohyponatremia, low anion gap, and type 2 (proximal) renal tubular acidosis with Fanconi syndrome. Virtually all patients with multiple myeloma have monoclonal immunoglobulins or light chains in the serum and urine. AKI occurs as a result of intraluminal precipitation of proteinaceous casts (cast nephropathy) and the resulting acute noninflammatory interstitial nephritis (myeloma kidney). Intratubular cast formation is facilitated by increased concentrations of calcium, sodium, and chloride (eg, after the use of a loop diuretic) in the urine; conditions that reduce flow rates (eg, intravascular depletion and the use of NSAIDs); and use of radiocontrast agents.

Treatment of cast nephropathy includes the following:

1. Vigorous hydration with normal saline

2. Correction of hypercalcemia

3. Avoidance of nephrotoxic or precipitating agents

4. Alkalinization of the urine to maintain pH >7 (possibly beneficial in some patients)

5. Plasmapheresis, which quickly removes light chains from the circulation and should be considered for patients with AKI and high serum levels of free light chains or hyperviscosity syndrome

- AKI in multiple myeloma occurs as a result of intraluminal precipitation of proteinaceous casts (cast nephropathy) and the resulting acute noninflammatory interstitial nephritis (myeloma kidney).

AMYLOIDOSIS

Amyloidosis is characterized by systemic extracellular deposition of antiparallel, β-pleated sheet, nonbranching, 8- to 12-nm fibrils that stain positive with Congo red (green birefringence with polarized light) or thioflavin T. Patients with primary (AL) amyloidosis are typically older than 50 years, and the kidneys are affected in 50% of patients. New advances in treatment of amyloidosis, including stem cell transplant, have improved the previously dismal prognosis. Secondary (AA) amyloidosis is most common in patients with rheumatoid arthritis, inflammatory bowel disease, chronic infection, familial Mediterranean fever, and drug users who inject heroin subcutaneously. The treatment of AA amyloidosis is directed at the underlying inflammatory process.

LIGHT CHAIN DEPOSITION DISEASE

Light chain deposition disease is characterized by immunoglobulin light chain deposition along the GBM. It is strongly associated with the development of myeloma, lymphoma, and Waldenström macroglobulinemia. Renal involvement is similar to that of amyloidosis, with proteinuria, nephrotic syndrome, and renal insufficiency. As in amyloidosis and multiple myeloma, treatment can lead to stabilization or improved renal function in some patients.

TUBULOINTERSTITIAL DISEASE

Acute and chronic interstitial inflammation can result in injury to renal tubules, leading to tubular dysfunction and, chronically, tubular atrophy. AIN is discussed earlier in this chapter in the "Intrinsic Renal AKI" section. Causes of chronic tubulointerstitial damage include analgesic nephropathy, uric acid, lithium, heavy metals, mercury, lead, and oxalates.

ANALGESIC NEPHROPATHY

Analgesic nephropathy is a slowly progressive chronic interstitial nephritis due to the long-term consumption of mixed analgesic preparations, frequently complicated by papillary necrosis and resulting in bilateral renal atrophy. Renal damage can develop from the use of acetaminophen in combination with aspirin and from long-term use of NSAIDs. Papillary necrosis may occur. Noncontrast computed tomography imaging of the kidneys has become the standard method for diagnosing analgesic nephropathy. No specific treatment is available. Patients with analgesic nephropathy are at an increased risk of uroepithelial tumors, particularly transitional cell carcinomas (renal pelvis, ureter, bladder, and proximal urethra). Tumors frequently occur simultaneously at different sites in the urinary tract, and close follow-up with regular urinary cytologic examination is recommended.

OTHER CAUSES

Other causes of chronic tubulointerstitial damage include the following:

1. Chronic uric acid nephropathy from chronic tophaceous gout results from interstitial crystal formation in the renal parenchyma. It has limited reversibility.

2. Lithium induces nephrogenic diabetes insipidus and microcystic changes in the renal tubules along with interstitial fibrosis.

3. Heavy metals (eg, cadmium, certain pigments and substances involved in manufacturing glass, plastic, metal alloys, electrical equipment, and some cigarettes) induce proximal renal tubular acidosis and tubulointerstitial nephritis.

4. Mercury in its organic salt form can induce chronic tubulointerstitial nephritis and MN or ATN.

5. Chronic lead intoxication can cause lead nephropathy, a chronic interstitial nephritis. The clinical presentation of patients with lead nephropathy includes hypertension, elevated SCr, little or no proteinuria, bland urinary sediment, and hyperuricemia. A history of nontophaceous gout is common.

6. Oxalate deposition from primary or secondary hyperoxaluria causes renal and extrarenal oxalate deposition. Secondary causes of oxalate deposition include ethylene glycol ingestion, methoxyflurane, high doses of ascorbic acid, vitamin B_6 deficiency, and enteric hyperoxaluria.

CLINICAL MANIFESTATIONS

Clinical manifestations in patients with tubulointerstitial disease include the following:

1. Tubular proteinuria (<1.5–2 g/1.73 m^2 per 24 hours)

2. Proximal tubule dysfunction

3. Distal tubule dysfunction

4. Medullary concentration defects

5. Abnormal urinary sediment

6. Azotemia and renal insufficiency

- Acute and chronic interstitial inflammation can result in injury to renal tubules, leading to tubular dysfunction and, chronically, tubular atrophy.

CYSTIC RENAL DISEASE

Autosomal dominant polycystic kidney disease (ADPKD) is the most common hereditary renal disease. It occurs in both males and females and is characterized by multiple, bilateral renal cysts and cysts in other organs (eg, liver, spleen, and pancreas). ADPKD is most often associated with mutations in 2 genes that code for interacting proteins found in renal tubular cells and in primary cilia:

1. *PKD1* gene, localized on chromosome 16p, encodes polycystin 1 (85%-90% of cases)

2. *PKD2* gene, localized on chromosome 4, encodes polycystin 2

Diagnosis is made through genetic testing. Additionally, the diagnosis of ADPKD can be made through renal imaging. Ultrasonographic criteria for diagnosis have been recently revised (age 15–39: 3 cysts in 1 or both kidneys; age 40–59: ≥2 cysts in each kidney; age ≥60: ≥4 cysts in each kidney).

Manifestations of renal involvement can include hypertension, flank or back pain, macroscopic hematuria, CKD, urinary tract infection, and inferior vena cava obstruction.

Extrarenal manifestations of ADPKD include polycystic liver disease (most common) and intracranial aneurysm (ICA). The incidence of ICA is 5% to 22%, depending on whether there is a positive family history of ICA. Risk of rupture depends on ICA diameter: if less than 5 mm, risk is minimal; if greater than 10 mm, risk is high. Screening all patients with ADPKD for ICA is not recommended. Screening should be reserved for patients with prior known ICA or family history of ICA or intracerebral bleeding; patients undergoing surgical procedures that may cause hemodynamic instability; and patients with occupations that may place others at risk (eg, aircraft pilots, bus drivers).

- ADPKD is the most common hereditary renal disease.

SUMMARY

- AKI denotes a rapid deterioration (within hours to weeks) of kidney function, resulting in the accumulation of nitrogenous metabolites and fluid, electrolyte, and acid-base imbalances.

- The key diagnostic tests for evaluating AKI are urinalysis with microscopy and renal ultrasonography.

- Nephritic syndrome is characterized by oliguria, edema, hypertension, proteinuria (usually <3.5 g/1.73 m^2 per 24 hours), and an active urinary sediment.

- Nephrotic syndrome is defined as the presence of urinary protein >3.5 g/1.73 m^2 per 24 hours, hypoalbuminemia (<3.0 g/dL), peripheral edema, hypercholesterolemia, and lipiduria.

- IgAN is the most common glomerulopathy worldwide.

- MPGN occurs as a complication of other systemic infectious and inflammatory diseases.

- FSGS is the most common form of idiopathic nephrotic syndrome in African Americans.

- MN is the most common cause of nephrotic syndrome in white adults.

- DN is the most common cause of ESRD in the United States.

EVALUATION OF KIDNEY FUNCTION AND CHRONIC KIDNEY DISEASE

Axel Pflueger, MD, PhD

GOALS

- Define normal kidney function.

- Cite methods to evaluate kidney function, including estimation of glomerular filtration rate (GFR), urinalysis, and renal imaging.

- Discuss the definition, causes, and treatment of chronic kidney disease (CKD).

NORMAL KIDNEY FUNCTION

The kidneys normally perform several essential functions:

1. Maintain a constant extracellular environment, which is required for adequate cell function and is achieved by excreting numerous metabolic waste products (eg, urea, creatinine, and uric acid) and by adjusting urinary excretion of water and electrolytes to match net intake and endogenous production. The kidneys regulate the excretion of water and solutes (eg, sodium, potassium, and hydrogen) by changing tubular reabsorption or secretion.

2. Secrete multiple hormones that participate in the regulation of systemic and renal hemodynamics (eg, renin, angiotensin II, adenosine, prostaglandins, nitric oxide, endothelin, and bradykinin); red blood cell production (erythropoietin); and calcium, phosphorus, and bone metabolism (1,25-dihydroxyvitamin D_3).

3. Catabolize peptide hormones.

4. Synthesize glucose (gluconeogenesis) in fasting conditions.

The kidneys help maintain normal body function and homeostasis by directly interacting with other organ systems, including the cardiovascular, nervous (eg, brain), gastrointestinal tract (eg, liver), blood, pulmonary, and muscular systems.

In patients with kidney disease, some or all of these functions may be diminished or entirely absent. As an example, patients with nephrogenic diabetes insipidus are less able to concentrate urine, but other functions are entirely normal. By comparison, all kidney functions may be significantly impaired in the patient with acute kidney injury, CKD, or end-stage renal disease (ESRD), thereby resulting in the retention of uremic toxins, marked abnormalities in fluid and electrolyte balance, anemia, and bone disease.

- The kidneys normally maintain a constant extracellular environment, secrete multiple hormones, and catabolize peptide hormones in fasting conditions.

EVALUATION OF KIDNEY FUNCTION

Kidney function is characterized by GFR and the functionality of the filtering structures of roughly 1 million nephrons in each kidney. Kidney function is assessed by the estimated and measured GFR. The functionality of the filtering structures is assessed by analysis of the urine (microscopic urine analysis and protein excretion) and by imaging studies of the kidney to determine structural abnormalities.

ESTIMATED GFR

The GFR can be estimated by measuring the concentration of molecules in the blood that are primarily filtered by the glomerulus. Typically, the concentration of serum creatinine is measured. In recent years, cystatin C has been used to estimate GFR.

The initial step in urine formation is the separation of an ultrafiltrate of plasma across the wall of the glomerular capillary. Fluid movement across the glomerulus is governed by Starling forces, which are proportional to the permeability of the membrane and to the balance between the hydraulic and oncotic pressure gradients:

$$GFR = LpS \times (\Delta \text{ Hydraulic Pressure} - \Delta \text{ Oncotic Pressure}),$$

where Lp is the unit permeability (or porosity) of the capillary wall, S is the surface area available for filtration, and Δ is change. The GFR in healthy adults is approximately 95±20 mL/min in women and 120±25 mL/min in men.

Serum Creatinine

Creatinine is an end product of muscle catabolism and is released in the circulation at a steady rate. It is not protein bound and is primarily filtered freely across the glomerulus (about 90%); a smaller portion is secreted by the tubules (about 10%). Therefore, the creatinine-based estimated GFR may overestimate the true GFR by about 10%. Several medications may inhibit tubular creatinine secretion and increase the serum creatinine level (Box 40.1). Other non-renal factors that increase the serum creatinine level include race or ethnicity (eg, African American), muscular build, and ingestion of creatine supplements. Factors that may decrease the serum creatinine level are older age, female sex, vegetarian diet, malnutrition, protein wasting, and limb amputation.

The creatinine-based estimated GFR (expressed in milliliters per minute per 1.73 m²) can be calculated by the Cockcroft-Gault (CG) estimation or the Modification of Diet in Renal Disease (MDRD) Study equation. Both formulas use 4 variables. Three of the variables are serum creatinine (SCr), age, and sex. Body weight is the fourth variable for the CG equation:

$$\text{GFR} = [140 - \text{Age (years)}] \times \text{Weight (kilograms)} \times 0.85$$
$$(\text{if Female})/\text{SCr} \times 72.$$

Race is the fourth variable for the MDRD equation:

$$\text{GFR} = 175 \times \text{SCr}^{-1.154} \times \text{Age}^{-0.203} \times 0.742$$
$$(\text{if Female}) \times 1.212 \text{ (if African American)}.$$

The MDRD Study equation has been found to have greater precision and accuracy than the CG formula, but it has not been validated in children, pregnant women, persons older than 70 years, and other racial and ethnic groups. Neither equation provides accurate results if patients have extreme levels of creatinine (eg, patients with muscle-wasting conditions, very high or low protein intake, an amputaed limb, or large or small body size).

Cystatin C

Cystatin C is a small protein excreted by all human nucleated cells, and it is filtered solely by the glomerulus. Therefore, it is less dependent on muscle mass and tubular function and has been shown to provide a more precise estimation of GFR than creatinine-based estimated GFR. It may eventually replace creatinine for estimating GFR.

MEASURED GFR

Clearance of *p*-aminohippurate is a measure of renal blood flow. Orthoiodohippurate is used in renal scans. The clearance rates of inulin, iothalamate, diethylenetriamine pentaacetic acid (DTPA), and creatinine are measures of the GFR.

Measurements of GFR are typically based on the urinary concentration of a glomerular-filtered substance (eg, SCr) divided by its plasma concentration expressed as follows:

$$\text{GFR} = [\text{Creatinine in Urine}]/[\text{Creatinine in Plasma}] \times$$
$$\text{Urine Volume (mL)}/\text{Collection Time},$$

where collection time is usually 24 hours, expressed in minutes (1,440 minutes).

- Kidney function is assessed by the estimated and measured GFR, by the functionality of the filtering structures through analysis of the urine (microscopic urine analysis and protein excretion), and by imaging studies of the kidney to determine structural abnormalities.

URINALYSIS

The causes of urine discoloration are listed in Table 40.1. Dysmorphic erythrocytes in the urinary sediment (if >80% of the erythrocytes) are indicative of glomerular injury, whereas hematuria without dysmorphic erythrocytes may be indicative of lower urinary tract bleeding (eg, neoplasm or bladder ulcer). Hansel stain is used to identify urinary eosinophils.

Normal urine osmolality varies in a wide range (eg, 40–1,200 mOsm/kg) and depends on the hydration status in a healthy person. In general, in a healthy person, urine osmolality should be similar to plasma osmolality. For example, in a euvolemic person with a plasma osmolality of 285 mOsm/L, urine osmolality would be expected to be similar; however, in a dehydrated person, urine osmolality may be higher than plasma osmolality. In patients with syndrome of inappropriate secretion of antidiuretic hormone, plasma osmolality is low and urine osmolality is high.

Table 40.1 CAUSES OF URINE DISCOLORATION

COLOR	CAUSE
Dark yellow or brown	Bilirubin
Brown-black	Homogentisic acid (ochronosis) Melanin (melanoma) Metronidazole Methyldopa/levodopa Phenothiazine
Red	Beets Rifampin Porphyria Hemoglobinuria or myoglobinuria Phenazopyridine hydrochloride (Pyridium) Urates
Blue-green	Indomethacin Amitriptyline
Turbid white	Pyuria Chylous fistula Crystalluria

Urine pH also varies (4–7.5 pH) and depends on the dietary intake in healthy persons. Acidic urine is indicative of a high-protein diet, acidosis, and potassium depletion. Alkaline urine is associated with a vegetarian diet, alkalosis (unless there is potassium depletion), and urease-producing bacteria. A urine pH less than 5.5 generally excludes type 1 renal tubular acidosis. A pH greater than 7 may suggest infection.

RENAL IMAGING

Radiography

Plain radiographs magnify the kidneys 30%. Normal renal size is 3.5 times the height of vertebra L2 (>11 cm). The left kidney is up to 1.5 cm longer than the right kidney. An enlarged kidney indicates obstruction, infiltration (eg, amyloidosis, leukemia, or diabetes mellitus), acute glomerulonephritis, acute tubulointerstitial nephropathy, renal vein thrombosis, or polycystic kidney disease. Calcifications are associated with stones, tuberculosis, aneurysms, and necrosis of the papillary tips.

Excretory Urography

Excretory urography provides a detailed definition of the collecting system and can be used to assess renal size and contour and to detect and locate calculi. It is also used to assess renal function qualitatively. Rapid sequence excretory urography is a poor screening test for renovascular hypertension. Complications include a large osmotic load (congestive heart failure) and reactions (5% of patients). An iodine load may occur and is a consideration if the patient has hyperthyroidism.

Ultrasonography

Ultrasonography is used to measure renal size (>9 cm) and to screen for obstruction, but the results may be negative early in the course of obstruction. Ultrasonography can be used to characterize mass lesions (eg, solid or cystic angiomyolipoma) and to screen for polycystic kidney disease. Ultrasonography may also be used to assess for renal vein thrombosis (ie, to assess for the presence or absence of blood flow), but it is not a screening test for renal artery stenosis.

Computed Tomography

Computed tomography shows calcification patterns. It is used to stage neoplasms, help determine the cause of obstruction (without contrast medium), and assess cysts, abscesses, and hematomas.

Magnetic Resonance Imaging

Magnetic resonance imaging may be used to identify adrenal hemorrhage and assess a mass in patients sensitive to contrast dyes. Magnetic resonance angiography is a promising screening method for renal artery stenosis. Extreme caution should be used to ensure that gadolinium-containing contrast material is not used in patients with stage 4 or 5 CKD, renal and hepatic transplant recipients, patients with severe acute renal insufficiency or hepatorenal syndrome, and intensive care unit patients.

Nephrogenic systemic fibrosis (also called nephrogenic fibrosing dermopathy) has been directly associated with exposure to gadolinium-containing contrast material in patients with stage 4 or 5 CKD. Nephrogenic systemic fibrosis is a painful skin disease characterized by thickening of the skin that can involve the joints and significantly limit motion within weeks to months.

The National Kidney Foundation recommends that alternative imaging techniques be attempted when patients have an estimated GFR of 30 mL/min per 1.73 m² or less and that if patients need a gadolinium-based contrast material, the lowest possible dose should be used. In patients with stage 5 CKD who are receiving dialysis, a reduced dose of gadolinium-based contrast material should be used only if absolutely unavoidable, and the patients should receive hemodialysis immediately afterward. Patients receiving peritoneal dialysis should not be given gadolinium.

- The choice of renal imaging technique is determined by the potential disease process being investigated.

Other Tests

Arteriography and venography are used to evaluate arterial stenosis, aneurysm, fistulas, vasculitis, and mass lesions and to assess living related donor transplants. Gallium and indium scans are used to evaluate acute interstitial nephritis, abscess, pyelonephritis, lymphoma, and leukemia. Diethylenetriamine pentacetic acid (also called pentetic acid or DTPA) and hippuran renal scanning are useful in assessing a transplanted kidney, obstruction (before and after furosemide), and infarct (presence or absence of blood flow).

CHRONIC KIDNEY DISEASE

More than 20 million people in the United States have CKD, including 11 million with stage 3 CKD (GFR <60 mL/min

Table 40.2 CAUSES OF CHRONIC KIDNEY DISEASE

CAUSE	CASES, %
Diabetes mellitus	42
Hypertension	26
Glomerulonephritis	11
Other or unknown	20

per 1.73 m²) (Table 40.2). The goals of recognizing and treating CKD are to prevent the morbidity and mortality associated with the progression of renal dysfunction, delay progression of kidney disease, and allow adequate time to educate the patients and their families about the patient's kidney disease and options for renal replacement therapy (RRT).

CKD has been categorized into 6 stages (Table 40.3). When renal function decreases to stage 3 (GFR 30–59 mL/min per 1.73 m²), the complications of CKD become evident. These complications include hypertension, cardiovascular disease, lipid abnormalities, anemia, metabolic bone disease, and electrolyte disturbances. To prevent the progression of CKD, therapy must be directed toward preventing these complications and achieving adequate glucose control in diabetic patients with CKD.

DIETARY RECOMMENDATIONS

Dietary adjustments are an important part of the care plan for patients with CKD. Dietary restrictions are directed at preventing electrolyte abnormalities and unwanted weight loss. As GFR decreases, the nephron is less able to handle potassium, phosphorus, sodium, and acid loads.

As their renal function changes, patients should be monitored for hyperkalemia and other electrolyte abnormalities, and their dietary prescription should be changed as indicated. Hyperkalemia usually occurs when the GFR is less than 20 mL/min per 1.73 m², but it can occur with higher GFRs when

Table 40.3 STAGES OF CHRONIC KIDNEY DISEASE

STAGE	DESCRIPTION	GFR, mL/min per 1.73 m²
0	At increased risk	>90 with chronic kidney disease risk factors
1	Kidney damage with normal or decreased GFR	≥90
2	Kidney damage with mildly decreased GFR	60–89
3	Moderately decreased GFR	30–59
4	Severely decreased GFR	15–29
5	Kidney failure	<15 or dialysis

Abbreviation: GFR, glomerular filtration rate.

renal tubular involvement is greater than glomerular involvement, such as in type 4 renal tubular acidosis. To prevent hyperkalemia, the recommended dietary potassium restriction is 70 mEq daily.

- Hyperkalemia usually occurs when the GFR is less than 20 mL/min per 1.73 m².

- Hyperkalemia can occur at higher GFRs when renal tubular involvement is greater than glomerular involvement, such as in type 4 renal tubular acidosis.

Sodium restriction of 90 mEq daily is recommended to prevent hypertension and fluid overload. In addition, usually after the patient's GFR has decreased to the range of stage 4 (GFR 15–29 mL/min per 1.73 m²) or stage 5 (GFR <15 mL/min per 1.73 m²) disease and urine output has decreased, the patient may also require fluid restriction.

Protein loading can lead to accumulation of acid, phosphorus, and uric acid. A protein restriction of 0.8 to 1.0 g/kg daily may be needed to prevent these complications. The benefits of protein restriction must be balanced against the morbidity and mortality associated with protein malnutrition. If the patient's protein stores are normal, a protein-restricted diet is recommended. If the patient becomes protein malnourished or the serum albumin decreases, the protein restriction should be liberalized.

- A protein restriction of 0.8 to 1.0 g/kg daily may be needed to prevent accumulation of acid, phosphorus, and uric acid in CKD.

Phosphorus retention can lead to metabolic bone disease and cardiovascular disease. If hyperphosphatemia develops, a dietary phosphorus limit of 1,200 mg daily is recommended. Decreased vitamin D production in CKD can lead to decreased calcium absorption and hypocalcemia. Maintaining a calcium intake of 1.0 to 1.2 g daily will help hypocalcemia and parathyroid stimulation. Unwanted weight loss, anorexia, and cachexia are complications of uremia and should be avoided by prescribing a diet that provides 35 kcal/kg daily.

- Phosphorus retention can lead to metabolic bone disease and cardiovascular disease.

TREATMENT OF CKD COMPLICATIONS AND PREVENTION OF PROGRESSION

Maximizing glucose control in diabetic patients, treating hypertension, and decreasing proteinuria are essential to preventing progression of CKD and its associated cardiovascular complications. Sodium retention and fluid overload contribute to hypertension in patients with CKD and progressive loss of renal function. In these patients, the use of diuretics is essential to controlling blood pressure. Thiazide diuretics are useful until the GFR is less than 45 mL/min per 1.73 m². At that point, loop diuretics should be used. In addition, angiotensin-converting enzyme inhibitors (ACEIs) and angiotensin receptor blockers (ARBs) are excellent choices for decreasing both systemic hypertension and proteinuria. The goal blood pressure is less than 130/80 mm Hg for patients with CKD and less than 120/75 mm Hg for those with CKD and proteinuria.

- Thiazide diuretics are useful until the GFR is <45 mL/min per 1.73 m^2.

- The goal blood pressure is <130/80 mm Hg for patients with CKD and <120/75 mm Hg for those with CKD and proteinuria.

Proteinuria is a marker of renal dysfunction and a risk factor for progression of CKD. ACEIs and ARBs are beneficial in delaying the progression of renal disease not only by controlling blood pressure but also by decreasing proteinuria. The goal is to decrease urinary protein excretion by 35% to 40% of the baseline level with an ideal goal of decreasing the urinary protein excretion to less than 0.3 g/1.73 m^2 per 24 hours.

- Proteinuria is a marker of renal dysfunction and a risk factor for progression of CKD.

- ACEIs and ARBs are beneficial in delaying the progression of renal disease not only by controlling blood pressure but also by decreasing proteinuria.

- Decreasing the urinary protein excretion to <0.3 g/1.73 m^2 per 24 hours is the ideal goal in CKD.

The use of ACEIs, ARBs, and β-blockers can lead to hyperkalemia, which may cause rhythm disturbances. Therefore, all patients with progressive renal dysfunction who are receiving these medications should be monitored for rhythm disturbances and electrolyte abnormalities.

Treating hyperlipidemia is also an important step in slowing the progression of CKD and in decreasing cardiovascular risks. Statins (3-hydroxy-3-methylglutaryl coenzyme A [HMG-CoA] reductase inhibitors) not only improve lipid profiles but also may slow the progression of ESRD; however, the data are inconclusive.

- Statins not only improve lipid profiles but also may slow the progression of ESRD.

Hyperphosphatemia and secondary hyperparathyroidism are risk factors for metabolic bone and mineral disease as well as for cardiovascular disease in persons with stage 3, 4, or 5 CKD. In addition, through a complex feedback system, renal disease leads to phosphate retention, hypocalcemia, acidosis, decreased 1,25-dihydroxyvitamin D production, and increased parathyroid hormone production. Relatively early in advancing renal insufficiency, hyperphosphatemia and a decreased level of 1,25-dihydroxyvitamin D begin the cascade leading to secondary hyperparathyroidism and the development of bone and systemic mineral disease. Osteitis fibrosa cystica is the classic form of renal failure–associated bone disease with overactive osteoclastic and osteoblastic activity.

- Hyperphosphatemia and secondary hyperparathyroidism are risk factors for metabolic bone and mineral disease as well as for cardiovascular disease in persons with stage 3, 4, or 5 CKD.

- Osteitis fibrosa cystica is the classic form of renal failure–associated bone disease with overactive osteoclastic and osteoblastic activity.

Recognizing and treating secondary hyperparathyroidism and vitamin D deficiency early in the course of CKD can prevent or minimize these complications. Treatment and prevention of renal osteodystrophy and CKD-associated mineral and bone disorders focus on the suppression of parathyroid hormone production by maintaining a normal calcium and phosphorus balance. Treatment begins with a low-phosphorus diet. If the serum level of phosphorus remains elevated, adding enteric phosphate binders is the next step. A low serum calcium level or a high parathyroid hormone level or both are indications for the addition of calcitriol or vitamin D analogues. An elevated calcium-phosphorus product has been associated with increased morbidity and mortality. The goal is a calcium-phosphorus product of less than 55. Further treatment of secondary hyperparathyroidism involves calcitriol, vitamin D analogues, or a calcimimetic agent to inhibit parathyroid hormone production. If the above measures fail to adequately suppress the parathyroid, a parathyroidectomy may be indicated.

Osteomalacia (low-turnover bone disease due to 1,25-dihydroxyvitamin D deficiency) is characterized by increased osteoid activity and diminished or absent osteoclastic and osteoblastic activity. Osteoporosis occurs rarely in ESRD and advanced CKD. Oversuppression of parathyroid hormone production with vitamin D analogues or calcimimetic agents is the most common cause.

- Osteomalacia results from 1,25-dihydroxyvitamin D deficiency.

With avoidance of aluminum phosphate binders and other aluminum-containing medications, aluminum bone disease occurs infrequently in CKD and ESRD. Aluminum bone disease is characterized by low levels of parathyroid hormone and 1,25-dihydroxyvitamin D in a patient presenting with microcytic anemia and bone fractures. Aluminum toxicity can also cause severe neurotoxicity. Thus, aluminum-containing medications should be avoided in all patients with stage 4 or stage 5 CKD. Aluminum osteodystrophy is diagnosed with an iliac crest bone biopsy and treated with deferoxamine chelation.

Anemia due to a decrease in erythropoietin production is another complication of CKD. This anemia is a normocytic normochromic anemia that is multifactorial; decreased erythropoietin production, hemolysis, and blood loss may help contribute to the low hemoglobin concentration. Bleeding is common in CKD because of platelet dysfunction, but treatment with desmopressin is helpful in reversing the bleeding tendency quickly. If the GFR decreases to less than 33 mL/min per 1.73 m², erythropoietin production by the renal parenchyma is not sufficient to prevent anemia.

Treatment with erythropoiesis-stimulating agents should be started if anemia develops in patients who have CKD and ESRD. Studies, however, have shown an increased risk of thromboembolic events when erythropoiesis-stimulating agents were given to patients who had hemoglobin levels of 11 g/dL or more. Other studies have shown decreased survival and progression of cancer when the target hemoglobin is between 12 and 14 g/dL in women with breast and ovarian cancer and in men and women with advanced head and neck cancer or with gastric and small cell lung cancer. On the basis of these findings, the recommended optimal hemoglobin target level is 10 to 12 g/dL. Erythropoiesis-stimulating agents have also been recognized as contributing to systemic nephrogenic fibrosis. Thus, the goal is to use the smallest possible dose of erythropoiesis-stimulating agents to achieve hemoglobin levels of 10 to 12 g/dL. Iron deficiency, which occurs in 25% to 38% of patients with CKD, is the most common cause of resistance to erythropoiesis-stimulating agents, so it should be corrected before starting erythropoiesis-stimulating therapy. Other causes of resistance to erythropoiesis-stimulating agents include inflammation, malignancy, secondary hyperparathyroidism, hematologic disorders, and increasing uremia.

- In anemia of CKD, the goal is to use the smallest possible dose of erythropoiesis-stimulating agents in CKD to achieve hemoglobin levels of 10–12 g/dL.

The complications of progressive renal dysfunction and uremia involve all organ systems. Uremic symptoms and signs may occur at different levels of GFR depending on the patient's comorbid illnesses and the management of the patient beginning dialysis.

Metabolic acidosis begins in the early phases of CKD, initially as a non–anion gap acidosis due to decreased ammonium secretion. As renal dysfunction progresses, phosphate and sulfate accumulate and the acidosis becomes a high anion gap acidosis.

Although hyperkalemia can occur with a GFR less than 20 mL/min per 1.73 m² and oliguria, hyperkalemia can also occur with a GFR much greater than 20 mL/min per 1.73 m² as a result of distal tubular dysfunction (type 4 renal tubular acidosis or aldosterone deficiency) and medications that interfere with potassium handling (ACEIs, ARBs, β-blockers, and potassium-sparing diuretics). Hyperkalemia associated with electrocardiographic changes should be treated emergently with intravenous calcium to protect the myocardium and then with an infusion of insulin to redistribute the potassium; however, if the patient has electrocardiographic changes and a low GFR, dialysis is indicated. Resins and dialysis are used to eliminate potassium. Chronic hyperkalemia can be treated with a scheduled dose of a resin, a low-potassium diet, and the avoidance of medications that interfere with potassium handling.

β₂-Microglobulin deposition occurs in persons with stage 4 or 5 CKD and results in carpal tunnel syndrome

and debilitating arthritis. Residual GFR is the most important factor in this phenomenon and is inversely related to β₂-microglobulin deposition. Pseudogout and periarthritis are other musculoskeletal complications in patients with stage 4 or 5 CKD.

- β₂-Microglobulin deposition occurs in persons with stage 4 or 5 CKD and results in carpal tunnel syndrome and debilitating arthritis.

Many abnormalities of the gastrointestinal tract can occur with advanced CKD, including gastritis, colitis, ileitis, constipation, peptic ulcer disease, and gastrointestinal tract bleeding. Anorexia is a multifactorial complication leading to protein and caloric malnutrition.

Neurologic complications commonly occur in persons with stage 3, 4, or 5 CKD. These include peripheral neuropathies, sleep disorders, restless legs, and eventually cognitive impairment and central nervous system irritability with seizures and coma in severe uremia.

CKD AND CARDIOVASCULAR DISEASE

Many large studies of patients with CKD have shown increased mortality and morbidity from cardiovascular disease. The nontraditional risk factors for cardiovascular disease associated with CKD include lipid abnormalities, endothelial dysfunction, anemia, inflammation, and abnormal metabolism of phosphorus and calcium. The presence of proteinuria is evidence of endothelial dysfunction and is an independent risk factor for cardiovascular disease. Lipid abnormalities associated with CKD begin with mild abnormalities in GFR. These lipid abnormalities include hypertriglyceridemia, decreased high-density lipoprotein, and increased levels of very low-density lipoprotein, remnant-like particles, intermediate-density lipoprotein, lipoprotein(a), and small dense low-density lipoprotein. As kidney disease progresses and approaches ESRD (stage 5 CKD), a progressive decrease in the total cholesterol level is associated with increased cardiovascular events and all-cause mortality. This is the low-cholesterol paradox of chronic malnutrition and signifies a state of inflammation. Stage 5 CKD is a state of increased levels of proinflammatory cytokines with elevated levels of C-reactive protein, increased oxidative stress, and decreased clearance of proinflammatory substances. This state of inflammation increases cardiovascular risks.

Additional factors contributing to increased cardiovascular risks include anemia and altered metabolism of calcium, phosphorus, and vitamin D. Anemia in patients with CKD contributes to the development of left ventricular hypertrophy. Vitamin D improves blood pressure and decreases inflammation, and decreased vitamin D production in CKD leads to increased cardiovascular risks. The mechanisms are thought to involve downregulation of the renin-angiotensin system and a decrease in cellular cytokine production. An elevated calcium-phosphorus product and hyperparathyroidism are associated with increased inflammation and systemic metastatic calcification leading to cardiovascular disease.

- Cardiovascular disease in CKD is multifactorial and is accompanied by lipid abnormalities, endothelial dysfunction, anemia, inflammation, and abnormal metabolism of phosphorus and calcium.

LONG-TERM DIALYSIS

The number of patients reaching ESRD and beginning dialysis continues to increase while diabetes mellitus and hypertension continue to be the leading causes of renal failure. Dialysis should be initiated before uremic symptoms develop. Indications for dialysis include fluid overload, systemic acidosis, hyperkalemia, and uremic symptoms.

If the GFR is less than 30 mL/min per 1.73 m², the patient should be told about options for RRT, which include in-center hemodialysis, home hemodialysis, peritoneal dialysis, and renal transplant. Innovative dialysis prescriptions include daily hemodialysis and nocturnal hemodialysis. The choice of dialysis type in chronic nonemergent renal failure depends on many clinical and mechanical factors and on patient choice. All types of dialysis can be done at home. Peritoneal dialysis offers a continuous ultrafiltration and solute clearance, avoiding rapid fluid shifts and hemodynamic instability. Hemodialysis offers more efficient clearance of solutes. Selected patients who have poor hemodialysis access options, cardiomyopathy, or a scheduled transplant may be candidates for peritoneal dialysis. Peritoneal dialysis will fail in patients with a history of recurrent abdominal operations or diseases that lead to fibrosis of the peritoneal lining. Frequent hemodialysis methods such as daily or nightly hemodialysis in a dialysis center or at home have been shown to improve blood pressure, control bone disease, and improve overall well-being.

- If the GFR is <30 mL/min per 1.73 m², the patient should be told about options for RRT.

Complications of Dialysis

Intradialytic hypotension is a common complication of hemodialysis. Rapid removal of fluid, osmolar shifts, and abrupt changes in calcium, bicarbonate, and potassium can lead to hemodynamic instability and arrhythmias. Rapid changes in electrolytes or fluid removal can also lead to nausea, vomiting, and muscle cramps.

The rapid removal of solutes, specifically urea in patients with high urea values, can lead to neurologic consequences known as dialysis dysequilibrium syndrome. The symptoms include headaches, nausea and vomiting, decreased or altered mental status, seizures, and death. This syndrome is thought to be caused by rapid shifts in urea and osmolality leading to fluid shifts into the central nervous system and cerebral edema. The best way to avoid this complication in patients with excessively high urea levels is to limit the efficiency of the dialysis session by dialyzing with low flows of blood and dialysate for short periods.

Allergic reactions to the hemodialyzer membrane can occur. Overt anaphylactic reactions are rare, but patients may complain of muscle cramps, pain (back, chest, or abdominal), nausea and vomiting, pruritus, or urticaria. These symptoms may be accompanied by fever, hypotension, or hypertension. Treatment is usually symptomatic and involves using another type of dialysis membrane.

All patients with ESRD are at increased risk of hepatitis B and C. They should receive hepatitis B vaccine. Infections involving the dialysis access are mostly seen with central venous catheters or arteriovenous grafts and peritoneal dialysis tunneled catheters. Early detection and treatment with antibiotics is critical. Complications specific to peritoneal dialysis include catheter leaks, obesity, hyperlipidemia, and hyperglycemia.

Selecting the appropriate medications in the appropriate doses for patients receiving dialysis is essential to avoid adverse reactions and accumulation of drugs leading to toxicity. Many drugs are not removed by hemodialysis or peritoneal dialysis and should be avoided or their doses adjusted as the patient's residual GFR decreases. Conversely, toxicity from some ingested drugs can be treated with hemodialysis (Box 40.2).

- Patients receiving dialysis should have all vaccinations up to date and be monitored carefully for concurrent infection.

Box 40.2 DIALYSIS AND OVERDOSES

Drugs removed with dialysis
  Methanol
  Aspirin
  Ethylene glycol
  Lithium
  Sodium
  Mannitol
  Theophylline
Drugs not removed with dialysis
  Tetracycline
  Benzodiazepines
  Digoxin
  Phenytoin
  Phenothiazines
Drugs to avoid in patients receiving dialysis
  Tetracycline
  Nitrofurantoin
  Probenecid
  Neomycin
  Bacitracin
  Methenamine
  Nalidixic acid
  Clofibrate
  Lovastatin
  Magnesium
  Oral hypoglycemic agents
  Antiplatelet drugs
  Renally excreted β-blockers

SUMMARY

- The kidneys normally maintain a constant extracellular environment, secrete multiple hormones, and catabolize peptide hormones in fasting conditions.

- Kidney function is assessed by the estimated and measured GFR, by the functionality of the filtering structures through analysis of the urine (microscopic urine analysis and protein excretion), and by imaging studies of the kidney to determine structural abnormalities.

- If the GFR is <30 mL/min per 1.73 m^2, the patient should be told about options for RRT.

PART X

ALLERGY

41.

ALLERGY[a]

Gerald W. Volcheck, MD

GOALS

- Categorize types of allergy testing and their indications.

- Describe diagnosis and treatment strategies for rhinitis.

- Compare and contrast urticaria and angioedema.

- Cite treatments for food, insect, and drug allergies.

ALLERGY TESTING

Standard allergy testing relies on identifying the IgE antibody specific for the allergen in question. Two classic methods of doing this are the immediate wheal-and-flare skin prick tests (a small amount of antigen is introduced into the skin and the site is evaluated after 15 minutes for the presence of an immediate wheal-and-flare reaction) and in vitro (blood) testing.

Allergy testing that does not have a clear scientific basis includes cytotoxic testing, provocation-neutralization testing or treatment, and "yeast allergy" testing.

PATCH TESTS AND PRICK (CUTANEOUS) TESTS

Patch testing of skin is not the same as immediate wheal-and-flare skin testing. Patch testing is used to investigate only contact dermatitis, a type IV hypersensitivity skin reaction. Patch tests require 72 to 96 hours for complete evaluation. Many substances cause contact dermatitis. Common contact sensitivities include nickel, formaldehyde, fragrances, and latex.

Inhalant allergens, in comparison, cause respiratory symptoms, such as allergic rhinitis and asthma, and are identified by skin prick testing. Their sources include dust mites, cats, dogs, cockroaches, molds, and tree, grass, and weed pollens. Food allergy is also assessed by skin prick testing.

- Patch testing is used to investigate contact dermatitis.

- Skin prick (immediate) testing is used to investigate respiratory allergy to airborne allergens and food allergy.

Prick and intradermal testing involve introducing allergen to the skin layers below the external keratin layer. The deeper techniques are more sensitive but less specific. With the deeper, intradermal tests, allergen is introduced closer to responding cells and at higher doses. Intradermal testing is used to evaluate stinging insect venoms and penicillin. Allergen skin tests performed by the prick technique adequately identify patients who have important clinical sensitivities without identifying a large number of those who have minimal levels of IgE antibody and no clinical sensitivity.

Drugs with antihistamine properties, such as H_1 receptor antagonists, and many anticholinergic and tricyclic antidepressant drugs can suppress immediate allergy skin test responses. Use of nonsedating antihistamines should be discontinued 5 days before skin testing. The H_2 receptor antagonists have a small suppressive effect. High-dose corticosteroids can suppress the delayed-type hypersensitivity and the immediate response.

- Intradermal skin tests are more sensitive but less specific than skin prick tests for airborne allergens.

- Intradermal skin testing is used to investigate allergy to insect venoms and penicillin.

IN VITRO ALLERGY TESTING

In vitro (blood) allergy testing initially involves chemically coupling allergen protein molecules to a solid-phase substance. The test is then conducted by incubating serum (from the patient) that may contain IgE antibody specific for the allergen that has been immobilized to the membrane for a standard time. The solid phase is then washed free of nonbinding materials from the serum and incubated in a second solution containing a reagent (eg, radiolabeled anti-IgE antibody). The measured radioactivity is correlated directly with the preparation of a standard curve in which known amounts of allergen-specific IgE antibody were incubated with a set of

[a] Portions previously published in Volcheck GW. Clinical allergy: diagnosis and management. Totowa (NJ): Humana; c2009. Used with permission of Mayo Foundation for Medical Education and Research.

standard preparations of a solid phase. Labeled anti-IgE can also be measured with colorimetry, fluorometry, or monoclonal and polyclonal anti-IgE antibodies.

This test only identifies the presence of allergen-specific IgE antibody in the same way that the allergen skin test does. Generally, in vitro allergy testing is not as sensitive as skin testing and has some limitations because of the potential for chemical modification of the allergen protein while it is being coupled to the solid phase. Generally, it is more expensive than allergen skin tests and has no advantage in routine clinical work. In vitro allergy testing may be useful clinically for patients who have been taking antihistamines and are unable to discontinue their use or for patients who have primary cutaneous diseases that make allergen skin testing impractical or inaccurate (eg, severe atopic eczema with most of the skin involved in a flare).

- Skin testing is more sensitive and less expensive than in vitro allergy testing.

CHRONIC RHINITIS

MEDICAL HISTORY

The differential diagnosis of chronic rhinitis is given in Box 41.1. *Nonallergic rhinitis* is defined as nasal symptoms occurring in response to nonspecific, nonallergic irritants. Vasomotor rhinitis is the most common form. Common triggers of vasomotor rhinitis are strong odors, respiratory irritants such as dust or smoke, changes in temperature, changes in body position, and ingestants such as spicy food or alcohol.

- *Nonallergic rhinitis* is defined as nasal symptoms occurring in response to nonspecific stimuli.

Historical factors favoring a diagnosis of *allergic* rhinitis include a history of nasal symptoms that have a recurrent seasonal pattern (eg, every August and September) or symptoms provoked by being near specific sources of allergens, such as animals. Factors favoring *vasomotor* rhinitis include symptoms provoked by strong odors and changes in humidity and temperature.

- Allergic rhinitis has a recurrent seasonal pattern and may be provoked by being near animals.

Box 41.1 **DIFFERENTIAL DIAGNOSIS OF CHRONIC RHINITIS**

Allergic rhinitis
Vasomotor rhinitis
Rhinitis medicamentosa
Sinusitis
Nasal polyposis
Nasal septal deviation
Foreign body
Tumor

- Triggers of vasomotor rhinitis include strong odors and changes in humidity and temperature.

Factors common to allergic rhinitis and nonallergic rhinitis (thus, without differential diagnostic value) include perennial symptoms, intolerance of cigarette smoke, and history of "dust" sensitivity. Factors that suggest fixed nasal obstruction (which should prompt physicians to consider other diagnoses) include unilateral nasal obstruction, unilateral facial pain, unilateral nasal purulence, nasal voice but no nasal symptoms, disturbances of olfaction without any nasal symptoms, and unilateral nasal bleeding. Further evaluation with computed tomographic (CT) scan of the sinuses or rhinolaryngoscopy is indicated.

- Perennial symptoms, intolerance of cigarette smoke, and history of "dust" sensitivity are common to allergic and nonallergic rhinitis.

- House dust mite sensitivity is a common cause of perennial allergic rhinitis.

- Rhinoscopy or CT scan of the sinuses should be performed to evaluate unilateral symptoms.

ALLERGY SKIN TESTS IN ALLERGIC RHINITIS

The interpretation of allergy skin test results must be tailored to the unique features of each patient.

1. For patients with perennial symptoms and negative results on allergy skin tests, the diagnosis is nonallergic rhinitis.

2. For patients with seasonal symptoms and appropriately positive allergy skin tests, the diagnosis is seasonal allergic rhinitis.

3. For patients with perennial symptoms, allergy skin tests positive for house dust mite suggest house dust mite allergic rhinitis. In this case, dust mite allergen avoidance should be recommended. Patients should encase their bedding with allergy-proof encasements, wash sheets and pillowcases in hot water weekly, and keep the relative humidity in the house at 40% to 50% or less.

CORTICOSTEROID THERAPY FOR RHINITIS

The need for systemic corticosteroid treatment for rhinitis is limited. Occasionally, patients with severe symptoms of allergic rhinitis may benefit greatly from a short course of prednisone (10 mg 4 times daily by mouth for 5 days). This may induce sufficient improvement so that topical corticosteroids can penetrate the nose and satisfactory levels of antihistamine can be established in the blood. Severe nasal polyposis may warrant a longer course of oral corticosteroids. Sometimes the recurrence of nasal polyps can be prevented by continued use of topical corticosteroids. Polypectomy may be required if nasal polyps do not respond to treatment with systemic and intranasal corticosteroids, but nasal polyps often recur after surgical intervention.

- Treatment of nasal polyposis can include oral prednisone, followed by topical corticosteroids.

In contrast to systemic corticosteroids, topical corticosteroid agents for the nose are easy to use and have few adverse systemic effects.

- Topical corticosteroid agents are helpful for allergic nasal congestion.

Long-term treatment with decongestant nasal sprays may have "addictive" potential (a vicious cycle of rebound congestion called *rhinitis medicamentosa* caused by topical vasoconstrictors). In contrast, intranasal corticosteroid does not induce this type of dependence.

- Unlike decongestant nasal sprays, intranasal corticosteroid does not induce tachyphylaxis and rebound congestion.

A substantial number of patients with nonallergic rhinitis also have a good response to intranasal (topical aerosol) corticosteroid therapy, especially if they have the nasal eosinophilia form of nonallergic rhinitis.

- Many patients with nonallergic rhinitis have a good response to topical intranasal corticosteroid therapy.

A patient who has allergic rhinitis and does not receive adequate relief with topical corticosteroid plus antihistamine therapy may need systemic corticosteroid treatment and immunotherapy. Unilateral symptoms suggest anatomical causes, including polyps, septal deviation, and tumor.

- If pharmacologic management fails, allergy immunotherapy should be considered for patients with allergic rhinitis.

An unusual side effect of intranasal corticosteroids is nasal septal perforation. Spray canisters deliver a powerful jet of particulates, and a few patients have misdirected the jet to the nasal septum.

- Rarely, topical corticosteroid nasal sprays cause perforation of the nasal septum.

ANTIHISTAMINES AND OTHER TREATMENTS

Antihistamines antagonize the interaction of histamine with its receptors. Histamine may be more causative than other mast cell mediators of nasal itch and sneezing. These are symptoms most often responsive to antihistamine therapy.

Pseudoephedrine is the most common decongestant agent in nonprescription drugs for treating cold symptoms and rhinitis and usually is the active agent in widely used prescription agents. Phenylpropanolamine has been removed from

the market because of its association with hemorrhagic stroke in women. Several prescription and nonprescription combination agents combine an antihistamine and a decongestant. Saline nasal rinses may provide symptomatic improvement in patients with chronic rhinitis by helping to remove mucus from the nares.

- Pseudoephedrine is the most common decongestant in nonprescription and prescription preparations.

In men who are middle-aged or older, urinary retention may be caused by antihistamines (principally the older drugs that have anticholinergic effects) and decongestants. Although there has been concern for years that decongestants may exacerbate hypertension because they are α-adrenergic agonists, a clinically significant hypertensive response is rare in patients with hypertension that is controlled medically.

- Antihistamines and decongestants may cause urinary retention in men.
- The elderly are more sensitive to the anticholinergic effects of antihistamines.

IMMUNOTHERAPY FOR ALLERGIC RHINITIS

Until topical nasal glucocorticoid sprays were introduced, allergen immunotherapy was considered first-line therapy for allergic rhinitis when the relevant allergen was seasonal pollen of grass, trees, or weeds. Immunotherapy became second-line therapy after topical corticosteroids were introduced because immunotherapy 1) requires a larger time commitment during the build-up phase and 2) carries a small risk of anaphylaxis to the immunotherapy injection itself. However, immunotherapy for allergic rhinitis can be appropriate first-line therapy for selected patients and is highly effective.

Immunotherapy is often reserved for patients who do not receive satisfactory relief from intranasal corticosteroids or who cannot tolerate antihistamines. Controlled trials have shown a benefit for pollen, dust mite, and cat allergies and a variable benefit for mold allergy. Immunotherapy is not used for food allergy or nonallergic rhinitis. Immunotherapy has been shown to decrease the incidence of the development of asthma in children with allergic rhinitis and to decrease the onset of new allergen sensitivities in those treated for a single allergen.

- Immunotherapy is often reserved for patients who do not receive relief from intranasal glucocorticoids or who cannot tolerate antihistamines.
- Controlled trials have shown that immunotherapy is very effective for allergic rhinitis and results in prolonged symptom improvement.
- Anaphylaxis is a risk of immunotherapy.
- Immunotherapy for allergic rhinitis can be first-line therapy for selected patients.

ENVIRONMENTAL MODIFICATION

House Dust Mites

Areas in the home harboring the most substantial mite populations are bedding and fabric-upholstered furniture (heavily used) and any area where carpeting is on concrete (when concrete is in contact with the ground). To decrease mite exposure, encase the bedding (and sometimes, when practical, furniture cushions) in dust-proof encasements. To some degree, this also prevents infusion of water vapor into the bedding matrix. These 2 factors combine to markedly decrease the amount of airborne allergen. In contrast, recently marketed acaricides that kill mites or denature their protein allergens have not proved useful in the home. Measures for controlling dust mites are listed in Box 41.2.

• Dust mites are an important source of respiratory allergen.

• The most substantial mite populations are in bedding and fabric-upholstered furniture.

• Impermeable encasements prevent egress of allergen.

• Chemical sprays (acaricides) capable of either killing mites or denaturing the protein allergens are not substantially helpful when applied in the home.

Pollen

Air conditioning, which enables the home to remain tightly closed, is the principal defense against pollinosis. Most masks purchased at local pharmacies cannot exclude pollen particles and are not worth the expense. Some masks can protect the wearer from allergen exposure. These are industrial-quality respirators designed specifically to pass rigorous testing by the Occupational Safety and Health Administration (OSHA) and the National Institute for Occupational Safety and Health (NIOSH) and certification for excluding a wide spectrum of particulates, including pollen and mold. These masks allow persons to mow the lawn and do yard work, which would be intolerable otherwise because of sensitivity to pollen allergen.

• Only industrial-quality masks are capable of excluding pollen particles.

Animal Dander

No measure for controlling animal dander can compare with getting the animal completely out of the house. If complete removal is not tenable, some partial measures must be considered. Recommendations include keeping the animal out of the bedroom entirely and attempting to keep the animal in 1 area of the home. A high-efficiency particulate air (HEPA) room air purifier should be placed in the bedroom. Naturally, the person should avoid close contact with the animal and should consider using a mask if handling the animal or entering the room where the animal is kept. Bathing cats about once every other week may reduce the allergen load in the environment.

• Complete avoidance is the only entirely effective way to manage allergy to household pets.

SINUSITIS

Sinusitis is closely associated with edematous obstruction of the sinus ostia (the osteomeatal complex). Poor drainage of the sinus cavities predisposes to infection, particularly by microorganisms that thrive in low-oxygen environments (eg, anaerobes). In adults, *Streptococcus pneumoniae*, *Haemophilus influenzae*, anaerobes, and viruses are common pathogens. In addition, *Branhamella catarrhalis* is an important pathogen in children.

Important clinical features of acute sinusitis are purulent nasal discharge, tooth pain, cough, and poor response to decongestants. Findings on paranasal sinus transillumination may be abnormal.

• Purulent nasal discharge, tooth pain, and abnormal findings on transillumination are important clinical features of sinusitis.

Physicians should be aware of the complications of sinusitis, which can be life-threatening (Box 41.3). Mucormycosis can cause recurrent or persistent sinusitis refractory to antibiotics. Allergic fungal sinusitis is characterized by persistent sinusitis, eosinophilia, increased total IgE, antifungal (usually *Aspergillus*) IgE antibodies, and fungal colonization of the sinuses. Wegener granulomatosis, ciliary dyskinesia, and hypogammaglobulinemia are medical conditions that can cause refractory sinusitis (Box 41.4).

Untreated sinusitis may lead to osteomyelitis, orbital and periorbital cellulitis, meningitis, and brain abscess. Cavernous sinus thrombosis, an especially serious complication, can lead to retrobulbar pain, extraocular muscle paralysis, and blindness.

Box 41.4 **CAUSES OF PERSISTENT OR RECURRENT SINUSITIS**

Nasal polyposis
Mucormycosis
Allergic fungal sinusitis
Ciliary dyskinesia
Wegener granulomatosis
Hypogammaglobulinemia
Tumor

Persistent, refractory, and complicated sinusitis should be evaluated by a specialist. Sinus CT is the preferred imaging study for these patients (Figure 41.1).

Amoxicillin (500 mg 3 times daily) or trimethoprim-sulfamethoxazole (1 double-strength capsule twice daily) for 10 to 14 days is the treatment of choice for uncomplicated maxillary sinusitis.

Plain radiography of the sinuses is less sensitive than CT (using the coronal sectioning technique). CT scans show greater detail about sinus mucosal surfaces, but CT usually is not necessary in acute uncomplicated sinusitis. CT is indicated, though, for patients being considered for a sinus operation and for those in whom standard treatment of sinusitis fails. However, patients with extensive dental restorations that contain metal may generate too much artifact for CT to be useful. For these patients, magnetic resonance imaging techniques are indicated.

- Sinus imaging is indicated for recurrent sinusitis.
- Sinus CT is preferred to sinus radiography for complicated sinusitis.

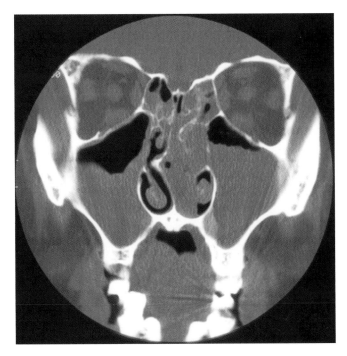

Figure 41.1 Sinusitis. Sinus computed tomogram shows opacification of the osteomeatal complex on the left, subtotal opacification of the right maxillary sinus, and an air–fluid level in the left maxillary antrum.

URTICARIA AND ANGIOEDEMA

DURATION OF URTICARIA

The distinction between *acute urticaria* and *chronic urticaria* is arbitrary and based on duration. If urticaria has been present for 6 weeks or longer, it is called chronic urticaria.

SECONDARY URTICARIA

Most patients simply have urticaria as a skin disease (*chronic idiopathic urticaria*). Many of these patients have an antibody that interacts with their own IgE or IgE receptor that produces the urticaria. Occasionally urticaria is the presenting sign of more serious internal disease. It can be a sign of lupus erythematosus and other connective tissue diseases, particularly the "overlap" syndromes that are more difficult to categorize. Thyroid disease, malignancy (mainly of the gastrointestinal tract), lymphoproliferative diseases, and occult infection (particularly of the intestines, gallbladder, and dentition) may be associated with urticaria. Immune-complex disease has been associated with urticaria, usually with urticarial vasculitis; hepatitis B virus has been identified as an antigen in cases of urticaria and immune-complex disease.

- Urticaria can be associated with lupus erythematosus and other connective tissue diseases, thyroid disease, malignancy, infection, and immune-complex disease.

A common cause of acute urticaria and angioedema (other than the idiopathic variety) is drug or food allergy. However, drug or food allergy usually does not cause chronic urticaria.

- Chronic urticaria and angioedema are often idiopathic.
- A common secondary cause of acute urticaria and angioedema is drug or food allergy.

RELATION BETWEEN URTICARIA AND ANGIOEDEMA

In common idiopathic urticaria, the hives last 2 to 18 hours, and the lesions itch intensely because histamine is the primary cause of wheal formation.

- Typical urticarial lesions last 2–18 hours and are pruritic.

The pathophysiologic mechanism is similar for urticaria and angioedema. The critical factor is the type of tissue in which the capillary leak and mediator release occur. Urticaria occurs when the capillary events are in the tissue wall of the skin—the epidermis. Angioedema occurs when the capillary events affect vessels in the loose connective tissue of the deeper layers—the dermis. Virtually all patients with the common idiopathic type of urticaria also have angioedema at some point.

C1 ESTERASE INHIBITOR DEFICIENCY

Hereditary angioneurotic edema (HANE) is characterized by recurrent episodes of angioedema, typically without urticaria. If HANE is strongly suspected, the diagnosis can be proved by the appropriate measurement of complement factors (decreased levels of C1 esterase inhibitor [quantitative and functional] and C4 [also C2, during an episode of swelling]).

- Levels of C1 esterase inhibitor and C4 are decreased in HANE.

Treatment of C1 esterase inhibitor dysfunction includes the following:

1. Plasma-derived C1 esterase inhibitor given intravenously—indicated for prophylaxis and acute attacks

2. Kallikrein inhibitor (ecallantide) given subcutaneously—indicated for acute attacks

3. Bradykinin B2 receptor antagonist (icatibant) given subcutaneously—indicated for acute attacks

The duration, size, and location of individual swellings vary. Many patients with HANE have also had symptoms resembling intestinal obstruction. These symptoms usually resolve in 3 to 5 days.

Lesions in HANE do not itch. The response to epinephrine is also a useful differential point: HANE lesions do not respond well to epinephrine, but common angioedema usually resolves in 15 minutes or less. Laryngeal edema almost never occurs in the common idiopathic type of disease (although it may occur in allergic reactions, most often in insect-sting anaphylaxis cases); however, it is relatively common in HANE (earlier articles cited a 30% mortality rate in HANE, with all deaths due to laryngeal edema). HANE episodes may be related to local tissue trauma in a high percentage of cases, with dental work often regarded as the classic precipitating factor.

- Many patients with HANE have been hospitalized for "intestinal obstruction."

- HANE lesions do not respond well to epinephrine.

- In HANE, laryngeal edema is relatively common.

- Dental work is the classic precipitating factor for HANE.

PHYSICAL URTICARIA

Heat, light, cold, vibration, and trauma or pressure can cause hives in susceptible persons. Obtaining the history is the only way to suspect the diagnosis, which can be confirmed by applying each of the stimuli to the patient's skin in the laboratory. Heat can be applied by placing coins (soaked in hot water for a few minutes) on the patient's forearm. Cold can be applied with coins kept in a freezer or with ice cubes. For vibration, a laboratory vortex mixer or any common vibrator can be used. A pair of sandbags connected by a strap can be draped over the patient to create enough pressure to cause symptoms in those with delayed pressure urticaria. Unlike most cases of common idiopathic urticaria, in which the lesions affect essentially all skin surfaces, many cases of physical urticaria seem to involve only certain areas of skin. Thus, challenges will be positive only in the areas usually involved and negative in other areas. Directing challenges to the appropriate area depends on the history.

- For physical urticaria, the history is the only way to suspect the diagnosis, which can be confirmed by applying stimuli to the patient's skin.

FOOD ALLERGY IN CHRONIC URTICARIA

Food allergy almost never causes chronic urticaria. However, urticaria (or angioedema or anaphylaxis) can be an acute manifestation of true food allergy.

- Food allergy almost never causes chronic urticaria.

- Food allergy may cause acute urticaria, angioedema, or anaphylaxis.

HISTOPATHOLOGY OF CHRONIC URTICARIA

Chronic urticaria is characterized by mononuclear cell perivascular cuffing around dermal capillaries, particularly involving the capillary loops that interdigitate with the rete pegs of the epidermis. Urticarial vasculitis shows the usual histologic features of leukocytoclastic vasculitis.

- The characteristic histopathologic feature of chronic urticaria is a mononuclear cell perivascular cuff around capillaries.

MANAGEMENT OF URTICARIA

The history is of utmost importance for discovering the 2% to 10% of cases of chronic urticaria due to secondary causes. A complete physical examination is needed, with particular attention paid to the skin (including testing for dermatographism) to evaluate for the vasculitic nature of the lesions and to the liver, lymph nodes, and mucous membranes. Laboratory testing need not be exhaustive but may include the following: chest radiography, a complete blood cell count with differential count (to discover eosinophilia), liver enzymes, tests for thyroid function and antibodies, erythrocyte sedimentation rate, serum protein electrophoresis (in patients older than 50), urinalysis, and stool examination for parasites. Allergy skin testing is indicated only if the patient has an element in the history suggesting an allergic cause. However, patients with idiopathic urticaria often have fixed ideas about an allergy causing their problem, and skin testing often helps to dissuade them of this idea.

- The history is of utmost importance in diagnosing chronic urticaria due to secondary causes.

- Laboratory testing may include chest radiography, eosinophil count, liver enzymes, tests for thyroid function and antibodies, erythrocyte sedimentation rate, serum protein electrophoresis, urinalysis, and stool examination for parasites.

Management of urticaria and angioedema consists of blocking histamine, beginning usually with nonsedating H_1 antagonists. The addition of leukotriene antagonists may be helpful. The role of H_2 antagonists is unclear; they may help a small percentage of patients. Tricyclic antidepressants, such as doxepin, have potent antihistamine effects and are useful. Systemic corticosteroids can be administered for acute urticaria and angioedema.

- Urticaria and angioedema: management is usually with H_1 antagonists.

- Urticaria and angioedema: systemic corticosteroids are used for acute cases.

ANAPHYLAXIS

There is no universally accepted clinical definition of *anaphylaxis*. The manifestations of anaphylaxis vary, depending on the severity, and can include any combination of urticaria, angioedema, flushing, pruritus, upper airway obstruction, lower airway obstruction, diarrhea, nausea, vomiting, syncope, hypotension, tachycardia, and dizziness. Approximately 90% of anaphylactic episodes include urticaria or angioedema. A cellular and molecular definition of *anaphylaxis* is a generalized allergic reaction characterized by activated basophils and mast cells releasing many mediators (preformed and newly synthesized). The dominant mediators of acute anaphylaxis are histamine and prostaglandin D_2. The serum levels of tryptase peak at 1 hour after the onset of anaphylaxis and may stay elevated for 5 hours. Physiologically, the hypotension of anaphylaxis is caused by peripheral vasodilatation and not by impaired cardiac contractility. Anaphylaxis is characterized by a hyperdynamic state. For these reasons, anaphylaxis can be fatal in patients with preexisting fixed vascular obstructive disease in whom a decrease in perfusion pressure leads to a critical reduction in flow (stroke) or in patients in whom laryngeal edema develops and completely occludes the airway.

- The clinical hallmarks of anaphylaxis are urticaria, flushing, hypotension, and tachycardia.

- Histamine and prostaglandin D_2 are the dominant mediators of acute anaphylaxis.

- Tryptase is an excellent marker of mast cell activation.

The most common causes of anaphylaxis are the following:

1. Foods (peanuts, tree nuts, fish, and shellfish)

2. Medications (antibiotics, neuromuscular blockers, and anticonvulsants)

3. Insect stings (bee, fire ant, and vespid)

4. Latex

5. Aspirin and other nonsteroidal anti-inflammatory agents

The vast majority of anaphylactic events occur within 1 hour, often within minutes, after exposure to the offending agent.

FOOD ALLERGY

CLINICAL HISTORY

The clinical syndrome of food allergy may include the following: Very sensitive persons experience tingling, itching, and a metallic taste in the mouth while the food is still in the mouth. Within 15 minutes after the food is swallowed, epigastric distress may occur. There may be nausea and rarely vomiting. Abdominal cramping is felt chiefly in the periumbilical area (small-bowel phase), and lower abdominal cramping and watery diarrhea may occur. Urticaria or angioedema may occur in any distribution, or there may be only itching of the palms and soles. With increasing clinical sensitivity to the offending allergen, anaphylactic symptoms may emerge, including tachycardia, hypotension, generalized flushing, and alterations of consciousness.

In extremely sensitive persons, generalized flushing, hypotension, and tachycardia may occur before the other symptoms. Most patients with a food allergy can identify the offending foods. The diagnosis should be confirmed by skin testing or in vitro measurement of allergen-specific IgE antibody.

- Allergic reactions to food usually include pruritus, urticaria, or angioedema.

COMMON CAUSES OF FOOD ALLERGY

Items considered to be the most common causes of food allergy are listed in Box 41.5.

FOOD-RELATED ANAPHYLAXIS

Food-induced anaphylaxis is the same process involved in acute urticaria or angioedema induced by food allergens, except that

---

Box 41.5 **COMMON CAUSES OF FOOD ALLERGY**

Eggs
Milk
Nuts
Peanuts
Shellfish
Soybeans
Wheat

---

the severity of the reaction is greater in anaphylaxis. Relatively few foods are commonly involved in food-induced anaphylaxis; the main ones are peanuts, shellfish, and nuts, although any food has the potential to cause anaphylaxis. In patients with latex allergy, food allergy can develop to banana, avocado, kiwifruit, and other fruits.

- Anaphylaxis to food can be life-threatening.

- There is cross-sensitivity between latex and banana, avocado, and kiwifruit.

ALLERGY SKIN TESTING IN FOOD ALLERGY

Patients presenting with food-related symptoms may have food allergy, food intolerance, irritable bowel syndrome, nonspecific dyspepsia, or a nonallergic condition. A careful and detailed history on the nature of the "reaction," the reproducibility of the association of food and symptoms, and the timing of symptoms in relation to the ingestion of food can help the clinician form a clinical impression.

In many cases, allergy skin tests to foods can be helpful. If the results are negative (and the clinical suspicion for food allergy is low), the patient can be reassured that food allergy is not the cause of the symptoms. If the results are positive (and the clinical suspicion for food allergy is high), the patient should be counseled about the management of the food allergy. The patient should strictly avoid the food or possible cross-reactive foods. These patients should also be given an epinephrine kit for self-administration in an emergency. Although some food allergies may be outgrown, peanut, tree nut, fish, and shellfish allergies are typically lifelong.

If the diagnosis of food allergy is uncertain or if the symptoms are mild and nonspecific, oral food challenges may be helpful. An open challenge is usually performed first. If the results are negative, the diagnosis of food allergy is excluded. If the results are positive, a blinded placebo-controlled challenge can be performed if there is suspicion about the positive result.

- Positive results on skin tests and double-blind food challenges can confirm the diagnosis of food allergy.

- If results of food skin tests are negative, food allergy is unlikely.

- Patients with anaphylaxis to food should strictly avoid the offending food and carry an epinephrine kit.

STINGING INSECT ALLERGY

In patients clinically sensitive to Hymenoptera, reactions to a sting can be either large local reactions or systemic, anaphylactic reactions. With a large local sting reaction, swelling at the sting site may be dramatic, but there are no symptoms distant from that site. Stings of the head, neck, and dorsum of the hands are particularly prone to large local reactions.

Anaphylaxis caused by allergy to stinging insects is similar to all other forms of anaphylaxis. Thus, the onset of anaphylaxis may be very rapid, often within 1 or 2 minutes. Pruritus of the palms and soles is the most common initial manifestation. Frequently, 1 or more of the following occur next: generalized flushing, urticaria, angioedema, or hypotension. The reason for attaching importance to whether a stinging insect reaction is a large local or a generalized one is that allergy skin testing and allergen immunotherapy are recommended only for generalized reactions. Patients who have a large local reaction are not at increased risk of future anaphylaxis.

- Two varieties of reaction to sting: large local and anaphylactic.

BEE AND VESPID ALLERGY

Yellow jackets, wasps, and hornets are vespids, and their venoms cross-react to a substantial degree. The venom of honeybees (family Apidae) does not cross-react with that of vespids. Thus, usually it is appropriate to conduct skin testing to honeybee and to each of the vespids. To interpret skin tests accurately, it is helpful to know which insect caused the sting producing the generalized reaction. Often, the circumstances of the sting can help determine the type of insect responsible. Multiple stings received while mowing the grass or doing other landscape jobs that may disturb yellow-jacket burrows in the ground are likely caused by yellow-jacket stings. A single sting received while near picnic tables or refuse containers at picnic areas is likely from a yellow jacket or possibly a hornet. Stings received while working around the house exterior (painting, cleaning eaves and gutters, or attic work) are most likely from wasps.

- Yellow jackets, wasps, and hornets are vespids, and their venoms cross-react.

- The venom of bees does not cross-react with that of vespids.

- It is helpful to know which insect caused the sting.

ALLERGY TESTING

Patients who have had a generalized reaction warrant allergen skin testing. Patients who have had a large local reaction to a Hymenoptera sting do not warrant allergen skin testing because they are not at significantly increased risk of future anaphylaxis.

- A generalized reaction warrants allergen skin testing.

- A large local reaction does not warrant allergen skin testing.

In many cases, skin testing should be delayed for at least 1 month after a sting-induced general reaction because tests conducted closer to the time of the sting have a substantial risk of producing false-negative results. Positive results that

Box 41.6 INDICATIONS FOR VENOM
IMMUNOTHERAPY

History of mild, moderate, or severe anaphylaxis to a sting
Positive results on skin tests to the venom that was implicated historically in the anaphylactic reaction
Urticaria distant from the site of the sting (adults only)

correlate with the clinical history are sufficient evidence for considering Hymenoptera venom immunotherapy.

- Skin testing should be delayed for at least 1 month after a sting-induced general reaction.

- Patients with clinical anaphylaxis and positive results on venom skin tests benefit from venom immunotherapy.

VENOM IMMUNOTHERAPY

The decision to undertake venom immunotherapy can be reached only after a discussion between the patient and the physician. General indications for venom immunotherapy are listed in Box 41.6. Patients must understand that after immunotherapy is begun, the injection schedule must be maintained and that there is a small risk of immunotherapy-induced allergic reaction. Patients also need to understand that despite receiving allergy immunotherapy, they must carry epinephrine when outdoors because of the possibility (from 2% with vespid stings to 10% with apid stings) that immunotherapy will not provide suitable protection. Most, but not all, patients can safely discontinue venom immunotherapy after 5 years of treatment.

- There is a small risk that venom immunotherapy will induce an allergic reaction.

- There is a 2%-10% chance that venom immunotherapy will not provide adequate protection.

AVOIDANCE

The warnings that every patient with stinging insect hypersensitivity should receive are listed in Box 41.7. A patient's specific circumstances may require additional entries to this list. Also, patients need to know how to use self-injectable epinephrine in its several forms. Many patients wear an anaphylaxis identification bracelet.

- All patients with stinging-insect sensitivity should carry an epinephrine kit.

DRUG ALLERGY

DRUG ALLERGY NOT INVOLVING IgE OR IMMEDIATE-TYPE REACTIONS

Patients with drug allergy not involving IgE or immediate-type reactions have negative results on skin prick and intradermal testing.

Avoid looking or smelling like a flower
Avoid flowered prints for clothes
Avoid cosmetics & fragrances, especially ones derived from flowering plants
Never drink from a soft-drink can outdoors during the warm months—a yellow jacket can land *on* or *in* the can while you are not watching, go inside the can, & sting the inside of your mouth (a dangerous place for a sensitive patient to be stung) when you take a drink
Avoid doing outdoor maintenance & yard work
Never reach into a mailbox without first looking inside it
Never go barefoot
Always look at the underside of picnic table benches & park benches before sitting down
Never attempt to eject a stinging insect yourself from the interior of a moving automobile; pull over, get out, & let someone else remove the insect

Stevens-Johnson Syndrome

Stevens-Johnson syndrome is a bullous skin and mucosal reaction; very large blisters appear over much of the skin surface, in the mouth, and along the gastrointestinal tract. Because of the propensity of the blisters to break down and become infected, the reaction often is life-threatening. Treatment consists of stopping use of the drug that causes the reaction, giving corticosteroids systemically, and providing supportive care. The patients are often treated in burn units. Penicillin, sulfonamides, barbiturates, diphenylhydantoin, warfarin, and phenothiazines are well-known causes. A drug-induced Stevens-Johnson reaction is an absolute contraindication to administering the causative drug to the patient in the future.

- Stevens-Johnson syndrome is life-threatening and is an absolute contraindication for rechallenge with the drug.

Toxic Epidermal Necrolysis

Clinically, toxic epidermal necrolysis is almost indistinguishable from Stevens-Johnson syndrome. Histologically, the cleavage plane for the blisters is deeper than in Stevens-Johnson syndrome. The cleavage plane is at the basement membrane of the epidermis, so even the basal cell layer is lost. This makes toxic epidermal necrolysis even more devastating than Stevens-Johnson syndrome because healing occurs with much scarring. Often, healing cannot be accomplished without skin grafting, so the mortality rate is even higher than for Stevens-Johnson syndrome. Patients with toxic epidermal necrolysis should always be cared for in a burn unit because of full-thickness damage over 80% to 90% of the skin. The very high mortality rate is similar to that for burn patients with damage of this extent.

- Toxic epidermal necrolysis is a life-threatening exfoliative dermatitis.

Morbilliform Skin Reaction

Morbilliform skin reaction is the most common dermatologic manifestation of a drug reaction. It is an immune-mediated drug rash without IgE involvement, manifested by a macular-papular exanthem. The rash can be accompanied by pruritus but has no other systemic symptoms. It typically occurs more than 5 days after use of a medication was begun. It is not associated with anaphylaxis or other serious sequelae.

- Morbilliform skin reaction is the most common dermatologic manifestation of a drug reaction and is not associated with anaphylaxis.

Ampicillin-Mononucleosis Rash

Ampicillin-mononucleosis rash is a unique drug rash that occurs when ampicillin is given to an acutely ill, febrile patient who has mononucleosis. The rash is papular, nonpruritic, and rose-colored. It occurs usually on the abdomen and feels granular when the fingers brush lightly over the surface of the involved skin. It is not known why the rash is specific for ampicillin and mononucleosis. This rash does not predispose to allergy to penicillin.

- Ampicillin-mononucleosis rash is papular, nonpruritic, and rose-colored, and it occurs on the abdomen.

- This rash does not predispose to penicillin allergy.

Fixed Drug Eruptions

Fixed drug eruptions are red to red-brown macules that appear on a certain area of the patient's skin; any part of the body can be affected. The macules do not itch or have other signs of inflammation, although fever is associated with their appearance in a few patients. The unique aspect of this phenomenon is that if a patient is given the same drug in the future, the rash develops in exactly the same skin areas. Resolution of the macules often includes postinflammatory hyperpigmentation. Except for cosmetic problems due to skin discolorations, the phenomenon does not seem serious. Antibiotics and sulfonamides are the most frequently recognized causes.

- In fixed drug eruptions, the same area of skin is always affected.

Erythema Nodosum

Erythema nodosum is a characteristic rash of red nodules about the size of a quarter, usually nonpruritic and appearing only over the anterior aspects of the lower legs. Histopathologically, the nodules are plaques of infiltrating mononuclear cells. Erythema nodosum is associated with several connective tissue diseases, viral infections, and drug allergy.

- Erythema nodosum rash is usually nonpruritic, appearing only over the anterior aspect of the lower legs.

- It is associated with several connective tissue diseases, viral infections, and drug allergy.

Contact Dermatitis

Contact dermatitis can occur with various drugs. Commonly, it is a form of drug allergy that is an occupational disease in medical or health care workers. In some patients receiving topical drugs, allergy develops to the drug or to various elements in its pharmaceutical formulation (eg, fillers, stabilizers, antibacterials, and emulsifiers). Contact dermatitis is a manifestation of type IV hypersensitivity. Clinically it appears as an area of reddening on the skin that progresses to a granular weeping eczematous eruption with some dermal thickening; the surrounding skin has a plaque-like quality. When patients are receiving treatment for dermatitis, and contact hypersensitivity develops to corticosteroids or other drugs used in treatment, a particularly difficult diagnostic problem arises unless the physician is alert to this possibility. When contact hypersensitivity to a drug occurs, it does not increase the probability of acute type I hypersensitivity and is not associated with serious exfoliative syndromes. However, exquisite cutaneous sensitivity of this type can develop in patients so that almost no avoidance technique in the workplace completely eliminates dermatitis; even protective gloves are only partly helpful. Thus, it can be occupationally disabling.

- Contact dermatitis is a form of drug allergy.

- It is a manifestation of type IV hypersensitivity.

DRUG ALLERGY INVOLVING IgE OR IMMEDIATE-TYPE REACTIONS

Penicillin Allergy

Penicillin can cause anaphylaxis in sensitive persons. It is an IgE-mediated process that can be evaluated with skin testing to the major and minor determinants of penicillin. Patients with positive results on skin testing and a clinical history of penicillin allergy can be desensitized to penicillin in a supervised setting.

- Penicillin can cause anaphylaxis.

- Both major and minor determinants of penicillin should be tested in suspected penicillin allergy.

- Patients can be desensitized under supervision.

Penicillin skin tests can be helpful in determining whether it is safe to administer penicillin to a patient with suspected penicillin allergy. About 85% of patients who give a history of penicillin allergy have negative results with skin tests to the major and minor determinants of penicillin. These patients are not at increased risk of anaphylaxis and can receive penicillin safely. If penicillin skin test results are positive, there is a 40% to 60% chance that an allergic reaction will develop if the patient is challenged with penicillin. These patients should avoid penicillin and related drugs. However, if there is a strong indication for penicillin treatment, desensitization can be performed. The desensitization procedure involves the administration of progressively increasing doses of penicillin. Desensitization can be accomplished by the oral or intravenous route and is usually performed in a hospital setting.

Ampicillin, amoxicillin, nafcillin, and other β-lactam antibiotics cross-react strongly with penicillin. Early studies suggested that up to 20% to 30% of patients with penicillin allergy were also allergic to cephalosporins. More recent studies have suggested that the cross-sensitivity of penicillin with cephalosporins is much less (about 5%). Most studies have suggested that aztreonam does not cross-react with penicillin.

- About 5% of patients with penicillin allergy are also allergic to cephalosporins.

- Aztreonam does not cross-react with penicillin.

Radiographic Contrast Media Reactions

Radiographic contrast media can cause reactions that have the clinical appearance of anaphylaxis. Estimates of the frequency of these reactions are 2% to 6% of procedures involving intravenous contrast media. The incidence of intra-arterial contrast-induced reactions is lower. Anaphylactoid reactions do not involve IgE antibody (thus, the reason for the term *anaphylactoid*). Radiocontrast media appear to induce mediator release on the basis of some other property intrinsic to the contrast agent. The tonicity or ionic strength of the media seems particularly related to anaphylactoid reactions. With the availability of nonionic or low-osmolar media, the incidence of reactions has been lower.

- The frequency of contrast media reactions is 2%-6% of procedures.

- The reaction does not involve IgE antibody.

- Nonionic or low-osmolar contrast media cause fewer anaphylactoid reactions than standard contrast media.

The frequency of radiocontrast media reactions can be decreased with the use of nonionic or low-osmolar media in patients with a history of asthma or atopy. Patients who have a history of reaction to radiocontrast media and who subsequently need procedures that use radiographic contrast media can be pretreated with a protocol of prednisone, 50 mg orally every 6 hours for 3 doses, with the last dose 1 hour before the procedure. At the last dose, 50 mg of diphenhydramine or an equivalent H_1 antagonist is recommended. Some studies show that the addition of oral ephedrine can be beneficial. Most studies show that the addition of an H_2 antagonist is unnecessary.

- Patients with a history of systemic reactions to radiocontrast media should be pretreated with systemic corticosteroids and an H_1 antagonist and should be offered nonionic contrast agents.

OTHER ALLERGIC OR IMMUNOLOGIC CONDITIONS

MASTOCYTOSIS

Systemic mastocytosis is a disorder of abnormal proliferation of mast cells. The skin, bone marrow, liver, spleen, lymph nodes, and gastrointestinal tract can be affected. The clinical manifestations vary but can include flushing, pruritus, urticaria, unexplained syncope, fatigue, and dyspepsia. Bone marrow biopsies with stains for mast cells (toluidine blue, Giemsa, or chloral acetate esterase) and immunochemical stains for tryptase are the most direct diagnostic studies. Serum levels of tryptase and urinary concentrations of histamine, histamine metabolites, and prostaglandins are typically increased.

Treatment initially consists of antihistamines. Cromolyn sodium given orally can be beneficial, especially in patients with gastrointestinal tract symptoms. Corticosteroids should be considered in severe cases, and interferon is a promising investigational treatment.

EOSINOPHILIA

Eosinophilia is idiopathic, primary, or secondary (reactive). Hypereosinophilia syndrome is an idiopathic eosinophilic disorder characterized by an absolute eosinophil count of more than 1.5×10^9/L; a course of 6 months or longer; organ involvement as manifested by eosinophilia-mediated tissue injury (cardiomyopathy, dermatitis, pneumonitis, sinusitis, gastrointestinal tract inflammation, left or right ventricular apical thrombus, or stroke); and no other causes of eosinophilia. The syndrome typically affects persons in the third through sixth decades of life; women are affected more often than men. Symptoms include fatigue, cough, shortness of breath, or rash. Cardiac involvement in hypereosinophilia syndrome is especially significant: endomyocardial fibrosis, mural thrombi, and mitral and tricuspid incompetence can occur. The clinical syndrome is manifested as restrictive cardiomyopathy with congestive heart failure. Echocardiography and endomyocardial biopsy are important diagnostic tests.

The primary clonal and monoclonal disorders include acute leukemia (myeloid and lymphoid); chronic myeloid leukemia; myelodysplastic syndrome and chronic myelomonocytic leukemia; classic and atypical myeloproliferative disorders (systemic mastocytosis); and unclassified (chronic eosinophilic leukemia).

Secondary causes include the following: infectious (tissue-invasive parasitosis); drugs; toxins; inflammation; atopy and allergies (asthma); malignancy (lymphoma, Hodgkin lymphoma, cutaneous T-cell lymphoma, and metastatic cancer); collagen vascular disease (eosinophilic vasculitis); pulmonary (hypereosinophilic pneumonitis and Löffler syndrome); and eosinophilic myalgia syndrome.

The clinical diagnostic approach is to exclude secondary eosinophilic disorders; to evaluate bone marrow aspirates and biopsy specimens with genetic and molecular studies; and to perform tests to assess eosinophilia-mediated tissue injury (chest radiography, pulmonary function tests,

Box 41.8 COMMON CAUSES OF EOSINOPHILIA

Atopic
    Allergic bronchopulmonary aspergillosis
    Asthma
    Atopic dermatitis
    Drug hypersensitivity
Pulmonary
    Eosinophilic pneumonia
    Löffler syndrome
Proliferative/neoplastic
    Idiopathic hypereosinophilic syndrome
    Eosinophilic leukemia
Vasculitis/connective tissue
    Churg-Strauss vasculitis
    Eosinophilic fasciitis
Eosinophilic gastroenteritis
Infectious
    Visceral larva migrans
    Helminth
Toxic
    Eosinophilia-myalgia syndrome
    Toxic oil syndrome

echocardiography, complete blood cell count, and liver enzyme and serum tryptase levels). The differential diagnosis of eosinophilia is given in Box 41.8.

Hypereosinophilia syndrome is treated with prednisone, 1 mg/kg daily, alone or in combination with hydroxyurea. Second-line therapy includes recombinant interferon-alfa.

COMMON VARIABLE IMMUNODEFICIENCY

Common variable immunodeficiency (CVID) affects males and females of all ages. It is the most common primary immunodeficiency in adults. Patients have recurrent sinopulmonary infections, primarily with encapsulated organisms. The primary laboratory abnormality is hypogammaglobulinemia (low IgG levels). IgA and IgM levels may be normal or decreased. Recurrent pyogenic infections include chronic otitis media, chronic or recurrent sinusitis, pneumonia, and bronchiectasis.

Patients with CVID often have autoimmune or gastrointestinal tract disturbances. About one-half of patients have chronic diarrhea and malabsorption. They may have steatorrhea, protein-losing enteropathy, ulcerative colitis, or Crohn disease. Other gastrointestinal tract problems associated with the disease are atrophic gastritis, pernicious anemia, giardiasis, and chronic active hepatitis. Pathologic changes in the gastrointestinal tract mucosa include loss of villi, nodular lymphoid hyperplasia, and diffuse lymphoid infiltration.

Autoimmune anemia, thrombocytopenia, or neutropenia is present in 10% to 50% of the patients and typically occurs before CVID is diagnosed. Inflammatory arthritis and lymphoid interstitial pneumonia are other associated conditions. Also, patients have an increased risk of a malignancy, particularly a lymphoid malignancy such as non-Hodgkin lymphoma.

The diagnosis of CVID should be considered if patients have recurrent pyogenic infections and hypogammaglobulinemia. Associated gastrointestinal tract or autoimmune disease and the exclusion of hereditary primary immunodeficiencies support the diagnosis. Treatment is with intravenous or subcutaneous γ-globulin. The typical dosage is 400 mg/kg monthly.

TERMINAL COMPLEMENT COMPONENT DEFICIENCIES

Patients with deficiency of the terminal complement component C5, C6, C7, or C8 have an increased susceptibility to meningococcal infections. The terminal complement components form the membrane attack complex that causes cell lysis; hence, deficiency of 1 of these components results in defective microbial killing. The terminal component C9 participates in membrane pore formation but is not essential for complement-mediated cell lysis. Thus, patients with the rare C9 deficiency have a limited increased susceptibility to infections.

Terminal complement component deficiency should be suspected if patients have recurrent meningococcal disease, a family history of meningococcal disease, systemic meningococcal infection, or infection with an unusual serotype of meningococcus. Diagnosis is confirmed with assay of total hemolytic complement and measurement of individual complement components.

SUMMARY

- Patch testing is used to investigate contact dermatitis.

- Skin prick (immediate) testing is used to investigate respiratory allergy to airborne allergens and food allergy.

- Allergic rhinitis has a recurrent seasonal pattern and may be provoked by being near animals.

- Triggers of vasomotor rhinitis include strong odors and changes in humidity and temperature.

- Urticaria and angioedema: management is usually with H_1 antagonists.

- Urticaria and angioedema: systemic corticosteroids are used for acute cases.

42.

ASTHMA[a]

Gerald W. Volcheck, MD

GOALS

- Recognize the pathophysiology and triggers of asthma.
- Categorize asthma by severity.
- Define testing and treatment strategies for asthma patients.

PATHOLOGY

The pathologic features of asthma have been studied chiefly in fatal cases; some bronchoscopic data are available for mild and moderate asthma. The histologic hallmarks of asthma include mucous gland hypertrophy, mucus hypersecretion, epithelial desquamation, widening of the basement membrane, and infiltration by eosinophils (Box 42.1).

- The histologic hallmarks of asthma include mucous gland hypertrophy, mucus hypersecretion, epithelial desquamation, widening of the basement membrane, and infiltration by eosinophils.

Box 42.1 HISTOLOGIC HALLMARKS OF ASTHMA

Mucous gland hypertrophy
Mucus hypersecretion
Alteration of tinctorial & viscoelastic properties of mucus
Widening of basement membrane zone of bronchial epithelial membrane
Increased number of intraepithelial leukocytes & mast cells
Round cell infiltration of bronchial submucosa
Intense eosinophilic infiltration of submucosa
Widespread damage to bronchial epithelium
   Large areas of complete desquamation of epithelium into airway lumen
   Mucous plugs filled with eosinophils & their products

PATHOPHYSIOLOGY

Bronchial hyperresponsiveness is common to all forms of asthma. It is measured by assessing pulmonary function before and after exposure to methacholine, histamine, cold air, or exercise. A decrease in forced expiratory volume in 1 second (FEV_1) of 20% or more with challenge is considered a sign of airway hyperreactivity.

Persons who have allergic asthma generate mast cell and basophil mediators that have important roles in the development of endobronchial inflammation and smooth muscle changes that occur after acute exposure to allergen. Mast cells and basophils are prominent during the immediate-phase reaction. In the late-phase reaction to allergen exposure, the bronchi show histologic features of chronic inflammation and eosinophils become prominent in the reaction.

Patients who have chronic asthma and negative results on allergy skin tests usually have an inflammatory infiltrate in the bronchi and histologic findings dominated by eosinophils when asthma is active. Patients with sudden asphyxic asthma may have a neutrophilic rather than an eosinophilic infiltration of the airway.

Important characteristics of cytokines are summarized in Table 42.1. Interleukin (IL)-1, IL-6, and tumor necrosis factor are produced by antigen-presenting cells and start the acute inflammatory reaction against an invader; IL-4 and IL-13 stimulate IgE synthesis; IL-2 and interferon-γ stimulate a cell-mediated response; and IL-10 is the primary anti-inflammatory cytokine.

- IL-4 stimulates IgE synthesis.
- IL-5 stimulates eosinophils.
- Helper T cells produce IL-4 and IL-5.

GENETICS

The genetics of asthma is complex and confounded by environmental factors. No "asthma gene" has been discovered. The gene encoding the β subunit of the high-affinity IgE receptor

---

[a] Portions previously published in Volcheck GW. Clinical allergy: diagnosis and management. Totowa (NJ): Humana Press; c2009. p. 189–278. Used with permission of Mayo Foundation for Medical Education and Research.

Table 42.1 **CHARACTERISTICS OF CYTOKINES**

CYTOKINE	MAJOR ACTIONS	PRIMARY SOURCES
IL-1	Lymphocyte activation Fibroblast activation Fever	Macrophages Endothelial cells Lymphocytes
IL-2	T- & B-cell activation	T cells (TH1)
IL-3	Mast cell proliferation Neutrophil & macrophage maturation	T cells Mast cells
IL-4	IgE synthesis	T cells (TH2)
IL-5	Eosinophil proliferation & differentiation	T cells (TH2)
IL-6	IgG synthesis Lymphocyte activation	Fibroblasts T cells
IL-8	Neutrophil chemotaxis	Fibroblasts Endothelial cells Monocytes
IL-10	Inhibition of IFN-γ & IL-1 production	T cells Macrophages
IL-13	IgE synthesis	T cells
IFN-α	Antiviral activity	Leukocytes
IFN-γ	Macrophage activation Stimulation of MHC expression Inhibition of TH2 activity	T cells (TH1)
TNF-γ	Antitumor cell activity	Lymphocytes Macrophages
TNF-β	Antitumor cell activity	T cells
GM-CSF	Mast cell, granulocyte, & macrophage stimulation	Lymphocytes Mast cells Macrophages

Abbreviations: GM-CSF, granulocyte-macrophage colony-stimulating factor; IFN, interferon; IL, interleukin; MHC, major histocompatibility complex; TH, helper T cell; TNF, tumor necrosis factor.

is located on chromosome 11q13 and is linked to total IgE, atopy, and bronchial hyperreactivity. Polymorphic variants of the β$_2$-adrenergic receptor are linked to bronchial hyperreactivity. The gene for IL-4 is located on chromosome 5q31 and is linked to total IgE.

OCCUPATIONAL ASTHMA

The incidence of occupational asthma is estimated to be 6% to 15% of all cases of adult-onset asthma. A large fraction of occupational asthma escapes diagnosis because physicians often obtain an inadequate occupational history. A wide range of possible industrial circumstances may lead to exposure and resultant disease. The most widely recognized causes of occupational asthma are listed in Box 42.2. Breathing tests

Box 42.2 **INDUSTRIAL AGENTS THAT CAN CAUSE ASTHMA**

Metals
  Salts of platinum, nickel, & chrome
Wood dusts
  Mahogany
  Oak
  Redwood
  Western red cedar (plicatic acid)
Vegetable dusts
  Castor bean
  Cotton
  Cottonseed
  Flour
  Grain (mite & weevil antigens)
  Green coffee
  Gums
Industrial chemicals & plastics
  Ethylenediamine
  Phthalic & trimellitic anhydrides
  Polyvinyl chloride
  Toluene diisocyanate
Pharmaceutical agents
  Phenylglycine acid chloride
  Penicillins
  Spiramycin
Food industry agents
  Egg protein
  Polyvinyl chloride
Biologic enzymes
  Bacillus subtilis (laundry detergent workers)
  Pancreatic enzymes
Animal emanations
  Canine or feline saliva
  Horse dander (racing workers)
  Rodent urine (laboratory animal workers)

performed in the workplace and away from the workplace aid in the diagnosis.

- Every patient evaluated for allergy or asthma must be asked to provide a detailed occupational history.

GASTROESOPHAGEAL REFLUX AND ASTHMA

The precise role of gastroesophageal reflux in asthma is not known. There appears to be a subgroup of asthma patients whose asthma is exacerbated by gastroesophageal reflux.

ASTHMA-PROVOKING DRUGS

It is important to recognize the potentially severe adverse response that patients with asthma may show to β$_1$- and β$_2$-blockers, including β$_1$-selective blockers such as atenolol.

Patients with asthma who have glaucoma treated with ophthalmic preparations of timolol or betaxolol may experience bronchospasm. β-Blockers are not absolutely contraindicated in asthma, but observation is warranted.

- β-Blockers, including those in eyedrops, can cause severe adverse responses in patients with asthma.

- β₁-Selective blockers such as atenolol may also provoke asthma.

A chronic, dry cough that mimics asthma may develop in persons taking angiotensin-converting enzyme inhibitor drugs. Wheeze and dyspnea, however, do not accompany the cough.

Aspirin ingestion can cause acute, severe, and fatal asthma in a small subset of patients with asthma. Most of the affected patients have nasal polyposis, hyperplastic pansinus mucosal disease, and moderate to severe persistent asthma. However, not all asthma patients with this reaction to aspirin fit the profile. Many nonsteroidal anti-inflammatory drugs can trigger the reaction; the likelihood correlates with a drug's potency for inhibiting cyclooxygenase. Only nonacetylated salicylates such as choline salicylate (a weak cyclooxygenase inhibitor) seem not to provoke the reaction. Leukotriene-modifying drugs may be particularly helpful in aspirin-sensitive asthma.

Traditionally, asthma patients have been warned not to take antihistamines because the anticholinergic activity of some antihistamines was thought to cause drying of lower respiratory tract secretions, further worsening the asthma. However, antihistamines do not worsen asthma, and some studies have shown a beneficial effect.

- Aspirin and other nonsteroidal anti-inflammatory drugs can cause acute, severe asthma.

- Asthma, nasal polyposis, and aspirin sensitivity form the "aspirin allergy triad."

- Leukotriene modifiers may be helpful in aspirin-sensitive asthma.

- Antihistamines are not contraindicated in asthma.

CIGARETTE SMOKING AND ASTHMA

A combination of asthma and cigarette smoking leads to accelerated chronic obstructive pulmonary disease. Because of the accelerated rate of irreversible obstruction, all asthma patients who smoke should be counseled to stop smoking.

Environmental tobacco smoke is an important asthma trigger. In particular, children with asthma who are exposed to environmental smoke have more respiratory infections and asthma attacks.

MEDICAL HISTORY

A medical history for asthma includes careful inquiry about symptoms, provoking factors, alleviating factors, and severity. Patients with marked respiratory allergy have symptoms when exposed to aeroallergens and often have seasonal variation of symptoms. If allergy skin test results are negative, one can be reasonably certain that the patient does not have allergic asthma. Respiratory infections (particularly viral), cold dry air, exercise, and respiratory irritants can trigger allergic and nonallergic asthma.

- In allergic asthma, symptoms can be perennial (eg, from dust mites or pets), or sporadic (eg, from seasonal pollens).

- Patients with allergic asthma are likely to react to many nonimmunologic triggers.

- Cold dry air and exercise can trigger asthma.

ASSESSMENT OF CONTRIBUTORS TO ASTHMA

The mnemonic *AIR-SMOG* provides a concise checklist of possible contributors to asthma (Box 42.3). In addition, patient compliance with medications and ability to use the inhaler correctly should be reviewed for all patients with persistent asthma.

ASSESSMENT OF SEVERITY

Asthma is *intermittent* if 1) the daytime symptoms are intermittent (<2 times weekly), 2) continuous treatment is not needed, and 3) the flow-volume curve during formal pulmonary function testing is normal between episodes of symptoms. Even for patients who meet these criteria, inflammation (albeit patchy) is present in the airways and corticosteroid inhaled on a regular basis diminishes bronchial hyperresponsiveness.

- Corticosteroid inhaled on a regular basis diminishes bronchial hyperresponsiveness.

Asthma is *mild persistent* or *moderate persistent* when 1) the symptoms occur with some regularity (>2 times weekly) or daily, 2) there is nocturnal occurrence of symptoms, or 3) asthma exacerbations are troublesome. For many of these patients, the flow-volume curve is rarely normal and complete pulmonary function testing may show evidence of hyperinflation, as indicated by increased residual volume or an increase

---

Box 42.3 *AIR-SMOG*: A MNEMONIC FOR A CHECKLIST OF CONTRIBUTORS TO ASTHMA

A—allergy
I—infection, irritants
R—rhinosinusitis
S—smoking
M—medications
O—occupational exposures
G—gastroesophageal reflux disease

above expected levels for the diffusing capacity of the lung for carbon dioxide. Asthma is *severe persistent* when symptoms are present almost continuously and the usual medications must be given in doses at the upper end of the dose range to control the disease.

Patients with mild, moderate, or severe persistent asthma should receive treatment daily with anti-inflammatory medications, usually inhaled corticosteroids. Most patients with severe asthma require either large doses of inhaled corticosteroid or oral prednisone daily for adequate control. A majority have been hospitalized more than once for asthma. The severity of asthma can change over time, and an early sign that asthma is not well controlled is the emergence of nocturnal symptoms.

- Patients with mild, moderate, or severe persistent asthma should receive treatment daily with anti-inflammatory medications.
- Nocturnal symptoms suggest that asthma is worsening.

METHACHOLINE BRONCHIAL CHALLENGE

If a patient has a history suggestive of episodic asthma but has normal results on pulmonary function tests on the day of the examination, the patient is a reasonable candidate for a methacholine bronchial challenge. The methacholine bronchial challenge is also useful in evaluating patients for cough if baseline pulmonary function appears normal. Positive results indicate that bronchial hyperresponsiveness is present, although results can be positive in conditions besides asthma (Box 42.4). Some consider isocapnic hyperventilation with subfreezing dry air (by either exercising or breathing a carbon dioxide–air mixture) or exercise testing as alternatives to a methacholine challenge.

Do not perform a methacholine challenge in patients who have severe airway obstruction or a clear diagnosis of asthma. Usually, a 20% decrease in FEV_1 is considered a positive result.

- Patients with suspected asthma and normal results on pulmonary function tests are candidates for methacholine testing.

Box 42.4 MEDICAL CONDITIONS ASSOCIATED WITH POSITIVE FINDINGS ON METHACHOLINE CHALLENGE

Current asthma
Past history of asthma
Chronic obstructive pulmonary disease
Smoking
Recent respiratory infection
Chronic cough
Allergic rhinitis

EXHALED NITRIC OXIDE

Exhaled nitric oxide has been studied as a noninvasive measure of airway inflammation. The fraction of nitric oxide in the exhaled air increases in proportion to inflammation of the bronchial wall, sputum eosinophilia, and airway hyperresponsiveness. Exhaled nitric oxide levels increase with deterioration in asthma control and decrease in a dose-dependent manner with anti-inflammatory treatment. The usefulness of measuring exhaled nitric oxide may be in monitoring asthma control, guiding therapy, and predicting response to corticosteroid therapy.

- Elevated exhaled nitric oxide levels are associated with eosinophilic respiratory inflammation and decreased asthma control.

DIFFERENTIAL DIAGNOSIS

The differential diagnosis of wheezing is given in Box 42.5.

MEDICATIONS FOR ASTHMA

Medications for asthma are listed in Box 42.6. They can be divided into bronchodilator compounds and anti-inflammatory compounds.

BRONCHODILATOR COMPOUNDS

Currently, the only anticholinergic drug available in the United States for treating asthma is ipratropium bromide, although it is approved for treating only chronic obstructive pulmonary

---

Box 42.5 DIFFERENTIAL DIAGNOSIS OF WHEEZING

Pulmonary embolism
Cardiac failure
Foreign body
Central airway tumors
Aspiration
Carcinoid syndrome
Chondromalacia or polychondritis
Löffler syndrome
Bronchiectasis
Tropical eosinophilia
Hyperventilation syndrome
Laryngeal edema
Vascular ring affecting trachea
Factitious (including psychophysiologic vocal cord adduction)
α_1-Antitrypsin deficiency
Immotile cilia syndrome
Bronchopulmonary dysplasia
Bronchiolitis (including bronchiolitis obliterans), croup
Cystic fibrosis

disease. Several short-acting β-adrenergic compounds are available, but albuterol, levalbuterol, and pirbuterol are prescribed most. More side effects occur when these medications are given orally rather than by inhalation. Nebulized β-agonists are rarely used long-term in adult asthma, although they may be used in acute attacks. For home use, the metered-dose inhaler or dry powdered inhalation is the preferred delivery system. Salmeterol and formoterol are 2 long-acting inhaled β-agonists. Both should be used only in combination with inhaled corticosteroids. Theophylline is effective for asthma, but it has a narrow therapeutic index, and interactions with other drugs (cimetidine, erythromycin, and quinolone antibiotics) can increase the serum level of theophylline.

- β-Agonists are best delivered by the inhaler route for long-term use.
- Theophylline is effective for asthma but has a narrow therapeutic index.

ANTI-INFLAMMATORY COMPOUNDS

Cromolyn and nedocromil are inhaled anti-inflammatory (mast cell stabilizing) medications that are appropriate for treatment of mild or moderate asthma. The 5-lipoxygenase inhibitor zileuton and the leukotriene receptor antagonists zafirlukast and montelukast are approved for treatment of mild persistent asthma. These agents work by decreasing the inflammatory effects of leukotrienes. Zileuton can cause increased liver function test results. Cases of Churg-Strauss vasculitis have also been linked to zafirlukast and montelukast, although a clear cause-and-effect relationship has not been established.

CORTICOSTEROIDS

Many experts recommend inhaled glucocorticoids for all severities of persistent asthma because of the potential long-term benefits of reduced bronchial hyperresponsiveness and reduced airway remodeling (fibrosis). Long-term use of β-agonist bronchodilators alone may adversely affect asthma; this also argues for earlier use of inhaled glucocorticoids. Asthma mortality has been linked to the heavy use of β-agonist inhalers. This association may simply reflect that patients with more severe asthma (who are more likely to die of an asthma attack) use more β-agonist inhalers. However, prolonged and heavy use of inhaled β-agonists may have a direct, deleterious effect on asthma. Asthma patients with regularly recurring symptoms should receive inhaled corticosteroids as part of the treatment.

- Prescribe inhaled glucocorticoids for mild, moderate, and severe persistent asthma.
- Long-term and heavy use of β-agonist bronchodilators may worsen asthma.

The inflammatory infiltrate in the bronchial submucosa of asthma patients probably depends on cytokine secretory patterns. Corticosteroids may interfere at several levels in the cytokine cascade, and they offer several benefits:

1. Corticosteroids reduce airway inflammation by modulating cytokines IL-4 and IL-5.
2. Corticosteroids can inhibit the inflammatory properties of monocytes and platelets.
3. Corticosteroids have vasoconstrictive properties.
4. Corticosteroids decrease mucous gland secretion.

The most common adverse effects of inhaled corticosteroids are dysphonia and thrush. These unwanted effects occur in about 10% of patients and can be reduced by using a spacer device and rinsing the mouth after administration. Usually, oral thrush can be treated successfully with oral antifungal agents. Dysphonia, when persistent, may be treated by decreasing or discontinuing the use of inhaled corticosteroids.

Detailed study of the systemic effects of inhaled corticosteroids shows that these agents are much safer than oral corticosteroids. Nevertheless, there is evidence that high-dose inhaled corticosteroids can affect the hypothalamic-pituitary-adrenal axis and bone metabolism. Also, high-dose inhaled corticosteroids may increase the risk of future development of glaucoma, cataracts, and osteoporosis. Inhaled corticosteroids can decrease growth velocity in children and adolescents. The effect of inhaled corticosteroids on final adult height is not known, but it appears to be minimal.

Poor inhaler technique and poor compliance can result in poor control of asthma. Therefore, all patients using a metered-dose inhaler or dry powder inhaler should be taught the proper technique for using these devices. Most patients using metered-dose inhaled corticosteroids should use a spacer device with the inhaler.

- The most common cause of poor results is poor inhaler technique.
- Patients should use a spacer device with metered-dose inhaled corticosteroids.

ANTI-IgE TREATMENT

Omalizumab is the first recombinant humanized anti-IgE monoclonal antibody approved for use in asthma. It blocks IgE binding to mast cells and is indicated for refractory moderate to severe persistent allergic asthma. It is approved for use in patients 12 years or older who have positive skin or in vitro allergy testing to relevant allergens. Dosing is based on the patient's IgE level and body weight. The dosage is typically 150 to 375 mg subcutaneously every 2 to 4 weeks.

- Omalizumab is approved for use in refractory moderate to severe persistent asthma.

ASTHMA MANAGEMENT

The goals of asthma management are listed in Box 42.7.

MANAGEMENT OF CHRONIC ASTHMA

Baseline spirometry is recommended for all patients with asthma, and home peak flow monitoring is recommended for those with moderate or severe asthma (Figure 42.1). Environmental triggers should be discussed with all asthma patients, and allergy testing should be offered to those with suspected allergic asthma or with asthma that is not well controlled. Although allergy immunotherapy is effective, it is recommended only for patients with allergic asthma who have had a complete evaluation by an allergist.

- Spirometry is recommended for all asthma patients.

Box 42.7 **GOALS OF ASTHMA MANAGEMENT**

No asthma symptoms
No asthma attacks
Normal activity level
Normal lung function
Use of safest & least amount of medication necessary
Establishment of therapeutic relationship between patient & provider

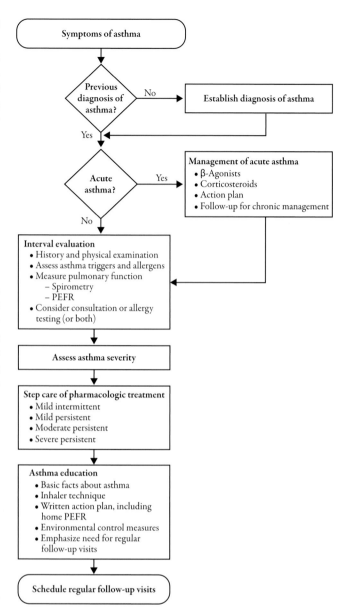

Figure 42.1 Diagnosis and Management of Asthma. PEFR indicates peak expiratory flow rate.

- Home peak flow monitoring is recommended for patients with moderate or severe asthma.

MANAGEMENT OF ACUTE ASTHMA

Inhaled β-agonists, measurements of lung function at presentation and during therapy, and systemic corticosteroids (for most patients) are the cornerstones of managing acute asthma (Figure 42.2). Generally, nebulized albuterol, administered repeatedly if necessary, is the first line of treatment. Delivery of β-agonist by metered-dose inhaler can be substituted in less severe asthma attacks. Inhaled β-agonist delivered by continuous nebulization may be appropriate for more severe disease.

It is important to measure lung function (usually peak expiratory flow rate but also FEV_1 whenever possible) at presentation and after administration of bronchodilators. These measurements provide invaluable information that allows the

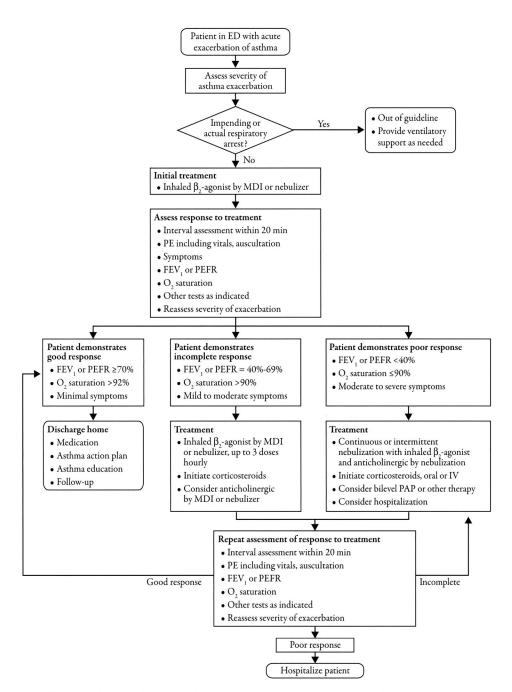

Figure 42.2 Management of Acute Asthma in Adults. ED indicates emergency department; FEV$_1$, forced expiratory volume in 1 second; IV, intravenous; MDI, metered-dose inhaler; O$_2$, oxygen; PAP, positive airway pressure; PE, physical examination; PEFR, peak expiratory flow rate. (Adapted from Sveum R, Bergstrom J, Brottman G, Hanson M, Heiman M, Johns K, et al. Diagnosis and management of asthma. 10th ed. Bloomington [MN]: Institute for Clinical Systems Improvement [updated 2012 Jul]. Available from: http://www.icsi.org/asthma__outpatient/ asthma__diagnosis_management_of__guideline_.html. July c2012. Used with permission.)

physician to assess the severity of the asthma attack and the response (if any) to treatment.

Patients who do not have a prompt and full response to inhaled β-agonists should receive a course of systemic corticosteroids. Patients with the most severe and poorly responsive disease (FEV$_1$ <50%, oxygen saturation <90%, and moderate to severe symptoms) should be treated on a hospital ward or in an intensive care unit.

- Measure pulmonary function at presentation and after giving bronchodilators.

- Most patients with acute asthma need a course of systemic corticosteroids.

ALLERGIC BRONCHOPULMONARY ASPERGILLOSIS

Allergic bronchopulmonary aspergillosis is an obstructive lung disease caused by an allergic reaction to *Aspergillus* in the lower airway. The typical patient presents with severe steroid-dependent asthma. Most patients with this

Box 42.8 DIAGNOSTIC FEATURES OF ALLERGIC BRONCHOPULMONARY ASPERGILLOSIS

Clinical asthma
Bronchiectasis (usually proximal)
Increased total serum IgE
IgE antibody to *Aspergillus* (by skin test or in vitro assay)[a]
Precipitins or IgG antibody to *Aspergillus*
Radiographic infiltrates (often upper lobes)
Peripheral blood eosinophilia

[a] Required for diagnosis.

condition have coexisting asthma or cystic fibrosis. The diagnostic features of allergic bronchopulmonary aspergillosis are summarized in Box 42.8. Fungi other than *Aspergillus fumigatus* can cause an allergic bronchopulmonary mycosis similar to allergic bronchopulmonary aspergillosis.

Chest radiography can show transient or permanent infiltrates and central bronchiectasis, usually affecting the upper lobes (Figure 42.3). Advanced cases show extensive pulmonary fibrosis. Allergic bronchopulmonary aspergillosis is treated with systemic corticosteroids. Total serum IgE may be helpful in following the course of the disease. Antifungal therapy alone has not been effective.

- Allergic bronchopulmonary aspergillosis develops in patients with asthma or cystic fibrosis.

SUMMARY

- Patients who have chronic asthma and negative results on allergy skin tests usually have an inflammatory infiltrate

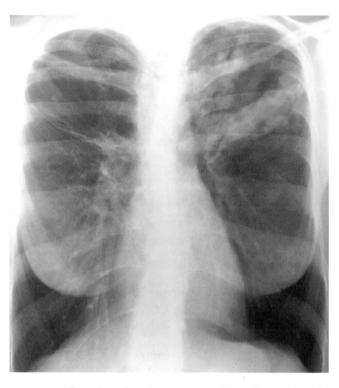

Figure 42.3 Allergic Bronchopulmonary Aspergillosis. Chest radiograph shows cylindrical infiltrates involving the upper lobes.

in the bronchi and histologic findings dominated by eosinophils when asthma is active.

- Patients with mild, moderate, or severe persistent asthma should receive treatment daily with anti-inflammatory medications.

- Baseline spirometry is recommended for all asthma patients; home peak flow monitoring is recommended for patients with moderate or severe asthma.

PART XI

PSYCHIATRY

43.

PSYCHIATRY

Brian A. Palmer, MD

GOALS

- Recognize common psychiatric disorders encountered by internists: mood disorders, anxiety disorders, somatoform disorders, factitious disorders, malingering, delerium, dementia, eating disorders, and substance abuse.

- Cite typical clinical scenarios of common psychiatric disorders.

- Summarize pharmacologic interventions for common psychiatric disorders.

This chapter reviews common psychiatric illnesses and emphasizes diagnosis and management. Since 30% to 40% of ambulatory primary care visits have a psychiatric component, successful patient management often hinges on successful treatment of comorbid psychiatric illness.

The key concept when assessing psychiatric symptoms is *whether the symptom interferes with a patient's functioning or causes distress*. For example, a patient may have a fear of heights. If this acrophobia never causes an alteration in activity, intervention is unnecessary. If, however, this acrophobia causes distress and interferes with the patient's functioning, intervention may be warranted.

MOOD DISORDERS

Mood disorders are common, with a prevalence of 8% in the general US population. The essential feature is disturbance of mood in a constellation of other symptoms (mood change alone, such as sadness, is not an illness). Mood disorders are accompanied by related cognitive, psychomotor, vegetative, and interpersonal difficulties. Mood disorders may be related to a general medical condition or be substance induced.

DEPRESSIVE DISORDERS

Major Depression

Major depression is a serious psychiatric disorder with primary symptoms that include 5 of the 9 criteria in Box 43.1 for at least 2 weeks. Acute mood changes (lasting <2 weeks) from medical causes, such as acute blood loss, are not major depression. The lifetime prevalence of depression is 20% for women and 12% for men. For women, the peak age at onset of depression is 33 to 45 years, and for men, more than 55 years.

If delusions or hallucinations are also present, they are usually less prominent than in schizophrenia, and the disorder is referred to as *major depression with psychotic features*. These features increase the likelihood of treatment resistance (although they predict a better response to electroconvulsive therapy [ECT]).

- Weight loss, fatigue, feelings of worthlessness, excessive guilt, loss of interest, and decreased ability to concentrate are hallmark symptoms of depression if they last >2 weeks.

Seasonal Affective Disorder

Seasonal affective disorder is a subtype of major depression characterized by the onset of symptoms in autumn or winter. It is twice as common among women compared with men and is associated with psychomotor retardation, hypersomnia, overeating (carbohydrate craving), and weight gain (resembling hibernation). Diagnosis requires 3 consecutive years of autumn or winter episodes that resolve by spring or summer. Treatment has relied primarily on phototherapy with a full-spectrum light source of 10,000 lux, which must be used for a minimum of 30 minutes daily. Antidepressant agents are also of benefit in treating this disorder.

- Recurrent depression in the winter must occur in 3 consecutive winters to be classified as seasonal affective disorder.

Postpartum Depression

Postpartum depression affects 10% of mothers. Although it occurs in all socioeconomic groups, single or poor mothers are at greatest risk. Untreated postpartum depression can adversely affect parent-child bonding. Treatment with antidepressants, although effective, must be balanced with the possible effect on a developing fetus or breast-fed infant, but it is generally accepted that in moderate to severe depression, the risks of not treating depression outweigh the risk of treatment with most antidepressants. Prescribing clinicians should be cognizant of the pregnancy category of the agent they prescribe in this patient group. Bipolar disorder is overrepresented in patients with postpartum mood disorders.

Dysthymia

Dysthymia is chronic depression that is milder in severity than major depression. It can be disabling for the person because the depressed mood is present most of the time during at least a 2–year period. Many patients have 1 or 2 associated vegetative signs, such as disturbance of sleep and appetite. Also, patients often feel inadequate, have low self-esteem, and struggle with interpersonal relationships. If onset is in late adolescence, the dysthymia may become intertwined with the person's personality, behavior, and general attitude toward life. Treatment is usually a combination of psychotherapy and pharmacotherapy. Pharmacotherapy may be particularly useful for patients with a family history of mood disorders or for those who have the early-onset form of dysthymia. In patients with dysthymia, superimposed major depressive episodes may develop.

- Dysthymia is characterized by disturbed sleep, appetite changes, low self-esteem, and issues with interpersonal relationships for ≥2 years.

Adjustment Disorder With Depressed Mood

Adjustment disorder with depressed mood is a reaction that develops in response to an identifiable psychosocial stressor (eg, divorce, job loss, or family or marital problems). The severity of the adjustment disorder (degree of impairment) does not always parallel the intensity of the precipitating event. The critical factor appears to be the relevance of the event or stressor to the patient and the patient's ability to cope with

the stress. In general, these reactions are relatively transient. Although patients generally can be managed by an empathetic primary care physician, the development of extreme withdrawal, suicidal ideation, or failure to improve as the circumstances improve may prompt psychiatric referral. Treatment includes supportive psychotherapy, psychosocial interventions, and, sometimes, use of antidepressant agents.

Principles of Depression Treatment

There are 3 common major groups of treatment modalities for depression: psychotherapy, pharmacotherapy, and ECT. Generally, these therapeutic modalities are used in some combination. Although internists rarely conduct formal psychotherapy, brief cognitive interventions, such as challenging overly perfectionistic beliefs, can be helpful.

The selection of medication is based on the side-effect profile of the medication and on the personal or family history of a good response to a particular agent. Initially, the patient should use a low dose, followed by titration to a therapeutic dose based on clinical assessment. Blood level determinations of a drug are meaningful only for tricyclic antidepressants used at higher doses. Treatment duration usually extends for a minimum of 6 to 12 months after the patient noticeably improves. Patients who have a severe depressive episode or who have experienced 2 or more depressive episodes are at high risk of symptom recurrence without prophylactic medication. Use of antidepressants should be tapered rather than stopped abruptly when treatment is discontinued. If the response to the first antidepressant agent is minimal, reevaluate the diagnosis, change to a different class of drug, or consider ECT.

MANIA AND BIPOLAR DISORDER

The essential features of a manic episode are the presence of an abnormally euphoric, expansive, or irritable mood associated with 3 of the criteria in Box 43.2 (4 criteria are required if the mood is only irritable). For a diagnosis of bipolar disorder, the patient must have had at least 1 episode of mania (bipolar I disorder) or hypomania (bipolar II disorder). Most patients with bipolar disorder have had recurrent depressive episodes in addition to manic episodes, although rarely patients have mania exclusively. The prevalence of bipolar disorder is estimated to be about 1%. Bipolar disorder occurs about as frequently in women as in men, and the usual age at onset is from the teens to 30 years. A family history of bipolar or other mood disorder is more common among patients with bipolar disorder than among patients with other mood disorders. Some patients do not experience a fully developed manic episode but have fewer symptoms. The term *hypomania* has been introduced to describe this form of bipolar disorder (bipolar II disorder), which generally is challenging to clinicians because its subtle features make it more difficult to recognize and it may be confused with other psychiatric disorders.

- A patient with mania may present with a euphoric mood, flight of ideas, decreased need for sleep, and unrestrained buying sprees.

Treatment is aimed at mood stabilization with medication and improved social and occupational functioning. Pharmacotherapy of mania includes lithium carbonate, valproic acid, other mood stabilizers, and atypical antipsychotics. Lithium has the added benefit of being useful in prevention or treatment of bipolar depression. Lamotrigine is also effective in treating bipolar depression. Patients with bipolar depression may be treated with ECT, lithium carbonate, lamotrigine, or an antidepressant (used simultaneously with a mood-stabilizing agent to help prevent mania).

MOOD DISORDERS CAUSED BY A GENERAL MEDICAL CONDITION

Mood disorders can be caused by medical illness. Many medical conditions may induce mood changes, so the clinical interview should identify coexisting symptoms such as excessive guilt, social withdrawal, or suicidal ideation, which are more specific for a primary depressive disorder. Medical conditions that may cause mood symptoms include endocrinopathies (Cushing syndrome, Addison disease, hyperthyroidism, hypothyroidism, hyperparathyroidism, and hypoparathyroidism), certain malignancies (lymphomas, pancreatic carcinoma, and astrocytomas), neurologic conditions (Parkinson disease, Huntington disease, and Alzheimer disease), autoimmune conditions (systemic lupus erythematosus), and infections (chronic hepatitis C, encephalitis, mononucleosis, and human immunodeficiency virus infection).

SUBSTANCE-INDUCED MOOD DISORDERS

The essential feature of a substance-induced mood disorder is a mood disturbance, either depressed or manic, due to the direct physiologic effects of a substance. Many substances can induce mood changes, including medications, toxins, and drugs of abuse. The mood symptoms may occur during the use of or exposure to the substance or during withdrawal from the substance. Medications that have been implicated in inducing mood disturbances include corticosteroids, interferon, reserpine, methyldopa, carbonic anhydrase inhibitors, stimulants, sedative hypnotics, benzodiazepines, and narcotics. Long-term use or abuse of alcohol or hallucinogens has also been implicated in inducing mood disturbances.

ANXIETY DISORDERS

Anxiety symptoms may be misinterpreted as those of medical illness because many of the symptoms overlap (eg, tachycardia, diaphoresis, tremor, shortness of breath, nausea, abdominal pain, and chest pain). Autonomic arousal and anxious agitation in a medically ill patient can also be attributed quickly to stress or anxiety when the symptoms may represent pulmonary embolus or cardiac arrhythmia. Common sources of anxiety in the medical setting are related to fears of death, abandonment, loss of function, pain, dependency, and loss of control. When to treat or to seek psychiatric consultation depends on the assessment of the degree of anxiety. Is the patient able to function in his or her role without distress or avoidance?

PANIC DISORDER AND AGORAPHOBIA

Panic disorder refers to recurrent, discrete episodes of extreme anxiety accompanied by various somatic symptoms such as dyspnea, unsteady feelings, palpitations, paresthesias, hyperventilation, trembling, diaphoresis, chest pain or discomfort, or abdominal distress. *Agoraphobia* refers to extreme fear of being in places or situations from which escape may be difficult or embarrassing. This may lead to avoidance, ultimately causing severe limitations in daily functioning for the patient. Panic disorder is more common in women (prevalence, 2%-3%) than in men (prevalence, 0.5%-1.5%). The usual age at onset is from the late teens to the early 30s. A history of childhood separation anxiety is reported in 20% to 50% of patients. The incidence is higher in first- and second-degree relatives. Most patients describe their first panic attack as spontaneous. They generally go to an emergency department after the first attack, believing that they are having a heart attack or a severe medical problem.

Patients with panic attacks may be prone to episodes of major depression. The differential diagnosis of panic disorder includes several medical disorders, such as endocrine disturbances (eg, hyperthyroidism, pheochromocytoma, and hypoglycemia), gastrointestinal tract disturbances (eg, colitis and irritable bowel syndrome), cardiopulmonary disturbances (eg, pulmonary embolism, exacerbation of chronic obstructive pulmonary disease, and acute allergic reactions), and neurologic conditions (especially conditions such as seizures that are episodic or are associated with paresthesias, faintness, or dizziness).

Several substances of abuse may cause or exacerbate anxiety symptoms. Stimulants (eg, cocaine, amphetamines, and caffeine) can fuel anxiety, as can withdrawal from sedating agents (eg, alcohol, benzodiazepines, and narcotics). Patients may use alcohol or benzodiazepines to prevent or treat panic symptoms, but regular or high-dose use may result in a cycle of tolerance and withdrawal, paradoxically causing an increase in anxiety symptoms.

Effective treatment for most patients includes the following, alone or in combination: antidepressants, cognitive behavioral therapy, or benzodiazepines (short-term). Alcohol and benzodiazepines may reduce the distress of panic attacks, but symptoms may rebound, potentially leading to substance abuse and paradoxically worsening anxiety.

POSTTRAUMATIC STRESS DISORDER

Posttraumatic stress disorder can be a brief reaction that follows an extremely traumatic, overwhelming, or catastrophic experience, or it may be a chronic condition that produces severe disability. The syndrome is characterized by the following:

1. Persistent reexperiencing (intrusive memories, flashbacks, nightmares)

2. Avoidance of reminders of the event and often a restricted range of affect

3. Persistently increased arousal (startle response, hypervigilance).

It may occur in adults or children. There is increased comorbidity with substance abuse, depression, and other anxiety disorders. Patients may be more prone to impulsivity, including suicide. As for other anxiety disorders, treatment is usually a combination of behavioral, psychotherapeutic, and, if necessary, pharmacologic interventions.

GENERALIZED ANXIETY DISORDER

Generalized anxiety disorder is characterized by chronic excessive anxiety and apprehension about life circumstances accompanied by somatic symptoms of anxiety, such as trembling, restlessness, autonomic hyperactivity, and hypervigilance. Treatment is usually a combination of cognitive-behavioral psychotherapy and psychopharmacologic modalities.

OBSESSIVE-COMPULSIVE DISORDER

Obsessive-compulsive disorder is characterized by 2 features:

1. Obsessions—distressing thoughts, ideas, or impulses experienced as unwanted

2. Compulsions—repetitive, intentional behaviors performed in response to an obsession, usually neutralizing the anxiety caused by the obsession

Prevalence rates are 2% to 3% and are about equal in men and women. The onset of this disorder is usually in adolescence or early adulthood. Obsessive traits are often present before onset of the disorder. The predominant neurobiologic theory for the cause of obsessive-compulsive disorder involves dysfunction of brain serotonin systems.

Pharmacologic treatment of this disorder is with antidepressants that are more selective for effects on the serotonin transmission system. These include clomipramine and selective serotonin reuptake inhibitors (SSRIs) (fluvoxamine, fluoxetine, paroxetine, and sertraline). Behavioral therapies and some forms of psychotherapy can also be helpful as primary or adjunctive therapy.

ADJUSTMENT DISORDER WITH ANXIOUS MOOD

Adjustment disorder with anxious mood is a maladaptive reaction to an identifiable environmental or psychosocial stress accompanied primarily by symptoms of anxiety that interfere with the patient's usual functioning. Treatment may include supportive counseling and help with identifying the stressor. However, in some cases, the anxiety may be so severe as to require short-term use of anxiolytic agents.

PSYCHOTIC DISORDERS

Psychosis is a generic term used to describe altered thought and behavior in which the patient is incapable of interpreting his or her situation rationally and accurately. Psychotic symptoms can occur in various medical, neurologic, and psychiatric disorders. Many psychotic reactions seen in medical settings are associated with the use of recreational or prescription drugs. Some of these drug-induced psychotic reactions are nearly indistinguishable from schizophrenia in terms of hallucinations and paranoid delusions (eg, amphetamine and phencyclidine [PCP] psychoses).

When evaluating psychotic patients, exploring temporal relationships between illness, medication, and the onset of symptoms is often helpful in determining the cause. As an example, it would be unusual for schizophrenia to initially manifest in a 70-year-old patient; thus, psychotic symptoms that develop at this age likely have a metabolic, medical, or substance-induced cause. Many brain regions may be involved with the production of psychotic symptoms, but abnormalities in the frontal, temporal, and limbic regions are more likely than others to produce psychotic features.

Various disorders throughout a person's life may be associated with schizophrenia-like psychoses, including the following examples:

1. Genetic abnormalities—a microdeletion of chromosome 22, the velocardiofacial syndrome

2. Childhood neurologic disorders—autism and epilepsy

3. Adult neurologic disorders—narcolepsy

4. Medical and metabolic diseases—infections, inflammatory disorders, endocrinopathies, nutritional deficiencies, uremia, and hepatic encephalopathy

5. Drug abuse

6. Psychologic stressors

Schizophrenia likely has many interrelated causes. Psychotic symptoms and altered interpersonal skills typically become evident initially in the teenaged years. Symptoms have been subdivided into positive (delusions and hallucinations) and negative (apathy and amotivational) symptoms. Diagnostic criteria include the presence of delusions and hallucinations; marked decrement in functional level in areas such as work, school, social relations, and self-care; and continuous signs of the disturbance for at least 6 months. Exclusion criteria include a consistent mood disorder component and evidence of an organic factor that produces the symptoms.

Brief psychotic disorder describes a primary psychotic illness lasting less than 1 month; *schizophreniform disorder* is a primary psychotic illness lasting 1 to 6 months.

SOMATOFORM DISORDERS, FACTITIOUS DISORDERS, AND MALINGERING

Somatoform disorders, factitious disorders, and malingering are manifested as medical symptoms that are excessive for the degree of objective disease. These conditions differ with regard to whether the symptoms and motivations for their persistence are conscious or unconscious.

SOMATOFORM DISORDERS

Somatoform disorders include somatization disorder, conversion disorder, hypochondriasis, chronic pain disorder, and body dysmorphic disorder. In all these conditions, the patient experiences physical complaints because of an effort to satisfy unconscious needs. These patients are not deliberately seeking to appear ill.

Somatization Disorder

Somatization disorder is a heterogeneous disorder that begins in early life, is characterized by recurrent multiple somatic complaints, and is seen more commonly in women. It is often best managed by collaborative work with an empathetic primary care physician and mental health professional. Regularly scheduled appointments with the primary care physician are a cost-effective strategy that lessens "doctor shopping" and frequent visits to an emergency department.

Conversion Disorder

Conversion disorder is a loss or alteration of physical functioning suggestive of a medical or, typically, a neurologic disorder that cannot be explained on the basis of known physiologic mechanisms. It is seen most often in the outpatient setting. Patients frequently respond to any of several therapeutic modalities that suggest hope of a cure. When conversion disorder becomes chronic, it carries a poorer prognosis and is difficult to treat. Treatment focuses on management of the symptoms rather than cure, much as in somatization or chronic pain disorder.

Chronic Pain Disorder

Chronic pain disorder (ie, somatoform, chronic pain syndromes) may occur at any age but most often develops in the 30s or 40s. It is diagnosed twice as often in women as in men and is characterized by preoccupation with pain for at least 6 months. No organic lesion is found to account for the pain, or if there is a related organic lesion, the complaint of pain or resulting interference with usual life activities is in excess of what would be expected from the physical findings. A thorough assessment is essential before this diagnosis can be established. Treatment is usually multidisciplinary (eg, primary care, psychiatry, psychology, and physiatry) and focused on helping the patient manage or live with the pain rather than continuing with the expectation of "cure." Avoidance of long-term dependence on addictive substances is an important goal.

- Patients with chronic pain disorder are preoccupied with pain for ≥6 months. The pain interferes with normal function, but no organic cause is found on careful medical evaluation.

Hypochondriasis

Hypochondriasis is an intense preoccupation with the fear of having a serious disease or the belief that one does have a serious disease despite the lack of physical evidence to support the concern. It tends to be a chronic problem for the patient. The differential diagnosis includes obsessive-compulsive disorder (somatic presentation) and delusional disorder (somatic type). Patients with hypochondriasis and obsessive-compulsive disorder tend to have fleeting insight into their excessive concern for their health, unlike patients with delusional thinking. The treatment of hypochondriasis, similar to that of obsessive-compulsive disorder, depends on a combination of serotonergic antidepressants and cognitive-behavioral psychotherapy.

FACTITIOUS DISORDERS

Factitious disorders are characterized by the *deliberate* production of signs or symptoms of disease. The diagnosis of these disorders requires that the physician maintain a high degree of awareness and look for objective data at variance with the patient's history (eg, surgical scars that are inconsistent with past surgical history). The more common form of factitious disorder generally occurs among socially conforming young women of a higher socioeconomic class who are intelligent, educated, and frequently work in a medically related field. The possibility of a coexisting medical disorder or intercurrent illness needs to be appreciated in the diagnostic and therapeutic management of these difficult cases. Factitious disorders are often found in patients with a history of childhood emotional traumas. The most extreme form of the disorder is Munchausen syndrome, which is characterized by the triad of simulating disease, pathologic lying, and wandering. This syndrome has been recognized primarily in men of lower socioeconomic class who have a lifelong pattern of poor social adjustment.

- Suspect factitious disorder in health professionals who have recurrent fevers but no other presenting signs or symptoms.

MALINGERING

Malingering persons intentionally produce symptoms that are false or exaggerated. The motivating factors vary (eg, avoiding a commitment, seeking money or drugs, or searching for a better place to live). Clues to malingering include situations with a medicolegal context that overshadows the clinical presentation, a marked discrepancy between what the person describes and the objective findings, uncooperative behavior for the diagnostic evaluation and for adherence with prescribed treatments, and the presence of an antisocial personality disorder. Malingering persons usually do not relate their symptoms to an emotional conflict.

DELIRIUM: AN ACUTE CONFUSIONAL STATE

The primary distinguishing feature between delirium and dementia is the retention and stability of alertness in dementia. Delirium is characterized by a fluctuating course of an altered state of awareness and consciousness. It may be accompanied by hallucinations (tactile, auditory, visual, or olfactory), illusions (misperceptions of sensory stimuli), delusions, emotional lability, paranoia, alterations in the sleep-wake cycle, and psychomotor slowing or hyperactivity. Delirium is usually reversible with correction of the underlying cause. It often is related to an external toxic agent, medication side effect, metabolic abnormality, central nervous system abnormality, or withdrawal of a medication or drug. Delirium is relatively common (range, 10%-30%) in medical or surgical inpatients older than 65 years. Patients may present with either agitation or withdrawal; withdrawal is more difficult to recognize. High-risk groups include elderly patients with medical illness (especially congestive heart failure, urinary tract infection, renal insufficiency, hyponatremia, dehydration, or stroke), postcardiotomy patients, and patients with dementia, drug withdrawal, severe burns, or AIDS.

Common causes of delirium in the elderly are infection and intoxication with psychotropic drugs, especially drugs with sedative and anticholinergic side effects. The first step in management is determining whether a specific cause can be identified. Comprehensive medical investigations are frequently warranted. After the cause of the delirium has been recognized, a treatment is selected that can reverse the underlying disease process. If the cause is unknown and the patient's behavior interferes with safety and medical care, several categories of intervention can be considered.

Management aspects include monitoring vital signs, electrolytes, and fluid balance and giving neuroleptic agents such as haloperidol. Orientation is aided with environmental supports such as calendars, clocks, windows, and family and other persons. Also, psychosocial support, including family or other care providers, is helpful. Severely agitated patients may require physical restraints to prevent injury to themselves or others if medications are not yet effective. To minimize injury, restraints should be avoided whenever possible.

- Suspect delirium with abrupt onset of visual hallucinations and paranoia accompanied by alteration of the sleep-wake cycle, impaired digit recall, and disorientation to time and date.

EATING DISORDERS

The 2 common eating disorders are *anorexia nervosa* and *bulimia*. Both are markedly more prevalent among women than men. Onset is usually in the teenaged or young adult years. Eating disorders are increasingly found across all income, racial, and ethnic groups. Both disorders have a primary symptom of preoccupation with weight and distortion of body image. For example, the patient perceives herself to look less attractive than an observer would. The disorders are not mutually exclusive, and about 50% of patients with anorexia nervosa also have bulimia. Many patients with bulimia previously had at least a subclinical case of anorexia nervosa. Eating disorders have the highest lethality of all psychiatric illnesses.

ANOREXIA NERVOSA

To meet the diagnostic criteria of anorexia nervosa, weight must be 15% below that expected for age and height. However, weight of 30% to 40% below normal is not uncommon and leads to the medical complications of starvation, such as depletion of fat, muscle wasting, bradycardia, arrhythmias, ventricular tachycardia and sudden death, constipation, abdominal pain, leukopenia, hypercortisolemia, and osteoporosis. Extreme cases are characterized by lanugo (fine hair on the body) and metabolic alterations to conserve energy. Thyroid effects include low levels of triiodothyronine (T_3), cold intolerance, and difficulty maintaining core body temperature. Reproductive effects include a pronounced decrease or cessation of the secretion of luteinizing hormone and follicle-stimulating hormone, resulting in secondary amenorrhea. Reinitiation of nourishment requires careful monitoring and supplementation of potassium, magnesium, and phosphate levels.

BULIMIA

Patients with bulimia frequently consume large quantities of food followed by purging. Physical complications of the binge-purge cycle may include fluid and electrolyte abnormalities, hypochloremic-hypokalemic metabolic alkalosis, esophageal and gastric irritation and bleeding, colonic abnormalities from laxative abuse, marked erosion of dental enamel with associated decay, parotid and salivary gland hypertrophy, and amylase levels 25% to 40% higher than normal. If bulimia is untreated, it often becomes chronic. Some patients have a gradual spontaneous remission of some symptoms.

SUBSTANCE USE DISORDERS

Alcohol and other substance use disorders are a major concern in all age groups and across all ethnic, socioeconomic, and racial groups. Despite high lifetime prevalence (up to 20%), less than 10% of persons with substance use disorders are involved in treatment (either self-help groups or professional care).

Several pharmacologic agents are available to help diminish the craving for alcohol and other drugs or to deter relapse. Although several medications, including disulfiram, acamprosate, and naltrexone, may help prevent relapse, they are adjunctive and not a substitute for treatment.

Substance dependence is typified by the following criteria (3 of the 7 are required for diagnosis):

1. Tolerance

2. Withdrawal

3. Increasing amount of use

4. Unsuccessful efforts to stop

5. Much time spent on activities to obtain the substance

6. Important social, occupational, or recreational activities are given up

7. Use continues despite consequences

Substance abuse includes 1 or more of the following without meeting the criteria for dependence:

1. Recurrent use resulting in failure to fulfill major role obligations (at work, school, or home)

2. Recurrent use when it is physically hazardous (eg, driving)

3. Recurrent legal problems

4. Continued use despite problems

ALCOHOL ABUSE AND DEPENDENCE

The CAGE questions (related to attempts to *c*ut down on alcohol use, other persons expressing *a*nnoyance, experiencing *g*uilt, and *e*arly-morning drinking) have excellent sensitivity and specificity for alcohol dependence. *Alcohol withdrawal* can range from mild to quite severe, beginning with tachycardia, hypertension, diaphoresis, and tremors and progressing to the occurrence of withdrawal seizures or delirium tremens (or both).

Psychologic functioning issues include impaired cognition and changes in mood and behavior. Interpersonal functioning issues include marital problems, child abuse, and impaired social relationships. Occupational functioning issues include academic, scholastic, or job problems. Legal, financial, and spiritual problems also occur.

BENZODIAZEPINE, SEDATIVE-HYPNOTIC, AND ANXIOLYTIC ABUSE AND DEPENDENCE

Benzodiazepines, sedative hypnotics, and anxiolytics are widely prescribed in many areas of medicine, so abuse and dependence often have an iatrogenic component. Five characteristics may help distinguish medical use from nonmedical use:

1. Intent: What is the purpose of the use?

2. Effect: What is the effect on the user's life?

3. Control: Is the use controlled by the user only or does a physician share in the control?

4. Legality: Is the use of the drug legal or illegal? Medical drug use is legal.

5. Pattern: In what settings is the drug used?

Withdrawal of the use of benzodiazepines and barbiturates, in particular, may be serious because of the increased risk of withdrawal seizures; slowly tapered doses are indicated, particularly for long-term use.

THE SUICIDAL PATIENT

Emergency medicine physicians are often the first to deal with patients who have suicidal ideation or who have attempted or completed suicide. The recognition of risk factors for suicide, a thorough assessment of the psychiatric and medical factors, and urgent intervention are critically important. Although the patient who overdoses with a benzodiazepine may be very serious about the intent to die, the person who overdoses with acetaminophen is more at risk of serious medical complications.

Recognition of a suicidal gesture is essential in evaluating a patient in an emergency department. Although drug overdoses are the commonest form, alcohol intoxication, single-vehicle accidents, and falls from heights may merit further investigation. Many suicidal patients see a physician the week before the attempt. Risk factors to be aware of include recent psychiatric hospitalization, an older divorced or widowed man, unemployment, poor physical health, past suicide attempts, family history of suicide (especially a parent), psychosis, alcoholism, drug abuse, chronic pain syndrome, sudden life changes, loneliness, and the anniversary of a significant loss. More than 50% of completed suicide attempts involve guns; access to firearms should be assessed as part of a standard suicide risk assessment.

PERSONALITY DISORDERS

While the *Diagnostic and Statistical Manual of Mental Disorders* (Fourth Edition, Text Revision) (*DSM-IV-TR*) recognizes 10 personality disorders, patients with borderline personality disorder (BPD) and other Cluster B disorders (antisocial, narcissistic, and histrionic) demand the most from internists. BPD is diagnosed with 9 criteria categorized as interpersonal (chaotic relationships, ideal and devalued; efforts to avoid abandonment), affective (lability, anger problems), self (identity confusion, emptiness), and behavioral (suicide attempts, self-injury, and impulsivity). The disorder is treatable and generally improves, despite common perceptions to the contrary. Internists can be most effective by balancing the need of the patient for adequate attention (increased frequency of short visits can be helpful) while maintaining appropriate limits (practicing safe and effective medicine).

PSYCHOPHARMACOLOGY

Medication alone is rarely the sole treatment of a psychiatric disorder but rather a component of a comprehensive treatment plan. Because psychoactive medications are used in various circumstances for many different indications, the major groups of these medications are discussed below in general terms. The choice of a medication usually is based on its side-effect profile and the clinical profile of the patient. There are many effective drugs in each major group, but they differ in terms of pharmacokinetics, side effects, and available routes of administration.

ANTIDEPRESSANTS: GENERAL PRINCIPLES

First-generation antidepressants include tricyclic antidepressants (TCAs) and monoamine oxidase inhibitors (MAOIs). Newer-generation antidepressants are not easily grouped by their chemical structure or function; SSRIs are the most widely used of this group.

Although older-generation antidepressants are effective in treating depression, they are associated with side effects that limit their use. TCAs are associated with orthostatic hypotension, anticholinergic side effects, and altered cardiac conduction. MAOIs are effective antidepressants but require special dietary restrictions and attention to interactions with other medications to avoid a hypertensive crisis caused by unmetabolized tyramine.

Antidepressants can be useful in depression, panic disorder, obsessive-compulsive disorder, generalized anxiety disorder, social anxiety disorder, posttraumatic stress disorder, enuresis, bulimia, and attention-deficit/hyperactivity disorder, among others. TCAs and duloxetine can be beneficial for treating certain pain syndromes.

A complete trial of antidepressant medication consists of 4 to 6 weeks of therapeutic doses before considering refractoriness. If improvement has occurred with the initial trial of the medication but the patient's condition has not returned to baseline, it may be appropriate to increase the dose of the medication, switch to another medication class, or augment it. After clinical improvement has been noted, the medication may need to be used for an extended period.

Concerns about antidepressants potentially causing an increase in suicidal thoughts or behavior have resulted in the development of a black box warning for all antidepressants. This topic is controversial since several studies have not corroborated this concern. The important clinical point to remember is that patients with depression should be assessed for suicidal thinking whether or not they are taking antidepressant medications.

ANTIPSYCHOTIC AGENTS

The most simple and direct mechanism of action of antipsychotic agents involves blockade of postsynaptic dopamine receptors; older agents are generally more potent dopamine blockers, with the "high-potency" neuroleptics providing the most direct blockade. The antipsychotic effects of these agents result from their actions on the dopaminergic neurons of the limbic system, midbrain tegmentum, septal nuclei, and mesocortical dopaminergic projections. Blockade of other dopaminergic pathways is responsible for side effects: nigrostriatal (motor activity) blockade leads to extrapyramidal symptoms; tuboloinfundibular (pituitary and hypothalamus) blockade can increase prolactin levels and cause changes in temperature and appetite regulation. Because they have less direct dopamine receptor blockade, atypical antipsychotic agents have a lower rate of extrapyramidal side effects, although they can still occur.

Side Effects

Several types of side effects are common and important:

1. *Acute dystonic reactions* occur within hours or days after treatment is initiated with antipsychotic drugs. Dystonia is an uncontrollable tightening of muscles, such as the sternocleidomastoid muscle (causing a neck twisting, torticollis), the extraocular muscles (oculogyric crisis), or the laryngeal muscles (respiratory difficulties). Treatment is with parenteral administration of an anticholinergic agent (eg, diphenhydramine).

2. *Akathisia* is an unpleasant feeling of restlessness and the inability to sit still, which generally occurs within days of initiating or increasing an antipsychotic dose. Akathisia is sometimes mistaken for exacerbation of psychosis. Treatment consists of decreasing the dose of the antipsychotic agent (if possible) or using a β-blocking agent such as propranolol.

3. *Neuroleptic malignant syndrome* is a potentially life-threatening disorder that may occur after the use of any antipsychotic agent, although it is more common with rapid increases in the dosage of high-potency antipsychotic agents. It is characterized by rigidity, fever, leukocytosis, tachycardia, tachypnea, diaphoresis, blood pressure fluctuations, and marked increase in creatine kinase levels because of muscle breakdown. Treatment consists of discontinuing use of the antipsychotic and providing life-support measures (ventilation and cooling). Pharmacologic interventions include dantrolene, a direct-acting muscle relaxant, or bromocriptine, a centrally acting dopamine agonist. ECT is effective.

4. *Parkinsonian symptoms* have a more gradual onset and can be treated with oral anticholinergic agents or decreased doses of an antipsychotic agent (or both).

5. *Tardive dyskinesia* has an incidence of 3% to 5% annually with first-generation neuroleptics and consists of

involuntary movements of the face, trunk, or extremities. The most consistent risk factors for its development are long-term medication use (>6 months) and older age. It is best if treatment with the antipsychotic agent can be discontinued at an early sign of tardive dyskinesia because the dyskinesia is sometimes reversible. It is rarer with atypical antipsychotics.

6. *Glucose intolerance, weight gain*, and *electrophysiologic cardiac changes* have been associated with atypical antipsychotics. Additionally, several studies have shown a lack of efficacy for off-label use in dementia patients, and safety concerns have arisen related to an increased risk of death among these patients.

7. *Clozapine side effects*: Clozapine is an atypical antipsychotic that can increase the risk of seizures, orthostasis, and myocarditis, and it has a 1% to 2% risk of producing agranulocytosis, which is reversible if use of the medication is withdrawn immediately. Because of this serious potential side effect, a specific requirement is that white blood cell counts be made regularly (weekly for the first 6 months).

BENZODIAZEPINES

Benzodiazepines are used most appropriately to treat time-limited anxiety or insomnia related to an identifiable stress or change in sleep cycle. After long-term use (>2–3 months), therapy with benzodiazepines and related substances should be tapered rather than discontinued abruptly to avoid relapse, rebound, and withdrawal.

Relapse is the return of the original anxiety symptoms, often after weeks to months. *Rebound* is the intensification of the original symptoms, which usually last several days and appear within hours to days after abrupt cessation of drug use. *Withdrawal* includes autonomic and central nervous system symptoms that are different from the original presenting symptoms of the disorder.

Several benzodiazepines have metabolites with long half-lives, so smaller doses are needed in the elderly, patients with cognitive dysfunction, and children. These patient groups, especially patients with known brain damage, are prone to paradoxical reactions (anxiety, irritability, aggression, agitation, and insomnia).

LITHIUM

Lithium is used for bipolar disorder and recurrent depression and as an adjunct for depression treatment after ECT. Peak levels occur in 1 to 2 hours, and its half-life is about 24 hours; levels are generally checked 10 to 12 hours after the last dose and 4 to 5 days after a dose change. Common side effects include resting tremor, diarrhea, polyuria, polydipsia, thirst, and nausea (give lithium on a full stomach). Use in the first trimester of pregnancy is associated with Ebstein anomaly. Renal effects generally can be reversed with discontinued use of lithium; renal function should be followed. A hematologic side effect is benign leukocytosis. Hypothyroidism is common, and thyroid function should be monitored.

Lithium has a narrow therapeutic index (typically 0.5–1.0 mEq/L), and toxicity (typically >1.5–2.5 mEq/L) can cause renal failure and death. Signs of toxicity include abdominal pain and vomiting, dry mouth, nystagmus and blurred vision, delirium, ataxia, hyperreflexia and fasciculations, and seizures.

Lithium levels are increased by angiotensin-converting enzyme inhibitors, thiazide diuretics, nonsteroidal anti-inflammatory drugs, dehydration, overheating or increased perspiration, and certain antibiotics (tetracycline, spectinomycin, and metronidazole). Levels can be decreased by caffeine and theophylline.

ELECTROCONVULSIVE THERAPY

ECT is the most effective treatment for severely depressed patients, especially those with psychotic features. It is also helpful in treating catatonia and mania and may be used in children and adults. ECT can be administered safely to pregnant women if fetal monitoring is available. A usual course of treatment is 6 to 12 sessions given over 2 to 4 weeks.

ECT no longer has any absolute contraindications, although it has several relative contraindications related to anesthesia risks, intracranial space-occupying lesions, and increased intracranial pressure. Before ECT is administered, the patient should be assessed for cardiovascular function, pulmonary function, electrolyte balance, neurologic status (eg, history of epilepsy), and previous experiences with anesthesia.

SUMMARY

- Weight loss, fatigue, feelings of worthlessness, excessive guilt, loss of interest, and decreased ability to concentrate are hallmark symptoms of depression if they last >2 weeks.

- Dysthymia is characterized by disturbed sleep, appetite changes, low self-esteem, and issues with interpersonal relationships for ≥2 years.

- A patient with mania may present with a euphoric mood, flight of ideas, decreased need for sleep, and unrestrained buying sprees.

- Patients with chronic pain disorder are preoccupied with pain for ≥6 months. The pain interferes with normal function, but no organic cause is found on careful medical evaluation.

PART XII

NEUROLOGY

44.

DIAGNOSIS OF NEUROLOGIC DISORDERS

Lyell K. Jones Jr, MD, Brian A. Crum, MD, Eduardo E. Benarroch, MD,

and Robert D. Brown Jr, MD

GOALS

- Review the clinical approach to patients with neurologic disease.

- Summarize tests commonly used in evaluating patients with neurologic disorders.

INTRODUCTION

Neurologic disorders are common, occurring in about 10% of patients in the ambulatory primary care setting. Approximately 25% of hospital inpatients have a neurologic diagnosis as a primary or secondary problem. Accordingly, primary care physicians must be familiar with common neurologic disorders, particularly as the population ages and cerebrovascular disorders, dementias, and Parkinson disease become more prevalent. Understanding neurologic disease in a patient depends on localizing the problem on the basis of the medical history and examination findings, considering a differential diagnosis, and correlating the clinical findings with abnormalities found on appropriate diagnostic testing.

- About 10% of patients in the ambulatory primary care setting have neurologic disorders.

- About 25% of inpatients have a neurologic disorder as a primary or secondary problem.

CLINICAL NEUROLOGIC EVALUATION

A careful history and neurologic examination are the most important components of the neurologic evaluation. The history should be clarified as precisely as possible for temporal profile, progression, and character of the symptoms (Box 44.1). Identifying positive and negative symptoms is

helpful; for example, patients with cerebral ischemia often present with negative symptoms such as weakness, aphasia, or anesthesia, while patients with seizures may present with positive symptoms such as paresthesia or abnormal movements. Symptoms that remain ill-defined despite attempted clarification are frequently, but not universally, nonneurologic.

If the history is suggestive of a neurologic disorder, the features of the symptoms in concert with the examination findings assist in localization (Box 44.2). Determine which levels of the nervous system may be affected:

1. Supratentorial (cerebral cortex and subcortical regions, including the basal ganglia, hypothalamus, and thalamus)

2. Posterior fossa (cerebellum, brainstem, and cranial nerves)

3. Spinal cord (including extramedullary, intramedullary, cauda equina, and conus medullaris lesions)

4. Peripheral (including spinal roots, plexi, peripheral nerves, neuromuscular junction, and skeletal muscle)

Consider in simple terms the geographic extent of the process. From the signs and symptoms, the lesion is determined to be on the right or left side or bilateral. Next determine whether the process is diffuse (affecting a whole level), focal, or multifocal. Then consider the temporal profile: acute (seconds to hours), subacute (days to weeks), or chronic (months to years). It is then possible to generate a differential diagnosis based on the suspicion of a focal or diffuse process (Table 44.1) and outline the appropriate diagnostic procedures, therapeutic options, and patient counseling.

- The history and examination findings suggest localization to the level and side of the nervous system.

- The temporal profile is then used to determine a differential diagnosis.

Temporal profile: When did the symptoms begin?
  Acute (seconds to hours)
  Subacute (days to weeks)
  Chronic (months to years)
Progression: How have the symptoms changed?
  Improving
  Static, unchanged, plateaued
  Progressive, worsening
  Fluctuating
  Episodic, spells
Character: What are the features of the symptoms?
  Positive symptoms (tremor or other abnormal movements, paresthesia, pain, behavioral outbursts)
  Negative symptoms (weakness, incoordination, anesthesia, amnesia, or cognitive deficit)
  Ill-defined symptoms (fatigue or imbalance, which frequently have a nonneurologic basis)

NEUROLOGIC DIAGNOSTIC TESTING

COMPUTED TOMOGRAPHY AND MAGNETIC RESONANCE IMAGING

Vascular Diseases

Computed tomography (CT) is a good initial test for evaluating a patient who may have cerebral ischemia (transient ischemic attack or stroke) because it can quickly identify acute hemorrhage in brain parenchyma or the subarachnoid space (Box 44.3). CT (even with contrast enhancement) often gives equivocal or negative results in the first 24 to 48 hours after an ischemic cerebral infarction. In these situations, magnetic resonance imaging (MRI) is the first neuroimaging test to show abnormalities during the evolution of an ischemic cerebral infarct. With diffusion and perfusion MRI scanning, cerebral ischemia can be delineated within minutes of the onset of symptoms, before CT or routine MRI shows any abnormality. In subacute and chronic stages of an ischemic cerebral

Box 44.2 LOCALIZATION OF NEUROLOGIC DISORDERS

Level of nervous system
  Supratentorial (cerebral hemispheres)
  Posterior fossa (brainstem and cerebellum)
  Spinal cord
  Peripheral (peripheral nerves, neuromuscular junction, & muscle)
Extent of the process
  Focal: Can the symptoms be explained with a single lesion?
  Multifocal: Can the symptoms be explained by multiple lesions at 1 or more levels?
  Diffuse: Does widespread dysfunction at 1 or more levels account for the symptoms?

infarction, MRI and CT provide roughly equivalent information. Vasculitic lesions or microinfarcts, as in systemic lupus erythematosus, are often seen on MRI but missed on CT. Subacute and chronic intracerebral hemorrhages are better defined by MRI, especially with gradient echo (GRE) MRI, which is sensitive for acute hemorrhage and old hemosiderin.

Magnetic resonance angiography (MRA) is noninvasive and has replaced standard angiography for many indications. It is quite sensitive in defining the degree of stenosis in the carotid or vertebrobasilar system. However, MRA does not adequately evaluate more distal intracranial arteries, and arteriography is required for this indication. MRA is also used as a screening study for aneurysms. Formal angiography still may be needed to examine the anatomical details of aneurysms or vascular malformations or when cerebral vasculitis is suspected. CT angiography is another sensitive test for determination of vascular disease and anatomical features.

- For evaluating acute hemorrhage in the brain and subarachnoid space, CT is better than standard MRI.

- During evolution of an acute ischemic cerebral infarct, MRI is better than CT.

- For evaluating subacute and chronic stages of an ischemic cerebral infarct, CT and MRI are equivalent.

- MRA and CT angiography are useful noninvasive studies to evaluate for vascular pathology.

Trauma

MRI is competitive with but not comparable to CT for assessing the brain after craniocerebral trauma. Soon after injury, CT is preferable because the examination time is shorter. Standard radiographic examination or CT is necessary to evaluate skull fractures because bone cortex is not well visualized with MRI.

CT is highly dependable for demonstrating subdural and other intracranial hematomas, which are also visualized with MRI. Coronal MRI sections are usually best for visualizing the size, shape, location, and extent of subdural hematomas. In traumatic brain injury (TBI) patients, conventional MRI can show changes from diffuse axonal injury that are not visible on CT. This is often the pathologic substrate for mental status changes or coma after head trauma when intracerebral hemorrhage is excluded. Newer MRI techniques, such as diffusion tensor imaging (DTI), may offer more sensitive assessments of TBI.

In adults and children with TBI, recovery of consciousness is unlikely after 12 months. Recovery is rare after 3 months in adults and children with nontraumatic brain injury.

- Soon after traumatic head injury, CT of the brain is recommended to exclude intracranial hemorrhage and skull fracture.

- CT is dependable for showing subdural and other intracranial hematomas.

- MRI is most sensitive in detecting diffuse axonal injury.

Table 44.1 FORMULATING A NEUROLOGIC DIFFERENTIAL DIAGNOSIS

PROCESS	ACUTE (SECONDS TO HOURS)	SUBACUTE (DAYS TO WEEKS)	CHRONIC (MONTHS TO YEARS)
Focal	Vascular (eg, MCA stroke) Migrainous Epilepsy (eg, complex partial seizure)	Infection (eg, cerebral abscess) Autoinflammatory (eg, multiple sclerosis)	Neoplasm (eg, low-grade glioma) Degenerative (eg, carpal tunnel syndrome)
Diffuse	Vascular (eg, SAH) Epilepsy (eg, GTC seizure) Metabolic (eg, hypoglycemic coma)	Infection (eg, bacterial meningitis) Autoinflammatory (eg, Guillain-Barré syndrome)	Degenerative (eg, Alzheimer dementia) Metabolic (eg, diabetic sensorimotor peripheral neuropathy)

Abbreviations: GTC, generalized tonic-clonic; MCA, middle cerebral artery; SAH, subarachnoid hemorrhage.

Intracranial Tumors

A wide spectrum of intracranial tumors is visualized with MRI and CT. Often MRI shows more extensive involvement (of 1 lesion or multiple smaller lesions) than CT, especially in gliomas or metastasis. MRI is superior in demonstrating diseases of the meninges (eg, carcinomatous meningitis). CT with a contrast agent and MRI with gadolinium are both excellent for detecting meningiomas. MRI is superior to CT for identifying all types of posterior fossa tumors and is the study of choice for identifying brainstem gliomas.

- MRI is favored over CT for the evaluation of tumors because it shows more anatomical detail and allows detection of smaller lesions.

- MRI is superior to CT for identifying posterior fossa tumors and brainstem gliomas.

White Matter Lesions

MRI is superior to CT in detecting abnormalities of the white matter, as may be seen in multiple sclerosis (in which lesions are most commonly periventricular white matter lesions and

---

Box 44.3 **COMPARISON OF COMPUTED TOMOGRAPHY (CT) AND MAGNETIC RESONANCE IMAGING (MRI) FOR NEUROLOGIC IMAGING**

CT advantages
    Evaluation of suspected acute hemorrhage
    Evaluation of skull fractures or bony spine trauma
    Lower cost
    Wider availability
MRI advantages
    Evaluation of subacute & chronic hemorrhage
    Evaluation of acute ischemic cerebral infarction
    Evaluation of primary & metastatic CNS tumors
    Diagnosis of multiple sclerosis
    Evaluation of posterior fossa & brainstem tumors & lesions
    Evaluation of the spine & spinal cord
    Safety (no ionizing radiation)

Abbreviation: CNS, central nervous system.

---

are often perpendicular to the lateral ventricles). MRI evidence of multiple subcortical ischemic cerebral infarctions may be the cause of adult-onset dementia. However, white matter changes in the elderly must be interpreted carefully because MRI shows some changes in the white matter of most neurologically normal elderly persons.

- MRI is the test of choice in multiple sclerosis, with periventricular white matter lesions (often perpendicular to the lateral ventricles) being the most common finding.

- MRI shows some changes in the white matter of most neurologically normal elderly persons.

Spinal Cord

A wide spectrum of lesions at the cervicomedullary junction and in the spinal cord can be seen more clearly with MRI because CT of these structures is obscured by bony artifact. Thus, MRI is the study of choice for assessing the cervicomedullary junction and spinal cord. Generally, MRI is better than CT for identifying intramedullary and extramedullary lesions of the spinal cord. CT can be helpful if bony detail is important (eg, fractures and spurs).

- MRI is superior to CT for assessing the cervicomedullary junction and spinal cord lesions.

Dementia

In assessing dementia, either CT or MRI can demonstrate potentially reversible lesions (ie, subdural hematoma, brain tumor, or hydrocephalus), but MRI is more sensitive for determining the presence of multiple infarcts in vascular dementia. MRI can assess atrophy more accurately, especially in the mesial temporal lobes, a common finding in Alzheimer disease. This is best viewed with thin-slice coronal imaging.

Spine

Protruding intervertebral disks are well visualized on MRI sagittal sections, which show the relation of the disk to the spine and nerve roots. CT myelography occasionally shows far lateral disk herniations that are not apparent with MRI, so that there are rare circumstances in which a clear radiculopathy with no structural cause evident on MRI would be apparent with CT myelography.

- MRI is the study of choice for most degenerative spinal disorders.

ELECTROMYOGRAPHY AND NERVE CONDUCTION STUDIES

Nerve conduction studies (NCS) involve electrically stimulating nerves and measuring certain electrophysiologic variables (amplitude of responses, conduction velocities, and distal latencies). Electromyography (EMG) is performed by inserting a small needle into the muscle and recording electrical activity at rest and with light muscle contraction. These tests are excellent for identifying diseases of the anterior horn cell, nerve root, peripheral nerve, neuromuscular junction, or muscle. They also assess the large-fiber sensory peripheral nervous system. They give little information, however, on small-fiber function, which requires specific testing of the autonomic nerves and sweating pathways. In addition, EMG does not thoroughly assess type 2 muscle fibers, which can be affected in myopathies caused by corticosteroid use or deconditioning. By helping to localize and to better define further diagnostic studies, EMG and NCS are an extension of the neurologic examination.

- NCS and EMG are valuable for identifying neuromuscular disorders affecting the anterior horn cell, nerve root, large-fiber sensory peripheral nerve, neuromuscular junction, or muscle.

- NCS and EMG do not exclude small-fiber dysfunction.

ELECTROENCEPHALOGRAPHY

Electroencephalography (EEG) is used mainly to study patients with suspected seizure disorders or encephalopathies. *Seizure disorder*, or *epilepsy*, is a clinical diagnosis and not an EEG diagnosis, and a normal EEG does not rule out epilepsy. EEG may show syndrome-specific abnormalities (such as in absence epilepsy), but it may show many nonspecific patterns that should not be overinterpreted.

Ambulatory EEG is available for detecting frequent unusual spells. Prolonged (inpatient) video EEG monitoring is helpful in defining epileptic surgical candidates, nonepileptic spells (pseudoseizures), and unusual seizures. EEG is imperative for diagnosing and treating nonconvulsive status epilepticus.

- EEG is specific in some forms of epilepsy, including typical absence epilepsy.

- Epilepsy is a clinical diagnosis, not an EEG diagnosis.

- A normal EEG does not rule out epilepsy.

- Prolonged video EEG monitoring is helpful in defining epileptic surgical candidates, nonepileptic spells, and unusual seizures.

EEG is valuable for evaluating various encephalopathies. Some drugs (especially benzodiazepines) cause an unusual fast pattern, and many metabolic encephalopathies cause a diffuse slow or triphasic pattern. Diffuse slow patterns are seen also in degenerative cerebral disease (eg, Alzheimer disease). Unusual, periodic, high-amplitude sharp wave activity helps define Creutzfeldt-Jakob disease and subacute sclerosing panencephalitis. EEG is often valuable in diagnosing certain infectious encephalopathies (eg, herpes simplex encephalitis).

EEG is essential for diagnosing various sleep disorders and is an *adjuvant* tool for diagnosing brain death. Brain death is a clinical diagnosis. EEG may be used as an intraoperative monitoring procedure (eg, during carotid endarterectomy).

By 24 to 48 hours after a hypoxic insult, the EEG assists in predicting the likelihood of neurologic recovery. Poor outcome is seen with alpha coma, burst suppression, periodic patterns, and electrocerebral silence.

- EEG is valuable in diagnosing certain infectious encephalopathies (eg, herpes simplex encephalitis).

- EEG is an adjuvant tool for diagnosing brain death.

- Brain death is a clinical diagnosis.

LUMBAR PUNCTURE AND CEREBROSPINAL FLUID ANALYSIS

Lumbar puncture should be performed only after a thorough clinical evaluation and after consideration of the potential value compared with the hazards of the procedure. Imaging of the brain (CT or MRI) is *mandatory* if there is any suspicion of a focal cerebral or cerebellar process.

Indications for Lumbar Puncture

Urgent lumbar puncture is performed for suspected acute meningitis, encephalitis, or subarachnoid hemorrhage (if suspected but not detected on CT) and for fever (even without meningeal signs) in infancy, acute confusional states, and neurologic manifestations in immunocompromised patients. Other indications for lumbar puncture may include unexplained subacute dementia, multiple sclerosis, myelopathy, peripheral neuropathy, and some headache disorders.

The IgG synthesis rate is increased in multiple sclerosis, but this finding is nonspecific, as is the finding of oligoclonal bands. A marked pleocytosis (based on the leukocyte count) should suggest a diagnosis other than multiple sclerosis.

Lumbar puncture is used to assess cerebrospinal fluid (CSF) pressure. High pressure occurs with pseudotumor cerebri (idiopathic intracranial hypertension); low pressure, with CSF hypovolemia from a CSF leak.

Lumbar puncture is indicated in cases of neurologic complications of infectious diseases, including AIDS, Lyme disease, and any suspected acute, subacute, or chronic infection (viral, bacterial, or fungal). Other indications for lumbar puncture are meningeal carcinomatosis, selected indications in non-Hodgkin lymphoma, and certain neuropathies (Guillain-Barré syndrome, acute inflammatory demyelinating polyneuropathy, and chronic inflammatory demyelinating polyradiculopathy).

Post–dural puncture headache occurs in approximately one-third of patients who undergo lumbar puncture. These headaches relate to some degree to the size of the needle used and the leakage of CSF through a dural rent or tear. A 20-gauge needle is recommended.

Contraindications for Lumbar Puncture

Suppuration in the skin and deeper tissues overlying the spinal canal, anticoagulation therapy, or bleeding diathesis are contraindications for lumbar puncture. A minimum of 1 to 2 hours should elapse between lumbar puncture and initiation of heparin therapy. If the platelet count is less than 20×10^9/L, platelets should be transfused before lumbar puncture is performed. The use of aspirin is not a contraindication to lumbar puncture. Use of other antiplatelet agents, such as clopidogrel, *may* increase the risk of bleeding; if possible to do so safely, discontinue use of the drug for 5 to 7 days before performing lumbar puncture. If this is not possible, lumbar puncture is still safe; we have not found any complications from this procedure in patients who are using clopidogrel or aspirin (or both).

Increased intracranial pressure due to a focal intracranial mass lesion is a contraindication. Lumbar puncture is dangerous when papilledema is due to an intracranial mass, but it is safe (and has been used therapeutically) in pseudotumor cerebri, in which the increased pressure is diffusely distributed and changes in the pressure due to CSF removal do not increase the risk of cerebral herniation. In complete spinal block or stenosis, lumbar puncture may aggravate the signs of spinal cord disease.

- Perform lumbar puncture only after a thorough clinical evaluation.
- Increased IgG synthesis and oligoclonal banding in the CSF are nonspecific findings, but they are most suggestive of multiple sclerosis.
- CSF pressure is high in pseudotumor cerebri (idiopathic intracranial hypertension).
- CSF pressure is low with CSF hypovolemia.
- Lumbar puncture is dangerous when an intracranial mass is present, with or without papilledema.
- Lumbar puncture is safe in pseudotumor cerebri, and it is therapeutic.
- Lumbar puncture aggravates the signs of spinal cord disease in complete spinal block.

SUMMARY

- The history and examination findings suggest localization to the level and side of the nervous system.
- The temporal profile is then used to determine a differential diagnosis.
- MRI is the study of choice for most degenerative spinal disorders.
- Epilepsy is a clinical diagnosis, not an EEG diagnosis.
- A normal EEG does not rule out epilepsy.
- CSF pressure is high in pseudotumor cerebri (idiopathic intracranial hypertension).
- CSF pressure is low with CSF hypovolemia.

45.

NEUROLOGIC DISORDERS CATEGORIZED BY ANATOMICAL INVOLVEMENT

Lyell K. Jones Jr, MD, Brian A. Crum, MD, Eduardo E. Benarroch, MD,

and Robert D. Brown Jr, MD

GOALS

- Review neurologic disease entities by anatomical level: supratentorial, posterior fossa, spinal cord, and peripheral nervous system.
- Recognize signs and symptoms of common neurologic disease entities.

SUPRATENTORIAL LEVEL: SYMPTOMS AND CLINICAL CORRELATIONS

The supratentorial region includes all structures of the nervous system inside the skull and above the tentorium cerebelli (ie, the top of the cerebellum), primarily the cerebral hemispheres. Symptoms and signs related to disorders of the cerebral cortex may include alterations in cognition and consciousness. Unilateral neurologic symptoms involving a single neurologic symptom (such as numbness [sensory system] or weakness [motor system]) commonly localize to the cerebral cortex. Abnormalities of speech and language are localized to the dominant cerebral hemisphere (typically the left side, even in most left-handers), whereas abnormalities of the nondominant hemisphere may lead to visuospatial deficits, confusion, or neglect of the contralateral side of the body. Abnormalities in the subcortical region may lead to weakness or numbness; they typically involve more than 1 limb. Abnormalities in the basal ganglia may lead to movement disorders, including tremor, bradykinesia (as in Parkinson disease), and chorea (as in Huntington disease). Disorders of the thalamus, another subcortical but supratentorial structure, typically cause unilateral sensory abnormalities, language problems, and cognitive changes. The hypothalamus is important in many functions that affect everyday steady-state conditions, including temperature regulation, hunger, water regulation, sleep, endocrine functions, cardiovascular functions, and regulation of the autonomic nervous system. Cortical and subcortical abnormalities may also lead to visual system deficits, usually homonymous visual defects of the contralateral visual field.

BRAIN DEATH

Brain death is the absence of function of the cerebral cortex and brainstem. Brain death is diagnosed clinically by showing lack of brainstem reflexes: pupillary response, corneal reflexes, oculocephalic (doll's eye) and oculovestibular (cold caloric) reflexes, gag reflex, and spontaneous respiration. Adjunctive tests include electroencephalography (EEG), somatosensory evoked potentials, and angiography.

MINIMALLY CONSCIOUS STATE

The minimally conscious state is a condition of severely altered consciousness in which minimal but definite behavioral evidence of self-awareness or environmental awareness is demonstrated. It is a disorder of limited responsiveness in which patients retain awareness, but their responses are so deficient that the evidence of their awareness may be difficult to detect. The minimally conscious state is distinguished from the vegetative state by the presence of behaviors associated with conscious awareness. The minimally conscious state may be a temporary state in a continuum from coma to vegetative state to minimally conscious state to normalcy, or, unfortunately, it may also be a permanent state.

In young people with traumatic brain injury, it is important to recognize the minimally conscious state early in the course of the disease since it carries a better prognosis than the vegetative state. However, the prognosis for both of these conditions depends on the age of the patient, the duration of the condition, and the cause (traumatic brain injury in the young carries the best prognosis, whereas hypoxic/ischemic or hypoglycemic brain injury at any age carries the worst).

PERSISTENT VEGETATIVE STATE

Persistent vegetative state is the absence of cerebral cortex function with normal brainstem function (deafferentated state). The patient has no detectable awareness and no purposeful interaction with the environment but, unlike a patient in a coma, is wakeful and has sleep-wake cycles.

LOCKED-IN SYNDROME

Locked-in syndrome is characterized by normal cerebral cortex function with no brainstem function. The lesion usually is in the pons and causes quadriplegia and the inability to speak, swallow, and move the eyes horizontally (ie, the de-efferentated state). The patient, however, is wakeful and aware but cannot communicate verbally because of the neurologic deficits. Often, though, these patients can communicate with eye blinks and vertical eye movements. This can also occur with severe neuromuscular weakness, such as in myasthenia gravis, Guillain-Barré syndrome, and botulism.

STUPOR AND COMA

For a person to stay awake, the cerebral hemispheres and reticular activating system must be intact. Patients with dysfunction of only 1 cerebral hemisphere have a focal neurologic deficit but are awake. Patients with a large unilateral cerebral lesion may go into stupor or coma if the lesion causes shifting and pressure changes in other parts of the brain, such as the opposite hemisphere or brainstem. These patients can have focal neurologic signs. Patients with brainstem lesions that directly affect the ascending reticular activating system are in coma but, again, have focal brainstem signs. Persons who feign coma have no focal signs, no abnormal reflexes, normal caloric responses, and a normal EEG. They account for a small percentage of patients with stupor and coma. The most common, potentially reversible causes of stupor and coma are toxic, metabolic, and infectious problems that affect both cerebral hemispheres diffusely (the famed "toxic/metabolic encephalopathy"). Thus, most patients in stupor or coma have an underlying systemic problem.

- Large unilateral cerebral lesions that cause a shift and pressure changes in the other hemisphere or brainstem produce focal neurologic signs together with coma.

- Brainstem lesions that cause coma also produce focal signs.

- Persons who feign coma have no focal signs, no abnormal reflexes, normal caloric responses, and a normal EEG.

- The most common reversible causes of stupor and coma are toxic, metabolic, and infectious problems that affect both cerebral hemispheres diffusely.

Patients with toxic or metabolic encephalopathies have changes in mental status and awareness before going into stupor or coma, but they typically have no focal neurologic signs. Corneal reflexes are lost early in the process, but pupillary reflexes remain. Ocular motility, tested with the doll's eye sign (oculocephalic reflexes) and the cold caloric response (oculo-vestibular reflex), is fully intact, at least early in the disease.

- Patients with systemic encephalopathies typically have no focal signs.

ACUTE CONFUSIONAL STATES

Acute confusional state is a manifestation of malfunction of the cerebral cortex and reticular activating system. Acute confusional states are abrupt, of recent onset, and often associated with fluctuations in the state of awareness and cognition. They are manifested by confusion, inattention, disorientation, and delirium. Thus, patients may be inattentive, dazed, stuporous, restless, agitated, or excited and may have marked autonomic dysfunction and visual and tactile hallucinations. Abnormal motor manifestations are common, including paratonia, asterixis, tremor, and myoclonus. The usual etiologic factors of acute confusional states are toxic, metabolic, traumatic, or infectious conditions; organ failure of any sort; or ictal or postictal encephalopathies. Withdrawal states from alcohol, benzodiazepines, and barbiturates are also important causes of acute confusion or delirium.

DEMENTIA

Dementia is chronic malfunction of the cerebral cortex or subcortical structures (or both) with normal function of the brainstem. It is a clinical state characterized by a marked loss of function in multiple cognitive domains and not resulting from an impaired level of arousal. Besides memory, other higher cognitive functions are impaired, including visuospatial, calculation, language, judgment, personality, and motor planning. The presence of dementia does not necessarily imply irreversibility, a progressive course, or any specific disease. Dementia is not a disease but an entity with various causes (Box 45.1). The most common causes of degenerative dementia are Alzheimer disease (AD), dementia with Lewy bodies, and frontotemporal dementias.

A small percentage of patients have reversible causes of dementia. These include the effects of medications, depression, thyroid disease, central nervous system (CNS) infections, vitamin deficiencies, and structural brain lesions (eg, neoplasms, subdural hematomas, and symptomatic hydrocephalus).

- Dementia is the potential result of many different diseases, a minority of which are reversible.

Alzheimer Disease

AD is the most common cause of dementia. Generally, patients present first with difficulties of memory (anterograde amnesia), but eventually difficulties develop in other cognitive domains, including aphasia, apraxia, or agnosia. These patients may also have various behavioral and psychiatric manifestations.

Mild cognitive impairment (MCI) consists of loss of memory (usually anterograde amnesia) or other cognitive function that is clearly evident at bedside testing but does not interfere with everyday function. In about 50% of patients, amnestic MCI progresses to AD within 4 years, and MCI eventually progresses to AD in almost all patients. Magnetic resonance imaging (MRI), with focus in the temporal lobes, may detect atrophy early in the mesial temporal lobe of MCI patients at risk of AD.

Pharmacologic treatment may transiently improve cognitive function in AD (Box 45.2). Some symptoms of AD are thought to be due to partial depletion of acetylcholine in the brain. Currently available, centrally active, noncompetitive, reversible cholinesterase inhibitors, including donepezil, rivastigmine, and galantamine, may improve symptoms slightly and slow the decline of cognitive function.

Lewy Body Disease

Patients with Lewy body disease typically exhibit parkinsonism, fluctuations of cognitive function, visual hallucinations, and rapid eye movement sleep behavior disorder. Antipsychotic medications may trigger a neuroleptic malignant-type syndrome in these patients. Cholinesterase inhibitors may improve hallucinations and other symptoms.

Frontotemporal Dementia

After AD, frontotemporal dementia is the second most common cause of degenerative dementia in patients younger than 65 years. These patients may present with difficulties with executive function, inappropriate behavior, or aphasia.

Normal-Pressure Hydrocephalus

Normal-pressure hydrocephalus (NPH) is a potentially reversible cause of cognitive dysfunction. The typical triad includes dementia, a gait disorder, and urinary incontinence, although sometimes only dementia and the gait disorder are present. A shuffling, magnetic gait (as if the feet are stuck to the floor) is most common. Computed tomography (CT) or MRI shows disproportionate enlargement of the ventricular system without any obstructive lesions.

Diagnosis of Dementia

The diagnosis of dementia is based primarily on a complete history and physical examination, including a mental status examination. Several bedside tests of mental status are used to help determine the primary cognitive domain affected, including memory, attention, language, semantic knowledge, and visuospatial function. For example, memory is affected early in AD, whereas executive, language, and visuospatial impairment may be the first manifestation of other dementias.

Neuroimaging should be done for all persons with dementia. MRI is preferred, although CT can exclude structural (and possibly reversible) causes of dementia (eg, NPH, tumor, subdural hematoma, and stroke). MRI has the advantage of detecting atrophy in mesial temporal lobes and hippocampal structures in AD. Neuropsychometric testing may also be considered, especially for cases that are mild, questionable, or atypical. Lumbar puncture may be indicated for persons who have had rapid onset of symptoms, persons younger than 55 years who have dementia, and persons with immunosuppression, possible CNS infection, reactive serum syphilis or Lyme serologic findings, or metastatic cancer without findings on an imaging study. EEG may be useful in evaluating rapidly progressive dementia, such as Creutzfeldt-Jakob disease. In these patients, fluid-attenuated inversion recovery (FLAIR) MRI techniques can also detect abnormalities in the cerebral

Box 45.3 CLASSIFICATION OF SEIZURES

Partial (focal) seizures
  Simple partial seizures
    Partial simple sensory
    Partial simple motor
    Partial simple special sensory (unusual smells or tastes)
    Speech arrest or unusual vocalizations
  Complex partial seizures
    Consciousness impaired at onset
    Simple partial onset followed by impaired consciousness
  Evolving to generalized tonic-clonic convulsions (secondary generalized tonic-clonic seizures)
    Simple evolving to generalized tonic-clonic
    Complex evolving to generalized tonic-clonic (including those with simple partial onset)
  True auras (actually, simple partial seizures)
Generalized seizures—convulsive or nonconvulsive (primary generalized seizures—generalized from onset)
  Absence and atypical absence
  Myoclonic
  Clonic
  Tonic
  Tonic-clonic
  Atonic
Unclassified epileptic seizures (includes some neonatal seizures)

cortex, basal ganglia, or thalamus when the findings of a standard MRI study are negative. The presence of increased levels of 14-3-3 protein or neuron-specific enolase in the cerebrospinal fluid (CSF), although a nonspecific finding, strongly supports the diagnosis of Creutzfeldt-Jakob disease.

SEIZURE DISORDERS

Seizures are electroclinical events, and *epilepsy* indicates a tendency for recurrent seizures. A classification of seizures is given in Box 45.3.

The proper treatment of epilepsy depends on accurate diagnosis of the seizure type, identification of the cause (if possible), and management of psychosocial problems. The EEG (preferably after the patient is sleep deprived) can be important in the classification of seizure type. MRI is also used to evaluate for focal or structural lesions. Much of the diagnosis rests on a supportive history. An aura and a period of altered mental status after the spell (*postictal confusion*) are highly suggestive of an epileptic seizure. The EEG is also important in deciding whether to treat a first unprovoked seizure. The risk of recurrent seizures is high if the initial EEG shows epileptiform activity and low if the EEG findings are normal.

Causes

Seizures occur at any age, but approximately 70% of all patients with epilepsy have their first seizure before age 20. Age distribution for the onset of epilepsy is bimodal, with the second most common group being the elderly population. Both the cause

and the type of epilepsy are related to age at onset. However, the cause may not be found in many patients. Neonatal seizures are often due to congenital defects or prenatal injury, and head trauma is often the cause of focal seizures in young adults. Brain tumors and vascular disease are major known causes of seizures in later life. Seizures often occur during withdrawal from alcohol, barbiturates, or benzodiazepines in young and old adults. Seizures also occur with the use of drugs such as cocaine, usually in young adults. Metabolic derangements (eg, hypoglycemia, hypocalcemia, hyponatremia, and hypernatremia) can occur at any age, as can infections (eg, meningitis and encephalitis). Metabolic abnormalities usually cause primary generalized tonic-clonic seizures and rarely focal or multifocal seizures. CNS infections usually cause partial and secondary generalized tonic-clonic seizures.

Pseudoseizures

Psychogenic spells (ie, pseudoseizures or nonepileptic seizures) are sudden changes in behavior or mentation not associated with any physiologic cause or abnormal paroxysmal discharge of electrical activity from the brain. They are often the cause of so-called intractable seizures. Effective treatment is elusive. A favorable outcome may be associated with an independent lifestyle, the absence of coexisting epilepsy, and a formal psychologic approach to therapy.

- Up to 70% of patients with epilepsy have their first seizure before age 20, although the fastest-growing population with epilepsy is the elderly.

- The cause and type of epilepsy are related to age at onset.

- Head trauma is a major cause of focal seizures in young adults.

- Brain tumors and vascular disease are major causes of seizures in older persons.

- Seizures occur with withdrawal from alcohol, barbiturates, and benzodiazepines.

- Seizures occur during the use of cocaine (usually in young adults).

- Pseudoseizures are often the cause of so-called intractable seizures.

Anticonvulsant Therapy

Drugs used to treat seizures are listed in Table 45.1. Monotherapy is the treatment of choice. The dosage of the drug may be increased as high as necessary and to as much as can be tolerated. The coadministration of antiepileptic drugs has not been shown to have more antiseizure efficacy than the administration of only 1 drug without concurrently increasing toxicity. In studies of a large population, a particular drug may be shown to be more efficacious and less toxic, but for a given patient, another drug may be more effective or have fewer side effects. Older antiepileptic drugs include phenytoin,

Table 45.1 GUIDANCE FOR USE OF ANTIEPILEPTIC DRUGS

CRITERIA	POSSIBILITIES	DRUG
Type of seizures	GTCSs	PHT, CBZ, VPA, lamotrigine, topiramate
	Partial seizures with or without secondary GTCSs	PHT, CBZ, VPA, PB, lamotrigine, topiramate, zonisamide, levetiracetam
	Absence seizures	Ethosuximide, VPA, lamotrigine
	Myoclonic seizures	VPA, clonazepam, lamotrigine, zonisamide
	Atonic, akinetic, or mixed seizures	VPA, felbamate, topiramate, lamotrigine
Use of other drugs metabolized in the liver	Drugs that do not affect metabolism of other drugs	Gabapentin, tiagabine, lamotrigine, zonisamide, levetiracetam
Avoidance of oral contraceptive pill failure	Drugs with no or minimal effect on contraceptive metabolism	VPA, clonazepam, gabapentin, tiagabine, lamotrigine, zonisamide, levetiracetam

Abbreviations: CBZ, carbamazepine; GTCS, generalized tonic-clonic seizure; PB, phenobarbital; PHT, phenytoin; VPA, valproic acid.

carbamazepine, valproic acid, benzodiazepines, and ethosuximide. Simple and complex partial seizures are most likely to be controlled with phenytoin and carbamazepine, whereas secondary generalized tonic-clonic seizures respond equally well to phenytoin, carbamazepine, or valproic acid. Idiopathic generalized epilepsy with absence seizures is well controlled with ethosuximide. Valproic acid controls all forms of generalized seizures. Extended-release formulations are available for carbamazepine and valproic acid, and a rectal formulation is available for diazepam.

The newer anticonvulsant drugs include gabapentin, tiagabine, lamotrigine, topiramate, felbamate, zonisamide, oxcarbazepine, levetiracetam, pregabalin, and lacosamide. These agents generally have less potential for drug interactions and fewer side effects than the older drugs. They are indicated as add-on therapy for partial seizures. Oxcarbazepine and levetiracetam are also commonly used as monotherapy for partial seizures. Lamotrigine and topiramate are commonly used as monotherapy for generalized seizures. Because the efficacy, cost, and dosing schedule (twice daily) are similar for many of these new anticonvulsants, tolerability is frequently the major determinant in choosing a particular drug.

Anticonvulsants have both neurologic and systemic side effects. Dose-initiation side effects such as fatigue, dizziness, incoordination, and mental slowing are common in most patients and can be prevented with slow introduction of the drug. Dose-related side effects may limit the use of a particular drug in a given patient. A dose-related side effect common to most drugs is cognitive impairment. Other neurologic side effects include cerebellar ataxia (phenytoin), diplopia (carbamazepine), tremor (valproic acid), and chorea or myoclonus (phenytoin and carbamazepine). Idiosyncratic side effects are rare, unpredictable, severe, and sometimes life-threatening. Idiosyncratic and systemic side effects are listed in Table 45.2.

Many antiepileptic drugs are metabolized in the liver and are responsible for important drug interactions. Liver enzyme inducers (eg, carbamazepine, phenobarbital, phenytoin, primidone, oxcarbazepine, felbamate, and topiramate) increase metabolism and decrease the efficacy of oral contraceptives in preventing pregnancy. Valproic acid and felbamate are enzyme inhibitors and increase the levels of other anticonvulsants.

Table 45.2 SYSTEMIC SIDE EFFECTS OF ANTIEPILEPTIC DRUGS

SIDE EFFECT	DRUG MOST COMMONLY INVOLVED
Skin rash & Stevens-Johnson syndrome	10% risk with lamotrigine, CBZ, or PHT; 5% risk with other AEDs; least risk with VPA *Note*: **Topiramate & zonisamide are contraindicated for patients with allergy to sulfa drugs**
Liver failure	Highest risk with VPA & felbamate Risk increased in infants with mental retardation & receiving polytherapy or with underlying metabolic disease or poor nutritional status
Bone marrow suppression	Highest risk with felbamate & CBZ
Gum hypertrophy, hirsutism, acne, osteoporosis	Phenytoin
Weight gain, hair loss, tremor	VPA
Weight loss	Felbamate, topiramate
Headache, insomnia	Felbamate
Behavioral & cognitive disturbances	Barbiturates, benzodiazepines, topiramte, levetiracetam
Kidney stones	Topiramate, zonisamide
Side Effect	Drug Most Commonly Involved
Hyponatremia	CBZ, oxcarbazepine
Atrioventricular conduction defect	CBZ, PHT
Neural tube defect	VPA > CBZ, but all AEDs are potentially teratogenic

Abbreviations: AED, antiepileptic drug; CBZ, carbamazepine; PHT, phenytoin; VPA, valproic acid.

Gabapentin has the advantage of fewer drug interactions because it is eliminated primarily by renal excretion. It may be safer than other anticonvulsants in the management of seizures in patients with porphyria.

Special issues must be considered when managing epilepsy in pregnancy. Seizure control is attempted first with monotherapy, with the lowest possible dose of anticonvulsant and monitoring of drug levels. Essentially all anticonvulsant drugs have the potential to cause developmental abnormalities. Valproic acid and, to a lesser extent, carbamazepine are selectively associated with an increased risk of neural tube defects.

- The treatment of choice for seizures is monotherapy.

- All anticonvulsant drugs have the potential to cause developmental abnormalities.

- Valproic acid (and, to a lesser extent, carbamazepine) is associated with a higher likelihood of birth defects than the other anticonvulsants.

When to Start and Stop Anticonvulsant Therapy

Decisions about when to start and stop anticonvulsant therapy are difficult and there is simply no easy algorithm on which to rely. The decision to begin anticonvulsant therapy after a first seizure should be individualized for each patient. The decision depends on the risk of additional seizures, the risk of seizure-related injury, the loss of employment or driving privileges, and other psychosocial factors. An important decision is whether a single generalized tonic seizure is provoked, for example, by sleep deprivation, alcohol, or concurrent illness. After the first seizure, the risk of recurrence ranges from 30% to 60%, with higher risks for patients with an abnormal EEG and a remote symptomatic cause (Box 45.4). After a second seizure, the risk of recurrence increases to 80% to 90%.

For many patients who have been seizure free for 1 to 2 years, anticonvulsant therapy can be discontinued. The benefit of discontinuing therapy should be weighed against the possibility of seizure recurrence and its potential adverse

---

Box 45.4 RISK FACTORS FOR RECURRENCE AFTER THE FIRST SEIZURE

Age >60 y
No precipitating factor identified (eg, no sleep deprivation or alcohol use)
Partial seizure
Abnormal neurologic examination
Abnormal electroencephalogram (spikes or nonspecific)
Abnormal imaging study
Other factors
    Family history of seizures (in first-degree relative)
    History of febrile seizures
    Onset during sleep
    Postictal Todd paralysis
Occupational risk

---

consequences. In adults, relapse occurs in 26% to 63% of patients within 1 to 2 years after therapy is discontinued. Predictors of relapse are an abnormal EEG before or during medication withdrawal, abnormal findings on neurologic examination, frequent seizures before entering remission, or mental retardation. To lessen the chance of seizures after discontinuing therapy, withdrawal should not proceed faster than a 20% reduction in dose every 5 half-lives.

Anticonvulsant Blood Levels

Measurement of anticonvulsant blood levels is readily available and helps attain the best control of seizures. It is important to remember that therapeutic levels are represented by a bell-shaped curve and that patients with well-controlled seizures are included under the bell-shaped curve. Seizures are well controlled in many patients who have anticonvulsant blood levels below or above the therapeutic range. The anticonvulsant dose should *never* be changed on the basis of blood levels alone. Remember that toxicity is a clinical phenomenon, *not* a laboratory phenomenon. Measurement of anticonvulsant blood levels ensures that patients are taking their medication and helps determine whether new symptoms might be related to toxicity from the medication.

- Therapeutic levels are represented by a bell-shaped curve.

- The dose of anticonvulsant should never be changed on the basis of blood levels alone.

- Toxicity is a clinical phenomenon, not a laboratory phenomenon.

If a patient is receiving therapy for epilepsy and has breakthrough seizures, several factors should be considered, including the following:

1. Compliance issues

2. Excessive use of alcohol or other recreational drugs

3. Psychologic and physiologic stress (eg, anxiety or lack of sleep)

4. Systemic disease of any type, organ failure of any type, or systemic infection

5. A new cause of seizures (eg, neoplasm)

6. Newly prescribed medication, including other anticonvulsants (ie, polypharmacy) and over-the-counter drugs

7. Toxic levels of anticonvulsants (with definite clinical toxicity)

8. Nonepileptic spells (eg, psychogenic spells)

9. Progressive CNS lesion not identified previously with neuroimaging or lumbar puncture

If no cause is found, the anticonvulsant dosage must be readjusted or the drug replaced with another.

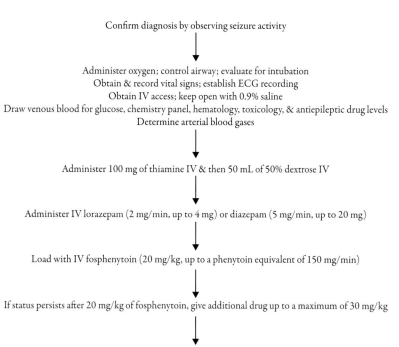

Confirm diagnosis by observing seizure activity

↓

Administer oxygen; control airway; evaluate for intubation
Obtain & record vital signs; establish ECG recording
Obtain IV access; keep open with 0.9% saline
Draw venous blood for glucose, chemistry panel, hematology, toxicology, & antiepileptic drug levels
Determine arterial blood gases

↓

Administer 100 mg of thiamine IV & then 50 mL of 50% dextrose IV

↓

Administer IV lorazepam (2 mg/min, up to 4 mg) or diazepam (5 mg/min, up to 20 mg)

↓

Load with IV fosphenytoin (20 mg/kg, up to a phenytoin equivalent of 150 mg/min)

↓

If status persists after 20 mg/kg of fosphenytoin, give additional drug up to a maximum of 30 mg/kg

↓

If status persists, transfer patient to ICU because intubation, ventilation, or vasopressor may be needed
Phenobarbital 20 mg/kg IV, up to 60 mg/min
If status persists, give general anesthesia with pentobarbital, midazolam, or propofol

Figure 45.1 Algorithm for the Management of Status Epilepticus. ECG indicates electrocardiographic; ICU, intensive care unit; IV, intravenous.

Status Epilepticus

Status epilepticus is a medical emergency and a life-threatening condition. It can be defined by the duration of the seizure (eg, >5 minutes) or by whether repetitive seizures occur without recovery between seizures. The most common causes of status epilepticus include stopping the use of an anticonvulsant agent, alcohol toxicity or withdrawal, recreational drug toxicity, and CNS trauma or infection. Rarely, status epilepticus is the initial presenting sign of epilepsy. The management of status epilepticus is summarized in Figure 45.1.

Nonconvulsive status epilepticus may cause an acute confusional state or stupor and coma, especially in the elderly. In these cases, there is often very subtle rhythmic motor activity in the limbs or face. EEG is a critical diagnostic tool because nonconvulsive status epilepticus must be treated as quickly and vigorously as convulsive status epilepticus.

- Status epilepticus is a life-threatening medical emergency.

- The seizure lasts >5 minutes, or there are repetitive seizures without recovery.

- Administer 100 mg of thiamine intravenously and then 50 mL of 50% dextrose intravenously.

- Slowly administer lorazepam intravenously.

- Antiepileptic treatment should begin with a loading dose of fosphenytoin.

- Cardiorespiratory monitoring is required if fosphenytoin or phenytoin is infused rapidly.

- Nonconvulsive status epilepticus may be a cause of acute confusional state and is manifest with subtle rhythmic motor activity; EEG is required for diagnosis.

Headache may indicate intracranial or systemic disease, but more commonly it is a primary disorder. Some headaches have a readily identified organic cause. Classic migraine and cluster headaches form distinctive and easily recognized clinical entities, although their pathophysiologic mechanisms are not fully understood. The major challenge is that often neither the location nor the intensity of the pain is a reliable clue to the nature of the problem. Episodic tension headache and migraine can be difficult to distinguish.

- Neither location nor intensity of headache pain is a reliable clue to the nature of the problem.

Conditions alerting physicians that a headache may have a serious cause are listed in Box 45.5. Chronic recurrent headaches are rarely, if ever, caused by eye strain, chronic sinusitis, dental problems, food allergies, high blood pressure, or temporomandibular joint syndrome. Headache without other neurologic signs or symptoms is rarely caused by a brain tumor. Serious causes of headache in which neuroimaging findings may be normal and lead to a false sense of reassurance are listed in Box 45.6.

- Any "worst headache of my life" or headache that is maximal at instantaneous onset warrants urgent evaluation.

- Headache with abnormal neurologic findings, papilledema, obscuration of vision, or diplopia warrants further evaluation.

- Headache without other neurologic signs or symptoms is rarely caused by a brain tumor.

"Worst headache of my life"

Headache that is maximal at instantaneous onset

Headache in a person not prone to headache, especially a middle-aged or elderly patient

Headache associated with abnormal neurologic findings, papilledema, obscurations of vision, or diplopia

Headache that changes with different positions or increases with exertion, coughing, or sneezing

Changes in headache patterns—character, frequency, or severity—in someone who has had chronic recurring headaches

Headache that awakens one from sound sleep

Headache associated with trauma

Headache associated with systemic symptoms (eg, fever, malaise, or weight loss)

Migraine and Tension Headache

Migraine is defined by multiple attacks of severe headache, often unilateral, which last several hours and are accompanied by photophobia, phonophobia, and osmophobia; nausea; a pounding quality to the headache; and an increase in the intensity with light activity. Most patients gravitate to a dark, quiet room and try to sleep. Many migraineurs experience an aura before the headache onset. The common auras are visual, with flashing lights, jagged lines, or scintillating scotomas. Tension headaches can be severe but are often bilateral, squeezing or tight in quality, and lack all the other associated symptoms that occur in migraine.

Pharmacotherapy along with psychologic and physical therapy are components of an approach to treating headache. An overview of pharmacologic treatment is shown in Box 45.7 and Table 45.3.

Abortive headache medications cover a wide range that includes simple analgesics, anxiolytics, nonsteroidal anti-inflammatory drugs, ergots, corticosteroids, major tranquilizers, and narcotics. Drugs that are effective in aborting acute migraine attacks include dihydroergotamine mesylate (DHE-45), sumatriptan, and related serotonin 1B/1D receptor agonists (the triptans: zolmitriptan, naratriptan, rizatriptan, almotriptan, eletriptan, frovatriptan, and others).

Giant cell or temporal arteritis

Glaucoma

Trigeminal or glossopharyngeal neuralgia

Lesions around sella turcica

Warning leak of aneurysm (sentinel bleed)

Inflammation, infection, or neoplastic invasion of leptomeninges

Cervical spondylosis

Pseudotumor cerebri

Low intracranial pressure syndromes (cerebrospinal fluid leaks)

Abortive medications

   Triptans

   Ergotamine

   Nonsteroidal anti-inflammatory drugs

   Dihydroergotamine mesylate (DHE-45)

   Prochlorperazine, metoclopramide, chlorpromazine

   Magnesium sulfate (1.0 g intravenously)

   Methylprednisolone

Prophylactic medications

   β-Blockers

   Tricyclic antidepressants

   Valproic acid

   Topiramate

   Gabapentin

   Verapamil

   Botulinum toxin type A

DHE-45 and sumatriptan can be administered parenterally or intranasally to patients who have severe nausea or vomiting. Sumatriptan and other vasoconstrictor drugs are contraindicated in patients with migraine associated with a focal neurologic deficit and in patients with symptomatic coronary artery disease.

Prophylactic medication should be given when the attacks occur more than 2 or 3 times weekly or even less frequently if they are incapacitating, associated with focal neurologic signs, or of prolonged duration. When prophylactic medication is indicated, the following should be observed:

1. Begin with a low dose and increase it slowly.

2. Perform an adequate trial of medication (1–2 months).

3. Confirm that the patient is not taking drugs that may interact with the headache agent (eg, vasodilators, estrogens, or oral contraceptives).

Table 45.3 **CHOICE OF TRIPTAN ACCORDING TO THE ATTACK**

PATTERN	DRUG OF CHOICE[a]
Daytime attack, moderate to severe	Almotriptan (12.5 mg) Eletriptan (80 mg) Rizatriptan (10 mg)
Severe nausea or vomiting	Rizatriptan (10 mg) Zolmitriptan (2.5 mg) Zolmitriptan NS (5 mg)
Pain that awakens the patient	Sumatriptan SC (6 mg) Zolmitriptan NS (5 mg)
Frequent, long-duration attacks	Frovatriptan (2.5 mg twice daily) Naratriptan (1–2.5 mg twice daily) Zolmitriptan (2.5 mg twice daily)

Abbreviations: NS, nasal spray; SC, subcutaneously.

[a] If tolerance is a concern, choose almotriptan (12.5 mg) or naratriptan (2.5 mg).

4. Determine that a female patient is not pregnant and that she is using effective contraception.

5. Attempt to taper and discontinue use of prophylactic medication after the headaches are well controlled.

6. Avoid polypharmacy and narcotic use.

7. Establish a strong doctor-patient partnership; emphasize that management of headache is often a team effort, with the patient having a role equal to that of the physician.

8. The best option is *no* medication.

Drugs used for migraine prophylaxis include β-blockers, calcium channel blockers, amitriptyline or nortriptyline, valproic acid, and other anticonvulsants (gabapentin or topiramate). The most widely used β-blocker is propranolol; others are atenolol, metoprolol, and timolol. Valproic acid is an excellent preventive agent, but its use may be limited because of weight gain and hair loss, and it is a less desirable choice for women of childbearing age. Amitriptyline is particularly useful in patients with migraine and chronic-type tension headache. Verapamil is a good alternative to β-blockers in athletes. There is evidence that topiramate is effective in prevention of migraine at a dosage of 50 mg twice daily. Botulinum toxin is also useful in some patients for preventive therapy.

Naproxen and other nonsteroidal anti-inflammatory drugs produce analgesia through alternate pathways that do not appear to induce dependence. They may be useful for the following headaches: migraine, for both acute attacks and prophylaxis; menstrual migraine (especially naproxen); benign exertional migraine and sex-induced headache (especially indomethacin); cluster variants (eg, chronic paroxysmal hemicrania, episodic paroxysmal hemicrania, and hemicrania continua); idiopathic stabbing headache, jabs-and-jolts, needle-in-the-eye, and ice-pick headaches (indomethacin is often effective); muscle contraction headaches; mixed headaches; and ergotamine-induced headache.

Cluster Headache

Cluster headache, unlike migraine, is uncommon and predominantly affects men. Its onset usually occurs in the late 20s but may occur at any age. The main feature is periodicity. On average, the cluster period lasts 2 to 3 months and typically occurs every 1 or 2 years. Attacks occur at a frequency of 1 to 3 times daily and tend to be nocturnal in more than 50% of patients. The average period of remission is about 2 years between clusters. Cluster headache is not associated with an aura. The pain reaches a peak in about 10 to 15 minutes and lasts 45 to 60 minutes. It is excruciating, penetrating, usually non-throbbing, and maximal behind the eye and in the region of the supraorbital nerve and temples. Typically, attacks of pain are unilateral. The autonomic features are both sympathetic paresis and parasympathetic overreaction. They may include 1) ipsilateral lacrimation, injection of the conjunctiva, and nasal stuffiness or rhinorrhea and 2) ptosis and miosis (ptosis may become permanent), periorbital swelling, and bradycardia. The scalp, face, and carotid artery may be tender. In contrast to migraineurs, patients with cluster headaches tend to be hyperactive during a headache.

- Cluster headache is uncommon and affects mostly men, with onset in the 20s.

- Periodicity is the main feature.

- The cluster period lasts 2–3 months.

- Cluster headache is not associated with an aura.

- The pain peaks in 10–15 minutes and lasts 45–60 minutes.

- The pain typically is unilateral, excruciating, penetrating, non throbbing, and maximal behind the eye.

- In >50% of patients, the pain is nocturnal.

- Autonomic features are present.

Abortive therapy includes oxygen inhalation (5–8 L/min for 10 minutes); sumatriptan; dihydroergotamine; ergotamine suppositories; corticosteroids (eg, 8 mg dexamethasone); local anesthesia (eg, intranasal 4% lidocaine); and capsaicin in the ipsilateral nostril. Sumatriptan is the drug of choice for management of an acute attack of cluster headache. Surgical intervention may be indicated under certain circumstances for chronic cluster headache but never for episodic headache.

Prophylactic treatment is the mainstay of cluster headache treatment. Calcium channel blockers (verapamil) are widely used. The usual daily dose of lithium is 600 to 900 mg in divided doses. Its effectiveness is known within 1 week. Topiramate has proved useful in cluster headache treatment. Methysergide is effective in the early course of the disease and least effective in later years. It must be used with caution because of the risk of retroperitoneal fibrosis. Ergotamine at bedtime is particularly beneficial for nocturnal attacks. Corticosteroids are helpful for short-term treatment, especially for patients resistant to the above drugs or to a combination of the above. The usual dosage is 40 mg prednisone daily tapered over 3 weeks. An effective treatment for chronic cluster headache is the combination of verapamil and lithium. Valproic acid may also be useful.

- Prophylaxis of cluster headaches is the mainstay of treatment.

- Calcium channel blockers are widely used.

- Methysergide is effective early in the disease but must be used with caution.

- Ergotamine is effective for nocturnal attacks.

- Corticosteroids are helpful short-term.

Typical Clinical Scenarios

- Migraine: A young patient has recurrent, episodic (about once monthly), and severe headaches. Often, the headache is unilateral and associated with nausea, vomiting, and photophobia. MRI findings are normal.

- Tension headache: A young patient has a 3-year history of headaches, which occur almost every month and last several days. They are bilateral and are not associated with any neurologic deficit, nausea, or vomiting.

- Cluster headache: A 27-year-old man has a 1-month history of severe, excruciating headaches that occur daily and last for approximately 1 hour. He had a similar episode 1 year ago, in which the headache lasted 3 months and then resolved completely. The pain is unilateral and worse behind the right eye. The right eye becomes red and teary during the headache.

Analgesic-Overuse Headache

Chronic daily headache may occur de novo, probably as a form of tension headache or, more importantly, it may be part of an evolution from periodic migraine or tension headache. Chronic daily headache is often accompanied by sleep disturbances, depression, anxiety, and overuse of analgesics; most patients with this disorder have a family history of headache. Episodic migraine and other episodic benign headaches can evolve into a daily refractory, intense headache. This syndrome is usually due to the overuse (>2–3 days weekly) of ergotamine tartrate, triptans, analgesics (especially analgesics combined with barbiturates), narcotics, and perhaps even benzodiazepines. To control the headache, the use of these medications has to be discontinued. Two points must be stressed: the overuse of these medications causes daily headache, and the daily use of these medications prevents other useful medications from working effectively.

The treatment of daily refractory headaches may require hospitalization and withdrawal of the overused medication, with repetitive intravenous administration of dihydroergotamine together with an antiemetic drug such as metoclopramide or prochlorperazine.

β-Blockers, calcium channel blockers, and tricyclic antidepressants do not cause transformation or withdrawal syndrome. Also, analgesic or rebound headache does not develop in patients who do not have headache but who take large amounts of analgesics for other conditions (eg, arthritis). Simple withdrawal of analgesics produces improvement in patients with chronic daily headache. A nonprescription medication can be withdrawn abruptly. However, prescription medications (eg, ergotamine tartrate, narcotics, and barbiturates) must be withdrawn gradually. When narcotics or compounds containing codeine and ergotamine tartrate are withdrawn, clonidine may be helpful in repressing withdrawal symptoms. Some physicians think that even simple analgesics (eg, aspirin and acetaminophen) taken for more than 2 to 3 days weekly can cause daily headache syndrome. The overuse (>3 days weekly for ≥2 weeks) of triptan drugs is now becoming a common cause of medication-overuse syndrome.

- Chronic daily headache is often accompanied by a family history of headache, sleep disturbances, depression, anxiety, and analgesic overuse.

- Migraine and other headaches can become a refractory, intense headache.

- Overuse of medications causes daily headache and prevents the effective action of other drugs.

- Nonsteroidal anti-inflammatory drugs, β-blockers, calcium channel blockers, and tricyclic antidepressants do not cause transformation or withdrawal syndrome.

Trigeminal Neuralgia

Patients with trigeminal neuralgia usually have symptoms in the second or third division of the trigeminal nerve. The idiopathic variety occurs in middle-aged and elderly patients and is heralded by a sharp, lancinating pain that usually can be triggered. Chewing, talking, or touching the skin or teeth often precipitates the pain of trigeminal neuralgia, and swallowing often precipitates the pain of glossopharyngeal neuralgia.

In the elderly, trigeminal neuralgia may be caused by an enlarged or tortuous artery (rarely a vein) that compresses the trigeminal nerve. This can be seen on MRI or magnetic resonance angiography. Importantly, in idiopathic trigeminal neuralgia, sensory and motor functions of the trigeminal nerve are normal. If there are signs or symptoms other than pain, evaluate for other compressive lesions (eg, neoplasm). Consider the possibility of multiple sclerosis if trigeminal neuralgia occurs in a young person or if it occurs bilaterally. Treatment options include carbamazepine, phenytoin, baclofen, gabapentin, and clonazepam. Carbamazepine is the most effective. Surgical treatment includes alcohol blocks, radiofrequency ablation of the gasserian ganglion (cranial nerve [CN] V), Gamma Knife radiosurgery, and an open craniotomy with microvascular decompression.

- Chewing, talking, or touching often precipitates pain in trigeminal neuralgia, as does swallowing in glossopharyngeal neuralgia.

- In idiopathic trigeminal neuralgia, there should be no other neurologic signs or symptoms when the patient is examined during an asymptomatic period.

- Consider multiple sclerosis if trigeminal neuralgia occurs in a young person or if it is bilateral.

INTRACRANIAL LESIONS

Leptomeningeal Lesions

Patients with inflammation, infection, or neoplastic invasion of the leptomeninges may present with similar signs and symptoms, as follows:

1. Cerebral—headache, seizures, and focal neurologic signs

2. Cranial nerve—any cranial nerve can be affected, especially CN III, IV, VI, and VII (CN VII is often affected in Lyme disease)

3. Radicular (radiculoneuropathy or radiculomyelopathy)— neck and back pain as well as radicular pain and spinal cord signs

Parasagittal Lesions

Because the cortical leg area and cortical area for control of the urinary bladder are located on the medial surface of each hemisphere, parasagittal lesions can cause spastic paraparesis with urinary problems and can, therefore, mimic a myelopathy. Meningioma is a common lesion in this location and may also cause seizures and headache.

- Parasagittal lesions may cause paraparesis with urinary problems.

- Meningioma may also cause seizures and headache.

Cortical Lesions

Cortical lesions produce focal signs. If the lesions are in the dominant hemisphere (usually the left), they cause language dysfunction, such as with encoding (eg, speaking) or decoding (eg, reading) the spoken or written word. Cortical lesions can also impair higher intellectual function, producing apraxia, agnosia, and neglect (ie, denial of illness or body parts), and they often impair cortical sensation (eg, joint position sense, traced figures, and stereognosis). A dense loss of primary sensation (eg, pinprick and touch) occurs with thalamic lesions.

- Cortical lesions may produce aphasia, apraxia, and agnosia.

- Thalamic lesions cause loss of primary sensation (eg, touch and pinprick).

Hydrocephalus

A combination of signs and symptoms—impaired mental status, gait disturbance, and urinary problems—suggests hydrocephalus.

Obstructive hydrocephalus (also called *noncommunicating hydrocephalus*) results from an obstructive lesion anywhere in the ventricular system. Patients with the obstructive type may have signs of increased intracranial pressure, including lethargy, nausea, vomiting, and headache; obscurations of vision are often associated with changes in position.

Communicating hydrocephalus includes the following 3 types:

1. Hydrocephalus ex vacuo—results from the loss of parenchyma, either gray or white matter, and is not associated with the signs listed above (if the cause of hydrocephalus is aging, the neurologic examination findings are normal; if the cause is AD, clinical examination shows signs of dementia)

2. NPH—due to decreased reabsorption of CSF

3. Hydrocephalus due to overproduction of CSF—rare and controversial; supposedly occurs with choroid plexus tumors

- NPH is due to decreased reabsorption of CSF and may be associated with urinary symptoms, gait disturbance, and memory dysfunction (see the "Dementia" subsection above).

POSTERIOR FOSSA LEVEL: SYMPTOMS AND CLINICAL CORRELATIONS

BRAINSTEM LESIONS

Brainstem lesions can produce crossed neurologic syndromes: cranial nerve signs are ipsilateral to the lesion, but long-tract signs (ie, corticospinal) are usually contralateral (ie, crossed syndrome). Other symptoms associated with brainstem lesions include impairment of ocular motility; medial longitudinal fasciculus syndrome (ie, internuclear ophthalmoplegia); rotary, horizontal, and vertical nystagmus (downbeat nystagmus is highly suggestive of a lesion at the cervicomedullary junction); ataxia; dysarthria; diplopia; vertigo; and dysphagia.

- Cranial nerve signs are ipsilateral to the brainstem lesion.

- Long-tract signs are usually contralateral to the brainstem lesion.

- Downbeat nystagmus is highly suggestive of a lesion at the cervicomedullary junction.

CEREBELLAR LESIONS

Problems with equilibrium and coordination suggest a cerebellar lesion. Lesions of the cerebellar hemisphere usually produce ipsilateral ataxia of the arm and leg. Lesions restricted to the anterior superior vermis, as in alcoholism, usually cause ataxia of gait (ie, a wide-based gait and heel-to-shin ataxia), with relative sparing of the arms, speech, and ocular motility. Lesions of the flocculonodular lobe cause marked difficulty with equilibrium and walking but not much difficulty with finger-to-nose and heel-to-shin tests if the patient is lying down.

VERTIGO AND DIZZINESS

Accurate visual, vestibular, proprioceptive, tactile, and auditory perceptions are necessary for normal spatial orientation. These inputs are integrated in the brainstem and cerebral hemispheres. The outputs are the cortical, brainstem, and cerebellar motor systems. The impairment of any of these functions or their input, integration, or output causes a complaint of "dizziness" (a sensation of altered orientation or space). Dizziness, vertigo, and dysequilibrium are common complaints. The results of diagnostic tests are often normal. Diagnosis depends mainly on the medical history, with physical examination findings required in some cases. Vestibular tests rarely provide an exact diagnosis. The types of dizziness are listed in Box 45.8.

Box 45.8 **TYPES OF DIZZINESS**

Vertigo
  Peripheral
  Central
Presyncopal light-headedness
  Orthostatic hypotension
  Vasovagal attacks
  Impaired cardiac output
  Hyperventilation
Psychophysiologic dizziness
  Acute anxiety
  Agoraphobia (fear & avoidance of being in public places)
  Chronic anxiety
Dysequilibrium
  Lesions of basal ganglia, frontal lobes, & white matter
  Hydrocephalus
  Cerebellar dysfunction
Ocular dizziness
  High magnification & lens implant
  Imbalance in extraocular muscles
  Oscillopsia
Multisensory dizziness
Physiologic dizziness
  Motion sickness
  Space sickness
  Height vertigo

Vertigo

Vertigo is an illusion of movement (usually that of rotation) and the feeling of vertical or horizontal rotation of either the person or the environment around the person. Most patients report this as "spinning" or "rotational" feelings. Others experience mainly a sensation of staggering. In contrast to vertigo, *dysequilibrium* is a feeling of unsteadiness or insecurity about the environment, without a rotatory sensation. Vertigo occurs when there is imbalance, especially acute, between the left and right vestibular systems. The sudden unilateral loss of vestibular function is dramatic; the patient complains of severe vertigo and nausea and vomiting and is pale and diaphoretic. With acute vertigo, the patient also has problems with equilibrium and vision, often described as "blurred vision," or diplopia. Autonomic symptoms are common—sweating, pallor, nausea, and vomiting—and occasionally can cause vasovagal syncope.

Ménière Disease

Fluctuating hearing loss and tinnitus are characteristic of Ménière disease. Abrupt complete unilateral deafness and vertigo occur with viral involvement of the labyrinth or CN VIII (or both) and with ischemia of the inner ear. Patients who slowly lose vestibular function bilaterally, as may happen with the use of ototoxic drugs, often do not complain of vertigo but have oscillopsia with head movements and instability with walking. Even if unilateral vestibular loss occurs slowly (eg, acoustic neuroma), patients usually do not complain of

vertigo; they typically present with unilateral hearing loss and tinnitus. Vertigo frequently occurs in episodes. Common vestibular disorders with a genetic predisposition include migraine, Ménière disease, otosclerosis, neurofibromatosis, and spinocerebellar degeneration.

Benign Positional Vertigo

Benign positional vertigo (BPV) is the most common cause of vertigo. Symptoms include brief episodes of vertigo that usually last less than 30 seconds with positional change (eg, turning over in bed, getting in or out of bed, bending over and straightening up, and extending the neck to look up). The usual cause is a misplaced otolith in a semicircular canal. In about half the patients who do not have BPV, no cause is found. For the other half, the most common causes are post-traumatic and postviral neurolabyrinthitis.

Typically, bouts of BPV are intermixed with variable periods of remission. Periods of vertigo rarely last longer than 1 minute, although after a flurry of episodes, patients may complain of more prolonged nonspecific dizziness that lasts hours to days (eg, light-headedness or a swimming sensation associated with nausea). Management includes reassurance, positional exercises (ie, vestibular exercises), and the canalith repositioning maneuver. Drugs are not very useful, but meclizine and promethazine may help with nausea and nonspecific dizziness. Rarely, in intractable cases, surgical treatment (section of the ampullary nerve) may be needed.

Cerebellar Lesions

Vertigo of CNS origin is caused by acute cerebellar lesions (hemorrhages or infarcts) or acute brainstem lesions (especially the lateral medullary syndrome [also called Wallenberg syndrome]). Vertebrobasilar arterial disease is also a cause, but vertigo by itself is almost never indicative of a transient ischemic attack. Other symptoms are necessary to make the diagnosis of vertebrobasilar insufficiency, such as dysarthria, dysphagia, diplopia, facial numbness, crossed syndromes, hemiparesis or alternating hemiparesis, ataxia, and visual field defects.

PRESYNCOPAL LIGHT-HEADEDNESS

Presyncopal light-headedness is best described as the sensation of impending faint. It results from pan cerebral hypoperfusion. Presyncopal light-headedness is not a symptom of focal occlusive cerebrovascular disease, but it may indicate orthostatic hypotension, usually due to decreased blood volume, chronic use of antihypertensive drugs, or autonomic dysfunction. Symptoms of vasovagal attacks are induced when emotions such as fear and anxiety activate medullary vasodepressor centers. Vasodepressor episodes can also be precipitated by acute visceral pain or sudden severe attacks of vertigo. Impaired cardiac output causes presyncopal light-headedness, as does hyperventilation. Chronic anxiety with associated hyperventilation is the most common cause of persistent presyncopal light-headedness in young patients. In most persons, a moderate increase in respiratory rate can decrease the $PaCO_2$ level to 25 mm Hg or less in a few minutes.

The following 5 types of syncopal attacks are especially common in the elderly:

1. Orthostatic—from multiple causes

2. Autonomic dysfunction—from peripheral (ie, postganglionic) or central (ie, preganglionic) involvement

3. Reflex—such as carotid sinus syncope or cough or micturition syncope

4. Vasovagal syncope—occurs less frequently in the elderly than in the young; however, the prognosis is worse for the elderly, with about 16% of them having major morbidity or mortality in the following 6 months compared with less than 1% of patients younger than 30 years (common precipitating events in the elderly include emotional stress, prolonged bed rest, prolonged standing, and painful stimuli)

5. Cardiogenic—from conditions such as arrhythmias or valvular disease

- Presyncopal light-headedness is the sensation of impending faint.

- It is not an isolated symptom of occlusive cerebrovascular disease.

- Vasovagal attacks occur less frequently in the elderly.

- In the young, a common cause of persistent presyncopal light-headedness is chronic anxiety with hyperventilation.

- The prognosis of vasovagal syncope is worse for the elderly; 16% have major morbidity or mortality within 6 months.

- In the elderly, vasovagal syncope may be precipitated by emotional stress, bed rest, prolonged standing, or pain.

Psychophysiologic Dizziness

Patients usually describe psychophysiologic dizziness as "floating," "swimming," or "giddiness." They also may report a feeling of imbalance, a rocking or falling sensation, or a spinning inside the head. The symptoms are not associated with an illusion of movement or movement of the environment or with nystagmus. Commonly associated symptoms include tension headache, heart palpitations, gastric distress, urinary frequency, backache, and a generalized feeling of weakness and fatigue. Psychophysiologic dizziness can also be associated with panic attacks.

Dysequilibrium

Patients who slowly lose vestibular function on 1 side, as with an acoustic neuroma, usually do not have vertigo but often describe a vague feeling of imbalance and unsteadiness on their feet. Dysequilibrium may be a presenting symptom of lesions involving motor centers of the basal ganglia and frontal lobe (eg, Parkinson disease, hydrocephalus, and multiple lacunar infarctions). The broad-based ataxic gait of persons with cerebellar disorders is readily distinguished from milder gait disorders seen with vestibular or sensory loss or with senile gait.

- Dysequilibrium may be a presenting symptom of basal ganglia, frontal lobe, or cerebellar lesions.

Multifactorial Dizziness and Imbalance

Multifactorial dizziness and imbalance is common in the elderly and especially in patients with systemic disorders such as diabetes mellitus. A typical combination includes, for example, mild peripheral neuropathy that causes diminished touch and proprioceptive input, decreased visual acuity, impaired hearing, and decreased baroreceptor function. In these patients, an added vestibular impairment, as from an ototoxic drug, can be devastating.

The resulting sensation of dizziness and imbalance is usually present only when the patient walks or moves and not when the patient is supine or seated. There is a feeling of insecurity of gait and motion. The patient is usually helped by walking close to a wall, using a cane, or by holding on to another person. Drugs should not be prescribed for this disorder. Instead, the use of a cane or walker is important to improve support and to increase somatosensory signals.

- Multifactorial dizziness and imbalance is common in elderly diabetic patients.

- Added vestibular impairment can be devastating.

- Do not prescribe drugs for this disorder.

SPINAL LEVEL: SYMPTOMS AND CLINICAL CORRELATIONS

Sensory levels, signs of anterior horn cell involvement (ie, atrophy and fasciculations), and long-tract signs in the posterior columns or corticospinal tract (or in both) suggest a spinal cord lesion. Extramedullary cord lesions are usually heralded by radicular pain. Intramedullary cord lesions are usually painless but may have an ill-described nonlocalizable pain, sensory dissociation, and sacral sparing. Conus medullaris lesions are often indicated by "saddle anesthesia" and early involvement of the urinary bladder.

- Extramedullary lesions are heralded by radicular pain.

- Intramedullary lesions are usually painless.

- Conus medullaris lesions are indicated by saddle anesthesia and early urinary bladder involvement.

CAUSES OF MYELOPATHY

A compressive or noncompressive spinal cord lesion may cause muscle weakness, which typically occurs in the arm and leg if the lesion is at the cervical level or only in the leg if the lesion is below the lower cervical level. The upper motor neuron pattern weakness is often bilateral and prominent in lower extremity flexors (iliopsoas, hamstrings, and anterior tibialis) and upper extremity extensors (triceps and wrist extensors). Bowel and bladder difficulties and numbness are frequently noted. The findings on examination include limb weakness, spasticity, and increased muscle stretch reflexes below the level of the lesion. Extensor plantar reflexes (Babinski signs) may also be elicited. Sensory findings are often noted.

The most common noncompressive lesion is transverse myelitis, usually of unknown cause. Some patients have a history of vaccination or symptoms suggestive of viral disease that usually precede the neurologic symptoms by a few days to 1 or 2 weeks. Up to 50% of these patients have antibodies, which were described from patients with neuromyelitis optica (NMO), to a water aquaporin channel (NMO IgG). They have recurrent episodes of severe myelitis and optic neuritis; consequently, long-term immunomodulatory therapy is usually indicated.

Compressive myelopathy is commonly due to degenerative spine or disk disease or to metastatic epidural neoplasm. The patients usually present with local vertebral column pain at the level of the spinal cord lesion. This symptom is present for weeks to months before the gross neurologic deficits occur, although occasionally bony pain may antedate other symptoms by only a few hours.

- Upper motor neuron pattern muscle weakness may be associated with a compressive or noncompressive spinal cord lesion.

- Transverse myelitis is the most common noncompressive lesion.

MOTOR NEURON DISEASE

Amyotrophic Lateral Sclerosis

Degenerative disorders that affect the motor neurons in the cerebral cortex and the anterior horn cells are called motor neuron diseases. The most common is amyotrophic lateral sclerosis (ALS). This disorder should be considered in any patient who has progressive, painless weakness. Typically, patients present with asymmetric weakness that begins distally and is associated with cramps and fasciculations. Footdrop and hand weakness are the most common first complaints. Often the initial (but incorrect) diagnosis is stroke, radiculopathy, carpal tunnel syndrome, or ulnar neuropathy. The diagnosis is often delayed. Bulbar weakness (eg, dysarthria and dysphagia) can be the presenting problem and is always eventually present. Bowel and bladder difficulties are very uncommon, and sensory abnormalities are rare. Findings on examination include weakness, atrophy, fasciculations, spasticity, and abnormal muscle stretch reflexes and extensor plantar responses. The hallmark is the mixture of both upper and lower motor neuron signs. Because of the progressive weakness affecting the limbs, bulbar muscles, and diaphragm, the disease is devastating, and patients have an average life span of about 3 years after the onset of symptoms.

ALS is sporadic in 80% to 90% of cases. In those that are familial, 10% of the patients harbor a mutation in the oxygen radical detoxifying enzyme superoxide dismutase (SOD-1). No drug has been found to be effective in reversing the progressive course of this disease. Some beneficial effect has been noted with riluzole, especially in patients with bulbar onset of the disease. This drug prolongs ventilator-free survival by 3 months.

Many drugs have been studied, including gabapentin, lamotrigine, insulinlike growth factor 1 (IGF-1), celecoxib, and lithium, but none have shown a benefit. Treatment of ALS focuses on rehabilitation issues, nutrition, mobility, and communication; a multidisciplinary approach is useful. Many agents hold promise and are being studied, including stem cells, although no clear indication exists for their use outside of a clinical trial.

Multifocal Motor Neuropathy

Multifocal motor neuropathy is a rare syndrome of purely lower motor neuron weakness that can mimic ALS. Treatment of multifocal motor neuropathy with intravenous immunoglobulin (IVIG) can be very effective in slowing the progression of weakness. It is often distal and asymmetrical, accompanied by motor conduction block on nerve conduction studies (NCS) and electromyography (EMG), and may be associated with high titers of serum antibodies to GM1 gangliosides. Kennedy disease (or spinobulbar muscular atrophy) is a pure lower motor neuron degenerative process that is X-linked and caused by an excess of CAG repeats in the androgen receptor gene. This most commonly affects elderly men and also leads to gynecomastia, diabetes mellitus, and a sensory peripheral neuropathy. Genetic testing is widely available. There is no effective treatment, although the disease is much more slowly progressive than ALS.

RADICULOPATHY

Nerve root lesions usually are indicated by pain that is often sharp and lancinating, follows a dermatomal or myotomal pattern, and is increased by increasing intraspinal pressure (eg, sneezing and coughing) or by stretching of the nerve root. Paresthesias and pain occur in a dermatomal pattern. Findings are in the root distribution and include weakness, sensory impairment, and decreased muscle stretch reflexes. Radiculopathies have many causes, including compressive lesions (eg, osteophytes, ruptured disks, and neoplasms) and noncompressive lesions (eg, postinfectious and inflammatory radiculopathies and metabolic radiculopathies, as in diabetes). Indications for emergent neurologic and neurosurgical consultation are increasing weakness, bowel or bladder dysfunction, or intractable pain with an appropriate lesion seen on MRI. Large disk protrusions can cause minimal symptoms and are not by themselves grounds for urgent surgical intervention.

- Nerve root lesions are indicated by sharp, lancinating pain with a dermatomal or myotomal pattern.

- Pain is increased by sneezing and coughing.

- Pain often has a dermatomal pattern.

- Findings are weakness, sensory impairment, and decreased muscle stretch reflexes.

- Radiculopathies have many causes.

- Surgery is considered for increasing weakness, bowel or bladder dysfunction, or intractable pain with an appropriate lesion seen on MRI.

DEGENERATIVE DISEASE OF THE SPINE

Cervical Spondylosis

MRI in combination with plain radiographs is the preferred approach for evaluating patients who have cervical spondylosis. Surgical results for the relief of symptoms of cervical radiculopathy are better when the cause is a soft disk herniation than when spondylitic radiculopathy and myelopathy are present. Cervical spondylitic myelopathy is a condition in which the spinal cord is damaged either directly by traumatic compression or indirectly by arterial deprivation or venous stasis as a consequence of proliferative bony changes in the cervical spine.

Lumbar Spine Disease

Asymptomatic bulging disks after the age of 30 years are common and are generally unlikely to cause nerve root compression. Bulging disks appear round and symmetrical compared with herniated disks, which appear angular and asymmetrical and extend outside the disk space. The criteria for surgical treatment of lumbar disk herniations include the presence of disk herniation on anatomical imaging; dermatome-specific reflex, sensory, or motor deficits; and failure of 6 to 8 weeks of conservative treatment.

The lateral recess syndrome is usually caused by an osteophyte on the superior articular facet and is characterized by the following:

1. Radicular pain is unilateral or bilateral with paresthesias in the distribution of L5 or S1

2. The pain is provoked by standing and walking and is relieved by sitting

3. The results of the straight leg raising test are usually negative

4. There is little or no back pain

Lumbar stenosis is characterized by the following:

1. Most patients are older than 50 years

2. Neurogenic intermittent claudication (pseudoclaudication) occurs

3. The symptoms are usually bilateral but can be asymmetrical or unilateral

4. The pain usually has a dull, aching quality

5. The whole lower extremity is generally involved

6. The pain is provoked while walking or standing

7. Sitting or leaning forward provides relief

8. There is often a "dead" feeling in the legs.

Bicycling causes little or no pain, unlike with vascular claudication. Decompressive operations for lumbar stenosis can be performed with low morbidity despite the advanced age of most patients. A very high initial success rate can be expected, although about 25% of patients become symptomatic again within 5 years. On reoperation, three-fourths of the patients ultimately have a successful outcome; failures result from progression of stenosis at levels not previously decompressed or restenosis at levels previously decompressed.

Musculoskeletal low back pain (without leg pain) is treated best with a formal program of physical therapy and exercise, weight reduction, and education on postural principles.

PERIPHERAL LEVEL: SYMPTOMS AND CLINICAL CORRELATIONS

PERIPHERAL NEUROPATHY

Peripheral neuropathies are usually characterized by distal weakness and distal sensory changes. They are usually symmetrical and more severe in the legs than in the arms. Weakness related to peripheral nerve disorders is typically worse distally, occasionally with footdrop. Clumsy gait is often associated with distal numbness and paresthesias. Examination findings include distal weakness, sensory loss, atrophy, and, sometimes, fasciculations. Muscle stretch reflexes usually are decreased. If a single plexus (lumbosacral or brachial) is involved, the weakness may be isolated to a single limb. However, the findings still are consistent with a "lower motor neuron" lesion, with decreased reflexes, weakness, atrophy, and sensory loss. Neuropathy has many causes, and the pattern of the neuropathy might suggest its cause (Table 45.4). The evaluation of peripheral neuropathy is summarized in Box 45.9. An extensive search usually uncovers the cause in 70% to 80% of cases. A high percentage of the

Table 45.4 **MAIN CLINICAL FEATURES AND DIFFERENTIAL DIAGNOSIS OF PERIPHERAL NEUROPATHIES**

PATTERN OF NEUROPATHY	COMMON OR IMPORTANT CAUSES
Mononeuropathy	Compressive neuropathy
	Idiopathic
	Tumor
	Trauma
	Diabetes mellitus
	HNPP
Mononeuropathy multiplex	Diabetes mellitus
	Vasculitis
	Lyme disease
	HIV neuropathy
	Sarcoidosis
	Leprosy
	Multifocal motor neuropathy
	HNPP
Acute motor polyradiculoneuropathy	AIDP (Guillain-Barré syndrome)
	Lyme disease
	HIV neuropathy
	Porphyria
	Toxins (arsenic, thallium)
	Carcinomatous or lymphomatous meningitis

(Continued)

Table 45.4 (CONTINUED)

PATTERN OF NEUROPATHY	COMMON OR IMPORTANT CAUSES
Chronic motor or sensorimotor polyradiculopathy	CIDP Paraproteinemia (eg, osteosclerotic myeloma) Hereditary neuropathy (eg, Charcot-Marie-Tooth disease) Lead toxicity Diabetes mellitus Amyloidosis
Length-dependent distal (stocking-and-glove) sensorimotor neuropathy	Diabetes mellitus Alcoholism Uremia Toxins (hexacarbons) Hereditary neuropathy Vitamin B$_{12}$ deficiency Hypothyroidism Gluten sensitivity Copper deficiency
Sensory ataxic neuropathy	Sjögren syndrome Paraneoplastic disorder Diabetes mellitus Paraproteinemia Vitamin B$_{12}$ deficiency HIV infection Cisplatin Vitamin B$_6$ excess Hereditary neuropathy
Painful peripheral neuropathy	Diabetes mellitus Vasculitis Hereditary amyloidosis Toxins (arsenic, thallium) Hepatitis C Cryoglobulinemia HIV neuropathy CMV polyradiculoneuropathy in HIV-positive patients Alcoholism Fabry disease

Neuropathy with prominent autonomic involvement	Acute or subacute
	  Guillain-Barré syndrome
	  Subacute pandysautonomia
	  Paraneoplastic pandysautonomia
	  Porphyria
	  Vincristine neuropathy
	  Botulism
	Chronic
	  Diabetes mellitus
	  Amyloidosis
	  Sjögren syndrome

Abbreviations: AIDP, acute inflammatory demyelinating polyradiculoneuropathy; CIDP, chronic inflammatory demyelinating polyradiculoneuropathy; CMV, cytomegalovirus; HIV, human immunodeficiency virus; HNPP, hereditary neuropathy with liability to pressure palsies.

cases of "idiopathic neuropathy" referred to specialty centers are in fact hereditary neuropathies. On examination, the finding of high arches (ie, pes cavus) or fallen arches (ie, pes planus) with hammertoe deformities is a clue to a long-standing or

Box 45.9 EVALUATION OF PERIPHERAL NEUROPATHY

Basic laboratory investigations
  CBC with platelets
  Erythrocyte sedimentation rate
  Fasting blood glucose
  Serum electrolytes
  Serum creatinine
  Liver function tests
  Serum & urine electrophoresis & immunoelectrophoresis
  Urinalysis
  Chest radiography
  Electromyography
Special investigations
  Thyroid function test
  Vitamin B$_{12}$
  Vitamin E
  Cholesterol & triglycerides
  HIV serology
  Lyme serology
  Hepatitis serology
  Cryoglobulins
  Angiotensin-converting enzyme
  Antineutrophil cytoplasmic antibodies
  Antinuclear antibodies
  Antibodies against extractable nuclear antigens
  Gliadin antibodies, endomysial & tissue transglutaminase antibodies
  Paraneoplastic antibodies
  GM1 antibodies
  Porphyrins
  Heavy metal screen
  Serum copper & ceruloplasmin
Investigations in selected cases
  Autonomic function tests
  Cerebrospinal fluid analysis
  Sural nerve biopsy
  Investigation for inborn errors of metabolism
  Genetic studies
  MRI of nerve roots or plexus

Abbreviations: CBC, complete blood cell count; HIV, human immunodeficiency virus; MRI, magnetic resonance imaging.

hereditary neuropathy. Also, examination or close questioning of family members may secure a diagnosis.

- The pattern of neuropathy and the time course suggest the cause.

- Peripheral neuropathy: distal weakness and sensory changes more in the legs than in the arms, usually symmetrical, and with distal muscle stretch reflexes impaired or absent.

- The cause of peripheral neuropathy is usually found in 70%-80% of cases; hereditary causes may explain many cases of "idiopathic neuropathy."

Mononeuropathy

Mononeuropathy is characterized by impairment of a single nerve. The usual cause is compression, as in compressive ulnar neuropathy at the elbow, compressive median neuropathy in the carpal tunnel, and compression of the peroneal nerve as it winds around the fibular head. Diabetes mellitus is a common underlying disorder in patients with multiple compression mononeuropathies.

Mononeuropathy Multiplex

Mononeuropathy multiplex consists of asymmetrical involvement of several nerves either simultaneously or sequentially. It suggests such causes as trauma or compression, diabetes mellitus, vasculitis, Lyme disease, human immunodeficiency virus (HIV) neuropathy, sarcoidosis, leprosy, tumor infiltration, multifocal motor neuropathies, or hereditary neuropathy with predisposition to pressure palsies.

- Common causes of mononeuropathy multiplex include diabetes mellitus, vasculitis, leprosy, sarcoidosis, and Lyme disease.

Acute Inflammatory Demyelinating Polyradiculoneuropathy

A progressive neuropathy of rapid onset that affects both distal and proximal nerves suggests acute inflammatory demyelinating polyradiculoneuropathy (AIDP), or Guillain-Barré syndrome. The weakness and paresthesias ascend over several days, often accompanied by severe back pain. On examination, the reflexes are absent. There may also be respiratory muscle weakness, cranial neuropathy (particularly facial palsy, which can be bilateral), and autonomic instability. Typically, it is associated with an increased CSF protein concentration but no pleocytosis. There are characteristic NCS and EMG findings with conduction block and temporal dispersion. About 50% of patients have a mild respiratory or gastrointestinal tract infection 1 to 3 weeks before the neurologic symptoms appear. In the other patients, the syndrome may be preceded by surgery, viral exanthems, or vaccinations. Also, the syndrome may develop in patients who have autoimmune disease or a lymphoreticular malignancy. This syndrome has no particular seasonal, age, or sex predilection. Either plasma exchange or IVIG is effective in AIDP. Corticosteroids are not effective. Attention must be paid to other complications of the disease: deep vein thrombosis, pain, constipation, back pain, tachyarrhythmias and hypertension, peptic ulcers, decubital ulcers, and accumulation of secretions in the respiratory tract and aspiration.

- In Guillain-Barré syndrome, 50% of patients have a mild respiratory or gastrointestinal tract infection 1–3 weeks before neurologic symptoms appear.

- Surgery, viral exanthems, or vaccinations may precede Guillain-Barré syndrome.

- The diagnosis is made clinically with support from NCS, EMG, and CSF analysis.

- Treatment is with either plasma exchange or IVIG, not corticosteroids.

Chronic Demyelinating Neuropathies

Chronic, predominantly motor or sensorimotor neuropathies include chronic inflammatory demyelinating polyradiculoneuropathy (CIDP), paraproteinemic neuropathies (eg, associated with POEMS syndrome, amyloidosis, or osteosclerotic myeloma), hereditary neuropathies, lead toxicity, and diabetes mellitus (which often has axonal features as well). Most neuropathies are length-dependent, but occasionally there is predominant proximal weakness, which suggests AIDP, CIDP, porphyria, or diabetic lumbosacral or cervical radiculoplexus neuropathies (referred to by numerous eponyms and collectively as proximal diabetic neuropathies). In sharp contrast to its lack of success in AIDP, corticosteroid therapy works well in CIDP. Plasma exchange and IVIG are also effective. Other potential causes are connective tissue diseases, vasculitis, vitamin B_{12} deficiency, copper deficiency, sarcoidosis, paraneoplastic syndromes, gluten sensitivity, and medications.

Most neuropathies associated with monoclonal gammopathies are not associated with underlying lymphoproliferative disorders, but some are associated with multiple myeloma, amyloidosis, lymphoma, or leukemia. These patients usually are older than 50 years and present early with symmetrical sensorimotor polyradiculoneuropathy. The CSF protein concentration is usually increased. IgM is more common than IgG or IgA and is generally more resistant to treatment. Plasma exchange can be effective therapy. Other immunosuppressive therapy, such as IVIG and perhaps rituximab, may also be effective.

Sensory Ataxic Neuropathy

Sensory ataxic neuropathies are characterized by severe proprioceptive sensory loss, ataxia, and areflexia. Some neuropathies are due to peripheral nerve demyelination and others to involvement of large dorsal root ganglion neurons. A predominantly sensory polyneuropathy suggests paraneoplastic disorder, Sjögren syndrome, diabetes mellitus, paraproteinemias, HIV infection, vitamin B_{12} deficiency, cisplatin toxicity, vitamin B_6 excess, or hereditary neuropathy.

Painful Neuropathy

Some peripheral neuropathies affect predominantly the small-diameter nociceptive fibers or their dorsal root ganglion neurons and are characterized by severe burning pain distally in the extremities. The examination findings are normal except for the distal loss of pain and temperature sensation. Typical causes are diabetes mellitus, vasculitis, amyloidosis, toxins, hepatitis C, cryoglobulinemia, some HIV-associated neuropathies, and alcoholism. Randomized, double-blind, placebo-controlled studies in diabetic neuropathy have shown that the following medications are helpful: amitriptyline, tramadol, gabapentin, pregabalin, and duloxetine. Others that are useful when these agents are not useful or when they lead to side effects include carbamazepine, lidocaine patch (5%), narcotics, lamotrigine, mexiletine, and venlafaxine.

Autonomic Neuropathy

Neuropathy with autonomic dysfunction (eg, orthostatic hypotension, urinary bladder and bowel dysfunction, and impotence) suggests Guillain-Barré syndrome, acute pandysautonomia, paraneoplastic dysautonomia, porphyria, diabetes mellitus, amyloidosis, or familial neuropathy.

Acute pandysautonomia is a heterogeneous, monophasic, usually self-limiting disease that involves the sympathetic and parasympathetic nervous systems. It may produce orthostatic hypotension, anhydrosis, diarrhea, constipation, urinary bladder atony, and impotence. The syndrome usually evolves over a few days to a few months, with a recovery that is generally prolonged and partial. This may be an immunologic disorder, but it is indistinguishable from paraneoplastic autonomic neuropathy. Some patients may have antibodies against the ganglion-type nicotinic acetylcholine receptor. IVIG treatment limits the duration and reduces the long-term disability of patients with acute pandysautonomia.

- Motor polyneuropathy: inflammatory demyelinating polyradiculoneuropathy, hereditary neuropathy, osteosclerotic myeloma, porphyria, and lead poisoning.

- Sensory polyneuropathy: diabetes mellitus, paraneoplastic disorder, Sjögren syndrome, dysproteinemias, HIV infection, vitamin B_{12} deficiency, cisplatin toxicity, vitamin B_6 excess, and some hereditary neuropathies.

- Neuropathy with autonomic dysfunction: amyloidosis, diabetes mellitus, Guillain-Barré syndrome, porphyria, and some familial neuropathies.

Diabetic Neuropathy

Diabetes mellitus may cause CN III neuropathy. Affected patients usually present with sudden diplopia, eye pain, impairment of the muscles supplied by CN III, and relative sparing of the pupil. With compressive CN III lesions, the pupil usually is involved early. Painful diabetic neuropathies include CN III neuropathy, acute thoracoabdominal (ie, truncal) neuropathy, acute distal sensory neuropathy, acute lumbar radiculoplexopathy, and chronic distal small-fiber neuropathy.

- Diabetes mellitus may cause CN III neuropathy, often with relative sparing of the pupil.

- The pupil is involved early in compression of CN III.

Acute or subacute muscle weakness can occur in various forms of diabetic neuropathy. Weakness, atrophy, and pain affect the pelvic girdle and thigh muscles (asymmetrical or unilateral—diabetic amyotrophy). This has been termed *diabetic polyradiculoplexus neuropathy* and is due to a microvasculitis of the nerve. Patients with diabetes (often mild and well controlled) may have bilateral proximal and pelvic girdle weakness, wasting, weight loss, and autonomic dysfunction. A course of intravenous corticosteroids may speed the recovery.

Neuromuscular Transmission Disorders

Patients with neuromuscular transmission disorders (classically, myasthenia gravis) present with fluctuating weakness manifested as fatigable weakness in the limbs, eyelids (ie, ptosis), tongue and palate (ie, dysarthria and dysphagia), and extraocular muscles (ie, diplopia). Sensation, muscle tone, and reflexes usually are normal except in Lambert-Eaton myasthenic syndrome (LEMS), in which the weakness is more constant and the reflexes are diminished. Drugs may cause problems at neuromuscular junctions; for example, penicillamine can cause a syndrome that appears similar to myasthenia gravis. Three major clinical syndromes of the neuromuscular junction are myasthenia gravis, LEMS, and botulism. Several drugs adversely affect neuromuscular transmission and may exacerbate weakness in these disorders. They include aminoglycoside antibiotics, quinine, quinidine, procainamide, propranolol, calcium channel blockers, and iodinated radiocontrast agents.

Myasthenia Gravis

Myasthenia gravis (MG) usually occurs in young women and older men and is often heralded by such cranial nerve findings as diplopia, dysarthria, dysphagia, and dyspnea. The deficits are usually fatigable, worsening with repetition or late in the day. However, muscle stretch reflexes, sensation, mentation, and sphincter function are normal. The diagnosis of MG is based on the detection of nicotinic acetylcholine receptor antibodies and the presence of decremental responses to repetitive electrical stimulation of motor nerves. Administration of a short-acting acetylcholine esterase inhibitor (eg, edrophonium) can immediately reverse weakness due to MG; this can be used as a diagnostic test. Acetylcholine receptor antibodies are rare in conditions other than MG (ie, they do not occur in patients with congenital MG and they occur in only about 50% of those with purely ocular MG). Striational antibodies are highly associated with thymoma in younger patients and sometimes occur in LEMS or small cell lung carcinoma. They can occur in penicillamine recipients, bone marrow allografts, and autoimmune liver disorders. Some myasthenic patients without acetylcholine receptor antibodies have muscle-specific kinase (MuSK) antibodies that are also diagnostic for MG. These patients may have more severe weakness, often bulbar, and may be more resistant to treatments. Of the 30% of patients who have MG without acetylcholine receptor antibodies, half have antibodies to MuSK.

Treatment strategies for MG include the use of anticholinesterase and immunomodulatory agents. Cholinesterase inhibitors, such as pyridostigmine bromide, are often given as initial therapy for MG. This therapy provides symptomatic improvement for most patients. Thymectomy is indicated (clinical trials are in progress) for selected patients younger than 60 years with generalized weakness and for all patients with thymoma. A CT chest scan should be performed in all patients with MG. Prednisone is the most commonly used immunomodulatory agent, but initial administration of high doses may exacerbate the weakness in about 10% of patients. Plasma exchange and IVIG are effective short-term therapies for patients with severe weakness and are particularly useful for a recent exacerbation, for preoperative preparation, or for initiating corticosteroid therapy.

Lambert-Eaton Myasthenic Syndrome

Patients with LEMS often have proximal weakness in the legs and absent or decreased muscle stretch reflexes (sometimes reflexes are elicited after brief exercise). This syndrome usually is diagnosed in middle-aged men who often have vague complaints such as diplopia, impotence, urinary dysfunction, paresthesias, mouth dryness, and other autonomic dysfunctions (eg, orthostatic hypotension). LEMS is due to the presence of antibodies directed against presynaptic voltage-gated P/Q-type calcium channels. It often is associated with small cell lung carcinoma. Treatment is focused on the cancer. Pyridostigmine can be helpful, like in MG, as can corticosteroids.

Botulism

Botulism should be suspected when more than 1 person has a syndrome that resembles MG or when 1 person has abdominal and gastrointestinal tract symptoms that precede a syndrome that resembles MG. Bulbar and respiratory weakness is common, and pupillary abnormalities are distinctive compared with findings in MG. Botulism occurs after the ingestion of improperly canned vegetables, fruit, meat, or fish contaminated with the exotoxin of *Clostridium botulinum*. Paralysis is caused by toxin-mediated inhibition of acetylcholine release from axon terminals at the neuromuscular junction. Although an antitoxin is available, treatment is mainly supportive, especially respiratory but also psychologic, because the signs and symptoms are reversible.

- Onset of MG: diplopia, dysarthria, dysphagia, dyspnea, and fatigability, often in young women and older men.

- Patients with LEMS often have proximal weakness in the legs and decreased or absent muscle stretch reflexes.

- LEMS occurs in middle-aged men who have vague complaints of diplopia, impotence, urinary dysfunction, and dry mouth.

- LEMS is often associated with small cell lung carcinoma.

- Botulism should be suspected if >1 person has a syndrome that resembles MG.

- Ingestion of the exotoxin of *C botulinum* causes botulism.

- In botulism, the release of acetylcholine is inhibited at the neuromuscular junction.

Miscellaneous Causes of Predominantly Motor Neuropathy

Other causes of subacute, predominantly motor neuropathy are Lyme disease, HIV- or cytomegalovirus-related polyradiculopathy, porphyria, organophosphate poisoning, hypoglycemia, toxins (lead, arsenic, and thallium), and paraneoplastic disease. Acute intermittent porphyria produces a severe, rapidly progressive, symmetrical polyneuropathy with or without psychosis, delirium, confusion, and convulsions. In most patients, weakness is most pronounced in the proximal muscles.

MUSCLE DISEASE

Patients with muscle disease typically present with symmetrical proximal weakness (legs more than arms) and with weakness of neck flexors and, occasionally, of cardiac muscle. Muscle stretch reflexes and sensory examination findings are usually normal. Common patient complaints are difficulty arising from a chair or raising the arms over the head. Dysphagia is uncommon. Some myopathies have more predominant distal involvement (eg, myotonic dystrophy, inclusion body myositis, and distal muscular dystrophies). In myotonic dystrophy, atrophy and weakness begin distally and in the face and especially in the sternocleidomastoid muscles. An interesting feature of this dystrophy is *myotonia* (ie, normal contraction of muscle with slow relaxation). Tests for myotonia include striking the thenar eminence with a reflex hammer and shaking the patient's hand, noting that the patient cannot let go quickly.

Muscle disease may be an acquired or progressive hereditary disease. *Myopathy* is a general term for muscle disease. If the disease is progressive and genetic, it is called *dystrophy*. However, patients with a muscular dystrophy may not have a family history positive for dystrophy. A classification of myopathies is given in Box 45.10. The diagnosis of myopathy is based on the history and physical examination, increased levels of creatine kinase, EMG, muscle biopsy results, and selected genetic testing. For many adults with acquired myopathy, no underlying cause is found.

Inflammatory Myopathy

Inflammatory myopathies include polymyositis, dermatomyositis, and inclusion body myositis. With inflammatory myopathies, especially dermatomyositis, an underlying cancer may also be present. Muscle biopsy should be used to confirm the diagnosis of an inflammatory myopathy, although it may be suggested by the history and examination findings, increased serum levels of creatine kinase, and EMG results. Inclusion body myositis (IBM) occurs mainly in men older than 60 years; they have asymmetrical weakness of proximal and distal muscles, with a predilection for quadriceps, biceps, and finger flexors (this pattern is highly suggestive of inclusion body myositis). IBM is not associated with collagen vascular diseases or neoplasms, and the creatine kinase level may be normal or slightly increased. IBM does not respond to immunosuppression.

Dystrophic myopathies (childhood or adult onset, progressive)

Congenital myopathies (congenital onset; slowly progressive or nonprogressive)

Inflammatory myopathies

    Infectious & viral—toxoplasmosis, trichinosis

    Granulomatous—sarcoidosis

    Idiopathic—polymyositis, dermatomyositis, IBM

    Inflammatory myopathy with collagen vascular disease

Metabolic myopathies

    Glycogenoses

    Mitochondrial disorders

    Defects of fatty acid oxidation

    Endocrinopathy

Periodic paralyses

Toxic—statin drugs, emetine, chloroquine, vincristine

Miscellaneous

    Amyloidosis

Abbreviation: IBM, inclusion body myositis.

Prednisone is the cornerstone for treatment of other inflammatory myopathies such as polymyositis and dermatomyositis. The most common pitfall in treating these conditions is treating with doses of prednisone that are too low and are given for an insufficient time. Dermatomyositis, unlike IBM or polymyositis, responds to IVIG. In both polymyositis and dermatomyositis, other immunomodulatory agents (including azathioprine, methotrexate, mycophenolate mofetil, cyclosporine, cyclophosphamide, and chlorambucil) are indicated if relapse occurs while the prednisone dose is being tapered, if unacceptable side effects develop from prednisone, or if there is no response to prednisone or the response is slow. Plasma exchange is ineffective for polymyositis, dermatomyositis, and inclusion body myositis. A regular exercise program is important, and it has been shown that physical therapy and exercise are not detrimental to patients with myopathies.

- *Myopathy* refers to muscle disease.

- If the disease is progressive and genetic, it is called *dystrophy*.

- Myotonic dystrophy: atrophy and weakness begin in the face and sternocleidomastoid muscles.

- Myotonia (ie, normal contraction with slow relaxation) is a feature of myotonic dystrophy; a patient with myotonia cannot let go quickly during a handshake.

- Acquired myopathy: no underlying cause is found in many adults.

- Patients with dermatomyositis: increased incidence of occult carcinoma.

- Causes of myopathies: collagen vascular disease, paraneoplastic changes, amyloidosis, endocrinopathy, sarcoidosis.

Acute Alcoholic Myopathy

Patients with acute alcoholic myopathy have acute pain, swelling, tenderness, and weakness of mainly proximal muscles. Gross myoglobinuria may cause renal failure.

- Gross myoglobinuria often occurs in acute alcoholic myopathy.

Statin-Induced Myopathy

Statin drugs (HMG-CoA reductase inhibitors) may produce an acute necrotizing myopathy characterized by myalgia, weakness, myoglobinuria, and a marked increase in creatine kinase. This toxic effect is potentiated by fibric acid–derivative drugs and cyclosporine. A more subacute to chronic myopathy can also occur with statins. Symptoms of cramps and myalgias can occur, occasionally with little or no muscle weakness or creatine kinase elevation. How soon symptoms abate after discontinuing use of the drug is unknown, although 3 to 6 months may be needed. It is also likely that in some patients statins unmask a presymptomatic acquired or genetic myopathy. The myopathic symptoms persist in some patients even after they discontinue the use of the statin medication.

Electrolyte Imbalance

Severe hypokalemia (<2.5 mEq/L) and hyperkalemia (>7 mEq/L) produce muscle weakness, as do hypercalcemia, hypocalcemia, and hypophosphatemia. Familial periodic paralysis of the hypokalemic, hyperkalemic, or normokalemic type consists of episodes of acute paralysis that last 2 to 24 hours and can be precipitated by a carbohydrate-rich meal or strenuous exercise; cranial or respiratory muscle paralysis does not occur. The diagnosis is difficult to make and is based on the potassium levels during an attack, family history, EMG, and, occasionally, genetic testing for certain sodium and calcium channel mutations.

Endocrine Diseases

Hyperthyroidism and hypothyroidism, hyperadrenalism and hypoadrenalism, acromegaly, and primary and secondary hyperparathyroidism cause muscle weakness.

ACUTE MUSCLE WEAKNESS

Physicians may overlook serious underlying diseases in patients whose chief or only complaint is weakness, especially if there are few or no obvious clinical signs. A delayed or missed diagnosis can lead to life-threatening complications, such as respiratory failure, irreversible spinal cord dysfunction, and acute renal failure. In some patients with neuromuscular weakness, respiratory muscles may be affected, although strength in the extremities is relatively normal. Patients with early Guillain-Barré syndrome may have distal paresthesias and increased respiratory effort and be given the diagnosis of hysterical hyperventilation.

Box 45.11 IMPORTANT CAUSES OF ACUTE MUSCLE WEAKNESS

Cerebral disease
    Hemiparesis
    Paraparesis—anterior cerebral artery
Spinal cord disease
    Transverse myelitis
    Epidural abscess
    Extradural tumor
    Epidural hematoma
    Herniated intervertebral disk
    Spinal cord tumor
Peripheral nerve disease
    Guillain-Barré syndrome
    Acute intermittent porphyria
    Arsenic poisoning
    Toxic neuropathies
    Tick paralysis
Neuromuscular junction disease
    Myasthenia gravis
    Botulism
    Organophosphate poisoning
Muscle disease
    Polymyositis
    Rhabdomyolysis-myoglobinuria
    Acute alcoholic myopathy
    Electrolyte imbalances
    Endocrine disease

Adapted from Karkal SS. Rapid accurate appraisal of acute muscular weakness. Updates Neurology. 1991, pp 31–9. Used with permission.

Tick paralysis is a rapid, progressive ascending motor weakness caused by neurotoxin injected by the female wood tick. It occurs endemically in the southeastern and northwestern United States. After an asymptomatic period (about 1 week), symptoms develop, usually with leg weakness.

- A missed diagnosis can lead to life-threatening complications: respiratory failure, irreversible spinal cord dysfunction, and acute renal failure.
- Early Guillain-Barré syndrome may be misdiagnosed as hysterical hyperventilation.

Acute, diffuse muscle weakness can be classified into 5 groups according to the anatomical location of the disorder: brain, spinal cord, peripheral nerve, neuromuscular junction, or muscle. Causes of acute muscle weakness are summarized in Box 45.11.

SUMMARY

- The most common reversible causes of stupor and coma are toxic, metabolic, and infectious problems that affect both cerebral hemispheres diffusely.
- Head trauma is a major cause of focal seizures in young adults.
- Brain tumors and vascular disease are major causes of seizures in older persons.
- Cranial nerve signs are ipsilateral to the brainstem lesion.
- Long-tract signs are usually contralateral to the brainstem lesion.
- Nerve root lesions are indicated by sharp, lancinating pain with a dermatomal or myotomal pattern.
- Motor polyneuropathy: inflammatory demyelinating polyradiculoneuropathy, hereditary neuropathy, osteosclerotic myeloma, porphyria, and lead poisoning.
- Sensory polyneuropathy: diabetes mellitus, paraneoplastic disorder, Sjögren syndrome, dysproteinemias, HIV infection, vitamin B_{12} deficiency, cisplatin toxicity, vitamin B_6 excess, and some hereditary neuropathies.

46.

NEUROLOGIC DISORDERS CATEGORIZED BY MECHANISM

Lyell K. Jones Jr, MD, Brian A. Crum, MD, Eduardo E. Benarroch, MD,

and Robert D. Brown Jr, MD

GOAL

Review neurologic diseases by pathophysiologic category:

- Cerebrovascular disease
- Neoplastic disease
- Movement disorders
- Inflammatory disorders
- Autoimmune disease

CEREBROVASCULAR DISEASE

ISCHEMIC CEREBROVASCULAR DISEASE

Pathophysiologic Mechanisms

The causes of ischemic cerebrovascular disorders, including transient ischemic attack (TIA) and cerebral infarction, can be classified according to the site of the source for the arterial blockage within the vascular system, from most proximal to distal:

1. *Cardiac source* (most proximal source of emboli): arrhythmias and structural disease (eg, valve disease, dilated cardiomyopathy, recent myocardial infarction); paradoxical emboli with a right-to-left shunt through a patent foramen ovale (PFO), although most patients with PFO are asymptomatic; the aorta

2. *Large-vessel disorders*: most commonly atherosclerosis or dissection in the carotid or vertebrobasilar system

3. *Small-vessel occlusive disease*: inflammatory or noninflammatory arteriopathies (eg, hypertension-induced disease, isolated central

nervous system [CNS] angiitis, and systemic lupus erythematosus)

4. *Hematologic disorders*: polycythemia, sickle cell anemia, thrombocytosis, severe leukocytosis (acute leukemia), antithrombin III deficiency, protein C deficiency, protein S deficiency, hereditary resistance to activated protein C, factor V Leiden mutation, anticardiolipin antibody syndrome, lupus anticoagulant positivity, and hypercoagulable states caused by carcinoma

Notably, illicit drug use is a common cause of stroke in young persons; it may cause arrhythmia, inflammatory arteriopathies, and a relative hypercoagulable state.

- Pathophysiologic mechanisms of ischemic cerebrovascular disease include a cardiac source, large-vessel disorders, small-vessel disorders, and hematologic causes.

- In young adults, illicit drug use is a risk factor for stroke.

Risk Factors

Risk factors for atherosclerotic occlusive disease are similar to those for coronary artery disease: hypertension, male sex, advanced age, cigarette smoking, diabetes mellitus, and hypercholesterolemia. Emboli from intracardiac mural thrombi also cause TIA and cerebral infarction. Proven cardiac risk factors are atrial fibrillation (including paroxysmal atrial fibrillation), atrial flutter, dilated cardiomyopathy, mechanical valve, rheumatic valve disease, recent myocardial infarction, and others (Box 46.1).

Hypertension is the most important modifiable risk factor for stroke, but other modifiable risk factors include cigarette smoking, diabetes mellitus, hypercholesterolemia, metabolic syndrome, sedentary lifestyle, obesity, obstructive sleep apnea, and, possibly, elevated homocysteine levels. Although low levels of alcohol consumption appear to have a protective effect for ischemic stroke, heavy alcohol consumption increases a person's risk for all types of stroke, particularly intracerebral and subarachnoid hemorrhage.

Transient Ischemic Attacks

Patients who experience TIA are at high risk for subsequent cerebral infarctions: 4% to 10% within 1 year to 33% within the patient's lifetime. Most TIAs last less than 15 minutes; about 90% resolve within 1 hour. Patients with cerebral infarcts, hemorrhages, and mass lesions can present with symptoms like those of TIAs.

Amaurosis fugax is defined as temporary, partial, or complete monocular blindness and is a classic symptom of carotid artery TIA. Glaucoma, vitreous hemorrhage, retinal detachment, papilledema, migrainous aura, temporal arteritis, and even ectopic floaters can mimic amaurosis fugax.

The long-term prognosis for patients who have TIA generally follows the rule of 3's: one-third will have cerebral infarction, one-third will have at least 1 more TIA, and one-third will have no more TIAs. The following features help to determine the risk of stroke after TIA: age older than 60 years, hypertension, weakness or speech disturbance with TIA, TIA duration more than 60 minutes, and diabetes mellitus.

- Most TIAs last <15 minutes.

- Patients with cerebral infarcts, hemorrhages, and mass lesions can present with symptoms like those of TIA.

- Amaurosis fugax is a classic symptom of carotid artery TIA.

- The rule of 3's for patients with TIA: one-third will have cerebral infarction, one-third will have ≥1 more TIA, and one-third will have no more TIAs.

Carotid Endarterectomy and Carotid Angioplasty With Stent Placement

Carotid endarterectomy markedly decreases the risk of stroke and death of *symptomatic* patients who have a 70% to 99% stenosis of the carotid artery. For a 50% to 69% stenosis, carotid endarterectomy is moderately efficacious in selected symptomatic patients. Medical treatment alone is better than carotid endarterectomy for patients with a stenosis of 49% or less. Symptoms must be those of a carotid territory TIA or minor stroke and must be of recent onset (<4 months). To have a favorable risk-benefit ratio, the perioperative complication rate must be low (<6%).

Carotid angioplasty with stent placement may be used as an alternative to carotid endarterectomy, particularly for high-risk patients, such as those who previously had carotid endarterectomy, radiotherapy to the neck, or neck dissection; those with a stenosis high in the internal carotid artery; or those otherwise deemed at high risk for the operation. The safety and durability of the endovascular approach compared with endarterectomy are not clear, and the available data are somewhat conflicting.

Selected patients with an *asymptomatic* carotid stenosis of at least 60% benefit from carotid endarterectomy (ie, they have a decreased risk of future ipsilateral stroke or related death). In the Asymptomatic Carotid Atherosclerosis Study (ACAS), medical patients were treated with aspirin and risk-factor reduction therapy. The risk of stroke was low for patients treated surgically and for those treated medically (5-year risk of ipsilateral stroke or death was 11% for those treated medically and 6% for those treated surgically). No trend was noted among the various degrees of stenosis, but the number of events was small in each stenosis subdivision. Surgeons and hospitals were chosen for having reported perioperative complication rates of less than 3% in asymptomatic patients. In the Asymptomatic Carotid Surgery Trial, the efficacy of surgery was similar to that noted in the ACAS trial outlined above. The primary end point was ipsilateral stroke or any perioperative stroke or death (within 30 days of the procedure or entry into the study). The risk was 12% over 5 years among patients treated medically and 6.4% among patients receiving surgical management.

Patients with asymptomatic carotid occlusive disease who require an operation for another reason (eg, coronary artery bypass graft or abdominal aortic aneurysm repair) usually can have that procedure performed without prophylactic carotid endarterectomy, because in this context the risk of stroke in asymptomatic persons is quite low. For patients with symptoms in the distribution of a stenotic carotid artery, the decision is more complicated. Generally, if a patient with an asymptomatic carotid stenosis has cardiac symptoms (eg, angina), coronary artery bypass grafting or angioplasty is performed first and carotid endarterectomy or angioplasty with stent placement is performed if the patient is otherwise a good surgical candidate.

Antiplatelet Agents

Aspirin, aspirin in combination with extended-release dipyridamole, and clopidogrel are all effective for secondary prevention of stroke. The optimal dose of aspirin is uncertain, with ranges recommended from 30 to 1,300 mg daily. Clopidogrel is given as a single dose, 75 mg daily. A combination of low-dose aspirin and extended-release dipyridamole is well tolerated and provides another useful alternative to aspirin for prevention of stroke. The combination may be slightly more effective than aspirin alone in secondary stroke prevention.

Ticlopidine is also an effective antiplatelet agent, but it is rarely given now because of associated neutropenia (thus, a complete blood cell count must be monitored every 2 weeks for the first 3 months of treatment) and thrombotic thrombocytopenic purpura, which has rarely been reported with clopidogrel.

There is evidence that the use of clopidogrel in combination with aspirin does not provide additional prevention for ischemic stroke but does increase the risk of significant bleeding; therefore, the combination is not commonly used for stroke prevention. When clopidogrel was compared with aspirin in combination with extended-release dipyridamole for the secondary prevention of stroke in a large randomized clinical trial, the study did not demonstrate any difference in effectiveness.

Warfarin

Warfarin is used for secondary prevention in selected patients who have TIA or cerebral infarction and 1) specific cardiac sources of embolus (eg, atrial fibrillation, left atrial or ventricular clot, dilated cardiomyopathy with markedly reduced ejection fraction, mechanical heart valves, recent myocardial infarction with left ventricular thrombus, valvular thrombus) or 2) hypercoagulable states. Warfarin may also be recommended for patients with TIA or cerebral infarction and aortic arch thrombus and for those with extracranial dissection; no clinical trial data support this treatment approach, though, and aspirin is sometimes recommended for these conditions instead of warfarin. In a clinical trial with patients who had symptomatic intracranial stenosis, warfarin was not more effective than aspirin in reducing ischemic stroke risk and was associated with a higher risk of hemorrhage.

Management of Acute Cerebral Infarction

If a patient has a severe neurologic deficit caused by an acute cerebral infarction, the immediate decision in the emergency department is whether the patient is a candidate for thrombolytic therapy (tissue plasminogen activator [tPA]). The initial therapeutic approach to ischemic infarction depends greatly on the time from the onset of symptoms to the presentation for emergency medical care. If the onset of symptoms was less than 3 hours before the evaluation, emergent thrombolytic therapy should be considered. If a patient awakens from sleep with the deficit, thrombolytic therapy should not be considered unless the duration of the deficit is clearly less than 3 hours. Some data do suggest, however, that patients may benefit from the use of tPA up to 4.5 hours after symptom onset.

Computed tomographic (CT) findings are important in selecting patients for tPA. CT should not show any evidence of intracranial hemorrhage, mass effect, early evidence of significant cerebral infarction (greater than one-third distribution of the cerebral hemisphere), or midline shift. Patients may be excluded by the following clinical criteria: rapidly improving deficit, obtunded or comatose status or presentation with seizure, history of intracranial hemorrhage or bleeding diathesis, blood pressure elevation persistently greater than 185/110 mm Hg, gastrointestinal tract hemorrhage or urinary tract hemorrhage within the previous 21 days, traumatic brain injury or cerebral infarction within 3 months, or mild deficit. Eligible patients should have marked weakness in at least 1 limb or severe aphasia. Laboratory abnormalities that may preclude treatment are heparin use within the previous 48 hours with an increased activated partial thromboplastin time, international normalized ratio (INR) greater than 1.5, or blood glucose concentration less than 50 mg/dL.

In a treatment trial of intravenous tPA, the efficacy in improving neurologic status at 3 months was defined for tPA compared with placebo, with the agent administered within 3 hours after the onset of symptoms. Although a greater proportion (about 12% greater) of subjects in the tPA group had minimal or no deficit at 3 months after the event, there was no increase in the proportion of persons who died. This is particularly important because there was an increased occurrence of symptomatic hemorrhage in the tPA group (6.4% compared with 0.6%).

Intravenous tPA should be given in a 0.9-mg/kg dose (maximum, 90 mg), with 10% given as a bolus and the rest over 60 minutes.

- Intravenous tPA should be considered for patients evaluated within 3 hours after the onset of symptoms of severe cerebral infarction.

- Do not treat with tPA if CT shows hemorrhage, mass effect, or midline shift.

Stroke Risks With Nonvalvular Atrial Fibrillation

Atrial fibrillation is associated with up to 24% of ischemic strokes and 50% of embolic strokes. The stroke rate for the entire cohort of patients with chronic atrial fibrillation is generally about 5% per year. However, patients younger than 60 with "lone atrial fibrillation" have a lower risk for stroke than other patients with atrial fibrillation and are often treated with only aspirin, depending on their CHADS2 score (congestive heart failure, hypertension, age >75 years, diabetes mellitus, and previous stroke) (see Table 2.8). Stroke risk factors with atrial fibrillation include a history of hypertension, recent congestive heart failure, previous thromboembolism (including TIAs), left ventricular dysfunction identified on 2-dimensional echocardiography, and increased size of the left atrium identified on M-mode echocardiography. Patients with atrial fibrillation who have 1 or more risk factors generally should receive anticoagulation with warfarin (INR, 2.0–3.0) and those at low risk should receive aspirin.

For patients receiving anticoagulant therapy, the dominant risk factor for intracranial hemorrhage is the INR, but age is another risk factor for subdural hemorrhage. An INR of 2.0 to 3.0 is probably an adequate level of anticoagulation for nearly all warfarin indications except for preventing embolization from mechanical heart valves. Generally, the lowest effective intensity of anticoagulant therapy should be given.

- Atrial fibrillation is associated with 24% of ischemic strokes and 50% of embolic strokes.

- The stroke rate is about 5% per year.

- Patients with "lone atrial fibrillation" have a lower risk for stroke.

HEMORRHAGIC CEREBROVASCULAR DISEASE

Intracerebral Hemorrhage

Hypertension commonly affects deep penetrating cerebral vessels, especially those supplying the basal ganglia, cerebral white matter, thalamus, pons, and cerebellum.

The following are common *misconceptions* of intracerebral hemorrhage:

1. The onset is generally sudden and catastrophic
2. Hypertension is invariably severe
3. Headache is always present
4. Reduced consciousness or coma is usually present
5. Cerebrospinal fluid (CSF) is always bloody
6. The prognosis is poor and mortality is high

None of these features, however, may be present and the prognosis depends on the size and location of the hemorrhage. Amyloid angiopathy is the second most common cause of intracerebral hemorrhage in older persons and often causes recurrent lobar hemorrhages.

- With intracerebral hemorrhage, the prognosis depends on the size and site of the hemorrhage.

Surgical evacuation of intracerebral hematomas may be necessary for patients who have signs of increased intracranial pressure or for those whose condition is worsening. However, apart from data for selected patients with lobar hemorrhages, there are no data that clearly show that surgery is beneficial for intracerebral hemorrhage.

Cerebellar Hemorrhage

It is important to recognize cerebellar hemorrhage because drainage may be lifesaving. The important clinical findings are vomiting and inability to walk. Long-tract signs usually are not present. Patients may have ipsilateral gaze palsy, ipsilateral cranial nerve (CN) VI palsy, or ipsilateral nuclear-type CN VII palsy (upper and lower facial weakness). They may or may not have headache, vertigo, and lethargy. Cerebellar hemorrhage may cause obstructive hydrocephalus.

- Vomiting and the inability to walk are important findings in cerebellar hemorrhage.

- Long-tract signs usually are not present.

- Cerebellar hemorrhage may cause obstructive hydrocephalus.

Subarachnoid Hemorrhage

Subarachnoid hemorrhage (SAH) accounts for about 5% of strokes, including about half of those in patients younger than 45 years, with a peak age range of 35 to 65 years. In up to 50% of cases, an alert patient with an aneurysm may have a small sentinel bleed with a warning headache, or the expansion of an aneurysm may cause focal neurologic signs or symptoms (eg, an incomplete CN III palsy). The prognosis is related directly to the state of consciousness at the time of intervention. Onset of the headache is characteristically sudden, and although one-third of SAHs occur during exertion, one-third occur during rest and one-third occur during sleep. The peak incidence of vasospasm associated with SAH occurs between days 4 and 12 after the initial hemorrhage. Other complications include hemorrhagic infiltration into the brain, ventricles, and even subdural space, which requires evacuation; hyponatremia associated with a cerebral salt-wasting syndrome or the syndrome of inappropriate secretion of antidiuretic hormone; and communicating hydrocephalus.

In addition to the initial hemorrhage, vasospasm and subsequent hemorrhage are the leading causes of morbidity and death among patients who have an SAH.

The outpouring of catecholamines may cause myocardial damage, with accompanying electrocardiographic abnormalities, pulmonary edema, and arrhythmias. Arrhythmias can be both supraventricular and ventricular and are most likely to occur during the initial hours or days after a moderate-to-severe SAH.

Initial treatment is supportive, often in an intensive care unit. Prevention of vasospasm is best achieved with maintaining normal or increased blood pressure and intravascular volume as well as using the calcium channel blocker nimodipine. If the SAH is from a ruptured aneurysm, an experienced team often does early intervention (surgical clipping or endovascular coiling).

The differential diagnosis of subtypes of hemorrhagic cerebrovascular disease is outlined in Table 46.1.

- About 5% of strokes are SAH.

- In 50% of cases, an alert patient with an aneurysm may have a small sentinel bleed.

- The prognosis is related directly to the state of consciousness at the time of intervention.

- Characteristically, the headache has a sudden onset.

NEOPLASTIC DISEASE

PRIMARY CNS NEOPLASMS

Brain tumors may manifest with focal progressive neurologic deficits, increased intracranial pressure (causing headache,

Hemorrhage into parenchyma
  Hypertension
  Amyloid angiopathy
  Aneurysm
  Vascular malformation
    Arteriovenous malformation
    Cavernous malformation
    Venous malformation (rare cause of hemorrhage)
  Trauma—primarily frontal & temporal
  Hemorrhagic infarction
  Secondary to brain tumors (primary & secondary neoplasms)
  Inflammatory diseases of vasculature
  Disorders of blood-forming organs (blood dyscrasia, especially leukemia & thrombocytopenic purpura)
  Anticoagulant or thrombolytic therapy
  Increased intracranial pressure (brainstem) (Duret hemorrhages)
  Illicit drug use (cocaine or amphetamines)
  Postsurgical
  Fat embolism (petechial)
  Hemorrhagic encephalitis (petechial)
  Undetermined cause (normal blood pressure & no other recognizable disorder)

Hemorrhage into subarachnoid space (subarachnoid hemorrhage)
  Trauma
  Aneurysm
    Saccular ("berry," "congenital")
    Fusiform (arteriosclerotic)—rarely causes hemorrhage
    Mycotic
  Arteriovenous malformation
  Many of the same causes listed under "Hemorrhage into parenchyma" above

Subdural & epidural hemorrhage (hematoma)
    Mainly traumatic (especially during anticoagulation)
    Many of the same causes listed under "Hemorrhage into parenchyma" above
Hemorrhage into pituitary (pituitary apoplexy)

vomiting, and papilledema), new-onset seizures, or progressive cognitive and behavioral changes. The most common primary brain tumors in adults are meningioma, astrocytoma, oligodendroglioma, and lymphoma.

The main risk factors associated with meningioma are sex steroid hormones and ionizing radiation. Treatment options vary according to patient age, comorbid conditions, and tumor size, location, progression, and histologic characteristics. Small asymptomatic tumors in older patients should be observed with follow-up CT or magnetic resonance imaging (MRI) every 6 to 12 months. If symptoms develop or there is clear tumor growth, surgical resection is indicated. Postoperative radiotherapy is indicated after incomplete resection or for tumors with aggressive histologic features (anaplastic or malignant meningiomas). Stereotactic radiosurgery is a treatment option in some cases.

Of all primary CNS neoplasms, 40% are gliomas, which occur in all areas of the brain and spinal cord. They are classified as grades I through IV according to their histologic features. Patients with gliomas, which are infiltrative tumors, may present with seizures. The prognosis depends on the patient's age at diagnosis and on the tumor type. Among patients with low-grade astrocytomas, median survival is 6 to 8 years; among patients with oligodendrogliomas, about 10 years. Clinical and radiologic observation is a reasonable approach for patients with stable lesions in a nonresectable area of the brain. Patients with large lesions and mass effect are candidates for surgical resection. The role of postoperative radiotherapy is still controversial.

High-grade astrocytomas, including anaplastic (grade III) astrocytoma and glioblastoma multiforme (grade IV) are associated with low survival (about 17.7% at 1 year). Surgical therapy is important for obtaining a tissue diagnosis, reducing the mass effect, and removing the majority of the lesion. Surgical therapy is followed by radiotherapy at the site of the lesion. Patients who receive concurrent temozolomide and radiotherapy have longer survival than those who receive radiotherapy alone.

Primary CNS lymphoma is becoming more common in patients with AIDS and in immunocompetent patients. Median survival has increased with the combination of radiotherapy and chemotherapy (mainly intravenous methotrexate).

NEUROLOGIC MANIFESTATIONS IN PATIENTS WITH SYSTEMIC CANCER

The most common neurologic symptoms of patients with systemic cancer are back pain, altered mental status, and headache. However, the most common neurologic complication of systemic cancer is metastatic disease, of which cerebral metastasis is most frequent. In patients with cancer and back pain, epidural metastasis and direct vertebral metastasis are common, but 15% to 20% of patients have no malignant diagnosis. Nonstructural causes are the most common reasons for headache. Identified causes include fever, side effects of therapy, lumbar puncture, metastasis (cerebral, leptomeningeal, or base of skull), and intracranial hemorrhage (thrombocytopenia or hemorrhage due to intracranial metastasis). The most common cause of altered mental status is toxic-metabolic encephalopathy, which is also the most common nonmetastatic manifestation of systemic cancer. Less common causes include intracranial metastatic disease (parenchymal and meningeal), paraneoplastic limbic encephalitis, intracranial hemorrhage, primary dementia, cerebral infarction, psychiatric disorder, known primary brain tumor, bacterial meningitis, and transient global amnesia.

Many neurologic problems in patients with cancer can be diagnosed from the medical history and findings on neurologic examination and require knowledge of both nonmetastatic- and noncancer-related neurologic illness.

Neurologic complications of systemic cancer are categorized as follows:

1. Metastatic: parenchymal, leptomeningeal, epidural, subdural, brachial plexus, lumbosacral plexus, and nerve infiltration; these complications are common

2. Infectious: unusual CNS infections because of immunosuppression

3. Complications of systemic metastases: hepatic encephalopathy

4. Vascular complications: cerebral infarction from hypercoagulable states, nonbacterial thrombotic endocarditis, and radiation damage to carotid arteries; cerebral hemorrhage (eg, from thrombocytopenia and hemorrhagic metastases)

5. Toxic-metabolic encephalopathies: usually from multiple causes, hypercalcemia, syndrome of inappropriate secretion of antidiuretic hormone, medications, and systemic infections

6. Complications of treatment (radiotherapy, chemotherapy, or surgery): radiation necrosis of the brain, radiation myelopathy, radiation plexopathy, fibrosis of the carotid arteries, neuropathies, encephalopathies, and cerebellar ataxia

7. Paraneoplastic (ie, nonmetastatic or "remote" effect of cancer): rare syndromes have been described from the cerebral cortex through the central and peripheral neuraxes to muscle

8. Miscellaneous: various systemic and neurologic illnesses unrelated to cancer

METASTASIS TO THE BRAIN

Brain metastases are the most common brain tumors. Approximately 30% of cancer patients have brain metastasis at presentation or later. Metastatic lung cancer is the most common (40%-50% of cases), followed by breast cancer, colon cancer, melanoma, and unknown primary cancer. Melanoma produces a disproportionate number of metastases in the CNS. Evaluation includes detailed history and examination, assessment of medical and neurologic performance status, and imaging studies (MRI of the brain with gadolinium; CT of the chest, abdomen, and pelvis; positron emission tomography). Brain metastases are frequently associated with surrounding edema. Dexamethasone (2 mg 2–4 times daily) is indicated in these cases, but additional treatment is required to prolong survival. Among untreated patients, median survival is 1 to 2 months; among treated patients, 2 to 10 months.

Survival depends on patient age, performance status, presence or absence of extracranial metastasis, and control of the primary tumor. Surgical resection of single accessible lesions increases survival among patients with good prognostic factors. Most patients receive postoperative whole-brain radiotherapy. Stereotactic radiosurgery can be used to treat multiple lesions in a single session in conjunction with whole-brain radiotherapy.

METASTASIS TO THE SPINAL CORD, LEPTOMENINGES, OR PERIPHERAL NERVES

Epidural spinal cord compression is the most common cause of spinal cord dysfunction in patients with cancer and is frequently preceded by vertebral metastasis. The most common causes are lung, breast, and prostate cancer, followed by non-Hodgkin lymphoma, multiple myeloma, and colorectal or renal carcinoma. About 60% of all cases involve the thoracic spine, and multiple sites are involved in one-third of the patients. The cardinal symptom is back pain, followed by weakness, sensory loss, and bladder or bowel dysfunction. Epidural spinal cord compression should be considered in all patients with any type of cancer and back or radicular pain.

Dexamethasone is highly effective at ameliorating symptoms. In many patients, radiotherapy is efficacious for preventing further tumor growth and neural damage. The therapeutic response is better with radiosensitive tumors (eg, multiple myeloma, lymphoma, and prostate, breast, and small cell lung carcinoma) than with relatively radioresistant tumors (eg, melanoma, renal cell carcinoma). Surgery is indicated for patients with spinal instability, bone impingement on the spinal cord, worsening deficits during or despite radiotherapy, radioresistant epidural tumors with limited tumor elsewhere, or a diagnosis that is in doubt.

Meningeal metastases occur in lung and breast cancer, melanoma, leukemia, and lymphoma. Patients typically present with symptoms and signs reflecting involvement at many levels of the nervous system: headache, encephalopathy, seizures, cranial nerve involvement (most commonly diplopia or facial weakness), back pain, or spinal root involvement. Diagnosis is suggested by the presence of meningeal enhancement on gadolinium MRI and is confirmed by CSF cytologic findings. Subsequent CSF samples may be necessary; the yield is 90% after the third lumbar puncture.

Intramedullary spinal cord metastases are much less frequent than epidural metastases and most commonly result from small cell lung carcinoma. Brachial plexus involvement is most frequent with lung and breast cancer. Colorectal cancer causes local pelvic metastasis and is the most frequent cause of neoplastic plexopathy. Head cancer and neck cancer are the most frequent sources of metastasis to the base of the skull.

- Cancers commonly causing neurologic problems are lung, breast, and colorectal cancers, leukemia, lymphoma, and melanoma.

- Common metastatic sites are the parenchyma of the cerebral hemispheres and cerebellum, leptomeninges, epidural and subdural spaces, brachial and lumbosacral plexuses, and nerves.

- Cerebral metastasis is the most common neurologic complication of systemic cancer.

- Epidural spinal cord compression should be considered for all patients with any type of cancer and back or radicular pain.

- The most frequent cause of tumor plexopathy is colorectal cancer.

- Melanoma produces a disproportionate number of metastases in the CNS.

- Toxic-metabolic encephalopathy is the most common nonmetastatic manifestation of cancer.

CLASSIFICATION OF PARANEOPLASTIC NEUROLOGIC DISORDERS

Central nervous system
  Encephalomyelitis
  Limbic encephalitis
  Cerebellar degeneration
  Brainstem encephalitis
  Opsoclonus-myoclonus
  Stiff person syndrome
  Chorea
  Necrotizing myelopathy
  Motor neuronopathy
Dorsal root ganglion & peripheral nerves
  Subacute sensory neuronopathy
  Gastroparesis or intestinal pseudo-obstruction
  Acute autonomic ganglionopathy
  Acquired neuromyotonia
  Neuropathy associated with plasma cell dyscrasia or lymphoma
  Vasculitis of nerve or muscle
Neuromuscular junction
  Lambert-Eaton myasthenic syndrome
  Myasthenia gravis
Muscle
  Dermatomyositis
  Polymyositis
  Acute necrotizing myopathy
Eye and retina
  Cancer-associated retinopathy
  Optic neuropathy

PARANEOPLASTIC DISORDERS

Paraneoplastic disorders are associated with increased levels of circulating antibodies (onconeural antibodies) directed against neoplastic cells and attacking membrane ion channels or intracellular (nuclear or cytoplasmic) proteins in neurons. The most common underlying malignancies are small cell lung carcinoma and breast cancer. Others include ovarian or testicular carcinoma, thymoma, Hodgkin disease, and parotid tumors. Paraneoplastic syndromes can affect any level of the CNS or peripheral nervous system (Box 46.2). Important examples include limbic encephalitis (characterized by behavioral and memory abnormalities and seizures), brainstem encephalitis, opsoclonus-myoclonus, cerebellar ataxia, myelopathy, peripheral neuropathy, stiff person syndrome (with axial and limb rigidity), sensory ganglionopathies, Lambert-Eaton myasthenic syndrome (LEMS), dermatomyositis, and retinopathy. These syndromes are characterized by an acute or subacute onset and increased levels of 1 or more antibodies (Table 46.2). A paraneoplastic neurologic syndrome precedes the diagnosis of cancer in 60% of cases and develops after tumor diagnosis or at tumor recurrence in 40%.

Treatment of the underlying neoplasm is the main factor associated with neurologic stabilization. Immunotherapy with corticosteroids, intravenous immunoglobulin, plasma exchange, cyclophosphamide, or rituximab may be helpful in

Table 46.2 **PARANEOPLASTIC ANTIBODIES ASSOCIATED WITH CANCER AND SYNDROMES**

ANTIBODY	ASSOCIATED CANCER	ASSOCIATED SYNDROMES
Anti-Hu (ANNA-1)	SCLC	Encephalomyelitis Limbic encephalitis Cerebellar degeneration SSN Autonomic ganglionopathy
Anti-Ri (ANNA-2)	Breast, gynecologic, SCLC	Ataxia Opsoclonus-myoclonus Brainstem encephalitis
Anti-Yo (PCA-1)	Breast, ovary	Cerebellar degeneration
CRMP-5	SCLC, thymoma	Chorea, myelopathy, optic neuritis, retinopathy, & others
Amphiphysin	Breast, SCLC	Stiff person syndrome Encephalomyelitis
Anti-Ma2	Testicular germinoma	Limbic encephalitis Brainstem encephalitis
P/Q type VGCC	SCLC	LEMS
Muscle nAChR	Thymoma	Myasthenia gravis
Ganglionic nAChR	SCLC	Autonomic ganglionopathy
Voltage-gated potassium channel	Thymoma, SCLC	Neuromyotonia Limbic encephalitis
NMDA receptor	Ovarian teratoma	Limbic encephalitis Rigidity Hypoventilation Dysautonomia

Abbreviations: ANNA, antineuronal nuclear antibody; CRMP, collapsin response mediator protein; LEMS, Lambert-Eaton myasthenic syndrome; nAChR, nicotinic acetylcholine receptor; NMDA, *N*-methyl-D-aspartate; PCA, Purkinje cell antibody; SCLC, small cell lung carcinoma; SSN, subacute sensory neuronopathy; VGCC, voltage-gated calcium channels.

paraneoplastic disorders related to antibodies against membrane antigens such as P/Q type voltage-gated calcium channels (LEMS) or voltage-gated potassium channels (limbic encephalitis).

- Paraneoplastic neurologic syndromes typically precede the diagnosis of the underlying cancer.

- A paraneoplastic syndrome should be suspected in any patient with a subacute inflammatory disorder affecting any level of the central or peripheral nervous system.

NEUROLOGIC COMPLICATIONS OF CANCER TREATMENT

Treatment of cancer with chemotherapeutic and biologic agents is frequently complicated by the development of neurotoxicity. Typical examples are listed in Table 46.3.

Table 46.3 EXAMPLES OF NEUROTOXICITY OF CHEMOTHERAPEUTIC AGENTS

AGENT	TYPICAL MANIFESTATIONS OF NEUROTOXICITY
Platinum compounds (cisplatin, oxaliplatin)	Sensory (large fiber) neuropathy (sensory ataxia) Autonomic neuropathy Ototoxicity Encephalopathy, cortical blindness, seizures Retrobulbar neuritis Retinal injury
Vinca alkaloids	Sensorimotor peripheral neuropathy Autonomic neuropathy
Taxanes (eg, paclitaxel)	Predominantly sensory peripheral neuropathy Occasional motor neuropathies Transient scotomata
Methotrexate	Acute chemical arachnoiditis (intrathecal administration) Acute, reversible, stroke-like syndrome Subacute encephalopathy Transverse myelopathy Chronic demyelinating encephalopathy
5-Fluorouracil	Cerebellar dysfunction Acute encephalopathy Subacute extrapyramidal syndrome Leukoencephalopathy (when combined with levamisole)
Cytarabine (ara-C)	Cerebellar dysfunction Cognitive impairment Necrotizing leukoencephalopathy Peripheral neuropathy Seizures, parkinsonism, myelopathy
Ifosfamide	Encephalopathy with agitation, visual & auditory hallucinations, behavioral & memory changes Hemiparesis, seizures, coma Cerebellar, extrapyramidal, or cranial nerve dysfunction
Nitrosoureas	Encephalopathy
Busulfan	Seizures
L-Asparaginase	Encephalopathy Cerebral venous thrombosis

MOVEMENT DISORDERS

TREMOR

Tremor is an oscillatory rhythmic movement disorder. A simple classification of tremor is rest tremor and action tremor. *Rest tremor* is observed while the patient is sitting with the arms lying in the lap or walking with the arms at the side. Rest tremor occurs in Parkinson disease. *Action tremor* occurs when there is muscle contraction. It includes postural tremor and kinetic tremor. *Postural tremor* affects the hands and is seen mainly with the arms outstretched, although there is often a kinetic component as well. Postural tremor is physiologic, but it is also noted pathologically in essential tremor. Drugs such as methylxanthines, β-adrenergic agonists, lithium, and amiodarone may produce postural tremor. *Kinetic tremor* is seen mainly in action, as in finger-to-nose testing. This type of tremor occurs with cerebellar disease and diseases of the cerebellar connections in the brainstem.

ESSENTIAL TREMOR

Essential tremor is the most common movement disorder and should be differentiated from tremor observed in Parkinson disease (Table 46.4). *Essential tremor* is a monosymptomatic condition manifested by rhythmic oscillations of various parts of the body. Middle-aged and older persons are most commonly affected, and there is often a genetic component. The hands are affected most, with the tremor present in the postural position and often having a kinetic component. The head and voice can be affected. Head tremor can be either horizontal ("no-no") or vertical ("yes-yes"). Head tremor almost never occurs in Parkinson disease, but parkinsonian patients may have tremor of the mouth, lips, tongue, and jaw. The legs and trunk (affected in orthostatic tremor) are affected less frequently in essential tremor. Essential tremor is a slowly progressive condition; its pathophysiologic mechanism is not known.

The agent most effective in decreasing essential tremor is alcohol. Drinking a beverage containing alcohol can substantially reduce the tremor for 45 to 60 minutes. Notably, the prevalence of alcoholism among patients with essential tremor is no different from that of the general population. Propranolol (80–320 mg daily), other β-blockers, and primidone (25–250 mg at bedtime) are also effective. Other drugs that have been prescribed are clonazepam, gabapentin, and topiramate. Deep brain stimulation (DBS) of the thalamus is effective for all

Table 46.4 DIFFERENTIAL DIAGNOSIS OF TREMOR

FEATURE	PARKINSON DISEASE	ESSENTIAL TREMOR
Tremor type & frequency	Rest >> postural; 3–5 Hz	Postural, kinetic; 8–12 Hz
Affected by tremor	Hands, legs, chin, jaw	Hands, head, neck, voice
Rigidity & bradykinesia	Yes	No
Family history	15%	60%
Alcohol response	Inconsistent	Consistent
Therapy	Levodopa, dopamine agonists, anticholinergics	Propranolol, primidone, gabapentin, botulinum toxin type A
Surgical treatment	Subthalamic stimulation	Thalamic (Vim) stimulation

Abbreviation: Vim, subnucleus ventralis intermedius.

types of tremor and is indicated for patients with functional disability that does not respond to drug therapy.

- Essential tremor affects the hands most and occurs mostly in middle-aged and older persons.

- There is often a genetic component.

- Head tremor almost never occurs in Parkinson disease.

PARKINSON DISEASE

Patients with Parkinson disease present with tremor (the initial symptom in 50%-70%, but 15% never have tremor), rigidity, and bradykinesia. The gait is unsteady, slow, and shuffling. Decreased blinking rate, lack of change in facial expression, small handwriting, and asymptomatic orthostatic hypotension are also common. Parkinson disease includes motor manifestations (Box 46.3) and nonmotor manifestations (Box 46.4). The classic motor manifestations of Parkinson disease, including rest tremor, muscle stiffness (rigidity), and slowness of movement initiation and execution (hypokinesia and bradykinesia), typically start asymmetrically and respond to levodopa therapy. Late motor manifestations, including difficulty swallowing, postural instability, and freezing of gait, are much less responsive to treatment. At late stages of the disease in patients who have received prolonged levodopa therapy, motor fluctuations develop. Some nonmotor manifestations may precede the diagnosis of Parkinson disease (Box 46.4).

The differential diagnosis of Parkinson disease includes disorders caused by drugs (Box 46.5) or toxins (eg, carbon monoxide, manganese), potentially treatable neurometabolic disorders (particularly Wilson disease in patients younger than 50 years), and other neurodegenerative disorders in which parkinsonism is a prominent feature ("Parkinson plus" syndromes) (Table 46.5). Conditions that should each suggest a disorder other than Parkinson disease as a cause of parkinsonism include the lack of response to levodopa, the presence of early postural instability or orthostatic hypotension, the detection of cerebellar findings (ataxia) or corticospinal signs

Box 46.3 MOTOR MANIFESTATIONS OF PARKINSON DISEASE

Early manifestations (typically asymmetric in onset & responsive to levodopa)
 Rest tremor
 Rigidity
 Bradykinesia
Late manifestations (less responsive to levodopa)
 Gait & postural instability
 Dysphagia
Motor fluctuations (in patients with severe disease & long-term levodopa therapy)
 "Wearing-off" & "on-off" phenomena
 Levodopa-induced dyskinesia

Box 46.4 NONMOTOR MANIFESTATIONS OF PARKINSON DISEASE

Autonomic
 Constipation[a]
 Orthostatic hypotension
 Bladder dysfunction
Sleep disorders
 Excessive diurnal somnolence
 Insomnia
 REM sleep behavior disorder[a]
 Periodic leg movement disorder
Cognitive symptoms
 Depression[a]
 Anxiety
 Hallucinations
 Abnormal behavior
Sensory symptoms
 Impaired olfaction[a]

Abbreviation: REM, rapid eye movement.

[a] May precede the diagnosis of disease.

(increased deep tendon reflexes, spasticity, or extensor plantar response), and early dementia. Although dementia is more frequent among patients with Parkinson disease, it is noted in only about 25% of those in whom the disease develops after age 60.

- Tremor does not occur in 15% of patients with Parkinson disease.

Box 46.5 DRUGS THAT INDUCE PARKINSONISM OR TREMOR

Antagonist of dopamine D_2 receptors
 Neuroleptics (haloperidol, risperidone, resperine, etc)
 Antiemetics (metoclopramide, prochlorperazine)
Other psychiatric drugs
 Selective serotonin reuptake inhibitors
 Tricyclics
 Lithium
Cardiovascular drugs
 Amiodarone
 Calcium channel blockers (flunarizine)
 Atorvastatin
Anticonvulsants
 Valproate
Others
 Cyclosporine
 Metronidazole
 Caffeine & other methylxanthines
 α-Adrenergic agonist
 Thyroxine
 Prednisone

Table 46.5 DIFFERENTIAL DIAGNOSIS OF PARKINSON PLUS SYNDROMES

MANIFESTATION	SUSPECT
Poor response to levodopa	Any Parkinson plus syndrome (MSA & PSP may respond)
Early falls	PSP or MSA
Severe OH, urologic symptoms, anosmia, or DEB	MSA
Cerebellar signs	MSA or spinocerebellar degeneration
Vertical gaze palsy	PSP
Asymmetric apraxia	Corticobasal degeneration
Early dementia	Lewy body dementia Creutzfeldt-Jakob disease

Abbreviations: DEB, dream enactment behavior; MSA, multiple system atrophy; OH, orthostatic hypotension; PSP, progressive supranuclear palsy.

- The effects of drugs should be excluded in all patients presenting with parkinsonism.
- Wilson disease should be considered in all patients younger than 50 years who present with parkinsonism (or dystonia, cerebellar ataxia, or cognitive or psychiatric manifestations).

- If ataxia, increased deep tendon reflexes, spasticity, extensor plantar responses, or lower motor neuron findings are present, consider "Parkinson plus" syndromes.

The treatment of the motor manifestations of Parkinson disease is summarized in Table 46.6. The initial treatment options include dopaminergic agonists and a combination of levodopa and carbidopa (Sinemet). Anticholinergic agents were used in the past for young patients with mild symptoms (predominantly tremor), but they are rarely used now and should not be given to patients older than 65 years because of the high incidence of side effects, such as memory loss, delirium, urinary hesitancy, and blurred vision.

Patients with disabling symptoms should receive carbidopa-levodopa. The initial dosage is a 25/100 tablet (25 mg carbidopa/100 mg levodopa) by mouth 3 times daily on an empty stomach. Although monotherapy with dopaminergic agonists carries a smaller risk of delayed motor complications than long-term levodopa therapy, these agents are less efficacious than levodopa. Dopaminergic agonists can be used as initial treatment in young patients to reduce the dose of levodopa. Dopaminergic agonists include pramipexole and ropinirole. Bromocriptine and pergolide, ergot derivatives, are no longer used because of the risk of retroperitoneal or cardiac valvular fibrosis. The main side effects of levodopa and dopaminergic agonists are nausea, orthostatic hypotension, and

Table 46.6 MANAGEMENT OF MOTOR MANIFESTATIONS OF PARKINSON DISEASE

TREATMENT[a]	INDICATION	CAVEATS/PROBLEMS
Carbidopa-levodopa Sinemet 25/100[b] Sinemet CR 50/200[c]	Most efficacious treatment Give early in patients with marked impairment	Nausea, vomiting, OH Motor fluctuations with long-term treatment
Dopaminergic agonists Pramipexole Ropinirole Rotigotine (patch)	Early use in young patients, either alone or associated with small dose of levodopa Motor fluctuation in patients taking Sinemet	Nausea, vomiting, OH More likely than Sinemet to produce excessive diurnal somnolence, impulse control disorder, hallucinations, or peripheral edema
COMT inhibitors Entacapone	Prolong the duration of action of levodopa in patients with wearing-off effect	Diarrhea
MAO-B inhibitors Selegiline Rasagiline	Delay the need to start levodopa therapy May be neuroprotective	Insomnia (with selegiline); nausea, hallucinations, confusion, dyskinesias, OH
Amantadine	Adjuvant treatment in patients with levodopa-induced dyskinesia	Dizziness, livedo reticularis, edema
Surgical treatment GPi or STN DBS Pallidotomy	Levodopa responsive, severe parkinsonism with unilateral symptoms, motor fluctuations & dyskinesia, normal cognitive function, & no psychiatric disease	Does not help gait instability Cognitive & psychiatric symptoms may follow STN DBS

Abbreviations: COMT, catechol O-methyltransferase; DBS, deep brain stimulation; GPi, globus pallidus, pars interna; MAO, monoamine oxidase; OH, orthostatic hypotension; STN, subthalamic nucleus.

[a] Anticholinergics (eg, trihexyphenidyl) are used only rarely and are contraindicated in patients older than 65 years owing to prominent autonomic and cognitive side effects.

[b] Carbidopa 25 mg, levodopa 100 mg.

[c] Controlled release formulation: carbidopa 50 mg, levodopa 200 mg.

hallucinations. An important side effect of all these agents is the development of unpredictable episodes of daytime sleepiness. An important side effect of dopaminergic agonists is the development of impulse dyscontrol, manifested as compulsive gambling, shopping, or hypersexuality. Patients and their spouses should be counseled about these problems before initiation of dopaminergic agonist therapy.

When given to a patient with newly diagnosed Parkinson disease, selegiline or rasagiline (monoamine oxidase type B inhibitors) may give mild symptomatic relief and delay the need to initiate levodopa therapy. Side effects include nausea, hallucinations, confusion, dyskinesias, and orthostatic hypotension.

Long-term high-dose levodopa monotherapy leads to dyskinesias and motor fluctuations. Management strategies include the use of smaller and more frequent doses of levodopa, long-acting levodopa preparations, dopaminergic agonists, and inhibitors of catechol *O*-methyltransferase. Apomorphine can be administered subcutaneously for severe, hypomobile, end-of-dose "wearing-off" times. A protein-restricted diet may decrease unpredictable off times. Amantadine, a glutamate receptor antagonist, is used as adjuvant treatment in patients with levodopa-induced dyskinesias.

A surgical approach, primarily DBS of the subthalamic nucleus or globus pallidus, is an option to relieve motor symptoms in eligible patients with levodopa-responsive Parkinson disease and severe motor fluctuations. Patient selection is critical to ensure maximal benefit of DBS. Patients who have cognitive or psychiatric disorders or who do not respond to levodopa are not eligible. Manifestations such as dysphagia, postural instability, and gait freezing do not respond to DBS. DBS of the subthalamic nucleus may result in transient cognitive or psychiatric manifestations: Suicide has been reported among some patients.

- Carbidopa-levodopa is the indicated treatment when patients have disabling motor symptoms or when the diagnosis of Parkinson disease is uncertain.

- Dopaminergic agonists are used as initial therapy in young patients to delay onset of levodopa-induced motor fluctuations.

- Before starting dopaminergic agonist therapy, patients and their spouses should be warned about the risk of falling asleep while driving and the possibility of compulsive gambling, shopping, or hypersexuality.

- DBS may be helpful in relieving motor symptoms in eligible patients with Parkinson disease, but patient selection is critical.

The management of nonmotor manifestations of Parkinson disease is summarized in Table 46.7. Orthostatic hypotension, constipation, bladder dysfunction, and other autonomic manifestations develop in many patients with parkinsonism. In these patients, Parkinson disease should be distinguished from multiple system atrophy. Findings suggestive of multiple system atrophy include lack of a predictable response to levodopa, the presence of cerebellar or pyramidal signs, severe orthostatic hypotension and urinary incontinence, sleep apnea, and laryngeal stridor. The management of orthostatic hypotension includes eliminating potentially offending drugs (eg, vasodilators, diuretics, dopaminergic agonists, and clozapine), increasing sodium and water intake, performing postural maneuvers, elevating the head of the bed, and wearing support stockings. Drug treatment includes fludrocortisone (0.1–1.0 mg daily) and vasoconstrictors such as midodrine (10–40 mg daily). Pyridostigmine can also be used for orthostatic hypotension in dosages similar to those used in myasthenia gravis (30–60 mg 3 times daily).

New-generation antipsychotic drugs, such as clozapine, olanzapine, and quetiapine, can be used to manage drug-induced psychosis because they have a lower risk of exacerbating parkinsonism in these patients.

OTHER MOVEMENT DISORDERS: BOTULINUM TOXIN THERAPY

Botulinum toxin, which blocks the neuromuscular junction, is effective therapy for cervical dystonia, blepharospasm, hemifacial spasm, spasmodic dysphonia, jaw-closing oromandibular dystonia, and limb dystonia, including occupational dystonias.

INFLAMMATORY AND AUTOIMMUNE DISORDERS

MULTIPLE SCLEROSIS

The most common inflammatory demyelinating disease of the CNS is multiple sclerosis, a disabling disorder that affects predominantly young adults, with an onset between ages 20 and 50 years. It affects women twice as often as men. Multiple sclerosis has a complex immunopathogenesis, variable prognosis, and an unpredictable course. Polygenic and environmental (possibly viral) factors probably have a substantial effect on susceptibility to multiple sclerosis. The disease attacks white matter and (in both early and late stages) axons of the cerebral hemispheres, brainstem, cerebellum, spinal cord, and optic nerve. Most patients (80%-85%) present with relapsing-remitting symptoms. In about 15% of patients, the disease is progressive from onset (primary progressive). Over time, in 70% of patients with the relapsing-remitting form, secondary progressive multiple sclerosis develops.

Symptoms reflect multiple white matter lesions disseminated in space and time. Typical syndromes include optic neuritis, myelopathy, brainstem syndromes, and paroxysmal attacks. Optic neuritis manifests with unilateral visual loss frequently associated with eye pain with movement. Myelopathy manifests with sensory symptoms, including a bandlike sensation in the abdomen and chest, spastic weakness of the limbs, and bladder and bowel dysfunction. Other typical symptoms include diplopia (due to internuclear ophthalmoplegia) and ataxia. Paroxysmal symptoms, including trigeminal neuralgia and hemifacial spasm, in a young patient should increase

Table 46.7 MANAGEMENT OF NONMOTOR MANIFESTATIONS OF PARKINSON DISEASE

MANIFESTATION	MECHANISM	MANAGEMENT
Orthostatic hypotension	Loss of sympathetic ganglion neurons & effects of dopaminergic agonists	Increase sodium & water intake Fludrocortisone, midodrine, pyridostigmine
Constipation	Loss of enteric neurons	Bulk agents, enema
Insomnia	Wearing off; PLMS	Nightly dose of levodopa
REM sleep behavior disorder	Early manifestation	Clonazepam, melatonin
Hallucinations	Medication effect (exclude DLB)	Discontinue use of anticholinergics, MAO-B inhibitors, & amantadine Reduce or discontinue use of dopamine agonists Quetiapine or olanzapine
Depression	Loss of serotonergic neurons?	SSRIs Optimize dopaminergic therapy
Anxiety	Akathisia, stressors	Optimize dopaminergic therapy
Cognitive impairment	Frontal lobe dysfunction Development of DLB	Cholinesterase inhibitors Optimize dopaminergic therapy
Impulse dyscontrol (compulsive gambling, shopping, hypersexuality)	Activation of dopamine D_3 receptors in limbic striatum	Warn the patients Reduce or discontinue use of dopaminergic agonist Quetiapine or SSRI may help
Fatigue	Multifactorial	Optimize dopaminergic therapy
Pain	Early morning dystonia Immobility	Increase levodopa Mobilization, physical therapy
Arm paresthesia	May reflect insufficient levodopa treatment	Increase levodopa Exclude other causes
Diplopia	Medication effect Poor convergence	Reading glasses or prisms instead of bifocals

Abbreviations: DLB, dementia with Lewy bodies; MAO, monoamine oxidase; PLMS, periodic leg movement disorder; REM, rapid eye movement; SSRI, selective serotonin reuptake inhibitor.

awareness of multiple sclerosis. Other important symptoms are memory and cognitive dysfunction and depression. Associated features that suggest multiple sclerosis include excessive unexplained fatigue and exacerbation of symptoms upon exposure to heat.

The diagnosis is primarily based on clinical and MRI data that show lesions disseminated in space and time. Abnormalities on MRI are most helpful and include multifocal lesions of various ages in the periventricular white matter, corpus callosum, brainstem, cerebellum, and spinal cord. Gadolinium-enhanced lesions are presumed to be active lesions of inflammatory demyelination. In patients with clinically isolated syndromes, such as optic neuritis, myelopathy, or brainstem syndrome, abnormal MRI findings are a strong predictor of the eventual clinical diagnosis of multiple sclerosis in the next 5 years. CSF findings include oligoclonal bands, increased IgG synthesis, and moderate lymphocytic pleocytosis (<50 mononuclear cells/μL). Visual and somatosensory evoked potential studies are less helpful.

Many other disorders mimic multiple sclerosis and should be considered when patients have atypical findings. Important examples include vasculitis, infections (eg, human immunodeficiency virus infection or Lyme disease), paraneoplastic disorders, neurosarcoidosis, systemic lupus erythematosus, Behçet disease, and lymphoma.

Predictors associated with a more favorable long-term course of multiple sclerosis include age younger than 40 years at onset, female sex, optic neuritis or isolated sensory symptoms as the first clinical manifestation, and relatively infrequent attacks. Prognostic factors associated with a poor outcome include age older than 40 years at onset, male sex, cerebellar or pyramidal tract findings at initial presentation, relatively frequent attacks during the first 2 years, incomplete remissions, and a chronically progressive course. However, no single clinical variable is sufficient to predict the course or outcome of this disease. There is evidence that a subset of multiple sclerosis patients has very benign disease; hence, not every patient with multiple sclerosis must receive long-term treatment.

The recommended therapy for acute exacerbations of multiple sclerosis is a 3- to 5-day course of a high dose of intravenous methylprednisolone (1.0 g daily). Severe or steroid-unresponsive exacerbations are treated with plasma exchange.

Interferon beta-1a, interferon beta-1b, and glatiramer acetate decrease the relapse rate and the intensity of relapse in patients with the relapsing-remitting type of multiple sclerosis. There is some evidence that these medications may also reduce disability. They are expensive, however, and significant side effects, including depression, can occur. For patients receiving interferon beta, periodic monitoring includes liver function tests and complete blood cell counts. In 5% to 30% of patients receiving interferon beta, neutralizing antibodies develop and block the effects of interferon beta.

Several drugs are used to treat specific symptoms of multiple sclerosis. Trigeminal neuralgia, flexor spasms, and other paroxysmal symptoms respond to carbamazepine, and spasticity responds to baclofen and tizanidine. Fatigue, a disabling symptom of multiple sclerosis, occasionally responds to amantadine, modafinil, or stimulants.

- Typical clinical scenario for multiple sclerosis: A 35-year-old woman has a history of rapid loss of vision in the right eye, with pain on eye movement. A similar episode occurred 2 years ago and involved the same eye; recovery was complete. She also has noticed weakness and paresthesias of both legs in the past 6 months. CSF analysis shows increased protein levels and oligoclonal bands on electrophoresis. Multiple T2 hyperintense areas consistent with demyelination are seen on MRI.

NEUROMYELITIS OPTICA

Neuromyelitis optica (NMO) is a recurrent severe demyelinating disease that may mimic multiple sclerosis. The diagnosis is based on the following: a) presence of severe optic neuritis or transverse myelitis, or both; b) MRI evidence of contiguous spinal cord lesions spanning more than 3 vertebral segments; c) absence of typical multiple sclerosis lesions on MRI of the brain; and d) presence of NMO-IgG antibodies that react against the water channel aquaporin 4. Unlike in multiple sclerosis, the CSF in NMO shows polynuclear pleocytosis (>50 cells/μL) and an absence of oligoclonal bands. Exacerbations may respond to intravenous methylprednisolone or plasma exchange. The presence of NMO-IgG antibodies indicates risk of recurrence and warrants long-term immunosuppression with azathioprine, cyclophosphamide, or rituximab.

- Not all acute demyelinating CNS disorders are multiple sclerosis.

- The diagnosis of multiple sclerosis is primarily based on clinical and MRI criteria showing dissemination in space and time.

- The presence of NMO-IgG is highly specific for NMO.

NEUROLOGY OF SEPSIS

The nervous system is commonly affected in sepsis syndrome. The neurologic conditions encountered are septic encephalopathy, critical illness polyneuropathy or myopathy (or both), cachexia, and panfascicular muscle necrosis. Neurologic complications also occur in intensive care units for critical medical illness. These complications include metabolic encephalopathy, seizures, hypoxic-ischemic encephalopathy, and stroke.

SEPTIC ENCEPHALOPATHY

Septic encephalopathy is brain dysfunction in association with systemic infection without overt infection of the brain or meninges. Early encephalopathy often begins before failure of other organs and is not due to single or multiple organ failure. Endotoxin does not cross the blood-brain barrier and so probably does not directly affect adult brains. Cytokines, important components of sepsis syndrome, may contribute to encephalopathy. Gegenhalten or paratonic rigidity occurs in more than 50% of patients, and tremor, asterixis, and multifocal myoclonus in about 25%. Seizures and focal neurologic signs are rare.

Electroencephalography is a sensitive indicator of encephalopathy. The mildest abnormality is diffuse excessive low-voltage theta activity (4–7 Hz). The next level of severity is intermittent rhythmic delta activity (<4 Hz). As the condition worsens, delta activity becomes arrhythmic and continuous. Typical triphasic waves occur in severe cases, especially in hepatic failure. In these cases, MRI and CT scans of the brain may be normal.

- Brain dysfunction is associated with systemic infection.

- Encephalopathy precedes failure of other organs.

- Cytokines are an important part of sepsis syndrome.

- More than 50% of patients have paratonic rigidity.

- Tremor, asterixis, and multifocal myoclonus occur in 25% of patients.

- Electroencephalography is a sensitive indicator of encephalopathy.

CRITICAL ILLNESS POLYNEUROPATHY

Critical illness polyneuropathy occurs in 70% of patients with sepsis and multiple organ failure. There is often an unexplained difficulty in weaning from mechanical ventilation. Nerve biopsy specimens show primary axonal degeneration of motor and sensory fibers without inflammation. Most patients also have concomitant myopathy. Recovery from critical illness polyneuropathy is satisfactory if the patient survives sepsis and multiple organ failure.

- In critical illness polyneuropathy, nerve biopsy specimens show primary axonal degeneration of motor and sensory fibers without inflammation.

- Recovery from critical illness polyneuropathy is satisfactory.

SUMMARY

- Pathophysiologic mechanisms of ischemic cerebrovascular disease include a cardiac source, large-vessel disorders, small-vessel disorders, and hematologic causes.

- Atrial fibrillation is associated with 24% of ischemic strokes and 50% of embolic strokes.

- Cerebral metastasis is the most common neurologic complication of systemic cancer.

- Tremor does not occur in 15% of patients with Parkinson disease.

- The diagnosis of multiple sclerosis is primarily based on clinical and MRI criteria showing dissemination in space and time.

PART XIII

DERMATOLOGY

47.

DERMATOLOGY

Carilyn N. Wieland, MD, and Lisa A. Drage, MD

GOALS

- Understand the natural history, diagnosis, and treatment of skin cancers, including malignant melanoma, squamous cell carcinoma, and basal cell carcinoma.

- Know how to diagnose and treat common skin conditions, including acne vulgaris, psoriasis, atopic dermatitis, and allergic contact dermatitis.

- Discern the autoimmune bullous diseases.

- Recognize serious skin conditions such as erythema multiforme and Stevens-Johnson syndrome.

- Know the dermatologic manifestations of drug reactions.

- Identify cutaneous signs of malignancy and common medical conditions.

GENERAL DERMATOLOGY

SKIN CANCER

Nonmelanoma skin cancers (basal cell carcinoma, squamous cell carcinoma) are the most common malignancies in the United States. Skin cancers will be diagnosed in more than 2 million people in the United States this year. The cure rate for nonmelanoma skin cancer is more than 90% with early detection and appropriate treatment. The incidence of nonmelanoma skin cancer is increasing because of a combination of increased exposure to ultraviolet light, changes in clothing style, increased longevity, and atmospheric ozone depletion.

Both basal cell and squamous cell carcinomas commonly occur on sun-exposed skin areas. The ratio of basal cell carcinoma to squamous cell carcinoma is 4:1 in immunocompetent people. Basal cell carcinomas are usually slow-growing and locally invasive. They may invade vital structures and can cause considerable disfigurement. Basal cell carcinomas rarely metastasize to regional lymph nodes. In contrast, the risk of metastases of squamous cell carcinoma in the general population is approximately 2%.

Organ transplant recipients have a high risk of nonmelanoma skin cancer and melanoma due to their immunosuppressed status. Squamous cell carcinoma is the most common skin cancer in solid organ transplant recipients and is more aggressive with a risk of metastasis of approximately 8%.

- Skin cancer is the most common cancer in the United States, accounting for almost half of all cancers.

- Basal cell carcinoma constitutes approximately 80% of all skin cancers in the general population.

- Basal cell carcinoma and squamous cell carcinoma occur on sun-exposed skin.

- The cure rate for nonmelanoma skin cancer is >90% with early detection and treatment.

- Organ transplant recipients have a high risk for squamous cell carcinoma of the skin.

MALIGNANT MELANOMA

In 2010, about 68,000 Americans received a diagnosis of cutaneous melanoma, and 8,700 died of the disease. The estimated lifetime risk of invasive melanoma is about 2% for Americans born in 2005.

The strongest risk factors for melanoma are a family history of melanoma, multiple benign or atypical nevi, and a previous melanoma. Additional risk factors include fair skin, blond or red hair, sun sensitivity, freckling, intermittent sun exposure, blistering sunburns, immunosuppression, human immunodeficiency virus (HIV) infection, and tanning bed use. Inherited mutations in *CDKN2A* and *CDK4* genes, which have been documented in some families with melanoma, are associated with a 60% to 90% lifetime risk of melanoma. The familial atypical mole-melanoma syndrome is transmitted by an autosomal dominant gene. Patients with either familial or nonfamilial atypical nevi have an increased risk for development of malignant melanoma. Other risk factors that have been identified include a personal or family history of melanoma or nonmelanoma skin cancer, a large number of benign pigmented nevi, giant pigmented congenital nevus, and immunosuppression.

Table 47.1 SURVIVAL IN MALIGNANT MELANOMA, BY TUMOR THICKNESS[a]

TUMOR, MM	5-YEAR SURVIVAL, %
<1.0	95.3
1.01–2.00	89.0
2.01–4.00	78.7
>4.00	67.4

[a] No nodal or distant metastasis.

The key to improved survival with malignant melanoma is early detection and diagnosis. A full skin examination is recommended for persons at risk, including an evaluation for *A*symmetry, *B*order irregularity, *C*olor variation, a *D*iameter more than 6 mm, and *E*volution (an ABCDE evaluation). Changing or symptomatic moles or moles that stand out from other moles should be biopsied. Pathologic staging of the primary melanoma guides prognosis and further surgical decisions.

Increase in thickness of a melanoma (Table 47.1), microscopic ulceration, and mitotic rate are all inversely correlated with survival. However, micrometastasis to the first draining lymph node is now the most powerful staging and prognostic tool.

- The key to improved survival with malignant melanoma is early diagnosis.

- Increased tumor thickness is associated with decreased survival.

- Micrometastasis to the first draining lymph node (sentinel lymph node) is the most powerful staging and prognostic tool.

Stages I and II malignant melanomas consist of the cutaneous lesion without lymph node involvement. Stage III consists of the primary skin lesion plus microscopic or macroscopic lymph node involvement, and stage IV represents distant metastasis. Surgical management is recommended for treatment of the primary melanoma and consists of excision with tumor-free margins of 1 to 3 cm. Sentinel lymph node biopsy, whereby the first draining lymph node(s) is identified (with blue dye injection and lymphoscintigraphy) and sampled, improves prognostic accuracy in intermediate and thick melanomas and identifies candidates for systemic adjuvant treatment. Adjuvant high-dose interferon alfa-2b increases relapse-free survival rates and may improve overall survival rates in select patients. New immune-based therapies have recently shown promise in select patients with advanced (distant metastases) disease. Ongoing therapeutic studies focus on vaccines, immunotherapy, and targeted chemotherapy.

- Surgical management of primary melanoma consists of excision with tumor-free margins of 1–3 cm.

- Node status, determined by sentinel lymph node biopsy, is the most powerful predictor of recurrence and survival.

- New immune-based therapies show promise in select patients with advanced disease.

PREVENTION OF MELANOMA AND NONMELANOMA SKIN CANCER

Dermatologists encourage regular use of sunscreens with a sun protection factor (SPF) of at least 30 and sun-protective clothing. Sun exposure during the first 18 years of life accounts for up to 80% of cumulative lifetime sun exposure. Persons with light skin types and people who spend time outdoors need to be particularly vigilant with sun protection.

CUTANEOUS T-CELL LYMPHOMA

Cutaneous T-cell lymphoma is a non-Hodgkin lymphoma characterized by expansion of malignant T cells within the skin. The most common clinical presentations are mycosis fungoides and Sézary syndrome. Mycosis fungoides generally presents with discrete or coalescing patches, plaques, or nodules on the skin. Mycosis fungoides may progress to involve lymph nodes and viscera. Once extracutaneous involvement is recognized, the median duration of survival is about 2.5 years. The course of patients with patch- or plaque-stage cutaneous lesions, without extracutaneous disease, is less predictable, but the median duration of survival is approximately 12 years. Sézary syndrome, the more aggressive leukemic form of cutaneous T-cell lymphoma, is characterized by generalized erythroderma, keratoderma of the palms and soles, and a Sézary cell count of more than $1,000/mm^3$ in the peripheral blood. Most patients have severe pruritus.

- Mycosis fungoides and Sézary syndrome are forms of cutaneous T-cell lymphoma.

- Mycosis fungoides may progress to involve lymph nodes and viscera.

- The median survival for patients with mycosis fungoides is 12 years, but it decreases to 2.5 years with extracutaneous involvement.

Both mycosis fungoides and Sézary syndrome are characterized by the presence of Sézary cells (enlarged atypical lymphocytes with convoluted nuclei) involving the epidermis (epidermotropism) and dermis. On immunohistochemical stains of cutaneous lesions, these malignant T cells usually express CD3 and CD4 antigens (T-helper cell markers), and molecular genetic studies show clonal rearrangement of the T-cell receptor gene in lymphocyte populations from skin biopsy, lymph node, and peripheral blood specimens of patients with cutaneous T-cell lymphoma.

- Mycosis fungoides and Sézary syndrome are T-cell lymphomas characterized by the presence of a clonal T-cell population in skin and peripheral blood.

Treatment of cutaneous T-cell lymphoma includes topical corticosteroids, topical nitrogen mustard, psoralen and ultraviolet A (PUVA), radiotherapy (electron beam, orthovoltage), and systemic chemotherapy. Interferons, retinoids, and monoclonal antibodies have also been used. Extracorporeal photopheresis has been used in the treatment of cutaneous T-cell lymphoma.

PSORIASIS

Psoriasis is a chronic, inflammatory, multisystem disease with considerable skin and joint signs that occurs in 2% of the US population. Onset is most common in the third decade of life, and about a third of patients have a family history of psoriasis. Psoriasis commonly presents with discrete red plaques covered with a silvery scale. Patterns of psoriasis include psoriasis vulgaris, which presents with plaques involving the elbows, knees, and scalp. Guttate psoriasis is an acute form that often follows streptococcal pharyngitis and presents with small, scaly papules of psoriasis on the trunk and limbs. Other, less common, forms of psoriasis include pustular psoriasis, which may be localized to the hands and feet or may be generalized. Approximately 50% of patients with psoriasis have nail abnormalities, most commonly onycholysis, pitting, and oil spots. Lesions of psoriasis may occur at previous sites of trauma (koebnerization). Medications such as lithium, β-adrenergic blockers, and antimalarials and discontinuation of the use of systemic corticosteroids can precipitate or exacerbate psoriasis. Psoriatic arthritis occurs in 5% to 8% of patients with skin psoriasis.

- The onset of psoriasis most often occurs in the third decade of life.

- One-third of patients have a family history of psoriasis.

- Psoriasis typically presents with red plaques with silver scale on elbows, knees, and scalp.

- About 50% of patients have nail abnormalities.

- Psoriasis occurs at sites of trauma (koebnerization).

The treatment of psoriasis includes topical corticosteroids, topical tar preparations, and phototherapy. Newer treatments for localized psoriasis include a topical synthetic vitamin D analogue, calcipotriene, and a topical retinoid, tazarotene.

Systemic agents used in the treatment of resistant psoriasis include methotrexate, acitretin, and cyclosporine.

Targeted Therapy in Psoriasis

Research into the pathogenesis of psoriasis has shown that the disease is T-cell–mediated. This knowledge has led to the development of several antibody-based or fusion protein–based targeted therapies. Infliximab, etanercept, and adalimumab (anti–tumor necrosis factor-α agents) have been effective in the treatment of psoriasis.

Phototherapy

Ultraviolet Light
Natural sunlight contains ultraviolet B (UVB, 280–320 nm), UVA (320–400 nm), and visible light. The UVB radiation causes sunburn reaction. It has been used in combination with tar for treating psoriasis. It also may benefit atopic dermatitis, lichen planus, and certain other inflammatory dermatoses.

Narrow-Band UVB
The wavelength of UVB with therapeutic effect for psoriasis has been identified in the 311-nm range. Light units producing this wavelength have been developed (narrow-band UVB) and have been shown to be more effective than traditional UVB for the treatment of psoriasis.

Psoralen and Ultraviolet A
Therapy with *PUVA* consists of ingestion of psoralen followed by exposure of the skin to UVA light. It has been used most commonly for therapy of generalized psoriasis, but it is also effective for the treatment of lichen planus, mycosis fungoides, urticaria pigmentosa, and vitiligo. This therapy is associated with minimal systemic adverse effects but is associated with an increased risk of cutaneous squamous cell carcinoma and melanoma in patients who have received long-term therapy.

- Ultraviolet light is commonly used for therapy of generalized psoriasis and other inflammatory dermatoses.

- PUVA, a form of phototherapy, consists of oral psoralen followed by UVA light exposure.

- Therapy with PUVA is associated with an increased risk of cutaneous squamous cell carcinoma and melanoma with long-term use.

ATOPIC DERMATITIS

Atopy is manifested by atopic dermatitis, asthma, and allergic rhinitis or conjunctivitis. Atopic dermatitis often presents in the neonatal period with scaling and erythema of the scalp and face, later spreading to the trunk. The distribution is often extensor in the older infant, and by the age of approximately 3 years distribution is the more classic flexural. In adolescence, facial involvement (perioral, eyelid, and forehead) is common. Generalized flares of eczema can occur at any age.

Disturbances in cell-mediated immunity lead to an increased incidence of bacterial and viral infections. Secondary colonization with *Staphylococcus aureus* presents as a weeping, crusting dermatitis (impetiginization). Eczema herpeticum is a secondary infection with the herpes simplex virus, which may be generalized. In patients with atopic dermatitis, infections with the human papillomavirus and molluscum contagiosum are also common and the lesions are more numerous.

- Eczema herpeticum, a generalized herpes simplex virus infection, may occur in patients with atopic dermatitis.

Emollients and topical corticosteroids have been the mainstay of treatment in atopic dermatitis.

ALLERGIC CONTACT DERMATITIS

Allergic contact dermatitis is a form of localized or generalized dermatitis that results from exposure to an antigen. This is a type 4 hypersensitivity reaction (delayed, cell-mediated). Recognition of antigens by T lymphocytes requires participation of Langerhans cells, which are the "antigen-presenting" cells of the epidermis. One must consider the anatomical location of the cutaneous lesions and environmental exposure to allergens, including occupational, household, and recreational contactants, to define the cause of the contact dermatitis.

- Allergic contact dermatitis is a type 4 hypersensitivity reaction (delayed, cell-mediated).

- Langerhans cells are the "antigen-presenting" cells of the epidermis.

Patch testing is performed by applying substances to a patient's back; each substance is placed under a small aluminum disk covered with adhesive tape. These are left on the patient's back for 48 hours, and the results are interpreted at 48 and 96 hours. Positive reactions occur most often to the following antigens: nickel sulfate, potassium dichromate, thimerosal, paraphenylenediamine, ethylenediamine, neomycin sulfate, benzocaine, thiuram, formaldehyde, and fragrance.

Nickel sulfate allergies are mainly associated with inexpensive jewelry. Paraphenylenediamine is present in hair dyes and other cosmetics; para-aminobenzoic acid in sunscreens is immunologically related to paraphenylenediamine. Potassium dichromate sensitivity is one of the most common types of occupational allergic contact dermatitis and occurs in construction workers exposed to cement, leathers, and certain paints. Formaldehyde is a common preservative in cosmetics and shampoos. Neomycin sulfate and benzocaine are components of many topical antimicrobial and analgesic preparations. Thimerosal is a commonly used preservative in contact lens solutions and in some intramuscular injections. Thiuram is a rubber accelerator and fungicide and therefore may correlate with occupational dermatitis related to wearing shoes containing rubber or rubber gloves. Allergic contact dermatitis to thiuram and other rubber accelerators is associated with rubber glove use in health care workers.

- Nickel sulfate allergies are associated with inexpensive jewelry.

- Potassium dichromate sensitivity occurs in construction workers exposed to cement, leathers, and certain paints.

- Formaldehyde is a common preservative in cosmetics and shampoos.

- Allergic contact dermatitis to thiuram and other rubber accelerators is associated with rubber glove use in health care workers.

Table 47.2 **TREATMENT OF ACNE VULGARIS**

TYPE OF ACNE	TREATMENT
Comedonal	Topical tretinoin, benzoyl peroxide
Papular or pustular	Same as above, plus topical or systemic antibiotics
Cystic	Systemic antibiotics; if severe, isotretinoin

ACNE VULGARIS

Acne vulgaris is one of the most common problems addressed in clinical dermatology. Acne occurs physiologically at puberty with varying degrees of severity but may persist into the second and third decades of life. The pathogenesis of acne is multifactorial; inheritance, increase in sebaceous gland activity, hormonal influences, disturbances of keratinization, and bacterial infection have all been implicated. The primary lesions of acne are noninflammatory and include microcomedones, closed comedones (whiteheads), and open comedones (blackheads). The secondary or inflammatory lesions include papules and pustules, nodules, and cysts. Treatment options for acne are given in Table 47.2.

Systemic Retinoid Use in Acne Vulgaris

Isotretinoin (13-*cis*-retinoic acid) is a synthetic vitamin A derivative used primarily for the treatment of severe nodulocystic acne vulgaris. The mechanism of action of 13-*cis*-retinoic acid in acne is probably multifactorial, including improvement in keratinization, decrease in sebum production, and decrease in inflammation. A 20-week course at a dosage of approximately 1 mg/kg per day is the standard regimen.

- Isotretinoin is used for the treatment of severe acne vulgaris.

The greatest risk associated with use of systemic retinoids is teratogenicity. Before isotretinoin is prescribed, female patients must be counseled on this adverse effect and use reliable contraception during therapy and for at least 1 month after use of the drug is discontinued.

- The greatest risk with the use of systemic retinoids is teratogenicity.

The systemic retinoids are associated with various adverse effects, including xerosis (dry skin), dermatitis, cheilitis, sticky skin, peeling skin, epistaxis, conjunctivitis, hair loss, and nail dystrophy. Symptoms of arthralgias and myalgias also may occur. Hyperlipidemia, including both hypertriglyceridemia and hypercholesterolemia, develops in most patients. Other potential laboratory abnormalities include increased liver enzyme values and leukopenia. Skeletal hyperostosis may occur, particularly in association with long-term use. Concerns regarding depression and suicidal ideation are being studied.

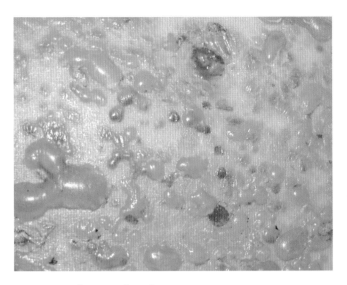

Figure 47.1 Bullous Pemphigoid.

- Adverse effects of systemic retinoids include xerosis, dermatitis, cheilitis, sticky skin, peeling skin, epistaxis, conjunctivitis, hair loss, and nail dystrophy. Concerns regarding depression and suicidal ideation are being studied.

AUTOIMMUNE BULLOUS DISEASES

Bullous pemphigoid (Figure 47.1) is the most common autoimmune blistering disease. The disease predominantly occurs in elderly patients and usually presents with large, tense bullae on an erythematous base with a predilection for flexural areas.

- Bullous pemphigoid is the most common autoimmune blistering disease.

- It occurs predominantly in elderly patients.

- It presents as large, tense bullae with a predilection for flexural areas.

Autoantibodies induce disruption at the skin's basement membrane zone, leading to subepidermal blisters. Immunofluorescence testing of a skin sample is important for the diagnosis of bullous pemphigoid. Direct immunofluorescence testing of perilesional skin shows deposition of C3 in a linear pattern at the basement membrane zone in almost all cases and of immunoglobulin (Ig) G in more than 90%. Indirect immunofluorescence testing of serum shows IgG anti–basement-membrane zone antibodies in approximately 70% of cases. Targeted antigens in bullous pemphigoid include bullous pemphigoid antigen 1 (BP230) and Bullous Pemphigoid Antigen 2 (BP180). These bullous pemphigoid antibodies can be measured with enzyme-linked immunosorbent assay.

- Immunofluorescence testing is important for the diagnosis of bullous pemphigoid.

- Almost all cases have deposition of C3 and IgG in a linear pattern at the basement membrane zone.

- BP230 and BP180 antibodies may be present in patients with bullous pemphigoid.

Treatment of bullous pemphigoid includes systemic corticosteroids, dapsone, azathioprine, cyclophosphamide, and mycophenolate mofetil.

Epidermolysis bullosa acquisita is another subepidermal bullous disease. It is characterized by blisters or erosions induced by trauma, which predominantly occur on distal locations. A small subset of patients has generalized lesions, which may be difficult to distinguish from bullous pemphigoid.

- Epidermolysis bullosa acquisita is characterized by blisters or erosions induced by trauma.

- It occurs predominantly on distal sites.

On direct immunofluorescence testing, epidermolysis bullosa acquisita has a pattern similar to that in bullous pemphigoid, namely, deposition of IgG and C3 in a linear pattern at the basement membrane zone. In contrast to bullous pemphigoid, C3 may be absent or IgG may be the dominant immunoreactant. Indirect immunofluorescence testing of serum shows IgG anti–basement-membrane zone antibodies in 25% to 50% of patients. Epidermolysis bullosa acquisita tends to be resistant to immunosuppressive therapy.

- On direct immunofluorescence, epidermolysis bullosa acquisita shows deposition of IgG and C3 in a linear pattern at the basement membrane zone.

- Epidermolysis bullosa acquisita tends to be resistant to immunosuppressive therapy.

Cicatricial pemphigoid is characterized by mucosal lesions, with limited or no cutaneous lesions. The disease predominantly affects oral and ocular mucous membranes and, less frequently, the genital, pharyngeal, or upper respiratory mucosa. This disease is also known as benign mucous membrane pemphigoid, which is a misnomer because untreated ocular involvement may lead to blindness. Patients may present with oral erosions or diffuse gingivitis.

- Cicatricial pemphigoid affects oral and ocular mucous membranes and, less frequently, genital, pharyngeal, or upper respiratory mucosa.

Treatment of cicatricial pemphigoid is similar to that of bullous pemphigoid, namely, systemic corticosteroids, dapsone, azathioprine, cyclophosphamide, and mycophenolate. Cyclophosphamide has been used particularly in patients with ocular involvement.

Herpes gestationis consists of intensely pruritic urticarial papules, plaques, or blisters, usually occurring in the latter half of pregnancy. The lesions are histologically characterized by a subepidermal bulla with eosinophils.

- Herpes gestationis consists of intensely pruritic urticarial papules, plaques, or blisters.

Direct immunofluorescence testing is particularly useful for the diagnosis of herpes gestationis because the other dermatoses of pregnancy (such as pruritic urticarial papules and plaques of pregnancy) are negative by immunofluorescence testing. The serum from approximately half of patients with herpes gestationis contains the HG factor, which is a complement-fixing IgG anti–basement-membrane zone antibody. The circulating antibody crosses the placenta, and the baby born to a mother with herpes gestationis may have a transient blistering eruption develop during the neonatal period.

- In herpes gestationis, direct immunofluorescence is useful because the other dermatoses of pregnancy are negative with such testing.

Linear IgA bullous dermatosis is characterized by vesicles or blisters on an erythematous base in a generalized distribution with a high rate of mucosal involvement. Drug-induced disease has occurred with vancomycin. This disease is characterized by the direct immunofluorescence finding of IgA deposition in a linear pattern at the basement membrane zone, with or without C3 or IgG deposition.

- In linear IgA bullous dermatosis, direct immunofluorescence shows IgA deposition in a linear pattern at the basement membrane zone.

Dermatitis herpetiformis (Figure 47.2) is characterized by extremely pruritic, grouped vesicles occurring predominantly over the elbows, knees, buttocks, back of the neck and scalp,

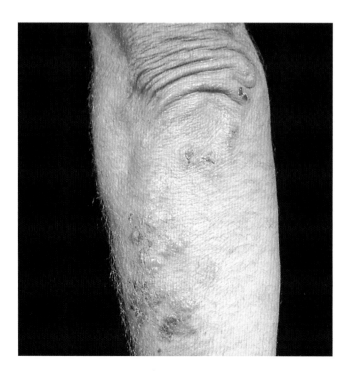

Figure 47.2 Dermatitis Herpetiformis.

and lower part of the back, usually beginning in the third or fourth decade of life. Although dermatitis herpetiformis is associated with thyroid disease, virtually all patients have some degree of gluten-sensitive enteropathy (celiac sprue), although it may be subclinical. This association is important in terms of management of dermatitis herpetiformis.

- In dermatitis herpetiformis, virtually all patients have some degree of gluten-sensitive enteropathy (celiac sprue).

The hallmark of the diagnosis of dermatitis herpetiformis is the direct immunofluorescence finding of IgA deposits in a stippled, granular, or clumped pattern along the basement membrane zone. Skin biopsy specimens should be obtained from an area 0.5 to 1 cm from an active lesion. The IgA deposits tend to persist in the skin over time. A small percentage of patients who strictly adhere to a gluten-free diet may show diminution in IgA deposits after many years, but IgA deposits in the skin are unaffected by pharmacologic therapy. Testing for tissue transglutaminase or endomysial antibodies is useful for both diagnosis and management of dermatitis herpetiformis, although these antibodies correlate with the degree of gluten-sensitive enteropathy rather than the skin lesions per se.

- In dermatitis herpetiformis, direct immunofluorescence shows IgA deposits in a stippled, granular, or clumped pattern.
- Testing for tissue transglutaminase or endomysial antibodies is useful for diagnosis and management.

The mainstay of treatment of dermatitis herpetiformis consists of dapsone and a gluten-free diet. Patients who strictly adhere to a gluten-free diet may have a decreased need for dapsone. Patients must adhere to the diet for at least 8 months before it is effective. Patients with gluten-sensitive enteropathy have an increased risk for small bowel lymphoma. Only adherence to a gluten-free diet will affect this risk. Systemic corticosteroids are not helpful for the treatment of dermatitis herpetiformis.

- Treatment of dermatitis herpetiformis consists of dapsone and a gluten-free diet.

Bullous eruption of systemic lupus erythematosus shares clinical and histologic features with dermatitis herpetiformis. The blisters were therefore originally thought to represent the coexistence of dermatitis herpetiformis and lupus erythematosus, but they are now established as a distinct subset of lupus.

Direct immunofluorescence testing shows deposition of IgG, IgM, IgA, or C3 in a linear or granular pattern at the basement membrane zone, similar to the classic lupus band.

- In bullous eruption of systemic lupus erythematosus, direct immunofluorescence shows deposition of IgG, IgM, IgA, or C3 in a linear or granular pattern at the basement membrane zone.

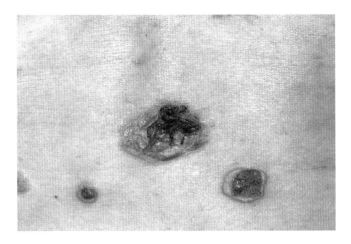

Figure 47.3 Pemphigus Foliaceus.

The clinical variants of pemphigus include pemphigus vulgaris and pemphigus foliaceus (with the subsets pemphigus erythematosus and fogo selvagem, the latter being an endemic form of pemphigus that occurs in South America). There is also a drug-induced variant of pemphigus, particularly associated with D-penicillamine, captopril, or other thiol-containing medications.

More than 50% of patients with pemphigus vulgaris present with oral lesions, and more than 90% have oral mucosal involvement at some point in the course of the disease. Pemphigus vulgaris is characterized by coalescing blisters and erosions, often with generalized involvement. In contrast, pemphigus foliaceus (Figure 47.3), considered to represent the superficial variant of pemphigus, may present with superficial scaling-crusting lesions of the head and neck area (in a seborrheic dermatitis-like pattern) or generalized distribution.

- Pemphigus vulgaris is characterized by coalescing blisters and erosions.

- Pemphigus foliaceus may present with superficial scaling-crusting lesions of the head and neck.

All types of pemphigus are characterized by the deposition of IgG and C3 at the intercellular space (epidermal cell surface) on direct immunofluorescence testing (intercellular substance [ICS] antibody). On indirect immunofluorescence testing, IgG anti-ICS antibodies are found in approximately 90% of cases. The titer of IgG anti-ICS antibodies is useful for both diagnosis and management of pemphigus.

- All types of pemphigus are characterized by the direct immunofluorescence finding of IgG and C3 deposition at the epidermal cell surface.

- The titer of IgG anti-ICS antibodies is useful for diagnosis and management.

High-dose corticosteroids generally are required to control pemphigus. Various steroid-sparing immunosuppressive agents have been used, including azathioprine, mycophenolate mofetil, cyclophosphamide, gold, and dapsone.

- High-dose corticosteroids generally are required to control pemphigus, followed by institution of a steroid-sparing agent.

ERYTHEMA MULTIFORME

Erythema multiforme (Figure 47.4) is an acute, usually self-limited eruption of maculopapular, urticarial, occasionally bullous lesions characterized morphologically by iris or target lesions. A subset of patients with erythema multiforme may have recurrent lesions. When erythema multiforme presents with extensive cutaneous and mucosal lesions, it is referred to as Stevens-Johnson syndrome. Various etiologic factors have been implicated in erythema multiforme. The most commonly cited precipitating factor is viral infection, particularly herpes simplex virus. This is responsible for a considerable percentage of recurrent erythema multiforme. Other infectious agents that have been noted to cause erythema multiforme include *Mycoplasma pneumoniae* and *Yersinia enterocolitica*. Drugs have been reported to induce erythema multiforme, particularly sulfonamides, barbiturates, and anticonvulsants. Erythema multiforme also may be associated with underlying connective tissue disease or malignancy. Erythema multiforme tends to involve the lips, buccal mucosa, and tongue, in contrast to pemphigus vulgaris, which typically involves the pharynx, buccal mucosa, and tongue, and pemphigoid, which most often involves gingivae. Neither pemphigus nor pemphigoid involves the lips.

- The most commonly cited precipitating factor for erythema multiforme is viral infection, particularly herpes simplex.

- Other infectious agents are *Mycoplasma pneumoniae* and *Yersinia enterocolitica*.

- Drugs also induce erythema multiforme: sulfonamides, barbiturates, and anticonvulsants.

ERYTHEMA NODOSUM

Erythema nodosum (Figure 47.5) typically presents as tender, erythematous, subcutaneous nodules localized to the

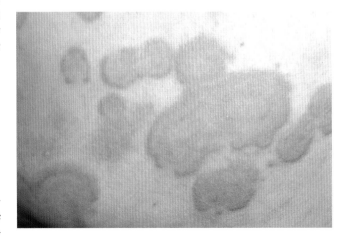

Figure 47.4 Erythema Multiforme.

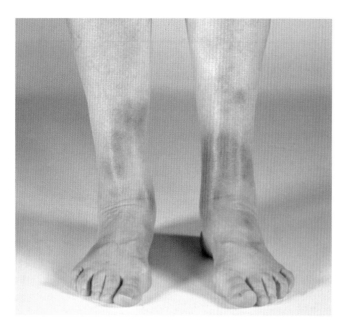

Figure 47.5 Erythema Nodosum.

pretibial areas. The nodules may be acute and self-limited or chronic, lasting for months to years. The most common cause is streptococcal pharyngitis. Other infectious agents that have been implicated in the development of erythema nodosum include *Yersinia enterocolitica*, *Coccidioides*, and *Histoplasma*. Drug-induced erythema nodosum most often is associated with oral contraceptives and sulfonamides. Other associations with erythema nodosum include sarcoidosis, inflammatory bowel disease, and Behçet syndrome.

- The most common cause of erythema nodosum is streptococcal pharyngitis.
- Drug-induced erythema nodosum most often is associated with oral contraceptives and sulfonamides.
- Other associations of erythema nodosum are sarcoidosis, inflammatory bowel disease, and Behçet syndrome.

DRUG REACTIONS

The morphologic spectrum of reactions that may be induced by medications is broad, and hundreds of drugs may produce a given cutaneous reaction. Types of cutaneous lesions induced by drugs include maculopapular eruptions, acne, folliculitis, necrotizing vasculitis, vesiculobullous lesions, erythema multiforme, erythema nodosum, fixed drug eruptions, lichenoid reactions, photosensitivity reactions, pigmentary changes, and hair loss.

Approximately 2% of hospitalized patients have cutaneous drug reactions, and penicillin, sulfonamides, and blood products are responsible for approximately two-thirds of such reactions. The most common types of clinical presentations (in descending order of frequency) are exanthematous or morbilliform eruptions, urticaria or angioedema, fixed drug eruptions, and erythema multiforme. Stevens-Johnson syndrome,

Table 47.3 CUTANEOUS REACTIONS TO DRUGS

TYPE OF SKIN REACTION	CAUSE
Urticarial	Aspirin, penicillin, blood products
Photoallergic	Sulfonamides, thiazides, griseofulvin, phenothiazines
Phototoxic	Tetracyclines
Slate-gray discoloration	Chlorpromazine
Slate-blue discoloration	Amiodarone
Yellow or blue-gray pigmentation	Antimalarials

exfoliative erythroderma, and photosensitive eruptions are less common. Table 47.3 outlines the types of cutaneous reactions to drugs.

- About 2% of hospitalized patients have cutaneous drug reactions.
- Penicillin, sulfonamides, and blood products are responsible for about two-thirds of drug reactions.
- Urticarial drug reactions are most often related to aspirin, penicillin, and blood products.
- Photoallergic reactions are most often associated with sulfonamides, thiazides, griseofulvin, and phenothiazines.
- Phototoxic reactions may be induced by tetracyclines.

Exanthematous or morbilliform eruptions are the most common type of cutaneous drug reaction. This type of eruption usually begins within a week of onset of therapy, but it may occur more than 2 weeks after initiation of the therapy or up to 2 weeks after use of the drug has been discontinued. Ampicillin, penicillin, and cephalosporins are commonly associated with morbilliform eruptions. A fixed drug eruption is one or several lesions that recur at the same anatomical location on rechallenge with the medication. The genital and facial areas are common sites of involvement. Phenolphthalein, barbiturates, salicylates, and oral contraceptives have been implicated in the cause of fixed drug eruptions. Lichenoid drug eruptions are morphologically similar to lichen planus (with violaceous papules of the skin) and most often have been associated with gold and antimalarial drugs, although various medications may induce this type of reaction.

- Exanthematous or morbilliform eruptions are the most common cutaneous drug reaction.
- A fixed drug eruption is one or several lesions that recur at the same location on rechallenge.
- Phenolphthalein, barbiturates, salicylates, and oral contraceptives are implicated in fixed drug eruptions.

CUTANEOUS SIGNS OF UNDERLYING MALIGNANCY

Cutaneous metastasis occurs in 1% to 5% of patients with metastatic neoplasms. The types of malignancy metastatic to the skin are lung, breast, kidney, gastrointestinal, melanoma, and ovary. Lesions usually present on the scalp, face, or trunk.

- Cutaneous metastasis occurs in 1%-5% of patients with metastatic neoplasms.

- Lesions usually present on the scalp, face, or trunk.

Paget disease of the nipple is an erythematous, scaly, or weeping eczematous eruption of the areola. Virtually all patients with Paget disease have an underlying ductal carcinoma of the breast. In contrast, extramammary Paget disease, a morphologically similar eruption that usually occurs in the anogenital region, is associated with underlying carcinoma in only about 50% of cases. Extramammary Paget disease may be associated with underlying cutaneous adnexal carcinoma or with underlying visceral carcinoma (particularly of the genitourinary or distal gastrointestinal tracts).

- Patients with Paget disease have underlying ductal carcinoma of the breast.

- Extramammary Paget disease may be associated with underlying carcinoma in only 50% of cases.

Acanthosis nigricans (Figure 47.6) consists of velvety brown plaques of the intertriginous regions, particularly the axillae and groin. It may be associated with adenocarcinoma of the gastrointestinal tract, particularly the stomach. It also occurs with insulin-resistant diabetes. Acanthosis nigricans also may be associated with obesity or certain medications (eg, prednisone and nicotinic acid). There is an autosomal dominant variant of acanthosis nigricans.

- Acanthosis nigricans may be associated with adenocarcinoma of the gastrointestinal tract, particularly the stomach.

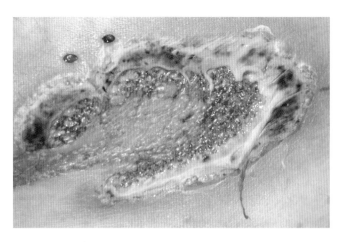

Figure 47.7 Pyoderma Gangrenosum.

- Acanthosis nigricans is most commonly associated with obesity and insulin-resistant diabetes.

Pyoderma gangrenosum (Figure 47.7) consists of ulcers with undermined, inflammatory, violaceous borders that heal with cribriform scarring. The lesions are most commonly associated with inflammatory bowel disease or rheumatoid arthritis. Pyoderma gangrenosum may be associated with malignancy of the hematopoietic system, particularly leukemia.

- Pyoderma gangrenosum is most commonly associated with inflammatory bowel disease or rheumatoid arthritis.

- Pyoderma gangrenosum may be associated with leukemia.

The skin lesions of glucagonoma syndrome (necrolytic migratory erythema) (Figure 47.8) consist of erosions, crusting, and peeling involving the perineum and perioral areas, but they may be generalized. The syndrome also includes stomatitis, glossitis (beefy tongue), anemia, diarrhea, and weight loss. It is associated with an islet cell (α) tumor of the pancreas.

- Glucagonoma syndrome consists of erosions, crusting, and peeling involving the perineum and perioral areas.

- It is associated with an islet cell tumor of the pancreas.

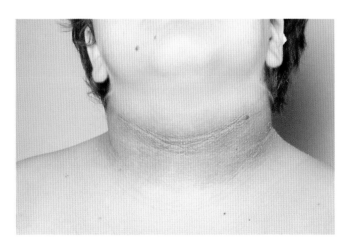

Figure 47.6 Acanthosis Nigricans.

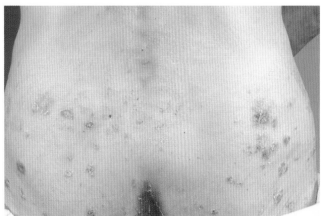

Figure 47.8 Glucagonoma Syndrome (Necrolytic Migratory Erythema).

Gardner syndrome is a hereditary (autosomal dominant) form of colon polyposis. Clinical features include adenomatous polyps of the colon, osteomas of the skull and face, scoliosis, soft tissue tumors (including dermoids, lipomas, and fibromas), and sebaceous (epidermal inclusion) cysts of the face and scalp. There is a high incidence of colon carcinoma. In approximately 60% of patients with Gardner syndrome, adenocarcinoma of the colon develops by age 40 years. Malignancies of other sites have been associated with this syndrome, including adrenal, ovarian, and thyroid.

- Gardner syndrome is a hereditary (autosomal dominant) form of colon polyposis.

- Clinical features are soft tissue tumors and sebaceous cysts of the face.

- There is a high incidence of colon cancer.

Acquired ichthyosis most often has been associated with Hodgkin disease, but it has been reported with other types of lymphoma, multiple myeloma, and various carcinomas.

- Acquired ichthyosis is associated with Hodgkin disease.

Hirsutism may reflect androgen excess due to an adrenal or ovarian tumor, but hypertrichosis is an increase in hair unrelated to androgen excess, such as hypertrichosis lanuginosa acquisita (growth of soft downy hair). It has been associated with carcinoid tumor, adenocarcinoma of the breast, lymphoma, gastrointestinal malignancy, and other types of neoplasms.

Sweet syndrome (acute febrile neutrophilic dermatosis) has skin lesions that consist of erythematous plaques and nodules, most commonly located on the proximal aspects of the extremities and face. The association is with leukemia, particularly acute myelocytic or acute myelomonocytic leukemia, although many other diseases also have been associated.

- Sweet syndrome is associated with leukemia (acute myelocytic or acute myelomonocytic).

Generalized pruritus is the presentation for many cutaneous and systemic disorders. Pruritus may be the presenting symptom in lymphoma.

- Pruritus may be the presenting symptom in lymphoma.

In dermatomyositis, the pathognomonic skin lesions are Gottron papules (Figure 47.9) involving the skin over the joints of the fingers, elbows, and knees. Poikilodermatous lesions or erythematous maculopapular eruptions may diffusely involve the face, particularly the periorbital area (heliotrope rash [Figure 47.10]), and the trunk and extremities. The cutaneous lesions are photosensitive and pruritic. The disease is characterized by proximal myositis. Although creatine kinase and aldolase levels usually are increased in patients with myositis, it is important to verify the diagnosis by obtaining an electromyogram or a muscle biopsy specimen.

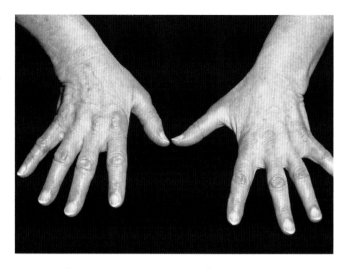

Figure 47.9 Dermatomyositis: Gottron Papules.

Dermatomyositis is associated with an increased incidence of underlying malignancy.

- Dermatomyositis may involve the periorbital area (heliotrope rash) or the dorsal aspect of the hands (Gottron papules).

- The lesions are photosensitive and pruritic.

- Dermatomyositis is characterized by proximal myositis.

- Dermatomyositis is associated with an increased risk of internal malignancy.

Amyloidosis may present clinically as macroglossia (Figure 47.11), waxy papules on the eyelids or nasolabial folds, pinch purpura, and postproctoscopic purpura (Figure 47.12). Amyloidosis may be associated with multiple myeloma.

- Amyloidosis may be associated with multiple myeloma.

Tylosis is a rare disorder characterized by palmar-plantar keratoderma associated with esophageal carcinoma. It has autosomal dominant inheritance.

- Tylosis is associated with esophageal carcinoma.

The autoimmune bullous diseases are a heterogeneous group of disorders characterized by antibody deposition at the basement membrane zone or epidermis. An association with malignancy has been found in several of these disorders.

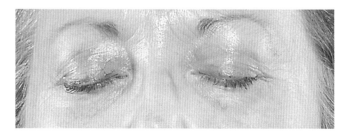

Figure 47.10 Dermatomyositis: Heliotrope Discoloration.

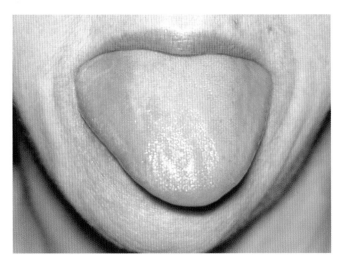

Figure 47.11 Amyloidosis: Macroglossia.

- Pemphigus is associated with thymoma with or without myasthenia gravis.
- Paraneoplastic pemphigus presents with clinical and histologic features of pemphigus and erythema multiforme and is associated with lymphoma and leukemia.
- Small bowel lymphoma rarely develops in patients with dermatitis herpetiformis.
- Epidermolysis bullosa acquisita is associated with amyloidosis and multiple myeloma.
- Bullous pemphigoid has not been associated with an increased risk of underlying malignancy.

DERMATOLOGY: AN INTERNIST'S PERSPECTIVE

PULMONARY

The skin is involved in 15% to 35% of patients with sarcoidosis. Lesions may present as 1) lupus pernio (red swelling of the nose), 2) translucent papules around the eyes and nasolabial folds, 3) annular lesions with central atrophy, 4) nodules on the trunk and extremities, and 5) scar sarcoid.

- The skin is involved in 15%-35% of patients with sarcoidosis.
- Lesions may present as lupus pernio (red swelling of the nose).

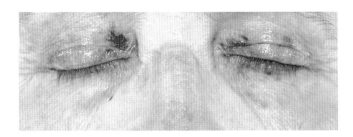

Figure 47.12 Amyloidosis: Postproctoscopic Purpura.

Acute sarcoidosis may present with a combination of erythema nodosum, bilateral hilar lymphadenopathy, fever, and arthralgias (Löfgren syndrome). Erythema nodosum (Figure 47.5) is a reactive condition that may be associated with acute sarcoidosis. Erythema nodosum typically presents as tender, erythematous, subcutaneous nodules localized to pretibial areas.

- Erythema nodosum may be associated with acute sarcoidosis (Löfgren syndrome).

In antineutrophil cytoplasmic autoantibody (ANCA)–associated granulomatous vasculitis, cutaneous involvement occurs in more than 50% of patients and is manifested by cutaneous infarction, ulceration, hemorrhagic bullae, purpuric papules, or urticaria. A skin biopsy may show hypersensitivity vasculitis or granulomatous vasculitis.

- In ANCA-associated granulomatous vasculitis, cutaneous involvement occurs in >50% of patients.
- Manifestations are ulceration, hemorrhagic bullae, purpuric papules, and urticaria.

Churg-Strauss granulomatosis (allergic granulomatosis) is characterized by a combination of adult-onset asthma, peripheral eosinophilia, and pulmonary involvement with recurrent pneumonia or transient infiltrates. Skin lesions have been reported in up to 60% of patients and consist of palpable purpura, cutaneous infarcts, and subcutaneous nodules.

- Skin lesions of Churg-Strauss granulomatosis occur in up to 60% of patients.
- Skin lesions include palpable purpura, cutaneous infarcts, and subcutaneous nodules.

In relapsing polychondritis, there is episodic destructive inflammation of cartilage of the ears, nose, and upper airways. There may be associated arthritis and ocular involvement. In the acute stage, the ears may be red, swollen, and tender. Later, they become soft and flabby. Nasal chondritis may lead to saddle-nose deformities. Relapsing polychondritis is mediated by antibodies to type II collagen.

- Relapsing polychondritis is characterized by episodic destructive inflammation of cartilage of ears, nose, and upper airways.
- Nasal chondritis may lead to saddle-nose deformities.

CARDIOVASCULAR

Pseudoxanthoma elasticum may be transmitted by autosomal dominant or autosomal recessive inheritance. Yellow xanthoma-like papules ("plucked-chicken skin") occur on the neck, axillae, groin, and abdomen. Angioid streaks may occur in the fundus of the eye. Skin biopsy shows degeneration of elastic fibers. Systemic associations include stroke, myocardial infarction, peripheral vascular disease, and gastrointestinal hemorrhage.

- Pseudoxanthoma elasticum is associated with stroke, myocardial infarction, peripheral vascular disease, and gastrointestinal hemorrhage.

Ehlers-Danlos syndrome includes 10 subgroups that vary in severity and systemic associations. Cutaneous findings are skin hyperextensibility with hypermobile joints and fish-mouth scars. Ehlers-Danlos syndrome is associated with angina, peripheral vascular disease, and gastrointestinal bleeding.

- Ehlers-Danlos syndrome is associated with angina, peripheral vascular disease, and gastrointestinal bleeding.

Erythema marginatum is one of the diagnostic criteria for acute rheumatic fever. This uncommon eruption occurs on the trunk and is characterized by erythematous plaques with rapidly mobile serpiginous borders.

- Erythema marginatum is one of the diagnostic criteria for acute rheumatic fever.

GASTROINTESTINAL

Osler-Weber-Rendu syndrome (hereditary hemorrhagic telangiectasia), an autosomal dominant disorder, is manifested by cutaneous and mucosal telangiectasias. Frequent nosebleeds and gastrointestinal bleeds may be a presenting feature. Pulmonary arteriovenous malformations and central nervous system angiomas are also features of this syndrome.

- Osler-Weber-Rendu syndrome has autosomal dominant inheritance.
- Features are cutaneous and mucosal telangiectasia, nosebleeds, gastrointestinal bleeds, pulmonary arteriovenous malformations, and central nervous system angiomas.

Acrodermatitis enteropathica is an inherited (autosomal recessive) or acquired disease characterized by zinc deficiency (failure of absorption or failure to supplement). The clinical features include angular cheilitis, a seborrheic dermatitis-like eruption, erosions, blisters, and pustules, with skin lesions particularly involving the face, hands, feet, and perineum. Alopecia and diarrhea are other features of this syndrome.

- Acrodermatitis enteropathica is an inherited (autosomal recessive) or acquired disease.
- The disease is characterized by zinc deficiency (failure of absorption or failure to supplement).

Peutz-Jeghers syndrome is an inherited (autosomal dominant) syndrome of intestinal polyposis. Patients have hamartomas, mostly involving the small bowel, and a slightly increased risk for carcinoma. Cutaneous lesions include macular pigmentation (freckles) of the lips, periungual skin, fingers, and toes and pigmentation of the oral mucosa.

- Peutz-Jeghers syndrome is an inherited (autosomal dominant) syndrome of intestinal polyposis.
- Patients have an increased risk for carcinoma.

Dermatitis herpetiformis (Figure 47.2) is an immune-mediated bullous disease that presents with intensely itchy vesicles on extensor surfaces (elbows, knees, buttocks, scapulae). Gluten-sensitive enteropathy occurs in almost all patients, although it may be subclinical. Gluten-sensitive enteropathy is associated with an increased risk of small B-cell lymphoma.

- Dermatitis herpetiformis is an immune-mediated bullous disease.
- Gluten-sensitive enteropathy occurs in almost all patients.
- Gluten-sensitive enteropathy is associated with an increased risk of small B-cell lymphoma.

Extensive aphthous ulceration may be associated with Crohn disease or gluten-sensitive enteropathy.

- Aphthous ulceration may be associated with Crohn disease or gluten-sensitive enteropathy.

Pyoderma gangrenosum (Figure 47.7) presents with ulceration, predominantly on the lower extremities, with inflammatory undermined borders. The lesions heal with cribriform scarring. The occurrence of the disease at sites of trauma (pathergy) is classic. Systemic disease associations include inflammatory bowel disease, rheumatoid arthritis, and paraproteinemia.

- Pyoderma gangrenosum occurs at sites of trauma.
- Associated diseases are inflammatory bowel disease, rheumatoid arthritis, and paraproteinemia.

Cutaneous Crohn disease may present as skin nodules with granulomatous histologic findings. Other manifestations include pyostomatitis vegetans (granulomatous inflammation of the gingivae), granulomatous cheilitis, oral aphthous ulceration, perianal skin tags, perianal fistulas, and peristomal pyoderma gangrenosum.

- A manifestation of Crohn disease is pyostomatitis vegetans (granulomatous inflammation of gingivae).

Bowel bypass syndrome presents with a flu-like illness with fever, malaise, arthralgias, myalgias, and inflammatory papules and pustules on the extremities and upper trunk. The disease is recurrent and episodic and occurs in up to 20% of patients after jejunoileal bypass. The condition responds to antibiotics or to reversal of the bypass procedure.

- Bowel bypass syndrome presents with a flu-like illness and inflammatory papules and pustules.
- Bowel bypass syndrome occurs in up to 20% of patients after jejunoileal bypass.

Gardner syndrome and glucagonoma syndrome are described earlier in this chapter.

NEPHROLOGIC

Partial lipodystrophy is associated with C3 deficiency and the nephrotic syndrome. Uremic pruritus is associated with end-stage renal disease and responds to UVB therapy.

NEUROCUTANEOUS

Fabry disease is an X-linked recessive disorder due to deficiency of the enzyme α-galactosidase A. The skin changes consist of numerous vascular tumors (angiokeratomas) in a "bathing-suit" distribution that develop during childhood and adolescence. Corneal opacities are present in 90% of patients. Systemic manifestations include paresthesias and pain due to involved peripheral nerves, renal insufficiency, and vascular insufficiency of the coronary and central nervous system.

- Fabry disease is a recessive disorder due to deficiency of α-galactosidase A.

- Systemic manifestations are paresthesias, renal insufficiency, and vascular insufficiency.

The clinical features of ataxia-telangiectasia include cutaneous and ocular telangiectasia, cerebellar ataxia, choreoathetosis, IgA deficiency, and recurrent pulmonary infections.

Tuberous sclerosis may be inherited in an autosomal dominant pattern (25%) or may occur sporadically (new mutation). Predominant cutaneous lesions include hypopigmented macules, adenoma sebaceum, subungual or periungual fibromas, and shagreen patch (connective tissue nevus) (Figure 47.13). This syndrome is associated with epilepsy (80%) and mental retardation (60%). Rhabdomyomas may occur in the heart in childhood. Angiomyolipomas occur in the kidneys in up to 80% of adults with this syndrome.

- Tuberous sclerosis may be inherited in an autosomal dominant pattern or be sporadic.

- It is associated with epilepsy (80%) and mental retardation (60%).

- Angiomyolipomas occur in the kidneys in up to 80% of affected adults.

Neurofibromatosis (von Recklinghausen disease) (Figure 47.14) occurs in 1 in 3,000 births. Inheritance is autosomal dominant, and approximately 50% of cases are new mutations. The major skin signs of the disease are café au lait spots, axillary freckling (Crowe sign), neurofibromas, and Lisch nodules of the iris.

- Neurofibromatosis is autosomal dominant.

- Major skin signs are café au lait spots, axillary freckling, neurofibromas, and Lisch nodules of the iris.

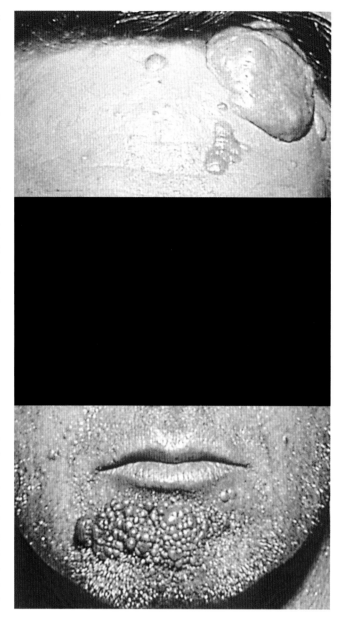

Figure 47.13 Tuberous Sclerosis: Adenoma Sebaceum and Forehead Plaque.

The associated central nervous system tumors include acoustic neuromas, optic gliomas, and meningiomas. Other associated tumors include pheochromocytoma, neuroblastoma, and Wilms tumor. Café au lait spots and neurofibromas frequently occur in the absence of neurofibromatosis. The diagnostic criteria for neurofibromatosis include 2 or more of the following:

1. Six or more café au lait macules more than 0.5 cm in greatest diameter in prepubertal patients, or more than 1.5 cm in diameter in adults

2. Two or more neurofibromas of any type, or 1 plexiform neurofibroma

3. Freckling of skin in axillary or inguinal regions

4. Optic gliomas

5. Lisch nodules

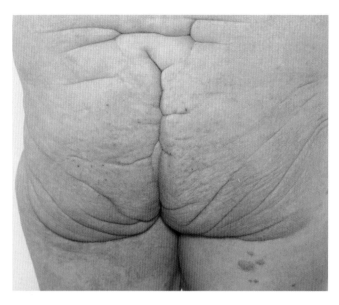

Figure 47.14 Neurofibromatosis: Plexiform Neurofibroma.

6. An osseous lesion such as sphenoid dysplasia or thinning of long bone cortex with or without pseudarthrosis

7. A first-degree relative with neurofibromatosis that meets the above diagnostic criteria

Sturge-Weber-Dimitri syndrome is characterized by capillary angioma (port-wine stain) in the distribution of the upper or middle branch of the trigeminal nerve. There may be associated meningeal angioma in the same distribution. Intracranial tramline calcification, mental retardation, epilepsy, contralateral hemiparesis, and visual impairment may be associated.

- Sturge-Weber-Dimitri syndrome is characterized by capillary angioma in the distribution of the upper or middle branch of the trigeminal nerve.

- Associated features are intracranial calcification, mental retardation, epilepsy, contralateral hemiparesis, and visual impairment.

RHEUMATOLOGIC

Psoriatic arthritis occurs in 5% to 8% of patients with cutaneous psoriasis. Several different patterns of arthritis occur. An asymmetric oligoarthritis occurs in 70% of patients. This group includes patients with "sausage digits" and monoarthritis. The second most common presentation is asymmetric arthritis clinically similar to rheumatoid arthritis, which occurs in 15% of patients with psoriatic arthritis. Distal interphalangeal involvement, arthritis mutilans, and a spinal form of arthritis similar to ankylosing spondylitis each occurs in 5% of patients with psoriatic arthritis.

- Psoriatic arthritis occurs in 5%-8% of patients with psoriasis.

- Asymmetric oligoarthritis is the most common pattern of psoriatic arthritis.

- Ankylosing spondylitis occurs in 5% of patients with psoriatic arthritis.

Reiter syndrome consists of the triad of urethritis, conjunctivitis, and arthritis. The disease usually affects young men. Two-thirds of patients have skin lesions, namely, circinate balanitis, consisting of erythematous plaques of the penis, and keratoderma blennorrhagicum, a pustular psoriasiform eruption of the palms and soles. Most patients are positive for HLA-B27.

- Reiter syndrome consists of the triad of urethritis, conjunctivitis, and arthritis.

- Skin signs of Reiter syndrome are circinate balanitis and keratoderma blennorrhagicum.

- Most patients with Reiter syndrome are positive for HLA-B27.

Erythema migrans is an annular, sometimes urticarial, erythematous plaque presenting as a manifestation of Lyme disease. The plaque develops subsequent to a tick bite. The deer tick *Ixodes scapularis* contains the spirochete *Borrelia burgdorferi*, which is responsible for the syndrome. Only 25% of patients recall a tick bite. Other acute features of Lyme disease include fever, headaches, myalgias, arthralgias, and lymphadenopathy. Arthritis is a late complication of Lyme disease. Weeks or months after the initial illness, meningoencephalitis, peripheral neuropathy, myocarditis, atrioventricular node block, or destructive erosive arthritis may develop.

- Erythema migrans presents as a manifestation of Lyme disease.

- The lesion develops subsequent to a tick bite.

- Only 25% of patients recall a tick bite.

In rheumatoid arthritis, rheumatoid nodules may occur over the extensor surfaces of joints, most commonly on the dorsal aspects of the hands and elbows. Rheumatoid vasculitis with ulceration may occur in the setting of rheumatoid arthritis with a high circulating rheumatoid factor.

During the late stages of gout, tophi (urate deposits with surrounding inflammation) occur in the subcutaneous tissues. Improved methods of treatment account for the decrease in the incidence of tophaceous gout in recent years.

- Gouty tophi may occur in subcutaneous tissues.

In lupus erythematosus (LE), cutaneous abnormalities occur in approximately 80% of patients. The skin manifestations of lupus can be classified into acute cutaneous LE (malar rash, generalized photosensitive dermatitis, or bullous LE), subacute cutaneous LE (annular or papulosquamous variants), and chronic cutaneous LE (localized discoid LE, generalized discoid LE, lupus panniculitis, tumid lupus, or chilblain lupus).

- In LE, cutaneous abnormalities occur in 80% of patients.

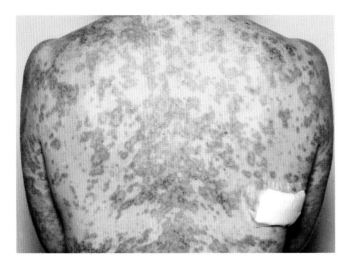

Figure 47.15 Subacute Cutaneous Lupus Erythematosus.

Skin lesions are present in up to 85% of patients with acute systemic LE. A butterfly rash with erythema involving the nose and cheeks is characteristic. Erythematous papules and plaques also may occur on the dorsal aspect of the hands, and the skin overlying the interphalangeal and metacarpal phalangeal joints is spared. Maculopapular erythema also may occur on sun-exposed areas.

Subacute cutaneous LE (Figure 47.15) usually presents with generalized annular plaques. The lesions may appear papulosquamous or vesiculobullous. Subacute cutaneous LE is characterized by the presence of anti-Ro (anti-SSA) antibodies in serum and photosensitivity. These antibodies cross the placenta, and children born to mothers with subacute cutaneous LE may develop congenital heart block or a transient photodistributed skin eruption during the neonatal period.

- Subacute cutaneous LE presents with annular plaques.

- Subacute cutaneous LE is characterized by the presence of anti-Ro (anti-SSA) antibodies and photosensitivity.

Discoid LE (Figure 47.16) is characterized by erythematous plaques with follicular hyperkeratosis and scale. It causes scarring. Localized discoid LE is usually not associated with progression to systemic LE. Discoid LE most commonly affects the face, scalp, and ears. Although most patients with discoid LE lack manifestations of systemic LE, approximately 25% of patients with systemic LE have had cutaneous lesions

of discoid LE at some point during the course of their illness. Circulating antinuclear antibodies are demonstrable in most patients with systemic LE and subacute cutaneous LE, but they are present in only a small percentage of patients with discoid LE.

- Discoid LE is characterized by erythematous plaques with follicular hyperkeratosis and scale. It causes scarring.

- Discoid LE most commonly affects the face, scalp, and ears.

- Approximately 25% of patients with systemic LE have had cutaneous manifestations of discoid LE.

The term *scleroderma* encompasses a wide spectrum of diseases ranging from generalized multisystem disease to localized cutaneous disease. The systemic end of the spectrum is represented by diffuse scleroderma and the CREST (calcinosis cutis, Raynaud phenomenon, esophageal involvement, sclerodactyly, and telangiectasia) syndrome. The middle area of the spectrum is represented by eosinophilic fasciitis and linear scleroderma, which may have systemic involvement. Localized scleroderma (also known as morphea) may be a single plaque or may be multiple plaques in a generalized distribution.

Systemic scleroderma consists of diffuse sclerosis associated with smoothness and hardening of the skin, with masklike face and microstomia. Sclerodactyly, periungual telangiectasia, telangiectatic mats, hyperpigmentation, and cutaneous calcification may be observed. Esophageal, pulmonary, renal, and cardiac involvement may be associated with systemic scleroderma. The CREST syndrome (Figure 47.17) is associated with circulating anticentromere antibodies.

- Systemic scleroderma may include sclerodactyly, periungual telangiectasia, telangiectatic mats, hyperpigmentation, and cutaneous calcification.

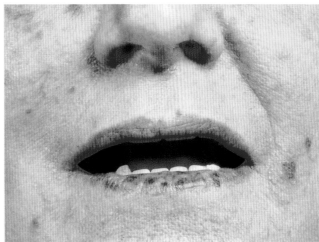

Figure 47.17 Scleroderma: CREST (*C*alcinosis Cutis, *R*aynaud Phenomenon, *E*sophageal Involvement, *S*clerodactyly, and *T*elangiectasia) Syndrome.

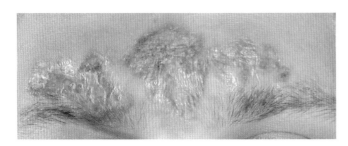

Figure 47.16 Discoid Lupus Erythematosus.

Eosinophilic fasciitis manifests as tightly bound thickening of the skin and underlying soft tissues of the extremities. Other features include arthralgias, hypergammaglobulinemia, and peripheral blood eosinophilia.

- Eosinophilic fasciitis manifests as tightly bound thickening of the skin and underlying soft tissue of the extremities.

Morphea manifests as discrete sclerotic plaques with a white, shiny center and erythematous or violaceous periphery. Localized or linear scleroderma may have various presentations depending on extent, location, and depth of sclerosis. Most lesions are characterized by sclerosis and atrophy associated with depression or "delling" of the soft tissue; underlying bone may be affected in linear scleroderma.

- Morphea manifests as discrete sclerotic plaques with a white, shiny center.
- Underlying bone may be affected in linear scleroderma.

HEMATOLOGIC

Graft-versus-host disease (GVHD) most commonly occurs after bone marrow transplant and represents the constellation of skin lesions, diarrhea, and liver enzyme abnormalities. GVHD occurs in 60% to 80% of patients who undergo allogeneic bone marrow transplant.

- GVHD commonly occurs after bone marrow transplant.
- GVHD includes skin lesions, diarrhea, and liver enzyme abnormalities.

GVHD generally occurs in 2 phases. Acute GVHD begins 7 to 21 days after transplant, and chronic GVHD begins within months to 1 year after transplant. One or both phases may occur in the same patient. Acute GVHD results from attack of donor immunocompetent T lymphocytes and null lymphocytes against host histocompatibility antigens. Chronic GVHD results from immunocompetent lymphocytes that develop in the recipient. The cutaneous abnormalities of acute GVHD include pruritus, numbness or pain of the palms and soles, an erythematous maculopapular eruption of the trunk, palms, and soles, and blisters that, when extensive, resemble toxic epidermal necrolysis. Acute GVHD also includes intestinal abnormalities resulting in diarrhea and liver function changes.

- Cutaneous abnormalities of acute GVHD are pruritus, numbness or pain of palms and soles, and erythematous maculopapular eruption of trunk, palms, and soles.

Chronic GVHD mainly affects skin and liver. Early chronic GVHD is characterized by a lichenoid reaction consisting of cutaneous and oral lesions that resemble lichen planus, with coalescing violaceous papules on the skin and white reticulated patches on the buccal mucosa. Late chronic GVHD is characterized by cutaneous sclerosis and scarring alopecia. The cutaneous infiltrate is composed predominantly of suppressor/cytotoxic T cells.

- Chronic GVHD is a lichenoid reaction consisting of cutaneous and oral lesions.

Mastocytosis (mast cell disease) can be divided into 4 groups, depending on the age at onset and the presence or absence of systemic involvement: 1) urticaria pigmentosa arising in infancy or adolescence without substantial systemic involvement, 2) urticaria pigmentosa in adults without substantial systemic involvement, 3) systemic mast cell disease, and 4) mast cell leukemia.

The cutaneous lesions may be brown to red macules, papules, nodules, or plaques that urticate on stroking. Less commonly, the lesions may be bullous, erythrodermic, or telangiectatic. The systemic manifestations are due to histamine release and consist of flushing, tachycardia, and diarrhea.

- Cutaneous lesions of mastocytosis are brown to red macules, papules, nodules, or plaques that urticate on stroking.
- Systemic manifestations of mastocytosis are due to histamine release.

Necrobiotic xanthogranuloma—indurated plaques with associated atrophy and telangiectasia with or without ulceration—may occur on the trunk or periorbital areas. Serum electrophoresis shows an IgG κ paraproteinemia or multiple myeloma.

ENDOCRINOLOGIC

Diabetes Mellitus

Several dermatologic disorders have been described in diabetes.

Necrobiosis lipoidica diabeticorum (Figure 47.18) classically occurs on the shins and presents as yellow-brown atrophic telangiectatic plaques that occasionally ulcerate. Two-thirds of patients with this skin disorder have diabetes mellitus.

- Necrobiosis lipoidica diabeticorum occurs on the shins.
- Two-thirds of patients have diabetes mellitus.

Granuloma annulare (Figure 47.19) is an asymptomatic eruption consisting of small, firm, flesh-colored or red papules in an annular configuration (less commonly nodular or generalized). The association with diabetes is disputed.

- Granuloma annulare consists of small, firm, flesh-colored or red papules in an annular configuration.

Rarely, patients with poorly controlled diabetes present with spontaneously occurring subepidermal blisters (bullosa diabeticorum) on the dorsal aspects of the hands and feet.

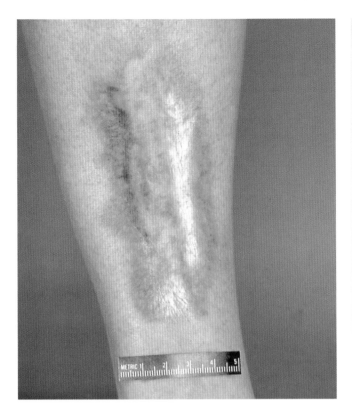

Figure 47.18 Necrobiosis Lipoidica Diabeticorum.

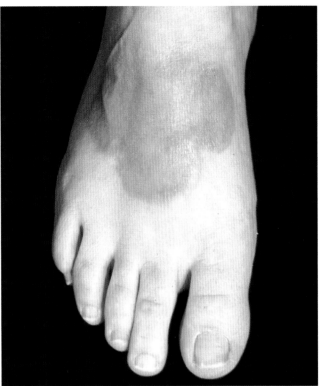

Figure 47.19 Granuloma Annulare.

The stiff-hand syndrome has been reported in juvenile-onset insulin-dependent diabetes. Patients have limited joint mobility and tight waxy skin on the hands. There is an increased risk of subsequent renal and retinal microvascular disease.

- Stiff-hand syndrome is associated with an increased risk of subsequent renal and retinal microvascular disease.

In scleredema, there is an insidious onset of thickening and stiffness of the skin on the upper part of the back and posterior aspect of the neck. The diabetes is often long-standing and poorly controlled.

- Scleredema is the onset of thickening of the skin on the upper part of the back and posterior aspect of the neck.

- In scleredema, diabetes is often long-standing and poorly controlled.

Thyroid

Pretibial myxedema and thyroid acropachy are cutaneous associations of Graves disease.

METABOLIC

The porphyrias are a group of inherited or acquired abnormalities of heme synthesis. Each type is associated with deficient activity of a particular enzyme. The porphyrias are usually divided into 3 types: erythropoietic, hepatic, and mixed.

Erythropoietic porphyria is a hereditary form (autosomal recessive) characterized by marked photosensitivity, blisters, scarring alopecia, hirsutism, red-stained teeth, hemolytic anemia, and splenomegaly. The skin lesions are severely mutilating. Onset is in infancy or early childhood.

- Erythropoietic porphyria is autosomal recessive.

- Skin lesions are severely mutilating.

Erythropoietic protoporphyria is an autosomal dominant syndrome that usually begins during childhood. It is characterized by variable degrees of photosensitivity and a marked itching, burning, or stinging sensation that occurs within minutes after sun exposure. It is associated with deficiency of ferrochelatase.

- Erythropoietic protoporphyria is autosomal dominant.

- It is associated with deficiency of ferrochelatase.

Porphyria cutanea tarda (Figure 47.20), one of the hepatic porphyrias, is an acquired or hereditary (autosomal dominant) disease associated with a defect in uroporphyrinogen decarboxylase. The disease may be precipitated by exposure to toxins (such as chlorinated phenols or hexachlorobenzene), alcohol, estrogens, iron overload, underlying hemochromatosis, and infection with hepatitis C. Porphyria cutanea tarda usually presents in the third or fourth decade of life. Clinical manifestations include photosensitivity, skin fragility, erosions and blisters (particularly on dorsal surfaces of the hands), hyperpigmentation,

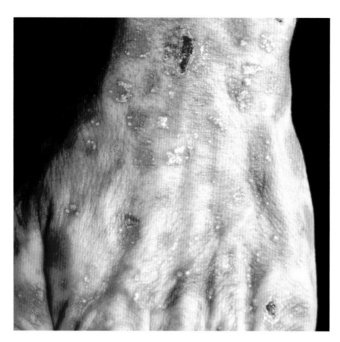

Figure 47.20 Porphyria Cutanea Tarda.

milia, hypertrichosis, and facial suffusion. Sclerodermoid skin changes develop in some patients. The diagnosis is confirmed by the finding of increased porphyrin levels in the urine. Treatment includes phlebotomy or low-dose chloroquine.

- Porphyria cutanea tarda is acquired or inherited (autosomal dominant).

- It is associated with a defect in uroporphyrinogen decarboxylase.

- It may be precipitated by exposure to toxins, infection with hepatitis C, or underlying hemochromatosis.

Acute intermittent porphyria lacks skin lesions and is characterized by acute attacks of abdominal pain or neurologic symptoms.

- Acute intermittent porphyria lacks skin lesions.

- It involves acute attacks of abdominal pain or neurologic symptoms.

Variegate porphyria (mixed porphyria) also follows autosomal dominant inheritance. Variegate porphyria is characterized by cutaneous abnormalities that are similar to those of porphyria cutanea tarda and by acute abdominal episodes, as in acute intermittent porphyria. Variegate porphyria tends to be precipitated by drugs such as barbiturates and sulfonamides.

- Variegate porphyria is autosomal dominant.

- It tends to be precipitated by drugs such as barbiturates and sulfonamides.

NAIL CLUES TO SYSTEMIC DISEASE

Onycholysis consists of distal and lateral separation of the nail plate from the nail bed. Onycholysis may be due to psoriasis, lichen planus, infection (such as *Candida* or *Pseudomonas*), a reaction to nail cosmetics, or a drug reaction. Drugs that have been noted to induce onycholysis include tetracycline and chlorpromazine. Association with thyroid disease (hyperthyroidism more than hypothyroidism) has also been noted.

- Onycholysis may be due to psoriasis, lichen planus, infection (*Candida* or *Pseudomonas*), nail cosmetics, or a drug reaction.

Pitting is a common feature of psoriatic nails. Graph-like pits have been associated with alopecia areata.

Terry nails consist of whitening of the proximal or entire nail as a result of changes in the nail bed. This abnormality is associated with cirrhosis.

- Terry nails are associated with cirrhosis.

Muehrcke lines consist of white parallel bands associated with hypoalbuminemia.

- Muehrcke lines are associated with hypoalbuminemia.

Half-and-half nails (Lindsay nails) are nails in which the proximal half is white and the distal half is red. This abnormality may be associated with renal failure.

- Half-and-half nails may be associated with renal failure.

Yellow nails are associated with chronic edema, pulmonary disease, pleural effusion, chronic bronchitis, bronchiectasis, and lung carcinoma.

Beau lines are transverse grooves in the nail associated with high fever, chemotherapy, systemic disease, and drugs.

Koilonychia (spoon nails) is associated with iron deficiency anemia, but it also may be idiopathic, familial, or related to trauma.

- Koilonychia is associated with iron deficiency anemia.

Blue-colored lunula is associated with hepatolenticular degeneration (Wilson disease) and argyria.

Mees lines are white bands associated with arsenic exposure.

- Mees lines are associated with arsenic exposure.

CUTANEOUS MANIFESTATIONS OF HIV INFECTION

Primary infection with HIV results in a flu-like illness and an exanthem in 30% to 60% of patients. The exanthem may be morbilliform, vesicular, or pityriasis rosea-like. Oral ulceration and erosions, genital erosions, and erosive esophagitis also may occur at this stage. The acute exanthem and enanthem are self-limited and often go undiagnosed.

In the early stage of the disease, cutaneous manifestations include genital warts, genital herpes, psoriasis, mild seborrheic dermatitis, xerosis, and pruritic papular eruption. With symptomatic HIV infection (CD4 count of 200–400/mcL), both infections and inflammatory dermatoses occur more frequently. These include psoriasis, seborrheic dermatitis, oral hairy leukoplakia, candidiasis, herpes zoster, drug reactions, herpes simplex, tinea pedis, and onychomycosis. In patients with a family history of atopy, atopic dermatitis may be a manifestation at this stage.

As the CD4 count decreases to less than 200/mcL, patients may present with a disseminated fungal infection, recurrent or severe herpes zoster, persistent herpes simplex, bacillary angiomatosis, and molluscum contagiosum. Bacillary angiomatosis consists of one or more vascular papules or nodules caused by the gram-negative bacteria *Bartonella quintana* and *Bartonella henselae*. Eosinophilic folliculitis, a pruritic eruption primarily involving the head, neck, trunk, and proximal extremities, is characteristic of symptomatic HIV infection.

With advanced HIV infection (CD4 counts of <50/mcL), overwhelming infection is characteristic. Infectious agents with skin manifestations include cytomegalovirus, *Cryptococcus*, *Acanthamoeba*, and extensive molluscum contagiosum.

Oral hairy leukoplakia is caused by Epstein-Barr virus infection of the oral mucosa and usually occurs in patients with advanced HIV infection.

Molluscum contagiosum, a common viral infection of otherwise healthy children, occurs in 10% to 20% of patients with HIV infection.

- Molluscum contagiosum occurs in 10%-20% of patients with HIV infection.

Epidemic Kaposi sarcoma usually presents as oval papules or plaques oriented along skin lines of the trunk, extremities, face, and mucosa. This presentation is in contrast to that of classic Kaposi sarcoma in elderly patients, which occurs predominantly on the distal lower extremities. Human herpesvirus 8 (HHV-8) has been identified in tissue from patients with both epidemic and classic Kaposi sarcoma.

- Epidemic Kaposi sarcoma presents as oval papules or plaques along skin lines of the trunk, extremities, face, and mucosa.

- It is most commonly associated with HIV infection.

SUMMARY

- Skin cancer is the most common cancer in the United States, accounting for almost half of all cancers.

- Micrometastasis to the first draining lymph node (sentinel lymph node) is the most powerful staging and prognostic tool for melanoma.

- Ultraviolet light is commonly used for therapy of generalized psoriasis and other inflammatory dermatoses.

- Immunofluorescence testing is important for the diagnosis of bullous pemphigoid.

- Penicillin, sulfonamides, and blood products are responsible for about two-thirds of drug reactions.

- Cutaneous metastasis occurs in 1%-5% of patients with metastatic neoplasms.

- In ANCA-associated granulomatous vasculitis, cutaneous involvement occurs in >50% of patients.

- Pseudoxanthoma elasticum is associated with stroke, myocardial infarction, peripheral vascular disease, and gastrointestinal hemorrhage.

PART XIV

CROSS-CONTENT AREAS

48.

GENETICS

C. Scott Collins, MD, and Christopher M. Wittich, MD

GOALS

- Review the application of genetic concepts to clinical practice.

- Recognize features of common genetic disorders that would be useful in providing primary care to patients with genetic disorders.

- Recognize when screening is indicated for family members of patients with genetic diseases.

Genetic factors play a role in the development of many human diseases. Genetic determinants include chromosome abnormalities, single gene defects, mitochondrial mutations, and multifactorial factors.

CHROMOSOME ABNORMALITIES

Chromosome abnormalities occur in 1 in 180 live births. One-third of these abnormalities are due to autosomal aneuploidy—an abnormal number of chromosomes. Risk factors for autosomal aneuploidy are maternal age 35 years or older and having had an affected child. The most common autosomal aneuploidy syndrome in term infants is Down syndrome. Approximately 35% of chromosome abnormalities in live-born infants involve sex chromosome aneuploidy. Klinefelter syndrome (47,XXY) and Turner syndrome (45,X) are 2 examples. Other chromosome abnormalities involve structural changes such as deletions, duplications, inversions, or translocations. Examples of common diseases caused by chromosome abnormalities are listed in Table 48.1.

SINGLE GENE DEFECTS

Single gene defects can be due to autosomal dominant, autosomal recessive, and X-linked recessive modes of inheritance. In autosomal dominant inheritance, 1 copy of the gene is sufficient for the trait to be expressed or for the disease to be present (ie, heterozygotes have the disease). There is a 50% chance that any child born to an affected person will inherit the abnormal gene. Penetrance varies in affected persons. In

autosomal recessive disease, 1 copy of the abnormal gene is not sufficient to cause disease, and heterozygotes (carriers) are not clinically different from the general population. When 2 persons who are heterozygotes for a given gene defect mate, the children are at 25% risk of inheriting the abnormal gene from both parents and, thus, of having the disease.

X-linked recessive diseases are caused by defects located on the X chromosome. Female heterozygotes that have 1 abnormal gene on 1 X chromosome and 1 normal gene on the other X chromosome usually are clinically normal. Males who inherit the abnormal gene have no corresponding genetic loci on the Y chromosome and therefore are referred to as hemizygotes and are clinically affected. Any male child born to a heterozygous female is at 50% risk for having the disease; female children are at 50% risk for inheriting the gene and being carriers.

- Categories of single gene defects are autosomal dominant, autosomal recessive, and X-linked recessive.

AUTOSOMAL DOMINANT DEFECTS

Table 48.2 lists important autosomal dominant conditions. *BRCA* mutations, hereditary spherocytosis, Huntington disease, low-density lipoprotein receptor deficiency (familial hypercholesterolemia), Lynch syndrome, multiple endocrine neoplasias types I, IIA, and IIB, polycystic kidney disease, and von Willebrand disease are other clinically important autosomal dominant conditions that are discussed in other chapters.

AUTOSOMAL RECESSIVE DEFECTS

Table 48.3 lists important autosomal recessive conditions. α_1-Antitrypsin deficiency, cystic fibrosis, hemochromatosis, sickle cell anemia, the thalassemias, and Wilson disease are common autosomal recessive conditions that are discussed in other chapters.

X-LINKED RECESSIVE DEFECTS

Table 48.4 lists 1 clinically important X-linked recessive condition. Hemophilia A and B are 2 other important X-linked recessive diseases that are discussed in other chapters.

Table 48.1 GENETIC DISORDERS CAUSED BY CHROMOSOME ABNORMALITIES

DISEASE	GENETIC ABNORMALITY	COMMENTS
Down syndrome	Trisomy 21	Risk when maternal age ≥35 years Congenital heart defects (VSD & AV canal defects) Early-onset Alzheimer dementia Mild to moderate mental retardation Median survival 60 years Increased risk for acute lymphocytic leukemia
Klinefelter syndrome	47,XXY	Tall, eunuchoid habitus Small testes Infertility Increased risk for germ cell tumors
Turner syndrome	45,X	Mentally normal Short stature, webbed neck Lack of secondary sex characteristics 30% risk of bicuspid aortic valve or aortic coarctation Increased ascending aortic aneurysm risk May have Y chromosome material (eg, 45,X/46,XY mosaicism) & increased risk for gonadal malignancy
Fragile X-linked mental retardation syndrome	Trinucleotide repeat (CGG) expansions on the X chromosome	May be physically normal or have a long, thin face, prominent jaw, large ears, & enlarged testes Mild to profound mental retardation

Abbreviations: AV, atrioventricular; VSD, ventricular septal defect.

Table 48.2 AUTOSOMAL DOMINANT GENETIC DISORDERS

DISEASE	GENETIC ABNORMALITY	COMMENTS
Ehlers-Danlos syndrome	Defect in gene coding for collagen. The defect varies based on the subtype of Ehlers-Danlos syndrome	Velvety textured, hyperextensible, & fragile skin Joints are hyperextensible & prone to dislocation Mitral valve prolapse occurs in many patients Most severe form results in tendency for arterial aneurysms & visceral organ rupture
Hypertrophic cardiomyopathy	Molecular defects in more than 20 different genes can cause hypertrophic cardiomyopathy	One of the most common causes of sudden death in adolescents & young adults All first-degree relatives should be evaluated Course is variable
Marfan syndrome	Defect in fibrillin-1 gene	Involves musculoskeletal, ocular, & cardiovascular systems Tall stature, scoliosis or kyphosis, & pectus deformities present Dislocations of the lens occur in 50%-80% All patients should have ophthalmologic evaluation Cardiovascular manifestations include mitral valve prolapse & dilatation of the ascending aorta β-Adrenergic blockers might delay progressive aortic dilatation Surgical treatment is often successful for mitral & aortic regurgitation & aortic dissection About 20% of cases arise by new mutation
Myotonic dystrophy	Triplet repeat expansion in myotonin protein kinase gene	Most common form of muscular dystrophy in adults Diagnosis is based on clinical findings & a typical electromyographic pattern characterized by prolonged rhythmic discharges Genetic counseling is warranted for patients & family members Age at onset is usually the second to third decade of life Myotonia, muscle atrophy & weakness, ptosis of eyelids, expressionless facies, & premature frontal baldness

(continued)

Table 48.2 (CONTINUED)

DISEASE	GENETIC ABNORMALITY	COMMENTS
		Testicular atrophy or menstrual irregularities, gastrointestinal symptoms Diabetes mellitus occurs in 6% Cardiac disease occurs in two-thirds of patients, & sudden death may occur Sleep-related central & respiratory muscle hypoventilation are very common
Neurofibromatosis 1 & 2	Multiple different mutations have been identified	Neurofibromatosis 1 has markedly variable expression but very high penetrance Malignancy (often peripheral nerve sheath tumors) develops in approximately 10% of patients Characteristics of neurofibromatosis 2 are vestibular schwannomas, nervous system gliomas, & subcapsular cataracts
Osler-Weber-Rendu disease (hereditary hemorrhagic telangiectasia)	Multiple genetic defects have been identified	Characterized by abnormal blood vessel formation in the skin, mucous membranes, lungs, liver, & brain Arteriovenous malformations occur in larger organs Nosebleeds & gastrointestinal bleeding are common
Tuberous sclerosis complex	One gene defect that causes tuberous sclerosis is located on chromosome 9 (hamartin) & another is located on chromosome 16 (tuberin)	About 50% of cases arise by new mutation Characterized by nodules of the brain & retina, seizures, mental retardation in <50%, depigmented "ash leaf" or "confetti" macules, facial angiofibromas, dental pits, subungual fibromas, & angiomyolipomas
Von Hippel-Lindau disease	The gene that causes von Hippel-Lindau disease (*VHL*) is localized to chromosome 3p25–26. The normal gene has a key role in cellular response to hypoxia & acts as a tumor suppressor	Typical case of von Hippel-Lindau disease: retinal, spinal cord, & cerebellar hemangioblastomas; cysts of kidneys, pancreas, & epididymis Renal cysts, hemangiomas, & benign adenomas are usually asymptomatic Retinal hemangioblastomas may be the earliest manifestation Periodic magnetic resonance imaging with gadolinium is recommended Renal cancer is a major cause of death

Table 48.3 AUTOSOMAL RECESSIVE GENETIC DISORDERS

DISEASE	GENETIC ABNORMALITY	COMMENTS
Friedreich ataxia	The gene involved, *FXN*, is localized to chromosome 9q13. The most frequent mechanism of mutation is expansion of a GAA trinucleotide repeat that results in abnormal accumulation of intramitochondrial iron	First sign of the disease is ataxic gait Mean age at onset is approximately 12 years Dysarthria, hypotonic muscle weakness, loss of vibration & position senses, & loss of deep tendon reflexes develop subsequently The major cause of death is cardiomyopathy
Gaucher disease	Deficiency of the enzyme glucocerebrosidase, which results in lipid storage in the spleen, liver, bone marrow, and other organs	Frequent in Ashkenazi Jews May be asymptomatic or present in childhood or adulthood with hepatosplenomegaly, thrombocytopenia, anemia, degenerative bone disease, osteoporosis, or pulmonary disease Enzyme replacement & substrate reduction therapies are effective for nonneuronopathic Gaucher disease

Table 48.4 X-LINKED RECESSIVE GENETIC DISORDER

DISEASE	GENETIC ABNORMALITY	COMMENTS
Glucose-6-phosphate dehydrogenase deficiency (G-6PD)	Abnormally low levels of glucose-6-phosphate dehydrogenase	G-6PD is important in red blood cell metabolism Most common human enzyme defect Patients may experience hemolytic anemia due to infection, fava ingestion, medications including antimalarials (primaquine & chloroquine), sulfa drugs, & isoniazid Heinz bodies on peripheral smear Coombs test negative

MITOCHONDRIAL MUTATIONS

Mitochondria contain several circular copies of their own genetic material called mitochondrial DNA. Mitochondrial disorders can arise as new mutations or be maternally inherited; in most cases, only the egg contributes mitochondria that persist in the zygote, and the sperm usually does not. Many mitochondrial enzymes, including most of the respiratory chain complex, are encoded by nuclear DNA and transported into the mitochondria. Mitochondrial DNA mutations cause Leber optic atrophy and the multisystem syndromes of mitochondrial myopathy, encephalopathy, episodes of lactic acidosis, and stroke (MELAS), myoclonic epilepsy with ragged red fibers (MERRF), and neuropathy, ataxia, and retinitis pigmentosa (NARP).

- Mitochondrial disorders are usually maternally inherited.

MULTIFACTORIAL CAUSATION

Multifactorial means that the disease or trait is determined by the interaction of environmental influences and a polygenic (many gene) predisposition. The multifactorial model predicts that there will be a tendency for familial aggregation of the condition but without a strict mendelian pattern of inheritance. Human conditions that may have multifactorial causation include many common birth defects (congenital heart defects, cleft lip and palate, and neural tube defects) and many common diseases (diabetes mellitus, asthma, hypertension, and coronary artery atherosclerosis).

- Common diseases such as diabetes mellitus, asthma, hypertension, and coronary artery atherosclerosis may have multifactorial causation.

IMPORTANCE OF AN ACCURATE CLINICAL DIAGNOSIS

Molecular genetic testing can be used for diagnosing a disorder in a patient who is suspected of having a specific disease. It also can be used for testing relatives who are at risk. The importance of a correct diagnosis in the index patient when diagnosis by DNA analysis for a relative is being contemplated cannot be overemphasized.

- Accurate clinical diagnosis is critical and supersedes laboratory testing.

SUMMARY

- Genetic factors play a role in the development of many common and uncommon human diseases. It is important to understand the basic genetic principles underlying the modes of inheritance of the above-described diseases. It is also important for the internist to know the natural history and clinical manifestations of these diseases in order to provide appropriate primary care and subspecialty referrals for patients.

49.

GERIATRICS

Margaret Beliveau, MD

GOAL

- Cite and give details of the components of geriatric assessment, including nutrition, depression, functional status, social support, advance directives, falls, vision, hearing, sexual function, memory impairment, delirium, pressure ulcers, urinary incontinence, and medications.

GERIATRIC ASSESSMENT

The assessment of elderly patients differs from that of younger adults. For assessment of the medical problems of elderly patients, it is also important to assess functional status, cognitive capacity, financial resources, and the safety and appropriateness of their domicile. Appropriate preventive screening should be a part of the assessment of elderly patients who are in good health. The subsequent sections of this chapter describe the components of a comprehensive assessment of the geriatric patient.

- The overall function of an elderly patient is influenced by factors in addition to medical problems.

- It is important to assess an elderly patient's functional status, cognitive capacity, financial resources, and the safety and appropriateness of their domicile.

- A thorough geriatric assessment should include the following areas: nutrition, depression, functional status, social support, advance directives, falls, vision, hearing, sexual function, memory impairment, delirium, pressure ulcers, urinary incontinence, and medications.

NUTRITION

Both undernutrition and obesity are common among the elderly and increase the risk of morbidity, mortality, and reduced functional status. Elderly patients should be asked about any weight changes during the past 3 months, and they should be weighed at every physician visit. Height should be checked annually. These measurements allow calculation of body mass index (weight in kilograms/height in meters squared). Laboratory markers that reflect undernutrition and have been correlated with increased mortality among the elderly include hypoalbuminemia and low serum levels of cholesterol.

DEPRESSION

Depression is common among the elderly and can reduce functional status. It also may result in considerable morbidity and mortality. Several effective screening tests, such as the Geriatric Depression Scale, are available. Unexplained weight loss may be a clue to depression.

FUNCTIONAL STATUS

How an elderly person functions in the environment is an important component of the assessment. Functional status represents a combination of the person's medical condition and his or her interactions with the social environment. It is important to remember that an elderly person's functional state may change quickly; for example, illness or prolonged hospitalization may cause a dramatic decline in functional status. The environment of the patient should be assessed to determine whether the patient's functional state allows him or her to live safely in that environment.

The functional state is evaluated in 3 tiers: 1) the basic activities of daily living are the most simple activities required to remain independent, such as eating, bathing, dressing, transferring, and toileting; 2) the instrumental activities of daily living are the more complex activities required to maintain a household, such as shopping, driving, managing finances, and performing routine household chores; and 3) the advanced activities of daily living are the ability to function in the community and include the ability to hold a job or to participate in recreational activities.

- Functional status should be evaluated as part of routine geriatric assessment.

SUPPORT

If an elderly patient has a compromised functional state, the degree of social support available for him or her should be determined. The physician needs to ascertain who is available to help with various tasks to keep the individual safe in an independent environment. Support usually includes family (most often an adult daughter), friends, and community services. A financial assessment should be made to determine whether the patient can afford treatments recommended by the physician or whether he or she qualifies for financial assistance from the government.

- A referral to social services may be needed to determine whether the patient meets the criteria for the benefits or services available.

ADVANCE DIRECTIVES

Advance directives should be discussed early with each elderly patient. It is important for the caregiver to know the patient's designated decision-maker and health care–related preferences should the patient become unable to make decisions. Living wills and a durable power of attorney for health care should be discussed and the directives reviewed periodically to determine whether the patient thinks they continue to reflect his or her wishes.

FALLS

Falls are a common cause of morbidity and an important contribution to mortality among the elderly. It is estimated that three-fourths of all deaths related to falls occur in persons older than 65 years. The increased frequency of falls among the elderly reflects multiple age-related changes, including decreased strength from loss of muscle mass, decreased visual and hearing acuity, decreased proprioception, and slowed reaction time. These changes can produce an alteration of gait and decreased balance in an elderly person.

Most falls (70%) occur in the person's home. An accident, usually related to hazards in the environment (throw rugs, slippery floors, lack of grab bars in bathtubs, and inadequate lighting), is the most common cause of falls among the elderly who live independently. Most accidental falls occur while the person is performing typical daily activities such as walking or changing position (eg, sitting to standing). The common risk factors for injuries related to falls include weakness of the legs (stroke or neuropathy), gait instability (Parkinson disease), balance disorder (vertigo or orthostatism), cognitive impairment (dementia), and the use of multiple medications (Box 49.1).

- Falls among the elderly usually reflect decreased strength from loss of muscle mass, decreased visual and hearing acuity, decreased proprioception, and slowed reaction time.

- Most falls (70%) occur in the person's home.

Box 49.1 RISK FACTORS FOR FALLS

Lower extremity weakness
History of falls
Gait deficit
Balance deficit
Use of assistive device
Visual deficit
Arthritis
Impaired activities of daily living
Depression
Cognitive impairment
Age >80 y
Multiple medications

EVALUATION OF FALLS

A thorough medical history is the most important component of the assessment of a fall. The history should include the patient's perception of the cause of the fall, any warning symptoms the patient experienced before the fall, and any associated symptoms that occurred with the fall. The patient also should be questioned about how he or she felt immediately after the fall. Loss of consciousness may suggest a cardiac or neurologic event.

The physical examination should include a neurologic examination that tests gait, balance, reflexes, sensory impairment, and extremity strength. Any sensory impairment should be noted. Because falls may be associated with acute illnesses, patients should be assessed for infections, myocardial infarction, and gastrointestinal tract hemorrhage. Orthostatic hypotension, although common among the elderly, also may indicate a medication effect or hypovolemia from hemorrhage or dehydration.

- A thorough medical history is the most important component of the assessment of a fall.

- The physical examination should include a neurologic examination that tests gait, balance, reflexes, sensory impairment, and extremity strength.

PREVENTION AND TREATMENT OF FALLS

The goal of the assessment of a fall is to decrease the likelihood of subsequent falls. The treatment plan is based on the findings of the assessment. However, more than 1 factor is often identified as contributing to falls. Potential interventions for the prevention of falls may include the following:

1. Reduction in environmental hazards: provide adequate lighting, remove obstacles from floors, eliminate slippery floors, and use appropriate footwear

2. Physical therapy: improves gait, balance, and strength, especially in the lower extremities

3. Assistive devices: improve gait and balance

4. Review of the medication program: avoid drug-drug interactions and eliminate potentially offending drugs

5. Treatment of medical problems that may contribute to falls (cataracts, postural hypotension, postprandial hypotension, Parkinson disease)

6. The most effective management strategies are multidimensional and individualized

VISION CHANGES

A combination of anatomical and physiologic changes related to aging and various disease states common in the elderly frequently cause decreased vision. Vision loss increases with advancing age, and more than 25% of those older than 85 years report marked visual impairment. More than 90% of the elderly wear eyeglasses, and it is estimated that 25% of nursing home residents are legally blind. The most common eye problem in the elderly is presbyopia (difficulty with close focus). Presbyopia is the result of decreased lens flexibility, which occurs with aging. Cataracts are also more common with advancing age; they begin forming early in life, but the progression varies from person to person. Cataract surgery with intraocular lens implantation is effective for restoring visual acuity.

GLAUCOMA

Glaucoma is characterized by increased intraocular pressure and associated optic nerve damage. The 2 major types of glaucoma are chronic open-angle and angle-closure.

Open-angle glaucoma is more common and occurs in up to 70% of adults with glaucoma. Chronic open-angle glaucoma produces a slow, progressive loss of peripheral vision that often is not appreciated by the patient until a considerable amount of vision is lost. Funduscopic examination shows atrophy and cupping of the optic disk. Visual field testing documents typical peripheral field defects.

Several options are available for the treatment of glaucoma, including surgery and medication. Medications are effective for decreasing the production of aqueous humor or for increasing its outflow. The goal of surgical treatment is to increase the flow of aqueous humor.

Acute angle-closure glaucoma is much less common than chronic open-angle glaucoma. Patients with acute angle-closure glaucoma present with symptoms of intense eye pain, blurred vision with halos around lights, headache, and nausea. Physical examination shows a slightly dilated pupil unresponsive to light. Urgent treatment is necessary to prevent permanent loss of vision.

MACULAR DEGENERATION

Macular degeneration is the leading cause of blindness in persons older than 50 years. Macular degeneration is associated with the gradual and progressive loss of central vision and

the sparing of peripheral vision. Although it initially tends to develop in 1 eye, it eventually becomes bilateral in many patients. It results in atrophy of the pigmented retinal epithelium. Impaired function of the photoreceptors eventually occurs, resulting in the characteristic loss of central vision and sparing of peripheral vision. The breakdown of the epithelium causes the deposition of drusen. The pathologic changes of macular degeneration generally can be seen on funduscopic examination. Laser treatment can be beneficial in some types of macular degeneration; however, the management of most patients with macular degeneration consists of devices used to assist vision, such as increased lighting and magnifying lenses.

- The most common eye problem in the elderly is presbyopia.

- Cataracts are very common in the elderly. Surgery with intraocular lens implantation can restore visual acuity.

- Glaucoma is characterized by increased intraocular pressure and associated optic nerve damage.

- Macular degeneration is associated with the gradual and progressive loss of central vision and the sparing of peripheral vision.

HEARING CHANGES

Notable hearing loss in the elderly is common and usually due to a central auditory processing disorder, which causes difficulty with speech perception. The prevalence of hearing loss, especially of high frequencies (presbycusis), increases markedly among persons older than 65 years and approaches 50% in those older than 80. Presbycusis is typically bilateral and associated with a high-frequency hearing loss.

Causes of conductive hearing loss include cerumen impaction, perforation of the tympanic membrane, cholesteatoma, Paget disease, and otosclerosis. Hearing aids may be beneficial. Hearing aids are most beneficial when used in an environment with minimal background noise, for example, a one-on-one conversation in a quiet room.

- The prevalence of hearing loss, especially of high frequencies (presbycusis), increases markedly in the elderly.

- Causes of conductive hearing loss include cerumen impaction, perforation of the tympanic membrane, cholesteatoma, Paget disease, and otosclerosis.

SEXUAL FUNCTION AND SEXUALITY

Multiple physical and social changes occur with aging that can result in changes in the desire and capacity of an older person for sexual activity. Although there is evidence that interest in sexuality is retained well into older age, for several reasons the frequency of sexual activity tends to be reduced with aging. One of the most important factors that may determine whether a person is sexually active is the availability of a partner who is capable of sexual activity. Painful conditions such as osteoarthritis also may contribute to diminishing desire for sexual activity.

Evidence suggests that androgens will increase sexual interest. Lack of estrogen can produce reduced vaginal lubrication and mucosal atrophy, which can cause dyspareunia.

- One of the most important factors that may determine whether a person is sexually active is the availability of a partner.

MEMORY IMPAIRMENT

MILD COGNITIVE IMPAIRMENT

Mild cognitive impairment is dysfunction in some cognitive domains, but it is not severe enough to interfere with activities of daily life. Mild cognitive impairment may be associated only with memory complaints or there may be impairments in multiple cognitive areas. Mild cognitive impairment is a risk factor for conversion to dementia. Nursing home placement rates are 2 to 3 times higher for the elderly with mild cognitive impairment. No medications have been shown to decrease the rate of conversion to dementia.

- Mild cognitive impairment is a risk factor for development of dementia.

DEMENTIA

Dementia is an acquired cognitive impairment that affects all spheres of the intellect. It is a gradually progressive disorder. Approximately 10% of the population older than 65 years has dementia. Cognitive functions that can be affected include judgment, abstract thinking, attention, ability to learn new material, and the recognition and production of speech.

The most common form of irreversible dementia is Alzheimer disease (50%-70%), followed by vascular dementia (15%-25%). The most common causes of potentially reversible dementia include depression, drugs, metabolic disorders, toxic agents, nutritional deficiencies, normal-pressure hydrocephalus, subdural hematoma, central nervous system (CNS) tumors, and CNS infections.

- The most common form of irreversible dementia is Alzheimer disease (50%-70%), followed by vascular dementia (15%-25%).
- Only 1%-2% of dementias are due to reversible causes.

ALZHEIMER DISEASE

The diagnosis of Alzheimer disease cannot be confirmed until postmortem examination. The clinical diagnosis is made primarily on the basis of the history. The disease is a gradually progressive impairment of cognition. It is characterized by gradually progressive difficulty learning new tasks and information. Loss of memory begins with recent events and eventually includes memory of distant events. Both receptive and expressive language difficulties develop in which the patient has difficulty naming familiar objects and understanding language. Patients may easily become lost, even in familiar surroundings. Calculation skills decline and patients may no longer be capable of such tasks as balancing a checkbook. Eventually behavioral problems develop in many patients, including the tendency to wander and to develop paranoia, agitation, delusions, or hallucinations.

Typically, patients with Alzheimer disease have little insight into the disease process. Driving safety is often impaired in persons with dementia, and the physician should play a prominent role in discussing this with the patient and his or her family. At times the physician may need to take steps to prevent the patient from driving if safety is an issue.

Pathologically, the CNS findings include neuronal plaques, which represent extracellular deposits of protein containing amyloid and neurofibrillary tangles. Alzheimer disease is associated with a decreased amount of CNS neurotransmitters such as acetylcholine, norepinephrine, and serotonin. Acetylcholine deficiency is especially prominent, as is a decrease in choline acetyltransferase activity.

Screening mental status examinations (such as the Mini-Mental State Examination, Mini-Cog test) often identify patients who may not have obvious cognitive impairment. If cognitive impairment is suspected but the mental status examination findings are normal, formal psychometric studies should be conducted. Normal findings on mental status examinations do not rule out dementia. The Mini-Mental State Examination is also used to follow future deterioration.

The medical evaluation consists of a medical history and physical examination and general laboratory tests. Accepted laboratory tests include a complete blood count, electrolytes, liver transaminases, blood urea nitrogen, creatinine, calcium, glucose, vitamin B_{12}, thyroid function, syphilis serology, chest radiography, and electrocardiography. CNS imaging study may be performed to rule out potentially reversible CNS processes such as mass lesions, normal-pressure hydrocephalus, or previous strokes. Electroencephalography, testing for human immunodeficiency virus, and lumbar puncture are performed only in specific clinical situations.

Until recently, the treatment of Alzheimer disease has been limited to controlling abnormal behavior with neuroleptic medications. However, none of the neuroleptic medications improve cognitive function and may worsen memory and orientation. Major tranquilizers may cause movement disorders (tardive dyskinesia) and can contribute to falls.

The recent availability of acetylcholinesterase inhibitors (tacrine, donepezil, rivastigmine, and galantamine) has given clinicians the first real options for treating Alzheimer disease. Although acetylcholinesterase inhibitors are not considered disease-modifying drugs, they may transiently delay cognitive decline and should be considered for patients who have mild to moderate dementia. The major benefit of these drugs is their potential to delay institutionalization. There may also be improvement in abnormal behaviors associated with dementia with the use of these drugs. The high prevalence of liver toxicity associated with tacrine has not been found with the other acetylcholinesterase inhibitors.

Memantine is an agent that may be disease-modifying in patients with Alzheimer disease. This drug blocks the effect of glutamate, an excitatory neurotransmitter in CNS neurons. Glutamate stimulates *N*-methyl-D-aspartate receptors, which are commonly involved in memory and learning. Excessive receptor stimulation can result in damage to the receptor. Memantine inhibits the activity of glutamate, protecting the *N*-methyl-D-aspartate receptors from damage. Memantine is recommended for patients with moderate to severe dementia. The most common adverse effect is dizziness. Increased confusion and hallucinations have been reported. Patients with Alzheimer disease can also be given a combination of an anticholinesterase medication and memantine.

- The diagnosis of Alzheimer disease is established on the basis of the history and determination of the cognitive status of the patient.

- Screening mental status examinations often identify patients who may not have obvious cognitive impairment.

- Accepted laboratory tests include a complete blood count, electrolytes, liver transaminases, blood urea nitrogen, creatinine, calcium, glucose, vitamin B$_{12}$, thyroid function, syphilis serology, chest radiography, and electrocardiography.

- Acetylcholinesterase inhibitors may delay institutionalization in patients with Alzheimer disease.

- Memantine may be disease-modifying in patients with dementia.

VASCULAR DEMENTIA

Vascular dementia is due to repeated cerebral infarcts. It can be difficult to differentiate from Alzheimer disease. The patient usually has a stepwise progression of cognitive impairment consistent with the multiple ischemic infarcts. Several types of vascular dementias are possible, including cortical multi-infarcts, subcortical multi-infarcts due to small- vessel thrombosis (lacunar strokes), and deep white matter small-vessel ischemia with demyelination (Binswanger disease). Amyloid angiopathy may cause cognitive impairment and is associated with cerebral hemorrhages. The presentation depends on which portion of the brain is affected by the ischemic insults. CNS imaging usually shows evidence of multiple strokes or white matter ischemia. Treatment consists of management of risk factors for cerebrovascular disease such as hypertension, diabetes mellitus, and hyperlipidemia. Also, antiplatelet therapy is usually given.

- Patients with vascular dementia usually have a stepwise progression of cognitive impairment.

DEMENTIA WITH LEWY BODIES

Patients with Lewy body dementia have cognitive impairments similar to those of Alzheimer disease. Lewy bodies are cytoplasmic inclusion bodies found in subcortical brain tissue. Patients have findings of parkinsonism with bradykinesia, extremity rigidity, and postural instability. Absence of a resting tremor is common (unlike Parkinson disease). Patients have difficulty maintaining attention. Also, they show marked day-to-day changes in cognitive status and may have hallucinations (visual and auditory). Patients are very sensitive to the effects of antipsychotic medications and frequently have adverse extrapyramidal reactions.

- Dementia with Lewy bodies is associated with cognitive impairment and findings of parkinsonism.

- Patients typically show marked day-to-day changes.

DEMENTIA WITH PARKINSON DISEASE

Up to 40% of patients with Parkinson disease develop dementia. These patients have features typical of Parkinson disease, including resting tremor, rigidity, and bradykinesia. In addition, they have the intellectual impairments of dementia. For some patients, effective treatment of Parkinson disease with dopamine improves cognitive status.

- Up to 40% of patients with Parkinson disease develop dementia.

FRONTOTEMPORAL DEMENTIA

Frontotemporal dementia is characterized by changes in personality and behavior due to prominent frontal lobe involvement. It has less effect on cognitive status and memory impairment. Onset of the disease tends to be somewhat earlier than for Alzheimer disease, often in the 50s and 60s. Patients frequently have poor personal hygiene and disinhibition and may demonstrate hypersexual behavior. Urinary incontinence is also common. Physical examination usually shows prominent frontal reflexes. CNS imaging shows the typical frontal and temporal lobe involvement. One type of frontotemporal dementia is Pick disease, characterized pathologically by intraneuronal inclusion bodies known as Pick bodies. Management of the behavioral disturbance is the most challenging aspect of the treatment of this condition.

- Pick disease is characterized by prominent changes in personality and behavior.

DELIRIUM

Delirium is an acute confusional disorder frequently mistaken for dementia. It is associated with a decreased level of consciousness, hallucinations, and delusions. Its several causes are listed in Box 49.2. It is important to differentiate delirium from dementia because of the potential for reversibility of

Drugs
  Sedative-hypnotics
  Anticholinergic agents
  NSAIDs
  Antipsychotic agents
Metabolic disturbances
  Hyperglycemia
  Hypoglycemia
  Hypercalcemia
Hypoxia
Hypotension
Medical illness
  Urinary tract infection
  Sepsis
  Pneumonia
Surgery
  Hip fracture repair
  Coronary artery bypass grafting
Trauma

Abbreviation: NSAID, nonsteroidal anti-inflammatory drug.

cognitive impairment associated with delirium. Patients with delirium frequently have a preexisting mild (often unrecognized) dementia.

Delirium is a medical emergency. It is important to find and treat the underlying cause, when possible. Work-up should be based on the history, often obtained from caregivers and family, and the physical examination. Laboratory evaluation should focus on fluid and electrolyte balance and signs of underlying cardiac, pulmonary, renal, and liver disease. All medications should be reviewed.

Treatment is largely supportive. The environment should be simplified as much as possible. Frequent orientation, clocks, and calendars are important. There are no drugs approved by the US Food and Drug Administration to treat delirium. There is no difference between haloperidol and newer antipsychotics for the treatment of delirium.

Delirium is associated with increased risk of morbidity and mortality.

- Delirium is a reversible cause of cognitive impairment and may be related to medications or acute medical conditions.

- Symptoms should be managed non-pharmacologically if possible.

- Haloperidol may be used for the treatment of symptoms.

PRESSURE ULCERS

Seventy percent of pressure ulcers occur in persons older than 70 years. Approximately 60% of pressure ulcers develop during hospitalization, 18% in nursing homes, and the rest at home. They are especially common among the elderly in intensive care units. The most important risk factor for the development of a pressure ulcer is immobility. Nutritional deficiencies, age-related changes in the skin, and urinary incontinence are also contributing risk factors. The common sites include the sacrum, greater trochanter, ischial tuberosity, calcaneus, and lateral malleolus.

Four factors are thought to be important in the development of pressure ulcers: pressure, shearing force, friction, and moisture. When the persistent pressure of skin overlying a bony prominence exceeds the capillary pressure, the blood supply to the tissues is impaired. Tissue ischemia can occur and result in skin ulceration.

- Risk factors for the development of pressure ulcers are immobility, nutritional deficiencies, age-related changes in the skin, and urinary incontinence.

Pressure ulcers can be classified into 1 of 4 stages (I-IV). They tend to be understaged because often the underlying tissue damage is not immediately apparent.

Stage I: Nonblanchable erythema of intact skin. There may be associated edema.

Stage II: Partial-thickness skin loss involving the epidermis or dermis or both. The ulcer is superficial and may present as an abrasion, a blister, or a shallow crater.

Stage III: Full-thickness skin loss with damage or necrosis of subcutaneous tissue. The damage may extend to the fascia. The ulcer is a deep crater.

Stage IV: Full-thickness skin loss with extensive destruction, tissue necrosis, or involvement of muscle, bone, or tendons. Sinus tracts may be present.

The most important component of pressure ulcer care is prevention. Preventive strategies include the following:

1. Repositioning patients at least every 2 hours

2. Use of pressure-reducing mattresses

3. Minimizing head elevation

4. Lifting instead of dragging the patient

5. Keeping the patient as dry as possible when incontinent

6. Keeping the skin moisturized to help maintain skin integrity

After a pressure ulcer has developed, the basic strategy for its treatment includes the following:

1. Relieving pressure over the ulcer

2. Débridement of nonviable tissue

3. Optimizing the wound environment (preventing wound maceration and avoiding friction and shearing forces) to promote the formation of granulation tissue

4. Management of other conditions (malnutrition or infection when present) that may delay wound healing

URINARY INCONTINENCE

Urinary incontinence is common among the elderly, affecting at least 15% of those living independently and about 50% of those in nursing homes. It is much more common in women than in men. It causes numerous medical, social, and economic complications and is a common reason for nursing home placement. The complications include urinary tract infection, skin breakdown, social isolation, and depression. Urinary incontinence also has been associated with an increased risk for falls in the elderly.

EVALUATION OF INCONTINENCE

The evaluation of urinary incontinence includes a thorough medical history, physical examination, and several selected laboratory tests. The history should include the amount of urine lost, duration of symptoms, precipitating factors, whether symptoms of obstruction exist, and the patient's functional status. Also, symptoms of neurologic disease, associated disease states, menstrual status and parity, and medications taken should be documented.

Physical examination of the abdomen should evaluate bladder distention and possible abdominal masses. Examination of the pelvis should include assessment for prolapse, atrophic vaginitis, and pelvic masses. The rectal examination should document any masses, fecal impaction, sphincter tone, and prostate enlargement or nodules. A neurologic examination should be performed. Patients should complete a voiding diary that records fluid intake, types of fluids ingested, and voiding (both continent and incontinent).

Laboratory tests commonly ordered in the investigation of urinary incontinence include urinalysis and urine culture, blood urea nitrogen, creatinine, calcium, and glucose. Occasionally, intravenous pyelography or renal ultrasonography may be necessary to check for hydronephrosis. A postvoid residual bladder volume test should be performed to determine the degree of bladder emptying.

Urodynamic studies are occasionally necessary to establish the diagnosis of incontinence. Urodynamic studies are indicated when patients have medically confusing histories or more than one type of urinary incontinence (mixed incontinence). Cystometry measures bladder volume and pressure and can be used to detect uninhibited detrusor muscle contractions, lack of bladder contractions, and bladder sensation. Voiding cystourethrography measures the urethrovesical angle and residual urine volume. Uroflow measures urinary flow rate and electromyography evaluates the external sphincter and detects detrusor-sphincter dyssynergia.

- The medical history is the most important part of the incontinence evaluation.

MEDICATIONS AFFECTING URINATION AND CONTINENCE

Many medications can have an effect on urinary continence. They may alter the ability of the brain to appreciate bladder fullness, alter the ability of the internal sphincter to contract and relax, or interfere with the function of the bladder. These medications include diuretics, anticholinergic agents, calcium channel antagonists, narcotics, sedative-hypnotics, and β-blockers.

TYPES OF INCONTINENCE

The 4 types of incontinence are overactive bladder (urge incontinence), outlet incompetence (stress incontinence), overflow incontinence, and functional incontinence (Table 49.1).

Overactive Bladder

Overactivity of the detrusor muscle (overactive bladder) is a common cause of incontinence, accounting for 40% to 70% of cases. When overactive bladder results in incontinence, it is known as urge incontinence. Overactive bladder causes early detrusor contractions at low bladder volumes. Symptoms include frequency, urgency, and loss of small-to-moderate urine volumes. Nocturia often occurs. Detrusor overactivity can occur with CNS disease (such as mass lesions, Parkinson disease, and stroke) or bladder irritation (such as urinary tract infection, benign prostatic hyperplasia, fecal impaction, and atrophic urethritis). There is no association between chronic asymptomatic bacteriuria and urinary incontinence.

- Overactivity of the detrusor muscle is a common cause of established incontinence.

- Symptoms include frequency, urgency, and loss of small-to-moderate urine volumes.

Outlet Incompetence

Outlet incompetence (stress incontinence) is common in middle-aged women and rare in men. It is caused by laxity of pelvic floor musculature and lack of bladder support. This may be caused by hypermobility of the urethra or intrinsic urinary sphincter insufficiency. The symptoms include loss of small amounts of urine with transient increases in intra-abdominal pressure (such as, cough, sneeze, laugh, or change in position). Some patients describe a combination of urge incontinence and stress incontinence. This is known as mixed urinary incontinence. In these patients, the history can be confusing because the patients describe symptoms of both urge incontinence and stress incontinence.

- Outlet incompetence (stress incontinence) is common in women.

- Symptoms include losses of small amounts of urine with transient increases in intra-abdominal pressure.

Table 49.1 TYPES OF ESTABLISHED URINARY INCONTINENCE

TYPE	CAUSE	SYMPTOMS	TREATMENT OPTIONS
Urge incontinence	Detrusor overactivity	Urgency, frequency, nocturia. Loss of small to moderate volumes of urine	Behavioral: urge suppression, elimination of bladder irritants, timed voiding Pharmacologic: antimuscarinic medications
Stress incontinence	Urinary outlet incompetence from intrinsic urethral sphincter insufficiency or hypermobility of the bladder	Losses of small amounts of urine associated with transient increases in intra-abdominal pressure (eg, cough, sneeze, laugh)	Behavioral: continence tampons, vaginal cones, urethral plugs, continence pessaries, pelvic floor exercises Surgical: urethral sling, tension-free vaginal tape, bladder suspension, injection of periurethral bulking agents, artificial urinary sphincter
Overflow incontinence	Urinary outlet obstruction or detrusor underactivity	Difficulty emptying bladder, low urine flow, straining to void, urinary dribbling	Relief of bladder outlet obstruction (TURP), α-adrenergic antagonists, indwelling or intermittent bladder catheterization

Abbreviation: TURP, transurethral resection of prostate.

Overflow Incontinence

Overflow incontinence is less common. It occurs with urinary outflow obstruction (benign prostatic hyperplasia, prostate cancer, or pelvic tumor) or detrusor underactivity-hypotonic bladder (autonomic neuropathy). This often occurs transiently in the elderly after surgery. Symptoms include difficulty emptying the bladder, low urine flow, and frequent dribbling. Patients give a history of difficulty starting urination and a weak urinary stream with hesitancy.

Functional Incontinence

Functional incontinence is the inability of normally continent patients to reach toilet facilities in time. Often, it is due to medications and limitation of mobility.

TREATMENT OF INCONTINENCE

All patients should be encouraged to drink an adequate volume of fluid, 40 to 60 oz daily. Behavioral training should be the initial treatment attempted. Often, it is successful for decreasing incontinent episodes. It includes eliminating bladder irritants (especially caffeine), urge suppression techniques (pelvic floor muscle contraction), scheduled toileting, and prompted voiding. When behavioral training is ineffective, pharmacologic therapy may be added. Medications that inhibit parasympathetic stimulation of the bladder muscle (antimuscarinics) are often effective. Drugs with antimuscarinic activity that are most commonly used include oxybutynin and tolterodine. Tricyclic antidepressants also have been used, but they have a higher risk of anticholinergic adverse effects. Topical estrogen therapy also may be effective in some women when atrophic urethritis is the cause of early contractions of the detrusor muscle.

- For urinary incontinence, nonpharmacologic therapy should be attempted initially.

- Medications that inhibit parasympathetic stimulation of the bladder muscle (antimuscarinics) are often effective.

- Topical estrogen therapy may be effective in some women.

For selected patients, surgical therapy may be effective. Internal sphincter bulking agents such as collagen may provide benefit. Occasionally a surgical procedure to provide an artificial urinary sphincter may be considered. For patients who have more severe symptoms of outlet incompetence, surgical suspension of the bladder and bladder neck sling therapy can restore continence.

- Patients with outlet incompetence should be instructed in pelvic floor exercises.

- For selected patients, surgical therapy may be effective.

The treatment of overflow incontinence is aimed at providing complete drainage from a bladder that either is not contracting adequately or has marked outflow obstruction. For a hypotonic bladder, treatment can include medications that increase the tone of the detrusor muscle. This may be effective for short-term use for a transient hypotonic bladder postoperatively. However, adverse effects are common in the elderly and limit its long-term use. Treatment of obstruction includes operation (transurethral resection of the prostate) and use of α-adrenergic antagonists (terazosin, doxazosin, or tamsulosin), which decrease the tone of the internal sphincter. Occasionally, an indwelling catheter or intermittent catheterization is necessary.

- Medications that increase the tone of the detrusor muscle can be tried for transient hypotonic bladder.

- Surgery is often necessary to relieve bladder outlet obstruction from benign prostatic hypertrophy.

- An indwelling catheter or intermittent catheterization is occasionally necessary.

URINARY TRACT INFECTIONS

Urinary tract infections are more common in the elderly. It is the most common infection in nursing home residents and the most common cause of sepsis. It is also a very common cause of delirium in the elderly. Incomplete emptying of the bladder, urinary instrumentation, and chronic catheterization all predispose the elderly to urinary tract infection.

The clinical presentation of bacteriuria in the elderly can vary tremendously. Many have no symptoms, and some have vague symptoms such as confusion, decreased appetite, and urinary incontinence. Pyuria is not a reliable indicator of bacteriuria in the elderly population.

Escherichia coli is a common cause of urinary tract infections in the elderly. Gram-negative organisms such as *Enterococcus* species, *Proteus* species, *Klebsiella* species, *Enterobacter* species, *Serratia* species, and *Pseudomonas* species are frequent in the elderly. Polymicrobial infections and resistant organisms are also common.

Asymptomatic bacteriuria becomes more common with age. Asymptomatic bacteriuria should not be treated unless there is a history of chronic urinary obstruction or if bladder instrumentation is planned.

- Urinary tract infection is the most common infection in nursing home residents and the most common cause of sepsis in the elderly.

- Because of the variety of organisms, the urine should be cultured when evaluating an elderly patient who has a urinary tract infection.

- Asymptomatic bacteriuria should not be treated unless there is a history of chronic urinary obstruction or if bladder instrumentation is planned.

MEDICATIONS

More than 30% of all prescriptions are written for persons older than 65 years. Medications are a common cause of iatrogenic disease in the elderly.

Pharmacokinetics in the elderly can be unpredictable. Drug absorption in the elderly can be altered due to decreased blood supply to the small bowel, villous atrophy, and decreased gastric acidity. Drug distribution has a major role in altered pharmacokinetics in the elderly. Volume of distribution can be variable in the elderly because of an increase in adipose tissue, a decrease in total body water and lean body mass, and a change in levels of plasma protein.

With advanced age, the ability of the liver to metabolize drugs decreases because of fewer functioning hepatocytes, reduced hepatic blood flow, and reduced hepatic enzymatic activity. Drug elimination is altered in the elderly because of decreased renal function. The serum level of creatinine is a poor measure of renal function in the elderly and tends to underestimate the degree of renal insufficiency. Because lean body mass decreases with advancing age, less creatinine is produced. Thus, an elderly patient who has as much as a 30% reduction in renal function may have a normal serum level of creatinine.

- Age-related changes occur in pharmacokinetics involving drug absorption, distribution, metabolism, and elimination.

- Serum creatinine level may underestimate the degree of renal insufficiency in the elderly.

Adverse drug reactions are common in the elderly. As a result of altered pharmacokinetics and pharmacodynamics with aging, medications need to be prescribed carefully for the elderly. Polypharmacy should be avoided whenever possible. Medications have been identified that have potentially greater risks in the elderly. These drugs should be prescribed with great caution for older patients.

Elderly patients often have limited organ reserve function and are unable to respond as younger persons can to an adverse effect. Drug-drug interactions tend to occur more commonly in the elderly and tend to be more serious. The likelihood of a drug-drug effect is related to the number of medications taken.

- Polypharmacy should be avoided in the elderly.

- Drug-drug interactions tend to occur more commonly in the elderly.

50.

PREVENTIVE MEDICINE

Amy T. Wang, MD, and Karen F. Mauck, MD, MSc

GOALS

- Explain key concepts in prevention and screening.

- Describe current guidelines for cancer screening.

- Understand updated recommendations for adult immunization.

- Identify appropriate preventive services and counseling in the prevention of chronic disease.

BURDEN OF DISEASE IN THE UNITED STATES

The leading causes of death in the United States are heart disease, cancer, and stroke. Accidents are the fifth leading cause of death. Mortality rates vary between groups of people:

1. Mortality rates from accidents, suicide, chronic liver disease, and assault are higher among men than women.

2. Mortality rates from diabetes mellitus and assault are higher among blacks and Hispanics than whites.

3. Mortality from suicide is highest among whites.

4. The mortality gaps between men and women and between blacks and whites have lessened slightly over time.

KEY CONCEPTS

Preventive medicine incorporates the principles of primary, secondary, and tertiary prevention in optimizing patient care.

TYPES OF PREVENTION

It is important to understand the differences between primary, secondary, and tertiary prevention.

1. *Primary prevention:* preventing disease before it occurs (eg, immunization to prevent disease, use of condoms to prevent sexually transmitted diseases) (Box 50.1).

2. *Secondary prevention:* detecting preclinical disease to start early treatment for better outcomes (eg, screening tests such as routine Papanicolaou [Pap] test, mammography, and colonoscopy) (Boxes 50.2 and 50.3).

3. *Tertiary prevention:* improving outcomes (quality of life, disease progression) in known disease (eg, use of aspirin after myocardial infarction to decrease recurrence, rehabilitation after a stroke).

- Screening tests are considered secondary prevention.

BIAS

To accurately use and interpret screening tests, sources of bias must be considered.

1. *Screening bias* can occur if the trial population used to study a screening test is not representative of the target population to be screened.

2. *Lead-time bias* can occur if the period between early detection and clinical presentation of disease is included in survival estimates. Inclusion of lead time can incorrectly increase survival for patients who underwent screening compared with patients who did not, even if early treatment has no benefit.

3. *Length-time bias* refers to a situation in which patients who have undergone screening may have a slowly progressing disease and a better prognosis, and they may seem healthier or live longer compared with patients who present with symptoms.

FEATURES OF AN IDEAL SCREENING TEST

It is important to understand the features of a good screening test.

1. Features of the disease:

    a. Be common.

    b. Cause significant morbidity and mortality.

Box 50.1 ROUTINE COUNSELING RECOMMENDATIONS

Stop tobacco use

Reduce harmful alcohol use

Dental health: Visit dental care provider regularly; brush & floss daily

Skin health: Use sunscreen

Vision & hearing: Use routine inquiry & simple tests to detect deficits in hearing & vision

Physical activity: Participate in moderate-intensity physical activity for ≥150 min weekly & muscle strengthening exercises at least twice weekly

Healthful dietary choices: Limit intake of saturated fats & processed foods, & increase intake of vegetables, fruits, & whole grains

Injury prevention

- Use safety belt in vehicles

- Use helmet with motorcycles, all-terrain vehicles, & bicycles

- Practice home safety measures, including use of smoke detectors & weapon safety

Chemoprophylaxis

- Women of childbearing age should take a multivitamin with folic acid daily

- Weigh risks & benefits of aspirin for primary prevention of cardiovascular events in adults at increased risk of coronary artery disease

c. Have a long preclinical phase (providing time to give treatments).

d. Have an effective and acceptable treatment that is readily available.

2. Features of the test:

a. Be safe, acceptable, and easy to perform.

b. Be highly sensitive.

c. Have a complementary, highly specific confirmatory test.

d. Have an acceptable rate of false-positive results.

e. Be inexpensive.

3. Features of the patient:

a. Be at risk for the specific condition.

b. Have access to testing.

c. Have adequate life expectancy and quality of life.

d. Be likely to follow through with additional testing and treatment.

CANCER SCREENING

While prostate and breast cancers are the most common cancers in men and women, respectively, lung cancer continues

Box 50.2 ROUTINE SCREENING RECOMMENDATIONS FOR ASYMPTOMATIC DISEASE

Abdominal aortic aneurysm: a 1-time abdominal ultrasonographic examination is recommended for men aged 65–75 who have ever smoked

Alcoholism: screen for alcohol use & dependence

Chlamydia: screening for all sexually active women 25 y or younger & others at increased risk

Depression: screen in practices with systems to support effective management

Diabetes mellitus, gestational: screening with glucose tolerance testing is recommended during pregnancy

Diabetes mellitus, type 2: screening is recommended for adults with hypertension

HIV: voluntary HIV testing should be offered to all adults

Hypertension: blood pressure screening at least every 2 y for all adults

Lipid disorders: routine screening is recommended every 5 y starting at age 35 for men & age 45 for women; if individuals have risk factors for coronary artery disease, start at age 20

Obesity: BMI calculation periodically

Osteoporosis: bone mineral density testing for women 65 y or older & for high-risk women younger than 65

Sexually transmitted diseases other than *Chlamydia* & HIV infections: screening for syphilis or gonorrhea (or both) in high-risk persons (consider local prevalence)

Tuberculosis: screening with TST or IGRA in high-risk groups

Abbreviations: BMI, body mass index; HIV, human immunodeficiency virus; IGRA, interferon-γ release assay; TST, tuberculin skin test.

to cause the most cancer-related deaths among both men and women. Although efforts in cancer prevention, screening, and treatment are attributed to an overall decrease in cancer mortality, cancer remains a leading cause of death.

LUNG CANCER

Lung cancer is the second most common cancer and the leading cause of cancer death among men and women. The mortality

Box 50.3 SCREENING INTERVENTIONS *NOT* ROUTINELY RECOMMENDED FOR ASYMPTOMATIC, AVERAGE-RISK PERSONS

Complete blood cell counts & routine urine tests

Thyroid disease testing

CAD screening

- Electrocardiography or cardiac stress testing

- Nontraditional markers of CAD risk: high-sensitivity C-reactive protein, ankle-brachial index, periodontal disease, carotid intima-media thickness, coronary artery calcification score on electron-beam computed tomography, homocysteine, and lipoprotein(a)

Abbreviation: CAD, coronary artery disease.

rate from lung cancer increased steadily from the 1930s until the 1980s, when it began to decrease in men. Incidence and mortality rates of lung cancer in women increased substantially in the 1960s until levelling off in the late 1990s.

Screening Recommendations

For asymptomatic persons, numerous lung cancer screening strategies, including chest radiography, sputum cytology, and low-dose computed tomographic (CT) scan, have been studied but have failed to *consistently* demonstrate a reduction in mortality. This is reflected in the most recent guidelines.

1. US Preventive Services Task Force (USPSTF), 2004:

   a. States that there is insufficient evidence to recommend for or against screening with any of the above modalities.

2. American College of Chest Physicians, 2007:

   a. Does not recommend low-dose CT scan except in the context of a well-designed clinical trial.

   b. Recommends against chest radiography and sputum cytology.

Future Directions

The National Lung Screening Trial (NLST) was a well-conducted randomized controlled trial (RCT) of low-dose CT scanning compared with chest radiography in current or former heavy smokers. In November 2010, the trial was stopped early owing to findings of 20% fewer lung cancer deaths in the low-dose CT group. Despite promising results, there are still many unanswered questions: Who should undergo screening and how often? How should overdiagnosis and high false-positive rates (>96%) be managed? What are the cost implications? Consequently, the findings are not yet reflected in clinical guidelines. However, the NLST and similar ongoing studies are likely to transform lung cancer screening recommendations in the coming years.

Lung Cancer Prevention

Smoking is the leading preventable cause of cancer in the United States and a leading cause of heart disease and stroke. Smoking causes 85% of all lung cancers. Smoking cessation decreases the risk of lung cancer in a former smoker by 20% to 90%. Physician advice to stop smoking, use of nicotine cessation aids and medications, and referral to smoking cessation programs have been shown to be helpful in smoking cessation. Population-based strategies, such as cigarette taxes and smoking restrictions in public places, have also been effective.

- Currently, guidelines recommend against screening for lung cancer in asymptomatic persons (with chest radiography, low-dose CT scan, or sputum cytology).

- Smoking is the leading preventable cause of cancer in the United States.

Breast cancer is the most commonly diagnosed cancer in women and the second leading cause of cancer death in women. The lifetime risk is estimated at 1 in 8 women. Of the women who receive a diagnosis of breast cancer, 10% to 15% have a first-degree relative who has been affected by breast cancer. The estimated 5-year breast cancer survival rate from the time of diagnosis is 89%. If a woman is a *BRCA1* or *BRCA2* carrier, she has a 50% to 85% lifetime risk of breast cancer.

Screening Tests

Mammography with or without clinical breast examination is the only recommended modality for breast cancer screening in average-risk, asymptomatic women. The American Cancer Society (ACS) recommends magnetic resonance imaging of the breast as an adjunct to screening mammography for women with a lifetime risk of breast cancer greater than 20% to 25%.

Screening Recommendations

Timing of initiation and frequency of breast cancer screening is a somewhat controversial topic. The USPSTF guidelines (updated in late 2009) are summarized as follows:

1. For women aged 40 to 49, the age to start screening mammography should be an individualized decision based on shared decision making.

2. For women aged 50 to 74, biennial screening mammography is recommended.

3. For women aged 75 or older, there is insufficient evidence to assess the benefits and harms of screening mammography.

4. There is insufficient evidence to recommend clinical breast examination.

5. The recommendation is against breast self-examination.

The American College of Physicians, American Academy of Family Physicians, and the Institute for Clinical Systems Improvement have adopted similar guidelines.

Other organizations such as the ACS, the American College of Radiology, and the American College of Obstetrians and Gynecologists (ACOG) recommend that annual mammography start at age 40. The National Cancer Institute recommends screening mammography every 1 to 2 years starting at age 40. Many of these organizations also recommend yearly clinical breast examinations and breast self-examinations.

Benefits of Screening Mammography

RCTs have shown a relative risk of 20% to 30% in breast cancer mortality attributed to screening mammography for women aged 50 to 69. Data on the potential benefit of screening among women aged 40 to 49 have shown a decrease in breast cancer mortality of 15%. Data showing screening benefits for women older than 70 are limited.

Potential Harms of Screening Mammography

Part of the controversy stems from the potential harms associated with screening mammography, which may affect women aged 40 to 49 more frequently than older women:

1. False-positive results: the high rate of false-positive results leads to additional testing, subsequent mammography, ultrasonography, or biopsy, which may lead to increased anxiety that may persist even after a woman learns that she does not have breast cancer

2. False-negative results: screening mammography misses up to 20% of breast cancers, especially in younger women owing to increased breast density, which may lead to a false sense of security

3. Other concerns: overdiagnosis, overtreatment, and radiation exposure must also be considered

Updated screening mammography recommendations of the USPSTF are as follows:

1. Ages 40–49: shared decision making to reach an individualized decision.

2. Ages 50–74: biennially.

3. Ages 75 or older: insufficient evidence for recommendation.

COLORECTAL CANCER

Colorectal cancer (CRC) is the second leading cause of cancer death and the fourth most commonly diagnosed cancer in the United States. Mortality from CRC has decreased owing to screening efforts and advances in treatment. Survival is inversely associated with stage at diagnosis; the 5-year survival rate is 80% to 90% among patients with localized CRC.

Most colorectal tumors are thought to develop from adenomatous polyps over a period of 10 years. The risk of a polyp becoming malignant is related to its size and histologic characteristics and to the number of polyps.

Factors that increase the likelihood of CRC developing include the following:

1. One or more polyps >10 mm.

2. One or more polyps with high-grade dysplasia.

3. One or more polyps with villous or tubulovillous morphology.

4. Three or more polyps.

Screening Tests

Multiple options are available for CRC screening among average-risk adults (those with no known risk factors other than age) starting at age 50:

1. Colonoscopy every 10 years.

2. Flexible sigmoidoscopy every 5 years (case-control data: 60%-80% decrease in CRC mortality; 60%-70% sensitivity compared with colonoscopy).

3. Double-contrast barium enema every 5 years (sensitivity, 48%-75%).

4. CT colonography every 5 years (sensitivity, 86%-92% depending on size of polyp).

5. Fecal occult blood test (FOBT) or fecal immunochemical test annually (FOBT RCT data: 15%-33% decrease in CRC mortality; sensitivity, 37%-79%).

Screening Recommendations

The USPSTF strongly recommends periodic CRC screening for average-risk asymptomatic men and women aged 50 to 75 years, with 1 of the following:

1. High-sensitivity FOBT annually.

2. Flexible sigmoidoscopy every 5 years *and* high-sensitivity FOBT every 3 years.

3. Colonoscopy every 10 years.

The USPSTF suggests that evidence is insufficient for using CT colonography or fecal DNA testing for CRC screening. The USPSTF does not recommend double-contrast barium enema as a screening modality.

An algorithm for CRC screening, based on age and risk factors for CRC, is shown in Figure 50.1. The following are special cases:

1. Family history of hereditary syndromes with a high risk of colon cancer, such as familial adenomatous polyposis and hereditary nonpolyposis CRC: recommendations vary according to the syndrome and counseling for genetic testing.

2. Family history of colon polyps or colon cancer in a first-degree relative or in 2 second-degree relatives: colonoscopy at age 40 or 10 years before the youngest case in the immediate family (whichever is first), then every 5 years.

3. Inflammatory bowel disease: colonoscopy 8 years after diagnosis if pancolitis (12–15 years if left-sided colitis) and then every 1 to 2 years.

• Asymptomatic persons should undergo CRC screening beginning at age 50 or earlier if they have a family history of colon polyps or colon cancer, hereditary syndromes, or inflammatory bowel disease.

• Screening can be done with colonoscopy, sigmoidoscopy, double-contrast barium enema, CT colonography, or FOBT at various intervals.

PROSTATE CANCER

Prostate cancer is the leading cancer diagnosis among men and the second most common cause of cancer death among

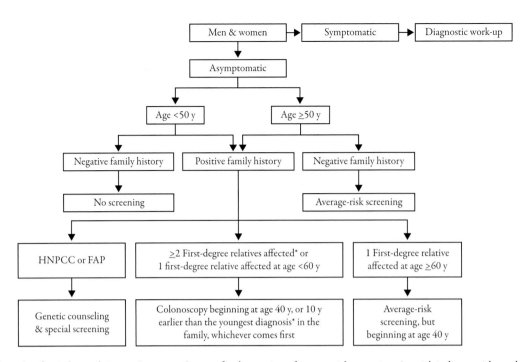

Figure 50.1 Algorithm for Colorectal Cancer Screening. See text for description of average-risk screening. Asterisk indicates either colorectal cancer or adenomatous polyp. FAP indicates familial adenomatous polyposis; HNPCC, hereditary nonpolyposis colorectal cancer. (Adapted from Winawer S, Fletcher R, Rex D, Bond J, Burt R, Ferrucci J, et al. Colorectal cancer screening and surveillance: clinical guidelines and rationale—update based on new evidence. Gastroenterology. 2003 Feb;124[2]:544–60. Used with permission.)

men, accounting for 10% of male cancer deaths annually in the United States. The mortality rate for prostate cancer has decreased, which may be attributable to earlier diagnosis and improved treatment strategies. Risk of prostate cancer is increased significantly for men with a family history of prostate cancer and for African American men.

Reviews of autopsy series have identified prostate cancer in 46% of men in their 50s, 70% of men in their 60s, and 83% of men in their 70s who died of other causes. This is reflected in the high lifetime risk of prostate cancer, which is estimated at 1 in 6 men. More than 90% of prostate cancers are localized at the time of diagnosis, which corresponds to a 5-year survival rate approaching 100%. However, only 1 in 34 men die of prostate cancer. Since prostate cancer has a high prevalence of nonclinically relevant disease, screening and subsequent management of low-grade prostate cancer are difficult.

Screening Tests

1. Digital rectal examination (DRE):

   a. Sensitivity and specificity of DRE vary with the examiner.

   b. RCT data show no mortality benefit.

   c. If prostate examination findings are suspicious, prostate biopsy is recommended.

2. Prostate-specific antigen (PSA):

   a. Sensitivity and specificity: A systematic review that used a cutoff of ≥4.0 ng/mL demonstrated a prostate cancer detection sensitivity of 21% and specificity of 91%; sensitivity was higher (51%) for detecting aggressive prostate cancers (Gleason score ≥8).

   b. Conflicting RCT mortality data: The Prostate, Lung, Colorectal, and Ovarian (PLCO) Cancer Screening Trial conducted in the United States did not show a mortality benefit; the European Randomized Study of Screening for Prostate Cancer (ERSPC) showed that PSA screening decreased the risk of death by 20%.

   c. PSA density, velocity, and doubling time and the ratio of free PSA to total PSA may improve sensitivity and specificity, but more data are needed.

   d. PSA levels are often increased in benign conditions such as prostatitis, urinary tract infection, and instrumentation.

3. Prostate imaging tests are *not* recommended for screening.

Potential Harms of Screening

Potential harms of screening include the following:

1. Additional testing, including biopsies, and potential complications of biopsies (bleeding, infection, physical discomfort, and prostate cancer–related anxiety).

2. Possibility of overdiagnosis and overtreatment, which may result in sexual dysfunction, urinary incontinence, or treatment-associated pain.

Screening Recommendations

1. ACS: Discuss risks and benefits of prostate cancer screening (PSA with or without DRE) when average-risk

men reach age 50; or beginning at age 45 for African American men or men with a family history of prostate cancer before age 65; or beginning at age 40 if multiple family members were affected before age 65.

2. USPSTF: Current evidence is insufficient for screening for prostate cancer at any age and a discussion of risks and benefits should occur before screening.

3. American Urological Association: Inform men of the risks and benefits of prostate cancer screening when they reach age 40 if their life expectancy is more than 10 years.

4. Despite controversy regarding recommendations for prostate cancer screening, there is consensus on the importance of considering prostate cancer screening after a discussion of risks and benefits with the patient.

CERVICAL CANCER

Cervical cancer screening has proved to be very effective, contributing to decreases in cervical cancer incidence and mortality of approximately 50% since the 1980s. Despite this success, racial and socioeconomic disparities in the burden of cervical cancer persist, with disproportionately higher rates of cervical cancer death in the underserved US population and in developing countries.

Human papillomavirus (HPV) infection is essential to the development of cervical cancer. HPV types 16 and 18 are thought to be responsible for approximately 70% of cervical cancer. The HPV vaccine, Gardasil, (discussed in more detail in the "Immunizations" section) is effective against the 4 most common virus strains (types 6, 11, 16, and 18).

Screening Tests

1. Pap smear:

   a. Sensitivity, 55%-80%; specificity, 80%-90%.

   b. Liquid-based cytology (eg, ThinPrep) improves sensitivity, but the USPSTF states that there is insufficient evidence to recommend for or against liquid-based cytology.

   c. Adequacy of the cervical sample affects the accuracy.

   d. No RCT data are available, but a wealth of evidence supports the mortality benefit of Pap testing.

2. HPV testing:

   a. Some studies have shown improved sensitivity with HPV testing alone and in conjunction with a Pap smear.

   b. More research is needed to learn how best to use HPV testing.

   c. USPSTF: there is insufficient evidence to recommend for or against HPV testing.

Screening Recommendations

1. USPSTF: Start screening for cervical cancer within 3 years of onset of sexual activity or age 21 (whichever comes first) and repeat screening at least every 3 years until age 65.

2. ACS: Same starting criteria as USPSTF; then annual screening until age 30 (every 2 years if using liquid-based cytology) and every 2 to 3 years thereafter, depending on past testing and risk factors, until age 70.

3. ACOG: Start screening at age 21, regardless of sexual history, and then screen every 2 years until age 30 and every 3 years thereafter until age 65 to 70 (in women with 3 consecutively negative Pap smears).

- Cervical cancer screening saves lives.

- Recommendations for age at initiation of screening and screening frequency vary, but there is general agreement for screening every 2–3 years after age 30 until age 65–70 (if patient has had previously normal Pap tests and no risk factors).

OVARIAN CANCER

Ovarian cancer is the fifth leading cause of cancer death among women. Unfortunately, 65% of ovarian cancers are diagnosed at a late stage with 5-year survival rates of 25%. Only 5% to 10% of ovarian cancer is associated with familial syndromes (lifetime risk of ovarian cancer is up to 25% for *BRCA1* carriers and up to 50% for *BRCA2* carriers). Pregnancy of any duration or the use of oral contraceptives reduces ovarian cancer risk.

Screening Tests

Pelvic examination may detect advanced disease, but sensitivity and specificity are not characterized. The following data are from the PLCO Cancer Screening Trial:

1. Cancer antigen 125: sensitivity, 20%-57%; specificity, 95%; positive predictive value, low (2%-3%).

2. Pelvic ultrasonography: sensitivity, 85%; specificity, 98%; positive predictive value, low (0.7%-1.7%).

Screening Recommendations

Routine screening for ovarian cancer is not recommended.

IMMUNIZATIONS

Immunization is one of the greatest successes of modern medicine for improving morbidity and mortality. Physicians who administer vaccines are required by law to keep permanent vaccine records and to report adverse events through the Vaccine Adverse Event Reporting System (VAERS). Providers are also required to give patients vaccine information handouts before vaccination as a mechanism for informed consent.

TYPES OF IMMUNITY

1. *Active immunity:* Antigen is presented to the host, which produces an immune response that lasts for years.

2. *Passive immunity:* Large amounts of preformed antibodies prevent or diminish the effect of infection (eg, tetanus immune globulin [TIG] and hepatitis B immune globulin [HBIG]); immune response lasts for months.

TYPES OF VACCINES

Live virus vaccines are generally contraindicated in pregnant women and in people who are severely immunocompromised or who are receiving immunosuppressive therapy. Human immunodeficiency virus (HIV)–infected persons who are immunocompetent and persons with leukemia in remission for at least 3 months may be vaccinated with some live vaccines. Examples of live virus vaccines include measles-mumps-rubella (MMR), varicella virus, and smallpox.

Inactivated vaccines are generally safe in pregnant women in whom they are indicated and in immunocompromised persons. The response may be decreased in immunocompromised persons.

ADVISORY COMMITTEE ON IMMUNIZATION PRACTICES (ACIP) RECOMMENDATIONS SUMMARY

The schedule for recommended adult immunizations is summarized in Figure 50.2.

Influenza Vaccination

Annual influenza vaccination is recommended for all adults:

1. Intranasally administered live, attenuated influenza vaccine (FluMist) is an option only for healthy, nonpregnant adults through age 49. Others should receive the trivalent inactivated vaccine.

2. If a person has an egg allergy but the reaction has been hives only, a provider familiar with egg allergy manifestations may administer inactivated influenza vaccine with observation for at least 30 minutes after vaccination. For other reactions (respiratory distress, angioedema, etc), patients should be referred to a physician with expertise in management of allergic conditions.

Tetanus-Diphtheria (Td) and Tetanus-Diphtheria-Acellular Pertussis (Tdap) Vaccination

1. Adults who have completed the primary vaccination series should receive a tetanus booster every 10 years.

2. Primary vaccination series should be completed in early childhood: the first tetanus-containing vaccine is given, the second vaccination occurs ≥4 weeks later, and the third occurs 6–12 months after the second.

3. Adults with an unknown or incomplete primary vaccination history should begin or complete the series.

Vaccine	Age Group				
	19-26 y	27-49 y	50-59 y	60-64 y	≥65 y
Influenza[a]	1 dose annually				
Tetanus, diphtheria, pertussis[a]	Substitute 1-time dose of Tdap for Td booster; then boost with Td every 10 y				Td booster every 10 y
Varicella[a]	2 doses				
Human papillomavirus (HPV)[a]	3 doses (females)				
Zoster				1 dose	
Measles-mumps-rubella (MMR)[a]	1 or 2 doses		1 dose		
Pneumococcal (polysaccharide)	1 or 2 doses				1 dose
Meningococcal[a]	1 or more doses				
Hepatitis A[a]	2 doses				
Hepatitis B[a]	3 doses				

[a]Covered by the Vaccine Injury Compensation Program.

For all persons in this category who meet the age requirements and who lack evidence of immunity (eg, lack documentation of vaccination or have no evidence of prior infection)

Recommended if some other risk factor is present (eg, on the basis of medical, occupational, lifestyle, or other indications)

No recommendation

Figure 50.2 Recommended Immunization Schedule for Adults—United States, 2011. Detailed footnotes accompanying this figure are published at http://www.cdc.gov/vaccines/recs/schedules/adult-schedule.htm. Td indicates tetanus-diphtheria; Tdap, tetanus-diphtheria-acellular pertussis.

4. A 1-time Tdap dose is *recommended* for adults regardless of when they last received a tetanus-containing vaccine.

    a. Adults younger than 65 years.

    b. May also be given to adults 65 years or older (according to a recent change in the guidelines).

    c. Persons 65 years or older who have close contact with an infant younger than 1 year.

5. Pregnant women can receive Td vaccine during the second or third trimester.

6. Recommendations for vaccination after an injury:

    a. If the primary vaccination status is complete and the wound is clean and minor, no further vaccination is needed.

    b. If the primary vaccination status is complete and the wound is contaminated, give Td booster if >5 years since the last booster.

    c. If the primary vaccination status is unknown or incomplete, give both Td and TIG.

Varicella Vaccination

1. Two doses are recommended for all seronegative adults unless there is a contraindication (eg, pregnancy, severe allergic reaction, severe immunodeficiency or immunosuppression).

2. Pregnant women without evidence of varicella immunity should be vaccinated in the immediate postpartum period.

HPV Vaccination

1. All females aged 11–26 years should be vaccinated with 3 doses (initial, second after 1–2 months, and third after 6 months after the initial dose).

2. In May 2010, the ACIP stated that the HPV vaccination may be given in males aged 9 to 26 but does not recommend routine vaccination.

3. HPV vaccine is available as either a quadrivalent vaccine (HPV4) against HPV 6, 11, 16, and 18 or a bivalent vaccine (HPV2) against HPV 16 and 18.

Herpes Zoster Vaccination

1. All persons 60 years or older should be vaccinated with zoster vaccine live (Zostavax) unless there is a contraindication (pregnancy, history of anaphylactic reactions to gelatin or neomycin, immunodeficiency, or immunosuppression).

2. In March 2011, the US Food and Drug Administration approved the use of Zostavax in adults aged 50 to 59. The ACIP stated that it is not issuing a recommendation for this age group at this time but that health care providers can offer vaccination to persons in this age group.

MMR Vaccination

1. Adults born after 1956 who do not have a medical contraindication should be vaccinated if they do not have documentation of at least 1 dose of MMR vaccine, physician documented disease, or an immune titer.

2. Adults who have never been vaccinated should receive 2 doses given at least 1 month apart.

3. Rubella immunity should be documented for women of childbearing age.

    a. If a nonpregnant woman is not immune to rubella, she should be vaccinated.

    b. If a pregnant woman is not immune to rubella, she should be vaccinated in the immediate postpartum period.

4. If an unvaccinated person is exposed to measles, vaccinate within 72 hours or give immune globulin within 6 days if the person is not a candidate for vaccine.

Pneumococcal Polysaccharide Vaccination

1. Vaccinate the following:

    a. Persons aged 65 or older.

    b. Persons with chronic cardiovascular or pulmonary disease (including asthma and smokers), diabetes mellitus, or chronic liver disease and persons who are immunocompromised (including patients with asplenia, chronic renal failure, or HIV infection).

2. Revaccinate as follows:

    a. If the person is immunocompromised, revaccinate after 5 years.

    b. If the person was vaccinated at least 5 years earlier *and* was younger than 65 at the time of primary immunization, revaccinate.

Meningococcal Vaccination

1. Vaccinate adults with asplenia, complement component deficiencies, or HIV.

2. Vaccination is also recommended for college freshmen living in dormitories and for military recruits.

Hepatitis A Vaccination

1. Vaccinate persons traveling to countries with high rates of hepatitis A virus infection, persons with chronic liver disease, injection drug users, and men who have sex with men.

2. A protective antibody level is induced within 4 weeks after hepatitis A vaccination.

3. Revaccinate at 6–12 months for long-lasting immunity.

Hepatitis B Vaccination

Efforts are being directed toward universal infant vaccination and catch-up vaccination for children and adolescents. Adult vaccination (3-dose series: initial dose, second dose 1 month after initial, and third dose 2 months after second dose) is recommended for high-risk groups, including the following:

1. Adults with high-risk behavior (persons with multiple sexual partners, persons with sexually transmitted diseases, men who have sex with men, and injection drug users).

2. Household and sexual contacts of persons with chronic hepatitis B virus infection.

3. Health care personnel with exposure to blood or body fluids.

4. Adults with chronic liver disease or HIV.

5. Adults receiving hemodialysis.

6. Travelers planning extended stays in endemic areas.

Haemophilus Influenza Type b Vaccination

Persons with asplenia, leukemia, or HIV infection should receive 1 dose.

Polio Vaccination

Vaccination is not recommended for adults unless they are traveling to an endemic area.

Rabies

Preexposure vaccination (3 doses) is recommended for veterinarians, animal handlers, and laboratory workers working with rabies virus. Vaccination may be considered for travellers to hyperendemic areas for at least 1 month and for persons whose activities involve exposure to potentially rabid animals. Postexposure prophylaxis requirements are as follows:

1. Persons with preexposure vaccination require 1 immediate dose of rabies vaccine and a second dose 3 days later.

2. Unimmunized persons require rabies immune globulin and 4 doses of rabies vaccine.

VACCINES FOR POTENTIAL BIOTERRORISM AGENTS

Smallpox (Vaccinia Virus) Vaccination

1. Enough live smallpox vaccine has been stockpiled to vaccinate everyone in the United States in an emergency.

2. Contraindications include pregnancy, atopic dermatitis or eczema, immunocompromise, and immunosuppressant therapy.

Anthrax Vaccination

Preexposure prophylaxis with anthrax vaccine is recommended only for certain military personnel and for laboratory personnel working directly with *Bacillus anthracis*.

Plague Vaccination

Vaccination is recommended only for persons at high risk of exposure, including persons working with *Yersinia pestis*.

51.

MEN'S HEALTH[a]

Thomas J. Beckman, MD, and Haitham S. Abu-Lebdeh, MD

GOALS

- Recognize key features of the history and physical examination of men with benign prostatic hyperplasia (BPH).

- Understand the interpretation and limitations of the prostate-specific antigen (PSA) test.

- Know the mechanisms of and indications for medications that are used to treat BPH.

- Identify risk factors for erectile dysfunction (ED).

- Discern the role of testosterone replacement therapy in men with ED.

BPH and ED are among the commonest diagnoses in a men's health practice.

BENIGN PROSTATIC HYPERPLASIA

BPH is common among older men. The prostate is the size of a walnut (20 cm^3) in men younger than 30 years and it gradually increases in size, leading to BPH in most men older than 60 years. BPH results from epithelial and stromal cell growth in the prostate, which in turn causes urinary outflow resistance. Over time, this resistance leads to detrusor muscle dysfunction, urinary retention, and lower urinary tract symptoms (LUTS), such as urgency, frequency, and nocturia. There is evidence that BPH progresses when left untreated. This progression is manifested as worsening prostate symptom scores (see below), decreasing urinary flow rates, and increased risk of acute urinary retention. Other complications of BPH include urinary tract infections, obstructive nephropathy, and recurrent hematuria.

Diagnosing BPH is challenging because prostate size correlates poorly with LUTS and numerous conditions other than BPH cause LUTS (Table 51.1). Nonetheless, assessing symptom severity, identifying prostatic enlargement on digital rectal examination (DRE), and documenting decreased urinary flow rates with increased postvoid residual volumes yield accurate diagnoses in most cases.

- Clinical BPH exists in most men aged 60 or older.

- Prostate size correlates poorly with symptoms of BPH.

- Complications of BPH include urinary tract infections, obstructive nephropathy, and recurrent hematuria.

HISTORY AND PHYSICAL EXAMINATION

When obtaining a history, consider the patient's age. Because prostate size increases with age, LUTS are most likely due to BPH in men older than 50 years and most likely due to other conditions in men younger than 40 years. Reviewing medications is also essential because many medications cause LUTS by affecting detrusor muscle and urinary sphincter function: 1) anticholinergic and antimuscarinic medications decrease detrusor muscle tone, 2) sympathomimetic medications increase urethral sphincter tone, and 3) diuretics increase urinary frequency (Table 51.1). Additionally, over-the-counter cold medications may cause LUTS by various mechanisms. When older men with subclinical BPH simply discontinue taking new medications, LUTS often resolve. Finally, a focused review of systems should identify fever, hematuria (indicating urothelial malignancy), urethral instrumentation or sexually transmitted diseases (suggesting the possibility of urethral stricture), sleep disturbances, patterns of fluid intake, and use of alcohol and caffeine.

The American Urological Association International Prostate Symptom Score (AUA/IPSS) is an objective measure of LUTS associated with BPH. The AUA/IPSS aids in diagnosing BPH and following the progression of BPH over time (Figure 51.1). Numerous studies have shown the reliability

[a] Portions previously published in Beckman TJ, Mynderse LA. Evaluation and medical management of benign prostatic hyperplasia. Mayo Clin Proc. 2005 Oct;80(10):1356–62. Errata in: Mayo Clin Proc. 2005 Nov;80(11):1533; and Beckman TJ, Abu-Lebdeh HS, Mynderse LA. Evaluation and medical management of erectile dysfunction. Mayo Clin Proc. 2006 Mar;81(3):385–90. Used with permission of Mayo Foundation for Medical Education and Research.

Table 51.1 DIFFERENTIAL DIAGNOSIS FOR LOWER URINARY TRACT SYMPTOMS

CATEGORY	EXAMPLES	COMMENTS
Malignant	Adenocarcinoma of the prostate Transitional cell carcinoma of the bladder Squamous cell carcinoma of the penis	Men should be offered PSA testing in conjunction with DRE With microhematuria on urinalysis, consider urothelial malignancies
Infectious	Cystitis Prostatitis Sexually transmitted diseases (eg, chlamydial infection & gonorrhea)	Urinalysis & urinary Gram stain are useful in evaluating for cystitis Prostatic massage specimens (VB3) assist in diagnosis of prostatitis Sexually transmitted diseases may cause LUTS from urethral scarring & stricture
Neurologic	Spinal cord injury Cauda equina syndrome Stroke Parkinsonism Diabetic autonomic neuropathy Multiple sclerosis Alzheimer disease	Primary mechanisms for neurologic causes of LUTS are detrusor weakness or uninhibited detrusor contractions (or both) Alzheimer disease can cause functional urinary incontinence
Medical	Poorly controlled diabetes mellitus Diabetes insipidus Congestive heart failure Hypercalcemia Obstructive sleep apnea	Medical conditions associated with urinary frequency are often overlooked causes of LUTS
Iatrogenic	Prostatectomy Cystectomy Traumatic urethrocystoscopic procedures Radiation cystitis	Surgery sometimes causes neurologic impairment Traumatic urethrocystoscopic procedures can cause scarring & urethral strictures
Anatomical	BPH Ureteral & bladder stones	Hematuria may be seen on urinalysis Consider urinary cytologic, cystoscopic, & renal imaging studies
Behavioral	Polydipsia Excessive alcohol or caffeine consumption	Consider assessing serum sodium level Voiding diary may provide useful information about fluid intake
Pharmacologic	Diuretics (eg, furosemide, hydrochlorothiazide) Sympathomimetics (eg, ephedrine, dextroamphetamine) Anticholinergics (eg, oxybutynin, amantadine) Antimuscarinics (eg, diphenhydramine, amitriptyline) Over-the-counter decongestants	Diuretics increase urinary frequency Sympathomimetic medications increase urethral resistance Anticholinergic & antimuscarinic medications decrease detrusor contractility Over-the-counter medications may cause LUTS by various mechanisms
Other	Overactive bladder	UDS can help distinguish BPH from isolated detrusor dysfunction

Abbreviations: BPH, benign prostatic hyperplasia; DRE, digital rectal examination; LUTS, lower urinary tract symptoms; PSA, prostate-specific antigen; UDS, urodynamic studies; VB3, voiding bottle 3 (postprostatic massage) urine specimen.

Adapted from Beckman TJ, Mynderse LA. Evaluation and medical management of benign prostatic hyperplasia. Mayo Clin Proc. 2005 Oct;80(10):1356–62. Erratum in: Mayo Clin Proc. 2005 Nov;80(11):1533. Used with permission of Mayo Foundation for Medical Education and Research.

and validity of the AUA/IPSS. The AUA/IPSS questionnaire asks 7 questions about the following symptoms: frequency, nocturia, weak stream, hesitancy, intermittency, incomplete bladder emptying, and urgency. Each question is answered on a 5-point scale. When the responses to the 7 questions are summed, a score of 0 to 7 represents mild symptoms of BPH, 8 to 19 represents moderate symptoms, and 20 to 35 represents severe symptoms.

- Diuretics and sympathomimetic and anticholinergic medications cause LUTS.

- Over-the-counter medications may cause LUTS.

- The AUA/IPSS is a reliable and valid assessment of bothersome LUTS.

Patients with LUTS should be evaluated for neurologic deficits, especially if the patients have a history or presenting symptoms that suggest a neurologic disorder. In such cases, useful findings include saddle anesthesia, decreased rectal sphincter tone, absent cremasteric reflex, or lower extremity neurologic abnormalities. On examination of the abdomen, masses resulting from a renal tumor, hydronephrosis, or bladder distention may be detected. The penis should be examined for pathologic changes. DRE findings most consistent with BPH are symmetrical enlargement and firm consistency, often likened to the thenar muscle or the tip of the nose. In contrast, findings consistent with adenocarcinoma of the prostate are prostate asymmetry, induration, and nodularity, often likened to the consistency of a knuckle or the forehead.

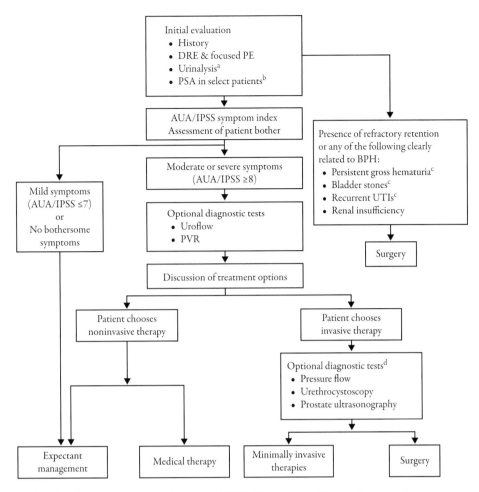

Figure 51.1 A Treatment Algorithm for Benign Prostatic Hyperplasia (BPH). Treatment decisions are based partly on patient symptom severity as determined with the American Urological Association International Prostate Symptom Score (AUA/IPSS). DRE indicates digital rectal examination; PE, physical examination; PSA, prostate-specific antigen; PVR, postvoid residual urine; UTI, urinary tract infection.

[a] In patients with clinically significant prostatic bleeding, a course of a 5α-reductase inhibitor may be used. If bleeding persists, tissue ablative surgery is indicated.

[b] Patients with at least a 10-year life expectancy for whom knowledge of the presence of prostate cancer would change management or patients for whom the PSA measurement may change the management of voiding symptoms.

[c] After exhausting other therapeutic options.

[d] Some diagnostic tests are used in predicting response to therapy. Pressure-flow studies are most useful in men before surgery.

(Adapted from AUA Practice Guidelines Committee. AUA guideline on management of benign prostatic hyperplasia [2003]. Chapter 1. Diagnosis and treatment recommendations. J Urol. 2003 Aug;170[2 Pt 1]:530–47. Used with permission.)

- Attempt to identify neurologic deficits on physical examination.

- The penis should be examined for pathologic changes.

- Prostate asymmetry, induration, and nodularity are consistent with prostate adenocarcinoma.

EVALUATION

A specimen for urinalysis should be obtained routinely when evaluating men who have LUTS. Urinalysis findings may include pyuria and bacteriuria, which suggest infection; hematuria, which suggests inflammation or urothelial malignancy; and active urine sediment, which suggests a possible postobstructive nephropathy.

Optional studies include measuring serum creatinine and PSA concentrations. The PSA measurement is optional because the results do not help discriminate BPH from adenocarcinoma of the prostate. Nevertheless, because LUTS may indicate prostate cancer, it is appropriate to routinely offer PSA testing. Although there is conflicting evidence regarding the utility of screening for prostate cancer with PSA, screening for prostate cancer with DRE and PSA may be appropriate for men aged 50 to 75 years, depending on the patient's preference after engaging in shared decision-making with his physician.

- Urinalysis is routinely used to evaluate men with symptoms of BPH.

- Measurement of serum creatinine and PSA levels is optional.

Serum PSA levels correlate with prostate volumes in men with BPH. Other causes of increased PSA levels are prostate carcinoma, bacterial prostatitis, acute urinary retention, instrumentation, prostate incision, and ejaculation. Conditions generally not believed to increase serum PSA levels are DRE, transrectal ultrasonography without biopsy, cystoscopy, and nontraumatic bladder catheterization.

- Other causes of increased PSA levels are prostate carcinoma, bacterial prostatitis, acute urinary retention, instrumentation, prostate incision, and ejaculation.

- Conditions that generally do not increase serum PSA levels are routine DRE, transrectal ultrasonography without biopsy, cystoscopy, and nontraumatic bladder catheterization.

There are different methods for interpreting serum PSA levels:

1. Cutoff value—the traditional cutoff is 4 ng/mL.

2. Age-adjusted values—age-adjusted normal limits are commonly used because prostate volume increases with age.

3. Ratio of free PSA to total PSA—the level of free (unbound) PSA is lower in men with adenocarcinoma of the prostate; therefore, a low ratio of free PSA to total PSA is more consistent with prostate adenocarcinoma than with BPH.

4. PSA velocity—a rapidly increasing PSA is more suggestive of carcinoma than BPH; in particular, an annual PSA velocity greater than 0.75 ng/mL is considered abnormal.

A uroflow study with ultrasonographic measurement of residual urine volume is an objective, noninvasive way to evaluate men presenting with LUTS. An accurate study requires urine volumes of at least 150 mL. Men with BPH often have peak flow rates less than 15 mL/s and increased residual urine volume (Figure 51.2). Notably, men with detrusor dysfunction

also have abnormal results. Consequently, as with any test, interpreting the results of uroflow studies depends on the pretest probability of disease. If the pretest probability of BPH is high, an abnormal test result is useful for confirming the diagnosis. But if the pretest probability is intermediate, an abnormal uroflow result is less useful. In such cases, patients may need to undergo complete urodynamic studies to further distinguish BPH from other causes of LUTS.

- Different methods for assessing PSA include use of a cutoff of 4 ng/mL, age-adjusted limits, the ratio of free PSA to total PSA, and the PSA velocity.

- A uroflow study is an objective, noninvasive assessment of LUTS.

MEDICAL MANAGEMENT OF BPH

Although this chapter focuses on the medical management of BPH, clinicians should recognize the indications for urologic referral and consideration of invasive therapy. These indications are moderate or severe symptoms, persistent gross hematuria, urinary retention, renal insufficiency due to BPH, recurrent urinary tract infections, and bladder calculi.

Expectant management is reasonable for patients with mild or moderate symptoms. These patients are monitored at least yearly or when new symptoms arise. In addition, these patients may be advised to practice scheduled voiding (every 3 hours during the day), to avoid excess evening fluid intake, and to be aware of potential adverse effects of over-the-counter decongestants.

Nearly all patients presenting with BPH are candidates for medical therapy. Moreover, medical therapy has replaced interventional therapy as the most common treatment of BPH. Prescription medications available for treating BPH are α_1-adrenergic antagonists (eg, tamsulosin) and 5α-reductase inhibitors (eg, finasteride).

- Expectant management is reasonable for patients with mild or moderate BPH.

- Available prescription medications are α_1-adrenergic antagonists and 5α-reductase inhibitors.

The α_1-adrenergic antagonist medications work on the dynamic component of bladder outlet obstruction by decreasing prostatic smooth muscle tone. They are the first line of medical therapy for most men with BPH. Although all α_1-adrenergic antagonist medications are equally efficacious in treating BPH, terazosin and doxazosin are more likely to cause side effects (mainly orthostatic hypotension) than other medications in this class. Other common side effects of α_1-adrenergic antagonists include dizziness, hypotension, edema, palpitations, ED, and fatigue.

The second class of prescription medications for treating BPH, the 5α-reductase inhibitors, act on the static (anatomical) component of bladder outlet obstruction. These medications decrease the conversion of testosterone to dihydrotestosterone in the prostate, thereby limiting prostate

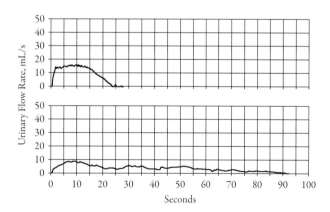

Figure 51.2 Uroflow Tracings. Top, Uroflow tracing from a young, asymptomatic male. Note the parabolic flow curve and peak flow rate >15 mL/s. Bottom, Uroflow tracing from an elderly man with benign prostatic hyperplasia. Note the prolonged voiding time and peak flow rate <10 mL/s. This patient's ultrasonographically measured residual urine volume was 100 mL. (Adapted from Beckman TJ, Mynderse LA. Evaluation and medical management of benign prostatic hyperplasia. Mayo Clin Proc. 2005 Oct;80[10]:1356–62. Erratum in: Mayo Clin Proc. 2005 Nov;80[11]:1533. Used with permission of Mayo Foundation for Medical Education and Research.)

growth. Two commonly prescribed 5α-reductase inhibitors are finasteride and dutasteride.

The following points about finasteride are important: it is most useful in men with severe BPH and large prostates (>40 cm³), it may need to be taken for more than 6 months before an optimal drug effect is apparent, and it can significantly decrease serum PSA. For this reason, experts recommend correcting the serum PSA value in men taking finasteride by multiplying the value by 2. Side effects with finasteride are uncommon. The most frequent side effects are related to sexual dysfunction and include decreased libido, ejaculatory dysfunction, and ED. Finally, evidence supports the use of α₁-adrenergic antagonists in combination with 5α-reductase inhibitors in men with inadequate responses to either drug alone.

- The α₁-adrenergic antagonists work on the dynamic component of bladder outlet obstruction.

- The 5α-reductase inhibitors work on the static component of bladder outlet obstruction.

- Use of α₁-adrenergic antagonists in combination with 5α-reductase inhibitors is often effective in patients with inadequate responses to monotherapy.

- Correct the serum PSA value in patients taking finasteride by multiplying the value by 2.

Herbal medications used to treat BPH include derivatives from African star grass, African plum tree bark, rye grass pollens, stinging nettle, and cactus flower. The most commonly used alternative treatment for BPH is saw palmetto (*Serenoa repens*). Many mechanisms for saw palmetto have been entertained, yet none are proven. Saw palmetto is considered safe, and studies including randomized trials and a meta-analysis have shown that it compares favorably with finasteride and that, compared with placebo, saw palmetto improves flow and decreases symptoms.

ERECTILE DYSFUNCTION

Male sexual dysfunction includes ED, decreased libido, anatomical abnormalities (eg, Peyronie disease), and ejaculatory dysfunction. *ED*, defined as the inability to achieve erections firm enough for vaginal penetration, affects millions of men in the United States. The Massachusetts Male Aging Study showed that the prevalence of ED increased by age: approximately 50% of men experienced ED at age 50, and nearly 70% at age 70.

- *ED* is defined as the inability to achieve erections firm enough for vaginal penetration.

Erectile physiology includes hormonal, vascular, psychologic, neurologic, and cellular components. Testosterone is primarily responsible for maintaining sexual desire (libido), and hypogonadism is sometimes associated with ED. Other hormonal causes of ED include hyperthyroidism and prolactinomas. The penile blood supply begins at the internal pudendal artery, which branches into the penile artery, ultimately giving rise to the cavernous, dorsal, and bulbourethral arteries. Psychogenic erections, triggered by fantasy or visual stimulation, are mediated by sympathetic input from the thoracolumbar chain (T11 through L2). Reflex erections are caused by tactile stimulation and are mediated by the parasympathetic nervous system (S2 through S4). Overall, parasympathetic signals are responsible for erection, and sympathetic signals are responsible for ejaculation.

- Testosterone is primarily responsible for maintaining libido.

- Psychogenic erections are mediated by the thoracolumbar chain, whereas reflex erections are mediated by sacral nerve roots S2 through S4.

- Parasympathetic signals control erection, and sympathetic signals control ejaculation.

Sexual arousal and parasympathetic signals to the penis initiate intracellular changes necessary for erection (Figure 51.3). Endothelial cells release nitric oxide, which in turn increases the level of cyclic guanosine monophosphate (cGMP). Increased levels of cGMP cause relaxation of arterial and cavernosal smooth muscle and increased penile blood flow. As the intracavernosal pressure increases, penile emissary veins are compressed, thus restricting venous return from the penis. The combination of increased arterial flow and decreased venous return results in erection. This process is reversed by the activity of cGMP phosphodiesterase (PDE) type 5 (PDE-5), which breaks down cGMP, resulting in cessation of erection.

Although ED is generally not an indicator of serious diseases, it is strongly associated with cardiovascular risk factors. In fact, the Health Professionals Follow-up Study showed that risk factors for ED and cardiovascular disease were nearly identical and that physically active men had a 30% lower risk of ED than inactive men. Therefore, men with diabetes mellitus, hypertension, and coronary artery disease are at increased

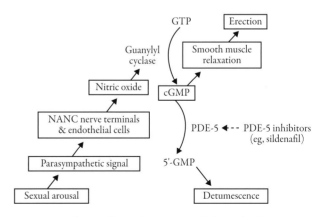

Figure 51.3 Mechanism for Penile Erection and the Molecular Activity of Phosphodiesterase Type 5 (PDE-5) Inhibitor Medications. cGMP indicates cyclic guanosine monophosphate; GMP, guanosine monophosphate; GTP, guanosine triphosphate; NANC, nonadrenergic noncholinergic. (Adapted from Beckman TJ, Abu-Lebdeh HS, Mynderse LA. Evaluation and medical management of erectile dysfunction. Mayo Clin Proc. 2006 Mar;81[3]:385–90. Used with permission of Mayo Foundation for Medical Education and Research.)

Table 51.2 QUESTIONS TO ASK WHEN TAKING A HISTORY FROM PATIENTS WITH ERECTILE DYSFUNCTION

QUESTION	COMMENT
Do you have difficulty achieving erections or difficulty with orgasms & ejaculation?	Sexual dysfunction includes various diagnoses, & it is important to determine whether the patient's primary complaint is ED
How often do you achieve erections? Are your erections firm enough for vaginal penetration?	Often patients are not satisfied with the quality of their erections, yet if patients can achieve erections adequately firm for vaginal penetration most of the time, their complaints are not classically defined as ED
Did your ED occur suddenly? Do you have nocturnal erections? Do you feel anxious or depressed? Do you & your partner have a satisfactory relationship?	The sudden onset of ED & the persistence of nocturnal erections indicate an inorganic (psychogenic) cause; in such cases, physicians should explore the psychosocial context of the patient's sexual history, such as whether the patient feels anxious or depressed or whether the patient is experiencing interpersonal relationship difficulties
Do you have a desire to engage in sexual activity?	Decreased sexual desire may indicate hypogonadism; if patients are not interested in sexual activity, serum testosterone levels should be assessed & mood disorders should be considered
Do you have penile curvature or pain with erections?	A positive response to this question may indicate Peyronie disease, which is sometimes detected on physical examination; identifying Peyronie disease is important because it precludes intraurethral alprostadil & penile injection therapy
Can you engage in vigorous physical activity without chest pain or unusual dyspnea?	PDE-5 inhibitor medications will be considered in most patients, & sexual activity is associated with cardiovascular stress; hence, a history should be obtained to identify undiagnosed ischemic heart disease or to assess the stability of known ischemic heart disease
What medications are you taking?	Numerous medications are associated with ED, especially antihypertensives & psychotropics; identify medications inhibiting cytochrome P450 (eg, ritonavir) because these medications increase plasma levels of PDE-5 inhibitor medications; an absolute contraindication to PDE-5 inhibitor medications is the concurrent use of nitrates (eg, isosorbide mononitrate); combining PDE-5 inhibitor medications with α_1-adrenergic antagonist medications can cause hypotension
How much alcohol do you consume? Do you use illegal drugs?	Substance abuse, including alcoholism, is commonly overlooked as a cause of ED
Which ED treatments have you already tried?	Knowing which medications patients have tried will help physicians decide the next therapeutic plan
Do you have a history of diseases involving your heart, blood vessels, nervous system, or hormones?	Identify common risk factors for ED
Do you have a history of hypertension, hyperlipidemia, diabetes mellitus, or tobacco abuse?	
Do you have a history of penile trauma or genitourinary surgery?	
Do you ride a bicycle regularly?	Prolonged & frequent bicycle riding can cause excessive pudendal pressure, leading to ED

Abbreviations: ED, erectile dysfunction; PDE-5, phosphodiesterase type 5.

Adapted from Beckman TJ, Abu-Lebdeh HS, Mynderse LA. Evaluation and medical management of erectile dysfunction. Mayo Clin Proc. 2006 Mar;81(3):385–90. Used with permission of Mayo Foundation for Medical Education and Research.

risk of ED. Not surprisingly, randomized controlled trial data show that erectile function significantly improves in obese men who lose weight through diet and exercise.

- Nitric oxide increases cGMP levels; increased cGMP levels cause cavernosal smooth muscle relaxation and erection.
- ED is strongly associated with cardiovascular risk factors.
- Weight loss may lead to improved erectile function in obese men.

EVALUATING PATIENTS WHO HAVE ED

History and Physical Examination

Certain questions should be asked routinely when taking a history from patients who have ED (Table 51.2). Especially important are questions about common ED risk factors such as cardiovascular disease, smoking, diabetes mellitus, hypertension, hyperlipidemia, prescription medications, alcohol use, recreational drug use, and mood disorders. In addition, validated questionnaires, such as the International Index of Erectile Function (IIEF), are useful for monitoring patients' responses to ED treatments.

A complete multisystem examination may identify indicators of cardiovascular disease (eg, obesity, hypertension, or femoral arterial bruits), endocrinopathies (eg, visual field defects, thyromegaly, or gynecomastia), or neurologic abnormalities (eg, decreased sphincter tone, absent bulbocavernosus reflex, or saddle anesthesia). The penis should be palpated in the stretched position to detect fibrous plaques consistent with Peyronie disease, which may be present on the dorsum and base of the penis. The testicles should be evaluated for masses (indicating malignancy) and decreased size and soft consistency (indicating hypogonadism). Finally, examining patients with ED is often a good opportunity to screen for prostate cancer and to assess for benign glandular enlargement.

- A careful history should identify ED risk factors, including cardiovascular disease.

- Fibrous plaques in the penis most likely indicate Peyronie disease.

- Small, soft testicles may indicate hypogonadism.

Laboratory Testing

Although disease-specific testing is favored, serum testosterone levels are frequently measured in a men's health practice. If a patient is hypogonadal, serum prolactin and luteinizing hormone (LH) levels should be assessed. If the prolactin level is elevated or the LH level is not elevated, magnetic resonance imaging (MRI) of the brain should be used to rule out a pituitary adenoma. Additional useful testing that pertains to ED risk factors includes measuring the levels of fasting glucose, fasting lipids, and thyrotropin.

- If the prolactin level is elevated or the LH level is not elevated, MRI of the brain should be used to rule out a pituitary adenoma.

MEDICAL MANAGEMENT OF ED

PDE-5 Inhibitors

PDE-5 inhibitor medications are the first line of therapy for most men with ED. PDE-5 inhibitors have revolutionized the treatment of ED since the introduction of sildenafil in 1998, and experts have observed that these medications have considerably affected (both positively and negatively) the sexual culture of older people. There were initial concerns about cardiovascular risks associated with PDE-5 inhibitors, but studies have shown that these medications are generally safe, even in patients with stable coronary artery disease who are not taking nitrate therapy.

Three commonly prescribed PDE-5 inhibitor medications are sildenafil (Viagra), vardenafil (Levitra), and tadalafil (Cialis). These medications inhibit cGMP PDE-5, thereby increasing cGMP levels and shifting the physiologic balance in favor of erection (Figure 51.3). In the absence of comparative clinical trials and meta-analyses, it appears that each of these medications is equally efficacious. Tadalafil has a longer half-life than sildenafil or vardenafil, which affords more spontaneity to tadalafil users (up to 36 hours). Patients should be instructed to take PDE-5 inhibitors at least 1 hour before sexual activity, and sildenafil should be taken on an empty stomach. Patients should also realize that PDE-5 inhibitors will not cause erections in the absence of sexual arousal (unlike intraurethral alprostadil and penile injection therapy).

- PDE-5 inhibitors are safe in patients with stable coronary artery disease who are not taking nitrate therapy.

- The PDE-5 inhibitor medications seem to be equally efficacious.

- PDE-5 inhibitors will not cause erections in the absence of sexual arousal.

The PDE-5 inhibitors have several common side effects due to the presence of PDE throughout the body: headache, flushing, gastric upset, diarrhea, nasal congestion, and light-headedness. A unique reaction to sildenafil is blue-tinged vision, which is probably related to the activity of sildenafil on PDE type 6 (PDE-6) in the retina. This reaction resolves with discontinuation of therapy. It is noteworthy that some varieties of retinitis pigmentosa have a PDE-6 gene defect. Consequently, patients with retinitis pigmentosa should not receive medications from the PDE-5 inhibitor class.

- Common side effects of PDE-5 inhibitors are due to the presence of PDE throughout the body.

- A unique reaction to sildenafil is blue-tinged vision, which is probably related to the activity of sildenafil on PDE-6 in the retina.

- Patients with retinitis pigmentosa should not receive medications from the PDE-5 inhibitor class.

A contraindication to the use of PDE-5 inhibitors is nitrate therapy. Indeed, patients treated for acute coronary syndromes should not receive nitrate therapy within 24 hours of taking sildenafil or vardenafil and within 48 hours of taking tadalafil. Physicians should also be cautious about prescribing PDE-5 inhibitors for patients with poorly controlled blood pressure or multidrug antihypertensive regimens. In patients with known or suspected ischemic heart disease, cardiac stress testing is useful for stratifying the risk of PDE-5 inhibitor therapy; patients who achieve 5 to 6 metabolic equivalent tasks without ischemia probably have a low risk of complications from engaging in sexual activity.

- Nitrate therapy is an absolute contraindication to the use of PDE-5 inhibitor medications.

- Cardiac stress testing helps stratify the risk of PDE-5 inhibitor therapy.

Treatment options for patients who have not had a response to PDE-5 inhibitors or who cannot take PDE-5 inhibitors include intraurethral alprostadil and penile injection therapy. These are generally more effective than PDE-5 inhibitors, but their obvious drawback is inconvenience. Contraindications for these treatments include blood cell dyscrasias (eg, sickle cell disease, leukemia, or multiple myeloma) and penile deformity, especially Peyronie disease. Anticoagulation is an additional contraindication to penile injection therapy. There is inadequate information on the safety of using PDE-5 inhibitors in combination with injection therapy, and hence, their coadministration is not advised.

Intraurethral Alprostadil

Intraurethral alprostadil (commercially available as MUSE [Medicated Urethral System for Erection]) is effective in men of all ages who have ED from various causes. Intraurethral alprostadil is inserted into the urethral meatus at the tip of the penis with an applicator. Patients should be instructed on the application technique. Additionally, owing to the risk of syncope, administration of the first dose should be supervised by a health care provider. The most common side effect is urethral and genital burning, and hypotension can occur. As for all medical ED treatments, patients are educated about priapism, and they are instructed to go to an emergency department if they have erections for more than 4 hours.

- The most common side effect of intraurethral alprostadil is urethral and genital burning.
- Hypotension and syncope may occur with alprostadil.

Intracavernosal Penile Injections

Intracavernosal penile injection, an efficacious and generally safe therapy, is the most effective medical treatment of ED. In practice, a triple-therapy combination of alprostadil, papaverine, and phentolamine is usually used. These medications increase penile blood flow. Specifically, alprostadil and papaverine cause relaxation of cavernosal smooth muscle and penile blood vessels, and phentolamine antagonizes α-adrenoreceptors. The use of intraurethral alprostadil requires patient instruction, and the initial dose is administered under the supervision of a health care provider. Although many patients are hesitant to attempt penile injection, this method is associated with minimal discomfort.

- Intracavernosal injections are the most effective medical therapy for ED.
- Initial doses of intraurethral and intracavernosal injections should be supervised by a health care provider.

Testosterone

Various hormonal therapies, including testosterone, were once widely used to treat ED. The penile nitric oxide pathway is testosterone dependent, and for this reason it is necessary to screen for low serum testosterone levels in men who have no response to medical therapy with sildenafil or whose presentation suggests hypogonadism. Hypogonadism is diagnosed by the presence of hypogonadal symptoms (such as decreased libido, cognitive decline, and generalized muscle weakness) and by morning fasting total testosterone levels less than 200 ng/dL on at least 2 separate occasions. In hypogonadal men, PDE-5 inhibitor therapy in combination with testosterone is often effective. Moreover, testosterone replacement alone increases sexual interest, nocturnal erections, and frequency of sexual intercourse. Nevertheless, testosterone replacement has not been shown to improve erectile function in men with normal serum testosterone levels.

- Hypogonadism is diagnosed by the presence of hypogonadal symptoms and morning fasting total testosterone levels <200 ng/dL on at least 2 separate occasions.
- Testosterone replacement has not been shown to improve erectile function in men with normal serum testosterone levels.

Testosterone is available by injection, skin patch, topical gel, or buccal oral tablets. Testosterone therapy is associated with potential risks. For example, prolonged use of high-dose, orally active 17α-alkyl androgens (eg, methyltestosterone) is associated with hepatic neoplasms, fulminant hepatitis, and cholestatic jaundice. Other risks of exogenous testosterone therapy include gynecomastia, alterations in the lipid profile (mainly decreased high-density lipoprotein cholesterol), erythropoietin-mediated polycythemia, edema, sleep apnea, hypertension, infertility (through suppression of spermatogenesis), and BPH. Exogenous testosterone also increases the risk of prostate carcinoma. Although testosterone replacement may not cause prostate carcinoma, it may stimulate the growth of existing occult prostate cancer. For this reason, all men should have screening for prostate cancer with DRE and serum PSA before using exogenous testosterone.

- Risks of testosterone therapy include hepatitis, cholestatic jaundice, hepatic neoplasms, gynecomastia, polycythemia, sleep apnea, and hypertension.
- Screening for prostate cancer is necessary before prescribing testosterone replacement.

The goal of testosterone replacement is to increase serum testosterone levels to the low or middle portion of the reference range. A recommended treatment is to apply topical testosterone, 1% gel at a starting dose of 5 g daily, to the shoulders, upper parts of the arms, or abdomen. A total testosterone level may be reassessed as soon as 14 days after starting treatment. The patient's therapeutic response and testosterone level are reassessed at 3 months, and decisions are then made about whether to continue using testosterone and whether to adjust the dose.

Although patients who receive testosterone replacement and have normal serum testosterone levels should not be at risk of adverse effects, monitoring patients during testosterone therapy is essential. Baseline determinations include whether the patient has a history of prostate cancer, BPH, obstructive sleep apnea, liver disease, hypertension, or hyperlipidemia. Baseline testing includes a complete blood cell count and levels of serum PSA, lipids, and liver transaminases. PSA levels and prostate-related symptoms should be assessed at 6 months and then annually, and patients with elevated or increasing PSA levels should not be treated with testosterone. The hematocrit and levels of lipids should be monitored biannually for the first 18 months and annually thereafter; the testosterone dose should be decreased or therapy discontinued if hematocrit values are greater than 50%. Finally, patient response to therapy and side effects are monitored quarterly during the first year of treatment.

- Patients receiving testosterone replacement require regular monitoring.

- Elevated or increasing PSA levels are an indication to stop therapy.

- Hematocrit values >50% are an indication to decrease the dose of testosterone or stop therapy.

NONMEDICAL TREATMENTS

Other ED treatments include topical vacuum pump devices and surgically inserted inflatable penile implants. Penile pumps work by creating a vacuum around the penis, thus drawing blood into the penis. When the penis is engorged with blood, an elastic ring is placed over the base of the penis and the pump is removed. Importantly, patients should use vacuum pump devices with vacuum limiters, which prevent negative pressure injury to the penis. Penile implants are generally not offered unless patients have no response to medical treatments, including maximal-strength injection therapy.

52.

WOMEN'S HEALTH

Nicole P. Sandhu, MD, PhD, and Lynne T. Shuster, MD

GOALS

- Review general health and medical issues unique to women, including gynecologic and breast health.

- Discuss medical conditions that present differently in women than in men, including cardiovascular disease.

MENSTRUATION AND MENOPAUSE

MENSTRUATION

The menstrual cycle is composed of 3 phases: follicular (proliferative), periovulatory, and luteal (secretory). At periovulation, the mature follicle triggers a surge in luteinizing hormone (LH) level, causing ovum release and stimulating the residual ovarian follicle to transform into a corpus luteum. Circulating estrogen and progestin levels increase. A thickened, enriched endometrium develops as a result of progestin secretion from the corpus luteum. In the absence of fertilization, the corpus luteum atrophies, circulating estrogen and progestin levels decline, follicle-stimulating hormone (FSH) release is stimulated, and the endometrium sloughs (menstruation). FSH then initiates follicle maturation, increasing estrogen production and endometrial growth. The duration of menstruation is, on average, 4 to 6 days. Most women's menstrual cycles last 24 to 35 days, but about 20% of women have irregular cycles. Women at the extremes of body mass index often have longer mean cycle lengths. Women within 5 to 7 years after menarche and 10 years before menopause have greater cycle variability.

- Menses occurs when fertilization does not occur; the corpus luteum atrophies, estrogen and progestin levels decline, and the endometrium sloughs.

- Menstrual cycle length is most variable at extremes of body mass index, closer to menarche, and closer to menopause.

PREMENSTRUAL SYNDROME

Premenstrual syndrome (PMS) is the cyclic occurrence of symptoms that interfere with quality of life and activities and appear with consistent and predictable relationship to the luteal phase. Typical symptoms include irritable mood, abdominal bloating, breast tenderness, back pain, headache, appetite changes, fatigue, and difficulty concentrating. Although up to 85% of menstruating women report at least one premenstrual symptom, only 5% to 10% have symptoms severe enough to interfere with life activities and thus meet the diagnostic criteria for PMS. Premenstrual dysphoric disorder (PDD) differs from PMS in that the severity of the emotional symptoms predominate over the physical symptoms. PDD may include markedly depressed mood, anxiety, anger or emotional lability, lethargy, difficulty concentrating, insomnia or hypersomnia, and a sense of being out of control. These symptoms occur during the last week of the luteal phase and resolve within a few days of menstruation. To meet the diagnostic criteria for PDD, symptoms must markedly interfere with work, school, or usual social activities and relationships with others. Other possible disorders must be considered before making the diagnosis of PDD, and prospective daily rating during at least 2 consecutive cycles should be completed to confirm the diagnosis.

- PMS consists of 1 or more menstrual cycle-related symptoms severe enough to interfere with quality of life and activities; only 5% to 10% of women have symptoms severe enough to meet diagnostic criteria for PMS.

- PDD differs from PMS in the severity of emotional symptoms; it is a diagnosis of exclusion.

- Symptoms must occur consistently and with a predictable relationship to the luteal phase to consider the diagnosis of PMS or PDD.

Reducing caffeine, salt, and alcohol intake while increasing complex carbohydrate intake during the luteal phase may help some women with mild to moderate premenstrual symptoms and PMS. Calcium carbonate seems to reduce symptom severity. Vitamin B_6 or magnesium may also help, but the evidence for these agents is less strong than that for calcium.

For women with more severe premenstrual symptoms, PMS, or PDD, selective serotonin reuptake inhibitors are the treatment of choice for emotional symptoms. They may be prescribed continuously or cyclically (luteal phase). Oral contraceptives may improve physical symptoms of PMS, but they do not seem to help mood. Dietary changes and calcium carbonate seem to reduce the severity of premenstrual symptoms.

- Selective serotonin reuptake inhibitors are the treatment of choice for severe PDD.

- Oral contraceptives may improve physical symptoms, but they do not help mood.

ABNORMAL UTERINE BLEEDING (IN WOMEN OF REPRODUCTIVE AGE)

Bleeding that is excessive or outside the normal cyclic bleeding pattern is called abnormal uterine bleeding (Box 52.1). The following are commonly used terms: *amenorrhea*, absence of bleeding for 3 usual cycles; *oligomenorrhea*, decreased frequency of menstrual periods; *menorrhagia*, excessive or prolonged bleeding at regular intervals of menstruation; *metrorrhagia*, light and irregular menstrual bleeding; and *menometrorrhagia*, heavy and irregular menstrual bleeding. Heavy menstrual bleeding that interferes with daily activities is the most common concern for women with abnormal uterine bleeding. Irregular bleeding is typically anovulatory and is most common at the extremes of reproductive age, whereas menorrhagia is typically ovulatory.

- Excessive bleeding or bleeding outside the normal cyclic pattern is called abnormal uterine bleeding.

Box 52.1 POSSIBLE CAUSES OF ABNORMAL UTERINE BLEEDING

Pregnancy
Anovulation or oligo-ovulation
Fibroids
Polyps, endometrial or endocervical
Adenomyosis
Endometriosis
Infection, including pelvic inflammatory disease
Endometrial hyperplasia
Endometrial carcinoma
Coagulation disorders
Hyperprolactinemia
Liver disease
Thyroid dysfunction
Obesity
Anorexia
Rapid fluctuations in weight
Corticosteroids
Hormonal contraceptives
Tamoxifen

The history directs evaluation and management and should include date of last period; timing, duration, and amount of bleeding; bleeding pattern; associated pain; evidence of ovulatory cycling (regular menses, cyclic symptoms); contraceptive history; medical conditions or history suggestive of a medical condition (eg, thyroid disease, celiac disease, and blood dyscrasias); medications; and the impact of bleeding on quality of life (which may help determine treatment options). The age and reproductive status of the patient assist with differential diagnosis.

Physical examination includes pelvic and breast examinations, assessing body habitus and hair distribution, and thyroid and skin examinations. Bleeding should be verified to be coming from the cervical os whenever possible. Mucosal lesions that may be the source of blood should be noted and evaluated appropriately. Obese women can have irregular, anovulatory bleeding due to increased circulating estrogen (androgen conversion in adipose tissue). Underweight patients may have oligomenorrhea due to hypothalamic dysfunction. Hirsutism suggests polycystic ovary syndrome, a cause of infrequent and sometimes very heavy menstrual periods associated with anovulation. Petechiae suggest abnormal clotting disorders. Vaginal atrophy and cervical lesions can cause postcoital spotting or bleeding. Pregnancy must be considered first when evaluating abnormal uterine bleeding. Ectopic pregnancy must be considered if a woman also has unilateral pelvic pain, particularly after an episode of amenorrhea. In the nonpregnant patient, further evaluation and management are guided by whether bleeding is irregular or menorrhagia. Management depends on the underlying cause, and medical causes should be considered (eg, thyroid or other endocrine disease, polycystic ovary syndrome, bleeding dyscrasias, or medication use). Treatment should focus on a defined medical or other underlying cause (eg, endocrine abnormality and uterine structural abnormalities) and impact on quality of life.

- The pattern of bleeding coupled with history and physical examination findings direct further evaluation of abnormal uterine bleeding.

- Medical problems (eg, thyroid and celiac disease) may cause abnormal uterine bleeding.

- Conservative management, including reassurance, monitoring, or hormonal agents, is often sufficient.

For irregular bleeding in women 35 years or older or at high risk of endometrial cancer, consider transvaginal ultrasonography or endometrial biopsy. If these tests are not indicated, therapy with oral contraceptives (or a progestin if oral contraceptives are contraindicated) may be initiated. If the response is inadequate, increase the dose and consider transvaginal ultrasonography or biopsy. In the setting of menorrhagia, oral contraceptives (or a progestin or nonsteroidal anti-inflammatory drug) as first-line therapy is appropriate. A levonorgestrel intrauterine device may be considered. If response is inadequate, transvaginal ultrasound or biopsy should be considered.

Definitive management should be considered for endometrial polyps or submucosal fibroids and for persistent bleeding inadequately responsive to medical therapy. Areas of hyperplasia should undergo biopsy. If there are no sonographic abnormalities and childbearing is complete, definitive therapy with endometrial ablation or hysterectomy or other appropriate treatment (eg, myomectomy) can be considered. If childbearing is incomplete, follow the menstrual pattern, observe the patient, and provide appropriate medical management. If transvaginal ultrasonography is inconclusive, hysteroscopy for direct visualization of the endometrial cavity may be considered. Additional measures should be directed at medical issues (eg, treatment of causative medical conditions, transfusion, intravenous fluids, and complete blood count).

- First-line therapy for irregular bleeding is medical (usually hormonal).

- Nonsteroidal anti-inflammatory drugs may also be used and help reduce blood flow.

- Endometrial biopsy is often unnecessary but is recommended in women ≥35 years old or with a high risk of endometrial cancer (eg, unopposed estrogen therapy).

- With inadequate response to hormonal agents, diagnostic testing (including hysteroscopy, transvaginal ultrasonography, or endometrial biopsy) may be indicated.

DYSFUNCTIONAL UTERINE BLEEDING

Abnormal, excessive uterine bleeding not due to a specific, identifiable cause is called dysfunctional uterine bleeding. It is most commonly observed at the extremes of reproductive age. Dysfunctional uterine bleeding is a diagnosis of exclusion. Useful therapies include hormonal contraception (usually combination oral contraceptive pills), cyclic oral progestins (most commonly medroxyprogesterone acetate), and nonsteroidal anti-inflammatory drugs (may reduce blood loss by up to 50%).

- Dysfunctional uterine bleeding is a diagnosis of exclusion.

CONTRACEPTION AND INFERTILITY

CONTRACEPTION

Contraceptive methods include hormonal (ie, oral, transdermal, vaginal, intrauterine, intradermal implant, and intramuscular injection), barrier, chemical, and physiologic approaches. None are 100% effective, and all are associated with some degree of risk (Table 52.1).

Factors to consider in counseling women regarding contraceptive methods include efficacy, convenience, duration of action, reversibility and time to return of fertility, effect

Table 52.1 **CONTRACEPTION OPTIONS**

CONTRACEPTIVE METHOD	RISKS	ADVERSE EFFECTS	BENEFITS
Combined hormonal contraceptives	DVT, stroke, MI, HTN, depression, hepatic adenoma; no STI prevention	Nausea, headaches, spotting, weight gain, mastalgia, mood changes	Reduced risk of dysmenorrhea; menorrhagia; anemia; ectopic pregnancy; PID; ovarian, endometrial, &, possibly, colorectal cancer; acne
Progestin-only pill	Less effective than combined OC for preventing pregnancy	Unpredictable spotting, bleeding	Safer than combination OCs with regard to HTN, CV disease, breast cancer, clotting. Does not interfere with lactation
IUD	STIs. Increased risk of ectopic pregnancy. Insertion-associated risks of infection & perforation	Spotting, cramping, back pain; longer, heavier periods	Levonorgestrel IUD reduces menorrhagia
Condom	None	Requires planning ahead; may decrease sensation	Protects against STIs
Depo-progestin	Depression, weight gain, bone loss, dyslipidemia	Menstrual changes, weight gain, headache	Lactation not disturbed; convenience; reduces seizures
Diaphragm	UTIs, toxic shock syndrome	Requires planning ahead; must be left in place for 6–8 h after sexual intercourse; vaginal discharge if left in too long	Avoids hormone-related side effects
Fertility awareness–based methods	Pregnancy risk estimated to be 9% with perfect use, 19% with typical use	Takes time to learn; requires abstaining from sexual intercourse or using barrier method during fertile window	Learning biomarkers of fertility can help a committed couple plan pregnancy or avoid pregnancy

Abbreviations: CV, cardiovascular; DVT, deep vein thrombosis; HTN, hypertension; IUD, intrauterine device; MI, myocardial infarction; OC, oral contraceptive; PID, pelvic inflammatory disease; STI, sexually transmitted infection; UTI, urinary tract infection.

on uterine bleeding, risk of adverse events, affordability, and protection against sexually transmitted infections. Balancing the advantages and disadvantages of each method guides individual decisions. Methods consistent with a woman's and a couple's values and lifestyle are most likely to be successful.

Effective contraceptive management requires education and counseling regarding appropriate use. It is particularly important for internists to be familiar with the medical aspects of hormonal contraceptives.

- Lifestyle, values, and other factors, such as risk of sexually transmitted infections, should guide contraceptive choice.

- Factors to consider include efficacy, convenience, cost, reversibility and time to fertility return, and risk of adverse events.

Hormonal contraceptives may include estrogen plus a progestogen or a progestogen alone. They come in various forms; the most common form is the combination estrogen-progestogen pill. Estrogen prevents ovulation by inhibiting pituitary release of gonadotropins, suppressing FSH and LH. Estrogens also alter endometrial secretion and local prostaglandin levels, contributing to corpus luteum degeneration. Progestogen effects inhibit ovulation by suppressing the midcycle LH and FSH peak. In addition, progestogens thicken cervical mucus and alter tubal motility, interfering with sperm transport, and lead to an atrophic endometrium, interfering with fertilized ovum implantation.

Combination estrogen-progestogen pills are highly effective (97%-99%) in preventing pregnancy when used correctly; the contraceptive failure rate is about 3 in 1,000 in the first year of use. However, with *typical* use, the failure rate is estimated to be 8%, due to pill-taking mistakes. Noncontraceptive benefits of oral contraceptives include reduced dysmenorrhea, menstrual flow, and functional ovarian cyst development; increased bone mineral density; reduced risk of ovarian cancer (40%-80% depending on duration of use) and endometrial cancer (50%); and reduced risk of pelvic inflammatory disease and ectopic pregnancy. Other benefits include treatment of acne, hirsutism, and perimenopausal symptoms.

- Estrogen and progestogen effects prevent ovulation and lead to other effects that inhibit pregnancy from occurring.

- Although these agents are highly effective when used correctly, typical use is associated with a failure rate of nearly 10%.

- Oral contraceptives have multiple noncontraceptive benefits, including reduced risk of ovarian cancer.

Estrogen-containing oral contraceptives are thrombogenic, but the absolute risk of venous thromboembolism is low. Lower-dose estrogen-containing oral contraceptives have lower associated risk. Excess risk declines after the first year of use. Women with inherited coagulopathies have a higher risk for venous thromboembolism. Screening for thrombophilias is not recommended in the absence of a personal or

---

Box 52.2 **CONTRAINDICATIONS TO USE OF ESTROGEN-CONTAINING ORAL CONTRACEPTIVES**

Absolute contraindications
  History of deep vein thrombosis or pulmonary embolism, unless defined nonhormonal cause
  History of arterial thromboembolism
  Active liver disease
  Cardiovascular disease such as congestive heart failure, myocardial infarction or coronary artery disease, atrial fibrillation, mitral stenosis, mechanical heart valve
  Systemic diseases that affect the vascular system (such as systemic lupus erythematosus, diabetes mellitus with retinopathy or nephropathy)
  Cigarette smoking by women >35 y
  Uncontrolled hypertension
  History of breast cancer
  Undiagnosed amenorrhea
Relative contraindications
  Classic migraine
  Hypertriglyceridemia
  Depression

---

strong family history of thrombotic events. Women older than 35 years who smoke cigarettes have a relative contraindication to combination oral contraceptives because of an increased risk of myocardial infarction and stroke (Box 52.2). Use of low-dose oral contraceptives by nonsmoking women without hypertension is not associated with a significantly increased risk of myocardial infarction or stroke. Oral contraceptives can also increase blood pressure, which should be monitored.

- Risk of thromboembolism is increased but overall is low unless a patient has a personal or family history of thrombosis.

- Oral contraceptives are contraindicated in smokers >35 years because of an increased risk of myocardial infarction and stroke.

Progestogens have adverse lipid effects, including decreased high-density lipoprotein cholesterol and increased low-density lipoprotein cholesterol. Lipid effect is related to amount and potency of the progestogen. Estrogens increase high-density lipoprotein cholesterol and decrease low-density lipoprotein cholesterol. Oral contraceptives with lower androgenic progestogens have less adverse effect on lipids. The net effect of these oral contraceptives is little or no change in total cholesterol, high-density lipoprotein cholesterol, or low-density lipoprotein cholesterol levels. However, the synthetic estrogen component may lead to substantial increases in triglyceride levels.

The relationship between use of oral contraceptives and breast cancer risk continues to be controversial. A slight increase may occur in breast cancer risk that decreases after discontinuation of contraceptive use. Progestogen-only pills are an option for women who need to avoid estrogen. They have a slightly higher failure rate than combination oral contraceptives and a higher frequency of breakthrough bleeding. Consider progestogen-only pills in women with migraine headaches, hypertension, diabetes mellitus, personal or family history of thromboembolism, cardiac or cerebrovascular disease, or hypertriglyceridemia and in women older than 35 years who are smokers.

- Progestogen-only pills have adverse effects on total, high-density lipoprotein, and low-density lipoprotein cholesterol levels, whereas the estrogen component in combination pills increases triglyceride levels.

- Consider progestogen-only pills in women with migraines, cardiovascular or cerebrovascular disease, diabetes, or history of blood clots and in women older >35 years who are smokers.

Table 52.1 has additional information on contraceptive methods.

INFERTILITY

Infertility is the inability to conceive after 1 year of intercourse without contraception and may be due to male or female factors or both. The cause may be difficult to identify. A woman's age is the most important determinant of a couple's fertility. Other common causes of female infertility are ovulatory disorders (eg, polycystic ovary syndrome, hypothyroidism, hyperprolactinemia, eating disorders, or extreme stress), endometriosis, pelvic adhesions, and tubal abnormalities. Declining oocyte quality with advanced age is a major cause of infertility.

Evaluation includes a careful history (duration of infertility; prior evaluation or interventions; menstrual history; sexual history; lifestyle factors including exercise, diet, stress, smoking, and substance abuse; medical and surgical history), partner semen analysis, documentation of ovulation through history and midluteal serum progesterone level, assessment of ovarian reserve (day 3 FSH and estradiol level measurements), assessment of fallopian tube patency with hysterosalpingography, and exclusion of endocrinologic causes by measurement of prolactin and thyrotropin levels.

- Infertility may be due to female or male factors or both; the cause is often elusive.

- Components of the work-up of infertility include biochemical studies to evaluate ovulation, assessment of fallopian tube patency with hysterosalpingography, and exclusion of endocrinologic causes through appropriate testing.

MEDICAL ISSUES OF PREGNANCY

PRECONCEPTION COUNSELING

Good prenatal care is associated with improved pregnancy outcomes. A healthful diet, exercise, and avoidance of tobacco and illicit drugs potentially harmful to the embryo should be addressed. Additional recommendations include adequate folic acid supplementation before conception (to decrease the risk of neural tube defect). Alcohol abuse during pregnancy is the third leading cause of mental retardation. It is associated with early spontaneous abortion, placental abruption, and fetal alcohol syndrome. The greatest negative impact is at the time of conception through the first month of pregnancy.

Smoking is associated with low birth weight, perinatal death, infertility, spontaneous abortion, ectopic pregnancy, placenta previa and placental abruption, and subsequent sudden infant death syndrome. Caffeine intake of 1 to 2 cups of coffee or other caffeinated beverage daily is not associated with miscarriage or birth defects.

- Folic acid supplementation before conception reduces the risk of neural tube defects.

- Alcohol abuse during pregnancy is the third leading cause of mental retardation and is associated with early spontaneous abortion and placental abruption.

- Smoking is associated with low birth weight, perinatal death, infertility, spontaneous abortion, ectopic pregnancy, placenta previa and placental abruption, and sudden infant death syndrome.

IMMUNIZATIONS AND PREGNANCY

Live vaccines should be avoided during pregnancy, but certain inactivated vaccines should be routinely administered during pregnancy, such as tetanus toxoid and the inactivated influenza vaccine (Box 52.3).

HYPERTENSION AND PREGNANCY

Hypertension complicates up to 10% of pregnancies and is an important cause of maternal and fetal morbidity and death. Hypertension may precede pregnancy or develop during pregnancy. The topics of hypertension during pregnancy and nursing are covered in Chapter 8, "Hypertension."

THROMBOEMBOLIC DISEASE AND PREGNANCY

Pregnancy creates a thrombogenic state, yet thromboembolism is uncommon during pregnancy. Women with hereditary thrombophilias are at high risk for thrombosis during pregnancy, with potentially serious complications. Women with antiphospholipid antibodies are prone to arterial or venous thromboembolism, placental infarction, recurrent pregnancy loss, preeclampsia, fetal growth retardation, or fetal death.

Low-molecular-weight heparin is the preferred treatment for thromboembolism during pregnancy or for prevention in high-risk women. Warfarin is teratogenic and increases the risk for spontaneous abortion and should be avoided during pregnancy. Aspirin is recommended before conception for women with antiphospholipid antibodies. After conception, additional treatment with heparin, glucocorticoids, or other medications may be indicated.

Inactivated vaccines

Hepatitis A: Vaccinate if at high risk for disease

Hepatitis B: Vaccinate if at risk

Human papillomavirus: Not recommended during pregnancy. Before or after pregnancy, vaccinate through age 26 y

Influenza: Vaccinate with inactivated flu vaccine all women who will be pregnant during the influenza season. *Avoid administration of nasal flu vaccine (FluMist), a live attenuated viral vaccine, during pregnancy*

Meningococcus: Administer if indicated. Vaccine should be administered to women at increased risk, such as those who are asplenic due to terminal complement component deficiencies, first-year college students living in a dormitory, military recruits & persons traveling to countries in which meningococcal disease is hyperendemic

Pneumococcus: Administer if indicated. Vaccine should be administered to women at increased risk, such as those who are asplenic and those with diabetes mellitus, cardiopulmonary or chronic kidney disease, or chronic liver disease

Toxoid vaccines

Td and Td plus acellular pertussis (Tdap): If last Td vaccination was ≥10 y previously, administer Td during second or third trimester. If last Td vaccination was <10 y previously, administer Tdap during immediate postpartum period. Acellular pertussis component of Tdap is safe in pregnancy

Live attenuated vaccines: Avoid during pregnancy

Influenza nasal vaccine (FluMist)

MMR: Avoid conception for 4 wk after MMR vaccination

Varicella: Avoid conception for 4 wk after varicella vaccination

Abbreviations: MMR, measles, mumps, & rubella; Td, tetanus/diphtheria.

- Women with thrombophilias are at increased risk for pregnancy-related thromboembolism.

- Low-molecular-weight heparin is the preferred treatment or prophylaxis for thromboembolism during pregnancy.

- Warfarin should be avoided because of its teratogenicity and risk for spontaneous abortion.

THYROID DISORDERS AND PREGNANCY

Maternal hypothyroidism is associated with infertility, miscarriage, stillbirth, placental abruption, preeclampsia, and motor and mental retardation in the infant. Thyrotropin should be measured early in pregnancy, and women taking thyroid hormone should be monitored regularly. About 20% require a dose increase. Thyrotropin levels are useful for detecting hypothyroidism or for monitoring thyroid hormone replacement.

Hyperthyroidism is the second most common endocrine disorder during pregnancy (after diabetes mellitus), but it occurs in only about 0.2% of pregnancies. Symptoms and signs may overlap with normal findings in pregnancy, and low weight gain may be the only clue. Poorly controlled hyperthyroidism may lead to spontaneous abortion, premature delivery, low birth weight, preeclampsia, and congestive heart failure. Propylthiouracil is the treatment of choice to prevent fetal goiter and hypothyroidism. In many women, the dose of propylthiouracil can be tapered or discontinued in the last trimester. Radioiodine is absolutely contraindicated during pregnancy and lactation. Surgery is sometimes necessary for gestational hyperthyroidism, but it should not be considered unless hyperthyroidism is refractory to medical therapy.

- Hypothyroidism during pregnancy poses risks to both mother and fetus.

- Inappropriately low weight gain should prompt thyroid evaluation.

- For poorly controlled hyperthyroidism, propylthiouracil is the treatment of choice.

- Radioiodine is absolutely contraindicated during pregnancy and lactation.

Postpartum thyroid dysfunction occurs in up to 10% of women during the year after delivery, mostly in women with goiters. Transient hyperthyroidism followed by hypothyroidism is typical. Hypothyroidism is often temporary, warranting thyroid hormone replacement for just several months.

- Postpartum thyroid dysfunction occurs in up to 10% of women within 1 year of delivery.

DISEASES OF THE UTERUS AND ADNEXA

ENDOMETRIOSIS

Endometriosis is defined as the presence of endometrial glands and stroma outside the endometrial cavity and uterine wall. The most common sites (decreasing frequency) are the ovaries, cul-de-sac, broad and uterosacral ligaments, uterus, fallopian tubes, sigmoid colon, appendix, and round ligaments. The most common symptom is pain, which may manifest as pelvic pain, chronic dyspareunia or dysmenorrhea, or cyclical bowel symptoms. Endometriosis is found in 20% to 40% of women with infertility and in up to 65% of women with chronic pelvic pain. Physical examination findings may be normal; localized tenderness in the cul-de-sac or uterosacral ligaments suggests endometriosis. Definitive diagnosis requires direct visualization and biopsy of endometriotic implants, ideally through laparoscopy. Imaging is rarely helpful for establishing the diagnosis or determining the disease extent. Blood cancer antigen 125 (CA 125) levels are often increased, but they should not be measured in this setting.

- Endometriosis is the presence of endometrial glands and stroma in non-endometrial sites (eg, ovaries, cul-de-sac, fallopian tubes, and colon).

- Pain is the most common symptom.

- Affected women may be infertile.

Table 52.2 TREATMENT OPTIONS FOR ENDOMETRIOSIS

SYMPTOM	TREATMENT OPTIONS	IMPACT ON ENDOMETRIOTIC IMPLANTS	ADVERSE EFFECTS
Mild pelvic pain	Analgesics (eg, NSAIDs)	Does not reduce endometriotic implants	Minimal
	Oral contraceptives	Evidence conflicts on whether therapy reduces implant size or inhibits progression of disease	Minimal
Moderate to severe pain Pain that does not respond to analgesics or oral contraceptives	GnRH agonist (eg, leuprolide, nafarelin, goserelin)	Reduces size of endometriotic implants	Menopausal symptoms, bone loss FDA approval for no more than 6 mo of continuous use Combination with progestins or low-dose estrogen-progestin therapy minimizes adverse effects & allows prolonged use
	Progestins (oral or depot medroxyprogesterone acetate)	Evidence unclear as to effect on implant size or inhibition of disease progression	Weight gain, irregular uterine bleeding, mood changes
	Danazol	Reduces size of endometriotic implants	Weight gain, muscle cramps, decreased breast size, acne, hirsutism, lipid changes, hot flushes, mood changes
Severe pain Pain unresponsive to medical management Advanced disease Large or symptomatic endometrioma	Surgery	Reduces size of endometriotic implants & adhesions	May lead to development of postsurgical adhesions

Abbreviations: FDA, US Food and Drug Administration; GnRH, gonadotropin-releasing hormone; NSAID, nonsteroidal anti-inflammatory drug.

- Direct visualization and biopsy are required for definitive diagnosis.

- Imaging is rarely helpful, and the level of CA 125 should not be measured.

Treatment is directed at symptom relief and may include medical or surgical therapy, or both (Table 52.2). Treatment choice depends on symptom severity, disease extent and location, desire for pregnancy, age of the patient, and response to prior therapies. A stepwise approach is usual. Empiric medical therapy with a nonsteroidal anti-inflammatory drug or oral contraceptive is reasonable in patients suspected to have endometriosis when other causes of pelvic pain have been excluded. If this therapy fails, in severe cases a diagnostic laparoscopy is often done. If endometriosis is confirmed, ablation and excision of endometriotic implants and adhesions can be performed. If pain persists, a trial of hormonal therapy with gonadotropin-releasing hormone agonists, danazol, or progestins should be used. There is no definite evidence that any one medical agent is superior for pain control. Oral contraceptive or other medical therapies may be used after surgery to maintain remission or in unresectable disease. Surgical therapy is reserved for severe symptoms, lack of response to medical management, or advanced disease. Conservative surgical therapy is usually attempted, with removal of the endometriotic implants and adhesions and preservation of the uterus and ovaries. Definitive surgical therapy involves hysterectomy and oophorectomy. The surgical approach depends on the severity of symptoms, the age of the patient, and the desire for fertility.

- Nonsteroidal anti-inflammatory drugs or oral contraceptives are used first for treatment of endometriosis, and progestins or danazol is used in more refractory cases.

- Conservative therapy is used first, moving to definitive surgery for the most severe, refractory cases.

UTERINE FIBROIDS

Uterine leiomyomas (fibroids or myomas) are benign monoclonal tumors that arise from the smooth muscle of the myometrium. There are 3 primary types: submucosal, intramural (most common), and subserosal. They are the most common female pelvic tumors, occurring in 50% to 80% of women. They are most prevalent during the reproductive years and usually regress after menopause. Approximately 25% of fibroids are symptomatic. The degree and type of symptoms depend on the number, size, and location of the fibroids. Fibroid-related symptoms are grouped into 3 categories: menstrual symptoms (eg, dysmenorrhea and menorrhagia), bulk-related symptoms (eg, pelvic pain, pelvic pressure, urinary frequency, constipation, and dyspareunia), and reproductive dysfunction (eg, recurrent miscarriage and obstetric complications). Fibroids that distort the endometrial cavity (primarily submucosal) increase infertility and risk for miscarriage. Large fibroids may increase the risk for premature labor, and a fibroid under the placenta increases the risk for placental abruption. Late menarche and increased parity are associated with a reduced risk for fibroids. The relative risk for fibroids is twofold to threefold greater in black women than in white women.

- Fibroids are the most common female pelvic tumor and are benign; most are asymptomatic.

- Fibroids are more common in black women than in white women and in women with early menarche and reduced parity.

An enlarged, irregularly shaped, firm, nontender uterus on pelvic examination suggests fibroids. Fibroids are often incidentally found on pelvic ultrasonography. Imaging should be done if the diagnosis is uncertain, especially if the adnexa cannot be palpated separately from the suspected fibroid. The most widely used imaging technique is transvaginal ultrasonography, which has high sensitivity for fibroids. Sonographically, they are symmetric, well-defined, hypoechoic, heterogeneous masses. Hysteroscopy may be used, particularly if myomectomy is planned. Magnetic resonance imaging provides very accurate imaging but is rarely used. It can be used to differentiate fibroids from other conditions (eg, adenomyosis) and to predict the outcome of uterine artery embolization. Annual pelvic examination should be done; further evaluation is warranted if symptoms change or uterine size increases. Consider a complete blood cell count in patients with prior anemia or menorrhagia. Routine surveillance imaging is not recommended.

- Clinically significant fibroids are identified on pelvic examination by finding an enlarged, irregular, firm, nontender uterus.

- Ultrasonographic features are well understood; magnetic resonance imaging is usually unnecessary, but it may be helpful if other conditions are possible or uterine artery embolization is being planned.

Treatment of fibroids is necessary only if they are symptomatic. Abnormal uterine bleeding is the most common symptom, typically causing prolonged or heavy menstruation but not intermenstrual bleeding. The bleeding pattern is primarily influenced by location of the fibroid; submucosal fibroids are more likely to cause heavy bleeding. A trial of medical therapy before surgical therapy is appropriate for symptomatic fibroids (anemia, heavy bleeding, or pain). Gonadotropin-releasing hormone agonists (eg, leuprolide) cause amenorrhea and reduce uterine size in most cases. They are used to reduce blood loss before definitive surgery, to reduce uterine size to allow less invasive surgical approach (vaginal or laparoscopic vs laparotomy), or as therapy for women approaching menopause who are expected to require no more than 6 months of treatment. Adverse effects, including reduced bone density, preclude long-term use. Pretreatment bleeding patterns and uterine size usually return rapidly after cessation of treatment. The role of oral contraceptives and progestins in the treatment of fibroids is controversial. In some women, these agents reduce menstrual bleeding and may inhibit formation of new fibroids; they do not reduce bulk-related symptoms. The levonorgestrel intrauterine device may also be effective for reducing menstrual blood loss and uterine size.

- Treatment of fibroids is reserved for those that are symptomatic.

- Medical therapy includes gonadotropin-releasing hormone agonists.

Surgical treatment of fibroids is indicated when symptoms persist despite medical treatment, when infertility or recurrent pregnancy loss is related to fibroids, or when malignancy is suspected. Surgery should be considered in a postmenopausal woman with a new or enlarging pelvic mass and pelvic pain and to exclude uterine sarcoma. Other risk factors for uterine sarcoma include prior pelvic irradiation, tamoxifen use, or the rare syndrome of hereditary leiomyomatosis and renal cell carcinoma.

Surgical options include myomectomy (if there is no suspicion of malignancy) or hysterectomy. Myomectomy involves removal of the myomas with uterine conservation and preserves childbearing potential. Disadvantages include high risk for new fibroid formation (about 50% at 5 years) and increased risk for uterine rupture in pregnancy. Less invasive options in women who have completed childbearing and in whom there is no suspicion of malignancy include endometrial ablation, myolysis (laparoscopic thermal coagulation or cryoablation of fibroids), uterine artery embolization, and magnetic resonance–guided focused ultrasound ablation.

- Surgery is indicated in symptomatic cases of fibroids refractory to medical therapy.

- Myomectomy preserves childbearing potential, whereas other less invasive options (eg, endometrial ablation, myolysis, uterine artery embolization, and magnetic resonance–guided ultrasound ablation) do not; such options are appropriate only when malignancy is not suspected.

ENDOMETRIAL CANCER

Endometrial cancer is the most common gynecologic malignancy in the United States. The incidence increases with age; average age at diagnosis is 60 years. Most cases (75%) occur in postmenopausal women. Fewer than 5% of cases occur in women before age 40 years. Most cases are due to excess estrogen stimulation without adequate progestin exposure. Box 52.4 lists other risk factors for endometrial cancer, including increasing age, nulliparity, chronic anovulation, late menopause, obesity, diabetes mellitus, and tamoxifen therapy.

The main genetic association is hereditary nonpolyposis colorectal cancer (Lynch syndrome II). Women with Lynch syndrome II have a lifetime risk for endometrial cancer of 27% to 71% and should undergo surveillance for this cancer and

Box 52.4 **FACTORS THAT AFFECT THE RISK OF ENDOMETRIAL CANCER**

Risk factors
    Increasing age
    Obesity
    Unopposed estrogen therapy
    Nulliparity
    Chronic anovulation (including polycystic ovary syndrome)
    Early menarche
    Late menopause
    Obesity
    Diabetes mellitus
    Hypertension
    Tamoxifen use
    First-degree relative with endometrial cancer
    Hereditary nonpolyposis colorectal cancer (Lynch syndrome II)
Protective factors
    Combination oral contraceptive therapy
    Smoking

for colorectal cancer or consider preventive surgery. In other populations, screening for uterine cancer in asymptomatic women is not warranted.

- Endometrial cancer is the most common gynecologic malignancy, and the majority of cases occur in postmenopausal women.
- Hereditary nonpolyposis colorectal cancer (Lynch syndrome II) is associated with a considerable lifetime risk of endometrial cancer, and affected women should undergo surveillance ultrasonography or preventive surgery once childbearing is complete.

The most common endometrial cancer is endometrioid adenocarcinoma. Clear cell and serous carcinomas are rarer and more aggressive. The classic symptom is abnormal uterine bleeding, occurring in 90% of cases. Endometrial cancer must be excluded in any postmenopausal woman with uterine bleeding (with the exception of predictable bleeding related to hormone therapy). Although atypical glandular cells on Papanicolaou smear are often due to benign conditions, underlying neoplasia in 9% to 38% of such women (including adenocarcinoma of the endometrium, cervix, ovary, and fallopian tube) may be identified, and evaluation should include colposcopy, endocervical sampling, testing for human papillomavirus, and endometrial assessment.

- Any postmenopausal woman with uterine bleeding not associated with hormone therapy should be evaluated for endometrial cancer.
- Although atypical glandular cells on Papanicolaou smear are usually due to benign conditions, underlying neoplasia and endometrial evaluation must be considered.

The initial diagnostic test to exclude endometrial cancer is endometrial biopsy. Alternatives include hysteroscopy with dilation and curettage or hysteroscopy with directed biopsy and curettage. Transvaginal ultrasonography is an acceptable initial step for postmenopausal women with uterine bleeding who cannot tolerate an endometrial biopsy or women for whom imaging of the adnexa is needed. In postmenopausal women, an endometrial thickness of less than 4 to 5 mm is associated with a low risk of endometrial disease; a thicker lining should prompt endometrial biopsy or hysteroscopy with dilation and curettage. Diffuse or focal increased echotexture or inadequate visualization of the endometrium on ultrasonography or persistent unexplained bleeding should also prompt hysteroscopy or endometrial biopsy. Transvaginal ultrasonography alone cannot exclude endometrial cancer in premenopausal women with abnormal uterine bleeding, given the cyclic variability in the thickness of the endometrium.

- Endometrial biopsy is used to exclude endometrial cancer.

ADNEXAL MASSES

The adnexa are the ovaries and fallopian tubes (the term also includes the uterine ligaments). Most adnexal masses are benign and can occur at any age. Differential diagnosis and management depend on the patient's age and menstrual status. The differential diagnosis of an adnexal mass includes ovarian and extraovarian masses; see Box 52.5 for examples.

A physiologic ovarian cyst is the most common adnexal mass in a premenopausal woman. In this population, less than 20% of adnexal masses are malignant. Ectopic pregnancy must

Box 52.5 **DIFFERENTIAL DIAGNOSIS OF ADNEXAL MASS**

Ovarian mass
    Physiologic cyst, simple or hemorrhagic
        Follicular
        Corpus luteum
    Polycystic ovary syndrome
    Benign ovarian neoplasm
    Leiomyoma (fibroid)
    Endometrioma
    Dermoid cyst (cystic teratoma); most common ovarian tumor in women in their second & third decades
    Cystadenoma
    Metatstatic carcinoma (ie, colon, endometrium, breast); non-Hodgkin lymphoma
    Ovarian carcinoma
Extraovarian mass
    Ectopic pregnancy
    Tubo-ovarian abscess
    Paraovarian cyst
    Peritoneal inclusion cyst
    Diverticular abscess
    Cancer of the fallopian tube

be excluded when a reproductive-age woman presents with an adnexal mass. In women 50 years or older, more than 30% of adnexal masses are malignant. In postmenopausal women, any solid enlargement of an ovary must be considered malignant until proved otherwise. Adnexal abnormalities, including masses, may cause pain. Associated features may help in diagnosis. Midcycle pain in premenopausal women suggests a follicular or corpus luteum cyst. Pain during or after intercourse may be related to a ruptured cyst. Ovarian torsion is suggested by sudden-onset severe pain, often with fever, nausea, and vomiting. Pelvic pain with fever may also be due to pelvic inflammatory disease, but appendicitis and diverticulitis should be considered. A tubo-ovarian abscess is most common in the setting of pelvic inflammatory disease but may develop after pelvic surgery or as a complication of appendicitis or diverticulitis. It usually presents with abdominal and pelvic pain, usually with fever and leukocytosis. Patients with ovarian cancer often present with vague symptoms (eg, back or pelvic pain, fatigue, gastrointestinal or urinary symptoms); most cases are diagnosed at late stage.

- Physiologic ovarian cysts are the most common adnexal masses in premenopausal women.

- Ectopic pregnancy must be excluded in a reproductive-age woman with an adnexal mass.

- Less than 20% of adnexal masses in premenopausal women are malignant, but more than 30% of adnexal masses in women ≥50 years are malignant.

- Malignancy must be excluded in any postmenopausal women with solid ovarian enlargement.

- Pain is a feature of various adnexal abnormalities, including masses; other features can help in the differential diagnosis.

Pelvic ultrasonography distinguishes cysts from solid adnexal lesions. Transvaginal ultrasonography better visualizes pelvic structures, and transabdominal ultrasonography better visualizes abdominal structures. Worrisome ultrasonographic features include septations, mural or septal nodules, thickened or irregular walls, and partially solid or solid masses.

Follicular and corpus luteum cysts are typically solitary, thin-walled, unilocular, and less than 10 cm in diameter. They may be associated with hemorrhage. In the premenopausal woman, a cyst that is less than 10 cm with no solid component can be reevaluated sonographically after several menstrual cycles. Approximately 70% resolve spontaneously. If the cyst is unchanged or larger, surgery should be considered. Oral contraceptives can prevent new cyst formation. Consider surgical exploration for cysts 10 cm or more (premenopausal women) and solid, fixed, or bilateral masses. Surgery should also be considered in women with ascites, symptoms suspicious for metastatic disease, or a family history of breast or ovarian cancer in a first-degree relative (potentially worrisome for *BRCA* mutation).

- A cyst <10 cm without suspicious features in a premenopausal woman can be reevaluated sonographically after several menstrual cycles; the majority spontaneously resolve.

- Surgical exploration should be considered for cysts ≥10 cm or with suspicious features.

Benign ovarian cysts may also occur in postmenopausal women, but the risk of ovarian cancer is higher. A simple unilocular cyst less than 5 cm on ultrasonography can be observed with serial ultrasonography and determination of serum CA 125 levels at 3-month intervals for 1 year. Most cysts resolve spontaneously within 1 year. Surgery should be considered for complex cysts, cysts 5 cm or more, or symptomatic adnexal masses. Surgery should also be considered in postmenopausal women with an adnexal mass and an increased serum CA 125 level, suspicion of metastatic disease, ascites, or a family history of breast or ovarian cancer in a first-degree relative (concerning for a *BRCA* mutation).

- Postmenopausal women may also have benign ovarian cysts, but the risk of malignancy is higher.

- Cysts <5 cm without suspicious features in postmenopausal women can be followed serially and usually resolve within 1 year.

- Surgery should be considered for ovarian cysts with any suspicious feature.

BRCA mutations are uncommon but are associated with increased risk for ovarian cancer. Other risk factors include early menarche and late menopause, white race, late parity, and prolonged hormone therapy. Protective factors include oral contraceptive use, early menopause, multiparity, tubal ligation, and breastfeeding.

The serum CA 125 level may be helpful in the evaluation of a suspicious adnexal mass, but it is not sufficient to establish or exclude a diagnosis of ovarian cancer and may result in false-positive or false-negative results. False-positive results may be due to endometriomas, uterine fibroids, pelvic inflammatory disease, nonadnexal malignancies, and gastrointestinal causes. The specificity is low in premenopausal women. However, in a postmenopausal woman, the combination of a suspicious finding on pelvic ultrasonography and an increased CA 125 level is highly specific and sensitive for ovarian cancer in postmenopausal women. The CA 125 test should not be used to screen for ovarian cancer in the general population. However, in women with a known *BRCA1* or *BRCA2* mutation, screening with transvaginal ultrasonography and serum CA 125 testing is appropriate because of the significant lifetime risk of ovarian cancer. The CA 125 level is most useful for surveillance in women with a diagnosis of ovarian cancer, particularly when the level was increased at the time of diagnosis.

- An increased serum CA 125 value is not sufficient to establish or exclude ovarian cancer.

- False-positives and false-negative findings lead to diagnostic errors.

- A suspicious result on pelvic ultrasonography and an increased CA 125 level are highly specific and sensitive for ovarian carcinoma in postmenopausal women.

- The only populations in whom CA 125 screening should be routinely undertaken are in women with known *BRCA* mutations or women with an established diagnosis of ovarian cancer.

CERVICAL CANCER SCREENING

Cervical cytologic screening has resulted in a decline of more than 50% in the incidence of cervical cancer in the past 3 decades. Approximately half of women in whom cervical cancer is diagnosed annually have not previously undergone cervical cytologic testing. High-risk human papillomavirus (HPV) subtype infection is necessary, but not sufficient, for development of squamous cervical neoplasia, including malignancy. In most HPV-infected women, cervical abnormalities of clinical significance will not develop. Although the virus is easily sexually transmitted, the immune response usually clears the infection or reduces viral load to undetectable levels 8 to 24 months after exposure. Infection and HPV-related cervical dysplasia are most common in young women (teens and early 20s), but they typically resolve spontaneously. Older women are more likely to have persistent infection, which correlates with increasing high-risk dysplasia with increasing age.

- High-risk HPV subtype infection is necessary, but insufficient, for cervical neoplasia.

- The immune system usually clears or sufficiently reduces the viral load within 2 years of exposure.

- HPV is sexually transmitted.

- Young women are most commonly infected, but infection and cervical dysplasia usually clear spontaneously in this group.

Liquid-based and conventional cervical cytologic methods are acceptable for screening, but conventional methods require avoidance of blood, discharge, and lubricant for accurate test results. The liquid-based method is more convenient, and gonorrhea and *Chlamydia* testing can be performed using the same preparation. However, it is more expensive and has decreased cytologic specificity.

- Both liquid-based and conventional cytologic methods are acceptable.

- Conventional methods have greater specificity.

In average-risk women, cervical cancer screening should begin at age 21 years (regardless of age of first sexual intercourse). Invasive cervical cancer is rare in women younger than 21 years (0.1% of cases). Screening at ages younger than 21 years is associated with more adverse effects from follow-up and unnecessary treatment. Although cervical dysplasia is common in women younger than 21 years, it rarely progresses to invasive cancer, and excisional treatment is associated with more subsequent premature births. The optimal frequency of cervical cytologic testing is every 2 years for women aged 21 to 29 years. Women aged 30 years or older with 3 prior normal cytologic results should undergo testing every 3 years. The rate of dysplasia decreases with increasing sequential negative testing. In the absence of high-risk factors, testing can be discontinued at age 65 to 70 years. Peak incidence of cervical cancer is during the fifth decade of life in white women, in the early 70s in Hispanic women, and in the late 70s in Asian-Pacific Islander women. The incidence increases during the lifespan of African American women. After total hysterectomy for benign indications and no prior high-risk cytologic findings, cervical cytologic testing can be discontinued (Obstet Gynecol. 2009 Dec;114[6]:1409–20).

- Begin cervical cytologic testing at age 21 years.

- Women 30 years or older without high-risk factors and with 3 consecutive normal test results should be tested every 3 years.

- In the absence of high-risk factors and with 3 consecutive normal results, discontinue testing at age 65–70 years.

- The incidence of cervical cancer varies among different ethnic populations.

- Cervical cytologic testing is not indicated after hysterectomy for benign indications in women without prior high-risk cytologic findings.

High-risk groups may require more frequent screening. These groups include women with human immunodeficiency virus (HIV) infection, women who are immunosuppressed (eg, transplant patients), women with in utero exposure to diethylstilbestrol, and women who have had treatment for high-grade intraepithelial lesions (J Low Genit Tract Dis. 2007 Oct;11[4]:223–39).

- High-risk groups may require testing more often than every 3 years.

Additional evaluation and treatment based on cervical cytologic findings depend on the abnormality (Table 52.3). As severity of dysplasia increases, likelihood of progression to cancer increases and time of progression decreases.

High-risk subtype HPV testing stratifies risk in women 21 years or older with atypical squamous cells of undetermined significance and postmenopausal women with a low-grade squamous intraepithelial lesion and is an adjunct to cervical cytologic testing in women 30 years or older. However, in premenopausal women with low-grade squamous intraepithelial neoplasia, HPV testing has very low specificity and should not be used to triage women to colposcopy. HPV testing is not recommended in women younger than 21 years; if done, results should not influence management. HPV testing has little utility when cytologic results show high-grade

CERVICAL CYTOLOGIC FINDING	SIGNIFICANCE	MANAGEMENT
ASC-US	Insufficient atypia to warrant squamous intraepithelial lesion designation	If HPV-negative, follow-up cytology in 12 mo *or* repeat cytology in 6 & 12 mo *or* colposcopy (not best first step) If HPV-positive, management is same as LSIL and consider colposcopy
ASC-H	Cytologic changes suggest but are insufficient to identify HSIL	Colposcopy; if no CIN 2, 3, then repeat cytology at 6 & 12 mo *or* HPV testing at 12 mo. If CIN 2, 3, see HSIL
LSIL	Indicator of probable HPV infection Prevalence of CIN 2 or higher >10%	Colposcopy; if no lesion or unsatisfactory, endocervical biopsy is preferred; with satisfactory colposcopy and lesion identified, biopsy is preferred. If no CIN 2 or 3, repeat cytology at 6 & 12 mo *or* HPV testing at 12 mo; if ASC or higher or HPV-positive, perform colposcopy; if normal, resume routine screening; if CIN 2 or 3, see HSIL
HSIL	High risk for significant cervical disease. High incidence of HPV positivity; therefore, cannot triage with HPV testing or cytology. Failure to detect CIN 2, 3 at colposcopy does not exclude the possibility	Loop electrosurgical excision or colposcopy with endocervical biopsy. If no CIN 2, 3, then colposcopy & cytology at 6 & 12 mo *or* diagnostic excision
AGC	Uncommon and usually benign; may be associated with adenocarcinoma of the cervix, endometrium, ovary, or fallopian tube	Colposcopy with endocervical biopsy. HPV testing *or* repeat cervical cytology every 6 mo until 4 consecutive normal results. If HPV-negative, repeat cytology at 12 mo; if HPV-positive, repeat cytology at 6 mo
CIN 1	Low risk for progression; usually spontaneously regresses	Repeat cytology at 6 & 12 mo *or* HPV testing. If cytology or HPV test negative, resume screening. If findings are greater than ASC or are HPV-positive, perform colposcopy
CIN 2, 3	CIN 2 has a higher likelihood to progress to CIN 3 but often regresses; CIN 3 is a cancer precursor	Colposcopy with excision or ablation then follow-up with cytology *or* cytology & colposcopy *or* HPV testing. If initial colposcopy is unsatisfactory *or* if recurrent CIN 2, 3, then diagnostic excision & follow-up with HPV *or* cytology with or without colposcopy

Abbreviations: AGC, atypical glandular cells (more likely associated with squamous and glandular abnormalities than ASC-US); ASC-H, atypical squamous cells, cannot exclude HSIL; ASC-US, atypical squamous cells, undetermined significance; CIN, cervical intraepithelial neoplasia (CIN 2 more likely to progress to CIN 3 and cancer than CIN 1, but often regresses spontaneously); HPV, human papillomavirus; HSIL, high-risk squamous intraepithelial lesion (includes moderate-severe dysplasia, CIN 2 & 3, & carcinoma in situ); LSIL, low-risk squamous intraepithelial lesion (includes low-grade dysplasia, HPV, & CIN 1).

intraepithelial lesion because results are expected to be positive in this group.

The combination of negative results of high-risk HPV testing and normal cervical cytologic results in women older than 30 years indicates a very low risk for development of a high-grade squamous intraepithelial lesion in the next 4 to 6 years; thus, cervical cytologic testing should not be done sooner than 3 years. Combination testing increases sensitivity but also decreases specificity and increases cost.

- Use of HPV results to triage to colposcopy depends on the population.

- HPV testing should not be done in women <21 years old.

- HPV test results are not useful when high-grade squamous intraepithelial lesion is the cervical cytologic result.

- Negative HPV test results and normal cytologic results in women >30 years old indicate low risk for development of a high-grade squamous intraepithelial lesion; repeat cytologic testing no sooner than 3 years.

Women previously treated for high-grade squamous intraepithelial lesion (cervical intraepithelial neoplasia 2 or 3) or cervical cancer remain at increased risk for at least 20 years after treatment, and initial posttreatment surveillance and annual cytologic screening should be done for at least 20 years.

- Women at high risk after treatment (high-grade squamous intraepithelial lesion or cervical cancer) remain at high risk of recurrence or residual disease for at least 20 years and should be followed annually.

VULVAR SKIN DISORDERS

Vulvar itching, burning, and pain are common genital symptoms. Symptoms may be acute or chronic, and skin changes may be visible; these features guide differential diagnosis (Box 52.6). Common causes of *acute* vulvar pruritus are vulvovaginal candidiasis and contact dermatitis. Causes of *chronic* vulvar pruritus include lichen sclerosus, lichen simplex chronicus, neoplastic conditions such as vulvar intraepithelial

Box 52.6 CONDITIONS COMMONLY ASSOCIATED
WITH VULVAR ITCHING

Acute
    Contact dermatitis
    Infections: fungal, trichomoniasis, molluscum, scabies
Chronic
    Dermatoses: contact dermatitis, lichen sclerosus, lichen planus,
        lichen simplex chronicus, psoriasis, genital atrophy
    Neoplasia: vulvar intraepithelial neoplasia, vulvar cancer, Paget
        disease
    Vulvar manifestations of systemic disease: eg, Crohn disease

Adapted from ACOG Practice Bulletin No. 93: diagnosis and management of
vulvar skin disorders. Obstet Gynecol. 2008 May;111(5):1243–53. Used with
permission.

neoplasia, squamous cell carcinoma, and Paget disease of the
vulva. Other causes are vulvar manifestations of systemic disease, such as Crohn disease. Vulvodynia is associated with
burning, stinging, rawness, or soreness, with or without pruritus. Typically, there are no visible vulvar skin changes and
pain mapping with cotton swab testing at the vaginal opening
is positive. Vulvar contact dermatitis may be acute (blisters,
itching, and weeping) or chronic (redness, burning, and swelling). Physical findings range from mild erythema and scaling
to intense erythema, fissures, erosions, and ulcers. Candidiasis
should be ruled out. Treatment is removal of the offending
irritant or allergen.

- Vulvar itching, burning, and pain are common and may be
  due to a wide variety of acute or chronic causes.

- Neoplastic conditions should be considered in the
  evaluation of chronic vulvar symptoms.

- Treatment of vulvar contact dermatitis is removal of the
  offending agent.

- Candidiasis should be excluded.

Vulvar lichen simplex chronicus may present with persistent intense itching, typically with scaling and lichenified
plaques that result from chronic rubbing or scratching. If the
condition is long-standing, vulvar skin may appear thickened
and leathery, with areas of hyperpigmentation or hypopig-
mentation. Consider eczema, psoriasis, atopic dermatitis, or
neurodermatitis.

- Not a primary skin disorder, vulvar lichen simplex
  chronicus is typically due to another (nongynecologic)
  condition.

Lichen sclerosus has the following features: thinned, whit-
ened, and crinkling skin; porcelain-white papules and plaques;
areas of ecchymoses or purpura; and possible agglutination of
tissues with fusion of the labia minora and phimosis of the
clitoral hood. The classic distribution is a figure-of-eight or
hourglass shape with perianal involvement. Biopsy should be

done to confirm the diagnosis before initiation of topical corticosteroids (typically clobetasol).

- Vulvar skin findings are often considerable and have a
  classic distribution, including perianal involvement.

- Biopsy before initiation of corticosteroid therapy to
  exclude malignancy.

Lichen planus is an inflammatory disorder with mucous
membrane findings ranging from white reticulate or
lacy-fernlike striae to deep, painful, erythematous erosions
and scarring resulting in obliteration of the vagina. The typical
findings are white, irregular lines and deep, painful erosions. In
erosive lichen planus, deep, painful, red erosions may be seen
at the posterior vestibule, often extending to the labia minora
and even extending into the vaginal epithelium. Treatment
options include topical and systemic corticosteroid, topical
and oral cyclosporine, topical tacrolimus, hydroxycholoro-
quine, methotrexate, azathioprine, and cyclophosphamide.
Lichen planus is chronic and tends to be treatment-resistant.

- An inflammatory disorder, lichen planus may cause
  considerable tissue changes.

- Multiple treatment options exist, but the condition is often
  refractory to therapy.

The common symptoms of vulvovaginal atrophy are vulvar
irritation and dryness. On examination, there is loss of labial
and vulvar fullness, pallor of urethral and vaginal mucosa, and
dryness. Diagnosis is based on the classic appearance and is
confirmed by an increased vaginal pH (6.0–7.5). Treatment is
with topical estrogen (cream, tablet, or vaginal ring).

- Vulvovaginal atrophy, due to estrogen depletion,
  commonly causes vulvar irritation and vaginal and vulvar
  dryness.

- The examination findings are fairly stereotypical, and
  treatment is with topical estrogen.

PERIMENOPAUSE

Perimenopause typically lasts several years and is characterized by erratic hormone levels and irregular menstrual periods.
Symptoms such as hot flushes, vaginal dryness, and sleep disturbances are common. Anovulatory cycles are common and
contribute to irregular menstrual bleeding. Despite reduced
fertility, pregnancy is possible until menopause is reached
(either 12 months of no menstrual periods or FSH levels consistently >30 mIU/mL).

Menstrual changes may include lighter or heavier bleeding, irregular bleeding duration, or skipped menstrual periods.
Certain patterns of bleeding warrant further evaluation: very
heavy flow, especially with clots; menstrual bleeding lasting
more than 7 days; bleeding intervals less than 21 days; intermenstrual spotting or bleeding; and postcoital bleeding.

- Perimenopause often lasts several years and is characterized by menstrual irregularity and symptoms including hot flushes, vaginal dryness, and sleep disturbance.
- Very heavy bleeding (especially with clots), more than 7 days of menstrual bleeding, intermenstrual bleeding, and postcoital bleeding warrant further evaluation to exclude an underlying abnormality, even in perimenopausal women.

Hormonal contraceptives may be useful for menstrual regulation, dysmenorrhea, menorrhagia, and hot flushes. Oral contraceptives are preferred over menopausal estrogen-progestogen therapy for treatment of hot flushes because postmenopausal hormone therapy does not suppress endogenous ovarian function and unscheduled vaginal bleeding is common.

The decision about when to stop use of oral contraceptives or switch to postmenopausal hormone therapy is not straightforward. Clinical signs of menopause are masked by use of hormonal contraceptives. FSH levels are labile in perimenopause, and unless they are consistently increased to more than 30 mIU/mL, menopause is not confirmed. Hormonal contraceptives may lower FSH levels, confounding interpretation. Measuring the FSH level on the seventh pill-free day is not sensitive for confirming menopause. FSH testing after a contraceptive pill-free interval of 1 to 2 months, while using alternative contraception, can help to establish menopause, if needed.

- Hormonal contraceptives may be useful for many perimenopausal symptoms.
- Postmenopausal hormone therapy is not sufficient to suppress ovarian function, and women may have unscheduled bleeding.
- Hormonal contraceptives mask signs of menopause.
- FSH levels are often unreliable for evaluation of menopause status because of labile levels during perimenopause; hormonal contraceptives may confound interpretation.

Terms related to menopause are defined in Box 52.7.

MENOPAUSE

Menopause is the permanent cessation of menses occurring when ovarian follicles are depleted. Natural menopause, a clinical diagnosis, is confirmed when a woman has no menses for 12 months and typically occurs between the ages of 42 and 58 years (average, 51 years). It often occurs earlier in smokers and nulliparous women. Menopause may also be induced by surgery, chemotherapy, or pelvic irradiation.

- Natural menopause, a clinical diagnosis, is confirmed when menses have not occurred for 12 months.
- Smoking and nulliparity often lead to earlier menopause.

Box 52.7 **MENOPAUSE-RELATED TERMS**

Natural/spontaneous menopause: the final menstrual period, confirmed after 12 consecutive mo of amenorrhea with no obvious pathologic cause

Induced menopause: permanent cessation of menstruation after bilateral oophorectomy or iatrogenic ablation of ovarian function

Perimenopause or menopausal transition: span of time when menstrual cycle changes & endocrine changes occur a few years before & 12 mo after the final menstrual period, resulting from natural menopause

Premature menopause: menopause reached at or before age 40 y

Premature ovarian failure: ovarian insufficiency occurring before age 40 y & leading to permanent or transient amenorrhea

Early menopause: natural or induced menopause occurring at or before age 45 y

---

- Surgery, chemotherapy, and pelvic irradiation are other possible causes of menopause.

The hallmark symptom of menopause is hot flushes or flashes (abrupt onset of warmth and red skin blotching involving the chest, face, and neck) often associated with transient anxiety, palpitations, and profuse sweating. Hot flushes and hot flashes are equivocal terms. Most menopausal women have hot flushes; 10% to 15% report that they are frequent or severe. Hot flushes often begin more than 2 years before menopause and usually peak within 2 to 3 years after menopause, but they continue in some women for many years after menopause. Frequency, duration, and intensity vary. Hot flushes coincide with declining estrogen levels, but they are not due to hypoestrogenism. The mechanism is attributed to dysfunction of the thermoregulatory center in the hypothalamus.

- Hot flushes are considered the hallmark of menopause and usually peak within 2–3 years.

Other postmenopausal symptoms include vaginal dryness and irritation, urinary urgency and frequency, dyspareunia, changes in sexual function, mood swings, and cognitive function changes. Menopausal symptoms tend to be more intense after surgically induced menopause than natural menopause.

When hot flushes occur in a healthy woman of typical menopausal age, no diagnostic testing is necessary. However, if the clinical scenario is atypical, testing for an increased FSH level may be helpful. In the setting of an atypical clinical scenario and normal premenopausal FSH and estradiol levels, other causes of hot flushes should be considered. These include thyroid dysfunction, infection, carcinoid syndrome, pheochromocytoma, autoimmune disorders, mast cell disorders, malignancies, and, rarely, seizure disorders.

- After menopause, any vaginal bleeding (with the exception of predictable bleeding associated with hormone therapy) is abnormal and needs diagnostic evaluation.

- In women presenting with hot flushes and a clinical scenario atypical for menopause, serum FSH and estradiol levels should be evaluated; in premenopausal women, consider nonmenopause-related causes of hot flushes.

POSTMENOPAUSAL BLEEDING

In postmenopausal women with bleeding not caused by vaginal or endometrial atrophy or cervical lesions, endometrial cancer must be ruled out, unless the patient is using cycling hormonal therapy. Endometrial cancer must be considered in the setting of any uterine bleeding in postmenopausal women (unless cyclic hormonal therapy is being used). Transvaginal ultrasonography or endometrial biopsy should be considered. If endometrial thickness is more than 4 mm on ultrasonography, there are other endometrial abnormalities (eg, a focal lesion), or bleeding is persistent, biopsy is indicated. Once malignancy is excluded, reassurance is usually sufficient.

- Postmenopausal bleeding requires evaluation to exclude malignancy.

- Transvaginal ultrasonography or endometrial biopsy should be considered for evaluation.

- Biopsy is indicated if transvaginal ultrasonography shows any abnormalities or if bleeding is persistent after normal findings on ultrasonography.

HORMONE THERAPY

Estrogen is the most effective treatment of hot flushes and other menopausal symptoms, but it is associated with potential risks (Box 52.8). Postmenopausal hormone therapy is appropriate only for women with moderate to severe symptoms of menopause interfering with quality of life or activities of daily living. It should be prescribed at the lowest dose that relieves symptoms and for the shortest duration needed for treatment goals. It is not indicated to treat osteopenia or osteoporosis in most women. In women with an intact uterus, unopposed estrogen increases the risk of uterine dysplasia and malignancy, and thus a cyclic progestogen must be used; women must be made aware that cyclic bleeding will occur in this setting.

- Systemic estrogen is the most effective therapy for menopausal symptoms but is associated with potential risks and is primarily indicated when symptoms are moderate to severe.

- The lowest dose of estrogen for the shortest duration to achieve symptom management is recommended.

- Systemic estrogen therapy is not indicated for management of osteopenia or osteoporosis in most women.

When estrogen therapy is indicated in the absence of significant contraindications (Box 52.2), the following general

---

Box 52.8 **BENEFITS AND RISKS OF HORMONE THERAPY**

Benefits
  Reduces hot flushes & night sweats
  Reduces vaginal dryness & dyspareunia
  Reduces postmenopausal osteoporotic fractures
  Reduces new onset of diabetes
  Associated with decreased risk of colon cancer (estrogen plus progestogen therapy, not estrogen therapy alone)
Risks
  Increases risk of venous thromboembolism
  Increases risk of coronary heart disease[a]
  Increases risk of ischemic stroke
  Increases risk of breast cancer[b]
  Increases risk of dementia when started in women >65 y[c]

[a] Hormone therapy may reduce coronary heart disease risk when initiated in younger & more recently postmenopausal women. Longer-duration hormone therapy is associated with reduced coronary heart disease risk & death & has been found to be associated with less accumulation of coronary artery calcium. Hormone therapy is not recommended as the sole or primary indication for coronary protection in women of any age.

[b] Breast cancer risk increases with estrogen plus progestogen therapy beyond 3-5 years. The increased events are rare: 4 to 6 additional cases per 10,000 women per year of estrogen plus progestogen therapy use beyond 5 years. No increased risk for women taking estrogen therapy alone, based on Women's Health Initiative data. Estrogen plus progestogen therapy reduces diagnostic interpretation of mammograms.

[c] Observational data report benefit of hormone therapy for reducing dementia when started in younger women & early in menopause. Hormone therapy is not recommended for cognitive protection in women of any age.

---

guidelines should be considered: 1) estrogen therapy alone is used when a woman has undergone hysterectomy; 2) combination estrogen-progestogen therapy is used in the setting of an intact uterus; 3) transdermal estrogen is associated with less risk for venous thromboembolism (in observational studies; no randomized controlled trials); 4) transdermal estrogen is preferred over oral in the clinical setting of hypertriglyceridemia, headaches, liver or gallbladder disease, or history of phlebitis; 5) topical, localized vaginal estrogen therapy is preferred over systemic estrogen for treatment of urogenital atrophy; and 6) extended-use hormone therapy should not be used to prevent bone loss or reduce fracture risk in women with osteopenia or osteoporosis unless alternative therapy is not possible, causes adverse effects, or its risk-benefit ratio is unfavorable.

- Combination estrogen-progestogen is indicated in the setting of an intact uterus, whereas estrogen alone can be used in women who have undergone hysterectomy.

- When vaginal symptoms prevail, vaginal estrogen (rather than systemic) is recommended.

- Transdermal estrogen is preferable in the setting of hypertriglyceridemia, liver or gallbladder disease, and history of phlebitis or headaches, and it seems to be associated with a reduced thromboembolic risk.

BREAST CONDITIONS

EVALUATION OF THE PALPABLE BREAST MASS

Breast lumps are common and usually benign. Benign characteristics are insufficient to exclude cancer; if clinical suspicion is high, negative findings on mammography and ultrasonography do not definitively exclude cancer.

- Negative results on breast imaging do not exclude cancer when clinical suspicion is high.

History should include location, duration, behavior related to menstrual cycle (premenopausal women), associated pain, skin or nipple changes (eg, discharge), and changes since noted. Risk factors should be considered, but a lack of defined risk factors does not exclude the possibility of cancer. Physical examination should include visual inspection for asymmetry, puckering, dimpling, nipple lesions or retraction, erythema, and peau d'orange. Palpation should include tissue from the clavicle to the inframammary area and from the sternum to the midaxillary line. The axillary, cervical, and supraclavicular nodal regions should be included.

Initial imaging evaluation includes diagnostic mammography and ultrasonography in women age 30 years or older and ultrasonography without mammography in women younger than 30 years. Mammography is useful in women younger than 30 years when the clinical suspicion of cancer is high, but its negative predictive value is limited in this setting. Ultrasonography reliably distinguishes solid from cystic masses and defines cystic features. No further evaluation is needed for a palpable mass or mammographic nodule corresponding to a simple cyst on ultrasonography. Symptomatic simple cysts can be aspirated. Nonbloody fluid does not require cytologic evaluation. A complex cyst should be aspirated to confirm complete resolution of the cyst.

- Lack of breast cancer risk factors does not exclude the possibility of cancer.

Tissue evaluation options are fine-needle aspiration (FNA), core needle biopsy, and excisional biopsy. FNA is inexpensive and can be done in an office setting, but the sensitivity and specificity are highly variable. A negative FNA result does not exclude cancer, particularly when clinical or imaging suspicion is high. Core needle biopsy provides enough tissue for histologic diagnosis and is often done with imaging guidance. Core needle biopsy has a higher sensitivity and better specimen quality than FNA. Concordance between core needle biopsy and excisional biopsy exceeds 90%. Excisional biopsy is reserved for cases in which FNA and core biopsy are technically unfeasible or when the findings on FNA or core biopsy are discordant with the physical examination or imaging findings. Core needle or excisional biopsy should be done when FNA shows atypical cells. Excisional biopsy should be done when core needle biopsy shows atypical ductal hyperplasia (to exclude malignancy) and should be considered when core

needle biopsy shows atypical lobular hyperplasia or lobular carcinoma in situ.

- FNA, core needle biopsy, or excisional biopsy may be performed, depending on the setting and circumstances.

- Core needle biopsy provides more reliable information than FNA and is highly concordant with excisional biopsy results.

- Excisional biopsy is generally not the first-line method for tissue evaluation.

EVALUATION OF NONPALPABLE MAMMOGRAPHIC ABNORMALITIES

Mammographic features of malignancy include soft tissue masses or clustered microcalcifications. The most specific mammographic feature of malignancy is a spiculated mass. Calcifications that are large and diffuse or scattered are usually benign, whereas those described as clustered punctate, fine pleomorphic, or fine linear branching suggest malignancy.

- Benign characteristics on history or physical examination do not exclude breast cancer.

- Negative findings on physical examination or mammography (with or without ultrasonography) do not exclude breast cancer.

- Descriptions of microcalcifications that suggest a malignant cause include clustered punctate, fine pleomorphic, and fine linear branching.

- The most specific mammographic finding for cancer is a spiculated mass.

BREAST PAIN

Breast pain (mastalgia) is classified into 3 categories: cyclic, noncyclic, and extramammary. Cyclic mastalgia occurs in premenopausal women and the pain begins in the luteal phase (2 weeks before the onset of menstruation) and resolves or substantially improves with menstruation. Pain is usually diffuse, bilateral, and concentrated in the upper outer aspect of the breasts, but it may be more severe in one breast.

Noncyclic mastalgia is not associated with the menstrual cycle; it can affect premenopausal and postmenopausal women. The cause of most cases of noncyclic breast pain is elusive, but it may be due to pregnancy, duct dilatation, cysts, fibroadenomas, injury, prior breast surgery, infection, or exogenous estrogen. Breast pain alone is due to cancer in less than 10% of cases, and less than 1% of women with breast pain and normal results on clinical examination and breast imaging have cancer. The evaluation of focal breast pain should include history and clinical examination, age-appropriate mammography, or ultrasonography. Ultrasonography alone should be used in women younger than 30 years who present with focal pain. In women whose history is consistent with cyclic pain and in whom results of clinical examination are negative, reassurance and pain management, depending on severity, is usually sufficient.

- Breast pain may be cyclic, noncyclic, or extramammary.
- In the setting of a history consistent with cyclic pain and negative results on physical examination, additional evaluation is not warranted; reassurance and pain management are adequate.
- Breast pain as the sole finding is very rarely related to breast cancer.

After appropriate evaluation, reassurance is often the only necessary treatment. For persistent or moderate to severe pain, initial treatment strategies for cyclic and noncyclic breast pain overlap: a well-fitted support brassiere (including nighttime use), heat or cold packs, gentle massage, dietary changes (eg, caffeine, sodium, and dietary fat), relaxation techniques, and exercise. Over-the-counter analgesics may be effective. Eliminating or adjusting exogenous estrogen doses may alleviate breast pain. Other hormonal agents may be effective in patients with severe cyclic breast pain unresponsive to conservative measures. Danazol is the only medication approved by the US Food and Drug Administration for mastalgia; adverse androgenic effects limit its utility. For noncyclic pain related to a nonmalignant breast cause, the above-listed methods and management of the underlying problem, if possible, are recommended (eg, treatment of an abscess and cyst aspiration).

- Conservative methods are usually sufficient to manage cyclic and noncyclic breast pain.
- Although danazol may be used for refractory cyclic mastalgia, adverse effects limit its utility.

NIPPLE DISCHARGE

Nipple discharge is common in reproductive-aged women and is usually benign. Evaluation to exclude breast cancer, a pituitary tumor, or infection should be considered on the basis of clinical presentation. Nipple discharge can be classified into 2 categories: due to ductal lesions or due to galactorrhea, defined as the discharge of milk or milk-like secretions 6 months or more postpartum in a non-breastfeeding woman. Galactorrhea presents as spontaneous, milky discharge from multiple ducts of both breasts as a result of increased serum prolactin. Evaluation and treatment of galactorrhea due to hyperprolactinemia are discussed in the "Endocrinology" section of this book. The patient with galactorrhea and a normal serum prolactin level does not require either visual field evaluation or brain imaging. Hypothyroidism should be considered. Treatment is offered only if the patient is bothered by the discharge, is unable to conceive, or has evidence of hypogonadism or low bone density. Prolactin levels should be monitored periodically in patients with persistent galactorrhea and previously normal prolactin levels.

- Nipple discharge is usually benign.
- Discharge may be due to ductal lesions or galactorrhea.
- In the setting of galactorrhea and a normal serum prolactin level, further evaluation is usually unnecessary.

Nipple discharge not due to galactorrhea may be benign or caused by ductal lesions, including malignancy. Benign nipple discharge typically is bilateral, nonbloody, and multiductal, but it may be unilateral. Green, gray, or blue is typical of fibrocystic breast change. Brown or yellow discharge is also usually benign. Clear (watery) discharge is usually benign, but malignancy must be excluded. Check thyrotropin and prolactin levels to exclude hypothyroidism and hyperprolactinemia if the discharge is milky. Pathologic discharge (which may be due to malignancy) is typically unilateral, uniductal, and spontaneous. It is typically bloody, serosanguineous, or, sometimes, watery or clear. The most common cause of bloody nipple discharge is a benign intraductal papilloma, followed by ductal ectasia (ductal dilatation with or without inflammation) and carcinoma. Ductal carcinoma in situ and papillary carcinoma are the most common types of breast cancer associated with bloody nipple discharge. Factors associated with a higher likelihood of cancer are detailed in Box 52.9.

- Nipple discharge features that are concerning for malignancy or other abnormality include it being unilateral, uniductal, spontaneous, and bloody, serosanguineous, or watery or clear.
- Green, gray, or blue nipple discharge is characteristic of fibrocystic change and requires no evaluation.

Mammography and ultrasonography should be done for all nonlactating women with nipple discharge who are older than 30 years unless it is clearly due to fibrocystic change. Ultrasonography alone should be done in women younger than 30 years. Galactography and ductoscopy are not routinely used in the evaluation of nipple discharge and should not be performed.

Patients with nipple discharge that is neither pathologic nor galactorrhea and with normal diagnostic breast imaging results can be reassured and observed. Patients with pathologic discharge that can be clinically localized to one duct should

---

Box 52.9 **FACTORS THAT INCREASE THE LIKELIHOOD OF CANCER ASSOCIATED WITH NIPPLE DISCHARGE**

Associated palpable mass
Age >40 y
Grossly bloody, guaiac-positive, serosanguineous, or watery or clear discharge
Unilateral
Spontaneous
Persistent
Single duct

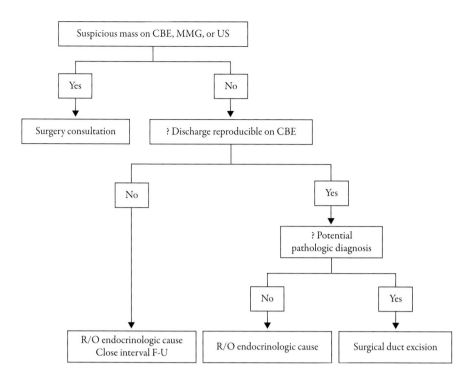

Figure 52.1 Algorithm for Evaluation of Spontaneous Nipple Discharge. CBE indicates clinical breast examination; F-U, follow-up; MMG, mammography; R/O, rule out; US, ultrasonography.

be considered for surgical duct excision, even when imaging results are negative. Patients who report bloody or watery nipple discharge with clinically nonreproducible discharge and normal results on imaging studies require close interval follow-up. Surgical duct excision should be performed if the involved duct subsequently can be identified. Subareolar duct excision can be considered if the discharge is persistent and bothersome to the patient, but it is not required. Figure 52.1 is a suggested algorithm for the evaluation of spontaneous nipple discharge.

- Galactography and ductoscopy should not be performed in the evaluation of nipple discharge.

- Reassurance is appropriate in the absence of galactorrhea or pathologic discharge with normal results of breast imaging (when appropriate to perform).

- Surgical duct excision should be performed if uniductal discharge and the duct can be clinically identified and in the setting of potentially pathologic discharge with negative imaging results as a means to exclude malignancy.

BENIGN BREAST DISEASE

Simple cysts are the most common cause of discrete benign breast lumps and occur most often between ages 35 and 50 years. Fibroadenomas are the most common solid, benign masses; the median age at diagnosis of fibroadenomas is 30 years, but they may also occur in postmenopausal women. There are many other histologic classifications of benign breast disease. The main significance lies in whether they confer an increased risk of breast cancer. Patients at significantly increased risk should be counselled about appropriate screening and risk reduction options. The magnitude of risk

varies depending on the histologic classification; the overall average relative risk is 1.56. The classification is detailed in Box 52.10.

- In premenopausal women, a simple cyst is the most common discrete breast lump and a fibroadenoma is the most common benign solid mass.

- Benign breast disease should be considered in the context of risk conferred for screening and counselling recommendations.

Box 52.10 **CATEGORIES OF BENIGN BREAST DISEASE**

Nonproliferative breast lesions (RR 1.27)
    Duct ectasia
    Fibroadenoma without proliferative epithelial changes
    Fibrosis
    Mastitis
    Mild hyperplasia without atypia
    Cysts
    Simple apocrine metaplasia
    Squamous metaplasia
Proliferative breast lesions without atypia (RR 1.88)
    Fibroadenoma with proliferative epithelial changes
    Moderate or florid hyperplasia without atypia
    Sclerosing adenosis
    Papilloma
    Radial scar
Atypia (RR 4.24)
    Atypical ductal hyperplasia
    Atypical lobular hyperplasia

Abbreviation: RR, relative risk.

BREAST CANCER RISK ASSESSMENT AND PREVENTION

Women at increased risk for breast cancer should be counselled about recommendations and options for screening and risk reduction. The most widely used risk assessment model for use in women older than 35 years without a history of breast cancer is the National Cancer Institute Risk Assessment Tool (Gail model). The tool cannot be applied to women 35 years or younger with a history of breast cancer (including ductal carcinoma in situ). It overestimates risk in women with numerous prior biopsies for nonproliferative (overall low risk) disease and women with high-risk lesions (eg, atypical hyperplasia) *and* a family history of breast cancer, and it underestimates risk in generations or cases of suspected inherited susceptibility. Alternative models are used in women whose predominant risk factor is family history. Current models do not account for breast density, an independent risk factor for breast cancer.

- The Gail model may underestimate or overestimate breast cancer risk.

Only 5% to 10% of all breast cancers are due to an inherited gene mutation. Both *BRCA1* and *BRCA2* mutations have autosomal dominant inheritance. Deleterious mutations confer a 55% to 80% lifetime risk of breast cancer and a 15% to 40% lifetime risk of ovarian cancer. Maternal and paternal family histories must be considered. Family history patterns concerning for a *BRCA* mutation include the following:

1. ≥2 first-degree relatives with breast cancer, one of whom received the diagnosis at age 50 years or younger

2. ≥3 first- or second-degree relatives with breast cancer regardless of age at diagnosis

3. Both breast and ovarian cancer among first- and second-degree relatives

4. A first-degree relative with bilateral breast cancer

5. ≥2 first- or second-degree relatives with ovarian cancer regardless of age at diagnosis

6. A first- or second-degree relative with both breast and ovarian cancer at any age

7. Breast cancer in a male relative

For women of Ashkenazi Jewish descent, a worrisome family history includes any first-degree relative (or 2 second-degree relatives on the same side of the family) with breast or ovarian cancer. Specific founder mutations exist in this and other populations. Several statistical models are available to estimate the probability of *BRCA1* or *BRCA2* mutation. Women with family histories suggestive of an inherited mutation should undergo genetic counseling and consideration of *BRCA* testing.

- Ashkenazi Jewish women are at increased risk of a mutation due to founder mutations.

- Women with a family history worrisome for a mutation should see a genetics counselor and consider gene mutation testing.

- Lifetime risk of breast (and ovarian) cancer is significant in *BRCA* mutation carriers.

MANAGEMENT OPTIONS FOR WOMEN AT INCREASED RISK OF BREAST CANCER

Options for surveillance and risk reduction should be discussed, depending on the woman's preferences and risk level.

Lifestyle Modifications

Factors associated with an increased risk include postmenopausal weight gain, alcohol intake in excess of 2 drinks per day, and physical inactivity. Corresponding lifestyle modifications in combination with healthy dietary choices may reduce risk. In general, it is prudent to try to avoid systemic hormone therapy in women at significant risk for breast cancer.

Careful Screening

Guidelines recommend that women with a known or suspected *BRCA* mutation begin monthly breast self-examination by age 18 to 21 years, annual or semiannual clinical breast examinations by age 25 to 35 years, and annual mammography beginning at age 25 to 35 years. Mutation carriers should begin annual or semiannual ovarian cancer screening with transvaginal ultrasonography and measurement of the CA 125 serum level at age 30 to 35 years. Women with a family history of breast cancer not consistent with a *BRCA* mutation should begin annual screening mammography 10 years before the age at diagnosis of the youngest affected relative but no later than age 40 years.

The American Cancer Society recommends consideration of annual breast magnetic resonance imaging (in addition to annual mammography) for women with any of the following characteristics: 1) known *BRCA* mutation, 2) unknown *BRCA* status and a first-degree relative with a known mutation, 3) lifetime risk of breast cancer of 20% to 25% (using an accepted breast cancer risk assessment model), or 4) chest irradiation between ages 10 and 30 years (eg, mantle radiation for lymphoma). Evidence was insufficient to recommend magnetic resonance imaging screening for women with 1) a prior history of breast cancer, 2) dense breast tissue, or 3) a history of atypical hyperplasia or lobular carcinoma in situ.

- Screening guidelines for breast cancer are affected by degree of risk.

- Magnetic resonance imaging as an adjunct to mammography can be considered in certain populations.

- Chest irradiation at a young age confers significant lifetime risk of breast cancer.

Chemoprevention

Tamoxifen and raloxifene are selective estrogen receptor modulators and are the only medications approved by the US Food and Drug Administration for risk reduction in women at high risk for breast cancer (Table 52.4). Tamoxifen is approved for risk reduction when 5-year predicted breast cancer risk (by the Gail model) is more than 1.66% or lifetime risk is more than 20% in premenopausal women older than 35 years and postmenopausal women, whereas raloxifene is approved in postmenopausal women only. *High risk* may also include at least one breast biopsy showing lobular carcinoma in situ or atypical hyperplasia.

Tamoxifen and raloxifene have overall low but similar incidences of ischemic heart and cerebrovascular events, osteoporotic fractures, and death. Both increase the risk of thromboembolism (both deep vein thrombosis and pulmonary embolus), but raloxifene is associated with a lower risk than tamoxifen. See Table 52.4 for further information regarding adverse effects. Overall, raloxifene is considered to have the more favorable adverse-effect profile. The evidence for use in women with *BRCA* mutations is not clear.

- Tamoxifen and raloxifene can be used for reduction of breast cancer risk in certain populations.
- Both medications have overall low but measurable adverse effects and adverse effects in clinical trials; these should be considered and discussed with the patients; risk:benefit consideration is essential.

Prophylactic Surgery

Prophylactic surgery is typically reserved for women at highest risk for breast cancer (primarily *BRCA* mutation carriers) and is associated with a more than 90% reduction in breast cancer risk. Bilateral oophorectomy in women younger than 40 to 45 years decreases both breast and ovarian cancer risk in *BRCA* mutation carriers.

- Women at significant lifetime risk should be counselled about preventive mastectomies.
- Preventive oophorectomy may be offered to premenopausal *BRCA* mutation carriers for reduction of breast and ovarian cancer risk once childbearing is complete.

CARDIOVASCULAR DISEASE IN WOMEN

Cardiovascular disease is the leading cause of death among women in the United States, and it is both underrecognized and undertreated in women. Risk factors, clinical presentation, diagnosis, and treatment differ between men and women (Table 52.5).

RISK FACTORS FOR CORONARY HEART DISEASE

Risk factors for men and women are similar but the magnitude of risk factor effect differs by sex. Compared with similarly aged men, premenopausal women have lower

---

Table 52.4 **COMPARISON OF RISKS, BENEFITS, AND ADVERSE EFFECTS OF RALOXIFENE AND TAMOXIFEN**

	AGENT	
CHARACTERISTIC	*Raloxifene*	*Tamoxifen*
Risk		
Deep vein thrombosis and pulmonary embolus	Increased risk (R<T)[a]	Increased risk (R<T)
Stroke	Increased risk (R=T)[b]	Increased risk (R=T)
Ischemic heart disease events	No change	No change
Uterine cancer	No change or decreased risk	Increased risk
Cataracts	Increased risk (R<T)	Increased risk (R<T)
Benefit		
Invasive breast cancer	Decreased risk (R=T)	Decreased risk (R=T)
Noninvasive breast cancer	No change	Decreased risk
Fractures	Decreased risk	Decreased risk
Adverse effects		
Hot flushes	Increased risk (R<T)	Increased risk (R<T)
Weight gain	Increased risk (R>T)[c]	Increased risk (R>T)
Leg cramps	Increased risk (R<T)	Increased risk (R<T)
Cognition	No change	May worsen cognition

Abbreviations: R, raloxifene; T, tamoxifen.

[a] R<T indicates that magnitude of risk is smaller for raloxifene than for tamoxifen.

[b] R=T indicates magnitude of risk is similar for raloxifene and tamoxifen.

[c] R>T indicates magnitude of risk is greater for raloxifene than for tamoxifen.

Table 52.5 **DIFFERENCES IN CARDIOVASCULAR DISEASE BY SEX**

FEATURE	DIFFERENCES IN CHARACTERIZING WOMEN RELATIVE TO MEN
Epidemiologic factors	Lower overall prevalence & incidence Later onset with respect to age
Risk factors	Before menopause, risk profile more favorable (lower blood pressure, lower LDL-C level, higher HDL-C level) After menopause, similar risk profiles Higher systolic blood pressure after age 45 y; more isolated systolic hypertension Higher fibrinogen, CRP levels Lower smoking rates Greater attributable risk for hypertension, diabetes mellitus, smoking
Pathogenesis	Less obstructive & less extensive epicardial disease Higher likelihood of microvascular disease
Clinical presentation	More likely to delay seeking evaluation & treatment after onset of symptoms More likely to present without chest pain More likely to present with unstable angina or non–ST-segment elevation MI Less likely to present with ST–segment-elevation MI Less likely to present with MI or sudden cardiac death as initial manifestation More likely to have hypertension & diabetes mellitus as comorbidities
Diagnosis	Lower sensitivity & specificity of exercise ECG Cardiac catheterization performed less often
Treatment	After MI, less likely to be admitted to monitored intensive care settings & to receive specialty care Less likely to receive early aspirin, β-blocker therapy, reperfusion therapy, & timely reperfusion Less likely to receive percutaneous coronary intervention or CABG after MI Lower utilization of cardiac rehabilitation
Prognosis	Higher short-term mortality rate from MI (in part due to older age at presentation & greater burden of comorbid disease) Women <50 y have twice the mortality rate due to MI compared with same-age men; narrowing mortality gap with advancing age Higher adjusted mortality rates after ST-elevation MI Higher short-term, but better long-term, mortality rate after CABG Increased complication rates after percutaneous coronary intervention

Abbreviations: CABG, coronary artery bypass grafting; CRP, C-reactive protein; ECG, electrocardiogram; HDL-C, high-density lipoprotein cholesterol; LDL-C, low-density lipoprotein cholesterol; MI, myocardial infarction.

low-density lipoprotein cholesterol and triglyceride levels and higher high-density lipoprotein cholesterol levels. However, these differences do not persist after menopause. Low levels of high-density lipoprotein cholesterol are more predictive of risk in women than high levels of low-density lipoprotein cholesterol. The total ratio of cholesterol to high-density lipoprotein cholesterol is most highly predictive of cardiovascular events among women. Serum C-reactive protein is a strong independent risk factor in women that adds to the predictive value of traditional risk factors. The relative risk of death from coronary heart disease is greater in females with diabetes mellitus than males. Smoking seems to confer a higher risk of coronary heart disease in women than men. Among patients with a first myocardial infarction, women are more likely to be older and to have a history of diabetes mellitus, hypertension, hyperlipidemia, or heart failure.

- Men and women share similar risk factors for coronary heart disease, but the magnitude of risk differs.

- After menopause, lipid abnormalities accumulate in women.

- Serum C-reactive protein is an independent risk factor for cardiovascular disease in women.

- Women with diabetes mellitus have a higher relative risk of death from coronary heart disease than men.

- Smoking confers greater risk in women than men.

PATHOGENESIS OF CORONARY HEART DISEASE

Women presenting with an acute coronary syndrome are less likely than age-matched men to have obstructive coronary artery disease, particularly triple-vessel or left main disease. Women referred for angiographic evaluation of presumed angina are more likely than men to have normal coronary arteries. Coronary microvascular dysfunction or myocardial infarction, or both, occurs in up to half of women with chest pain and normal coronary arteries. Proposed mechanisms for the absence of detectable coronary artery disease on angiography include diffuse atherosclerosis not detectable by angiography, rapid clot lysis, coronary vasospasm, coronary microvascular dysfunction, or reduced myocardial perfusion due to high left ventricular filling pressures related to hypertension or diastolic dysfunction.

Left ventricular apical ballooning is an uncommon, but increasingly recognized, form of acute, reversible left ventricular dysfunction associated with ST-segment elevation without obstructive coronary artery disease. It typically occurs in postmenopausal women after intense emotional or physiologic stress. It appears to be triggered by catecholamine-mediated myocardial stunning and is usually self-limited.

CLINICAL PRESENTATION OF CORONARY HEART DISEASE

Women having a myocardial infarction may have multiple presenting symptoms or absence of chest pain. Up to 50% of women have non–chest pain symptoms of heart disease and myocardial infarction, which may include neck, shoulder, upper back, or abdominal discomfort; indigestion; belching; "gas" pains; nausea or vomiting; weakness; unexplained fatigue; dyspnea; or a sense of doom. Because women tend to be older when symptoms develop, comorbid conditions (eg, arthritis) may mask cardiac symptoms.

- Women having a myocardial infarction often present with symptoms different from the typical ones observed in men; hence, a high degree of clinical suspicion is necessary.

CARDIOVASCULAR STRESS TESTING

Treadmill exercise testing has a lower sensitivity and specificity in women than men, possibly due to the increased prevalence of nonobstructive coronary artery disease and single-vessel disease in women. The false-positive rate is higher in women than men, particularly in young women with a low likelihood of coronary artery disease. The false-negative rate is also higher in women, in part because they are commonly older at presentation and thus less likely to be able to achieve an adequate workload on treadmill exercise testing. Despite these limitations, guidelines still support the use of exercise testing in women at intermediate pretest risk of coronary artery disease (based on symptoms and risk factors) who have normal results on resting electrocardiograms and are capable of maximal exercise. Exercise electrocardiography has a high negative predictive value in women with a low pretest probability of coronary artery disease.

- Stress testing may help in risk stratification for coronary artery disease in women, but treadmill testing has lower sensitivity and specificity in women and a high false-positive and false-negative rate.

Exercise stress echocardiography or nuclear perfusion scanning can be considered for symptomatic women with an intermediate to high pretest probability of coronary artery disease or an abnormal resting electrocardiogram. Pharmacologic stress testing with echocardiographic or nuclear imaging is recommended for women unable to exercise adequately. Imaging stress tests have similar sensitivity and specificity in women and men.

- Exercise echocardiography or nuclear perfusion scanning provides more reliable results in women, particularly in those with intermediate to high probability of disease or abnormal resting electrocardiographic findings.

SEX-BASED DIFFERENCES IN CORONARY HEART DISEASE MANAGEMENT AND OUTCOMES

Despite guidelines, after a myocardial infarction, women are less likely to receive standard of care such as early aspirin and β-blocker therapy, and they are less likely to receive early revascularization (reperfusion or percutaneous coronary intervention) or coronary artery bypass grafting (CABG). In-hospital mortality rate after CABG is higher in women than in men, largely due to older age and greater number of comorbidities. However, long-term outcomes after CABG appear to be slightly better for women than men. Women with multivessel disease who are treated with CABG have better long-term survival than women treated medically.

- Women are less likely to receive standard of care medical therapy or early revascularization after a myocardial infarction.
- Women appear to have better long-term outcomes after CABG, but the in-hospital survival rate after surgery is higher.

Although women with myocardial infarction are more likely than men to survive to reach the hospital, their in-hospital and 30-day mortality rates exceed those for men, as do long-term mortality rates. These trends are due, in part, to the increased age and comorbidities of women presenting with a myocardial infarction relative to men, but underrecognition of symptoms and less aggressive diagnostic and therapeutic approaches likely contribute. The mortality rate from coronary artery disease is higher in black women than in white women.

Women with normal coronary arteries and persistent nonspecific chest pain have a higher risk of future adverse coronary events than women with normal arteries and nonspecific chest pain that resolves. The absence of obstructive disease on angiography cannot definitively exclude ischemia in women with persistent symptoms suggestive of ischemia or positive results on stress testing. Further diagnostic evaluation, risk factor modification, symptom management, and measures to improve microvascular and macrovascular function should be considered.

- Women with normal coronary arteries and persistent chest pain have a higher risk of future adverse coronary events than women with normal arteries and pain that resolves.
- Normal results on angiography do not definitively exclude ischemia in women with suspicious clinical or stress test results.

PRIMARY AND SECONDARY PREVENTION

Low-dose aspirin has not been shown to prevent first myocardial infarction or death from cardiovascular causes in women, but it was associated with a significant reduction in stroke incidence in women 65 years or older. Aspirin is effective for acute treatment of myocardial infarction and for secondary prevention of cardiovascular disease in both men and women. Bleeding risk is similar for women and men.

Statins appear to be equally effective in women and men for primary prevention. For secondary prevention, statin therapy is at least equally effective in women as in men. Postmenopausal hormone therapy should *not* be used for primary or secondary prevention of coronary artery disease. Hormone therapy should be discontinued if a cardiovascular disease event occurs. Lipid alterations associated with hormone therapy include both favorable and unfavorable changes (see "Hormone Therapy" section, this chapter). Oral, but not transdermal, estrogen increases C-reactive protein levels.

- Hormone therapy should not be used for the purpose of primary or secondary prevention of cardiovascular disease.

HEART FAILURE IN WOMEN

Women account for nearly 50% of hospital admissions for heart failure, which usually develops at an older age in women than in men. During the past 50 years, the incidence of heart failure has declined among women but not among men. Women with heart failure are more likely to have hypertension, diabetes mellitus, obesity, tobacco use, or atrial fibrillation, whereas men are more likely to have coronary artery disease and left ventricular systolic dysfunction. Women are more likely to have diastolic heart failure with preserved systolic function. Women with heart failure usually survive longer than men with heart failure, but they have more dyspnea on exertion and functional impairment. Depression, often associated with heart failure, is more common in women than in men.

- Nearly 50% of heart failure-related hospital admissions occur in women.

- Women more commonly have hypertension, diabetes, obesity, tobacco use, or atrial fibrillation than men, whereas men are more likely to have coronary artery disease and left ventricular systolic dysfunction.

- Women are more likely to have diastolic dysfunction with preserved systolic function.

Peripartum cardiomyopathy, in which left ventricular systolic dysfunction and heart failure symptoms occur between the last month of pregnancy and the first 5 months postpartum, has unknown cause. It is a diagnosis of exclusion. Medical management is similar to that of other forms of dilated cardiomyopathy (see the "Cardiology" section of this book).

- Peripartum cardiomyopathy is a diagnosis of exclusion and is managed like other forms of dilated cardiomyopathy.

ATRIAL FIBRILLATION IN WOMEN

Although atrial fibrillation is less common in women than men, women are at higher risk for stroke. This difference may be due to women being less likely to receive treatment with anticoagulation (see the "Cardiology" section of this book).

DEPRESSION AND ANXIETY IN WOMEN

The lifetime prevalence of depression is higher in women than men, and the peak age at onset is 33 to 45 years in women and older than 55 years in men. Women are less likely to commit suicide but twice as likely to make an attempt, and white women are twice as likely as African American women to commit suicide. The lifetime prevalence of dysthymia is slightly higher in women than in men. There is no sex difference for bipolar disorder.

- Women are more likely to have depression, and it occurs at a younger age than in men.

- Men are more likely to commit suicide, but women are twice as likely to make an attempt.

- African American women are at lower risk of suicide.

The risk of depressive symptoms and clinical depression increases during perimenopause. There is no association between natural or surgical menopause and rate of depression. Hormone therapy leads to improved Beck Depression Inventory scores in nondepressed women but not in clinically depressed women. Postmenopausal estrogen may improve mild depressive symptoms, but it is not sufficient for treatment of clinical depression.

- Depression increases during perimenopause.

- Postmenopausal estrogen helps mild symptoms but not clinical depression.

Postpartum depression affects 10% to 15% of women and develops in the first month after childbirth. It is often unrecognized. Risk factors include prior major or postpartum depression, depression during pregnancy, unmarried status, or unplanned pregnancy. It is essential to evaluate thyroid function in postpartum women with depressive symptoms because of overlap in presentation. Psychosis develops in few women with postpartum depression; it usually requires acute hospitalization.

- Postpartum depression is not uncommon and is often unrecognized.

- Evaluate thyroid function in postpartum women with depression symptoms.

Anxiety disorders that are more prevalent in women include panic disorder, agoraphobia, social phobia, generalized anxiety disorder, and posttraumatic stress disorder. Women with panic disorder may have a comorbid psychiatric condition. An anxiety disorder may underlie persistent somatic complaints. If non-pharmacologic measures are inadequate, combined medication and cognitive behavioral therapy should be offered.

- Multiple anxiety disorders are more common in women.
- Persistent somatic complaints may be due to underlying anxiety disorder.

The risks and benefits of pharmacologic therapy need to be considered in pregnant or nursing women. Tricyclic antidepressants and some selective serotonin reuptake inhibitors seem to be relatively safe, although there are isolated adverse reports of infants exposed to these agents through breast milk.

- Pharmacologic therapy is often safe during pregnancy, but risk of therapy must be balanced with benefit of treatment and risk of no medical therapy.

INTIMATE PARTNER VIOLENCE

Intimate partner violence is intentional controlling or violent behavior. Controlling behavior may include physical or emotional abuse, sexual assault, economic control, or social isolation of the victim. In 95% of reported cases, a male is the perpetrator and a female is the victim. At least 1 in 3 US women is assaulted by a partner during her lifetime. Female victims most often present for care indirectly related to abuse injuries. Battered women use health services 6 to 8 times more than nonbattered women and have an increased incidence of headaches, sexually transmitted diseases, irritable bowel syndrome, depression, and anxiety. Suggestive aspects of the history include depression, chronic pain syndromes, gastrointestinal complaints, an overprotective partner, injuries during pregnancy, frequent visits for injuries, and a history of childhood abuse. All women should be asked about intimate partner violence. Routine prenatal screening for intimate partner violence is particularly important because abuse occurs in 1 of 6 pregnancies and often begins or escalates in early pregnancy.

- Intimate partner violence is common.
- Victims may present with symptoms not directly attributable to injury, and a high degree of clinical suspicion is necessary.

Suggestive physical examination findings include injuries incompatible with the history, multiple injuries in various healing stages, injuries suggestive of a defensive posture (eg, ulnar fractures), and pattern injuries (eg, burns, choking or bite marks, or wrist or ankle abrasions).

Documentation in the medical record is essential and may provide evidence to help the victim separate from the perpetrator. If the victim consents, injury photographs should be obtained. Physical evidence should be preserved.

Victims need treatment of injuries, support, safety assessment, and referral to appropriate resources to prevent further abuse. A safety assessment by a victim's advocate, social worker, or law enforcement personnel is critical. When these persons are not available, a trained physician or nurse should perform a safety assessment. Immediate psychiatric referral should be arranged for patients expressing suicidal or homicidal intentions. The assessment must include inquiries regarding children in the home, and any child abuse must be reported to child abuse authorities. Some jurisdictions require reporting to the child abuse authorities any intimate partner violence in a home where children reside. Because intimate partner violence homicides are more likely to occur immediately after separation, ensuring the safety of the victim during separation is critical.

- Aspects of the history that may suggest intimate partner violence include depression, chronic pain syndromes, gastrointestinal complaints, an overprotective partner, injuries during pregnancy, frequent visits for injuries, and a history of childhood abuse.
- Victims of intimate partner violence should be provided with treatment of their injuries; validation, support, and counselling; safety assessment; referral to appropriate resources to prevent further abuse; and medical and legal documentation of abuse.

SEXUAL ASSAULT

Sexual assault is any sexual act performed without consent. Most cases are unreported, and about half of victims have some acquaintance with their attacker. A sexual assault victim should be evaluated by a trained sexual assault nurse examiner or health care professional with equivalent training.

53.

GENERAL INTERNAL MEDICINE: PREOPERATIVE EVALUATION[a]

Karen F. Mauck, MD, MSc, and Margaret Beliveau, MD

GOALS

- Use the American College of Cardiology and American Heart Association (ACC/AHA) guidelines to estimate cardiac risk, choose the appropriate noninvasive test to further stratify cardiac risk, and recommend risk reduction strategies.

- Understand perioperative management of antiplatelet agents in patients with coronary stents.

- Identify the perioperative risk of pulmonary complications and recommend risk reduction strategies.

- Use appropriate deep vein thrombosis (DVT) prophylaxis in the surgical patient according to risk.

- Recommend appropriate preoperative testing.

More than 33 million US residents (about 10% of the US population) undergo surgery annually. This number is projected to increase substantially by 2020. Internists commonly evaluate the fitness of patients for surgery and help manage their comorbidities in the perioperative period.

GOALS OF PREOPERATIVE EVALUATION

The goals of a preoperative evaluation include the following:

1. Evaluate, assess, and quantify the risk of anesthesia and surgery and communicate this risk to the patient, the anesthesiologist, and the surgeon to allow for informed decision making.

2. Coordinate perioperative care in an attempt to minimize this risk.

Both patient- and surgery-specific risks contribute to overall perioperative risk. Although the most frequent types of major perioperative risks are cardiac, pulmonary, and thromboembolic, patients may have other types of risks. The following sections cover perioperative evaluation, including general risks of anesthesia and surgery and specific risk assessment and management strategies.

STANDARD ASPECTS OF THE PREOPERATIVE EVALUATION

HISTORY AND REVIEW OF SYSTEMS

Include a careful cardiovascular history, focusing on clinical predictors outlined in the ACC/AHA guidelines (Box 53.1). Functional status, based on the patient's report, can be estimated in metabolic equivalent tasks (METs) (Table 53.1). Patients' pulmonary, anesthetic, thrombotic, and bleeding histories should be reviewed. Document the presence and status of any medical illness (eg, glaucoma, diabetes mellitus, hypertension, thyroid disease, sleep apnea, renal insufficiency, cognitive impairment). Ask about corticosteroid use in the past year. Include screening questions for sleep apnea. Consider the possibility of pregnancy in any woman of childbearing age.

Document all previous surgical procedures with approximate dates, type of anesthesia, and complications. Include a comprehensive list of the patient's past medical diagnoses. Include relevant smoking, alcohol, or drug history, including extent of past use and most recent use. Family history should be limited to first-degree relatives with serious anesthetic (eg, malignant hypertension) or bleeding complications.

Perhaps the greatest contribution that the internist can make to the preoperative assessment is the compilation of an accurate and complete medication list. Full dosing information should be included for all prescription and nonprescription drugs, dietary supplements, and herbs. Confirm the allergy list and ask about latex allergy.

[a] Portions previously published in Mauck KF, Litin SC. Clinical pearls in perioperative medicine. Mayo Clin Proc. 2009 Jun;84(6):546–550. Used with permission of Mayo Foundation for Medical Education and Research.

Box 53.1 CLINICAL PREDICTORS OF INCREASED PERIOPERATIVE CARDIOVASCULAR RISK (MYOCARDIAL INFARCTION, HEART FAILURE, AND DEATH)

Active Cardiac Conditions

Unstable coronary syndromes

Acute or recent MI with evidence of important ischemic risk by clinical symptoms or noninvasive study[a]

Unstable or severe angina[b] (CCS class III or IV)[c]

Significant arrhythmias

High-grade atrioventricular block

Symptomatic ventricular arrhythmias in the presence of underlying heart disease

Supraventricular arrhythmias with uncontrolled ventricular rate

Severe valvular disease

Decompensated heart failure

Clinical Risk Factors[d]

History of ischemic heart disease (including patients with pathologic Q waves on ECG)

History of compensated or prior heart failure (systolic or diastolic)

History of cerebrovascular disease (TIA or stroke)

Diabetes mellitus requiring insulin

Renal insufficiency (preoperative serum creatinine >2 mg/dL)

Abbreviations: CCS, Canadian Cardiovascular Society; ECG, electrocardiogram; MI, myocardial infarction; TIA, transient ischemic attack.

[a] *Recent* MI means that MI occurred more than 7 days previously but within 30 days; *acute* MI, within 7 days.

[b] May include "stable" angina in patients who are unusually sedentary.

[c] Campeau L. Grading of angina pectoris. Circulation. 1976 Sep;54(3):522–3.

[d] From the revised cardiac risk index: Lee TH, Marcantonio ER, Mangione CM, Thomas EJ, Polanczyk CA, Cook EF, et al. Derivation and prospective validation of a simple index for prediction of cardiac risk of major noncardiac surgery. Circulation. 1999 Sep 7;100(10):1043–9.

Adapted from Fleisher LA, Beckman JA, Brown KA, Calkins H, Chaikof E, Fleischmann KE, et al. ACC/AHA 2007 guidelines on perioperative cardiovascular evaluation and care for noncardiac surgery: a report of the American College of Cardiology/American Heart Association Task Force on Practice Guidelines (Writing Committee to Revise the 2002 Guidelines on Perioperative Cardiovascular Evaluation for Noncardiac Surgery). J Am Coll Cardiol. 2007 Oct 23;50(17):e159–242 and Fleisher LA, Beckman JA, Brown KA, Calkins H, Chaikof E, Fleischmann KE, et al. ACC/AHA 2007 guidelines on perioperative cardiovascular evaluation and care for noncardiac surgery: a report of the American College of Cardiology/American Heart Association Task Force on Practice Guidelines (Writing Committee to Revise the 2002 Guidelines on Perioperative Cardiovascular Evaluation for Noncardiac Surgery): developed in collaboration with the American Society of Echocardiography, American Society of Nuclear Cardiology, Heart Rhythm Society, Society of Cardiovascular Anesthesiologists, Society for Cardiovascular Angiography and Interventions, Society for Vascular Medicine and Biology, and Society for Vascular Surgery. Circulation. 2007 Oct 23;116(17):e418–99. Epub 2007 Sep 27. Errata in: Circulation. 2008 Aug 26;118(9): e143–4. Circulation. 2008 Feb 5;117(5):e154. Used with permission.

PHYSICAL EXAMINATION

Include blood pressure, temperature, and pulse and respiratory rates. The head and neck examination should include neck range of motion, evaluation of the airway (Figure 53.1), carotid auscultation, and assessment of the jugular veins. The cardiopulmonary examination should focus on murmurs,

Table 53.1 ESTIMATED REQUIREMENTS FOR VARIOUS ACTIVITIES

REQUIREMENT	ACTIVITY
1 MET	Can you take care of yourself?
	Eat, dress, or use the toilet?
	Walk indoors around the house?
	Walk a block or 2 on level ground at 2–3 mph (3.2–4.8 kph)?
	Do light work around the house like dusting or washing dishes?
4 METs	Climb a flight of stairs or walk up a hill?
	Walk on level ground at 4 mph (6.4 kph)?
	Run a short distance?
	Do heavy work around the house like scrubbing floors or lifting or moving heavy furniture?
	Participate in moderate recreational activities such as golf, bowling, dancing, doubles tennis, or throwing a baseball or football?
>10 METs	Participate in strenuous sports such as swimming, singles tennis, football, basketball, or skiing?

Abbreviations: kph, kilometers per hour; MET, metabolic equivalent task; mph, miles per hour.

Adapted from Eagle KA, Brundage BH, Chaitman BR, Ewy GA, Fleisher LA, Hertzer NR, et al. Guidelines for perioperative cardiovascular evaluation for noncardiac surgery. Report of the American College of Cardiology/American Heart Association Task Force on Practice Guidelines (Committee on Perioperative Cardiovascular Evaluation for Noncardiac Surgery). Circulation. 1996 Mar 15;93(6):1278–317 and Eagle KA, Brundage BH, Chaitman BR, Ewy GA, Fleisher LA, Hertzer NR, et al. Guidelines for perioperative cardiovascular evaluation for noncardiac surgery. Report of the American College of Cardiology/American Heart Association Task Force on Practice Guidelines (Committee on Perioperative Cardiovascular Evaluation for Noncardiac Surgery). J Am Coll Cardiol. 1996 Mar 15;27(4):910–48. Used with permission.

gallops, rales, rhonchi, and wheezes. Perform a brief abdominal examination for features such as organomegaly and scars. Examine the extremities for palpable distal pulses and evidence of peripheral edema. Perform a limited neurologic examination that includes mental status and a gross sensory and motor evaluation (ie, identify baseline cognitive or neurologic problems).

IMPRESSION AND PLAN

Summarize your assessment of perioperative risk and any additional testing and management recommendations based on this risk. This usually includes the following statement: "The patient is medically optimized for the planned surgical procedure." Avoid using the expression "cleared for surgery," which implies a guarantee of no problems and can be easily misinterpreted. For completeness, it is often helpful to divide this section into the following categories:

1. Cardiac risk: Include important factors that led to your recommendations, such as active cardiac conditions, clinical risk factors, functional capacity, and the urgency and type of operation planned. Include your rationale and plan for additional testing if indicated and a plan for perioperative management and surveillance.

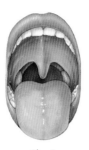 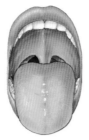 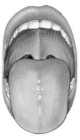 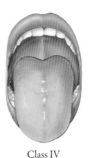

| Class I | Class II | Class III | Class IV |

Figure 53.1 Mallampati Classification. The Mallampati Classification is based on the structures visualized with maximal mouth opening and tongue protrusion in the sitting position. (This test was originally described without phonation, but some have suggested that Mallampati Classification with or without phonation correlates with intubation difficulty: higher Mallampati scores are more likely to indicate greater intubation difficulty.)

2. Pulmonary risk: Include risk factors for perioperative pulmonary complications, the rationale for additional testing if indicated, and a plan for perioperative management for risk reduction.

3. DVT risk: Include risk factors for DVT risk and the rationale for a perioperative prophylaxis regimen.

4. Perioperative management of medical comorbidities: List other medical comorbidities that will affect perioperative care, and comment on management recommendations (for diabetes mellitus, seizure disorder, renal insufficiency, corticosteroid dependence, sleep apnea, hypertension, etc).

5. Perioperative management of medications: Include a plan for continuing or discontinuing use of medications and a recommendation for the timing of the administration of the medications.

6. Perioperative alerts: Include alerts for allergies, personal or family history of serious anesthetic complications, concern for difficult intubation, pacemaker dependence, defibrillator, known aortic stenosis, concern for neck instability in rheumatoid arthritis or Down syndrome patients, etc.

RISKS OF ANESTHESIA AND SURGERY

Mortality associated with anesthesia and surgery has decreased markedly in the past several decades. Today the overall mortality is 1:250,000 even though more complex surgical procedures are performed on sicker patients. The American Society of Anesthesiologists (ASA) classification, with broadly defined categories, is used to estimate overall risk of mortality within 48 hours postoperatively (Table 53.2). Although this classification system is quite subjective, it has stood the test of time and reproducibility in broadly estimating overall risk.

Neuraxial anesthesia and general anesthesia are not associated with significantly different outcomes for mortality and cardiac events. Many anesthesiologists recommend one type of anesthetic technique over another, depending on the surgical procedure performed and the comorbidities of the patient, but even though spinal, regional, and general anesthesia have different risks and benefits, the internist should not recommend a particular anesthetic technique or agent. This decision is best left to the anesthesia team at the time of surgery.

The type of operation performed is also an important determinant of cardiovascular morbidity and mortality (Table 53.3). However, the importance of comorbid disease in determining surgical risk may outweigh the nature of the procedure or the type of anesthesia used in predicting outcome. The following sections discuss 1) cardiac and pulmonary risk assessment and management strategies and 2) prophylaxis of thromboembolism and management of anticoagulants in the perioperative period.

CARDIAC RISK ASSESSMENT AND RISK REDUCTION STRATEGIES

Coronary artery disease (CAD) is a frequent cause of perioperative cardiac mortality and morbidity after noncardiac surgery. Perioperative myocardial infarction (MI) occurs in approximately 1% of general surgical procedures and in up to 3.2% of vascular surgical procedures. Among patients who have a perioperative MI, the hospital mortality rate is 15% to 25%, and those who survive to dismissal from the hospital have an increased risk of another MI and cardiovascular death during the ensuing 6 months postoperatively. Perioperative

Table 53.2 **AMERICAN SOCIETY OF ANESTHESIOLOGISTS CLASSIFICATION OF ANESTHETIC MORTALITY WITHIN 48 HOURS POSTOPERATIVELY**

CLASS	PHYSICAL STATUS	MORTALITY AT 48 H
I	Healthy person younger than 80 y	0.07%
II	Mild systemic disease	0.24%
III	Severe but not incapacitating systemic disease	1.4%
IV	Incapacitating systemic disease that is a constant threat to life	7.5%
V	Moribund patient not expected to survive 24 h, regardless of surgery	8.1%
E	Suffix added to any class to indicate emergency procedure	Doubles risk

Adapted from Pinnock C, Lin T, Smith T, Jones R. Fundamentals of anaesthesia. 2nd ed. London (UK): Greenwich Medical Media; c2003. Used with permission.

Table 53.3 CARDIAC RISK STRATIFICATION FOR NONCARDIAC SURGICAL PROCEDURES

REPORTED CARDIAC RISK[a]	PROCEDURE
High—often >5%	Emergent major operations, particularly in the elderly Aortic & other major vascular procedures Peripheral vascular procedures Anticipated prolonged surgical procedures associated with large fluid shifts or blood loss (or both)
Intermediate—generally <5%	Carotid endarterectomy Head & neck operations Intraperitoneal & intrathoracic procedures Orthopedic procedures Prostate operations
Low—generally <1%[b]	Endoscopic procedures Superficial procedures Cataract extraction Breast operation

[a] Combined incidence of cardiac death and nonfatal myocardial infarction.

[b] Further preoperative cardiac testing is not generally required.

Adapted from Fleisher LA, Beckman JA, Brown KA, Calkins H, Chaikof E, Fleischmann KE, et al. ACC/AHA 2007 guidelines on perioperative cardiovascular evaluation and care for noncardiac surgery: a report of the American College of Cardiology/American Heart Association Task Force on Practice Guidelines (Writing Committee to Revise the 2002 Guidelines on Perioperative Cardiovascular Evaluation for Noncardiac Surgery). J Am Coll Cardiol. 2007 Oct 23;50(17):e159–242 and Fleisher LA, Beckman JA, Brown KA, Calkins H, Chaikof E, Fleischmann KE, et al. ACC/AHA 2007 guidelines on perioperative cardiovascular evaluation and care for noncardiac surgery: a report of the American College of Cardiology/American Heart Association Task Force on Practice Guidelines (Writing Committee to Revise the 2002 Guidelines on Perioperative Cardiovascular Evaluation for Noncardiac Surgery): developed in collaboration with the American Society of Echocardiography, American Society of Nuclear Cardiology, Heart Rhythm Society, Society of Cardiovascular Anesthesiologists, Society for Cardiovascular Angiography and Interventions, Society for Vascular Medicine and Biology, and Society for Vascular Surgery. Circulation. 2007 Oct 23;116(17):e418–99. Epub 2007 Sep 27. Errata in: Circulation. 2008 Aug 26;118(9): e143–4. Circulation. 2008 Feb 5;117(5):e154. Used with permission.

death attributed to cardiac causes is less prevalent and occurs in 1% to 2% of all surgical procedures.

CARDIAC RISK ASSESSMENT

A stepwise approach is used for perioperative cardiac assessment as outlined in the "ACC/AHA 2007 Guidelines on Perioperative Cardiovascular Evaluation and Care for Noncardiac Surgery" (Figure 53.2). These guidelines present a framework for determining which patients are candidates for further testing on the basis of patient-related and surgery-related risk factors.

1. Surgical or percutaneous intervention is rarely necessary simply to lower the risk of surgery unless the intervention is indicated irrespective of the preoperative context.

2. No testing should be performed unless the results will influence patient treatment.

3. The guideline is intended to assist clinical decision making, not to replace clinical judgment.

4. The ultimate decision about the care of a particular patient must be made by the physician and the patient in light of all the specific clinical circumstances.

There are patient-specific factors and surgery-specific factors that contribute to cardiac risk. The patient-specific risk factors are clinical predictors (including the patient's relevant clinical history) and the patient's functional status. The surgery-specific risks are most often related to urgency, duration, and type of surgery.

Assessing Patient-Specific Risk

Clinical predictors of increased perioperative risk of MI, heart failure, and death are classified into 2 categories (active cardiac conditions and clinical risk factors) on the basis of the pretest probability of cardiac disease (Box 53.1).

Functional capacity is estimated from the patient's history and is expressed in METs. One MET is a unit of sitting or resting oxygen uptake per kilogram of body weight per minute. Oxygen uptake is considered the best measure of cardiovascular fitness and exercise capacity. Table 53.1 outlines the estimated energy requirements for various activities. A clinically useful cutoff is 4 METs. Perioperative cardiac and long-term risks are increased in patients who are unable to meet a 4-MET demand during most normal daily activities.

Assessing Surgery-Specific Risk

The surgery-specific cardiac risk of noncardiac surgery is related to 2 important factors: 1) the type of surgery itself, which may identify a patient with a greater likelihood of underlying heart disease (eg, vascular surgery), and 2) the degree of hemodynamic cardiac stress associated with the surgery. Certain operations may be associated with, for example, pain, blood loss, and profound alterations in heart rate, blood pressure, and vascular volume. Types of procedures and their surgery-specific risks of cardiac death and nonfatal MI are outlined in Table 53.3.

A STEPWISE APPROACH

With the above information, use the ACC/AHA guidelines in your decision process (Figure 53.2).

Step 1. Does the patient need emergency noncardiac surgery? If the answer is yes, the patient should be taken to the operating room without delay, and risk stratification and surveillance should be done postoperatively.

Step 2. Does the patient have an active cardiac condition (Box 53.1)? If an active cardiac condition exists, the patient should be evaluated according to ACC/AHA guidelines. If there are no active cardiac conditions, proceed to step 3.

Step 3. Is the patient undergoing low-risk surgery (ie, a skin, eye, or breast procedure)? If so, the patient can proceed to the operating room without further cardiac evaluation. If not, proceed to step 4.

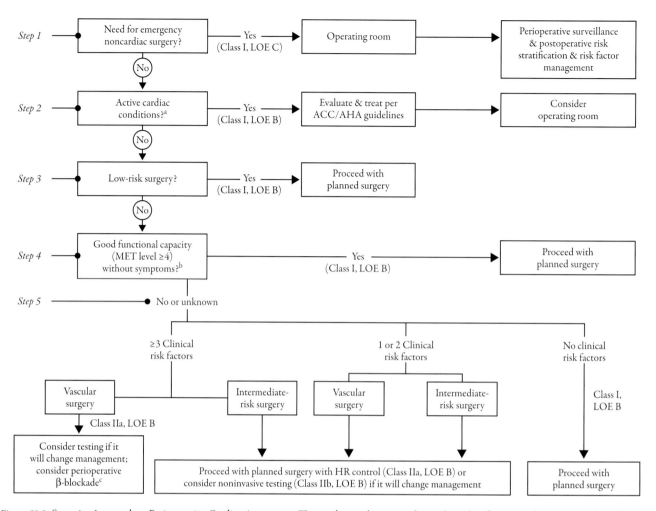

Figure 53.2 Stepwise Approach to Perioperative Cardiac Assessment. This cardiac evaluation and care algorithm for noncardiac surgery is based on active clinical conditions, known cardiovascular disease, and cardiac risk factors for patients 50 years or older as outlined in "ACC/AHA 2007 Guidelines on Perioperative Cardiovascular Evaluation and Care for Noncardiac Surgery." Clinical risk factors include ischemic heart disease, compensated or prior heart failure, diabetes mellitus, renal insufficiency, and cerebrovascular disease. Superscript letters indicate the following: [a], see Box 53.1; [b], see Table 53.1; [c], see Table 53.4. HR indicates heart rate; LOE, level of evidence; MET, metabolic equivalent task. (Adapted from Fleisher LA, Beckman JA, Brown KA, Calkins H, Chaikof E, Fleischmann KE, et al. ACC/AHA 2007 guidelines on perioperative cardiovascular evaluation and care for noncardiac surgery: a report of the American College of Cardiology/American Heart Association Task Force on Practice Guidelines [Writing Committee to Revise the 2002 Guidelines on Perioperative Cardiovascular Evaluation for Noncardiac Surgery]. J Am Coll Cardiol. 2007 Oct 23;50[17]:e159–242 and Fleisher LA, Beckman JA, Brown KA, Calkins H, Chaikof E, Fleischmann KE, et al. ACC/AHA 2007 guidelines on perioperative cardiovascular evaluation and care for noncardiac surgery: a report of the American College of Cardiology/American Heart Association Task Force on Practice Guidelines [Writing Committee to Revise the 2002 Guidelines on Perioperative Cardiovascular Evaluation for Noncardiac Surgery]: developed in collaboration with the American Society of Echocardiography, American Society of Nuclear Cardiology, Heart Rhythm Society, Society of Cardiovascular Anesthesiologists, Society for Cardiovascular Angiography and Interventions, Society for Vascular Medicine and Biology, and Society for Vascular Surgery. Circulation. 2007 Oct 23;116[17]:e418–99. Epub 2007 Sep 27. Errata in: Circulation. 2008 Aug 26;118[9]: e143–4. Circulation. 2008 Feb 5;117[5]:e154. Used with permission.)

Step 4. Does the patient have a good functional capacity (≥4 METs) without symptoms? If yes, the patient should proceed to surgery without further evaluation. If the functional capacity is unknown or less than 4 METs, proceed to step 5.

Step 5. Does the patient have any clinical risk factors (Box 53.1)?

1. With no clinical risk factors, the patient should proceed to surgery.

2. With 1 or 2 clinical risk factors, the patient should proceed to surgery with a β-blocker dosage that controls the heart rate at less than 65 beats per minute. Noninvasive testing should be performed only if the results will change management.

3. With 3 or more risk factors, the type of surgery needs to be considered.

   a. For an intermediate-risk procedure, the patient should proceed to surgery with a β-blocker dosage that controls the heart rate at less than 65 beats per minute. Noninvasive testing should be performed only if the results will change management.

b. For vascular surgery, noninvasive or invasive testing should be considered if the results will change management. Often, heart rate control with β-blockers is the best course of action even in the highest-risk patients.

If the decision has been made, based on risk assessment, that further cardiac testing is advisable, the next step is to choose the appropriate testing modality. There are many options for noninvasive testing, including exercise stress testing without imaging, exercise testing with imaging (nuclear or echocardiographic), and pharmacologic stress testing with imaging (nuclear or echocardiographic). Some tests are contraindicated in certain populations; some tests may be more useful than others, depending on the clinical situation.

Choose the Method of Myocardial Stress

Exercise

1. If patients can achieve 85% of the maximal predicted heart rate for their age and do not have left bundle branch block (LBBB), a regular Bruce exercise stress test is the most cost-effective test for preoperative cardiac risk stratification.

2. Avoid exercise if a patient has baseline LBBB (because of false-positive results on imaging).

3. If the patient cannot exercise, myocardial stress can be achieved with either a vasodilator (dipyridamole or adenosine) or an inotropic catecholamine (dobutamine).

Vasodilator (Dipyridamole or Adenosine)

1. Avoid in patients who have second- or third-degree heart block, sick sinus syndrome, symptomatic bradycardia, hypotension, critical carotid disease (cerebral ischemia), or bronchorestrictive or bronchospastic disease.

2. Favor in patients with LBBB, multiple wall motion abnormalities at baseline, history of coronary artery bypass graft (CABG) surgery, severe hypertension, or symptomatic arrhythmias (atrial fibrillation with rapid ventricular response, paroxysmal supraventricular tachycardia, etc).

Inotropic Catecholamine (Dobutamine)

1. Avoid in patients who have clinically significant hypertension or hypotension or LBBB (because of the association with false-positive results).

2. Favor in patients with borderline-low or low blood pressure, bradycardia, bronchospastic or bronchorestrictive disease, or heart block.

Choose the Method of Myocardial Imaging

1. If the patient meets appropriate criteria (ie, normal baseline electrocardiogram [ECG], no pacemaker, no use of digoxin, no history of percutaneous intervention or CABG surgery, and no LBBB), no additional imaging is needed.

2. Imaging can be achieved with nuclear agents (sestamibi or thallium) or with echocardiography:

   a. Nuclear imaging.

      1) More appropriate in patients who have poor echocardiographic windows, multiple wall motion abnormalities at baseline, or a history of multivessel revascularization.

   b. Echocardiographic imaging.

      1) Preferred in patients with valvular dysfunction, known decreased ejection fraction, or large breasts that might be associated with false-positive results in nuclear imaging studies.

      2) Gives additional anatomical and functional information beyond what nuclear imaging can give and is generally more cost effective.

3. In general, the diagnostic accuracy is similar between nuclear perfusion imaging and echocardiography.

Although routine perioperative evaluation of left ventricular function is not recommended, it is reasonable in some clinical situations to obtain a resting echocardiogram before planned elective surgery. These situations may include patients with dyspnea of unknown cause or patients with current heart failure or a prior history of heart failure who have worsening dyspnea or a change in clinical status. If patients are clinically stable, routine echocardiography is not recommended unless a valvular abnormality or other clinically significant cardiac abnormality is suspected from the clinical examination.

Recent evidence suggests that surgical or percutaneous intervention is rarely necessary simply to decrease the surgical risk unless the intervention is indicated irrespective of the preoperative context. Because percutaneous or surgical intervention is also associated with risk of adverse cardiac outcomes, a morbidity and mortality advantage has not been shown for most patients when these interventions are performed before noncardiac surgery. The exception, however, is patients who would have been referred for intervention irrespective of the preoperative context (eg, left main CAD, severe 3-vessel disease). In general, preoperative revascularization is beneficial in patients who have any of the following:

1. Clinically significant left main CAD.

2. Stable angina and 3-vessel disease.

3. Coronary artery stenosis and either an ejection fraction <50% or demonstrable ischemia on noninvasive testing.

4. High-risk, unstable angina or non–ST-segment elevation MI.

5. Acute ST-segment elevation MI.

The expected timing of the planned surgical procedure also needs to be considered when deciding on the type of revascularization procedure. Surgery performed within 30 days of CABG surgery is associated with an increased risk of postoperative cardiac complications. Percutaneous interventions with angioplasty alone or in conjunction with stent placement also require an appropriate course of dual antiplatelet therapy during vessel injury healing and reendothelialization. To decrease the risk of adverse cardiac outcomes and death, nonemergent surgery should be postponed for at least 2 weeks after balloon angioplasty, 4 to 6 weeks after bare metal stent placement, and 1 year after drug-eluting stent placement.

β-Blockers have been reported to decrease the risk of perioperative cardiac complications in patients who are at risk. This subject is controversial because recent data have shown mixed results. However, until additional studies are completed, the ACC/AHA guidelines published in 2007 are the best resource (Table 53.4). Patients receiving β-blockers, regardless of the indication, should continue taking them in the perioperative period to avoid a rebound effect on blood pressure and pulse. Patients receiving β-blockers for perioperative cardiac risk reduction should begin taking them a few days preoperatively so that the dose can be adjusted to achieve a resting heart rate of 55 to 65 beats per minute. The dose must be adjusted in the postoperative period (2–5 days) to keep the heart rate at 55 to 65 beats per minute and to achieve maximal benefit for risk reduction.

Recent data have not supported the practice of avoiding use of β-blockers in patients who have a diagnosis of chronic obstructive pulmonary disease (COPD). However, instituting β-blockade in these patients should be done cautiously. For most patients, administration of a perioperative β-blocker is not associated with an increase in pulmonary symptoms.

There is insufficient evidence to suggest that the perioperative use of calcium channel blockers or nitrates reduces cardiac outcomes. In several studies, statins improved perioperative outcomes in vascular surgery patients, so statin use should continue throughout the perioperative period. Use of aspirin should not be stopped in high-risk patients unless it is absolutely necessary from a perioperative bleeding standpoint; aspirin withdrawal is associated with a rebound in platelet adhesiveness in the perioperative period, which puts the patient at increased risk of perioperative MI.

MONITORING FOR PERIOPERATIVE ISCHEMIA

Patients who have CAD or major risk factors for CAD are at higher risk of perioperative myocardial ischemia or MI. Although most perioperative ischemic events usually occur within 48 hours after surgery, many occur during anesthesia recovery or shortly thereafter owing to many ischemia-provoking stimuli (tachycardia, hypertension, hypercoagulability, sympathetic discharge, pain, etc).

Table 53.4 **PERIOPERATIVE β-BLOCKADE RECOMMENDATIONS BASED ON PUBLISHED RANDOMIZED CONTROLLED TRIALS**

SURGERY	NO CLINICAL RISK FACTORS[a]	≥1 CLINICAL RISK FACTORS[a]	CAD OR HIGH CARDIAC RISK	PATIENTS CURRENTLY TAKING β-BLOCKERS
Vascular	May consider	May consider	Yes[b] Reasonable to consider[c]	Yes
High-risk or intermediate-risk	Insufficient data	May consider	Reasonable to consider	Yes
Low-risk	Insufficient data	Insufficient data	Insufficient data	Yes

Abbreviation: CAD, coronary artery disease.

[a] Clinical risk factors: history of ischemic heart disease (including pathologic Q waves on electrocardiography); history of compensated heart failure or prior heart failure (systolic or diastolic); history of cerebrovascular disease (transient ischemic attack or stroke); diabetes mellitus requiring insulin; or renal insufficiency (preoperative serum creatinine >2 mg/dL).

[b] For patients found to have coronary ischemia on preoperative testing or patients found to have CAD.

[c] For patients without ischemia or no previous testing.

Adapted from Fleisher LA, Beckman JA, Brown KA, Calkins H, Chaikof E, Fleischmann KE, et al. ACC/AHA 2007 guidelines on perioperative cardiovascular evaluation and care for noncardiac surgery: a report of the American College of Cardiology/American Heart Association Task Force on Practice Guidelines (Writing Committee to Revise the 2002 Guidelines on Perioperative Cardiovascular Evaluation for Noncardiac Surgery). J Am Coll Cardiol. 2007 Oct 23;50(17):e159–242 and Fleisher LA, Beckman JA, Brown KA, Calkins H, Chaikof E, Fleischmann KE, et al. ACC/AHA 2007 guidelines on perioperative cardiovascular evaluation and care for noncardiac surgery: a report of the American College of Cardiology/American Heart Association Task Force on Practice Guidelines (Writing Committee to Revise the 2002 Guidelines on Perioperative Cardiovascular Evaluation for Noncardiac Surgery): developed in collaboration with the American Society of Echocardiography, American Society of Nuclear Cardiology, Heart Rhythm Society, Society of Cardiovascular Anesthesiologists, Society for Cardiovascular Angiography and Interventions, Society for Vascular Medicine and Biology, and Society for Vascular Surgery. Circulation. 2007 Oct 23;116(17):e418–99. Epub 2007 Sep 27. Errata in: Circulation. 2008 Aug 26;118(9): e143–4. Circulation. 2008 Feb 5;117(5):e154. Used with permission.

Perioperative cardiac ischemia is often not associated with major or classic symptoms. Instead, it is usually associated with non–ST-segment elevation and non–Q-wave events. The most cost-effective approach to ischemia monitoring in high-risk patients is to evaluate serial ECGs obtained preoperatively, immediately postoperatively, and on postoperative days 1 and 2. Patients who do have ST-segment changes suggestive of ischemia are at significantly increased risk of future MI and other adverse cardiac events. Diligent postoperative follow-up with additional testing and risk factor modification is indicated if perioperative ischemia or infarction is identified.

Biochemical evidence of myocardial injury is common in the perioperative period. Troponins are both sensitive and specific for myocardial injury, and troponin levels should be determined in patients who have signs, symptoms, or ECG evidence of ischemia. However, troponin determination as a surveillance method for perioperative ischemia is not cost-effective and should be reserved for patients at high risk of cardiac complications and who are undergoing a major surgical procedure.

PATIENTS WITH CORONARY STENTS

The "ACC/AHA 2007 Guidelines on Perioperative Cardiovascular Evaluation and Care for Noncardiac Surgery" also recommend an approach to patients who have had coronary stent placement in the past. This is an important issue because premature discontinuation of dual antiplatelet therapy markedly increases the risk of catastrophic stent thrombosis and death or MI.

Approximately 5% of patients who undergo coronary stenting require a surgical procedure within 1 year after stent placement. For patients with bare metal stents, elective or nonurgent surgery should be delayed for 30 to 45 days after placement. After 30 to 45 days of dual antiplatelet therapy, surgery should be done with the patient receiving aspirin. Patients with drug-eluting stents should have elective or nonurgent surgery delayed at least 365 days after placement. After 1 year of dual antiplatelet therapy, surgery should be done while the patient is receiving aspirin. If urgent or emergent surgery is needed within the required dual antiplatelet therapy window, a difficult choice has to be made. The generally accepted policy is to stop antiplatelet therapy 7 to 10 days before a surgical or endoscopic procedure because of the possibility of excessive bleeding. However, premature discontinuation of antiplatelet therapy markedly increases the risk of stent thrombosis, a catastrophic event that frequently leads to myocardial infarction or death. Premature discontinuation of antiplatelet therapy results in a perioperative cardiac death rate that is increased 5 to 10 times, with an average incidence of death of about 30%. The case fatality rate is 45% for patients in whom stent thrombosis develops. This obviously puts internists, surgeons, and patients in a difficult situation. In this case, it is best to compare the risks and benefits of continuation of the antiplatelet therapy with discontinuation.

What is the risk of surgical bleeding with antiplatelet agents? Aspirin increases the rate of bleeding complications by 1.5 times; however, for most surgical procedures, this is not associated with an increase in the severity of bleeding complications or in the mortality due to bleeding complications. The exceptions are for intracranial neurosurgical procedures and transurethral prostate procedures. Compared with aspirin alone, aspirin in combination with clopidogrel is associated with a 30% to 50% increase in relative risk (0.4%-1.0% absolute risk) of major bleeding perioperatively. In studies of perioperative patients with drug-eluting stents, dual antiplatelet therapy did not result in increased surgical mortality (except during intracranial neurosurgery) but was associated with a slight increase in the need for reoperation and a 30% increase in the need for transfusion.

If the surgery presents minimal bleeding risk (cataract surgeries, dermatologic procedures, etc), some experts have advocated that the patient continue dual antiplatelet therapy in the perioperative period. If the surgical bleeding risk is too high, the antiplatelet therapy can be stopped, but it should be resumed as soon as possible postoperatively (preferably requiring the patient to stop the antiplatelet therapy for only 5 days or less, if possible).

Stent thrombosis is a serious risk in the perioperative period, and any decision to stop dual antiplatelet therapy before the full recommended course should not be made until after a detailed discussion with the patient and the family about the risk of a potentially catastrophic outcome should stent thrombosis occur while antiplatelet therapy is interrupted.

PULMONARY RISK ASSESSMENT AND RISK REDUCTION STRATEGIES

Pulmonary complications (respiratory failure, atelectasis, and pneumonia) are as common as cardiac complications in patients undergoing noncardiothoracic surgery, with an overall rate of approximately 6%. These complications account for an increase in hospital length of stay and for an increase in perioperative morbidity and mortality.

PULMONARY RISK ASSESSMENT

Pulmonary risk can be divided into patient-related risk factors and procedure-related risk factors (Table 53.5). Although it seems intuitive that obesity, asthma, restrictive lung disease, and obstructive sleep apnea (OSA) would be associated with an increased incidence of perioperative pulmonary complications, there is not good evidence that this is the case. Clinical studies have not shown an increased risk of postoperative pulmonary complications in obese patients, even if they are morbidly obese. Patients with mild or moderate asthma have not been shown to have increased risk, nor have patients with chronic restrictive lung disease or restrictive physiologic characteristics (neuromuscular disease or chest wall deformities). OSA increases the risk of airway management problems, but its influence on postoperative pulmonary complications has not been well studied. OSA has been shown, however, to be associated with increases in the number of unplanned

Table 53.5 RISK FACTORS FOR PERIOPERATIVE PULMONARY COMPLICATIONS

RISK FACTORS	ODDS RATIO (95% CI)
Patient-Related	
ASA class ≥II	4.9 (3.3–7.1)
Chronic obstructive pulmonary disease	2.4 (1.9–2.9)
Age, y	
50–59	1.5 (1.3–1.7)
60–69	2.3 (1.9–2.8)
70–79	3.9 (2.7–5.7)
≥80	5.6 (4.6–6.9)
Functional dependence	
Total dependence	2.5 (2.0–3.2)
Partial dependence	1.7 (1.4–2.0)
Congestive heart failure	2.9 (1.0–8.4)
Serum albumin <35 g/L	2.5 (2.0–2.6)
Impaired sensorium	1.4 (1.1–1.8)
Cigarette use	1.4 (1.2–1.7)
Procedure-Related	
Surgical site or type of procedure	
Open abdominal aortic repair	6.9 (2.7–17.4)
Thoracic	4.2 (2.9–6.2)
Abdominal	3.1 (2.5–3.8)
Neurosurgical	2.5 (1.8–3.5)
Head & neck	2.2 (1.6–2.7)
Vascular	2.1 (0.8–5.4)
Emergency surgery	2.5 (1.7–3.8)
Prolonged surgery (>3 h)	2.3 (1.5–3.5)
General anesthesia	2.4 (1.8–3.1)
Transfusion >4 units	1.5 (1.3–1.7)

Abbreviation: ASA, American Society of Anesthesiologists.

Adapted from Smetana GW, Lawrence VA, Cornell JE; American College of Physicians. Preoperative pulmonary risk stratification for noncardiothoracic surgery: systematic review for the American College of Physicians. Ann Intern Med. 2006 Apr 18;144(8):581–95. Used with permission.

intensive care unit transfers, serious complications, and length of hospital stay in the postoperative period.

- Significant patient-related risk factors include COPD, age older than 60 years, ASA class ≥II, functional dependence, congestive heart failure, and serum albumin <35 g/L.

- Obesity, mild or moderate asthma, and restrictive lung disease are not significant risk factors for postoperative pulmonary complications.

- Procedure-related risk factors include prolonged surgery (>3 hours), open aortic aneurysm repair, abdominal surgery, thoracic surgery, head and neck surgery, vascular surgery, emergency surgery, and general anesthesia.

PULMONARY TESTING

Historically, the common practice was to evaluate patients with spirometry testing and chest radiography during the routine preoperative evaluation as a way to predict the risk of pulmonary complications. Although consensus exists on the value of spirometry before lung resection or CABG surgery, the value of spirometry before extrathoracic surgery has not been shown. Similarly, routine chest radiography has not been shown to influence perioperative management in patients undergoing nonthoracic surgery. Spirometry and chest radiography may be appropriate in patients undergoing extrathoracic surgery who have a previous diagnosis of COPD or asthma or who have respiratory symptoms identified during the preoperative evaluation. Additionally, some evidence suggests that chest radiography may be helpful if patients have cardiopulmonary disease or if they are older than 50 years and are undergoing upper abdominal, thoracic, or abdominal aortic aneurysm surgery. Although a low serum albumin level has been identified as a powerful predictor of risk of postoperative pulmonary complications, obtaining albumin levels routinely in the preoperative evaluation has not been the standard of care.

- Spirometry and chest radiography may be appropriate in patients undergoing extrathoracic surgery who have a previous diagnosis of COPD or asthma or who have respiratory symptoms identified during the preoperative evaluation.

- Some evidence suggests that chest radiography may be helpful if patients have cardiopulmonary disease or if they are older than 50 years and are undergoing upper abdominal, thoracic, or abdominal aortic aneurysm surgery.

RISK REDUCTION STRATEGIES

All patients who are identified as having an increased risk of postoperative pulmonary complications should receive both of the following interventions postoperatively:

1. Deep breathing exercises or incentive spirometry (positive airway pressure for patients unable to perform these).

2. Selective use of a nasogastric tube (as needed for postoperative nausea and vomiting, inability to tolerate oral intake, or symptomatic abdominal distension).

The following procedures should not be used for the purpose of reducing postoperative pulmonary complications:

1. Right heart catheterization.

2. Total parenteral or enteral nutrition (for patients who are malnourished or have low serum albumin levels).

VENOUS THROMBOEMBOLIC PROPHYLAXIS

Although all surgical patients are at increased risk of venous thromboembolic (VTE) disease, certain patients form a

Table 53.6 LEVELS OF THROMBOEMBOLISM RISK AND RECOMMENDED THROMBOPROPHYLAXIS IN HOSPITAL PATIENTS[a]

LEVEL OF RISK	APPROXIMATE DVT RISK WITHOUT THROMBOPROPHYLAXIS, %[b]	SUGGESTED THROMBOPROPHYLAXIS OPTIONS
Low		
Minor surgery in mobile patients	<10	No specific thromboprophylaxis
Medical patients who are fully mobile		Early and "aggressive" ambulation
Moderate		
Most general, open gynecologic or urologic surgery patients	10–40	LMWH (at recommended doses), LDUH 2 or 3 times daily, fondaparinux
Medical patients (bed rest or sick)		
Moderate VTE risk plus high bleeding risk		Mechanical thromboprophylaxis[c]
High		
Hip or knee arthroplasty, hip fracture surgery	40–80	LMWH (at recommended doses), fondaparinux, oral vitamin K antagonist (INR 2–3)
Major trauma, spinal cord injury		
High VTE risk plus high bleeding risk		Mechanical thromboprophylaxis[c]

Abbreviations: DVT, deep vein thrombosis; INR, international normalized ratio; LDUH, low-dose unfractionated heparin; LMWH, low-molecular-weight heparin; VTE, venous thromboembolic.

[a] The descriptive terms are purposely left undefined to allow individual clinician interpretation.

[b] Rates are based on objective diagnostic screening for asymptomatic DVT in patients not receiving thromboprophylaxis.

[c] Mechanical thromboprophylaxis includes intermittent pneumatic compression or venous foot pump, with or without graduated compression stockings; consider switching to anticoagulant thromboprophylaxis when high bleeding risk decreases.

Adapted from Geerts WH, Bergqvist D, Pineo GF, Heit JA, Samama CM, Lassen MR, et al. Prevention of venous thromboembolism: American College of Chest Physicians Evidence-Based Clinical Practice Guidelines (8th Edition). Chest. 2008 Jun;133(Pt 6 Suppl):381S–453S. Used with permission.

high-risk subset, including those who are elderly and those who have prolonged anesthesia, previous VTE, hereditary disorders of thrombosis, prolonged immobilization or paralysis, malignancy, obesity, varicosities, or pharmacologic estrogen use. The American College of Chest Physicians released the eighth edition of its antithrombotic and thrombolytic therapy guidelines, which includes a section on prevention of venous thromboembolism. This guideline is lengthy and provides group-specific recommendations for patients undergoing surgery. A simplified classification system is outlined in Table 53.6.

General principles to keep in mind include the following:

1. Aspirin alone is not recommended as prophylaxis against VTE for any patient group.

2. Patients undergoing an operation for hip or knee replacement, hip fracture, or malignancy are at particularly high risk. In these patient populations, prophylaxis is more aggressive and data suggest that prophylaxis should continue after hospital dismissal (from 10 days to 1 month).

3. Consider renal impairment when deciding on doses of low-molecular-weight heparin, fondaparinux, and other antithrombotic drugs that are renally excreted, particularly for elderly patients and those who are at high risk of bleeding. Many of these drugs are contraindicated in dialysis patients.

4. In all patients undergoing neuraxial anesthesia or analgesia, use special caution when using anticoagulants

for DVT prophylaxis—it may be best to wait until the catheter is removed.

5. Some patients should continue a prolonged course of DVT prophylaxis well after hospital dismissal. Patients undergoing major surgery for malignancy, hip or knee replacement, or hip fracture repair require 2 to 6 weeks of DVT prophylaxis postoperatively. Details on specific duration and recommended methods are described in the American College of Chest Physicians guidelines.

PREOPERATIVE TESTING GUIDELINES

Results of routine laboratory and diagnostic tests, while often obtained, usually have little effect on perioperative management. Therefore, routine tests are often not necessary before many surgical procedures unless a specific indication is present.

COAGULATION STUDIES

Prothrombin time and international normalized ratio are recommended for patients who have a known coagulation abnormality or a history suggestive of coagulation problems (chronic liver disease, malnutrition, excessive bleeding with past procedures, etc). Additionally, patients who are taking anticoagulants or who will receive full doses of anticoagulants postoperatively should have coagulation studies preoperatively. Partial thromboplastin time and bleeding time are rarely indicated for these patients preoperatively.

COMPLETE BLOOD CELL COUNT

Hemoglobin measurement is recommended for patients with a history of anemia, diseases known to cause anemia, a history of recent blood loss, or physical signs suggestive of anemia (ie, tachycardia and pallor). Additionally, patients who are undergoing operations in which clinically significant blood loss is anticipated (cardiac procedures, major vascular surgery, major spinal surgery, etc) should have a baseline hemoglobin measurement. Often, it is requested if the patient's blood is being typed and crossmatched.

A *white blood cell count* is appropriate for patients who have conditions known to affect the white blood cell count, who are taking medications known to affect the white blood cell count, or who have symptoms of infection at the preoperative evaluation.

Platelet counts are recommended for patients with a history of platelet abnormalities or myeloproliferative disease and for patients who are taking medications known to alter platelet counts. Of course, if the history and physical examination identify concerns for altered hemostasis, platelet counts would also be indicated preoperatively.

ELECTROLYTES

Measurement of the *potassium* level should be considered for patients who are taking digoxin, diuretics, angiotensin-converting enzyme inhibitors, angiotensin receptor blockers, or other medications known to alter electrolytes. It is recommended for any patient with a history of renal insufficiency or renal failure.

Measurement of the *sodium* level should be considered for patients who are undergoing urologic procedures that involve bladder irrigation or patients who have conditions associated with hyponatremia or hypernatremia (congestive heart failure, liver failure, syndrome of inappropriate secretion of antidiuretic hormone, etc).

CREATININE

Measurement of the creatinine level is recommended for patients with any of the following: renal insufficiency, age older than 50 years, diabetes mellitus, hypertension, cardiovascular disease, plans to undergo major surgery, or use of medications that may affect renal function.

GLUCOSE

Glucose determination is recommended only for patients who have risk factors for diabetes mellitus or who are known to have diabetes and need to assess glucose control.

LIVER TESTS

Liver tests are rarely helpful preoperatively unless there is clinical concern that the test results might be relevant to the decision to proceed with surgery.

URINALYSIS

Urinalysis is recommended only for patients with urologic symptoms at the preoperative evaluation or before a urologic procedure or certain orthopedic procedures. Orthopedic surgeons often request that a urinalysis be done before the placement of hardware to ensure that there is no potential focus of infection that could possibly seed the new hardware.

ELECTROCARDIOGRAPHY

An ECG is recommended before intermediate- or high-risk surgery for men older than 40 years, or women older than 50. Additionally, an ECG is recommended for any patient (regardless of age) with known CAD or for those who are at increased risk of CAD because they have a history of diabetes mellitus, cerebrovascular disease, hypertension, chest pain, congestive heart failure, smoking, peripheral vascular disease, inability to exercise, or morbid obesity. An ECG is recommended for any patient with any new cardiovascular symptoms or with signs and symptoms of new or unstable cardiac disease. An ECG performed within 6 months preoperatively is adequate if clinical symptoms have not changed in the interim.

CHEST RADIOGRAPHY

Chest radiography is recommended for patients older than 50 years, patients who have known cardiac or pulmonary disease, and patients who have symptoms or physical examination findings suggestive of new or unstable cardiopulmonary disease.

HOSPITAL MEDICINE

Majid Shafiq, MD, Neel B. Shah, MB, BCh, and James S. Newman, MD

GOALS

- Recognize the signs of alcohol withdrawal.

- Recognize the importance of medication reconciliation.

- Understand nutritional assessment and replacement in hospitalized patients.

- Discern complications that are commonly associated with hospitalization and surgery.

- Comprehend the importance of patient satisfaction and quality improvement.

INTRODUCTION

Technologic advancements and other innovative efforts to improve the quality of hospital-based care have resulted in large, complicated networks of personnel, information systems, devices, medications, and countless other resources. In parallel with these changes, the medical acuity of the typical hospitalized patient has increased. The field of hospital medicine emerged in response to this combination of increasing hospital complexity, patient acuity, and professional demands.

HOSPITAL ADMISSION

On admission to the hospital, there are opportunities to identify issues that, if not addressed, may lead to poor outcomes. These include the following:

1. Recognizing cultural and other barriers to communication

2. Identifying substance abuse and nutritional status

3. Most importantly, reconciling medication

CROSS-CULTURAL AWARENESS

A person's education level, social habits, employment and occupational history, and cultural background contribute to shaping the patient-physician relationship, the style of communication used, the risk of complications, and the management strategy.

For example, at least one-sixth of the people in the United States speak a language other than English in their homes. If language barriers are not addressed, a patient with limited English proficiency may be at higher risk of an adverse event. Accordingly, all health care facilities that receive federal funding are obligated to provide interpreter services for patients who do not speak English and for patients who are deaf.

A patient's religious beliefs may also need to be incorporated into the management plan. For example, for a patient who is a Jehovah's Witness, acknowledging, reconfirming, and abiding by a refusal to accept blood transfusions is essential to appropriate care. For a patient with dietary restrictions, the most important intervention from a patient satisfaction viewpoint may be provision of meals that are kosher (Jewish), halal (Muslim), or beef-free (Hindu).

PATIENTS WITH INTELLECTUAL DISABILITY

Compared with the general population, patients who have intellectual disability (ID) are more likely to use the US health care system. Annually, 30% of patients with ID are seen in emergency departments and 16% are hospitalized.

Patients with trisomy 21 have an increased likelihood of congenital heart disease, hearing deficits, seizures, depression, premature Alzheimer disease, hypothyroidism, celiac disease, type 1 diabetes mellitus, obstructive sleep apnea, and atlanto-axial instability (which may complicate endotracheal intubation). In addition, patients with ID may be at increased risk of aspiration due to neuromuscular dysfunction.

Assessment of patients with ID may be complicated by their associated behavioral abnormalities. Self-injurious behavior may be a clue to uncontrolled pain, especially in nonverbal individuals. Screening for occult fractures, corneal abrasions, and other possible sources of pain may be indicated.

Many patients with ID have surrogate decision makers (relatives or court-appointed guardians), and ethical issues may arise. In addition, these patients (and their care providers) may have additional socioeconomic needs compared with patients who do not have ID.

TREATMENT OF ALCOHOL WITHDRAWAL

Alcohol abuse in hospitalized patients is underrecognized. Patients with alcohol withdrawal are best treated as inpatients, especially if they have a history of seizures, delirium tremens, psychiatric disease, or multiple medical comorbidities. Delirium tremens occurs in up to 20% of untreated patients with alcohol withdrawal.

Patients in early withdrawal, within 48 hours of the last drink, may have mild hypertension and tachycardia, mild hyperthermia, fine tremors, agitation, slightly impaired orientation, and early visual and auditory hallucinations. Seizures may occur during early withdrawal and may be the presenting complaint for admission. Seizures can occur in up to one-third of the patients and should be considered in patients who have had withdrawal seizures previously. Other causes or cofactors to exclude are hyponatremia, hypoglycemia, central nervous system trauma, and infection. Alcohol withdrawal seizures are best treated with benzodiazepines.

It is hard to predict which patients will progress to late withdrawal (ie, delirium tremens). Risk factors include older age, concomitant medical disease, prior delirium tremens, and abnormal liver function test results. This condition is characterized by tachycardia, hyperthermia, gross tremors, delirium, disorientation, and hallucinations. Nausea and vomiting may lead to aspiration. Fluctuations in blood pressure may predispose the patient to cardiac and cerebrovascular events. Patients with arrhythmias need to be monitored, and often a bed in the intensive care unit is required if the patient is severely affected and may need intubation. Severe withdrawal carries a significant risk of death.

Patients with alcohol withdrawal are evaluated with the revised Clinical Institute Withdrawal Assessment (CIWA), a symptom-based nurse-administered scale for assessing nausea and vomiting, tremulousness, diaphoresis, anxiety, agitation, paresthesias, auditory and visual disturbances, headache, and disorientation. The results are used for determining the benzodiazepine dosage. Patients who have had severe withdrawal previously should receive a loading dose of benzodiazepines, preferably one with a longer half-life, such as chlordiazepoxide. Phenobarbital can be used if withdrawal is refractory to benzodiazepines; however, patients receiving both of these agents may not be able to protect their airway. Alcoholic patients should routinely receive chemical dependency counseling and psychiatric evaluation. Notably, these patients are at risk of Wernicke encephalopathy, which is seen in thiamine-deficient patients and is characterized by palsy of the abducens nerve (cranial nerve VI), nystagmus, ataxia, and disorientation. The usual replacement dosage of thiamine is 100 mg daily. Hypomagnesemia should be treated since a low magnesium level may decrease the seizure threshold.

- Alcohol abuse in hospitalized patients is often underrecognized.
- The revised CIWA is a symptom-based scale for assessing nausea and vomiting, tremulousness, diaphoresis, anxiety, agitation, paresthesias, auditory and visual disturbances, headache, and disorientation.

- Delirium tremens occurs in up to 20% of untreated patients with alcohol withdrawal.
- Wernicke encephalopathy, seen in thiamine-deficient patients, is characterized by palsy of the abducens nerve (cranial nerve VI), nystagmus, ataxia, and disorientation.

MEDICATION RECONCILIATION

Medication reconciliation involves comparing a patient's medication orders or prescriptions with the list of medications that the patient has actually been taking. This process must occur with each transition of care to decrease the risk of duplications, incorrect dose or frequency, omissions, and drug interactions—errors that occur too easily during transitions of care and lead to considerable morbidity and mortality. All medications should be reviewed for ongoing indications. For example, proton pump inhibitors, which are often prescribed for prophylaxis at admission are commonly continued afterward without an indication.

Polypharmacy is common among geriatric patients and patients receiving treatment for psychiatric conditions. Each year, patients older than 65 years fill an average of 12 prescriptions in addition to buying over-the-counter and herbal medications. Medication reconciliation becomes even more crucial for these patients since the risk of adverse events increases with the number of medications.

The use of electronic health records (EHRs) does not eliminate the need for careful medication reconciliation; an outdated EHR itself can be the source of serious medication errors and provide a false sense of security. Arguably, the most important innovation for applying EHRs to The Joint Commission's National Patient Safety Goal is improved interoperability of medication lists across organizations and EHRs.

NUTRITIONAL ASSESSMENT AND PROVISION IN THE HOSPITAL

Up to 40% of patients admitted to the hospital may be malnourished. While hospitalization offers opportunities to correct this condition, a patient's nutritional status can also worsen malnutrition since the acute illness that led to hospitalization may trigger a hypermetabolic state. If the digestive tract is functioning properly, and the person can eat, malnourishment may be the consequence of impaired access to adequate food. Patients most at risk of malnutrition include those with gastrointestinal tract dysfunction (eg, xerostomia, dysphagia, malabsorption, pancreatitis, and diarrhea), malignancy, infection, chronic lung disease, alcoholism, and depression. Micronutrient deficiencies are often associated with specific signs and symptoms (Table 54.1).

Patients who cannot eat enough to satisfy metabolic demand should be evaluated for a mechanical feeding problem, malabsorption, or causes of increased metabolic requirements. Mechanical feeding problems may require altering the consistency of food and nutritional supplements.

Table 54.1 NUTRITIONAL DEFICIENCIES[a]

NUTRIENT	SIGNS, SYMPTOMS, & ASSOCIATED CONDITIONS
Onset After Short-term (Weeks) Deficiency	
Vitamin B$_1$ (thiamine)	Wet beriberi—congestive heart failure, edema Dry beriberi—neurologic disease
Vitamin B$_2$ (riboflavin)	Sore throat, hyperemic mucosae, normocytic normochromic anemia May be due to phenothiazines, tricyclic antidepressants
Vitamin B$_6$ (pyridoxine)	Seizures, glossitis, cheilosis May be due to isoniazid, cycloserine, penicillamine
Vitamin C	Petechial & gingival hemorrhage, corkscrew hair, spongy gums with tooth loss, poor wound healing
Magnesium	Muscle stiffness, tetany
Zinc	Acrodermatitis, poor wound healing
Essential fatty acids	Alopecia, thrombocytopenia, anemia, dermatitis Consider in patients receiving parenteral nutrition
Onset After Mid-term (Months) Deficiency	
Copper	Hypochromic microcytic anemia
Vitamin K	Bleeding, high prothrombin time, & international normalized ratio
Vitamin B$_3$ (niacin)	Pellagra (diarrhea, dermatitis, dementia)
Onset After Long-term (Years) Deficiency	
Vitamin A	Night blindness (may progress to permanent blindness)
Vitamin D	Rickets, osteomalacia, elevated parathyroid hormone level Calcium level may initially be normal
Vitamin E	Areflexia, decreased vibrational & positional sense
Selenium	Myalgias, cardiomyopathy, hemolytic anemia
Chromium	Glucose intolerance, peripheral neuropathy
Iron	Anemia, restless legs syndrome
Cobalt	Anemia
Vitamin B$_{12}$ (cobalamin)	Macrocytic anemia, smooth tongue, subacute combined degeneration of the spinal cord, bilateral paresthesias, impaired proprioception & vibrational sense, spastic ataxia, central scotomata, dementia, weakness, hyperreflexia, bilateral extensor plantar responses

[a] Many complications are frequently attributed to micronutrient deficiencies that are still controversial, especially when complications occur without classic features and with measured nutrient levels near or within the reference range (eg, putative associations of vitamin D deficiency).

Nutrition should be delivered enterally whenever possible. Notably, enteral feeding decreases the risk of stress ulcer bleeding. A long-term need for enteral feeding may require a percutaneous transabdominal gastric or jejunal tube. Patients with problems with gastric emptying or aspiration may benefit from a nasojejunal feeding tube. A nasogastric tube does not prevent aspiration.

Parenteral nutrition may be provided through a peripheral (short-term) or central (long-term) intravenous catheter. The core components of parenteral nutrition are amino acids, vitamins, electrolytes, and fat. The electrolytes depleted most commonly in the hospital are magnesium, potassium, phosphorous, and calcium. Refeeding syndrome may lead to hypophosphatemia.

GERIATRIC ASSESSMENT

All hospitalized geriatric patients should be evaluated for overall functional capacity and home safety, including consideration of the following: home environment; evidence of abuse; mobility, fall risk, and the need for assistive devices; neuropsychiatric issues; bowel and bladder problems; pain; and nutritional issues. Functional assessment begins with evaluation of activities of daily living (ADL) and instrumental ADL (Box 54.1).

Assessment of elder abuse is a vital but frequently missed intervention for the hospitalized geriatric patient. According to a nationwide study by Adult Protective Services, there were more than 250,000 reports of abuse of adults aged 60 years or

Box 54.1 ACTIVITIES OF DAILY LIVING (ADL) AND INSTRUMENTAL ACTIVITIES OF DAILY LIVING (IADL)

ADL
 Bathing
 Dressing
 Using toilet
 Mobility
 Continence
 Feeding self
IADL
 Using telephone
 Shopping
 Preparing meals
 Housekeeping
 Laundry
 Transportation
 Taking medicine
 Managing money

older, which translated into 832.6 reports for every 100,000 people over the age of 60 in 2006.

Mobility and fall risk assessment should include evaluating the need for assistive devices such as walkers, toilet seats with arms, and appropriate footwear. The history of recent falls and the circumstances associated with them should be obtained. Physical therapy and occupational therapy guidance should be sought if needed. Several simple mobility scales are available.

Neuropsychiatric evaluation should include screening for depression, delirium, and dementia. Depression is a common problem that can be assessed with the Geriatric Depression Scale. Delirium is common in hospitalized patients and results from various causes, including medication, infections, and opiates. Patients can be assessed with the Confusion Assessment Method (Box 54.2). The Mini-Cog assessment, the Folstein Mini-Mental State Examination, and other tests are available to screen for dementia. Screening for alcoholism also is essential. Visual and auditory deficits may exacerbate cognitive problems, depression, and barriers to education.

Assessment for urinary incontinence, urinary retention, and problems with bowel function should occur at admission and before discharge.

Nutritional issues specific to geriatric patients include problems related to dentition, dentures, the risk of dysphagia and aspiration, reduced appetite, and recent weight changes.

Box 54.2 CONFUSION ASSESSMENT METHOD[a]

1. Acute onset with fluctuating course
2. Inattention
3. Disorganized thinking
4. Altered level of consciousness

[a] Diagnosis of delirium requires the presence of 1 *and* 2, along with either 3 *or* 4.

Data from Inouye SK, van Dyck CH, Alessi CA, Balkin S, Siegal AP, Horwitz RI, et al. Clarifying confusion: the confusion assessment method. A new method for detection of delirium. Ann Intern Med. 1990 Dec 15;113(12):941–8.

COMPLICATIONS OF HOSPITALIZATION

Complications of hospitalization may be *iatrogenic* (caused by medical examination or treatment) or *nosocomial* (originating in the hospital). Some adverse outcomes are predictable, and others are not. Adverse events related to the hospital environment itself include falls, thrombosis, debility, pressure ulcers, sleep deprivation, and aspiration pneumonia. Infections related to the hospital include health care–associated pneumonia, catheter-related bloodstream infections, *Clostridium difficile* colitis, and the development of resistant organisms. Discontinuity of patient care caused by poor communication during patient handoffs and dismissals can lead to preventable injury and error. In addition, health care workers are exposed to risks of occupational injury while taking care of hospitalized patients.

PRESSURE ULCERS

Pressure ulcers result from soft tissue being compressed between bone and an external surface, leading to tissue necrosis. Ulcers are staged according to their degree of penetration. Several factors may contribute to the formation of pressure ulcers. Patient-specific risk factors include immobility, malnutrition, impaired cognition, circulatory dysfunction, immunosuppression (eg, diabetes mellitus), and sensory impairment. External factors include pressure, shearing forces (such as when a patient slides in a bed or chair, leading to stretching and angulation of the underlying subcutaneous tissue and impaired lymphatic and capillary flow), friction, and moisture.

Prevention of ulcers is of utmost importance. The first step in management is to identify patients at risk and modify their risk factors. Sites most at risk are the heels and the sacrum. Frequent turning, maintaining skin hygiene, and maintaining nutritional integrity are essential. Underlying pressure must be relieved, and various pressure-relieving devices, including heel boots and specialty mattresses, are available.

The wound should be débrided by surgical, chemical, mechanical, or biotherapeutic means. Superficial wounds are treated with semipermeable membranes; deeper wounds may require either hydrocolloids or hydrogels. Deep wounds may be treated surgically with skin grafts or flaps. The cornerstone of ulcer treatment is to keep the wound moist and the surrounding skin dry. Adjunctive therapy may include vacuum-assisted closure, larval therapy, or growth factors. Routine antibiotics are not indicated unless the ulcer is complicated by soft tissue infection or osteomyelitis.

FALLS

Falls among hospitalized patients are common and may lead to serious injury or death. The outcome of a fall can vary with patient-specific and environmental factors. For example, it is important to recognize that the outcome of an otherwise simple fall may be worse for a patient receiving anticoagulation.

Risk factors for in-hospital falls include debility, toileting, orthostatic hypotension, altered mental status, sedation, history of previous falls, recent environmental changes, binders (such as urinary catheters), restraints, poor communication

Table 54.2 RISK FACTORS FOR IN-HOSPITAL FALLS AND PREVENTION

RISK FACTOR	ASSESSMENT	PREVENTION
Debility	Functional musculoskeletal assessment	Physical therapy; early mobilization
Binders	Routinely assess need for urinary catheter, oxygen, & intravenous lines	Remove unneeded binders; avoid physical restraints
Delirium	Determine CAM score for admitted patients (Box 54.2)	Identify & address risk factors (electrolytes, medications, etc)
Medications	Review medication list for medications with anticholinergic properties	Avoid tricyclic antidepressants & other drugs that increase fall risk
Inadequate records	Obtain fall history	Identify patients at risk
Insufficient education	Assess patient's knowledge of call lights & assistive devices	Education of patients & families
Inadequate staff	Monitor ratio of number of staff to number of falls	Provide adequate staff for high-risk patients

Abbreviation: CAM, Confusion Assessment Method.

between providers, depression, sensory impairment, and incontinence. Falls tend to occur in periods of lower staffing (eg, nights and weekends). Interventions to prevent falls include identifying at-risk patients, avoiding excess binders, encouraging early mobilization, and providing physical therapy (Table 54.2).

VENOUS THROMBOEMBOLISM

Venous thromboembolism (VTE) is a common complication of hospitalization. Even among patients receiving standard-of-care pharmacologic prophylaxis, the risk of VTE in some populations may be as high as 7% to 10%. That risk may be 15% or higher (*much* higher after knee, hip, pelvic, and other orthopedic operations) among patients who do not receive appropriate prophylactic care. Unsuspected pulmonary embolism may be associated with 5% to 10% of hospital deaths.

Medical conditions that predispose a patient to VTE include acute infectious disease, congestive heart failure, acute myocardial infarction, cerebrovascular accident, rheumatic disease, and inflammatory bowel disease. Specific risk factors include age older than 75 years, previous VTE, immobility, recent trauma or surgery, estrogen use, obesity, and hypercoagulable states. Patients with malignancy—particularly pancreatic cancer and other mucin-positive adenocarcinomas—are at especially high risk. Patients with a cerebrovascular accident are also at higher risk but carry a putative increased risk of intracranial hemorrhage.

Among nonpharmacologic means of VTE prophylaxis, ambulation is the most easily accomplished. In postoperative nonambulatory patients, graduated compression stockings have been shown to decrease the rate of VTE by 50%. Isolated ankle exercises are also helpful in increasing lower extremity venous blood flow. These nonpharmacologic approaches are especially important in patients for whom anticoagulation is contraindicated.

Pharmacologic prevention with heparin, low-molecular-weight heparin, or fondaparinux (a factor Xa inhibitor) appears to be effective, although the rates of risk reduction and the rates of use vary by center. Other anticoagulants continue to be studied and compared with these more established ones. Ximelagatran, a direct thrombin inhibitor, has been shown to have an efficacy and side-effect profile comparable to those of warfarin.

HOSPITAL-ACQUIRED INFECTIONS

Since Semmelweis understood the cause of puerperal fever in the hospital, hand washing has been encouraged to reduce hospital-acquired infection. Although hand hygiene is a simple, readily available intervention, it still fails to reach 100% adherence. There has been extensive debate about factors that contribute to deficient hand hygiene and options to improve compliance. These include the health beliefs of health care workers (eg, the provider's belief about the potential risk of infection, relating to both the body site and the patient's assumed cleanliness), time constraints, established care practices, and demonstration by example of senior staff.

CATHETER-RELATED BLOODSTREAM INFECTIONS

Each year, 150 million central or peripheral intravenous catheters are placed (an average of 5 per patient). They result in around 850,000 infections (<0.6%), including about 250,000 catheter-related bloodstream infections (CRBIs) that result in septic thrombophlebitis, bacteremia, and endocarditis. CRBIs lead to increased morbidity, mortality, and health care costs and to longer hospitalizations.

The risk of CRBI is related to the type of catheter, the location, placement (who places the catheter and the technique used) and the length of time the catheter remains in place. The highest risk is with peripheral catheters placed by surgical cutdown. The next highest risks are with peripheral steel needles, intra-aortic balloon pumps, and short-term hemodialysis catheters. Nasal carriers of *Staphylococcus aureus* have a higher risk of CRBI than noncarriers. Use of simple infection control procedures can decrease the risk of infection by 65%.

Safety checklists and specialized teams that use a standardized approach have been shown to significantly decrease rates. Specific measures include changing peripheral catheter sites every 72 to 96 hours to reduce the risk of infection and patient discomfort associated with superficial phlebitis. Control and prevention guidelines from the Centers for Disease Control and Prevention (CDC) are given in Box 54.3.

HEALTH CARE–ASSOCIATED PNEUMONIA

Health care–associated pneumonia (HCAP) is defined as pneumonia in a patient who has been hospitalized in an acute care facility for 2 or more days within the past 90 days, has resided in a nursing home or long-term care facility, has received recent intravenous antibiotic therapy or chemotherapy or wound care within 30 days of the current infection, or is receiving hemodialysis.

Bacteria frequently involved in HCAP include *Streptococcus pneumoniae*, methicillin-sensitive *S aureus*, and methicillin-resistant *S aureus* (MRSA); antibiotic-sensitive gram-negative bacilli such as *Escherichia coli*, *Klebsiella pneumoniae*, *Enterobacter* species, *Proteus* species, and *Serratia marcescens*; and multidrug-resistant (MDR) enteric gram-negative bacilli such as *Pseudomonas aeruginosa* and *Acinetobacter*. Fungal pathogens such as *Candida* and *Aspergillus* may need to be considered in immunosuppressed patients. Although a viral pathogen is less frequent, the most common virus is *Influenzavirus A*. Risk factors for infection with MDR pathogens include the following: recent antibiotic therapy, current hospitalization of more than 5 days, high local resistance rates, and an immunosuppressed state. MDR pathogens are most frequent in intensive care units and transplant patients.

Treatment of HCAP should include early recognition, initial broad-spectrum coverage with subsequent de-escalation based on culture results, attempts at bacteriologic diagnosis, avoidance of the overuse of antibiotics, and application of prevention strategies. Hospitalized patients, especially those with impaired mentation or neuromotor deficits, may be at risk of aspiration. These patients should be kept in a semirecumbent position (30°–45°), especially when receiving enteral feeding.

HOSPITAL-ACQUIRED DIARRHEA

One of the most common hospital-acquired infections and the most common cause of diarrhea among hospitalized patients is *C difficile*. It is a frequent cause of morbidity and mortality among elderly hospitalized patients. The spectrum of disease includes asymptomatic carrier, mild to moderate diarrhea, pseudomembranous colitis, and toxic megacolon. Symptoms usually occur after 5 to 10 days of antibiotic treatment, but they may develop as early as 1 day into treatment or as late as 10 weeks after its cessation. Presenting manifestations may include fever, abdominal pain, and a prominent leukocytosis. Diagnosis is made by demonstrating *C difficile* toxin in the stool, although patients may need to have direct colon imaging in unclear cases.

Nonpharmacologic treatment of *C difficile* infection includes correcting fluid losses and electrolyte imbalances and avoiding the use of antiperistaltic agents. Strict observation of contact isolation precautions and hand washing with soap and water are essential.

Pharmacologic treatment of *C difficile* infection includes use of the following:

1. Metronidazole—first-line antibiotic for mild infection

2. Oral vancomycin—for severe resistant infections and during pregnancy

3. Rifaximin, intravenous immune globulin, and fecal transplant—possible adjuncts in refractory infection

4. Probiotics (eg, *Lactobacillus* species and *Saccharomyces boulardii*)—useful for decreasing the incidence of antibiotic-associated diarrhea but not reliably useful for preventing *C difficile* infection

Indications for surgical intervention include poor clinical response to antibiotics, progressive fever, rigors, peritoneal signs, bacteremia, persistent leukocytosis, or computed tomographic (CT) evidence of significant pericolonic inflammation with increasing bowel wall edema. The recommended surgical procedure is subtotal colectomy with ileostomy, which may be converted to ileorectal anastomosis later.

CATHETER-ASSOCIATED URINARY TRACT INFECTIONS

Catheter-associated urinary tract infections (CAUTIs) are the most common type of health care–associated infection (Box 54.4). Approximately 900,000 CAUTIs are reported each year. They are responsible for an estimated $500 million in additional expense annually, and they increase the patient length of stay by 2 to 4 days. Over 10,000 deaths are attributable to CAUTIs annually; CAUTIs are the leading cause of secondary bloodstream infections, with approximately 10% mortality. Other negative repercussions of CAUTIs are the additional antibiotic use and the associated risks of resistance. The CDC recommends the following evidence-based measures for reducing the incidence of CAUTIs:

1. Insert catheters only for appropriate indications.

2. Only trained personnel should insert catheters.

3. Leave catheters in place only as long as needed, and reassess the need daily.

4. Maintain catheters properly with a closed drainage system and with unobstructed urine flow.

5. Practice hand hygiene procedures and Standard Precautions at all times.

COMPLICATIONS OF SURGERY

The following section deals with some of the common medical issues in postoperative patients, including ileus; delirium; alterations in pulmonary, renal, and cardiac function; and the complications of bariatric surgery.

ILEUS

Postoperative ileus is a nonmechanical disruption of normal gastrointestinal tract motility. Physiologically, gastric motility and small-bowel motility normalize several hours postoperatively; colon motility normalizes at 24 to 48 hours. Postoperative ileus can cause discomfort, adversely affect nutrition, increase the risk of infection, compromise wound healing, increase catabolism, and increase the risk of need for parenteral nutrition by delaying oral feeding. Signs include abdominal distention, diffuse abdominal pain, nausea and vomiting, absence of flatus, and inability to tolerate an oral diet. The cause most likely is a combination of neurologic mechanisms, including inhibitory neural reflexes, inflammation from manipulation, and neurohumoral peptides. There are no standardized preventive strategies, although limiting opiates, using minimally invasive surgery, and using epidural anesthesia may be of benefit.

Ischemia or perforation of the bowel should be excluded; an elevated leukocyte count or metabolic acidosis may be suggestive of this. Liver function tests and pancreatic enzymes should be checked to exclude secondary causes such as pancreatitis. A flat and upright plain film of the abdomen may show multiple dilated loops of bowel, air fluid levels, and diminished colonic gas. CT scan of the abdomen can help differentiate ileus from small-bowel obstruction. If there is still doubt, consider CT enterography.

Neither pharmacologic treatment nor early ambulation has proved to be curative. Primary therapy should be aimed at bowel rest, hydration, and avoidance of drugs that have antiperistaltic effects such as opiates.

One form of postoperative ileus is acute colonic pseudo-obstruction (Ogilvie syndrome). Plain radiography should be used to estimate cecal diameter; surgeons should be involved if this measurement exceeds 10 cm, the threshold for colonic perforation. Emergent decompressive colonoscopy also may be considered. Success has been reported with intravenous neostigmine, although mechanical obstruction must first be excluded. Cardiac monitoring is imperative during neostigmine administration.

POSTOPERATIVE DELIRIUM

Risk factors for postoperative delirium include uncontrolled pain, intraoperative hypoxia or hypoperfusion, pharmacologic agents used for anesthesia and analgesia, and nonoperative factors, including infection and ischemia (Box 54.5).

Postoperative delirium among elderly patients may be associated with poor outcomes, including impaired cognitive and functional recovery, institutionalization, and death. Delirium may develop in almost 25% of elderly patients, with

---

Box 54.5 RISK FACTORS FOR POSTOPERATIVE DELIRIUM

Uncontrolled pain
Geriatric patient
Preexisting cognitive impairment
Cerebrovascular & neurodegenerative disease
History of delirium
Alcohol abuse & withdrawal
Narcotic or benzodiazepine dependence
Anticholinergic medications
Hypoxia
Anemia
Hyperglycemia & hypoglycemia
Electrolyte abnormalities
Infection & sepsis
Myocardial ischemia

---

even higher rates associated with vascular and orthopedic surgery (around 60%).

Initial management is nonpharmacologic and involves identifying and eliminating the likely cause along with providing supportive measures such as frequent orientation, a quiet environment (especially at night), and adequate hydration. Restraints and binders should be avoided if possible.

Antipsychotic drugs (eg, haloperidol, olanzapine, quetiapine) may be used, but caution should be taken with patients who have long QT intervals and a risk of torsades de pointes. Benzodiazepines exacerbate delirium in the elderly and should not be used.

STRESS GASTROINTESTINAL TRACT ULCERS

Routine stress gastrointestinal tract ulcer prophylaxis is not indicated. Certain conditions in critically ill patients carry a higher risk of upper gastrointestinal tract ulcers. These include thrombocytopenia, respiratory failure, liver failure, multisystem organ failure, and a previous history of ulcer and recent corticosteroid use. Proton pump inhibitor use should be discontinued at hospital discharge if the need for prophylaxis no longer exists.

OLIGURIA

Postoperative acute kidney injury with acute oliguria (urine output <400 mL daily) is a common surgical complication that may be caused by several factors (Box 54.6).

PULMONARY COMPLICATIONS

Pulmonary complications of surgery are as common as cardiac complications and as important clinically for mortality, morbidity, and length of hospital stay. Pulmonary complications include the following:

Box 54.6 FACTORS CAUSING ACUTE OLIGURIA POSTOPERATIVELY

Prerenal causes
  Decreased cardiac preload from blood loss, extravasation of fluid, & inadequate hydration
  Cardiac events (eg, myocardial infarction) that may cause hypotension & decrease perfusion pressure
  Vasodilation due to sepsis, drugs, or anaphylaxis
  Arterial obstruction with thrombosis or embolism secondary to the procedure
Acute tubular necrosis due to perioperative ischemia
Intravenous radiologic contrast-induced nephropathy
Transfusion-related myoglobinuria
Rhabdomyolysis
Postrenal causes
  Opioid-related urinary retention
  Ureteral obstruction
  Urethral obstruction or blocked urinary catheter

---

1. *Upper airway obstruction*, manifested as stridor, is a medical emergency. Causes include laryngeal edema, vocal cord injury, and obstruction by the tongue.

2. *Atelectasis* is best managed with incentive spirometry, which is relevant to both prevention and treatment. It is dependent on user compliance, though.

3. *Bronchospasm* can be caused by aspiration, drug reactions, or activation of an underlying pulmonary disease. Treatment is similar to nonpostoperative management.

4. *Pleural effusions*, common in patients who have had abdominal surgery, usually resolve spontaneously. An effusion in combination with fever or leukocytosis, especially after abdominal surgery, raises the possibility of a subphrenic abscess.

5. *Chemical pneumonitis* results from aspiration of gastric contents (exacerbated by diminished upper airway reflexes perioperatively in combination with anesthetic medications) and is usually manifested as infiltrates on chest imaging.

6. *Postoperative pneumonia*, which is nosocomial by definition and should be treated as an HCAP, is caused by either *S pneumoniae* or *Haemophilus influenzae* in 20% to 30% of the patients. The risk of *S aureus*, which may be MRSA, is increased in neurosurgical patients, in patients who have chronic renal failure or diabetes mellitus, and in intravenous drug abusers. *Pseudomonas* is more common in late infections after prolonged intubation. Other organisms to consider are *Acinetobacter* and anaerobes.

7. *Pulmonary edema* can result from excessive fluid administration in the perioperative setting.

POSTOPERATIVE FEVER

Most fever in the first days after surgery is related to inflammation. If the fever is persistent, a search is indicated for surgical site infections or other common hospital-related infections such as urinary tract infection, aspiration pneumonia, ventilator-related pneumonia, or line infection. Noninfectious causes include drug fever and, less commonly, deep vein thrombosis, malignant hyperthermia, gout, transfusion reactions, thyroid storm, and atelectasis. The type of fever and the timing may aid in the diagnosis. Neurosurgical procedures may cause meningitis. Abdominal surgery may result in deep abdominal abscess formation, and fever after transplant should lead to a search for unusual causes in a newly immunosuppressed patient.

- Persistent postoperative fever may be from surgical site infection, urinary tract infection, aspiration or ventilator-related pneumonia, or line infection.

- Noninfectious causes of fever include drug fever and, less commonly, deep vein thrombosis, malignant hyperthermia, gout, transfusion reactions, thyroid storm, and atelectasis.

POSTOPERATIVE MYOCARDIAL INFARCTION

Postsurgical myocardial infarction carries substantial morbidity and mortality. Patients may present in an atypical fashion, without chest pain (masked by pain medications or anesthetics). The infarction tends to occur within the first 5 days postoperatively and is diagnosed in the usual fashion. Serial electrocardiograms are not recommended postoperatively but may be warranted in patients at increased risk of ischemia. The preoperative use of β-blockers in certain patients at increased risk may decrease the risk of perioperative infarction.

COMPLICATIONS OF BARIATRIC SURGERY

Obesity has reached epidemic status in the United States, and increasing numbers of patients are turning to bariatric surgery. Bariatric surgical procedures reduce caloric intake by modifying the anatomy and function of the gastrointestinal tract.

The types of procedures can be characterized as restrictive or malabsorptive. The most common restrictive procedures include gastroplasty and adjustable gastric banding. Biliopancreatic diversion is a malabsorptive procedure. The Roux-en-Y gastric bypass is a combination of both.

The mortality rate is 0.1% to 2%, depending on the facility, and is higher for the malabsorptive procedures. The most common causes of mortality are pulmonary embolism and anastomotic leaks (Box 54.7). Nonfatal surgical complications include thromboembolism, anastomotic leaks, bleeding, incidental splenectomy, hernias, and small-bowel obstruction. Nausea and vomiting occur in 50% of patients with restrictive procedures. Dumping syndrome occurs in 70% of patients after a Roux-en-Y procedure.

Box 54.7 COMPLICATIONS OF BARIATRIC SURGERY

Perioperative surgical complications
  Anastomotic leaks
  Pulmonary embolism
  Hemorrhage
  Incidental splenectomy
  Hernia
  Small-bowel obstruction
Nutritional complications
  With restrictive surgery
    Calcium
    Folate
    Vitamin B_{12}
  With malabsorptive surgery
    Protein malabsorption
    Fat-soluble vitamin deficiency (vitamins A, D, E, & K)
Gastrointestinal tract complications
  Dumping syndrome: flushing, palpitations, light-headedness, fatigue, & diarrhea
  Strictures
  Cholelithiasis
  Dehydration
  Ulcers

Table 54.3 SELECTED QUALITY MEASURES

CONDITION	SELECTED QUALITY MEASURES
Acute MI	Aspirin at arrival & discharge ACE inhibitor or ARB for LV systolic dysfunction β-Blocker at arrival & discharge Statin at discharge Thrombolytic within 30 min of arrival at hospital Primary PCI within 120 min of arrival at hospital Smoking cessation advice & counseling 30-d risk-standardized acute MI mortality & readmissions
Heart failure	Discharge instructions LV function assessment ACE inhibitor or ARB for LV systolic dysfunction Smoking cessation advice & counseling 30-d risk-standardized heart failure mortality & readmissions
Pneumonia	Oxygenation assessment Pneumococcal vaccination status Influenza vaccination status Blood culture performed in emergency department before administration of first antibiotic in hospital Initial antibiotic received within 4 h of arrival at hospital Appropriate initial antibiotic selection Smoking cessation advice & counseling 30-d risk-standardized pneumonia mortality & readmissions

Abbreviations: ACE, angiotensin-converting enzyme; ARB, angiotensin receptor blocker; LV, left ventricular; MI, myocardial infarction; PCI, percutaneous coronary intervention.

Data from Centers for Medicare and Medicaid Services/Hospital Quality Alliance [database on the Internet]. Baltimore (MD). [Updated 2006 Dec 13; cited 2012 Jul 30]. Available from: https://www.cms.gov/HospitalQualityInits/downloads/HospitalHQA2004_2007200512.pdf.

THE QUALITY MOVEMENT AND HOSPITAL CARE

The Agency for Healthcare Research and Quality has defined *quality health care* as "doing the right thing, at the right time, in the right way, for the right person—and having the best possible results." Organizations involved in inpatient quality assessment (eg, The Joint Commission) have defined key measures believed to reflect the effectiveness and efficiency of care, and hospital physicians are expected to work toward them (Table 54.3).

Achieving these quality-related goals in the hospital requires multidisciplinary provider participation, adoption of several approaches (Box 54.8), and the practice of continuous quality improvement (CQI). The practice of CQI applies the scientific method to measure and evaluate the implementation of changes in clinical practice. CQI involves identifying a goal, defining a change that may help achieve the goal, delineating indexes to measure success, and evaluating the implementation of the change before repeating the cycle again to allow continuous incremental improvements.

PATIENT SATISFACTION

Patient satisfaction is a vital measure of the quality of health care and correlates with a physician's communication skills. Patients' satisfaction with their care may have both financial and legal implications.

Inpatient physicians should be aware of the patient satisfaction indexes that increasingly are being assessed by oversight organizations. These indexes cover patients' perceptions of the frequency with which physicians and nurses treat them with courtesy and respect, listen carefully, respond promptly to a call light (particularly for assistance with bed pans and other toileting needs), explain things clearly (including information about side effects and indications before administration of medications), clarify details of postdismissal follow-up, and provide adequate pain control.

During end-of-life care, communication is especially important. Frequent updates, culturally competent education, and empathy are essential to patients and families as they deal with impending death. The most important elements of end-of-life care from a patient satisfaction viewpoint include control of pain, dyspnea, secretions, toileting, and anxiety.

PATIENT SAFETY

Patient safety refers to freedom from accidental or preventable injury. A report in 1999 from the Institute of Medicine highlighted the issue of patient safety in the hospital. Awareness of this issue has been raised by the often-quoted estimate of 44,000 to 98,000 deaths annually related to medical errors in US hospitals. Among hospitalized patients, 1% to 5% sustain a major injury related to their medical care.

Errors in the hospital may result from failure to complete a planned action or, alternatively, from the wrong approach to achieve an aim. *Adverse events* are untoward incidents, therapeutic misadventures, iatrogenic injuries, or other adverse occurrences that result directly from care or services provided and not from the underlying disease or condition of the patient. A *near miss* (or *close call*) is an event or situation that could have resulted in an accident, injury, or illness but did not happen because of chance or a timely intervention.

A *sentinel event*, as defined by The Joint Commission, is any unanticipated event in a health care setting resulting in death or serious physical or mental injury and not related to the natural course of the patient's disease. The term *sentinel event* is not synonymous with *error*. The goal is to focus attention on potentially deleterious factors that lead to the event and induce change in systems, procedures, and culture. Hospitals are required to report, identify, and respond to these events. Not all sentinel events are caused by medical error, and not all errors are sentinel events. *Errors of commission* are the result of an action taken (committed), such as a patient being given the wrong drug, a drug by the wrong route, or a drug with the wrong timing; surgical procedures performed on the wrong patient or at the wrong site; and blood crossmatch errors. *Errors of omission* result from an action not taken (omitted), such as a delay in an indicated procedure, a missed or delayed medication dose, a suicide due to a lapse in a procedure, or a lack of provision of an interpreter.

- A sentinel event is any unanticipated event in a health care setting resulting in death or serious physical or mental injury and not related to the natural course of the patient's disease.

- Common sentinel events include suicide, wrong-site surgery, medication errors, and delay in treatment.

- Errors can be of commission (eg, wrong site surgery) or omission (eg, delay in treatment).

A common method for identifying the source of an error is root cause analysis (RCA), a collection of problem-solving methods designed to isolate the root causes of untoward events. The focus is on systems and procedures as opposed to individual error. The goal is to learn from errors and avoid repeating them. RCA is an important tool of CQI. Multidisciplinary teams review the causes and suggest ways to prevent events. With the use of a plan-do-study-act (PDSA) cycle, the effect of these changes can be monitored and modified.

- RCA is a common approach to identifying the source of error.

- A PDSA cycle is a method for responding to a sentinel event.

Several major national safety initiatives target certain harmful events and call for increased efforts to eliminate them (Box 54.9). *Never events* are particular medical errors that should never occur. Hospital payment and reporting have been linked to these events. Those most applicable to internists are listed in Box 54.10.

MEDICATION SAFETY

Initiation of medication therapy and withdrawal can lead to drug errors, drug-drug and drug-disease interactions, and side effects. Adverse drug events (ADEs) are common, expensive, dangerous, and frequently preventable. They affect an estimated 5% to 7% of hospitalized patients. Medication-related errors for hospitalized patients cost roughly $2 billion annually. As many as 40% of serious ADEs are preventable. About one-half of all medication errors occur during ordering, and one-third during administration.

Errors may involve the incorrect choice of medication for a condition: either the drug is prescribed inappropriately or the wrong drug is administered. Drug-drug interactions can cause error, too. Fluoroquinolones, for example, may inhibit the metabolism of warfarin and lead to an increase in the international normalized ratio. Missed drug allergies can lead to fatal consequences. Drug-disease interactions also are common; use of hepatically metabolized drugs, for example, should be avoided in patients with liver failure. Certain abbreviations, such as *qod* (for *every other day*) and *U* (for *units*), may be misread and should not be used. An ADE resulting from a drug administered in the hospital may occur after patient discharge.

Drugs and drug classes that are associated with a particularly high risk of adverse outcomes include narcotics, anticoagulants (including heparin and warfarin), sedatives, and insulin. Several medications are often responsible for electrolyte and other pathophysiologic abnormalities (Table 54.4).

Even if a medication is generally well tolerated by a patient in a healthy state, the medication may cause severe adverse effects if that person is ill or has compromised oral intake. Common culprits include long-acting oral hypoglycemic agents, diuretics, and other antihypertensives.

Certain supplements and over-the-counter medications may have clinically significant side effects. Herbal remedies may affect coagulation (eg, dong quai, ginseng, and ginkgo), lead to hepatoxicity (eg, kava), or interact with warfarin. Commonly used over-the-counter medications that may cause various unintended consequences include nonsteroidal anti-inflammatory drugs (which may cause peptic ulcers and gastrointestinal tract bleeding) and antihistamines (which may cause altered mental status and urinary retention).

A single medication may cause many potential adverse events. Subtherapeutic dosing of heparin, for example, may potentiate thrombosis, whereas its overdosage could lead to hemorrhage. Appropriate dosing of heparin still could induce thrombocytopenia with associated paradoxical thrombosis. Heparin may also cause hyperkalemia by inhibiting aldosterone secretion. A key to providing safe pharmacologic treatment in the hospital lies in one's awareness of the potential complications associated with each drug's use. Knowledge of cytochrome P450 interactions has become increasingly important in polypharmaceutic management (Table 54.5).

RISKS TO HEALTH CARE WORKERS

Hospitals employ approximately 4.5 million of the 8 million health care workers in the United States or about 4% of the total US workforce. The hospital is a complex environment. Both students and experienced personnel function in a high-stress environment replete with various hazards, including radiation, toxic chemicals, biologic hazards, and needles. Needlestick injuries are a constant threat to hospital workers. The CDC estimates that health care workers (HCWs) in hospitals receive 385,000 needlestick injuries (NSIs) annually. The rate of NSI is higher in teaching hospitals; one-third occur in the operating room, and another one-fourth in the patient's room. The hollow-bore syringe is the most frequent cause. Nurses have the highest rate among HCWs (approximately 35%), and residents and fellows have almost the same rate as attending physicians (10%). Phlebotomists have a fairly low rate (5%). There have been documented cases of transmission of viruses (eg, Ebola, herpes simplex virus, varicella-zoster virus) and of brucellosis, blastomycosis, leptospirosis, malaria, Rocky Mountain spotted fever, syphilis, toxoplasmosis, and tuberculosis. HCWs also have viral and bacterial exposures from animals in teaching institutions with research programs (herpesvirus B from primates, human T-lymphotropic virus, and various bacterial infections).

- NSIs are more frequent in teaching hospitals; one-third occur in the operating room and another one-fourth occur in the patient's room.

ELECTROLYTE IMBALANCE	DRUG	PATHOPHYSIOLOGIC CHANGE
Hypokalemia	Diuretics	Urinary potassium wasting
	Laxatives	Fecal potassium loss
Hyperkalemia	β-Blocker, heparin	Hyporeninemic aldosterone synthesis
		Decreased cellular uptake of potassium
	Cyclosporine	Hypoaldosteronism
	Digoxin	Induced chloride shunt
		Impaired cellular uptake
		Reduced renal excretion
	Pentamidine, trimethoprim	Altered sodium transport (increased in HIV infection)
	NSAIDs	Hyporeninemic hypoaldosteronism
	Succinylcholine	Intracellular leakage of potassium
Hyponatremia	ACE inhibitor, amiodarone, chemotherapy (vincristine, cisplatin, cyclophosphamide), ciprofloxacin, SSRIs	SIADH
	Carbamazepine	Increased ADH sensitivity in renal tubules
	Chlorpropamide	Increased number of ADH receptors
	Thiazide diuretics	Distal renal tubular loss
Hypernatremia	Amphotericin B, foscarnet	ADH deficiency
	Cisplatin	
	Carbamazepine, lithium	Suppressed ADH (drug-induced diabetes insipidus)
Hypocalcemia	Bisphosphonates	Inhibit osteoclastic activity
	Citrate (transfusion plasma exchange)	Decreased ionized calcium from deposition
	Foscarnet	Possibly due to binding of foscarnet to ionized calcium (associated in patients with CMV & HSV)
	Phenytoin	Increased vitamin D metabolism
	Phosphate enemas	Decreased ionized calcium from intravascular binding
Hypercalcemia	Hypervitaminosis A, retinoic acid, levothyroxine	Increased bone resorption
	Lithium	Altered PTH set-point
	Thiazide diuretics	Renal tubular calcium resorption
Hypomagnesemia	Diuretics, cisplatin	Renal wasting

Abbreviations: ACE, angiotensin-converting enzyme; ADH, antidiuretic hormone; CMV, cytomegalovirus; HIV, human immunodeficiency virus; HSV, herpes simplex virus; NSAID, nonsteroidal anti-inflammatory drug; PTH, parathyroid hormone; SIADH, syndrome of inappropriate secretion of antidiuretic hormone; SSRI, selective serotonin reuptake inhibitor.

- The syringe is the most frequent cause of NSIs.

- Nurses have the highest rate among HCWs (approximately 35%), and residents and fellows have almost the same rate as attending physicians (10%).

Before the use of hepatitis B virus (HBV) vaccine, the rate of HBV infection was more than 10,000 per year. The rate of infection in unvaccinated HCWs is 10% to 30%. Postexposure prophylaxis is required after HBV exposure from NSI or mucous membrane contact involving a patient with known or suspected positive status for hepatitis B surface antigen (HBsAg). For an unvaccinated HCW, treatment with hepatitis B immune globulin (HBIG) and HBV vaccine is indicated. An HCW who is a known responder to vaccine does not need treatment. An HCW who is a nonresponder (ie, received treatment but did not mount an antibody response) should receive HBIG or HBIG and another vaccination. For the HCW who has been vaccinated but has an unknown antibody response, test the status immediately and proceed accordingly.

- Hepatitis B exposure from NSI or mucous membrane contact involving a patient with known or suspected HBsAg-positive status requires evaluation for postexposure prophylaxis.

- For an unvaccinated HCW, treatment with HBIG and HBV vaccine is indicated.

- An HCW who is a nonresponder (ie, received treatment but did not mount an antibody response) should receive HBIG or HBIG and another vaccination.

Hepatitis C virus (HCV) seroconversion after an NSI from an infected person is approximately 0% to 5%. No cases have been reported from blood exposure to intact skin, but cases have been reported from conjunctival exposure. Routine testing recommended after exposure includes the following:

1. Baseline testing for anti-HCV, HCV RNA, and alanine aminotransferase

Table 54.5 FREQUENTLY ENCOUNTERED CYTOCHROME P450 INTERACTIONS

CYTOCHROME P450 ISOZYME	DRUG	EFFECT ON METABOLISM	
		Increased	*Decreased*
1A2	Amitriptyline Cyclobenzaprine Haloperidol Acetaminophen Propranolol Verapamil Warfarin	Broccoli Charbroiled meat Brussels sprouts Nafcillin Insulin Omeprazole Tobacco	Amiodarone Fluoroquinolones
2C19	Proton pump inhibitors Phenytoin Propranolol Warfarin	Carbamazepine Prednisone Rifampin	Fluoxetine Ketoconazole Omeprazole
2C9	NSAIDs Glipizide ARBs Sulfonylureas Amitriptyline Celecoxib Fluoxetine Phenytoin Rosiglitazone Tamoxifen Warfarin	Rifampin	Amiodarone Fluconazole Isoniazid Sertraline Sulfamethoxazole Voriconazole
2D6	Carvedilol Metoprolol Amitriptyline Paroxetine Haloperidol Metoclopramide Ondansetron Oxycodone Tramadol	Dexamethasone Rifampin	Amiodarone Bupropion Citalopram Duloxetine Escitalopram Fluoxetine Metoclopramide Methadone Paroxetine Ranitidine Sertraline Diphenhydramine Hydroxyzine
3A4, 3A5, 3A7	Macrolides (excluding azithromycin) Benzodiazepines Cyclosporine Tacrolimus HIV antivirals Calcium channel blockers HMG-CoA reductase inhibitors (excluding pravastatin) Fentanyl Dapsone Dexamethasone Haloperidol Ondansetron Quetiapine Risperidone Trazodone Zolpidem	HIV antivirals Barbiturates Carbamazepine Glucocorticoids Phenytoin Rifampin St John's wort	HIV antivirals Amiodarone Macrolides (excluding azithromycin) Diltiazem Azole antifungals Verapamil

Abbreviations: ARB, angiotensin receptor blocker; HIV, human immunodeficiency virus; NSAID, nonsteroidal anti-inflammatory drug.

2. Follow-up testing for HCV RNA at 4 to 6 weeks after exposure

3. Follow-up testing for anti-HCV, HCV RNA, and ALT at 4 to 6 months after exposure

Treatment with immune globulin after exposure is not recommended; however, effective treatment is available for HCWs who have an acute HCV infection (pegylated interferon with an antiviral such as ribavirin).

- HCV seroconversion after an NSI from an infected person is approximately 0%-5%.

Human immunodeficiency virus transmission is even less likely with exposure (0.3%); however, postexposure prophylaxis with a combination regimen of antiretroviral therapy is indicated.

DISCHARGE FROM THE HOSPITAL

Each year, 35 million patients are discharged from US hospitals. The majority of these patients are older than 75 years; of those older than 85, one-third transition from hospitals to long-term care facilities. A premature dismissal may lead to ADEs or to other safety issues, decreased satisfaction, and an increased risk of readmission. For approximately 20% of patients, adverse events occur after dismissal from the hospital; at least one-third of these events are preventable, and another third can be made less severe by timely intervention. Of these, ADEs are the most common.

Discharge from the hospital is a critical period of transition. As the health care setting changes from the hospital to a home, assisted living center, nursing home, hospice facility, or rehabilitation center, care providers change, as may the patient's diet, level of activity, and routes of medication administration. This culmination of the hospital stay has the potential to affect patient satisfaction, safety, medical outcome, and cost of care. Patients at highest risk are the elderly and those with multiple medical conditions.

The discharge process should begin at admission. In an era of increasing costs and pressures to limit the use of resources, a successful hospital discharge must be planned in detail. Prolonged or unnecessary hospitalization may increase the risk of hospital-associated adverse outcomes such as infections, falls, debility, loss of independence, and overall dissatisfaction.

- Discharge from the hospital is a critical transition in care.

- The discharge process should begin at admission.

- Elderly patients and those with complex medical issues are at highest risk.

- After discharge, 20% of patients have adverse events; many of these are preventable.

A safe discharge from the hospital depends on excellent communication. Patient and family education should take into account possible barriers to learning such as health illiteracy and dementia. Key elements of this education may include indications for medications, the natural course of a disease, and the signs of disease progression. For example, the patient with congestive heart failure who recognizes the early warning signs of exacerbation can seek care before reaching extremis. An accurate and clear discharge summary can be useful for the patient and for outpatient health care providers. Written or oral interprofessional communication of key details may also be helpful; these include the patient's condition at discharge, recent or expected changes, and plans for follow-up. Provision of discharge instructions is a Joint Commission core performance measure.

- As part of any handoff, accurate information should be provided about a patient's care, treatment and services, present condition, and any recent or expected changes.

- Provision of discharge instructions is a Joint Commission core performance measure.

From the hospital, all patients should return to a safe environment. Patients who have had long hospitalizations almost invariably are debilitated and may require short-term rehabilitation. A predischarge evaluation should include assessment for risk of falling, particularly for older patients. Before discharge, arrangements should be made for home health care, home infusion therapy, or physical therapy when indicated. Other predischarge considerations include the patient's functional status (ADL), cognitive status, caregiver capacity, knowledge deficits, and environmental factors. Preserving independence and continuing to live at home safely are important goals.

Some disease-specific guidelines recommend initiating certain interventions before discharge (eg, medications for myocardial infarction, counseling for tobacco dependence). Such changes in management may require close follow-up after discharge.

Many medications carry a high risk of adverse events after hospital discharge (Box 54.11). Appropriate warfarin dosing, for example, depends on drug interactions, diet, and a patient's sensitivities. Corticosteroid use is accompanied by short-term risks (eg, hypertension, delirium, hyperglycemia) and long-term effects (eg, osteoporosis, immunosuppression). Medication reconciliation before discharge is essential.

Box 54.11 **HIGH-RISK DRUGS AT HOSPITAL DISCHARGE**

Antiarrhythmics
Antihypertensives
Corticosteroids
Diuretics
Narcotics
Oral hypoglycemic agents & insulin
Warfarin

- Many discharge-related adverse events are the consequence of medication errors.

- Some higher-risk drugs may require extensive education and plans for follow-up and monitoring.

- Medication reconciliation at all transitions of care, including discharge, is essential.

DEPARTURE FROM THE HOSPITAL AGAINST MEDICAL ADVICE

Departures of patients from the hospital against medical advice account for 1% to 2% of all "discharges" and are more common in urban settings. Inner-city hospitals may have rates as high as 6% in the general medical population. Risk factors include human immunodeficiency virus, lack of a primary care provider, substance abuse, prior discharge against medical advice, and prior emergency department admission. When a person wants to leave the hospital against medical advice, it is essential to assess and document that person's decision-making capacity and to discuss and document the risks associated with premature departure. Persons who lack the ability to make informed decisions and who want to depart against medical advice may pose a risk to themselves or to others and may be best served by temporary involuntary retention in the hospital. In all circumstances, efforts should be made to provide follow-up care.

GENERAL INTERNAL MEDICINE AND QUALITY IMPROVEMENT

Christopher M. Wittich, MD, and Thomas J. Beckman, MD

GOALS

- Counsel and treat patients who use tobacco.

- Define commonly encountered otorhinolaryngologic (ear, nose, and throat) disorders encountered in an ambulatory internal medicine practice.

- Define common causes of red eye and recognize when it is an emergency.

- Categorize the common types of kidney stones and describe their management.

- Cite commonly used quality improvement methodologies and tools used in health care.

SMOKING CESSATION

Tobacco use is the leading cause of preventable death and the cause of most lung cancers in the United States. The US Preventive Services Task Force (USPSTF) recommends tobacco use screening for all patients. Brief behavioral counseling and pharmacologic interventions have been shown to improve cessation rates.

The USPSTF recommends the 5 *A*'s approach to behavioral counseling:

1. Ask about tobacco use

2. Advise to quit

3. Assess willingness to quit

4. Assist the patient in quitting

5. Arrange follow-up

US Food and Drug Administration (FDA)–approved medications for smoking cessation include nicotine replacement, bupropion, and varenicline. Nicotine replacement is available in several forms, including transdermal patches, gum, nasal spray, inhalers, and lozenges. Transdermal patches provide continuous release of nicotine and are applied daily, improving adherence. Immediate-release nicotine products have the advantage of allowing as-needed administration for the treatment of urges.

Bupropion is an antidepressant medication that is FDA approved for smoking cessation. The patient should be instructed to pick a quit date within 2 weeks of starting bupropion therapy to allow for a steady state to be achieved. Bupropion should not be used in patients with seizures, eating disorders, or alcohol abuse.

Varenicline is a nicotine receptor partial agonist that helps to reduce nicotine craving. Varenicline frequently causes nausea, so patients should be counseled to take the medication with a full glass of water and on a full stomach. Varenicline should be used with caution in patients with psychiatric disorders.

- The 5 *A*'s approach (ask, advise, assess, assist, arrange) can be used to counsel patients who smoke.

- FDA-approved medications for smoking cessation include nicotine replacement, bupropion, and varenicline.

OTORHINOLARYNGOLOGY

RHINOSINUSITIS

According to the American Academy of Otolaryngology, *acute rhinosinusitis* is defined as up to 4 weeks of purulent nasal discharge with nasal obstruction and facial pain or pressure. The diagnosis of *viral rhinosinusitis* should be made if symptoms are present for less than 10 days and are not worsening. *Acute bacterial rhinosinusitis* should be diagnosed if symptoms are present for more than 10 days and if there is worsening of symptoms after initial improvement.

Radiographic imaging is not recommended unless an alternative diagnosis is in question. Treatment should be supportive and tailored to the symptoms. Watchful waiting with no antibiotics is an appropriate option for patients with acute bacterial rhinosinusitis if the patient is afebrile and has only mild pain. If antibiotics are chosen, the first-line agent is amoxicillin. If there is no response within 10 days, therapy with an alternative antibiotic should be initiated.

Patients who have *chronic rhinosinusitis* have had symptoms for more than 12 weeks. In these patients, sinus imaging with computed tomography may be indicated. Allergy testing and immune function testing may also be appropriate.

- Radiographic imaging for *acute* rhinosinusitis is not recommended unless an alternative diagnosis is in question.

OTITIS EXTERNA

Acute Otitis Externa

Acute otitis externa, also known as swimmer's ear, is an infection of the external auditory canal. A moist environment, eczematous dermatitis, repeated insertion of foreign bodies (eg, cotton swabs), and psoriasis can predispose to otitis externa. Most patients present with otalgia and otorrhea. On examination, the tympanic membrane appears normal, but the external auditory canal is erythematous, often with exudate. Typical examination findings include pain with pressure on the tragus and with traction of the pinna. Management of otitis externa includes avoidance of excessive water exposure and application of topical antibiotics and corticosteroids.

- Several conditions can mimic acute otitis externa; unlike patients with those conditions, though, most patients with acute otitis externa present with otalgia and otorrhea.

Malignant Otitis Externa

Malignant otitis externa is a feared complication of acute otitis externa in diabetic patients and other immunocompromised patients. It is typically caused by *Pseudomonas aeruginosa*. The infection can penetrate the cartilaginous structures of the ear canal into the temporal bone, where it causes osteomyelitis. Patients present with severe pain, fever, and possibly cranial neuropathies. On examination, granulation tissue is often present in the external auditory canal. The condition requires emergent care with intravenous antibiotics and sometimes surgical débridement of the skull base osteomyelitis.

- Malignant otitis externa is typically caused by *P aeruginosa*.
- Malignant otitis externa causes severe pain, fever, and symptoms of skull base osteomyelitis, possibly cranial neuropathies.
- Granulation tissue is often present in the external auditory canal.

PHARYNGITIS

Most cases of pharyngitis are viral. The goal is to identify patients with group A β-hemolytic streptococcal (GABHS)

pharyngitis and to treat them to prevent rheumatic fever. With the Centor clinical prediction criteria for the diagnosis of GABHS, 1 point is assigned for each of the following:

1. Fever
2. Anterior cervical lymphadenopathy
3. Tonsillar exudates
4. Absence of cough

With the modified Centor criteria, a point is added if the patient is younger than 18 years and subtracted if the patient is older than 44 years. Patients who have no more than 1 Centor criterion have a low probability of GABHS pharyngitis and should be observed. Most guidelines suggest rapid streptococcal antigen testing and treating with antibiotics only if test results are positive and 2 or 3 criteria are present. If all 4 criteria are present, empirical antibiotics are indicated. If the patient has accompanying fever and posterior cervical adenopathy, the diagnosis of infectious mononucleosis should be considered.

- The Centor clinical prediction criteria for the diagnosis of GABHS assign 1 point each for fever, anterior cervical lymphadenopathy, tonsillar exudates, and absence of cough.

OPHTHALMOLOGY

RED EYE

The red eye is a common ocular complaint. While the majority of causes are benign, the clinician should be able to recognize the syndromes on examination to determine when an emergent referral to an ophthalmologist is indicated.

Subconjunctival Hemorrhage

Subconjunctival hemorrhage is typically unilateral and painless. It may follow trauma, coughing, straining, or emesis. Subconjunctival bleeding also occurs in patients with uncontrolled arterial hypertension, in patients who are receiving anticoagulants or antiplatelet agents, and in patients with intrinsic disorders of coagulation. It resolves spontaneously and requires only reassurance.

Conjunctivitis

Conjunctivitis can result from allergic, viral, and bacterial causes. Patients with allergic conjunctivitis present with bilaterally red, itchy eyes with excessive tearing. Other allergic symptoms, such as sneezing and nasal congestion, typically accompany the eye symptoms. Systemic or topical antihistamines are usually effective for managing symptoms.

Viral conjunctivitis causes bilateral ocular redness, irritation, and excessive tearing. Preauricular lymphadenopathy may be present. Viral conjunctivitis is usually caused by an adenovirus and is highly contagious. It is a self-limited condition, and no antimicrobials are warranted.

Patients with bacterial conjunctivitis usually present with acute unilateral redness, irritation, and discharge. The infection warrants topical antibacterial therapy. Failure to resolve within 7 to 10 days should prompt consultation with an ophthalmologist. Chlamydial and gonorrheal conjunctivitis should be suspected in high-risk patients.

Blepharitis

A *hordeolum*, or *stye*, is an infectious, painful, erythematous, localized nodule of the eyelid. An *external hordeolum* is caused by a blockage and subsequent infection of the glands of the eyelid. An *internal hordeolum* is caused by infection of the meibomian glands. *Staphylococcus aureus* is responsible for the majority of these infections. Although most of the lesions drain spontaneously, some require incision and drainage by an ophthalmologist. Application of warm compresses may assist in spontaneous drainage. Antibiotics are not generally required unless the infection has spread beyond the nodule.

A *chalazion* is a more chronic, rarely painful, and always internal noninfectious eyelid disorder. It is caused by granulomatous inflammation in the meibomian glands. It may be removed if bothersome or large.

Episcleritis

Patients with episcleritis (Figure 55.1) present with sectorial injection of the episcleral vessels. Most cases are idiopathic, but sometimes there is an associated disease. Typically, the diseases are the same disorders that are associated with scleritis. The condition is usually self-limited and an oral nonsteroidal anti-inflammatory medication is usually sufficient to relieve symptoms.

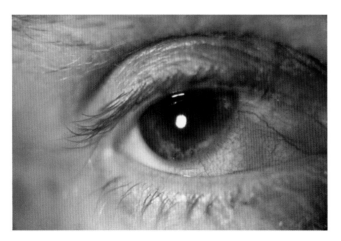

Figure 55.1 Episcleritis. (Adapted from McDonald FS. Mayo Clinic images in internal medicine: self-assessment for board exam review. Rochester [MN]: Mayo Clinic Scientific Press and Boca Raton [FL]: CRC Press; c2004. p. 123. Used with permission of Mayo Foundation for Medical Education and Research.)

Scleritis

Scleritis manifests as an intense, deep pain in the eye caused by scleral inflammation. The pain worsens with movement of the eye and may be referred to the ipsilateral temple. On examination, the scleral vessels are dilated and the eye appears red. Many patients with scleritis have an associated systemic disorder, such as polyarteritis nodosa, systemic lupus erythematosus, Wegener granulomatosis, seronegative spondyloarthropathies (eg, ankylosing spondylitis), and rheumatoid arthritis. Successful therapy requires treatment with topical corticosteroids, cycloplegics, and systemic therapy for any underlying disease.

Iritis

Iritis, also called acute anterior uveitis, is inflammation of the iris and ciliary body. Patients typically present with erythema, photophobia, pain, and blurred vision. Disorders associated with iritis include autoimmune diseases. Patients with HLA-B27 are at an increased risk of iritis. The diagnosis requires a slit-lamp examination, and immediate referral to an ophthalmologist is necessary.

Angle-closure Glaucoma

The development of acute angle-closure glaucoma is a medical emergency. Patients with angle-closure glaucoma present with abrupt ocular pain, headache, visual blurring, and often nausea. Frequently, there is diffuse redness of the eye, and the cornea is hazy. It is more common in the elderly. Patients with angle-closure glaucoma should be immediately referred to an ophthalmologist.

- Although the majority of causes of red eye are benign, the clinician should be able to recognize the syndromes on examination to determine when an emergent referral to an ophthalmologist is indicated.

GLAUCOMA

Glaucoma is a form of optic neuropathy caused by elevated intraocular pressure. Risk factors for open-angle glaucoma include age, being African American, and having diabetes mellitus. The majority of patients with glaucoma are treated with ocular hypotensive drops. Patients who cannot tolerate topical medications or those who progress despite treatment are candidates for surgical therapies, such as laser trabeculectomy.

AGE-RELATED MACULAR DEGENERATION

Age-related macular degeneration (ARMD) is a common cause of visual impairment in older adults. Women and cigarette smokers are at higher risk for ARMD. There are 2 forms of the disease: dry ARMD is characterized by soft drusen and pigmentary changes, whereas wet ARMD is characterized by exudative and choroidal neovascular changes. Patients with dry ARMD typically present with more gradual loss of central vision, central scotoma, visual distortion, and color changes. In wet ARMD, the changes often occur more abruptly. A National Institutes of Health study showed that, for certain patients with intermediate to advanced dry ARMD, vitamins C and E, β-carotene, zinc, and copper may decrease the risk of vision loss. Differentiating between dry and wet ARMD guides therapy.

UROLITHIASIS

Patients with urolithiasis typically present with renal colic. Symptoms may include waves of pain in the abdomen or flank, nausea, hematuria, and dysuria. Urinalysis typically shows red blood cells. Calcium-containing stones are radiodense. Computed tomography has become the imaging study of choice to determine size and location of the stone.

CALCIUM OXALATE STONES

Calcium oxalate stones are the most common type of urolith. Risk factors include hypercalcemia, hypercalciuria, hyperoxaluria, and hypocitraturia. Additionally, bariatric surgery causes hyperoxaluria; it is believed that oxalate reabsorption requires an intact gut.

Conservative treatment includes correcting dietary stresses and increasing urine volume. Pharmacologic interventions include potassium citrate for hypocitraturia, neutral phosphates for idiopathic calcium urolithiasis, thiazides for hypercalciuria, and allopurinol for hyperuricosuria.

Primary hyperoxaluria is the most aggressive stone disease. Treatment includes fluids, pyridoxine (alters glycine metabolism, an oxalate precursor), neutral phosphates, or liver transplant.

- Calcium oxalate stones are the most common type of urolith.
- Bariatric surgery predisposes to oxalate stones.

CALCIUM PHOSPHATE STONES

Calcium phosphate stones are the second most common type of urolith. The formation of calcium phosphate stones occurs in a relatively alkaline urine pH. Primary hyperparathyroidism is a risk factor for formation of calcium phosphate stones. Type 1 renal tubular acidosis (RTA) is an additional risk factor. Patients with type 1 RTA have nephrocalcinosis, a urine pH greater than 5.3, and a hyperchloremic hypokalemic normal anion gap acidosis with hypocitraturia. The primary treatment is correction of the acidosis with alkali. Other conditions associated with calcium phosphate stones are medullary sponge kidney and the use of absorbable alkalis (eg, Tums, Rolaids).

- The presence of calcium phosphate stones indicates a relatively alkaline urine pH.

URIC ACID STONES

Most patients with uric acid urolithiasis have normal levels of uric acid in the serum and urine. Patients with type 2 diabetes mellitus or metabolic syndrome have an increased risk of uric acid stone formation. An excess of dietary protein also can predispose to uric acid stones. Patients with chronic diarrhea, colectomies, or ileostomies form uric acid stones because diarrhea causes the urine volume to decrease and urine acidity to increase. Uric acid urolithiasis is treated with preventive measures such as increased intake of fluid and decreased intake of protein. Alkalizing the urine to pH 6.5 helps to prevent and dissolve uric acid renal stones. Allopurinol may be helpful for patients with hyperuricosuria and for dissolving stones.

- Type 2 diabetes mellitus and diarrhea are risk factors for uric acid stone formation.

STRUVITE STONES

Struvite stones are associated with urease-producing bacteria, including *Proteus*, *Staphylococcus*, *Klebsiella*, *Enterobacter*, *Yersinia*, and *Pseudomonas*. These stones typically have a staghorn shape, and 50% occur bilaterally. Treatment includes surgical removal of the stone and administration of antibiotics postoperatively to eradicate infection. Failure to remove all stones requires antibiotic suppression.

- Struvite stones are associated with urease-producing bacteria.
- Treatment is surgical removal and antibiotics.

STONE EXPULSION

Stone size is a strong predictor of spontaneous passage. Typically, stones smaller than 5 mm in diameter will pass spontaneously. Larger stones may require medical or surgical therapy. Medical therapy can include α-blockers such as tamsulosin to aid in stone expulsion. Patients with 1 kidney, infection, bilateral stones, large stones, or intractable pain may require prompt surgical evaluation.

QUALITY IMPROVEMENT AND PATIENT SAFETY

Since the publication of the Institute of Medicine's report, "To Err is Human," increased attention has been paid to making health care safer. The report estimated that medical errors may contribute to the deaths of nearly 100,000 hospitalized patients annually. Quality improvement methodologies have been adapted from industry and applied to medicine.

QUALITY IMPROVEMENT METHODOLOGIES

LEAN (developed by Toyota Motor Corp) is a quality improvement methodology designed to remove waste from a system, including waiting time, transportation of patients

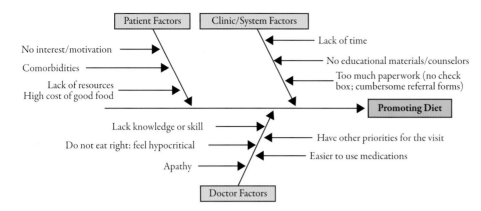

Figure 55.2 Cause-and-Effect (Fish Bone) Diagram. (Adapted from Fluker SA, Whalen U, Schneider J, Cantey P, Bussey-Jones J, Brady D, et al. Incorporating performance improvement methods into a needs assessment: experience with a nutrition and exercise curriculum. J Gen Intern Med. 2010 Sep;25[Suppl 4]:S627–33. Used with permission.)

and equipment, and defects. In health care, the most common type of waste is patient waiting time. The goal of LEAN is to eliminate waste and make the system "lean."

Six Sigma (invented by Motorola Inc) is a quality improvement methodology designed to remove defects and variation from a system. The name Six Sigma refers to 6 standard deviations from the mean, which represents 3.4 defects per 1 million opportunities. Six Sigma uses a stepwise approach called DMAIC (Define, Measure, Analyze, Improve, and Control).

- LEAN is a quality improvement methodology designed to eliminate waste.

- Six Sigma is a quality improvement methodology that seeks to decrease defects and variation.

QUALITY IMPROVEMENT TOOLS

Root Cause Analysis

Root cause analysis is a process to identify the nature of a problem or error. A cause-and-effect diagram (Figure 55.2) is a quality improvement tool that organizes root causes of a problem. These diagrams are also known as fish bone diagrams because of their visual appearance. The "backbone" of the diagram is the problem being studied. Root causes are grouped together and displayed as the "ribs."

Control Chart

A control chart (Figure 55.3) plots variation in a process over time. The chart includes a line representing the mean in the center and lines representing upper and lower control limits based on 3 standard deviations from the mean. A control chart is used to determine whether variation in a process is from a common (predictable) or special (unpredictable) cause.

Value Stream Map

Value stream maps (Figure 55.4) are used in the LEAN process to identify areas of waste. Value stream maps visually display each step in a process, including people, material flow, and information flow, from the patient's perspective. The goal is to identify waste and non–value-added steps.

Pareto Chart

Pareto charts (Figure 55.5) are used to graphically display sources of a problem in order of frequency. The objective is to identify and fix the most common causes of the problem. The 80–20 rule states that 80% of the problem is attributable to 20% of the root causes.

- Quality improvement tools include cause-and-effect diagrams, control charts, value stream maps, and Pareto charts.

PATIENT SAFETY

Medical errors occur. Patient safety principles state that the system should be examined to determine ways to prevent future errors. In medicine in general, procedures are a common source of error. In internal medicine, medication errors, infections, and falls are a frequent threat to patient safety.

Computerized physician order entry systems have helped to decrease medication errors. Medications that commonly interact with other medications include warfarin, cimetidine, antibiotics, phenytoin, HMG-CoA reductase inhibitors, lithium, and antifungals. Medications with common adverse events include those that can prolong the QT

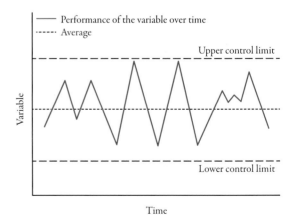

Figure 55.3 Control Chart. (Adapted from Varkey P, Reller MK, Resar RK. Basics of quality improvement in health care. Mayo Clin Proc. 2007 Jun;82[6]:735–9. Used with permission of Mayo Foundation for Medical Education and Research.)

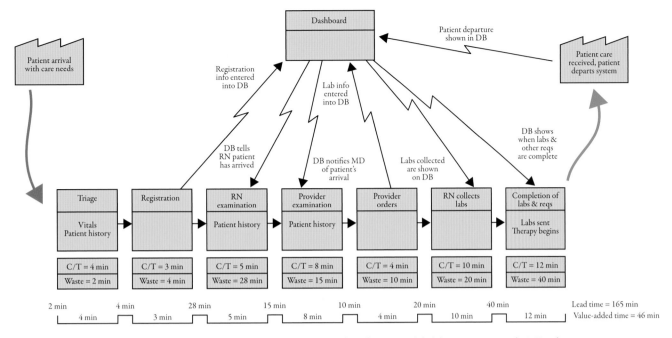

Figure 55.4 Value Stream Map. C/T indicates cycle time; DB, dashboard; info, information; lab, laboratory test result; MD, physician; reqs, requisitions; RN, registered nurse. (Adapted from Dickson EW, Singh S, Cheung DS, Wyatt CC, Nugent AS. Application of lean manufacturing techniques in the Emergency Department. J Emerg Med. 2009 Aug;37[2]:177–82. Epub 2008 Aug 23. Used with permission.)

interval (eg, amiodarone, methadone, quinolones), warfarin, heparin, insulin, antibiotics, and narcotics and those with a low therapeutic index (eg, digoxin, lithium). When any of these medications are prescribed, special care should be taken to prevent errors.

Infections, including central line–associated bloodstream infections and catheter-associated urinary tract infections have been a major focus of quality improvement in hospitals. Hand washing initiatives and standardized orders have been instituted at many hospitals to prevent these infections.

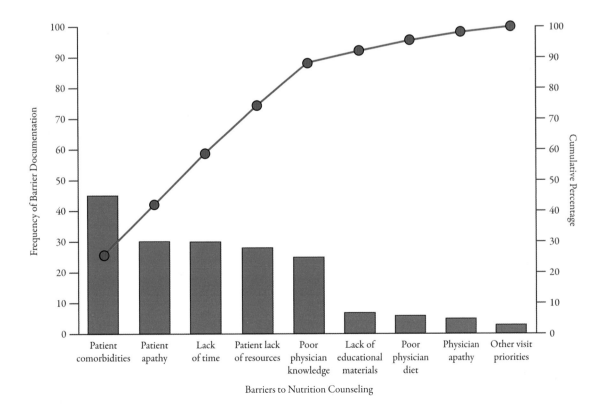

Figure 55.5 Pareto Chart. (Adapted from Fluker SA, Whalen U, Schneider J, Cantey P, Bussey-Jones J, Brady D, et al. Incorporating performance improvement methods into a needs assessment: experience with a nutrition and exercise curriculum. J Gen Intern Med. 2010 Sep;25[Suppl 4]:S627–33. Used with permission.)

Falls are another focus of patient safety endeavors. To improve patient care, patients at risk of falling have been identified and prevention strategies have been instituted.

Human factors include how people interact with their environment. Eliminating human factor errors through engineering is an approach to improve patient safety. Techniques to eliminate human factor errors include memory aids, checklists, standardization, mistake proofing, redundancy, computerized systems, medication reconciliation, and patient education.

- Medical errors should be examined from a systems perspective.
- Medication errors, infections, and falls are common sources of patient safety issues.
- Human factors should be considered to improve patient safety.

56.

GENERAL INTERNAL MEDICINE: CLINICAL EPIDEMIOLOGY

Scott C. Litin, MD, and John B. Bundrick, MD

GOALS

- Describe the diagnostic test characteristics of sensitivity and specificity.

- Demonstrate the influence of disease prevalence on positive and negative predictive values.

- Illustrate how clinicians may use likelihood ratios to analyze the results of a diagnostic test.

- Review common measures for reporting the magnitude of benefit and harm from a therapeutic intervention.

INTERPRETATION OF DIAGNOSTIC TESTS

Diagnostic tests are tools that either increase or decrease the likelihood of disease. When a diagnostic test is applied to a population at risk of a particular disease, patients in the studied population can be assigned to 1 of 4 groups on the basis of disease status and the test result. Table 56.1 illustrates the concept.

By convention, the 4 groups are assigned the letters *a* for true positive (TP), *b* for false positive (FP), *c* for false negative (FN), and *d* for true negative (TN) (Table 56.2). On the basis of this table (called a *2×2 table*), the following test characteristics can be defined:

1. *Sensitivity*

   a. Positive (test) in disease

   b. TP rate—proportion of patients with the disease who have a positive test result:

$$\text{Sensitivity} = \frac{\text{TP}}{\text{TP}+\text{FN}}.$$

   c. The 2×2 table definition: a/(a+c)

   d. Rules to remember:

      1) *SN out*—if a test has 100% sensitivity, a negative test rules *out* the disorder

      2) Screening tests are used to maximize sensitivity and avoid missing a person who has the disease

      3) Characteristic of test—not affected by the prevalence of disease in the population

2. *Specificity*

   a. Negative (test) in health

   b. TN rate—proportion of patients without the disease who have a negative test result:

$$\text{Specificity} = \frac{\text{TN}}{\text{TN}+\text{FP}}.$$

   c. The 2×2 table definition: d/(b+d)

   d. Rules to remember:

      1) *SP in*—if a test has 100% specificity, a positive test rules *in* the disorder

      2) Confirmatory tests are used in follow-up to maximize specificity and avoid incorrectly labeling a healthy person as having disease

      3) Characteristic of test—not affected by the prevalence of disease in the population

3. *Positive predictive value*

When a patient's illness is evaluated by interpreting a diagnostic test, the 2×2 table is read horizontally, not vertically. One really wants to know whether a patient with positive test results actually has the disease; that is, how well the test results predict a disease compared with the reference standard for that disease. Thus, in the 2×2 table, the horizontal rows for the diagnostic test result

Table 56.1 FOUR OUTCOMES OF A DIAGNOSTIC TEST

OUTCOME	DISEASE STATUS	TEST RESULT
True positive	Present	Abnormal
False positive	Absent	Abnormal
False negative	Present	Normal
True negative	Absent	Normal

are of primary interest. Among all patients with a positive diagnostic test result (TP+FP), in what proportion, $\frac{TP}{TP+FP}$, has the diagnosis been predicted correctly or ruled in? This proportion is the *positive predictive value* (PPV).

- PPV is the proportion of patients who have the disease among all the patients who test positive for the disease.

- PPV provides information most useful in clinical practice.

- PPV is affected by the prevalence of the disease in the population.

- The 2×2 table definition: PPV = $\frac{TP}{TP+FP}$ = a/(a + b).

4. Negative predictive value

It is also important to know the percentage of patients with a negative test result (FN+TN) who actually do not have the disease. This proportion, $\frac{TN}{FN+TN}$, is the *negative predictive value* (NPV).

Table 56.2 2×2 TABLE

		TARGET DISORDER		
		Present	*Absent*	
Diagnostic Test Result	Positive	True positive ⟶ a	b ⟵ False positive	a+b
	Negative	c ⟵ False negative	d ⟶ True negative	c+d
		a+c	b+d	a+b+c+d

Prevalence = (a+c)/(a+b+c+d)
Test characteristics
  Sensitivity = a/(a+c)
  Specificity = d/(b+d)
Frequency-dependent properties
  Positive predictive value = a/(a+b)
  Negative predictive value = d/(c+d)

- NPV is the proportion of patients who do not have the disease of interest among all the patients who test negative for the disease.

- NPV is affected by the prevalence of disease in the population.

- The 2×2 table definition: NPV = $\frac{TN}{FN+TN}$ = d/(c + d).

5. Prevalence

Prevalence is defined as the proportion of persons with the disease in the population to whom the test has been applied. In terms of the 2×2 table, prevalence is written as follows:

$$\frac{TP+FN}{TP+FP+FN+TN} = \frac{a+c}{a+b+c+d}.$$

HOW TO CONSTRUCT A 2×2 TABLE

The sensitivity, specificity, and predictive values of normal and abnormal test results can be calculated with even a limited amount of information. For example, assume that a new diagnostic test is positive in 90% of patients who have the disease and is negative in 95% of patients who are disease-free. The prevalence of the disease in the population to which the test is applied is 10%. This provides the following information:

Sensitivity = 90%,

Specificity = 95%, and

Prevalence = 10%.

This test is now ready to be applied to a group of patients by filling in a 2×2 table (Table 56.3). The calculation is often easier if the test is applied to a large number of patients. For example, if it is applied to 1,000 patients, a+b+c+d = 1,000.

Because the prevalence of the disease is 10%, 100 patients have the disease (0.1×1,000 = 100, or a+c = 100). Of the patients, 90%, or 900, are disease-free (0.9×1,000 = 900, or b+d = 900).

Sensitivity of 90% means that 90% of the 100 patients with disease have a positive test result (a = 0.9×100 = 90) and 10% have a negative result (c = 0.1×100 = 10).

Specificity of 95% means that 95% of the 900 patients who are disease-free have a negative test result (d = 0.95×900 = 855) and 5% have a positive test result (b = 0.05×900 = 45).

The 2×2 table in Table 56.3 shows that 135 patients (a+b) have a positive test result; however, only 90 of these 135 patients actually have the disease. Therefore, the PPV of a positive test is $\frac{a}{a+b} = \frac{90}{135} = 66.7\%$. That is, only two-thirds of all patients with a positive test result will actually have the disease. Similarly, one can determine that 865 patients (c+d) have a negative test result; 855 of these 865 patients are disease-free.

Therefore, the NPV of the test is $\frac{d}{c+d} = \frac{855}{865} = 98.8\%$.

		DISEASE PRESENT	DISEASE ABSENT	
Diagnostic Test Result	Positive	90 a	45 b	135 a+b
	Negative	c 10	d 855	c+d 865
		a+c 100	b+d 900	a+b+c+d 1,000

Prevalence = (a+c)/(a+b+c+d) = 100/1,000 = 10%
Test characteristics
    Sensitivity = a/(a+c) = 90/100 = 90%
    Specificity = d/(b+d) = 855/900 = 95%
Frequency-dependent properties
    Positive predictive value = a/(a+b) = 90/135 = 66.7%
    Negative predictive value = d/(c+d) = 855/865 = 98.8%
Likelihood ratio (LR) for a positive test result:
    LR+ = Sensitivity/(1 − Specificity) = 90%/5% = 18
Likelihood ratio for a negative test result:
    LR− = (1 − Sensitivity)/Specificity = 10%/95% = 0.11
Pretest odds = Prevalence/(1 − Prevalence) = 10%/90% = 0.11
Posttest odds = Pretest odds × LR
Posttest probability = Posttest odds/(Posttest odds + 1)

Clinicians should be able to perform these simple calculations. Clinical decision making by internists is more likely to depend on the PPV and NPV of test results for a given population than on the sensitivity or specificity of the test.

For example, if the prevalence of the disease in the clinician's population is 2% instead of 10%, the PPV and NPV can be recalculated. The PPV of abnormal test results decreases to 26.9%, which is quite different from 66.7% (based on a prevalence of 10%), although the test's sensitivity (90%) and specificity (95%) have not changed (Table 56.4).

- An important factor in interpreting a patient's test result is knowledge of the prevalence of the disease in the population being tested.

- High-risk populations (high prevalence of disease) tend to improve the PPV of an abnormal test result.

- Low-risk populations (screening tests) make the NPV of a normal test result look impressive.

USE OF ODDS AND LIKELIHOOD RATIOS

Some physicians prefer interpreting diagnostic test results by using the likelihood ratio. This ratio takes properties of a diagnostic test (sensitivity and specificity) and makes them more helpful in clinical decision making. It helps the clinician determine the probability of disease in a specific patient after a diagnostic test has been performed.

The formula for a likelihood ratio for a positive test result (LR+) is

$$LR+ = \frac{\text{Positive Test in Disease}}{\text{Positive Test in No Disease}} = \frac{\text{Sensitivity}}{1 - \text{Specificity}}.$$

The formula for a likelihood ratio for a negative test result (LR−) is

$$LR- = \frac{\text{Negative Test in Disease}}{\text{Negative Test in No Disease}} = \frac{1 - \text{Sensitivity}}{\text{Specificity}}.$$

For example, if test A has a sensitivity of 95% and a specificity of 90%,

$$LR+ = \frac{\text{Sensitivity}}{1 - \text{Specificity}} = \frac{95}{10} = 9.5 \text{ and}$$

$$LR- = \frac{1 - \text{Sensitivity}}{\text{Specificity}} = \frac{5}{90} = 0.06.$$

However, if test B has a sensitivity of 20% and a specificity of 80%, then

$$LR+ = \frac{\text{Sensitivity}}{1 - \text{Specificity}} = \frac{20}{20} = 1 \text{ and}$$

$$LR- = \frac{1 - \text{Sensitivity}}{\text{Specificity}} = \frac{80}{80} = 1.$$

As a general rule, diagnostic tests with an LR+ greater than 10 or an LR− less than 0.1 have a greater influence on the posttest probability of disease (ie, they are better tests) than diagnostic

Table 56.4 2×2 TABLE FOR TEST WITH 90% SENSITIVITY, 95% SPECIFICITY, AND 2% PREVALENCE

		DISEASE PRESENT	DISEASE ABSENT	
Diagnostic Test Result	Positive	18 a	49 b	67 a+b
	Negative	c 2	d 931	c+d 933
		a+c 20	b+d 980	a+b+c+d 1,000

Prevalence = (a+c)/(a+b+c+d) = 20/1,000 = 2%
Test characteristics
  Sensitivity = a/(a+c) = 18/20 = 90%
  Specificity = d/(b+d) = 931/980 = 95%
Frequency-dependent properties
  Positive predictive value = a/(a+b) = 18/67 = 26.9%
  Negative predictive value = d/(c+d) = 931/933 = 99.8%

tests with likelihood ratios between 10 and 0.1. In the 2 examples above, test A is more likely to rule in or rule out disease than test B.

Sample likelihood ratios are provided in the example below and in Table 56.5.

Example

A 40-year-old man is admitted to the hospital for pneumonia. He says that he consumes 2 six-packs of beer each week. On the basis of this history and your clinical judgment, you assume that he has a pretest probability of 20% for a diagnosis of alcoholism. You ask him questions from the CAGE (*c*ut down, *a*nnoyed, *g*uilty, *e*ye opener) questionnaire, and his responses are positive for all 4 questions. The LR+ for 3 or more CAGE questions is 250.

At this point, you have 2 choices. The first is to use a nomogram (Figure 56.1) and, with a straightedge, connect the pretest probability of 20% and the LR+ of 250 to the posttest probability. This shows that the posttest probability for a diagnosis of alcoholism is 99%.

The second option should be used when there is no nomogram for performing this simple calculation. Without a nomogram, the following steps must be done:

1. Convert the pretest probability to pretest odds.

2. Multiply the pretest odds by the likelihood ratio to obtain the posttest odds.

Table 56.5 EXAMPLES OF SYMPTOMS, SIGNS, AND TESTS AND THE CORRESPONDING LIKELIHOOD RATIO (LR)

TARGET DISORDER	PATIENT POPULATION	HEALTH CARE SETTING	SYMPTOM, SIGN, TEST	NO. OF SIGNS OR SYMPTOMS	LR
Alcohol abuse or dependency	Patients admitted to orthopedic or medical services over a 6-mo period	US teaching hospital	Yes to ≥3 questions on CAGE questionnaire		250
Sinusitis (by further investigation)	Patients with nasal complaints	US teaching hospital	Maxillary toothache, purulent nasal secretion, poor response to nasal decongestants, abnormal transillumination, or history of colored nasal discharge	≥4 3 2 1 0	6.4 2.6 1.1 0.5 0.1
Ascites	Male veteran patients	US veterans' hospital	Presence of fluid wave (done by internal medicine residents)		9.6

Abbreviation: CAGE, *c*ut down, *a*nnoyed, *g*uilty, *e*ye opener (screening questionnaire for potential alcoholism).

Data from Bush B, Shaw S, Cleary P, Delbanco TL, Aronson MD. Screening for alcohol abuse using the CAGE questionnaire. Am J Med. 1987 Feb;82(2):231–5; Williams JW Jr, Simel DL. Does this patient have sinusitis? Diagnosing acute sinusitis by history and physical examination. JAMA. 1993 Sep 8;270(10):1242–6; Williams JW Jr, Simel DL, Roberts L, Samsa GP. Clinical evaluation for sinusitis: making the diagnosis by history and physical examination. Ann Intern Med. 1992 Nov 1;117(9):705–10; Williams JW Jr, Simel DL. The rational clinical examination: does this patient have ascites? How to divine fluid in the abdomen. JAMA. 1992 May 20;267(19):2645–8; and Simel DL, Halvorsen RA Jr, Feussner JR. Quantitating bedside diagnosis: clinical evaluation of ascites. J Gen Intern Med. 1988 Sep–Oct;3(5):423–8.

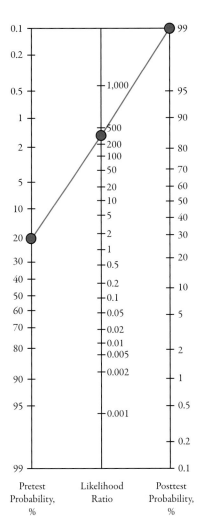

Figure 56.1 Nomogram.

3. Convert the posttest odds to posttest probability.

Probability and odds can be converted somewhat interchangeably with the following formulas:

$$\text{Odds} = \frac{\text{Probability}}{1 - \text{Probability}} \quad \text{and}$$

$$\text{Probability} = \frac{\text{Odds}}{1 + \text{Odds}}.$$

In the example, step 1 involves converting pretest probability to pretest odds. In this case, you estimated that the pretest probability of alcoholism is 20%. With the formulas above,

$$\text{Pretest Odds} = \frac{0.20}{1 - 0.20} = 0.25.$$

Therefore, 0.25 is the pretest odds of having the condition. Step 2 involves determining the posttest odds for a positive test. This can be determined by multiplying the pretest odds (0.25) by the LR+ for 3 or more positive questions on the CAGE questionnaire (250): 0.25×250 = 62.5. Step 3 allows

conversion of posttest odds to posttest probability by placing the numbers in the following formula:

$$\text{Posttest Probability} = \frac{\text{Odds}}{1 + \text{Odds}} = \frac{62.5}{63.5} = 98.4\%.$$

In conclusion, the posttest probability for the diagnosis of alcoholism for this patient is 98.4%, which is close to the value obtained from the nomogram.

INTERPRETATION OF THERAPEUTIC RESULTS

Physicians often make treatment decisions on the basis of the results of randomized controlled trials (RCTs). To understand whether the results of such trials are impressive, the physician is required to translate these results into language understandable to both physicians and patients. This terminology can also be used to compare various therapies for the disease of interest. Several authors have coined terms and derived useful equations to help physicians make sense of RCTs concerned with therapy.

RELATIVE RISK REDUCTION

The results of RCTs of anticoagulant therapy to prevent stroke in patients with atrial fibrillation have been published and summarized. In primary prevention studies, the average 1-year risk of stroke in the placebo group was 5% per year. Because no therapy was administered to that group, this can be called the *control event rate* (CER). In these studies of patients with atrial fibrillation treated with adjusted-dose warfarin (international normalized ratio [INR], 2.0–3.0), the approximate stroke risk was reduced to 2% per year. This can be called the *experimental event rate* (EER) because the patients received a particular therapy.

The traditional measure often used to report the difference between the treated and untreated groups is the *relative risk reduction* (RRR), which is calculated as $\frac{\text{CER} - \text{EER}}{\text{CER}}$. This easure relates the reduction in risk of the outcome event with the intervention to the baseline risk rate (ie, the CER). In this example, the RRR is = $\frac{5\% - 2\%}{5\%}$ 60%. Therefore, anticoagulant therapy reduced the yearly risk of a stroke in patients with atrial fibrillation by 60% compared with the baseline risk of a stroke with no therapy. However, the RRR often is not clinically helpful because the number itself does not provide information about the baseline risk rate (ie, the CER). For example, even if only a very small percentage of control patients (0.005%) and patients receiving anticoagulation (0.002%) experience stroke, the RRR is unchanged: $\frac{0.005\% - 0.002\%}{0.005\%}$ = 60%. Therefore, the RRR often is not useful to the clinician or patient, although a large RRR can be used to make a dramatic endorsement for therapy by proponents of that therapy.

- $RRR = \dfrac{CER - EER}{CER}$.

- Often RRR is not clinically useful because it does not provide information about the baseline risk rate.

ABSOLUTE RISK REDUCTION

In the example above, it would be useful for the physician and patient to know the absolute difference in rates of stroke between the control group and the atrial fibrillation group given anticoagulants (CER−EER). This measure is called the *absolute risk reduction* (ARR). In the combined Stroke Prevention in Atrial Fibrillation (SPAF) trials, the ARR or (CER−EER) = (5%−2%) = 3% per year.

- ARR = (CER−EER).

- ARR is clinically more useful for interpreting therapeutic results.

NUMBER NEEDED TO TREAT

The physician and patient often want to know the number of patients needed to treat (NNT) with a therapy to prevent 1 additional bad outcome. That number can be calculated as $\dfrac{1}{ARR}$. The NNT to prevent 1 stroke by using the adjusted dose of warfarin in patients with atrial fibrillation would be $\dfrac{1}{0.03} = \dfrac{1}{3\%} = 33$. Therefore, the NNT would be 33 patients; that is, 33 patients would need to be treated with warfarin (INR, 2.0–3.0) for 1 year to prevent 1 additional stroke.

- NNT identifies the number of patients who need to be treated with a therapy to prevent 1 additional bad outcome.

- $NNT = \dfrac{1}{ARR}$.

NUMBER NEEDED TO HARM

Conversely, if the rate of adverse events caused by the experimental therapy is known and compared with the rate of adverse events in the placebo group, the number needed to harm (NNH) can be calculated. This useful number tells the physician how many treated patients it takes to produce 1 additional harmful event. In the SPAF trials, the average risk of intracranial hemorrhage for the group given warfarin was 0.3% per year, compared with 0.1% per year for the placebo group. Therefore, the NNH can be calculated as the reciprocal of the absolute risk increase (ARI). The ARI is calculated by subtracting the harm CER from the harm EER or, in this case, 0.3%−0.1% = 0.2%. In this example, $NNH = \dfrac{1}{0.2\%} = \dfrac{1}{0.002} = 500$. Therefore, 500 patients would need to be treated with anticoagulant for 1 year to cause 1 additional intracranial hemorrhage, compared with the control group.

- NNH identifies how many treated patients are needed to produce 1 additional harmful event.

- $NNH = \dfrac{1}{Harm\ EER - Harm\ CER}$.

57.

MEDICAL ETHICS[a]

Keith M. Swetz, MD, C. Christopher Hook, MD, and Paul S. Mueller, MD

GOALS

- Identify the 4 prima facie principles of medical ethics.
- Relate the tension among the 4 principles to common ethical dilemmas in clinical medical practice.
- Investigate the intersection of medical ethics and the law by examining major cases.
- Examine ethical principles governing medical care at the end of life.

Medicine is first and foremost a relationship—a coming together of a patient, who is ill or has specific needs, and a physician, whose goal is to help the patient. The physician-patient relationship is a *fiduciary* relationship; physicians have knowledge, skills, and privileges that patients do not have. In turn, patients trust that physicians act in their patients' best interests.

Medical ethics consists of a set of principles and systematic methods that guide physicians on how they ought to act in their relationships with patients and others and how to resolve moral problems that arise in the care of patients. These principles and methods are based on moral values shared by both the lay society (which may vary from culture to culture) and the medical profession.

- The physician-patient relationship is a *fiduciary* relationship; physicians have knowledge, skills, and privileges that patients do not have. As a result, patients trust that physicians act in their patients' best interests.
- Medical ethics consists of a set of principles and systematic methods that guide physicians on how they ought to act in their relationships with patients and others.

ETHICAL DILEMMAS

An ethical dilemma is a predicament caused by conflicting moral principles in which there is no clear course to resolve a problem (ie, credible evidence exists both for and against a certain action). Advances in medical science and the ever-changing social and legal milieu are responsible for dynamic changes, challenges, and ethical dilemmas in medical practice. Even when ethically challenging situations and dilemmas are resolved, physicians may still experience distress due to conflicting values and personal conscience.

- An ethical dilemma is a predicament caused by conflicting moral principles in which there is no clear course to resolve a problem.
- Advances in medical science and the ever-changing social and legal milieu are responsible for dynamic changes, challenges, and ethical dilemmas in medical practice.

PRINCIPLES OF MEDICAL ETHICS

A widely used framework for medical ethics is principalism, which delineates 4 prima facie principles that encompass most clinical ethical concerns. These principles are 1) beneficence, 2) nonmaleficence, 3) respect for patient autonomy, and 4) justice. *Beneficence* refers to the duty to do good, *nonmaleficence* refers to the duty to prevent or do no harm, *respect for patient autonomy* refers to the duty to respect persons and their rights of self-determination, and *justice* refers to the duty to treat patients fairly (free of bias and based on medical need). No principle has ethical priority over another. Although beneficence is a primary motivating ethical principle for most physicians, the other principles contextualize and inform our orientation to accomplish the good (Figure 57.1). In clinical practice, these principles can be at odds with each other. For example, a beneficent physician may recommend an intervention with minimal risks of harm. However, the patient may exert his or her autonomy and decline the intervention.

[a] Portions previously published in Mueller PS, Hook CC, Fleming KC. Ethical issues in geriatrics: a guide for clinicians. Mayo Clin Proc. 2004 Apr;79(4):554–62. Used with permission of Mayo Foundation for Medical Education and Research.

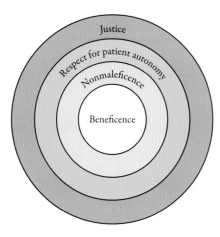

Figure 57.1 The 4 Principles of Medical Ethics.

BENEFICENCE

Beneficence is acting to benefit patients by preserving life, restoring health, relieving suffering, and restoring or maintaining function. The physician is obligated to help patients attain their own interests and goals as determined by the patient, not the physician. This principle may be viewed on several levels of benefit, including how an intervention may 1) biomedically or physiologically benefit a patient, 2) personally benefit the patient (ie, waiting for family to arrive before withdrawing a ventilator), or 3) ultimately benefit the patient (ie, in respect to a patient's belief system or world view).

NONMALEFICENCE AND PRACTICAL APPLICATIONS IN CLINICAL PRACTICE

Nonmaleficence closely couples with beneficence and requires that physicians should not harm (or should prevent harm to) patients. This principle has roots in the Hippocratic corpus, "as to diseases, help, but at least do no harm." This principle also addresses unprofessional behavior, such as verbal, physical, and sexual abuse of patients or uninformed and undisclosed interventions or experimentation on patients.

Nonabandonment

Abandonment is the act of leaving the patient (for whom the physician has provided health care in the past) without providing for immediate or future medical care. Abandonment of patients is contrary to the fiduciary nature of the physician-patient relationship and is a legally punishable act. In contrast, nonabandonment denotes an ethical obligation to provide ongoing medical care once the patient and physician mutually concur to enter into an alliance. Nonabandonment is closely related to the principles of beneficence and nonmaleficence and is fundamental to the long-term physician-patient relationship. Patient noncompliance, in terms of taking medications or following a physician's instructions, is not grounds for abandonment. Physicians should strive to respond to a patient's needs over time, but they should not trespass their own values in the process.

- Nonabandonment is an ethical obligation to provide ongoing care once the patient and physician mutually concur to enter into an alliance.

Conflict of Interest

Physicians should refrain from activities that are not in patients' best interests. Nevertheless, physicians may have conflicts of interest. Such conflicts may unduly influence physicians' practices (eg, prescribing, ordering of tests, or therapeutic recommendations). For example, accepting a gift from a representative of a pharmaceutical company constitutes a conflict of interest if the physician accepting the gift writes prescriptions for drugs manufactured by that company.

- Conflict of interest is contrary to the principles of beneficence and nonmaleficence.

The Impaired Physician

According to the American Medical Association, the impaired physician is one who is "unable to practice medicine with reasonable skill and safety to patients because of physical or mental illness, including deteriorations through the aging process, or loss of motor skill, or excessive use or abuse of drugs including alcohol." Impairment is distinct from competence, which specifically concerns the physician's knowledge and skills to adequately perform his or her duties as a physician. Impairment and incompetence both may compromise patient care and safety. Physicians have a moral, professional, and legal obligation to report impaired and incompetent colleagues to the appropriate authority. Specifics of reporting vary by state, but all states have a reporting requirement. Typical authorities to contact include the institutional chief of staff or impairment program, local or state medical society impairment programs, or the state licensing body. It is important that reporting the behavior of a colleague be based on objective evidence rather than supposition.

- Physicians have an obligation to report impaired colleagues.

The Rule of Double Effect (Beneficence vs Nonmaleficence)

In managing patients, pursuing beneficence may lead to injury or death. Classic examples of such include 1) a terminally ill patient who may require high doses of opioids for adequate analgesia yet such doses risk the potential for respiratory depression and earlier death, 2) taking patients to surgery with the risk of anesthetic or surgical complications and death, or 3) giving chemotherapy for malignant disease with the risk of possible treatment-related mortality. The rule of double effect attempts to resolve the conflict. The rule of double effect states that 1) the act itself must be good or morally neutral, 2) the act or agent intends only the good effect, 3) the bad effect must not be a means to the good effect (eg, death is the only way to achieve the

Table 57.1 OPTIONS AT THE END OF LIFE: HOW DO THEY DIFFER?

	OPTION				
	Life-Sustaining Treatment		*Palliative Sedation and Analgesia*	*Physician-Assisted Death*	*Euthanasia*
	Withhold	*Withdraw*			
Cause of death	Underlying disease	Underlying disease	Underlying disease[a]	Intervention prescribed by physician & used by patient	Intervention used by physician
Intent/goal of intervention	Avoid burdensome intervention	Remove burdensome intervention	Relieve symptoms	Termination of patient's life	Termination of patient's life
Legal?	Yes[b]	Yes[b]	Yes	No[c]	No

[a] Palliative sedation & analgesia may hasten death ("double effect").

[b] Several states limit the power of surrogate decision makers regarding life-sustaining treatment.

[c] Legal only in Oregon, Washington, & Montana.

desired outcome), and 4) the good effect must outweigh the bad effect. By the reasoning of double effect and the beneficent goal of mitigating patient suffering, adequate analgesia to relieve suffering should always be given even if death is hastened. Analgesics should be dosed and administered with the primary intent of relieving pain and not hastening death. If death occurs after analgesia is given in this careful fashion, it is not equivalent to euthanasia, in which the central intent is termination of a patient's life (Table 57.1). Adequate analgesia, particularly in patients at life's end, is the responsibility of the physician.

- Analgesics should be dosed and administered to patients with the primary intent of relieving pain and not hastening patient death. Furthermore, if dosed and administered appropriately, opioids are rarely associated with hastening death by respiratory depression.

RESPECT FOR PATIENT AUTONOMY

The word *autonomy* derives from the Greek words *auto* ("self") and *nomos* ("rule"). The principle of respect for patient autonomy is the concept that persons have the right to establish, pursue, and maintain their values and goals (the right to self-determination). For patients to be fully autonomous, they must be informed (see below), have liberty (free from coercion and duress), and have decision-making capacity. Notably, decision-making capacity is not the same as the legal term *competence*. Capacity is a physician's clinical determination of a patient's ability to understand his or her situation and make appropriate decisions for treatment, whereas competence is the legal determination and status that an individual has the right to make life-affecting decisions (not only health-related decisions but also, for example, financial decisions).

- Respect for autonomy is the concept that persons have the right to establish, pursue, and maintain their values and goals (the right to self-determination).
- Autonomy requires decision-making capacity.

- Capacity is the physician's clinical determination of the patient's ability to understand his or her situation and make appropriate decisions for treatment.
- Competence is the legal determination and status that an individual has the right to make life-affecting decisions.

In clinical practice, the lack of decisional capability should be proved, not presumed. Confusion, disorientation, psychosis, and other cognitive changes caused by diseases, metabolic disturbances, and medical interventions can affect decision-making ability. Decisionally capable patients have the right to refuse all medical interventions, even at the risk of death.

- The lack of decisional capability should be proved, not presumed.

Several clinical standards are used to assess decision-making capacity: 1) the patient can make and communicate a choice; 2) the patient understands the medical situation and prognosis, the nature of the recommended care, available alternative options, and the risks, benefits, and consequences of each; 3) the patient's decisions are stable over time; 4) the decision is consistent with the patient's values and goals; and 5) the decision is not due to delusions.

The ethical principle of respect for patient autonomy and numerous court decisions, from the Quinlan (1976) and Cruzan (1990) cases to the Schiavo (2005) case (Table 57.2), establish a patient's right to refuse medical treatment, even if death inevitably follows such refusals.

Liberty allows a patient the freedom and opportunity to influence the course of one's life and medical treatments.

- The principle of respect for patient autonomy, particularly as it affects an individual's right to refuse life-sustaining treatments, has been affirmed by ethicists and the courts.

Promoting and Preserving Patient Autonomy

Physicians commonly care for patients who lack or lose decision-making capacity. To preserve their autonomy,

Table 57.2 PERTINENT LEGAL RULINGS

CASE, YR	LEGAL ISSUE	COURT	DECISION
Salgo, 1957	Informed consent	California Court of Appeals	First used term "informed consent"
Brooks, 1965	Jehovah's Witness refusal of blood	Illinois District Court	Patients have right to personal treatment on religious grounds
Canterbury, 1972	Degree of disclosure required for adequate informed consent	US District Court	Established "prudent patient test"
Quinlan, 1976	PVS—discontinuation of mechanical ventilation, previously articulated directive	New Jersey Supreme Court	Discontinuation (based on right to privacy)
Brophy, 1986	PVS—discontinuation of gastrostomy feedings, previously articulated directive	Massachusetts Supreme Court	Discontinue feedings (based on autonomy)
Bouvia, 1986	Severely impaired, refusal of nasogastric tube feedings by a decisionally capable patient	California Court of Appeals	Removal of nasogastric tube (based on autonomy)
Corbett, 1986	PVS—discontinuation of nasogastric tube feedings, no predefined directive(s)	Florida Court of Appeals	Discontinue feedings (based on right to privacy)
Cruzan, 1990	PVS—state of Missouri required "clear & convincing" evidence of individual's wishes before allowing withdrawal of life support	US Supreme Court	States have right to restrict exercise of right to refuse treatment by surrogates; decisionally capable patients may refuse life-sustaining therapy, including hydration, nutrition, & mechanical ventilation
Wanglie, 1991	PVS—family wished continued support despite objections to continue life-sustaining therapy by physicians & institution	Minnesota District Court	Continuation (based on autonomy, substituted judgment)
Quill, Lee, 1997	Assisted suicide	US Supreme Court	States have the right to make laws prohibiting or allowing physician-assisted suicide & euthanasia
Schiavo, 2005	PVS—family conflict over withdrawal of feeding tube	Florida District Court of Appeals, Florida Supreme Court, US Supreme Court	Upheld the right of surrogates to withdraw a feeding tube if acting in accord with patient's wishes
Gonzales, 2006	Assisted suicide	US Supreme Court	Upheld the Constitutional legitimacy of the Oregon assisted suicide law

Abbreviation: PVS, persistent vegetative state.

patients who lose capacity nonetheless may communicate through 2 means to express their wishes: advance directives and surrogate decision makers.

Advance Directive

An advance directive is a document in which a person either states choices for medical treatments or designates an individual who should make treatment choices when the patient does not possess decision-making capacity. The term also can apply to oral statements from the patient to the caregivers, given at a time when the patient was decisionally capable. Oral statements to a physician regarding a patient's desires should be recorded in the medical record at the time of the communication. Advance directives can take several forms: 1) the living will, 2) the durable power of attorney for health care (DPAHC), 3) a document appointing a health care surrogate (in jurisdictions that do not formally recognize a DPAHC), 4) an advance treatment-specific directive, and 5) the health care directive that combines elements of the living will and the DPAHC. Laws concerning advance directives vary from jurisdiction to jurisdiction, and physicians should be familiar with their local statutes.

- An advance directive is a document in which a person either states choices for medical treatments or designates an individual who should make treatment choices when the patient does not possess decision-making capacity.
- Legal requirements for advance directives vary from state to state.

The traditional *living will* requires that 2 conditions be present before it takes effect: 1) the patient must be terminally ill, and 2) the patient must lack decision-making capacity. Like the laws concerning advance directives, the determination of terminally ill varies from jurisdiction to jurisdiction. Because of these requirements, the living will is more restrictive and may not be useful in circumstances in which a patient lacks decision-making capacity but is not necessarily terminally ill. When activated, the living will provides guidance to the caregivers about what treatments the patient does or does not desire. It is, however, ineffective if vaguely written or applied to patients with uncertain prognoses.

- The living will requires that a patient be terminally ill before it takes effect.

The *DPAHC* is a document that designates a surrogate decision maker should the patient lose decision-making capacity. It does not require that the patient be terminally ill, and therefore it is more broadly useful than the living will. Within the DPAHC, the patient can make specific directives concerning different treatments such as cardiopulmonary resuscitation and artificial nutrition and hydration. The major value of the DPAHC, however, is that it identifies an individual who can dynamically interact with the health care team.

- The DPAHC designates a surrogate decision maker should the patient lose decision-making capacity.

An *advance treatment-specific medical care directive* is useful for patients who have specific desires never to receive certain forms of therapy. For instance, many Jehovah's Witnesses do not want blood or blood products under any circumstances. Other individuals may refuse dialysis or some other intervention regardless of the circumstance. The advance treatment-specific medical care directive is a document that states this categorical refusal for a specific treatment. For example, it may take the form of a no-transfusion card or a MedicAlert bracelet or necklace.

- The advance treatment-specific medical care directive typically addresses 1 medical intervention.

In response to the Cruzan decision (Table 57.2), the United States Congress passed the *Patient Self-Determination Act*, which attempts to ensure that patients are informed of their rights to accept or refuse medical interventions and to create and execute an advance directive. This act requires that hospitals, nursing homes, hospices, managed care organizations, and home health care agencies provide this information to patients at the time of admission or enrollment. The organizations are required to 1) document whether patients have advance directives, 2) establish policies to implement the advance directives, and 3) educate their staff and community about advance directives and these policies. The Patient Self-Determination Act, however, does not require patients to have advance directives.

- The Patient Self-Determination Act requires that all health care providers, at the time of admission, provide information to patients about their rights to accept or refuse interventions and to create an advance directive.

Surrogate Decision Making

A surrogate is a person who represents the patient's interests and previously expressed wishes, should the patient be unable or unwilling to do so for himself or herself. The surrogate is optimally designated by the patient before he or she loses decisional capacity. One type of surrogate is the DPAHC, in which an individual is designated to speak on a patient's behalf. The second type of surrogate is the patient's family or the court. The third type is a moral surrogate (usually a family member) who best knows the patient and has the patient's interests at heart. Difficulties may arise when the moral surrogate is not the legal surrogate.

- A surrogate represents the patient's interests and previously expressed wishes in the context of the medical issues.
- Optimally, a surrogate is designated by the patient before he or she loses decisional capacity.

In the absence of explicit directives, the surrogate should decide to the best of his or her ability, based on the patient's beliefs and values. Applying choices that the patient would make were he or she able to speak for himself or herself (not what the surrogate would choose) is referred to as substituted judgment. Physicians can guide surrogates by asking "If your loved one could wake up for 15 minutes, understand his or her situation, and then had to return to it, what would he or she choose?" (N Engl J Med. 2005 Apr 21;352[16]:1630–3. Epub 2005 Mar 22). In some circumstances the surrogate may not have engaged in adequate communication with the patient to be able to project how the patient would decide. In these circumstances, the surrogate's and clinician's obligations are to try to decide in the patient's best interests.

Advance directives are often lacking, and jurisdictions vary regarding which individuals may serve as surrogate if one has not been appointed. Physicians should be aware, in the absence of an advance directive, of which individuals should be approached about the surrogate role. Indeed, this variability underscores the value and importance of encouraging patients to formally designate a surrogate through an advance directive.

- In the absence of explicit directives (written or oral), surrogates should use substituted judgment (what the choices would be if the patient were able to speak for himself or herself).

- If substituted judgment is not possible, the surrogate should make choices in the patient's best interest.

Patients may also delegate decision making to a surrogate, even while still possessing decisional capacity. This situation arises in certain cultural contexts in which decision-making authority is given to a certain member of the family or to a community leader. It is respectful of the patient's autonomy to accept his or her delegation of decision making to another.

- A patient may delegate decision-making authority to a surrogate, even while still possessing decision-making capacity himself or herself.

Situations may arise in which a surrogate's decisions or instructions to physicians conflict with a patient's previously expressed directive or with those of other family members. Because the physician's primary responsibility is to the patient, the physician should determine as best as possible what the patient would choose for himself or herself. When the physician is unable to resolve the conflict, it may be helpful to involve an independent third-party arbitrator, such as an ethics consultant or committee or legal counsel. Once it has been established what the patient would want, it is the obligation of the treating physician(s) to comply with those wishes, even in the face of disagreement with surrogates. Only if clear evidence can be provided that the advance directive does not reflect what the patient really desired can the directive be overruled.

- The primary responsibility of the physician is to serve the patient's interest.

Informed Consent and Exceptions

A derivative of the principle of respect for patient autonomy (and nonmaleficence) is informed consent (and refusal): the voluntary acceptance (or refusal) of physician recommendations by decisionally capable patients, or their surrogates, who have been provided sufficient information regarding the risks, benefits, and alternatives of the proposed interventions. There are 3 required elements of informed consent: 1) patient decision-making capacity, 2) patient voluntariness, and 3) accurate and sufficient information. The amount of information shared with the patient should be guided not only by what the physician believes is adequate (professional practice standard) but also by that which the average, prudent person would need in order to make an appropriate decision (reasonable person standard). Discussion of available alternatives to the proposed treatment, including doing nothing, should be included.

- Informed consent (and refusal) requires patient decision-making capacity and voluntariness and accurate and sufficient information.

- The amount of information shared with a patient should be guided by the reasonable person standard: what an average prudent person would need to make an informed decision.

In shared decision making, the physician should present the patient with recommendations that the patient can accept or reject. Simply laying out a menu of choices before the patient may lead to confusion or the perception by the patient that the physician is unconcerned with his or her welfare. If the patient refuses the recommended treatment and chooses one of the alternatives, the physician should respect the patient's choice. The final plan should reflect an agreement between a well-informed patient and a well-informed, sympathetic, and unbiased physician.

- The physician should provide all alternatives, followed by specific recommendations.

- If the patient refuses the recommended treatment, the physician should respect the patient's choice.

In rare exceptions, the physician can treat a patient without informed consent (eg, in an emotionally unstable patient who requires urgent treatment, when informing the patient of the details may produce further problems). The principle of implied consent is invoked when true informed consent is not possible because the patient (or surrogate) is unable to express a decision regarding treatment. This situation often occurs in emergencies in which physicians are compelled to provide medically necessary therapy, without which harm would result. Implied consent and duty to assist a person in urgent need of care have been legally accepted (eg, Good Samaritan laws) and provide the physician a legal defense against battery (although not negligence).

Informed consent from surrogates is necessary to perform an autopsy (except in certain instances such as coroners' cases) or to practice intubation, placement of intravascular lines, or other procedures on the newly dead.

- Implied consent is invoked when true informed consent is not possible, such as in emergency situations.
- Informed consent from surrogates is necessary to perform an autopsy.

Truth Telling and Therapeutic Privilege

The physician must provide decisionally capable patients with truthful information to assist them in making informed medical decisions. Without the receipt of sufficient, accurate, and true information, patients cannot make autonomous decisions. Occasionally, the physician may withhold part or all of the truth if it is believed that telling the truth is likely to cause considerable injury, a concept known as therapeutic privilege. The decision for intentional nondisclosure must be fully recorded in the medical record. Although invoking therapeutic privilege may be ethically justified in some circumstances, legal protection for less-than-full disclosure is not guaranteed.

Some decisionally capable patients may forgo complete disclosure, referring the receipt of information and decision making to others. Waiver of complete disclosure may occur by individual preference or in the context of cultural norms. Regardless, this preference should be respected as the patient's autonomous choice.

- The physician must provide patients with truthful information to assist them in making autonomous decisions.

Medical Errors

Errors committed in the course of treatment require full, honest disclosure, because patients deserve to know the truth in this regard. Frank disclosure helps to preserve or restore trust in the physician-patient relationship. Physicians often fear that if they disclose errors they will be sued, but the opposite is true. Patients are more likely to pursue legal action if they suspect something has gone awry or subsequently discover the error but were not told. Studies have shown that many patients sue physicians primarily to discover the truth.

- Medical errors should be quickly and honestly reported to the patient.

Confidentiality

Privacy is integral to respect persons and to protect an individual's autonomy. Confidentiality respects the right to privacy and provides the patient with security to keep sensitive, personal information within the realm of the physician-patient relationship. The physician is ethically and legally obliged to maintain a patient's medical information in strict confidence, a tradition dating back to the Hippocratic Oath. Ensuring confidentiality encourages complete communication of all relevant information that may affect the patient's health.

However, the obligation to protect patients may be overridden when serious bodily harm to the patient or others may result if reasonable steps are not taken. In some instances, a patient's data must be shared with public health care agencies. Examples include certain infectious diseases, physical abuse, gunshot wounds, and other concerns to the public health and welfare. There is state-to-state variability in reporting requirements, and physicians should be aware of local statutes.

Notably, the Genetic Information Nondiscrimination Act (2008), a federal law, prohibits discrimination by employers and health insurers on the basis of genetic information. Employers are prohibited from requesting, requiring, or purchasing genetic information from or about potential or existing employees. Insurers are prohibited from 1) requiring genetic testing as a condition for eligibility for insurance and 2) adjusting premiums or contribution amounts for a group on the basis of genetic information.

- A physician is obliged to maintain medical information in strict confidence.
- Certain exceptions to confidentially are justified because of overriding ethical and social concerns (eg, mandatory reporting requirements).

Futility or Demands for Nonbeneficial Interventions

Patients have the right to refuse any and all medical therapies. But does the principle of respect for autonomy give patients, or their surrogates, the right to demand treatments? This question arises when patients or families request treatments that have little chance of resulting in survival or meaningful recovery. May physicians unilaterally withhold or withdraw medical interventions if, in their opinion, the intervention is futile? The conflict seemingly is between patient autonomy and the professional judgment, moral autonomy, and integrity of the caregivers. Physicians are also moral agents and should not be forced to violate their ethical beliefs.

A futile intervention is one that cannot achieve specified goals no matter how many times it is repeated. From this definition, physicians are not required to provide treatments that have no pathophysiologic rationale, that have previously failed in a given patient, or that cannot achieve the goals of care agreed on by the physician and patient or surrogate. However, many so-called futility conflicts arise clinically when an intervention is *possible* but is *unlikely* to benefit the patient or in which there is a conflict about the goals of treatment (such as maintaining physiologic life vs restoration of independent functioning or survival to dismissal). Because of the diverse nature of situations labeled futile, a more accurate label might be nonbeneficial interventions. There have been many attempts to create functional definitions of futility that would cover these circumstances, but all have the flaw of establishing arbitrary thresholds that are value-laden.

When treatments of disputed efficacy are being requested by patients or surrogates or when physicians have varying opinions regarding the benefit of treatment, all attempts at maximizing the process of shared decision making should be undertaken. This approach often takes the form of ongoing, regular assessment of goals of care, exploring where fundamental disagreements regarding care are occurring, and involving external experts (eg, palliative medicine consultants and ethics consultants) when appropriate. If differences cannot be resolved, efforts at intra-institutional or inter-institutional transfer may need to be arranged.

- A futile intervention is one that cannot achieve the goals of intervention no matter how many times it is repeated.

- As much as possible, resolution of futility conflicts should be attempted by using a due-process approach.

Conscientious Objection

Another conflict between patient and physician (and other health care providers) occurs when the patient requests an intervention that may be legally sanctioned but is morally unacceptable to the physician. In this situation, the ethical issue centers on moral acceptability of the intervention and not on efficacy. An objector may believe so strongly against the intervention that he or she considers the intervention as commission of evil.

Historically, dating back to the Hippocratic Oath, medical ethics has recognized that physicians, in their obligations to protect life, may conscientiously object to acts involving the deliberate taking of human life. Many states have conscience laws protecting health care providers from being forced to be complicit in acts that would violate their conscience.

What constitutes an issue of conscience? In medicine, the issue of objection must regard a specific act. Claims of conscience regard acts, not persons. Claims of conscience that intrinsically involve discrimination against a given individual (eg, race, color, sexual preference, nationality, religion) are not legitimate and violate the principle of justice (see "Justice" below). Furthermore, the conscientious objector is restricted to forgoing participation only in the specific objectionable act, not in the rest of the patient's care as such. To do otherwise would be an act of abandonment. For example, a physician may refuse to participate in performing an abortion (including providing anesthesia and those actions directly and immediately involved in the act), but a physician may not decline postoperative care of a patient who might experience complications of the procedure. Although the conscientious objector has the right to decline participation in the requested intervention, he or she should not berate or obstruct the patient in receiving that intervention from others. Health care organizations may legitimately expect the physician to refer the patient to another provider, or at least to institutional resources that can assist the patient in securing legally sanctioned interventions, such as a patient affairs office or an administrator.

- Health care professionals have a right of conscience and to decline from participation in acts that violate deeply held religious and philosophical principles, but they do not have a right to discriminate against persons.

- The physician and medical institutions should provide alternative means for patients to secure legally sanctioned interventions if requested.

JUSTICE

The principle of justice expresses that every patient deserves and must be fairly provided optimal care as warranted by the underlying medical condition and within the constraints of available resources. The identification of optimal medical care should be based on the patient's medical need and the perceived medical benefit to the patient. The patient's social status, ability to pay, or perceived social worth should not dictate the quality or quantity of medical care. The physician's clear-cut responsibility is to the patient's well-being (beneficence). Physicians should not make decisions about individual patient care based on larger societal needs, because the bedside is not the place for general policy decisions. Nevertheless, physicians should be conscious of larger societal needs and should be leaders in developing fair policies to regulate the allocation of scarce or costly resources, but these endeavors should take place away from the bedside and an individual physician-patient relationship.

- Justice is allocation of medical resources fairly and according to medical need.

- Physicians should be conscious of larger societal needs and should be leaders in developing fair policies to regulate the allocation of scarce or costly resources, but these involvements must take place away from the bedside and the individual physician-patient relationship.

ETHICAL CONSIDERATIONS AT THE END OF LIFE

INCURABLE DISEASE AND DEATH

Transitioning from full therapeutic efforts against illness to comfort care for patients inevitably approaching death can be difficult. Nevertheless, compassionate, ongoing care for patients at the end of life is critical. The patient and family (if the patient so desires) should be provided ample opportunity to talk with the physician and ask questions. An unhurried openness and willing-to-listen attitude on the part of the physician are critical for a positive outcome.

The physician should assume responsibility for furnishing and arranging for physical, emotional, and spiritual support. Adequate pain control, respect for human dignity, and ongoing contact with the patient and family are crucial. The emotional and spiritual support available through hospital chaplains or local clergy (as appropriate, given the patient's personal beliefs) and efforts to avoid dehumanization of the patient are important. These nonpharmacologic interventions often are invaluable for alleviating patient suffering as opposed to a firm reliance on sedation.

- Adequate pain control, respect for human dignity, and close contact with the family are crucial at the end of life.

WITHHOLDING AND WITHDRAWING LIFE-SUSTAINING TREATMENTS

Carrying out patients' requests to withhold or withdraw unwanted medical treatments is legal and ethical and is not the same as physician-assisted suicide or euthanasia. In assisted suicide, the patient personally terminates his or her life by using an external means provided by a clinician (eg, lethal prescription). In euthanasia, the clinician directly terminates the patient's life (eg, lethal injection). In assisted suicide and euthanasia, a new intervention is introduced (eg, drug), whose sole intent is the patient's death. In contrast, when a patient dies after an intervention is withheld or withdrawn, the underlying disease remains the cause of death (Table 57.2). The intent is freedom from interventions that are perceived as burdensome.

The right to refuse medical treatments is not so much a "right to die," as it has been frequently described, but rather a "right to be left alone," or a "freedom from unwanted touching." Notably, there is no ethical or legal distinction between withholding treatment in the first place and withdrawing a treatment once begun. The right of a decisionally capable person to refuse artificial hydration and nutrition was upheld by the US Supreme Court (Table 57.2), but a surrogate decision maker's right to refuse treatment for decisionally incapable persons may have restrictions in some states. Some states require "clear and convincing evidence" that withdrawing and withholding of life-sustaining treatment would be the patient's desire. The value of each medical therapy (risk:benefit ratio) should be assessed for each patient. When appropriate, the withholding or withdrawal of life support is best accomplished with input from more than one experienced clinician.

- Withholding or withdrawing life-sustaining treatments does not conflict with the principles of beneficence, nonmaleficence, and autonomy.

- Patients have the right to refuse medical treatment at any point in the course of treatment if they view the treatment as more burdensome than beneficial.

DO-NOT-RESUSCITATE ORDERS

Do-not-resuscitate (DNR) orders affect administration of cardiopulmonary resuscitation (CPR) only; other therapeutic options should not be influenced by the DNR order. A DNR order can be compatible with maximal forms of treatment (eg, elective intubation, elective cardioversion, surgery). Every person whose medical history is unclear or unavailable should receive CPR in the event of cardiopulmonary arrest.

Of paramount importance are the patient's knowledge of the extent of disease and the prognosis, the physician's estimate of the potential efficacy of CPR, and the wishes of the patient (or surrogate) regarding CPR as a therapeutic tool.

The appropriateness of a DNR order should be reviewed frequently because clinical circumstances may dictate other measures (eg, a patient with terminal cardiomyopathy who had initially turned down heart transplant and had DNR orders may change her or his mind and now opt for the transplant). Optimally, physicians should discuss the appropriateness of CPR or DNR in the outpatient setting, during the initial period of hospitalization, periodically during hospitalization, and during care transitions. DNR orders (and rationale) should be entered in the patient's medical records.

- DNR orders affect CPR only.

- A DNR order can be compatible with maximal forms of treatment.

- In the absence of a DNR order, universal consent for CPR is presumed.

- DNR orders should be reviewed frequently.

PERSISTENT VEGETATIVE STATE

Persistent vegetative state is a chronic state of unconsciousness (loss of self-awareness) lasting for more than a few weeks, characterized by the presence of wake-sleep cycles, but without behavioral or cerebral metabolic evidence of cognitive function or of being able to respond in a willful manner to external events or stimuli. The body retains functions necessary to sustain physiologic survival (eg, respiration, circulation, endocrine function) if provided nutritional and other supportive measures. Many patients in persistent vegetative state require only artificially administered nutrition and hydration, in addition to routine nursing care, to continue to physically survive. However, without the medical intervention of placing a feeding tube or giving intravenous nutrition and hydration, the patient will die of the underlying disorder that prevents receipt of adequate hydration and nutrition. Thus, artificial nutrition and hydration are medical therapies that may be refused or discontinued by a surrogate decision maker, just as any other medical intervention, if consistent with a patient's previously stated desires (Table 57.1).

- Persistent vegetative state is unconsciousness (loss of self-awareness) lasting for more than a few weeks.

- There is no distinction between artificially administered nutrition and hydration and mechanical ventilation or other interventions in terms of being medical treatments.

PHYSICIAN-ASSISTED DEATH

All 4 principles of medical ethics have an impact on the issue of physician-assisted suicide (sometimes referred to as physician aid in dying) and euthanasia. Historically, the medical profession has taken a strong stand against physicians directly killing patients, but this prohibition has been challenged on the basis of patient autonomy, beneficence or compassion, and other grounds. The American Medical Association, the American

College of Physicians, and other large professional medical groups have maintained a stance against physician-assisted suicide and euthanasia.

In 1997, the US Supreme Court ruled that states may maintain laws prohibiting euthanasia and assisted suicide but may also pass laws allowing these practices. Although the Court did not find a right to physician-assisted death, it emphasized the patient's right to adequate, aggressive pain control, even if it might shorten the patient's life. In 1997, the people of the state of Oregon reiterated their support for physician-assisted suicide by reapproving a referendum first passed in 1994 legalizing assisted suicide but prohibiting euthanasia. The Oregon law requires that the patient 1) have a terminal condition, 2) be decisionally capable, 3) has initiated 2 verbal requests and 1 written request for a prescription for a lethal overdose, 4) undergo a second-opinion consultation, 5) receive appropriate psychiatric intervention if perceived to be depressed, and 6) undergo a 15-day waiting period after the request has been made to allow the patient to change his or her mind. Similar decisions have been made in Washington and Montana. At the time of publication, assisted suicide is illegal in the 47 other states and euthanasia is illegal throughout the United States.

Regardless of one's position on physician-assisted suicide and euthanasia, physicians are obligated to address the underlying concerns that lead patients and physicians to believe that assisted suicide and euthanasia are necessary. Physicians should be acquainted with appropriate means of pain management and palliative care and treat patients' distressing symptoms.

- Euthanasia is legally prohibited in the United States.

- Physician-assisted suicide is permitted only in the states of Oregon, Washington, and Montana.

- Physicians should strive to provide optimal symptom management and to promote dignity in dying patients in all locations.

DEFINITION OF DEATH

Death is the irreversible cessation of circulatory and respiratory function or the irreversible cessation of all functions of the entire brain, including the brainstem. Clinical criteria (at times supported by electroencephalographic testing or assessment of cerebral perfusion) permit the reliable diagnosis of brain death.

The family should be informed of brain death but should not be asked to decide whether further medical therapy should be continued. One exception is when the patient's surrogate (or the patient, via an advance directive) permits certain decisions, such as organ donation, in the case of brain death.

Once it is ascertained that the patient is "brain dead" and that no further therapy can be offered, the primary physician, preferably after consultation with another physician involved in the patient's care, may withdraw supportive measures. This approach is accepted throughout the United States, with the exception of the states of New Jersey and New York, which have modified their definition-of-death statutes to allow a religious exemption for groups (such as Orthodox Jews) that do not accept brain death as a valid criterion for death. In these states, continued care may be requested of the caregivers until circulatory and respiratory function collapses.

- Death is defined as the irreversible cessation of circulatory and respiratory function or the irreversible cessation of all functions of the entire brain, including the brainstem.

AUTHORS' NOTE

This review is meant as a guide; individual practitioners are referred to their state medical societies for further information regarding state-specific mandates and laws.

INDEX

Note: Page numbers followed by b, f, or t indicate a box, figure, table, respectively

ventricular tachycardia (*Cont.*)
   refractory ventricular tachycardia, 28
   sustained ventricular tachycardia, 14*t*
ventricular tachycardia and fibrillation,
   27–28
verapamil, 23, 61, 78
vertebral infections, 354
vespid allergies, 584
Vibrio cholerae, 163, 302*t,* 305
Vibrio parahaemolyticus, 163, 164, 305
Vibrio vulnificus, 165, 350, 353
viral arthritis, 353, 405–406
viral diarrhea, 305–306
viral hemorrhagic fevers, 252*t*
viral pathogens, in AIDS
   adenovirus, 129
   cytomegalovirus, 128
   herpes simplex virus, 128–129
viral pneumonia, 272
viridans group streptococci, 345
visceral leishmaniasis, 271
vitamin C deficiency, 498
vitamin D deficiency, 571
von Hippel-Lindau disease, 119, 677*t*
von Willebrand disease, 513–515
   biochemistry, 514
   classification, 513
   clinical features, 514
   definition, 513
   function of, 514
   inheritance of, 515
   laboratory testing, 514
   management, 515

   stepwise assessment approach, 514*t*
   variables affecting vWF levels, 514–515
vulvar skin disorders, 717–718
vulvovaginal candidiasis, 301

W
Waldenström macroglobulinemia, 534
warfarin therapy
   acquired coagulation deficiencies, 517*t*
   for antiphospholipid antibody
     syndrome, 400
   contraindication in pregnancy, 56
   for dilated cardiomyopathy, 74
   for ischemic cerebrovascular disease, 639
   for mitral valve prolapse, 49*t*
   for venous thromboembolism, 527
water balance disorders. *See* diabetes
   insipidus; hypernatremia;
   hyponatremia; osmotic diuresis
Wegener granulomatosis (granulomatosis
   with polyangiitis), 215–216,
   369–370, 580
Wells model for predicting pulmonary
   embolism, 525*t*
West Nile virus encephalitis, 4*t*
Whipple disease, 165–166, 407
Wilson disease, 180–182, 384
Wiskott-Aldrich syndrome, 522
Wolff-Parkinson-White syndrome, 11
   adenosine/verapamil contraindication,
     13
   with atrial fibrillation, 21
   atrial fibrillation in, 26–27

   conduction of sinus impulses in, 27*f*
   definition, 25–26
   supraventricular tachycardia in, 26*f*
   treatment, 25–26
women's health, 706–729. *See also* breast
   cancer; contraceptives, hormonal;
   contraceptives, oral; infertility
   (female); menopause; pregnancy
   abnormal uterine bleeding, 707–708,
     707b, 713, 714
   adnexal masses, 714–716, 714b
   anxiety and depression, 728–729
   breast conditions
     benign breast disease, 723
     nipple discharge, 722–723
     nonpalpable mass evaluation, 721
     pain, 721–722
     palpable mass evaluation, 721
   cardiovascular disease
     atrial fibrillation, 728
     clinical presentation, 727
     gender-based management, outcomes,
       727
     heart failure, 728
     pathogenesis, 726–727
     primary/secondary prevention,
       727–728
     risk factors, 725–726
     stress testing, 727
   cervical cancer screening,
     716–717
   contraception options, risks, 708–710,
     708*t*

   dysfunctional uterine bleeding, 708
   intimate partner violence, 729
   menopause
     hallmark symptoms, 719–720
     hormone therapy, 720
     postmenopausal bleeding, 720
     related terms, 719b
   menstruation, 706
   perimenopause, 718–719
   premenstrual syndrome, 706–707
   sexual assault, 729
   uterine diseases
     endometrial cancer, 713–714, 714b
     endometriosis, 711–712
     uterine fibroids, 712–713
   vulvar skin disorders, 717–718

X
X-linked lymphoproliferative syndrome,
   266

Y
yellow jacket stings, 584
yellow nail syndrome, 218
Yersinia enterocolitica, 164, 264, 305
Yersinia pestis (plague), 252*t,* 254

Z
zanamivir, 273
Zenker diverticulum, 146, 148, 151
zoledronic acid, 465, 479, 489
Zollinger-Ellison syndrome, 144,
   153–154